SIDE EFFECTS OF DRUGS
ANNUAL 22

Complementary to this volume:

SIDE EFFECTS OF DRUGS ANNUALS 1–21 (1977–1998)
Edited by M.N.G. Dukes (Annuals 1–16) and J.K. Aronson (Annuals 15–21)

MEYLER'S SIDE EFFECTS OF DRUGS, 13th EDITION (1996)
Edited by M.N.G. Dukes

UNWANTED EFFECTS OF COSMETICS AND DRUGS USED IN DERMATOLOGY, 3rd EDITION (1994)
A.C. de Groot, J.W. Weyland and J.P. Nater

DRUGS AND HUMAN LACTATION, 2nd Edition (1996)
P.N. Bennett

PHARMACOLOGICAL AND CHEMICAL SYNONYMS, 10th Edition (1994)
E.E.J. Marler

A MANUAL OF ADVERSE DRUG INTERACTIONS, 5th Edition (1997)
J.P. Griffin and P.F. D'Arcy

A DICTIONARY OF PHARMACOLOGY AND ALLIED TOPICS (1998)
D.R. Laurence and J. Carpenter

SIDE EFFECTS OF DRUGS ANNUAL 22

A worldwide yearly survey of new data and trends

EDITOR

J.K. ARONSON M.A., D.PHIL., M.B., F.R.C.P.

Clinical Reader in Clinical Pharmacology
University Department of Clinical Pharmacology
Radcliffe Infirmary, Oxford, United Kingdom

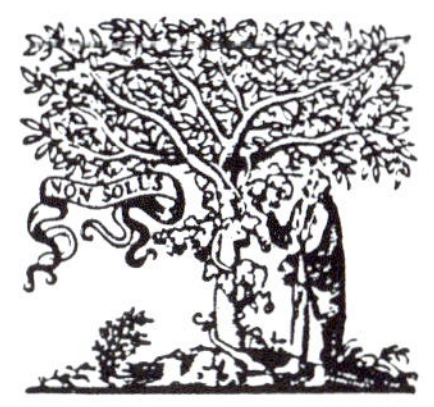

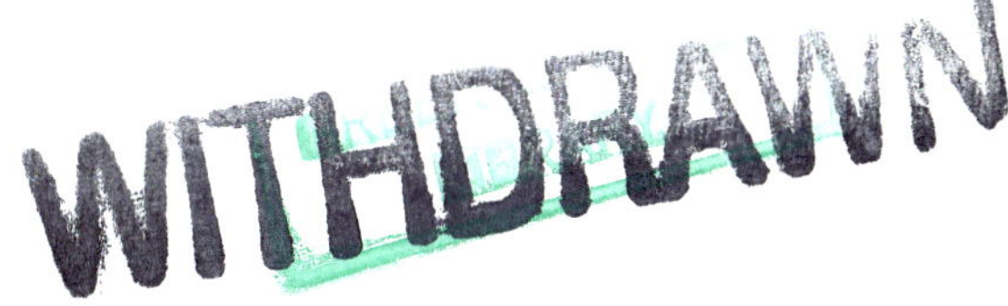

1999

ELSEVIER

Amsterdam – Lausanne – New York – Oxford – Shannon – Singapore – Tokyo

ELSEVIER SCIENCE B.V.
Sara Burgerhartstraat 25
P.O. Box 211, 1000 AE Amsterdam, The Netherlands

First edition 1999

ISBN: 0-444-50092-8
ISSN: 0378-6080
Library of Congress Cataloging Card Number: 78-644057 (ISSN 0378-6080)

∞ The paper used in this publication meets the requirements of ANSI/NISO Z39.48-1992 (Permanence of Paper).
Printed in The Netherlands.

Contributors

J.K. ARONSON, M.A., M.B.CH.B., D. PHIL., F.R.C.P.
University Department of Clinical Pharmacology, Radcliffe Infirmary, Woodstock Road, Oxford OX2 6HE, U.K.

I. AURSNES, M.D.
University of Oslo, Department of Pharmacotherapeutics, P.O. Box 1065 Blindern, N-0316 Oslo, Norway

J. BARNES, B.PHARM., M.R.PHARM.S., M.I.F.A.
Department of Complementary Medicine, Division of Community Health Science, School of Postgraduate Medicine and Health Sciences, University of Exeter, 25 Victoria Park Road, Exeter EX2 4NT, U.K.

A.G.C. BAUER, M.D.
Havenziekenhuis, Haringvliet 2, 3011 TD Rotterdam, The Netherlands

P. BROWN, F.R.C.S., F.R.C.R.
Department of Diagnostic Imaging, Northern General Hospital NHS Trust, Sheffield S5 7AU, U.K.

A. BUITENHUIS, M.D.
Department of Clinical Pharmacology & Pharmacotherapy, Academic Medical Center, Meibergdreef 9, 1105 AZ Amsterdam, The Netherlands

A. CARVAJAL, M.D., PH.D.
Instituto de Farmacoepidemiología, Facultad de Medicina, 47005 Valladolid, Spain

G. CHEVREL, M.D.
Service de Rhumatologie et Immunologie Clinique, Hôpital Edouard Herriot, 5 Place d'Arsonval, 69437 Lyon Cédex 03, France

N.H. CHOULIS, M.D., PH.D.
School of Pharmacy, University of Athens, P.O. Box 4315, Athens 102 10, Greece

P. COATES, M.B., B.S., F.R.A.C.P.
Department of Endocrinology, Royal Adelaide Hospital, North Terrace, South Australia, Australia 5000

J. COSTA, M.D.
Clinical Pharmacology Department, Hospital Universitari Germans Trias i Pujol, Universitat Autònoma de Barcelona, Ctra de Canyet, 08916 Badalona, Spain

P.J. COWEN, M.D.
University Department of Psychiatry, Warneford Hospital, Oxford OX3 7JX, U.K.

S. CURRAN, B.SC., M.B.CH.B., M.R.C.PSYCH., M.MED.SC., PH.D.
Fieldhead Hospital, Ouchthorpe Lane, Wakefield WF1 3SP, U.K.

A.C. DE GROOT, M.D., PH.D.
Department of Dermatology, Carolus-Liduina Hospital, P.O. Box 1101, 5200 BD 's-Hertogenbosch, The Netherlands

M.D. DE JONG, M.D., PH.D.
Department of Medical Microbiology, Academic Medical Center, University of Amsterdam, P.O. Box 22700, 1100 DE Amsterdam, The Netherlands

A. DEL FAVERO, M.D.
Istituto di Medicina Interna e Science Oncologiche, Policlinico Monteluce, 06122 Perugia, Italy

J. DESCOTES, M.D., PHARM.D., PH.D.
Laboratoire de Pharmacologie, Toxicologie Médicale et Medecine de l'Environment, Faculté de Médecine Lyon-RTH Laënnec, rue Guillaume Paradin, 69372 Lyon cedex 08, France

H.J. DE SILVA, M.B.B.S., M.D.
Department of Medicine, Faculty of Medicine, University of Kelaniya, P.O. Box 6, Ragama, Sri Lanka

F.A. DE WOLFF, PH.D.
Toxicology Laboratory, Department of Clinical Chemistry, Pharmacy and Toxicology, Leiden University Medical Center, P.O. Box 9600, 2300 RC Leiden, The Netherlands

S. DITTMANN, M.D., D.SC.MED.
World Health Organisation, Regional Office for Europe, 8 Scherfigsvej, 2100 Copenhagen O, Denmark

R.E. EDWARDS, M.B.B.S., F.R.C.A.
Consultant in Anaesthesia and Intensive Care, 4 Heathfield Road, Seaford, East Sussex BN25 1TH, U.K.

H.W. EIJKHOUT, M.D.
Central Laboratory of the Netherlands Red Cross Blood Transfusion Service, Plesmanlaan 125, 1066 CX Amsterdam, The Netherlands

C.J. ELLIS, M.D., F.R.C.P.
Department of Communicable and Tropical Diseases, East Birmingham Hospital, Bordesley Green East, Birmingham B9 5ST, U.K.

E. ERNST, M.D., PH.D.
Department of Complementary Medicine, Division of Community Health Science, School of Postgraduate Medicine and Health Sciences, University of Exeter, 25 Victoria Park Road, Exeter EX2 4NT, U.K.

M.A. FAIGAN, M.B., CH.B.
Department of Pharmacology and Clinical Pharmacology, Faculty of Medicine and Health Science, The University of Auckland, Private Bag 92019, Auckland, New Zealand

M. FARRÉ, M.D.
Department de Farmacologia i Toxicologia, Institut Municipal d'Investigació Mèdica, Universitat Autònome de Barcelona, Doctor Aiguader 80, 08003 Barcelona, Spain

R.E. FERNER
West Midlands Centre for Adverse Drug Reactions Reporting, City Hospital, Birmingham B18 7QH, U.K.

P.I. FOLB, M.D., F.R.C.P.
Department of Pharmacology, University of Cape Town Medical School, Groote Schuur Hospital, Observatory 7925, Cape Town, South Africa

J.A. FRANKLYN, M.D.
Department of Medicine, University of Birmingham, Queen Elizabeth Hospital, Edgbaston, Birmingham B15 2TH, U.K.

M.G. FRANZOSI, PH.D.
Department of Cardiovascular Research, Istituto di Richerche Farmacologiche Mario Negri, Via Eritrea 62, 20157 Milano, Italy

A.H. GHODSE, M.D., PH.D., F.R.C.P., F.R.C.PSYCH.
Center for Addiction Studies, St. George's Hospital Medical School, 6th Floor, Hunter Wing, Cranmer Terrace, London SW17 0RE, U.K.

A.I. GREEN, M.D.
Commonwealth Research Center and Massachusetts Mental Health Center, Harvard Medical School, Boston, MA 02115, U.S.A.

A.H. GROLL, M.D.
Immunocompromised Host-Section, Pediatric Oncology Branch, National Cancer Institute, National Institutes of Health, Bldg. 10, Rm. 13N240, 10, Center Drive MSC, Bethesda, MD 20891, U.S.A.

R.G. IRWIN, M.D.
Immunocompromised Host-Section, Pediatric Oncology Branch, National Cancer Institute, National Institutes of Health, Bldg. 10, Rm. 13N240, 10, Center Drive MSC, Bethesda, MD 20891, U.S.A.

J.W. JEFFERSON, M.D.
Madison Institute of Medicine, Inc., 7617 Mineral Point Road, Suite 300, Madison, WI 53717, U.S.A.

H.M.J. KRANS, M.D.
Department of Endocrinology and Metabolic Diseases, Leiden University Medical Center, Albinusdreef 2, Building 1, C4-R, 2333 ZA Leiden, The Netherlands

S. KRISHNA, B.A., D.PHIL., F.R.C.P.
Division of Infectious Diseases, Department of Cell and Molecular Sciences, St. George's Hospital Medical School, Cranmer Terrace, London SW17 0RE, U.K.

S. LALLY, B.SC., M.B.CH.B.
Division of Psychiatry and Behavioural Sciences, Level 5, Clinical Sciences Building, St. James's University Hospital, Leeds LS9 7TF, U.K.

R. LATINI, M.D.
Department of Cardiovascular Research, Istituto di Ricerche Farmacologiche Mario Negri, Via Eritrea 62, 20157 Milano, Italy

M. LEUWER, M.D., PH.D.
Department of Anesthesiology, Hannover Medical School, D-30625 Hannover, Germany

K.M. LULICH, B.SC., PH.D.
Department of Pharmacology, University of Western Australia, Nedlands WA 6907, Australia

P. MAGEE, B.SC., M.SC., M.R.PHARM.S.
Director of Pharmaceutical Services, Walsgrave Hospitals NHS Trust, Clifford Bridge Road, Walsgrave, Coventry CV2 2DX, U.K.

A.P. MAGGIONI, M.D.
Department of Cardiovascular Research, Istituto di Ricerche Farmacologiche Mario Negri, Via Eritrea 62, 20157 Milano, Italy

L.H. MARTÍN ARIAS, M.D., PH.D.,
Instituto de Farmacoepidemiología, Facultad de Medicina, 47005 Valladolid, Spain

G.T. McINNES, B.SC., M.D., F.R.C.P., F.F.P.M.
University Department of Medicine and Therapeutics, Gardiner Institute, Western Infirmary, Glasgow G11 6NT, U.K.

R.H.B. MEYBOOM, M.D.
Bremhoeven 1, 5244 GV Rosmalen, The Netherlands

T. MIDTVEDT, M.D., PH.D.
Laboratory of Medical Microbial Ecology, Karolinska Institute, Box 285, S-171 77 Stockholm, Sweden

S.K. MORCOS, F.R.C.S., F.F.R.R.C.S.I., F.R.C.R.
Department of Diagnostic Imaging, Northern General Hospital NHS Trust, Sheffield S5 7AU, U.K.

A.N. NICHOLSON, O.B.E., D.SC., M.D.(H.C.), PH.D., F.R.C.P.(EDIN. & LOND.), F.R.C.PATH., F.F.O.M.
Centre for Human Sciences, Defence Evaluation and Research Agency, Farnborough, Hampshire, GU14 0LX, U.K.

J.K. PATEL, M.D.
Commonwealth Research Center and Massachusetts Mental Health Center, Harvard Medical School, Boston, MA 02115, U.S.A.

J.W. PATERSON, B.SC., M.B.B.S., F.R.C.P., F.R.A.C.P., F.R.C.P.A.
Department of Pharmacology, University of Western Australia, Nedlands WA 6907, Australia

K. PEERLINCK, M.D.
Center for Molecular and Vascular Biology and Division of Bleeding and Vascular Disorders, University of Leuven, Herestraat 49, B-3000 Leuven, Belgium

E. PERUCCA, M.D., PH.D.
Clinical Pharmacology Unit, University of Pavia, Piazza Botta 10, 27100 Pavia, Italy

B.C.P. POLAK, M.D.
Department of Ophthalmology, Free University Hospital, P.O. Box 7057, 1007 MB Amsterdam, The Netherlands

P. REISS, M.D., PH.D.
National AIDS Therapy Evaluation Center and Department of Infectious Diseases, Tropical Medicine and AIDS, Academic Medical Center, University of Amsterdam, P.O. Box 22700, 1100 DE Amsterdam, The Netherlands

H.D. REUTER, PH.D.
Siebengebirgsallee 24, D-50939 Köln, Germany

I. RIBEIRO, M.D.
Division of Infectious Diseases, Department of Cell and Molecular Sciences, St. George's Hospital Medical School, Cranmer Terrace, London SW17 0RE, U.K.

J.E. RITCHIE, M.B.CH.B.
Section of Anaesthetics, Department of Pharmacology, University of Auckland, Private Bag 92019, Auckland, New Zealand

M. SCHACHTER, M.D.
Department of Clinical Pharmacology, Imperial College School of Medicine, St. Mary's Hospital, London W2 1NY, U.K.

S.A. SCHUG, M.D., F.A.N.Z.C.A., F.F.P.M.A.N.Z.C.A.
Section of Anaesthetics, Department of Pharmacology, University of Auckland, Private Bag 92019, Auckland, New Zealand

R.P. SEQUEIRA, PH.D.
Department of Pharmacology and Clinical Pharmacology, College of Medicine and Medical Sciences, Arabian Gulf University, P.O. Box 22979, Manama, Bahrain

T.G. SHORT, M.B., CH.B., M.D.
Department of Pharmacology and Clinical Pharmacology, Faculty of Medicine and Health Science, The University of Auckland, Private Bag 92019, Auckland, New Zealand

A. STANLEY, PH.D., M.R.PHARM.S.
Birmingham Oncology Centre, St. Chad's Unit, City Hospital, Dudley Road, Birmingham B18 7QH, U.K.

W.G. VAN AKEN, M.D.
Central Laboratory of the Netherlands Red Cross, Blood Transfusion Service, Plesmanlaan 125, 1066 CX Amsterdam, The Netherlands

C.J. VAN BOXTEL, M.D., PH.D.
Department of Clinical Pharmacology & Pharmacotherapy, Academic Medical Center, Meibergdreef 9, 1105 AZ Amsterdam, The Netherlands

G.B. VAN DER VOET, PH.D.
Toxicology Laboratory, Department of Clinical Chemistry, Pharmacy and Toxicology, Leiden University Medical Center, P.O. Box 9600, 2300 RC Leiden, The Netherlands

R. VERHAEGHE, M.D.
Center for Vascular and Molecular Biology, University of Leuven, Herestraat 49, 3000 Leuven, Belgium

J. VERMYLEN, M.D.
Center for Molecular and Vascular Biology and Division of Bleeding and Vascular Disorders, University of Leuven, Herestraat 49, B-3000 Leuven, Belgium

T. VIAL, M.D.
Centre Anti-Poisons, Centre de Pharmacovigilance, Hôpital Edouard Herriot, 5 Place d'Arsonval, 69437 Lyon Cédex 03, France

T.J. WALSH, M.D.
Immunocompromised Host-Section, Pediatric Oncology Branch, National Cancer Institute, National Institutes of Health, Bldg. 10, Rm. 13N240, 10, Center Drive MSC, Bethesda, MD 20891, U.S.A.

E.J. WONG, M.D.
Massachusetts Mental Health Center, Harvard Medical School, Boston, MA 02115, U.S.A.

C. WOODROW, M.A., M.R.C.P.
Division of Infectious Diseases, Department of Cell and Molecular Sciences, St. George's Hospital Medical School, Cranmer Terrace, London SW17 0RE, U.K.

F. ZANNAD, M.D., PH.D., F.E.S.C.
Clinical Pharmacology and Cardiology, Centre d'Investigation Clinique INSERM-CHU and Centre de Dépistage et de Prévention du Risque Cardiovasculaire, Hôpital Jeanne d'Arc, Dommartin les Toul, Université Henri Poincaré, Nancy, France

O. ZUZAN, M.D.
Department of Anesthesiology, Hannover Medical School, D-30625 Hannover, Germany

Contents

Special reviews

Cumulative index of special reviews, Annuals 16–21

Index of drugs

Note: the format 19.211 refers to SEDA 19, p. 211

Index of side effects

How to use this book

THE SCOPE OF THE 'ANNUAL'

The Side Effects of Drugs Annual has been published each year since 1977. It is designed to provide a critical and up-to-date account of new information relating to adverse drug reactions and interactions from the clinician's point of view. The *Annual* can be used independently or as a supplement to the standard encyclopedic work in this field, *Meyler's Side Effects of Drugs*, the 13th edition of which was published in December, 1996; the 14th edition is scheduled to appear in the year 2000.

SPECIAL REVIEWS

As new data appear, older findings may be discredited and existing concepts may require revision. The 'special reviews' deal critically with such topics, interpreting conflicting evidence and providing the reader with clear guidance. Special reviews are identified by the traditional prescription symbol and are printed in italic type. Older papers cited in these reviews are either listed by name or via cross-references to previous Annuals or past editions of Meyler's Side Effects of Drugs, which can be found in most medical libraries.

SELECTION OF MATERIAL

In compiling the *Side Effects of Drugs Annual* particular attention is devoted to those publications which provide essentially new information or throw a new light on problems already recognized. In addition, some authoritative new reviews are listed. Publications which do not meet these criteria are omitted. Readers anxious to trace all references on a particular topic, including those which duplicate earlier work, are advised to consult *Adverse Reactions Titles*, a monthly bibliography of titles from approximately 3400 biomedical journals published throughout the world, compiled by the Excerpta Medica International Abstracting Service.

PERIOD COVERED

The present *Annual* reviews all reports presenting significant new information on adverse reactions to drugs from January 1997 – March 1998. During the production of this *Annual*, more recent papers have been included.

CLASSIFICATION

Drugs are classified according to their main field of application or the properties for which they are most generally recognized. In borderline cases, however, some supplementary discussion has been included in other chapters relating to secondary fields of application. Fixed combinations of drugs are dealt with according to their most characteristic component.

DRUG NAMES

Drug products are in general dealt with in the text under their most usual non-proprietary names; where these are not available, chemical names have been used; fixed combinations usually have no proprietary connotation and here trade names have been used as necessary.

SYSTEM OF REFERENCES

References in the text are coded as follows:

R: In the original paper, the point is *reviewed* in some detail with reference to other literature.

r: The original paper *refers* only briefly to the point, on the basis of evidence adduced by other writers.

C: The original paper presents *detailed original clinical evidence* on this point.

c: The original paper provides *clinical evidence*, but only *briefly or anecdotally*.

The code has not been applied to animal pharmacological papers.

The various Editions of *Meyler's Side Effects of Drugs* are cited in the text as SED-11, SED-12 etc.; *SED Annuals 1–20* are cited as SEDA-1, SEDA-2 etc.

INDEXES

Index of drugs: this index provides a complete listing of all references to a drug for which side effects and/or interactions are described.

Index of side effects: this index is necessarily selective, since a particular side effect may be caused by very large numbers of compounds; the index is therefore mainly directed to those side effects which are particularly serious or frequent, or are discussed in special detail. Before assuming that a given drug does not have a particular side effect, one should consult the relevant chapters.

For *interactions*, the reader should refer to the *Index of drugs* where all interactions are listed under the drugs concerned, irrespective of the chapter in which they appear.

It should be borne in mind that American spelling has been used throughout, e.g. anemia, estrogen etc. (instead of anaemia, oestrogen etc.).

Errors in prescribing, preparing, and giving medicines: definition, classification, and prevention

Robin E. Ferner* and Jeffrey K. Aronson

INTRODUCTION

After the event, an error in prescribing, making up, or giving a drug can be only too clear. The 'red man' ('red neck') syndrome of vasodilatation that follows the over-rapid administration of vancomycin, when a characteristic effect follows shortly after the commission of a well-recognized error, is a case in point (SEDA-17, 312). This error represents one, visible, manifestation of 'medication errors', potentially preventable deviations from ideal treatment. The extent to which such errors occur, their nature, their classification, and the possible ways of intervening to prevent them, are the subjects of this essay.

DEFINITIONS

Barker et al. (1) defined a medication error as a dose administered to the patient that deviates from the physician's orders, such as an omission, wrong dosage, or unauthorized drug. An example would be when one patient was given one of the doses intended for another. We assume that the authors meant that an error was an act of administering a deviant dose, rather than the dose itself. This restrictive definition examines only that part of the process subsequent to the physician's writing his or her prescription. It also classifies as 'errors' what are in fact corrections to errors perpetrated by the physician. For example, an 'error' would be committed if a nurse deliberately (and correctly) administered 250 μg of digoxin, rather than the 250 mg of digoxin that a physician had prescribed.

In 1993 the American Society of Hospital Pharmacists (2) published a list of 'types of medication error', with definitions. This list included an interesting category of 'compliance error', defined as inappropriate patient behavior regarding adherence to a prescribed medication regime. The implicit definition of 'medication error' as a mistake in prescribing, dispensing, or planned medication administration does not include non-compliance; and whilst failure to give any or adequate instructions on how to use a medicine would clearly be an error, deliberate failure on the patient's part to take the medicine would be a rather different form of therapeutic problem.

The National Coordinating Council for Medication Error Reporting and Prevention (NCC MERP) provided an even more inclusive definition: A medication error is any preventable event that may cause or lead to inappropriate medication use or patient harm while the medication is in the control of the health care professional, patient, or consumer. Such events may be related to professional practice, health care products, procedures, and systems, including: prescribing; order communication; product labelling, packaging, and nomenclature; compounding; dispensing; distribution; administration; education; monitoring; and use (3).

*This year's guest author, Robin Ferner, MSc, MD, FRCP, is Director of the West Midlands Centre for Adverse Drug Reaction Reporting, City Hospital, Birmingham B18 7QH, UK.

The WHO definition of an adverse drug reaction (ADR) (4) does not include ADRs that arise through error, and Bates et al (5) therefore used the more inclusive term 'adverse drug event' (ADE) to cover both ADRs and errors. They defined an adverse drug event as an injury resulting from medical intervention related to a drug.... For example, oversedation and aspiration pneumonia resulting from a ten-fold overdose of a drug would not be considered an ADR according to the [World Health Organization] definition, but would be an ADE. There are two problems with this definition.

The first problem is the dichotomy between adverse drug reactions and other, unclearly specified, adverse drug events. Adverse drug reactions can be due to error; for example, when fetal malformation results from the treatment of maternal acne with aromatic retinoids. However, they can also be inevitable, either because they are unpredictable, or because the action of a drug, such as a cytotoxic drug, includes unavoidable undesirable consequences, such as bone marrow suppression. However, in considering medication errors, it is only the (potentially) avoidable events that are of interest.

The second problem is that the definition excludes errors that do not translate into harm. For example, a child who received a single 10-fold overdose of penicillin might suffer no ill effects, and such an error, whilst potentially very serious with another drug, or in a patient with severe renal insufficiency, would go undetected. A satisfactory definition would also explicitly include errors that cause harm but are not detected. For example, a patient who had suffered a cardiac arrest might be given 10 times too much adrenaline, without those present being aware of the error; such an error could prevent successful resuscitation, but go undetected.

For the purposes of this essay, therefore, we propose to define a medication (drug) error as follows:

> a medication error is a failure in the treatment process that leads to, or has the potential to lead to, harm to the patient.

We use the word 'failure' to signify that the process has fallen below some attainable standard. The 'treatment process' starts after the decision to adopt treatment for symptoms or their causes, or to investigate or prevent disease or physiological changes (and so includes not only therapeutic drugs, but also, for instance, oral contraceptives, hormones used in replacement therapy, and radiographic contrast media). It includes the monitoring of therapy, but is not directly concerned with success or failure in reaching the therapeutic goal. Our definition does not specify who makes the error—it could be a doctor, a nurse, a pharmacist, a carer, the patient, or another.

Errors in diagnosis are not considered: they tend to be very different in form from the errors that occur after a plan of treatment has been decided upon. This is because diagnostic decisions are always based on probabilities of the association of an abnormality or group of abnormalities with a particular diagnosis. Patients are sometimes harmed by errors in the manufacture or storage of drugs, but these errors are not considered here.

CLASSIFYING MEDICATION ERRORS

Previous classifications

Classifying errors allows observers to identify broad categories of error, to quantify them, and, if the classification is related to some underlying model of the way in which errors occur, to predict and prevent them (6). Several attempts have been made to classify medication errors.

A model of drug therapy, such as the one outlined by Barker et al. (1), consists of a linear sequence: diagnosis ∅ prescription written ∅ prescription received and processed (by a pharmacist) ∅ drug dispensed ∅ drug administered ∅ patient receives drug ∅ 'patient gets well'. Barker et al. considered that the outcome of each stage was 'error' or 'no error'. This scheme makes several basic facts plain: (1) there are many steps in the process; (2) the steps often involve several different people, with different expertise and training; (3) at each step there is scope for several errors; (4) errors at any step can potentially be injurious; (5) whilst some errors made at one step could be found and corrected during a later step, others can escape detection until harm is done.

The scheme also suggests some ways in which the number of errors could be reduced, the propagation of errors from one step to the next could be held in check, and injury could be prevented. An obvious example is the problem that the doctor's handwriting is so bad that it is misread by the dispensing pharmacist or nurse. The advent in general practice in the UK of computer-generated typed prescriptions has made illegibility less likely, and has reduced the chances of an error in dispensing as a result of misreading.

Parenthetically, some errors can be propagated through the system (writing the wrong dosage, for example), whilst others are bound to be discovered before administration (omission of the drug name, for example). There are fewer subsequent checks on errors that occur later in the process, and this makes recovery from the error difficult or impossible (picking up the wrong syringe is an example of a late error).

Betz and Levy (7) considered three major groups of errors, namely those in prescribing, dispensing, and administering drugs. Each group was then subdivided into several rather specific categories. At this rather more detailed level, each step in the process can be examined to see what errors could occur. Such lists can appear repetitive; for instance, Tesh and Beeley (8) included dose omitted, frequency omitted, route omitted, and prescription unsigned as separate categories of error. A more etiological, or theological, classification might regard all these as sins of omission. Barker et al. (1) and Lesar et al. (9) had a single category of 'omission' or 'missing information', but distinguished among several subcategories: 'wrong drug', 'wrong route', and 'wrong dosage form', or 'wrong patient', all of which could be classified as identification errors.

Lists like those of Ferner (10) can be based on the potential weaknesses of the process, but in practical terms some especially common or especially dangerous errors are more important than others. The American Society of Hospital Pharmacists (2), for example, listed the following common errors: (1) ambiguous strength designation on labels or in packaging; (2) drug product nomenclature (look-alike or sound-alike names); (3) equipment failure or malfunction; (4) illegible handwriting; (5) improper transcription; (6) inaccurate dosage calculation.

However, this classification says nothing about why the errors occurred.

The NCC MERP proposed classifying errors into one of nine categories, according to the harm they caused, the so-called Medication Error Index (11). For example, Category A included 'circumstances or events with the capacity to cause error', Category G 'an error that resulted in permanent patient harm', and Category I included errors that resulted in death. However, this classification is not very helpful in terms of prevention, since it deals with outcome, not cause.

Parallels with other error-prone processes

Leape et al. (12) considered the parallel between errors in prescribing and major incidents, such as the nuclear accident at the Three Mile Island generating station. Investigation of that and other serious events has suggested that they occur as the end of a chain of events in a poorly designed system that induces errors, or makes them difficult to detect. Poor systems, such as working in an environment in which frequent interruptions distract the worker, create 'accidents waiting to happen.' Leape et al. (12) pointed out that, whilst in medicine attempts are made to reduce the number of errors by 'training, exhortation, rules, and sanctions', this approach is not favored by those who have investigated errors in other contexts. They maintained that it is more effective to redesign a system so that individuals are less likely to commit errors, and so that errors are more easily detected and rectified before they result in harm.

Engineers interested in the safety of industrial processes have developed sophisticated methods of analysing and quantifying the risks of human errors. For example, Kirwan (6) lists the nominal likelihood that errors will occur during the performance of tasks of different sorts. These likelihoods are estimated from observing either the operation of real processes, or simulations, or by asking experts to judge them. For example, in an experiment in which subjects were asked to enter 40 seven-digit telephone numbers on a keypad, errors occurred once every 30 keypresses. The probability of an error in 'a routine operation where care is required' is estimated as 0.01, but for a 'complicated nonroutine task, with stress', it is 30 times higher. The nominal likelihood is increased by 'error-producing conditions', such as 'unfamiliarity with a situation which is potentially important, but which only occurs infrequently', 'a mismatch between perceived and real risk', or 'little or no independent checking or testing of output', all of which apply only too clearly to some circumstances in which medication errors occur.

Leape et al (12), in considering how errors arise in the system for giving drug treatment, introduced the idea that there is a 'proximal cause', in the technical language that they used, for an error. By this they meant a broad category into which a group of systems analysts divided the 'reasons' for the medication errors they observed. Such categories included errors due to inadequate knowledge (of the drug or the patient), rule violations, slips, lapses of memory, and faults in identifying or checking drugs.

This attempt by pharmacists and others to use the systematic description of human errors and errors in systems that psychologists and others have built up over the last century or so was prefigured by anesthetists, notably in the Australian Incident Monitoring Study (13), in which errors ('when a planned sequence of mental or physical activities fails to result in the intended outcome') were investigated in anesthesia. Its authors defined only a small number of categories of active error, namely: (1) knowledge-based errors; (2) rule-based errors; (3) technical errors; (4) slips or lapses.

This classification rests heavily on psychological foundations.

Psychological aspects of human error: mistakes and slips

The psychological aspects of human error have been lucidly reviewed (6), (14). Briefly, psychologists consider an error to be a disorder of intentional acts, and they distinguish between errors in planning an act and errors in its execution. If a prior intention to reach a specified goal leads to action, and the action leads to the goal, then all is well. If the plan of action contains some flaw (for example, planning to give a medicine to a child, but failing to realize that children require different doses from adults), then that is a 'mistake'; if an error occurs in carrying out the action, that is a 'slip or lapse'. A slip is a form of human error defined to be 'the performance of an action that was not what was intended' (15). A slip of the pen, when a doctor intends to write chlorpromazine but distractedly writes chlorpropamide, is an example. Lapses are covert slips, particularly errors of memory. Slips and lapses are errors due to failures of skill—for example, picking the wrong medicine from a shelf, or administering the medicine to the wrong Mr Brown, when two patients have the same surname.

Technical errors, in which the correct rules are applied correctly, but the result is still not what is desired, are important in anesthesia and surgery, but hardly relevant to prescribing, preparing, and giving drugs, except when the last requires great technical expertise—for instance, stellate ganglion blockade and the like. They can in any case be considered a subset of slips (skill-based errors).

Norman (15) developed a classification of slips, based on their presumed causes. Underpinning the classification is the theoretical view that actions are controlled by a form of knowledge called a schema, which is an organized memory 'template'. Slips can occur as early as that point at which an intention to act is formed, if the situation that demands action is misclassified, and so the wrong schema is chosen. A practical example might be starting cardiopulmonary resuscitation on a patient who was merely asleep. There can also be slips in acting according to the schema, an important example being the 'capture' of one schema by the sequence of actions belonging to another, more familiar, schema. The classic example is of the man who went to his bedroom to change for dinner, and subsequently found himself in bed in his pyjamas. A prescriber who habitually used pethidine 100 mg as a postoperative analgesic might specify the dosage of morphine as 100 mg as the result of such a capture error. Errors in carrying out the sequence of events specified in the schema, such as omitting or duplicating some step, are a further important class of slips. An example would be when a nurse, having already added 20 mmol of potassium chloride to a bag of infusion fluid, forgot having done so and added a further 20 mmol of potassium chloride. There can, in addition, be faults in activation of the schema that lead to slips. For example, when several things are happening at the same time, two schemata can become confused. A verbal slip that illustrates this is when a person may be thinking of both 'closed' and 'shut' and say 'clut'.

One important consequence of this analysis is that slips cannot easily be prevented by exhortation. Norman (15) has expressed the view that slips can be detected only if there is feedback at several levels.

Slips and lapses (that is, skill-based errors) are distinguished from mistakes. These can be subdivided into those that are due to lack of expertise (knowledge-based errors), when there is ignorance of the rule required and thus a need to plan an action from first principles; and those due to a failure of expertise (rule-based errors), when rules are applied inappropriately. An expansion of the ideas of skill-based and rule-based errors is founded on the psychological notion that, if they can, people recognize a pattern and act according to a schema applied to the pattern, rather than calculating or analysing each new problem separately. This leads to 'strong-but-wrong' errors, where people are strongly impelled to use a familiar strategy, even if it is applied in the wrong circumstances. Rule-based errors can further be categorized as the misapplication of good rules, and the application of bad rules. Reason (14) combined the ideas of skill-based, rule-based, and knowledge-based errors against a background of schemata and of the tendency to reach for ready-made solutions into the Generic Error Modelling System (GEMS).

The models used to explain the occurrence of human error can also be used as the basis for a classification of them. Kirwan (6) has considered the advantages of having such a taxonomy, but also points out two major pitfalls:

(1) an incomplete classification may mean that important errors are omitted from the analysis of a process;
(2) an incorrect or superficial classification can obscure important differences or similarities between different observed errors, and reduce the ability of the classification to predict or avoid future errors.

Kirwan has also provided a flow chart to identify tasks with 'cognitive-error potential'. For example, the potential for cognitive error is indicated by an answer of 'yes' to any of the following questions: (1) does the task involve any problem-solving, judgement, or diagnosis? (2) will the operator have to resort to theory or abstract knowledge to derive a solution? (3) does the task have any highly unusual or novel aspects not covered by procedures or training?

And, for non-routine tasks, answers of 'no' to these questions: (1) do operators unambiguously understand the task? (2) do procedures cover the case? (3) are operators trained so they understand the task?

The chilling thing about this flow chart is that the tasks associated with prescribing, making up, dispensing, and administering medicines are quite clearly liable to cognitive errors.

THE EPIDEMIOLOGY OF ERRORS

The medical literature contains a large number of case reports of medication errors, and various authors, particularly Cohen in the US and Cousins and Upton in the UK, have collected salutary examples of the genre (see http://www.ismp.org/ISMP/Novel.html).

Until quite recently, the medical defence organizations in Britain knew of all errors that led to legal action against doctors, and their annual reports were also important catalogues of the sorts of prescribing problem that can occur. In the UK this is still true of errors in General Practice, but not in National Health Service hospitals, each of which now has its own catalogue of errors.

Systematic attempts to count the number of medication errors are beset by the problem that errors (for example, in the dosage written on a prescription) that are detected and corrected before they lead to harm may in any event have been detected, or may not have led to harm; conversely, not all errors that cause harm will be detected. With these limitations, several attempts have been made to examine the frequency of errors in hospital practice.

- A partly retrospective audit of prescription charts in the 1970s (8) found deviations from the ideal in 30% of all prescriptions.
- Observers of prescribing in long-stay homes and hospitals in the 1980s found medication errors on about 12% of those occasions on which it was possible to commit them (1).
- This rate was similar to the error rate found in a hospital outpatient pharmacy in the early 1980s, although only 1.5% of errors were classified as potentially serious (16).
- A decade later, rates of all errors (12.5%) and potentially serious errors (1.5%) in hospital out-patient dispensing had hardly changed (17).
- An error rate of 4.4% was observed for a system of unit-dose dispensing by pharmacy technicians, designed to reduce error rates; although 'wrong-time errors', when the drug was given more than 90 min before or after the scheduled time, accounted for about two-thirds of all the errors (18).
- In a 1-year study by pharmacists of prescribing errors by physicians in an American teaching hospital, 905 errors were detected in 289 411 prescriptions, with a rate of potentially severe or fatal errors of 1.8 per 1000 prescriptions. First-year physicians were nearly five times more likely to make a severe error than fourth-year physicians (9).
- A careful prospective analysis of drug-related harm in two teaching hospitals, covering 4031 medical admissions, detected 70 adverse events due to errors (1.7% of all patients), and 143 potential errors in the use of drugs. Seven preventable adverse drug events left the patient with residual disability at the time of discharge. The highest rates of adverse events were found on medical intensive care units (5).
- This last result was borne out by an intensive care study that showed that preventable adverse drug events were substantially more common in medical than surgical intensive care units (19).
- Human error accounted for the vast majority of the medication errors reported in a neonatal intensive care unit, where the risk of an incident was 13.4 per 1000 patient days (20).
- Another study, of over 1000 administrations to children in hospital, detected errors in 5%; a substantial reduction from the rate found in the same institution several years before (21).
- An analysis of coroner's investigations into deaths from adverse drug events suggested that about 20% of such fatalities result from errors rather than adverse reactions (22).

In summary, prescribing errors, sometimes serious, are still quite frequent in hospital practice. Errors that cause patients to receive treatment that was not as intended may occur about 1% of the time, although detected errors that lead to harm are relatively rare, occurring in perhaps one in 1000 patients.

The rates of medication error outside hospitals were investigated in one study that estimated prescribing errors to occur in 5% of general practice prescriptions presented to community pharmacists, who spent a great deal of time telephoning prescribers to clarify prescriptions (23).

In a study of 263 consecutive patients receiving prehospital advanced cardiac life support for cardiac arrhythmias associated with cardiac arrest, treatment errors made by paramedics and physicians in telemetric communication with them occurred in 120 patients (46%) (24).

EXAMPLES OF IMPORTANT MEDICATION ERRORS

Human error analysis, which investigates and tries to quantify the risk of future errors

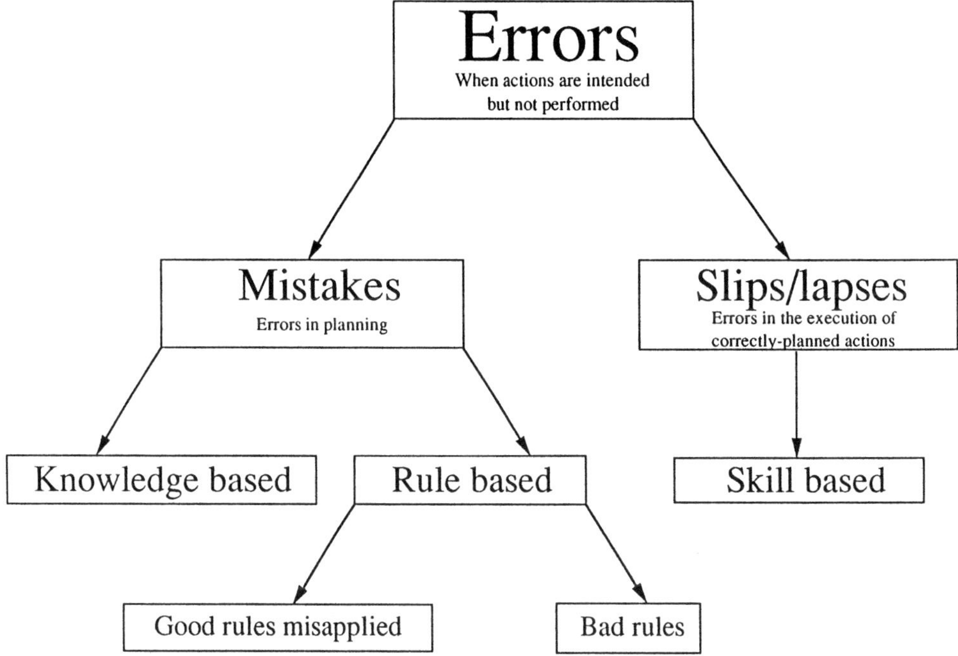

Figure 1. *A classification of types of errors, suitable for classifying medication errors. For examples in each category see the text.*

from general rules (like those of Williams referred to above) and specific examples of error, has not, as far as we know, formally been applied to medication errors. Some insight can still be gained by an examination of errors reported in the past with a view to reducing or preventing their future occurrence, but there is the risk that a great deal of time and effort will be spent on avoiding errors that are vanishingly rare, or alternatively, failing to take precautions against errors so common that they are rarely reported.

The classification of errors discussed here is shown in Figure 1. The different categories are illustrated by the following examples.

Errors in prescribing

Knowledge-based errors

Prescribers can make mistakes because they do not know enough about a patient—for example, that she is asthmatic or that he is allergic to a particular drug.

A woman was found to have raised blood pressure at a nurse-run well-woman clinic; the general practitioner prescribed propranolol and the patient died from an acute attack of asthma after the first tablet. The doctor was unaware that the patient suffered from asthma (25).

A busy house officer prescribed trimethoprim by telephone for a surgical patient whom the ward sister reported to have symptoms of a urinary tract infection; the patient suffered an allergic reaction and died after a single tablet. The notes and drugs chart both stated that the patient was allergic to trimethoprim, but this was not noticed (26).

These errors were certainly due to insufficient knowledge, but ignorance might have been avoided by applying better rules. For example, the rule always ask about drug allergy before prescribing would have prevented the trimethoprim tragedy, if it had been applied.

Knowledge-based errors also arise through ignorance of the prescribed drug, or its interactions with other drugs.

Ten heroin addicts died within 2–4 days of starting a methadone maintenance programme. The average starting dose was methadone 53 mg daily. High concentrations of methadone were found in the blood of several of the patients after they had died. Lack of appreciation of the long half-life of methadone, difficulty in assessing the degree of opiate tolerance in individuals, and the existence of liver disease, which may have reduced methadone clearance, were all possible factors in these deaths (27).

Failure to appreciate that the opioid antagonist naloxone has a very short half-life leads from time to time to deaths, when patients poisoned with opiate analgesics are given naloxone, wake up, are left unobserved, and develop renewed respiratory depression as the naloxone wears off.

A man taking warfarin developed gout, was given azapropazone, and had a fatal hemorrhage (22). Azapropazone augments the anticoagulant effect of warfarin.

A further form of knowledge is also required, and that is knowledge of what others will know or understand.

Before histamine H2 receptor antagonists were introduced, patients with peptic ulcers were sometimes treated by slowly instilling milk into the stomach via a nasogastric tube. In 1973 (unpublished observation), a young woman suffered a fat embolus when an inexperienced nurse, asked to set up a 'milk drip', took a bottle of milk from the ward refrigerator, warmed it in a saucepan, and then administered it intravenously using a glass giving-set.

Rule-based errors in prescribing

Published examples of rule-based errors, when, for example, the prescriber correctly applies a faulty algorithm, are hard to find. One example is the habit of starting warfarin therapy with two successive daily doses of warfarin 10 mg followed by one of 5 mg ('ten, ten, five'), which often leads to over- or under-anticoagulation. An 'intelligent' algorithm, in which the dose on each succeeding day is adjusted according to the coagulation result from the previous day, is better at ensuring therapeutic anticoagulation in a specified time (28).

The high incidence of neutropenia that attended the use of captopril shortly after it was marketed was the result of a bad rule: to use very high doses. The 1981–2 Data Sheet for Capoten® stated that in adults "The usual dose range of Capoten (captopril) is 25–150 mg t.i.d. The maximum recommended daily dose is 450 mg". The recommended starting dose in hypertension today is 12.5 mg twice daily, with a maximum daily dose in severe hypertension of 150 mg. Neutropenia, which is dose-dependent, is now very rarely encountered.

A rather literal example of a faulty algorithm is the following:

A man with a sore throat consulted the practice nurse. He told her he was allergic to penicillin. She prescribed, by computer, 'Deteclo', which contains a combination of tetracyclines. The patient took 'Deteclo' and developed a rash. The computer, although containing the information that the patient had previously been allergic to 'Deteclo', failed to display it because of a fault in the computer program (25).

Skill-based errors (slips and lapses)

Writing illegibly has traditionally been a prerogative of doctors. The consequences can be difficulties in interpretation for the pharmacist who is to dispense a prescription, and since pharmacists may pride themselves on their ability to read doctors' handwriting, they may also feel a need to resolve the difficulties without reference to the prescriber. This leads to a propagated error. For example:

A doctor scrawled a prescription for the antibacterial 'Amoxil' (amoxicillin); the pharmacist read it as 'Daonil' (glibenclamide); the patient developed severe hypoglycemia that led to permanent brain damage (29).

A patient who took a toxic dose of methotrexate was given a prescription for folinic acid as rescue therapy, but the scribbled prescription was read by the nurses as folic acid, which is ineffective. After several doses of folic acid, the error was discovered, folinic acid was given, and the patient's bone marrow eventually recovered (30).

The number of separate drugs runs to several thousand, even in countries such as the UK, which has relatively few licensed medical products. Since some of us cannot consistently call our children by their correct names, it is not surprising that drug names become confused (31), (32). Slips, such as confusing chlorpropamide with chlorpromazine (33) and 'Lasix' with 'Losec' (34), are probably common, and would be expected, as the schema for writing one name captures the schema for writing a similar, less commonly written name. A comparable slip would be writing the year 1998 on prescriptions (or cheques) written in early January 1999.

Lambert (35) has described simple linguistic methods for predicting whether two drug names are likely to be confused, one of which is based on what is known as the Levenshtein distance: the number of changes (including additions or deletions) that you would have to make to change one name into another. If the distance is less than five such steps, the two names are likely to be confused.

Similar slips result when a prescriber writes, say, the habitual dosage appropriate for ibuprofen when, exceptionally, prescribing indomethacin.

A large dose of haloperidol (5 mg three times daily) was transcribed as the more commonly used dose of haloperidol (0.5 mg three times daily), with fatal consequences (22).

The dosage, units of dose, and route of administration are also sensitive to handwriting errors. Sometimes there is confusion among them. For example, 100U can be read as 1000 [units]; and IU can be read as IV.

An important class of skill-based errors is those that relate to inaccurate calculations of dosage. The arithmetical skill required is usually not high, but the process seems to be very prone to error in the stressful setting of acute medical care. Doses in children, commonly calculated on the basis of body weight or body surface area, are especially hard for clinical staff to get right.

A premature infant was given 1 mg/kg of pancuronium bromide instead of 0.1 mg/kg and required ventilation for 2 days (36).

When formally tested on their skills in dosage calculation, pediatric nurses made 10-fold errors once in 12 sums, and pediatricians once in 26 sums on average; experience made no difference to accuracy, but experienced nurses felt more certain of their results (37).

Errors sometimes come from confusing volume and amount.

A baby died when given 2.5 ml/kg per day of potassium chloride solution, instead of 2.5 mmol/kg per day (1.25 ml/kg per day) (22).

Errors in dispensing and making up drugs

Knowledge-based errors

One of the paradoxes of the medication process is that pharmacists, who have a thorough knowledge of many aspects of the process, do not usually apply it when dispensing, except to check for errors in prescribing. Knowledge-based errors can sometimes occur in drug preparation if a pharmacist is not involved.

A 70-year-old man suffered severe diarrhea, nausea, and vomiting after drinking a herbal tea brewed by his wife. She had for many years collected the comfrey leaves she used for the tea, 'knitbone', but on this occasion had mistakenly gathered foxglove (*Digitalis purpurea*), not recognizing the difference, or knowing the dangers (38).

Rule-based errors

A hypothetical example of a rule-based error in dispensing is the systematic labelling of antibacterial formulations Complete the treatment course unless otherwise directed. In some circumstances (the *British National Formulary* cites diarrhea during treatment with clindamycin), the patient will be encouraged to take a medicine that is responsible for a serious adverse effect, and come to harm as a result.

Skill-based errors (slips and lapses)

Many dispensing errors are slips that occur when the name of one drug is read as the name of another, either on the prescription or on the stock bottle.

Three pharmacists reported that dispensers had taken vials of 'Zofran' (ondansetron) injection when 'Zantac' (ranitidine) had been prescribed (39).

A pharmacist dispensed 'Norflex' (orphenadrine) when norflox[acin] had been written; the patient became dizzy and unable to move. She had taken the medicine exactly as prescribed, four tablets twice a day. (40).

Making assumptions about the contents of a vial of a particular shape or in a particular place can also lead to slips.

A child was poisoned with theophylline when a pharmacy worker tidied a vial of theophylline solution into a stock box that contained very similar vials of dextrose solution, and another worker dispensed the theophylline instead of dextrose (39).

A pharmacy stocked metronidazole close to mivacurium (a curare-like muscle relaxant), and a technician prepared four intravenous infusions containing the muscle relaxant instead of the antibacterial drug. One patient died and one almost died when given the wrong infusions (41).

Failure to check the drug name on an ampoule probably led a New Zealand anesthetist to administer dopamine hydrochloride in place of doxapram hydrochloride; the patient died. The ampoule had been taken from a drawer intended only for ampoules of doxapram. The anesthetist was nevertheless convicted of manslaughter (42).

Skill is needed to make up solutions of medicines accurately.

A study of the concentrations of sympathomimetic drugs made up by nurses in an intensive care unit showed substantial variation between the prescribed concentration and the concentration measured in samples of infusate (43).

Errors in giving drugs

Errors in administering drugs extend to every aspect of the process, and range from giving the correct drugs to the wrong patient to giving the wrong drug to the right patient. Errors in dose and strength, and in route, time, and frequency of administration, are all well-recognized.

Knowledge-based errors

Failure to appreciate that calcium gluconate forms a milky-white precipitate of calcium carbonate when injected into alkaline solution, such as sodium bicarbonate solution, would be an example of a knowledge-based error of administration.

Rule-based errors

An important danger of intramuscular injection is damage to the sciatic nerve, and rules of administration have evolved to prevent this happening. The standard teaching at one time was for such injections to be given into the 'upper, outer quadrant' of the buttock, but injuries to the nerve running through the buttock still occurred. In consequence, doctors and nurses are now taught that the preferred route for intramuscular injection is the outer side of the anterior of the thigh muscle (44). This rule ensures that major motor nerves are distant from the site of injection. However, some formulations for injection are sufficiently toxic to the skin or subcutaneous tissues that the only safe way to administer them is into a very bulky muscle, and so from time to time patients develop skin necrosis after injections into the thigh, for example, when some non-steroidal anti-inflammatory drugs are given (45).

Some drugs are intrinsically dangerous, and their safe use requires adherence to well-defined rules.

A patient treated with gentamicin for presumed infective endocarditis suffered vestibular damage. This was almost certainly the result of excessive doses of the drug, and the fact that therapy was monitored only by measuring trough concentrations, not both peak and trough concentrations, and not at all in the last week of treatment. The patient failed to win damages for negligence, as an expert had testified that at the time she was treated, he would not have measured peak gentamicin concentrations (46).

Better rules for monitoring gentamicin, based on once-a-day therapy, have now been devised (47).

A more subtle rule-based error is illustrated by the following case:

Labetalol was prescribed for a young woman with osteogenesis imperfecta and hypertension, but her ward had none. A nurse was sent to another ward and returned with a small pot containing 10 tablets of labetalol 100 mg. The pot carried a hand-written adhesive label saying 'labetalol 100 mg'. Later, another nurse, asked to administer the treatment, took the label to mean that the total dose of the 10 tablets in the pot was 100 mg, and gave all of them to the patient, who died.

Failure to have, or observe, adequate rules regarding the transfer of medicines from one ward to another, and their labelling, combined with use of a medicine unfamiliar to the patient or nurse, led to this fatal error.

A doctor asked a nurse to fetch some 'flushing solution' for an intravenous cannula (unpublished observation). The nurse returned with a bottle marked 'F/S' (?flushing solution), which the doctor injected. The patient developed a severe inflammatory response to the Formol Saline.

This illustrates the serious errors that can arise from ignoring the golden rule of ascertaining unequivocally what you are about to inject.

Skill-based errors (slips and lapses)

Slips at this stage are potentially very dangerous. Once a syringe filled with potassium chloride strong solution has been injected by mistake, the patient's life is in jeopardy. This can happen as a result of an error earlier in the process, such as drawing up the wrong drug, or mislabelling drugs. It can also happen when pre-prepared syringes are inadvertently confused.

The Australian Incident Monitoring Study received reports of 70 'syringe swap' errors in the first 2000 reports of anesthetic incidents; of these, eight involved the administration of suxamethonium instead of fentanyl, or the reverse (48).

It seems almost impossible to prevent slips in which medicines intended for administration by one route are given by another route. For example:

Intravenous vincristine and intrathecal methotrexate are often prescribed together, and deaths have occurred when the routes of administration have been inadvertently interchanged. Intrathecal vincristine causes an arachnoiditis that is usually fatal (49).

This type of error has on occasion led doctors to be charged with manslaughter. This error could also be classified as rule-based, since it suggests that the doctors administering the drugs had not observed the implicit rule, mentioned in the section on 'Rule-based errors in giving drugs' above, that only unambiguously specified medicines should be injected.

In a similar case, undoubtedly a slip, daunorubicin solution (which is red) was injected intrathecally when cytosine arabinoside solution (clear) should have been given; the patient died (50).

In this case, the pharmacist who drew up the solutions transposed the labels affixed to the syringes, and no-one noticed the discrepancy in color.

On three occasions confusion arose between intravenous cannulae and either intra-arterial or intra-epidural cannulae (51).

The authors of this last report suggested that a specific and standardized male–female connector should be used for arterial lines, so that they could not be confused with other lines.

Sometimes drugs are given by the wrong route as a result of deficiencies of technical skill. For example, a cannula for intravenous injection can inadvertently be sited in an artery, with serious consequences. This error may have an incidence of one in 4000 cannulations (52). The consequences of this error are more apparent with some formulations, notably barbiturates, some benzodiazepines, and phenytoin (53), than with others, and so the error may be more easily recognised if those drugs are given.

A subcutaneous reservoir for the pump of an intrathecal infusion system for morphine administration was refilled by percutaneous puncture. The patient became very drowsy when, in error, morphine 450 mg was injected beside the reservoir and not into it (54).

Another example of a deficiency of skill led to censure of the anesthetist involved by the Conduct Committee of the General Medical Council.

A 22-year-old woman had teeth extracted under general anesthesia in a dental surgery. Whilst she was anesthetized, the consultant anesthetist inserted a diclofenac suppository for pain relief, and the anesthetist explained this to the patient and her husband after the surgery was over. Subsequently, the woman noted a vaginal discharge which led her to fear that she had been raped whilst under anesthetic, and the police became involved. It transpired that the anesthetist had erroneously inserted the suppository into the vagina, not the rectum. The anesthetist was brought before the professional conduct committee of the General Medical Council and found guilty of treatment without informed consent and of assault (55). The dentist was also found guilty of assault (56).

MAKING TREATMENT SAFER

Errors of all forms are common in the process of prescribing, drawing up, and giving drugs, and they can have serious consequences. They arise, not just at every stage in the process, but from all the hypothesized roots of error: insufficient knowledge; inadequate or misapplied rules; and failures of skill (slips and lapses). No single change is likely to reduce the prevalence of all these forms of error. There is a set of changes, related to 'feed-back', or checking, which would be likely to improve matters generally. This set of changes includes:

(1) asking all involved to report any error to a single person or group within an organization—for example, to a designated pharmacist in a hospital; this can only happen effectively if there is no censure of those who report their own errors;
(2) making all people in the chain from prescriber to patient responsible for previous stages in the chain and for not giving a medicine until the rules have been complied with—for example, making nurses responsible for drawing to the attention of a doctor any failure to write a prescription in the agreed fashion;
(3) making it clear that people require to be taught the skills of prescribing and giving drugs in a formal fashion, rather than by apprenticeship.

A more specific treatment for failures of skill—inability to prepare concentrations of the required solution, for example—would be to make sure that a subset of hospital staff, probably pharmacists or their technicians in this specific example, was trained to a standard sufficient for the purpose, and was available to perform the skilled task when needed.

Slips and lapses are more likely when there are competing tasks, when the task is unfamiliar, or when the operator is tired. These are common conditions of work for doctors and nurses. Reducing the extent to which tasks depend upon them may help. For example, many slips in prescribing could be detected, or their presence suspected, by a suitably programmed computer. In such a fashion, any discrepancy between a patient's age, sex, weight, current medication, or drug allergy history, and the drug name, dose, or form, could be signalled automatically. A more sophisticated system might be able to link knowledge from hospital information systems to improve the process still further. Some progress has been made in this direction, and two recent reports have shown the reduction in serious incidents that can be achieved by constraining physicians to prescribe by computer (57), (58). For example, Raschke's system (58) would warn a physician if his or her patient were receiving heparin treatment and the platelet count fell below 50×10^{12}/l, arousing the suspicion of heparin-induced thrombocytopenia.

Slips that commonly result from the confusion of one drug for another are apparently difficult to eradicate. There are two schools of thought as to what might be done to reduce drug confusion at the level of drawing up drugs. One proposes that all drugs for intravenous administration should be packaged in ampoules of the same size and character, so that they could only be distinguished one from another by careful attention to the label (59). The other school proposes that especially dangerous or important medicines should be packaged in conspicuous and clearly differentiated packaging (60), (61). More experimental psychology is needed to decide between these opposing alternatives, neither of which is entirely satisfactory (62).

Since a number of slips would be prevented by meticulous application of rules, such as always write prescriptions legibly, always ask patients about drug allergies, and always make sure that someone else checks that you are drawing up and injecting the correct drug, some thought needs to be given to making rules that are generally observable. Perhaps changes in society that have reduced the fear of breaking rules have worked against the interests of patients in this area.

A further problem that sometimes arises is that a dispenser substitutes one drug by another (usually less expensive) drug, from a different manufacturer, and often entirely different in respect of size, shape, and color, the last two being largely determined by fashion and convenience. One way forward for oral medication might be to assign a code word to every formulation and strength of a particular drug, made up of five letters (yielding almost 12 million possible combinations, using a 26-letter alphabet), so that every formulation of every product can at least carry a consistent code, regardless of manufacturer, brand-name, color, or shape.

There is a paradox in the fact that those who are most likely to administer drugs—nurses and junior doctors—are less well trained in the skills of doing so than pharmacists, who have specific expertise in the problems of drug treatment. All three professional groups are motivated to help patients, but the people most motivated of all are the patients. When they have been taking medicines at home for many years, they or their carers are likely to be more expert in administering their treatment than the professionals.

We shall have to wait for 'intelligent' computer prescribing, although it may not be far off. In the meantime, methods to encourage reporting of slips and mistakes, and of preventing their propagation, should help. We should also ask whether a system in which pharmacists or patients make up and administer drugs might be best.

REFERENCES

1. Barker KN, Mikeal RL, Pearson RE, Illig NA, Morse ML. Medication errors in nursing homes and small hospitals. Am J Hosp Pharm 1982;39:987–91.
2. American Society of Hospital Pharmacists. ASHP guidelines for preventing medication errors. Am J Hosp Pharm 1993;50:305–14.
3. Anonymous. National Council focuses on coordinating error reduction efforts. USP Quality Rev 1997;(57).
4. World Health Organization. International drug monitoring: the role of national centres. Technical Report Series No 498. Geneva: WHO, 1972.
5. Bates DW, Cullen DJ, Laird N, Petersen LA, Small SD, Servi D, Laffel G, Sweitzer BJ, Shea BF, Hallisey R, VanderVliet M, Nemeskal R, Leape LL. Incidence of adverse drug events and potential adverse drug events. Implications for prevention. ADE Prevention Study Group. J Am Med Assoc 1995;274:29–34.
6. Kirwan B. A Guide to Practical Human Reliability Assessment. London: Taylor and Francis, 1994.
7. Betz RP, Levy HB. An interdisciplinary method of classifying and monitoring medication errors. Am J Hosp Pharm 1985;42:1724–32.
8. Tesh DE, Beeley L. Errors of drug prescribing. Br J Clin Pharmacol 1975;2:403–9.
9. Lesar TS, Briceland LL, Delcoure K, Parmalee JC, Masta Gornic V, Pohl H. Medication prescribing errors in a teaching hospital. J Am Med Assoc 1990;263:2329–34.
10. Ferner RE. Forensic Pharmacology. Oxford: Oxford University Press, 1996.
11. Hartwig SC, Denger SD, Schneider PJ. Severity-indexed, incident report-based medication error-reporting program. Am J Hosp Pharm 1991;48:2611–16.
12. Leape LL, Bates DW, Cullen DJ, Cooper J, Demonaco HJ, Gallivan T, Hallisey R, Ives J, Laird N, Laffel G, et al. Systems analysis of adverse drug events. ADE Prevention Study Group. J Am Med Assoc 1995;274:35–43.
13. Runciman WB, Sellen A, Webb RK, Williamson JA, Currie M, Morgan C, Russell WJ. Errors, incidents and accidents in anaesthetic practice. Anaesth Intensive Care 1993;21:506–19.
14. Reason JT. Human Error. New York: Cambridge University Press, 1990.
15. Norman DA. Categorization of action slips. Psychol Rev 1981;88:1–15.
16. Guernsey BG, Ingrim NB, Hokanson JA, Doutre WH, Bryant SG, Blair CW, Galvan E. Pharmacists' dispensing accuracy in a high-volume outpatient pharmacy service: focus on risk management. Drug Intell Clin Pharm 1983;17:742–6.
17. Kistner UA, Keith MR, Sergeant KA, Hokanson JA. Accuracy of dispensing in a high-volume, hospital-based outpatient pharmacy. Am J Hosp Pharm 1994;51:2793–7.
18. Jozefczyk KG, Schneider PJ, Pathak DS. Medication errors in a pharmacy-coordinated drug administration program. Am J Hosp Pharm 1986;43:2464–7.
19. Cullen DJ, Sweitzer BJ, Bates DW, Burdick E, Edmondson A, Leape LL. Preventable adverse drug events in hospitalized patients: a comparative study of intensive care and general care units. Crit Care Med 1997;25:1289–97.
20. Vincer MJ, Murray JM, Yuill A, Allen AC, Evans JR, Stinson DA. Drug errors and incidents in a neonatal intensive care unit. A quality assurance activity. Am J Dis Child 1989;143:737–40.
21. Nahata, MC. Paediatric drug therapy II: drug administration errors. J Clin Pharm Ther 1988;13:399–402.
22. Ferner RE, Whittington RM. Coroner's cases of death due to errors in prescribing or giving medicines or to adverse drug reactions: Birmingham 1986–1991. J R Soc Med 1994; 87:145–8.
23. Neville RG, Robertson F, Livingstone S, Crombie IK. A classification of prescription errors. J R Coll Gen Pract 1989;39:110–12.
24. Peacock JB, Blackwell VH, Wainscott M. Medical reliability of advanced prehospital car-

diac life support. Ann Emerg Med 1985;14:407–9.
25. Ferner RE. More errors in prescribing and giving medicines. J Med Defence Union 1995; 11:80–2.
26. Cousins DH, Upton DR. Medication errors. When words fail us. Hosp Pharm Pract 1993;September:466.
27. Drummer OH, Opeskin K, Syrjanen M, Cordner SM. Methadone toxicity causing death in ten subjects starting on a methadone maintenance program. Am J Forensic Med Pathol 1992; 13:346–50.
28. Fennerty A, Dolben J, Thomas P, Backhouse G, Bentley DP, Campbell IA, Routledge PA. Flexible induction dose regimen for warfarin and prediction of maintenance dose. Br Med J Clin Res Ed 1984;288:1268–70.
29. Brahams D. Uninsured pharmacists and illegible prescriptions. Lancet 1989;i:510.
30. Cousins DH, Upton DR. Medication errors. Where are the pharmacists? Hosp Pharm Pract 1994;May:219–20.
31. McNulty H, Spurr P. Drug names that look or sound alike. Br Med J 1979;2:836.
32. McNulty H, Spurr P. Drug names which look or sound alike. Pharm J 1982;December 11:686–8.
33. Stocks AE, Martin FI. Hypoglycaemia due to erroneous drug ingestion. Med J Aust 1972; 1:1256–8.
34. Raffalli J, Nowakowski J, Wormser GP. 'Vira something': a taste of the wrong medicine. Lancet 1997;350:887.
35. Lambert BL. Predicting look-alike and sound-alike medication errors. Am J Health Syst Pharm 1997;54:1161–71.
36. Koren G, Barzilay Z, Greenwald M. Tenfold errors in administration of drug doses: a neglected iatrogenic disease in pediatrics. Pediatrics 1986; 77:848–9.
37. Perlstein PH, Callison C, White M, Barnes B, Edwards NK. Errors in drug computations during newborn intensive care. Am J Dis Child 1979;133:376–9.
38. Bain RJ. Accidental digitalis poisoning due to drinking herbal tea. Br Med J Clin Res Ed 1985;290:1624.
39. Cohen MR. Medication error reports. Hospital Pharmacy 1991;26:626–32.
40. Pincus JM, Ike RW. Norflox or Norflex? New Engl J Med 1992;326:1030.
41. Mohseni IE, Wong DH. Medication errors analysis is an opportunity to improve practice. Am J Surg 1998;175:4–9.
42. Collins DB. Medical manslaughter. NZ Med J 1991;104:318–19.
43. Allen EM, Van Boerum DH, Olsen AF, Dean JM. Difference between the measured and ordered dose of catecholamine infusions. Ann Pharmacother 1995;29:1095–100.
44. Aronson JK. Routes of drug administration: 5. Intramuscular. Prescr J 1995;35:32–6.
45. Giovannetti M, Machado MA, Borrelli Junior M, Ikejiri CI, Alonso N, Branco PD. Necrose tecidual: efeito colateral do diclofenaco de sodio, relato de casos e discussao da fisiopatologia. Rev Hosp Clin Fac Med Sao Paulo 1993;48:39–42.
46. Brahams D. Dosage of gentamicin and monitoring of blood levels: an action fails. Lancet 1986;i:1395–6.
47. Nicolau DP, Freeman CD, Belliveau PP, Nightingale CH, Ross JW, Quintiliani R. Experience with a once-daily aminoglycoside program administered to 2,184 adult patients. Antimicrob Agents Chemother 1995;39:650–5.
48. Currie M, Mackay P, Morgan C, Runciman WB, Russell WJ, Sellen A, Webb RK, Williamson JA. The Australian Incident Monitoring Study. The 'wrong drug' problem in anaesthesia: an analysis of 2000 incident reports. Anaesth Intensive Care 1993;21:596–601.
49. Dyke RW. Treatment of inadvertent intrathecal injection of vincristine. New Engl J Med 1989;321:1270–1.
50. Mortensen ME, Cecalupo AJ, Lo WD, Egorin MJ, Batley R. Inadvertent intrathecal injection of daunorubicin with fatal outcome. Med Pediatr Oncol 1992;20:249–53.
51. McAnulty GR, Sutton B. A case for anticonfusion devices in parenteral catheters. Anaesthesia 1994;49:557–8.
52. Rees M, Dormandy J. Accidental intra-arterial injection of diazepam. Br Med J 1980; 281:289–90.
53. Sintenie JB, Tuinebreijer WE, Kreis RW, Breederveld RS. Digital gangrene after accidental intra-arterial injection of phenytoin (Epanutin). Eur J Surg 1992;158:315–16.
54. Wu CL, Patt RB. Accidental overdose of systemic morphine during intended refill of intrathecal infusion device. Anesth Analg 1992;75:130–2.
55. Mitchell J. A fundamental problem of consent. Br Med J 1995;310:43–6.
56. Laljee MM. A fundamental problem of consent. Dentist is aggrieved at outcome. Br Med J 1995;310:935.
57. Bates DW, Leape LL, Cullen DJ, Laird N, Petersen LA, Teich JM, Burdick E, Hickey M, Kleefield S, Shea B, Vander Vliet M, Seger DL. Effect of computerized physician order entry and a team intervention on prevention of serious medication errors. J Am Med Assoc 1998;280:1311–16.
58. Raschke RA, Gollihare B, Wunderlich TA, Guidry JR, Leibowitz AI, Peirce JC, Lemelson L, Heisler MA, Susong C. A computer alert system to prevent injury from adverse drug events: development and evaluation in a community teaching hospital. J Am Med Assoc 1998; 280:1317–20.
59. Nunn DS. Ampoule labelling: the way forward. Pharm J 1992;March 14:361.
60. Orser BA, Oxorn DC. An anaesthetic drug error: minimizing the risk. Can J Anaesth 1994; 41:120–4.
61. Hill G. The KCl killer. J Med Defence Union 1990;(Spring):10–11.
62. Ferner RE. Misleading drug packaging. Br Med J 1995;311:514.

Reginald P. Sequeira

1 Central nervous system stimulants and drugs that suppress appetite

METHYLXANTHINES *(SED-13, 1; SEDA-19, 1; SEDA-20, 1; SEDA-21, 1)*

Caffeine

Caffeine reinforcement can be augmented as a result of two distinct mechanisms: (a) an acute stimulant effect and (b) withdrawal symptoms. The DSM-IV criterion for defining psychoactive drug dependence is that the substance is taken to relieve or avoid withdrawal symptoms (1[R]). Recent studies have provided further support for the view that in those who consume caffeine in moderate or high amounts, caffeine is used primarily to relieve or avoid withdrawal symptoms (2[C]), (3[C]) (see SEDA-20, 1).

Interactions The effect of *cimetidine* on caffeine metabolism has been investigated in 11 children aged 2.5–15 years, by giving them oral ^{13}C-labelled caffeine, followed by measurement of ^{13}C-labelled CO_2 in the expired air (4[c]). Cimetidine did not inhibit the metabolism of caffeine. These results contrast with inhibition of the metabolism of caffeine (5[c]) and theophylline (6[c]) by cimetidine in adults.

The combination of caffeine (200 mg) with *ephedrine* (20 mg), used as an aid to slimming, has been evaluated in 136 patients with a basal metabolic index above 25 kg/m^2, to determine their safety in hypertensives. There were no changes in blood pressure acutely or during treatment for 6 weeks, either in normotensive or hypertensive obese patients. Furthermore, the antihypertensive effect of β-blockade was not attenuated by caffeine–ephedrine (7[C]).

Side Effects of Drugs, Annual 22
J.K. Aronson, ed.

Theophylline

Interactions The individual and combined effects of *cimetidine* and *ciprofloxacin* on theophylline metabolism have been studied in healthy young and elderly male and female smokers (8[C]). In healthy male and female smokers, the basal oxidative metabolism of theophylline falls with age but is unaltered by sex. Cimetidine and ciprofloxacin impaired the elimination of theophylline. In therapeutic doses, concomitant administration of both drugs caused greater inhibition of theophylline clearance and metabolite formation than with either drug alone. Neither age nor sex affected the inhibition of theophylline metabolism by cimetidine and ciprofloxacin.

These findings may have significant clinical implications for the use of theophylline in old people. Age is the best predictor of major toxicity in cases of chronic theophylline overmedication, and elderly patients have a significantly higher risk of serious adverse effects from theophylline toxicity than younger patients, even at similar plasma concentrations (9[c]), (10[c]). Nevertheless, although cimetidine and ciprofloxacin had similar effects on theophylline metabolism in both age groups, lower baseline theophylline clearance as a result of age-related changes may increase the likelihood of drug–drug interactions in elderly people, necessitating careful monitoring.

A case of apparent theophylline toxicity induced by *fluvoxamine* has been reported (11[c]).

A 40-year-old woman had depression with psychotic features, successfully treated with fluvoxamine 100 mg/day and olanzapine 10 mg/day. Five days after she started to take theophylline 300 mg bd for chronic obstructive pulmonary disease she developed nausea, vomiting, confusion, insomnia, poor appetite, and lack of energy. About 12 h after the last dose of theophylline, her plasma theophylline concentration was 144 mmol/l. The elimination half-life was 35 h. Theophylline was withdrawn and her condition resolved over the next 5 days.

Theophylline toxicity in this patient was probably due to inhibition of CYP1A2, the major enzyme involved in theophylline detoxification, of which fluvoxamine is an inhibitor (12), (13[cr]). Several previous reports (14[c])–(16[c]) have documented this interaction.

In another study, fluvoxamine reduced the total clearance of theophylline from 80 to 24 ml/min and prolonged the elimination half-life from 6.6 to 22 h. The clearances of the theophylline metabolites, 1-methyluric acid, 3-methyluric acid, and 1,3-dimethyluric acid also fell (17[C]).

In the same study *griseofulvin* increased the clearance of theophylline in four subjects but had no effect in eight others (16[C]). The elimination half-life fell in all the subjects, but the fall was more pronounced in the four subjects in whom there was increased clearance. It is therefore possible that some subjects are more susceptible to induction by griseofulvin of the gene encoding for CYP1A2.

In 12 volunteers *grepafloxacin*, a fluoroquinolone, inhibits theophylline metabolism (18[c]). Grepafloxacin (600 mg/day for 10 days) increased the C_{max} and AUC of theophylline and reduced the apparent total clearance by about 50%.

STIMULANTS AND ANORECTIC AGENTS *(SED-13, 13; SEDA-19, 2; SEDA-20, 2; SEDA-21, 2)*

Cocaine *(SED-13, 14)*

Cardiovascular A young man had an *acute inferior myocardial infarction* following the application of cocaine as a topical anesthetic for nasal surgery. Coronary angiography showed occlusion of both posterior descending and posterolateral arteries, which were resistant to intracoronary glyceryl trinitrate and verapamil, a finding consistent with thrombotic occlusion. An angiogram 3 months later showed no residual lesion (19[c]).

Interactions Coronary artery vasospasm occurred in a patient who was given *ephedrine* intravenously to correct hypotension during spinal anesthesia (20[c]). The authors speculated that the coronary vasospasm was due to cocaine use 4 days before, causing upregulation of α-adrenoceptors in vascular smooth muscle and an exaggerated response to endogenous catecholamines; studies in dogs support this hypothesis (21). However, other causes, such as severe hypotension or acute thrombus formation could not be excluded. The authors recommended the use of glyceryl trinitrate, calcium antagonists, or α-adrenoceptor antagonists to control α-adrenoceptor agonist-precipitated coronary artery vasospasm and to avoid β-blockers, since these could worsen vasospasm (SEDA-21, 4).

Interference with laboratory tests The effect of several abused drugs and cocaine metabolites on cocaine and cocaethylene binding to human serum proteins in vitro has been investigated using equilibrium dialysis technique (22). Binding of cocaine was enhanced by codeine, methamphetamine, and cocaethylene, whereas morphine and benzylecgonine reduced it. These findings have important implications for laboratory screening of drugs in blood, because multidrug abuse is common among abusers.

Fenfluramine, dexfenfluramine, and phentermine *(SEDA-12, 9; SEDA-19, 2; SEDA-20, 2; SEDA-21, 2)*

Cardiovascular *Vasospasm* causing ischemic necrosis of the fingers had been attributed to dexfenfluramine (23[c]).

A 44-year-old non-insulin-dependent diabetic developed pain and discoloration of the left index and small fingers. Three months before he had started to take dexfenfluramine 15 mg bd for mild obesity. Angiography showed occlusion of both digital arteries of the index and small fingers; one digital artery was occluded in each of the other fingers. Vasospasm in the carpal arch abated with an injection of tolazoline. Dexfenfluramine was discontinued, but despite therapy with local transdermal nitrate, local sympathetic blockade with bupivacaine, and oral nifedipine, the lesion progressed to necrosis, and amputation of the involved distal phalanges was required. Pathological examination showed thrombosis of the digital arteries with gangrenous necrosis but no vasculitis or emboli. He was instructed to avoid dexfenfluramine. However, some weeks later he developed mild discoloration of several fingers of the right hand after he took dexfenfluramine again.

Dexfenfluramine can interfere with serotonin turnover (24[cr]), and it could be argued that serotonin-induced vasospasm was responsible for this adverse event. Lower extremity arterial ischemia has also been reported in a patient who took dexfenfluramine and minocycline (25[c]). Coronary vasospasm can also be produced by dexfenfluramine, producing myocardial infarction (26[cr]). Pulmonary hypertension is a well-known complication of dexfenfluramine.

Cardiac valvulopathies in patients taking fenfluramine and related drugs

During the past year several reports have provided evidence linking valvular heart disease to the use of a combination of widely used drugs, fenfluramine and phentermine.

Phentermine was approved by the FDA in 1959 for single-drug, short-term treatment of obesity. Subsequently in 1973, fenfluramine was approved on a similar basis. Dexfenfluramine was approved in 1976 as a single-drug, prescription-only appetite suppressant for longer term use in moderately obese people, with a warning that its safety beyond 1 year of use had not been established. Recently, both fenfluramines have been used in combination with phentermine and for periods longer than a few weeks. Since 1995 more than 14 million prescriptions have been written for either fenfluramine or dexfenfluramine. Most of the use was in women and people aged over 60 years. Based on a median treatment course of 3–12 months, an estimated 1.2–4.7 million people in the US have been exposed to these drugs.

Reports and demographic features *Echocardiography in 24 women who were taking fenfluramine–phentermine showed unusual valvular morphology and regurgitation. Both right- and left-sided heart valves were involved. Eight of these patients also had newly documented pulmonary hypertension. The heart valves had a glistening white appearance and the histopathological features were identical to those seen in carcinoid or ergotamine-induced valve disease (27[C]).*

These descriptions are limited by a lack of pathological confirmation in the majority of cases. Many of these patients continue to be treated medically and have not undergone invasive investigation. Consequently, neither direct inspection or histopathological evaluation has been carried out in most cases. In addition, no routine pretreatment echocardiographic baseline studies were performed. In the absence of a control group or a case–control study, definitive statements about a true association of valvular heart disease with fenfluramine–phentermine therapy cannot be made.

However, following this landmark publication, several other reports have substantiated these observations. Between October 1994 and July 1997, the Belgian Centre for Pharmacovigilance received 43 reports of valvular heart disease among women who had used anorectic drugs. Echocardiographic confirmation was available in 31 of these patients, who had had past exposure to anorectic drugs such as fenfluramine ($n = 8$), fenfluramine and diethylpropion ($n = 18$), fenfluramine and phentermine ($n = 1$), and fenfluramine, diethylpropion, and phentermine ($n = 3$). The mean duration of exposure was estimated in 25 patients to be 40 months, and the mean age of the patients was 42 years. The aortic valve was most frequent involved (in 18 cases). Thirteen patients presented with symptoms such as dyspnea ($n = 6$), primary pulmonary hypertension ($n = 2$), and chest pain, chest discomfort, angina, pulmonary edema, and peripheral edema in one patient each (28[C]).

In July 1997 the FDA issued a Public Health Advisory asking that other cases be reported. In response, the FDA received 28 additional reports from the US with similar disease; the median age was 45 years and all were women (29[CR]). The median daily dose of fenfluramine was 60 mg and of phentermine 30 mg; the median duration of therapy before diagnosis of valvular disease was 10 months. Six patients underwent valve replacement surgery, of whom one died.

In a further update, by 30 September 1997 the FDA had received 144 individual spontaneous reports (including the 24 cases reported earlier) involving fenfluramine or dexfenfluramine with or without phentermine, in association with valvulopathy (30[CR]). Valvulopathy was defined as "documented aortic regurgitation of mild or greater severity and or mitral regurgitation of moderate or greater severity after exposure to these drugs". Of these 144 spontaneous reports 132 had complete information and 113 met the case definition. Of these 113 cases, 98% occurred among women; the median age was 44 years. Out of these 113 cases 2% had used fenfluramine alone; 14% dexfenfluramine alone; 79% a combination of fenfluramine with phentermine; and 5% a combination of all three drugs; none had taken phentermine alone. The median duration of drug use was 9 months (range 1–39). Overall, 87 (77.1%) of the 113 cases were symptomatic. A total of 27 (24%) patients required cardiac valve replacement and three died after surgery.

Mechanism *It has been postulated that fenfluramine and phentermine potentiate the effect or concentration of circulating serotonin and could contribute to the development of valvular injury, similar to that seen in patients with carcinoid syndrome or in those taking ergot derivatives. Serum serotonin and urinary 5-hydroxyindole acetic acid (5-HIAA) have been measured in seven subjects taking fenfluramine and phentermine for a mean duration of 11 months as adjunct therapy in type 2 diabetes mellitus. None of these subjects had raised concentrations of serum serotonin or urinary 5-HIAA (31[C]). Thus, direct implication of serotonin has not been substantiated.*

Two patients with valvular heart disease associated with fenfluramine–phentermine were also taking a selective serotonin reuptake inhibitor (SSRI) (27[C]). The suggestion that fluoxetine is a safer alternative to fenfluramine in the medical treatment of obesity (32[C]) should be viewed with scepticism.

Valves affected *Although most of these patients had either dyspnea or evidence of congestive heart failure, 14% were asymptomatic. The mitral valve was affected in 24 (86%), the aortic valve in 19 (69%), the tricuspid valve in 11 (39%), and the pulmonary valve in one (4%). A left-sided valve was involved in all cases, and two or more valves were involved in 78%. Pulmonary hypertension was reported in 10 patients, four of whom had left-sided valvular lesions only. Valvular disease did not resolve in any patient after withdrawal of the appetite suppressants.*

Risk factors *Factors that are potentially associated with cardiac valvulopathy, but not yet determined, are:*

(1) The natural history of these lesions, including the relation between the development of the lesions and the duration of drug use, and whether the lesions generally resolve, progress, or remain unchanged on drug withdrawal;
(2) The clinical importance of mild valvulopathy in asymptomatic people without audible murmurs; and
(3) The characteristics, if any, that might predispose someone to develop cardiac valve abnormalities during exposure to these drugs.

Monitoring and prevention *Color-flow Doppler echocardiographic surveillance of all persons being treated with appetite suppressants, particularly asymptomatic women, has been recommended (33[C]). However, the optimal timing of follow-up echocardiography to determine the progression, regression, or stabilization of valvular lesions is currently unknown.*

The US Department of Health and Human Services has issued the following interim recommendations for people previously exposed to fenfluramine or dexfenfluramine with cardiac valvulopathies (30[R]):

(1) All people exposed to fenfluramine for any period of time, either alone or in combination with other anorectic agents, should undergo a medical history and cardiovascular examination by their physician to determine the presence or absence of cardiopulmonary signs and symptoms.
(2) Echocardiography should be performed

on all people who have been exposed to fenfluramine or dexfenfluramine for any period of time, either alone or in combination with other agents, and who have cardiopulmonary signs, including a new murmur or symptoms suggestive of valvular disease, such as dyspnea.

(3) *Any echocardiographic findings that meet the American Heart Association (AHA) criteria for antimicrobial prophylaxis for endocarditis, regardless of whether they are attributable fenfluramine or dexfenfluramine, should be recognized as an indication for antimicrobial prophylaxis. For emergency procedures for which cardiac evaluation cannot be performed, empirical antibiotic prophylaxis should be administered according to AHA guidelines.*

(4) *Because of the prevalence of minimal degrees of regurgitation in the general population, the current definition of drug-associated valvulopathy should include exposed patients with echocardiographically demonstrated aortic regurgitation of mild or greater severity and/or mitral regurgitation of moderate or greater severity, based on published criteria.*

Respiratory *Pulmonary hypertension* has been reported in patients taking fenfluramine hydrochloride and phentermine hydrochloride (34[c]), (35[c]).

A 30-year-old woman had a basal metabolic index of 28 kg/m^2, but no history of pulmonary disease, drug abuse, HIV infection, recent pregnancy, immunological disease, or other drug use. After taking fenfluramine and phentermine for 4 weeks, she began to have dyspnea and stopped taking the anorexiants. Six months later she developed progressive dyspnea on exertion and edema and had a syncopal episode. Echocardiography showed right ventricular hypertrophy and dilatation. Cardiac catheterization confirmed the presence of severe pulmonary hypertension. She was given prostacyclin and warfarin. A few months later she died, and at post mortem examination the cause of death was attributed to pulmonary hypertension associated with the use of fenfluramine–phentermine.

Severe plexogenic pulmonary arteriopathy developed in a 29-year-old woman who had taken fenfluramine and phentermine for 23 days. She probably had not had any pre-existing disease, and the histological age of the lesion was consistent with the time elapsed since she had taken the drugs.

In both of these cases, the short duration of drug exposure is worth noting (SEDA-18, 7; SEDA 21, 2).

Nervous system *Cerebral hemorrhage* has been attributed to fenfluramine with phentermine (36[c]).

A 56-year-old woman suddenly developed weakness and clumsiness of her right leg and right arm. She had taken dl-fenfluramine 20 mg/day and phentermine 15 mg/day for obesity for 6 months. CT and MRI scans showed a hemorrhage in the medial aspect of the left motor cortex with a small amount of surrounding edema. Fenfluramine and phentermine were withdrawn. Her right hemiparesis gradually resolved over 3 months, when MRI showed complete resolution.

Although the authors of this report suggested that fenfluramine–phentermine may have contributed to the development of cerebral hemorrhage, other causes, particularly cryptic arteriovenous malformations, could not be completely excluded. The intermittent aspirin the patient was using for back pain could also have contributed (37[R]).

Psychiatric Various psychiatric adverse effects of dexfenfluramine have been reported (38[c]), (39[c]). In the first case *psychotic episodes* associated with dexfenfluramine were probably due to an interaction of dexfenfluramine with doxepin (38[c]). In the second a direct effect of dexfenfluramine was suggested (39[c]).

A 56-year-old white woman with bipolar depression developed distinct mood cycles 2 weeks after starting to take dexfenfluramine. Her symptoms included anger, homicidal thoughts, racing thoughts, and labile moods. She was unable to control her mood. Her sleep changed minimally with continued use of zolpidem. She reverted to a long-quiescent pattern of alcohol abuse. The dexfenfluramine was withdrawn and the dosage of alprazolam was increased to 2 mg bd. Her other medications (divalproex, carbamazepine, molindone, zolpidem) were unchanged. Within 3 days her mixed-manic, rapid-cycling state improved and in 2 weeks she achieved baseline status.

In another case *psychotomania* occurred after treatment with fenfluramine and phentermine in a depressed woman (40[c]). On two separate occasions she experienced similar symptoms with fenfluramine and phentermine.

These reports emphasize the need to use appetite suppressants judiciously in patients with pre-existing psychiatric illness, although it is difficult to establish a definite association between these adverse effects and use of anorectic drugs (SEDA-19, 2).

Interaction Attention has been drawn to a possible interaction between fenfluramine and *imipramine*, mediated via the inhibition of cytochrome P450 (41[c]).

A 55-year-old woman had generalized anxiety, in remission with imipramine 350 mg/day. During this period she also took hyoscyamine sulfate, 0.375 mg/day, and levothyroxine sodium 0.15 mg/day. Her imipramine concentration at the end of each of the previous years of treatment was 145–218 mg/l. Four weeks after the addition of fenfluramine, 20 mg tds, she complained that she had momentarily fallen asleep while driving. Her imipramine plus desipramine concentration was 704 mg/l. Fenfluramine was withdrawn, and no further episodes of daytime sleepiness were reported. Her blood concentration of imipramine and desipramine 2 weeks later was 252 mg/l.

Imipramine metabolism depends on CYP1A2, CYP2C, CYP2D6, and CYP3A4 (42[R]). Although fenfluramine might inhibit some of these isoenzymes, there is no published evidence that it does. It is prudent to be aware of the potential for fenfluramine–imipramine interaction.

Ephedrine and pseudoephedrine *(SED-13, 350; SEDA-21, 5)*

Skin and appendages A non-pigmentary *fixed drug reaction* has been attributed to ephedrine and pseudoephedrine (43[c]). A patch test and oral rechallenge produced eruptions at the same site. The dermis, rather than the epidermis, is the primary site of the drug sensitivity response in this type of dermatitis (44[c]).

Effects on laboratory tests Clinical doses of β-adrenoceptor agonists, including ritodrine and ephedrine, cause *hypersecretion of salivary amylase* in about one-third of women with pre-term labor contractions (45[C]).

Methylphenidate *(SEDA-20, 3; SEDA-21, 6)*

Recent studies (46[c])–(48[c]) have addressed the safety issues related to the use of methylphenidate in children with attention deficit hyperkinetic disorder (ADHD). Nearly 80% of children treated with methylphenidate experienced appetite suppression, affecting body weight and height. However methylphenidate also *exacerbated tics*. In patients with marked *anxiety*, *agitation*, or *psychotic disorders* these symptoms may be precipitated methylphenidate. Patients with mental retardation and children under 6 years old are at risk of adverse effects such as *irritability* and *depressed mood*. The most common adverse effects of methylphenidate include *sleep problems*, *anorexia*, *stomach ache*, and *headache* (for a comprehensive review see (49[R]), (50[R])).

Interactions An interaction of methylphenidate with *sertraline* has been described (51[c]).

A 13-year-old white man with a history of ADHD and a depressive disorder had taken methylphenidate 1.8 mg/kg per day for nearly 10 months. Because of worsening of his mood disturbances, sertraline 25 mg/day was added. One week later he had a tonic–clonic seizure. Sertraline was withdrawn and methylphenidate continued unchanged. There was no recurrence.

Although this may be first reported case of seizure activity in someone taking sertraline and methylphenidate, this report does not provide convincing evidence of an interaction, particularly because blood concentrations were not determined. The possibility of a cytochrome P450-mediated drug interaction as an underlying mechanism has yet to be explored.

Prolintane

Prolintane hydrochloride is available mainly in formulations containing multivitamin supplements in many European countries, Australia, and South Africa. It has structural and pharmacological properties similar to dextroamphetamine. Its adverse effects include *insomnia*, *nervousness*, *irritability*, *euphoria*, *headache*, *dizziness*, and *psychotic reactions*. Acute overdosage can cause *cardiorespiratory arrest* and *death*.

A patient who developed a *panic attack* after taking Katovit® (prolintane with multivitamins) has been reported to the Spanish Drug Surveillance Scheme (52[c]). The authors pointed out that none of the 30 physicians questioned about this formulation was aware that prolintane is related to amphetamine. They urged that in countries in which prolintane is marketed in combination with vitamins, this irrational combination should be withdrawn in view of the public health risk.

OTHER CENTRALLY ACTING DRUGS *(SEDA-19, 4, 148; SEDA-20, 4; SEDA-21, 6)*

Pemoline *(SEDA-21, 6)*

There is considerable interest in giving pemoline to children with ADHD who do not respond to methylphenidate (53[c]), (54[c]). However, troubling adverse effects occurred when the maximum recommended dose was used. Among seven children, two developed *tics* and one *hallucinations* (54[c]).

Liver The available data on pemoline-associated *hepatotoxicity* have been reviewed and the need to establish an adverse reactions registry has been emphasized (55[R]). A 19-year-old woman with ADHD was treated with methylphenidate and pemoline and developed reversible hepatitis (56[c]). There is no evidence that methylphenidate predisposed her to pemoline hepatotoxicity. However, there is no indication for using multiple stimulants to treat ADHD.

Tacrine *(SEDA-19, 4; SEDA-20, 4; SEDA-21, 6)*

The American Psychiatric Association has published practice guidelines for the treatment of patients with Alzheimer's disease and other dementias of late life (57[R]).

The FDA has described a 'Treatment-Investigational New Drug (TIND)' protocol, whereby large volumes of data related to clinical trials can be handled rapidly and effectively (58[CR]). Serious adverse events have been reported directly to trained operators and summarized on a weekly basis for reporting to the FDA: 1951 physicians agreed to participate and 10 187 patients were enrolled; 9861 (96.8%) of these were taking tacrine. One or more serious adverse events were reported by 1148 (12%) patients (1206 events in all), the most frequently reported adverse event being a raised AlT (337 patients). A comprehensive review of risk:benefit assessment of tacrine in the treatment of Alzheimer's disease, including treatment guidelines for prescribing tacrine and recommendations for monitoring toxicity, has been described (59[R]).

Since only about one-third of patients with Alzheimer's disease respond favorably to tacrine, the search for predictors of favorable/unfavorable responses continues. Patients with white matter low attenuation, also known as leukoaraiosis (periventricular hypodense areas on CT scan), can still respond to tacrine, although the rate of withdrawal from treatment is much higher in these patients (60[C]). The small number of patients in this study ($n = 72$) precludes firm conclusions as to whether leukoaraiosis is a predictor of the efficacy and tolerability of tacrine.

Psychiatric Two cases of tacrine-associated *depression* have been reported (61[c]).

Two elderly women (aged 82 and 70 years) had taken tacrine hydrochloride 40 mg/day for at least 1 month. They developed symptoms of depression and had Hamilton Depression Rating Scale Scores of 27 and 29. The 82-year-old did not respond to fluoxetine 200 mg/day for 35 days, but improved with a course of ECT; the other improved with fluoxetine alone. Tacrine was withdrawn.

Based on the evidence provided, it is difficult to accept with any degree of certainty that indeed there is an association between tacrine treatment and depression. Considering the use of tacrine in a large number of patients with Alzheimer's disease, the association, if any, is probably very weak.

Interactions Antidepressants, such as *fluvoxamine*, are often given to patients with Alzheimer's disease who are also given tacrine. The interaction between them has therefore been investigated in 13 healthy volunteers in a double-blind, randomized crossover comparison of the effects of fluvoxamine (100 mg/day for 6 days) and placebo on the pharmacokinetics of a single dose of tacrine (40 mg) (62[C]). Fluvoxamine reduced the apparent non-renal clearance of tacrine and increased the plasma concentrations of its three monohydroxylated metabolites. These results are attributable to inhibition by fluvoxamine of CYP1A2, which is responsible for the biotransformation of tacrine to its inactive hydroxylated metabolites and its reactive metabolites, which are potentially toxic if not conjugated with glutathione (63[R]). Five subjects had gastrointestinal adverse effects, but the clinical consequences of concomitant prescription of tacrine and inhibitors of CYP1A2, such as fluvoxamine (12), in patients with Alzheimer's disease cannot be extrapolated from this study.

REFERENCES

1. American Psychiatric Association. Diagnostic and Statistical Manual of the Mental Disorders, 4th edition. Washington DC: American Psychiatric Association 1994:175–272.
2. Schuh KJ, Griffiths RR. Caffeine reinforcement: the role of withdrawal. Psychopharmacology 1997;130:320–6.
3. Phillips-Bute BG, Lane JD. Caffeine withdrawal symptoms following brief caffeine deprivation. Physiol Behav 1997;63:35–9.
4. Parker AC, Pritchard P, Preston T, Dalzell AM, Choonara I. Lack of inhibitory effect of cimetidine on caffeine metabolism in children using the caffeine breath test. Br J Clin Pharmacol 1997;43:467–70.
5. Broughton LJ, Rogers HJ. Decreased systemic clearance of caffeine due to cimetidine. Br J Clin Pharmacol 1981;12:155–9.
6. Roberts RK, Grice J, Wood L, Petroff V, McGuffie C. Cimetidine impairs the elimination of theophylline and antipyrine. Gastroenterology 1981;81:19–21.
7. Ingerslev J, Svendsen TL, Mork A. Is ephedrine caffeine treatment contraindicated in hypertension? Int J Obes 1997;21:666–73.
8. Loi CM, Parker BM, Cusack BJ, Vestal RE. Aging and drug interactions. III. Individual and combined effects of cimetidine and ciprofloxacin on theophylline metabolism in healthy male and female nonsmokers. J Pharmacol Exp Ther 1997;280:627–37.
9. Shannon M. Predictors of major toxicity after theophylline overdose. Ann Intern Med 1993; 119:1161–7.
10. Shannon M, Lovejoy FH Jr. The influence of age vs. peak serum concentration on life-threatening events after chronic theophylline intoxication. Arch Intern Med 1990;150:2045–8.
11. Devane CL, Markowitz JS, Hardesty SJ, Mundy S, Gill HS. Fluvoxamine-induced theophylline toxicity. Am J Psychiatry 1997;154:1317–18.
12. Brosen K, Skelbo E, Rasmussen BB. Fluvoxamine is a potent inhibitor of cytochrome P4501A2. Biochem Pharmacol 1993;45:1211–14.
13. Rasmussen BB, Maenpaa J, Pelkonen O, Loft S, Poulssen HE, Lykkesfeldt J, Brosen K. Selective serotonin reuptake inhibitors and theophylline metabolism in human liver microsomes: potent inhibition by fluvoxamine. Br J Clin Pharmacol 1995;39:151–9.
14. Diot P, Jonville AP, Gerard F, Bonnelle N, Autret E, Breteau M, Lemarie E, Lavandier M. Possible interaction between theophylline and fluvoxamine. Thérapie 1991;46:170–1.
15. Sperber AD. Toxic interaction between fluvoxamine and sustained release theophylline in an 11-year-old boy. Drug Saf 1991;6:460–2.
16. Van der Breckel AM, Harrington L. Toxic effects of theophylline caused by fluvoxamine. Can Med Assoc J 1994;151:1289–90.
17. Rasmussen BB, Jeppesen U, Gaist D, Brosen K. Griseofulvin and fluvoxamine interaction with the metabolism of theophylline. Ther Drug Monit 1997;19:56–62.
18. Efthymiopoulos C, Bramer SL, Maroli A, Blum B. Theophylline and warfarin interaction studies with grepafloxacin. Clin Pharmacokinet 1997;33(Suppl 1):39–46.
19. Williams MJA, Stewart RAH. Serial angiography in cocaine-induced myocardial infarction. Chest 1997;111:822–4.
20. Lustik SJ, Chhibber AK, Van Vliet M, Pomerantz RM. Ephedrine induced coronary artery vasospasm in a patient with prior cocaine use. Anaesth Analg 1997;84:931–3.
21. Jones LF, Tacket RL. Chronic cocaine treatment enhances the responsiveness of the left an-

terior descending coronary artery and the femoral artery to vasoactive substances. J Pharmacol Exp Ther 1990;255:1366–70
22. Bailey DN. Effect of drugs and cocaine metabolites on cocaine and coca-ethylene binding to human serum in vitro. Ther Drug Monit 1997; 19:427–30.
23. Marinella MS, Barrettoni BA. Digital necrosis associated with dexfenfluramine. New Engl J Med 1997;337:1776–7.
24. McCann UD, Seiden LS, Rubin LJ, Ricaurte GA. Brain serotonin neurotoxicity and primary pulmonary hypertension from fenfluramine and dexfenfluramine: a systematic review of the evidence. J Am Med Assoc 1997;278:666–72.
25. Prate B, Spreux A, Chichmanian RM. Ischémie subaiguë distale du membre inférieur gauche au cours et traitment associant dexfenfluramine et minocycline. Thérapie 1992; 47: 438–9.
26. Evard P. Myocardial infarction associated with dextrofenfluramine. Br Med J 1990; 301:1050.
27. Connolly HM, Crary JL, McGoon MD, Hensrud DD, Edwards BS, Edwards WD, Schaff HV. Valvular heart disease associated with fenfluramine-phentermine. New Engl J Med 1997;337:581–8.
28. Kurz X, Van Ermen A. Valvular heart disease associated with fenfluramine-phentermine. New Engl J Med 1997;337:1772–3.
29. Graham DJ, Green L. Further cases of valvular heart disease associated with fenfluramine-phentermine [1]. New Engl J Med 1997;337:635.
30. Bowen R, Glicklich A, Khan M, Rasmussen S, Wadden T, Bilstadt J, Graham D, Green L, Lumpkin M, O'Neil R, Sobel S, Hubbard VS, Yanovski S, Sopko G. Cardiac valvulopathy associated with exposure to fenfluramine or dexfenfluramine: US Department of Health and Human Services Interim Public Health Recommendations, November 1997. J Am Med Assoc 1997;278:1729–31.
31. Redmon B, Raatz S, Bantle JP. Valvular heart disease associated with fenfluramine-phentermine. New Engl J Med 1997;337:1773–4.
32. Anchors M. Fluoxetine is a safer alternative to fenfluramine in the medical treatment of obesity. Arch Intern Med 1997;157:1270.
33. Rasmussen S, Corya BS, Glasman RD. Valvular heart disease associated with fenfluramine-phentermine. New Engl J Med 1997;337:1773.
34. Dillon KA, Putnam KG, Avorn JL. Death from irreversible pulmonary hypertension associated with short use of fenfluramine and phentermine. J Am Med Assoc 1997;278:1320.
35. Mark EJ, Patalas EO, Chang HT, Evans RJ, Kessler SC. Fatal pulmonary hypertension associated with short-term use of fenfluramine and phentermine. New Engl J Med 1997; 337: 602–6.
36. Wen PY, Feske SK, Teoh SK, Stieg PE. Cerebral hemorrhage in a patient taking fenfluramine and phentermine for obesity. Neurology 1997;49:632–3.
37. Kase CS. Bleeding disorders. In: Kase CS, Caplan LR, eds. Intracerebral Hemorrhage. Boston: Butterworth-Heinemann 1994:117–53.
38. Preval H, Pakyurek AM. Psychotic episode associated with dexfenfluramine. Am J Psychiatry 1997;154:1624–5.
39. Bowden CL, Dickson J Jr. Mania from dexfenfluramine. J Clin Psychiatry 1997;58:548–9.
40. Raison CL, Klein HM. Psychotic mania associated with fenfluramine and phentermine use. Am J Psychiatry 1997;154:711.
41. Fogelson DL. Fenfluramine and the cytochrome P450 system. Am J Psychiatry 1996; 154:436–7.
42. Nemeroff CB, DeVane CL, Pollock BG. Newer antidepressants and the cytochrome P450 system. Am J Psychiatry 1996;153:311–20.
43. Garcia-Ortiz JC, Terron M, Bellido J. Non-pigmentary fixed exanthema from ephedrine and pseudoephedrine. Eur J Allergy Clin Immunol 1997;52:229–30.
44. Shelley WB, Shelley ED. Nonpigmentary fixed drug eruption as a distinctive reaction pattern: examples caused by sensitivity to pseudoephedrine hydrochloride and tetrahydrozoline. J Am Acad Dermatol 1987;17:403–7.
45. Takahashi T, Minakami H, Tamada T, Sato I. Hyperamylasemia in response to ritodrine or ephedrine administered to pregnant women. J Am Coll Surg 1997;184:31–6.
46. Effron D, Jarman F, Barker M. Side effects of methylphenidate and dexamphetamine in children with attention deficit hyperactivity disorder: a double blind, crossover trial. Pediatrics 1997; 100:662–6.
47. Musten LM, Firestone P, Pisterman S, Bennett S, Mercer J. Effects of methylphenidate on preschool children with ADHD: cognitive behavioral functions. J Am Acad Child Adolesc Psychiatry 1997;36:1407–15.
48. Schachar RJ, Tannock R, Cunningham C, Corkum PV. Behavioral, situational and temporal effects of treatment of ADHD with methylphenidate. J Am Acad Child Adolesc Psychiatry 1997;36:754–63.
49. Cantwell D. Attention deficit disorders. A review of the past 10 years. J Am Acad Child Adolesc Psychiatry 1996;35:978–87.
50. Rappley MD. Safety issues in the use of methylphenidate. An American perspective. Drug Saf 1997;17:143–8.
51. Feeney DJ, Klykylo WM. Medication induced seizures. J Am Child Adolesc Psychiatry 1997; 36:1018–19.
52. Martinez-Mir I, Catalan C, Palop V. Prolintane: a masked amphetamine. Ann Pharmacother 1997;31:256.
53. Pelham WE, Swanson JM, Furman MB, Swindt H. Pemoline effects on children wth ADHD: a time response analysis on classroom measures. J Am Acad Child Adolesc Psychiatry 1995;34:1504–13.

54. Winsberg B, Barbato M. Pemoline in ADHD. J Am Acad Child Adolesc Psychiatry 1997; 36:1649–50.
55. Shevell M, Schreiber R. Pemoline associated hepatic failure: a critical analysis of the literature. Pediatr Neurol 1997;16:14–16.
56. McCurry L, Cronquist S. Pemoline and hepatotoxicity. Am J Psychiatry 1997;154:713–14.
57. American Psychiatry Association. Practice guidelines for the treatment of patients with Alzheimer's disease and other dementias of late life. Am J Psychiatry 1997;Suppl 154:1–39.
58. Symons JP, Ibara M, Kraemer DF, Luscombe FA. Tacrine hydrochloride treatment IND: methods for rapid physician patient enrolment and data retrieval. Pharmacoepidemiol Drug Saf 1997;6:409–16.
59. Samuels SC, Davis KL. A risk:benefit assessment of tacrine in the treatment of Alzheimer's disease. Drug Saf 1997;16:66–77.
60. Amar K, Wilcock GK, Scot M, Lewis T. The presence of leukoaraiosis in patients with Alzheimer's disease predicts poor tolerance to tacrine, but does not discriminate responders from non-responders. Age Aging 1977;26:25–9.
61. Pancrazi-Boyer MP, Arnaud-Castiglioni R, Michel B, Azorin JM. Tetraaminotacrine treatment and depression. Alzheimer's Res 1997; 3:115–17.
62. Becquemont L, Regueneau I, Le Bot MA, Riche C, Funck-Brentano C, Jallon P. Influence of the CYP1A2 inhibitor fluvoxamine on tacrine pharmacokinetics in humans. Clin Pharmacol Ther 1997;61:619–27.
63. De Vane CL, Gill HS. Clinical pharmacokinetics of fluvoxamine: applications to dosage regimen design. J Clin Psychiatry 1997;58 Suppl:7–14.

P.J. Cowen

2 Antidepressant drugs

TRICYCLIC ANTIDEPRESSANTS *(SED-13, 42; SEDA-19, 7; SEDA-20, 6; SEDA-21, 10)*

Risk factors The use of psychotropic drugs is associated with a greater risk of falls and hip fracture in *elderly people*. Tricyclic antidepressants have sedative and autonomic effects that might predispose to falls, while selective serotonin re-uptake inhibitors (SSRIs) are relatively free from these effects. In a case–control study of 8239 patients admitted to hospital for hip fracture over a 1-year period, current use of SSRIs was associated with a 2.4 times increase in the risk of hip fracture (95% CI 2.0–2.7) relative to untreated controls (1[R]). The risk was the same with tricyclic antidepressants that are secondary amines (such as nortriptyline) (2.2, CI 1.8–2.8) and lower with tricyclic antidepressants that are tertiary amines (such as amitriptyline) (1.5, CI 1.3–1.7).

These findings are somewhat surprising, given that tertiary tricyclic antidepressants, such as amitriptyline, would be expected to have more sedative and hypotensive effects than secondary tricyclics or SSRIs. However, dosage estimates showed that while most of the patients taking SSRIs were rated as having adequate antidepressant doses this was the case for only a minority of those taking tricyclic antidepressants. So, adequate dosages of tricyclic antidepressants might have led to a greater incidence of fractures. It is also possible that depression itself rather than antidepressant drug treatment predisposes to accidents and falls, but in that case one would have to suppose that those taking SSRIs had not responded well to adequate doses. From this study it appears that routine use of SSRIs in place of tricyclic antidepressants will not necessarily lead to a reduced incidence of hip fracture in elderly people.

Interactions *Valproic acid*, which is being increasing used as a mood stabilizing drug, increases plasma concentrations of amitriptyline and its metabolite nortriptyline in healthy volunteers (SEDA-21, 10). There has now been a report that it can increase plasma clomipramine concentrations too (2[C]).

A 43-year-old woman had history of epilepsy but had had no seizures for 3 years while taking valproic acid. She started taking clomipramine 75 mg daily for depression, but 12 days later developed generalized clonic–tonic seizures that did not respond to diazepam 10 mg intravenously. She was admitted as an emergency and was in status epilepticus for 2 h, responding eventually to intravenous phenytoin and phenobarbital. The plasma clomipramine concentration was 341 ng/ml (target range 68–272 ng/ml). The authors did not give any information about withdrawal or rechallenge in this case.

Clomipramine, like other tricyclic antidepressants, can predispose to seizures, but the plasma concentrations seen here were higher than expected, particularly for a dose of 75 mg daily. It seems likely that valproate increases concentrations of tricyclic antidepressants through inhibition of cytochrome P450 enzymes.

SELECTIVE SEROTONIN RE-UPTAKE INHIBITORS (SSRIs) *(SED-13, 65; SEDA-19, 9; SEDA-20, 7; SEDA-21, 11)*

The increasing use of SSRIs is matched by the growing numbers of reports of adverse reactions and drug interactions. While SSRIs are all potent inhibitors of the re-uptake of serotonin, their detailed pharmacological profiles and pharmacokinetics show a number of contrasts. It is important to establish whether

Side Effects of Drugs, Annual 22
J.K. Aronson, ed.

these pharmacodynamic and pharmacokinetic distinctions are reflected in important clinical differences between individual SSRIs. In the past year there has been particular focus on drug interactions and discontinuation syndromes.

Nervous system and psychiatric In a thorough search of the published literature 28 reports were found, involving 42 patients who experienced an *extrapyramidal movement disorder* in association with SSRI treatment over the period 1990–6 (3[R]). A full clinical spectrum of disorders was reported, including acute dystonic reactions, akathisia, parkinsonism, tardive dyskinesia, and neuroleptic malignant syndrome. Each disorder was reported in conjunction with the use of SSRIs alone, but often pharmacokinetic and pharmacodynamic interactions with other drugs, notably dopamine receptor antagonists, played a contributory role. On other occasions individual predisposition, for example pre-existing brain damage or Parkinson's disease, was judged important.

The majority of reports involved fluoxetine, but this is likely to reflect its widespread use, rather a truly greater propensity to produce movement disorders compared with other SSRIs. From the relatively small number of reports, extrapyramidal reactions appear to be rare in patients without predisposing factors who are taking SSRIs alone. The mechanism of SSRI-induced movement disorders is believed to involve serotonin-mediated inhibition of dopamine pathways in the substantia nigra and the ventral tegmental area.

Like other antidepressants SSRIs can induce *mania*, but it is uncertain whether the incidence of manic switch with SSRIs is different to that of tricyclic antidepressants. While previous reports of SSRI-induced mania have implicated fluoxetine and fluvoxamine, mania has been reported in six patients, five of whom were taking citalopram and one paroxetine (4[r]). In three patients concomitant lithium treatment failed to prevent the manic episode, although these subjects were taking particularly high doses of SSRIs.

Endocrine *Breast enlargement* is common in women taking antipsychotic drugs, but less so with tricyclic antidepressants. In a series of 59 patients, 23 (39%) reported some degree of breast enlargement while taking SSRIs or venlafaxine (5[C]). The highest rate was with paroxetine, which also produced a significant increase in plasma prolactin concentration. The breast enlargement was associated with generalized weight gain but did not correlate with age or duration of treatment. Presumably increases in plasma prolactin play a role in breast enlargement with SSRIs.

Sexual function SSRI treatment can lead to *impaired sexual function*. In a retrospective questionnaire survey of 107 men and women taking fluoxetine (37), paroxetine (21), sertraline (27), or bupropion (22), all three SSRIs lowered libido and sexual arousal and increased the time needed to achieve orgasm; intensity of orgasm was also reduced (6[C]). One or more adverse sexual effects were noted by 73% of patients taking SSRIs, but by only 14% of those taking bupropion. In contrast, 77% of the patients taking bupropion reported one or more positive effects on sexual function.

The results of this study must be interpreted with caution, because the patients who returned the questionnaire (107/320) might have been more troubled by unwanted sexual effects than those who did not. However, the survey does suggest that SSRIs commonly produce sexual dysfunction. The positive effect of bupropion on sexual function is interesting and may reflect its ability to facilitate dopamine neurotransmission.

Withdrawal Discontinuation symptoms are not uncommon after abrupt withdrawal of SSRI treatment. The most common symptoms are *dizziness*, *nausea*, *lethargy*, and *headache*. However, other symptoms can occur, including *anxiety*, *paresthesia*, *confusion*, *tremor*, *sweating*, *irritability*, *insomnia*, *memory problems*, and *anorexia* (7[R]). Symptoms after sudden SSRI discontinuation usually last about 1–2 weeks, but some patients can experience difficulties for longer periods.

A retrospective review has suggested that discontinuation symptoms are most common after paroxetine and fluvoxamine (8[R]). Similarly, among reports of withdrawal reactions to the WHO Collaborating Center for International Drug Monitoring there were significantly more reports with paroxetine than sertraline and fluoxetine (9[r]). In a double-blind study in which long-term SSRI treatment was substituted by placebo for 5–8 days there were significantly more discontinuation symptoms in patients taking paroxetine and sertraline than in those taking fluoxetine (10[C]). Discontinuation symptoms after fluoxetine withdrawal are uncommon, perhaps because of the long half-life of its active metabolite, norfluoxetine. If withdrawal symptoms are experienced it may be some weeks after fluoxetine has been stopped.

The greater likelihood of withdrawal reactions with paroxetine may be attributable to its relatively short half-life or perhaps to antagonist effects at muscarinic cholinergic receptors, which might produce cholinergic rebound on discontinuation. There have been few reports to date of withdrawal reactions after citalopram discontinuation, but it is uncertain whether this reflects a truly lower propensity to cause withdrawal symptoms.

Drug interactions with SSRIs

Mechanisms *SSRIs have been implicated in many pharmacokinetic interactions with other drugs, because of their ability to inhibit certain cytochrome P450 (CYP) enzymes (Table 1).*

Citalopram has the least inhibitory effect on cytochrome P450 enzymes and thus far has not been associated with clinically significant interactions with other CNS drugs.

In contrast, fluoxetine and paroxetine are potent inhibitors of CYP2D6 and can produce clinically significant increases in plasma concentrations of antipsychotic drugs, such as haloperidol, perphenazine, risperidone, and thioridazine, particularly in subjects who are extensive metabolizers of these drugs. Extrapyramidal effects and cognitive impairment can result.

Table 1. *Cytochrome P450 isozymes inhibited by SSRIs (11[R])*

SSRI	Cytochrome P450 isozyme(s) inhibited
Citalopram	CYP2D6 (weakly)
Fluoxetine (and active metabolite norfluoxetine)	CYP2D6 CYP2C19 CYP3A3/4
Fluvoxamine	CYP1A2 CYP2C19 CYP3A3/4
Paroxetine	CYP2D6
Sertraline (and active metabolite desmethylsertraline)	CYP2D6

Interactions with other CNS drugs *Interactions of SSRIs with other CNS drugs are important, because of the frequency of combined therapy and the risks of CNS toxicity. Interactions between SSRIs and a number of other psychotropic drugs, including antipsychotic agents, tricyclic antidepressants, and mood stabilizers, have been reviewed (12[R]).*

Antipsychotic drugs *Fluvoxamine does not inhibit CYP2D6, but it is a potent inhibitor of CYP1A2 and produces substantial increases in concentrations of clozapine and other antipsychotic drugs, such as haloperidol.*

Although clozapine is mainly metabolized through CYP1A2, a secondary metabolic pathway involves CYP2D6, and fluoxetine, paroxetine, and sertraline treatment can increase clozapine concentrations (SEDA-21, 12; (13[C])).

Benzodiazepines *Benzodiazepines are often co-administered with SSRIs in the treatment of anxiety disorders. Both fluoxetine and fluvoxamine inhibit CYP3A and can increase plasma concentrations of alprazolam and diazepam, while sertraline has smaller effects. Paroxetine and citalopram are unlikely to increase benzodiazepine concentrations. Both fluoxetine and fluvoxamine, as inhibitors of CYP3A, can increase concentrations of carbamazepine (12[R]).*

Drugs acting on cholinergic pathways *In 13 healthy volunteers, oral fluvoxamine (100 mg/day for 6 days) significantly increased plasma concentrations of the cholinesterase inhibitor tacrine and reduced its clearance; concentrations of its active metabolites were also increased (14[C]). The authors attributed this interaction to the inhibitory effect of fluvoxamine on CYP1A2, which is responsible for the metabolism of tacrine. Increased tacrine concentrations could cause adverse gastrointestinal effects and an increased risk of hepatotoxicity.*

In another case paroxetine caused delirium when added to the muscarinic antagonist benztropine (15[c]).

A 17-year-old boy was taking haloperidol 5 mg/day, benztropine 2 mg bd, valproate 1750 mg/day, gabapentin 300 mg/day, and buspirone 5 mg bd. Paroxetine 20 mg/day was added and 8 days later he reported dry mouth and nausea and was disorientated in time, disorganized, and amnesic. The serum benztropine concentration was 36 ng/ml (toxic concentration >25 ng/ml). Two days after withdrawal of haloperidol, benztropine, valproate, and paroxetine his symptoms had completely resolved.

The presentation in this case was consistent with an anticholinergic syndrome due to high benztropine concentrations. It is likely that inhibition of CYP2D6 activity by paroxetine led to reduced benztropine metabolism. The modest anticholinergic properties of paroxetine could also have contributed. Benztropine should be used cautiously in conjunction with fluoxetine, paroxetine, or sertraline.

Drugs that facilitate brain 5HT neurotransmission *The combined effects of SSRIs with other drugs that can facilitate 5HT neurotransmission can lead to serotonin toxicity, known as the serotonin syndrome. The antimigraine drug sumatriptan is a $5HT_{1D}$ receptor antagonist, and it has been recommended that it should not be given with SSRIs. Thus far there has been no clinical evidence of important interactions, but a recent case report supports this suggestion (16[c]).*

A 48-year-old woman, taking sertraline 100 mg/day for recurrent depression, received an injection of subcutaneous sumatriptan (dose not specified) for the treatment of acute headache. Within 10 min she became agitated, ataxic, and disoriented. She had incoordination and hyper-reflexia in all four limbs. Improvement in her psychiatric and neurological symptoms began within 3 h and was complete within 24 h.

No other cause of this episode could be established. The symptoms and signs met criteria for the serotonin syndrome.

Two other patients have been described who experienced signs of serotonin toxicity while taking sumatriptan. One had taken sumatriptan alone, while the other had taken sumatriptan, lithium, and sertraline. However, there have been other reports that sumatriptan can be combined safely with SSRIs (17[c]), and the mechanism of this adverse effect is unclear.

Tramadol *Tramadol is an analgesic with some ability to inhibit 5HT re-uptake, and a serotonin syndrome has been reported in a patient taking tramadol and sertraline (18[c]).*

A 42-year-old woman who had been taking sertraline 100 mg/day for over a year for the treatment of major depression was treated with tramadol 300 mg/day. After 3 weeks she developed confusion, agitation, tremor, and sweating, and a diagnosis of serotonin syndrome was made. Her symptoms settled within 36 h after withdrawal of tramadol and reduction of the sertraline dosage to 50 mg/day.

This patient was taking several other medications, so it is not entirely clear that this reaction was attributable to the combination of sertraline with tramadol. However, the use of SSRIs in combination with tramadol is probably not uncommon, because patients with chronic pain often suffer from major depression. Further data are required on the possible risks of this combination.

Tricyclic antidepressants *Through CYP2D6 inhibition, both paroxetine and fluoxetine increase plasma concentrations of co-administered tricyclic antidepressants sufficient to lead to adverse effects such as dry mouth, cognitive impairment, and seizures (12[R]). Fluvoxamine increases plasma concentrations of tertiary tricyclics, such as amitriptyline, through inhibition of CYP1A2, but the effects of citalopram are modest and probably not clinically significant (12[R]). Sertraline inhibits CYP2D6 less than paroxetine or fluoxetine, but in dosages of 150 mg/day it produced clinically significant increases in plasma concentrations of imipramine and desipramine in 12 healthy men (19[C]). A similar finding was reported in 14 elderly depressed patients, in whom the addition of sertraline 100 mg/day or more produced a median increase of 40% in plasma nortriptyline concentrations; in contrast sertraline 50 mg/day increased nortriptyline concentrations by only 2% (20[C]).*

Interactions of SSRIs with other drugs

Fluoxetine *It has been suggested that fluoxetine should be used with caution with certain drugs that have a narrow therapeutic index and are metabolized via CYP3A. Examples include astemizole, cisapride, and terfenadine, which can cause cardiac dysrhythmias at the toxic plasma concentrations that be caused by drug interactions. However, fluoxetine (60 mg/day for 9 days) did not inhibit the metabolism of terfenadine in 12 healthy men (21[C]), suggesting a lack of effect of fluoxetine on CYP3A.*

These results nevertheless need to be received with caution, because some patients take fluoxetine in regimens that would lead to higher plasma concentrations of fluoxetine and norfluoxetine than were seen in this study. It is also worth noting that the active metabolite of fluoxetine, norfluoxetine, is a more potent inhibitor of CYP3A than fluoxetine itself and has a long half-life (about 7 days), making it accumulate slowly. Supporting evidence that fluoxetine can inhibit CYP3A4 comes from a report that fluoxetine may have inhibited the metabolism of nifedipine, another substrate for CYP3A; the patient experienced weakness, tachycardia, and hypotension, which resolved on withdrawal of fluoxetine (22[c]).

Fluvoxamine *Fluvoxamine pre-treatment (100 mg/day for 8 days) inhibited the transformation of the antimalarial drug chloroguanide to cycloguanil in extensive but not poor metabolizers (23[C]). This transformation is carried out by CYP2C19, suggesting that fluvoxamine inhibits this enzyme. The effect of fluvoxamine may be clinically significant, because chloroguanide acts as a pro-drug for cycloguanil, and the efficacy of antimalarial therapy with chloroguanide could therefore be compromised by concomitant fluvoxamine treatment.*

Sertraline *Treatment for 26 days with sertraline (maximum dosage 200 mg/day) in 12 healthy volunteers produced a small increase in prothrombin time when it was co-administered with warfarin (24[C]). Although the increase was not thought to be clinically important, the authors recommended that the prothrombin time be carefully monitored when sertraline and warfarin are given together. The mechanism was probably displacement of warfarin from protein binding sites. Warfarin is metabolized by CYP2C9/10, and the authors concluded that sertraline appears to have a fairly modest inhibitory effect on this enzyme.*

A similar regimen of sertraline treatment slightly but significantly reduced the clearance of tolbutamide, another substrate for CYP2C9/10, in 12 healthy men (25[C]). The increase in tolbutamide concentrations was not thought to be clinically significant. Fluoxetine and fluvoxamine are rather more potent inhibitors of CYP2C9 (12[R]) and might therefore be expected to have a greater potential than sertraline to interact with warfarin and tolbutamide.

Fluoxetine

Cardiovascular Although there have been reports that fluoxetine can be helpful in the treatment of *Raynaud's phenomenon*, it has also been attributed to fluoxetine (26[c]).

A 54-year-old woman was taking fluoxetine 40 mg/day for major depression. When the dosage was increased to 60 mg/day she developed fixed Raynaud's phenomenon in both hands. The dosage of fluoxetine was reduced to 40 mg/day and the Raynaud's phenomenon resolved, although digital plethysmography of her hands showed cold-induced, reversible, painless vasoconstriction. When the dosage of fluoxetine was increased to 60 mg/day she again started to have spontaneous attacks of Raynaud's phenomenon, after which the fluoxetine was withdrawn. Seven weeks later there was no evidence of spontaneous Raynaud's phenomenon and no abnormality on plethysmography.

Hematological Fluoxetine has been associated with severe *neutropenia* in a 79-year-old man (leukocyte count 2.8×10^9/l) with granulocytopenia and monocytosis (0% segmented cells, 11% band cells, 2% metamyelocytes, 45% lymphocytes, 36% monocytes, and 6% eosinophils) (27[c]). Other hematological indices were unchanged. While the patient was taking other medications (warfarin, glipizide, and diphenhydramine) the neutrophil count returned to normal within 10 days of fluoxetine withdrawal and occurred again within a few days of fluoxetine re-introduction; when fluoxetine was withdrawn once again the neutropenia rapidly resolved. This reaction must be very rare but did seem to be convincingly associated with fluoxetine in this case.

Liver Fluoxetine has rarely been associated with increased concentrations of hepatic aminotransferases. In a 35-year-old man fluoxetine treatment was associated with severe *chronic hepatitis*, which mimicked autoimmune hepatitis (28[c]). Withdrawal of fluoxetine led to normalization of liver function tests and subsequent investigation showed that the abnormal tests correlated well with the use and withdrawal of fluoxetine.

Gastrointestinal Two women had *stomatitis* while taking fluoxetine; in one the stomatitis recurred on rechallenge (29[c]).

Paroxetine

Cardiovascular Tricyclic antidepressants can cause postural hypotension, and SSRIs may therefore be preferred in patients with a history of cardiovascular disease. However, *postural hypotension* has been reported with paroxetine (30[c]).

A 75-year-old woman who had undergone coronary bypass surgery 6 months before started to take paroxetine 10 mg/day for depression. Her other medication (quinine bisulfate, fluvastatin, and temazepam) was unchanged. After 14 days the paroxetine was increased to 20 mg/day, and 6 days later she became dizzy, with marked postural hypotension (blood pressure 170/90 mmHg lying and 90/60 standing). Paroxetine was withdrawn and the postural hypotension settled, but recurred when paroxetine was re-introduced in a dose of 10 mg/day.

Special senses The report of an association between paroxetine and *acute angle closure glaucoma* (SEDA-21, 13) has been followed by two further case reports (31[c]), (32[c]). It is uncertain whether this effect of paroxetine is linked to its anticholinergic activity or whether facilitation of serotonin neurotransmission can itself cause acute angle closure in some individuals.

Sertraline

Endocrine In 11 patients taking thyroxine replacement therapy, *TSH concentrations rose* and increased doses of thyroxine maintenance therapy (16–50%) were required when sertraline was added. The mechanism is unclear, but this effect can occur with other antidepressant drugs. *Hypothyroidism* has also been reported in patients taking sertraline who were not taking thyroxine supplements (33[C]).

OTHER ANTIDEPRESSANTS

Nefazodone *(SED-13, 61; SEDA-20, 9)*

Psychiatric Nefazodone treatment appeared to produce *a manic episode* in a patient with no previous history of bipolar disorder (34[c]).

A 55-year-old woman had a 13-year history of recurrent unipolar depression. Trials of nortriptyline and fluoxetine had been ineffective, but she responded well to desipramine and later to sertraline. When depression recurred on sertraline treatment she was given paroxetine instead, but did not respond. She then received nefazodone 100 mg bd, and within a week developed a manic episode, with racing thoughts, hypersexuality, and grandiose ideas. Nefazodone was withdrawn, but over the next 4 weeks her condition deteriorated, with mixed affective features that did not respond to valproic acid. Eventually her mood became more stable with carbamazepine and sertraline, but some depressive symptoms remained.

As with all manic switches it is difficult to know how much of a role nefazodone played in this presentation. However, the patient had not apparently developed mania with a variety of other antidepressant drugs.

Endocrine, metabolic A 54-year-old woman with insulin-dependent diabetes mellitus suffered *hypoglycemia* after starting to take nefazodone (35[c]). Over the next month her insulin requirements fell and she lost weight. While these effects were beneficial for this particular patient, this report suggests that careful monitoring of blood glucose may be needed when diabetic patients are treated with nefazodone.

Interactions The pharmacokinetics of nefazodone have been reviewed (36[R]). It is a weak inhibitor of CYP2D6 and does not inhibit CYP1A2. It does, however, inhibit CYP3A4. This produces clinically significant interactions between nefazodone and substrates for CYP3A4, such as *triazolam*, *alprazolam*, *cyclosporin*, and *carbamazepine*. There is also potential for interactions with *astemizole*, *cisapride*, and *terfenadine*, with the risk of cardiac dysrhythmias.

Venlafaxine *(SED-13, 64; SEDA-20, 9; SEDA-21, 13)*

Withdrawal effects Discontinuation of venlafaxine can result in withdrawal symptoms, including *flu-like symptoms*, *dizziness*, *nausea*, *abdominal pain*, and *agitation* (SEDA-21, 13). Two patients had *visual hallucinations* after abrupt discontinuation of venlafaxine (37^c). During the 3 days after treatment discontinuation there were withdrawal reactions after abrupt discontinuation of modified-release venlafaxine (75 mg) in seven of nine patients taking venlafaxine, but only two of nine taking placebo (38^C). The most common withdrawal symptoms were *dizziness or light-headedness*, *sweating*, *irritability*, *dysphoria*, and *insomnia*. These results suggest that both immediate-release and modified-release venlafaxine should be tapered gradually when treatment is discontinued.

Overdosage Preliminary data suggest that venlafaxine is safer in acute overdose than tricyclic antidepressants. A patient who took about 3 g of venlafaxine in a suicide attempt had *clonic–tonic seizures* and *abnormal liver function tests* (39^c). While seizure activity has been reported previously in association with venlafaxine overdose, abnormal liver function tests have not. It is probably worth monitoring liver function after overdosage of venlafaxine.

REFERENCES

1. Liu B, Anderson G, Mittmann N, To T, Axcell T, Shear N. Use of selective serotonin-reuptake inhibitors or tricyclic antidepressants and risk of hip fractures in elderly people. Lancet 1998;351:1303–8.
2. DeToledo JC, Haddad H, Ramsay RE. Status epilepticus associated with the combination of valproic acid and clomipramine. Ther Drug Monit 1997;19:71–3.
3. Caley CF. Extrapyramidal reactions and the selective serotonin-reuptake inhibitors. Ann Pharmacother 1997;31:1481–9.
4. Vesely C, Fischer P, Goessler R, Kasper S. Mania associated with serotonin selective reuptake inhibitors. J Clin Psychiatry 1997;58:88.
5. Amsterdam JD, Garcia-Espania F, Goodman D, Hooper M, Hornig-Rohan M. Breast enlargement during chronic antidepressant therapy. J Affect Disord 1997;46:151–6.
6. Modell JG, Katholi CR, Modell JD, DePalma RL. Comparative sexual side effects of bupropion, fluoxetine, paroxetine, and sertraline. Clin Pharmacol Ther 1997;61:476–87.
7. Haddad P. Newer antidepressants and the discontinuation syndrome. J Clin Psychiatry 1997; 58:17–21.
8. Coupland NJ, Bell CJ, Potokar JP. Serotonin reuptake inhibitor withdrawal. J Psychopharmacol 1996;16:356–62.
9. Stahl MMS, Lindquist M, Pettersson M, Edwards IR, Sanderson JH, Taylor NFA, Fletcher AP, Schou JS. Withdrawal reactions with selective serotonin re-uptake inhibitors as reported to the WHO system. Eur J Clin Pharmacol 1997;53:163–9.
10. Rosenbaum JF, Fava M, Hoog SL, Ascroft RC, Krebs WB. Selective serotonin reuptake inhibitor discontinuation syndrome: a randomized clinical trial. Biol Psychiatry 1998;44:77–87.
11. Caccia S. Metabolism of the newer antidepressants. An overview of the pharmacological and pharmacokinetic implications. Clin Pharmacokinet 1998;34:281–302.
12. Sproule BA, Naranjo CA, Bremner KE, Hassan PC. Selective serotonin reuptake inhibitors and CNS drug interactions. A critical review of the evidence. Clin Pharmacokinet 1997;33:454–71.
13. Armstrong SC, Stephans JR. Blood clozapine levels elevated by fluvoxamine: potential for side effects and lower clozapine dosage. J Clin Psychiatry 1997;58:499.
14. Becquemont L, Ragueneau I, Le Bot MA, Riche C, Funck-Brentano C, Jaillon P. Influence of the CYP1A2 inhibitor fluvoxamine on tacrine pharmacokinetics in humans. Clin Pharmacol Ther 1997;61:619–27.
15. Armstrong SC, Schweitzer SM. Delerium associated with paroxetine and benztropine combination. Am J Psychiatry 1997;154:581–2.
16. Mathew NT, Tietjen GE, Lucker C. Serotonin syndrome complicating migraine pharmacotherapy. Cephalalgia 1996;16:323–7.
17. Wing YK, Clifford EM, Sheehan BD, Campling GM, Hockney RA, Cowen PJ. Paroxetine treatment and the prolactin response to sumatriptan. Psychopharmacology 1996;124:377–9.
18. Mason BJ, Blackburn KH. Possible serotonin syndrome associated with tramodol and sertraline coadministration. Ann Pharmacother 1997;31: 175–7.
19. Kurtz DL, Bergstrom RF, Goldberg MJ, Cerimele BJ. The effect of sertraline on the pharmokinetics of desipramine and imipramine. Clin Pharmacol Ther 1997;62:145–56.
20. Solai LK, Mulsant BH, Pollock BG, Sweet RA, Rosen J, Kai Y, Reynolds CF. Effect of sertraline on plasma nortriptyline levels in depressed elderly. J Clin Psychiatry 1997;58:440–3.
21. Bergstrom RF, Goldberg MJ, Cerimele BJ,

Hatcher BL. Assessment of the potential for a pharmacokinetic interaction between fluoxetine and terfenadine. Clin Pharmacol Ther 1997; 62:643–51.
22. Azaz-Livshits TLT, Danenberg HD. Tachycardia, orthostatic hypotension and profound weakness due to constant use of fluoxetine and nifedipine. Pharmacopsychiatry 1997;30:274–5.
23. Jeppsen U, Buur-Rasmussen B, Brosen K. Fluvoxamine inhibits the CYP2C19-catalyzed bioactivation of chloroguanide. Clin Pharmacol Ther 1997;62:279–86.
24. Apseloff G, Wilner KD, Gerber N, Tremaine LM. Effect of sertraline on protein binding of warfarin. Clin Pharmacokinet 1997;32:37–42.
25. Tremaine LM, Wilner KD, Peskorn SH. A study of the potential effect of sertraline on the pharmokinetics and protein binding of tolbutamide. Clin Pharmacokinet 1997;32:31–6.
26. Rudnick A, Modai I, Zelikovski A. Fluoxetine-induced Raynaud's phenomenon. Biol Psychiatry 1997;41:1218–21.
27. Vilinsky FD, Lubin A. Severe neutropenia associated with fluoxetine hydrochloride. Ann Intern Med 1997;127:573–4.
28. Johnston DE, Wheeler DE. Chronic hepatitis related to use of fluoxetine. Am J Gastroenterol 1997;92:1225–6.
29. Palop V, Sancho A, Morales-Olivas FJ, Martinez-Mir I. Fluoxetine associated stomatitis. Ann Pharmacother 1997;31:1478–80.
30. Andrews C, Pinner G. Postural hypertension induced by paroxetine. Br Med J 1998;316:595.
31. Lewis CF, DeQuardo JR, DuBose C, Tandon R. Acute angle-closure glaucoma and paroxetine. J Clin Psychiatry 1997;58:123–4.
32. Kirwan JF, Subak-Sharpe I, Teimory M. Bilateral acute angle closure glaucoma after administration of paroxetine. Br J Ophthalmol 1997;81:252.
33. McCowen KC, Garber JR, Spark R, Clary CM, Harrison WM. Elevated serum thyrotropin in thyroxine treated patients with hypothyroidism given sertraline. New Engl J Med 1997;337:1010–11.
34. Dubin H, Spier S, Giannandrea P. Nefazdone-induced mania. Am J Psychiatry 1997;154:578–9.
35. Warnock JK, Biggs F. Nefazodone-induced hypoglycemia in a diabetic patient with major depression. Am J Psychiatry 1997;154:288–9.
36. Greene DS, Barbhaiya RH. Clinical pharmacokinetics of nefazodone. Clin Pharmacokinet 1997;33:260–75.
37. Agelink MW, Zitzelsberger A, Kleiser E. Withdrawal syndrome after discontinuation of venlafaxine. Am J Psychiatry 1997;154:1473–4.
38. Fava M, Mulroy R, Alpert J, Nierneberg AA, Rosenbaum JF. Emergence of adverse events following discontinuation of treatment with extended release venlafaxine. Am J Psychiatry 1997;154:1760–2.
39. Zhalkovsky B, Walker D, Bourgeois JA. Seizure activity and enzyme evaluations after venlafaxine overdose. J Clin Psychopharmacol 1997;17:490–1.

J.W. Jefferson

3 Lithium

Evidence continues to accrue that the benefits of long-term lithium therapy with regard to reduced morbidity and mortality outweigh the risks of adverse effects and toxicity (1[R])–(3[R]), although agreement is not universal (4[R]). The same cannot be said for other mood stabilizers (e.g. carbamazepine, valproate, lamotrigine, gabapentin), because of a paucity or absence of adequate long-term follow-up data (5[R])–(7[R]).

In a randomized, but not blinded, multicenter maintenance comparison of lithium (n = 74) with carbamazepine (n = 70) over 2 years, there were similar numbers of hospitalizations and recurrences, but when factors such as concomitant medication and severe adverse effects were also considered, lithium was the superior drug (8[C]). Milder adverse effects, such as *tremor*, *polydipsia*, *polyuria*, and *diarrhea*, were more common with lithium, while pruritus was more common with carbamazepine. The only suicide and only suicide attempt occurred in the carbamazepine group. In a double-blind crossover study two of 42 patients discontinued lithium because of adverse effects (acne and psoriasis), while 10 of 35 did so with carbamazepine (mostly because of rash) during the 1-year treatment periods (9[C]).

Reports from two major Italian lithium clinics (in Naples and Sardinia) have further substantiated a remarkable reduction in manic-depressive morbidity during lithium treatment of many years duration (10[C]), (11[C]). In addition, further evidence has appeared to support an association between long-term lithium therapy and reduced risks of suicide and suicidal behavior. Suicidal acts per 100 patient years were 2.30 before lithium, 0.36 during lithium, 7.11 in the first year after discontinuation, and 2.29 at later times (12[CR]). Rapid withdrawal of lithium was associated with a 1.96 times greater risk of suicidal behavior than gradual withdrawal (a non-significant trend). This observation is in keeping with an increasing body of evidence of reduced affective morbidity with gradual (15–30 days) versus rapid (1–14 days) withdrawal of lithium (13[C]), (14[C]), (15[CR]). However, withdrawal of lithium does increase the risk of recurrence, and concern has been expressed that some patients may not respond when retreated (16[c]), (17[c]). Two more recent reports have been reassuring in this regard, finding no evidence of such treatment resistance when lithium was resumed (18[C]), (19[C]).

In a randomized, non-blind comparison of lithium (n = 43) and carbamazepine (n = 47) for maintenance treatment of schizoaffective disorder over 30 months, dropout rates overall (32 vs 12%) and because of adverse effects (9 vs 2%) were greater for carbamazepine, while more patients taking lithium had slight to moderate adverse effects (42 vs 27%) (20[C]). Adverse effects evaluated after the first 6 months of treatment that occurred significantly more often in patients taking lithium were *tremor*, *appetite increase*, *weight gain*, *fatigue*, *weakness*, *difficulty in concentrating*, *dry mouth*, *polyuria*, *sweating*, *difficulty falling asleep*, and *retarded thought processes*. On the other hand, there were no suicide attempts in the lithium group but four in those taking carbamazepine. Mean serum concentrations with both drugs were relatively low: lithium 0.58 mmol/l; carbamazepine 27 μmol/l (6.4 μg/ml).

ORGANS AND SYSTEMS

Cardiovascular An 80-year-old man with a lithium concentration of 2.7 mmol/l had *sinus bradycardia* (30–40 bpm) and *hypotension* (85/50 mmHg) (21[c]). The sinus bradycardia with occasional premature ventricular contractions evolved into atrial fibrillation, which

Side Effects of Drugs, Annual 22
J.K. Aronson, ed.

was treated with a temporary pacemaker, digoxin, and quinidine. As the lithium toxicity resolved, sinus rhythm returned and the pacemaker and antidysrhythmic drugs were withdrawn. The report somewhat contradictorily stated that the patient had no history of cardiopulmonary problems before the episode and also mentioned a history of paroxysmal atrial fibrillation. Nevertheless, the case serves as a reminder that lithium toxicity can cause cardiac dysrhythmias (as can therapeutic concentrations of lithium in susceptible individuals) (22[cR]), (23[c]).

Nervous system A review of irreversible neurotoxicity associated with lithium both alone and in conjunction with other drugs, particularly neuroleptic drugs, was supplemented by seven case vignettes that emphasized the predominantly cerebellar nature of the residua (24[cR]). In keeping with these observations, a 52-year-old woman who died 24 days after admission for lithium intoxication (serum lithium 3.2 mmol/l), despite repeated hemodialysis, at autopsy had severe *cerebellar atrophy* involving the internal granule and Purkinje cell layers together with Bergmann gliosis (25[c]).

Clinical manifestations of lithium toxicity (*ataxia*, *intention tremor*, *slurred speech*) in a 72-year-old woman also included prominent orolingual-facial and abdominal dyskinesias and choreiform movements of the fingers and toes (serum lithium 1.1 mmol/l) (26[c]). When lithium was withdrawn, the cerebellar findings resolved quickly, but the *chorea* and *dyskinesias* persisted (since follow-up duration was not specified, one cannot equate persistence with permanence). Because she had taken lithium for over 20 years in the absence of neuroleptic drugs or other dopamine antagonists, the tardive dyskinesia was attributed to lithium (although long-term tricyclic antidepressant use could also have played a role).

Central pontine myelinolysis has been linked to a wide variety of medical disorders, including over-rapid correction of hyponatremia, but it had not been previously associated with lithium toxicity (27[c]).

A 63-year-old man who had taken lithium for 35 years became dehydrated and hypernatremic (serum sodium 155 mmol/l), with a serum lithium concentration of 1.9 mmol/l that "remained high for more than 2 weeks despite stopping lithium". When the concentration fell to 0.9 mmol/l, he was discharged taking lithium carbonate 300 mg/day, only to return 6 weeks later with severe neurological impairment, a serum lithium concentration of 1.5 mmol/l, and an MRI scan showing acute pontine demyelination consistent with a diagnosis of CPM. Four months later he remained impaired neurologically and the MRI findings were unchanged.

Other case reports have described *choreoathetosis* (28[c]) and transient *aphasia* (29[c]) in association with lithium toxicity. Choreoathetosis has been described before, but this report serves as a reminder that all neurotoxicity is not cerebellar. The latter involved a 66-year-old woman with a lithium concentration of 3.0 mmol/l who had a reversible Wernicke's aphasia in the absence of delirium or dementia.

A general review of drug-induced movement disorders included little detail about lithium but provided useful references (30[R]). The following rating system was used: (1) well-documented or frequent; (2) relatively well-documented or relatively frequent; (3) not well-documented, or anecdotal.

Lithium received the following ratings: postural tremor (well-documented); myoclonus (relatively well-documented); parkinsonism, chorea, tardive dyskinesia, and akathisia (not well-documented).

Endocrine, metabolic *Thyroid* Two brief reviews of the relation between lithium and the thyroid have appeared in the German literature (31[r]), (32[r]) and one more extensive review in English (33[R]). The latter discussed the effects of lithium on thyroid physiology, the hypothalamic–pituitary axis, cellular metabolism, and thyroid hormone action, as well as clinical effects on goiter, hypothyroidism, and hyperthyroidism.

A study of 23 lithium-treated patients involved baseline and periodic (at intervals of 6–12 months) thyroid ultrasound and laboratory testing (T_4, T_3, TSH, antithyroid antibodies) (34[C]). The results suggested that preexisting thyroid abnormalities were predictive of lithium-associated thyroid dysfunction, and that lithium does not cause autoimmune thyroiditis de novo.

However, thyroiditis has been described in a patient taking lithium (35[c]).

A goiter resected in a 29-year-old woman who had taken lithium for 5 years had histological findings consistent with thyroiditis which, in conjunction with positive serum antithyroglobulin and antimicrosomal antibodies, led to a diagnosis of lithium-associated autoimmune thyroiditis (baseline antibody titers had not been measured). Although she was euthyroid at surgery, she had been diagnosed as having Graves' disease almost 3 years before, and despite treatment with methimazole (lithium was continued) her thyroid function tests were in the hyperthyroid range 18 months later.

Hyperthyroidism during lithium treatment has been described previously and has always been something of a paradox in view of lithium's more usual thyroid suppressing effects. In fact, lithium was shown to be useful in conjunction with propylthiouracil for treating amiodarone-induced thyrotoxicosis ($n = 9$) (36[C]).

Parathyroid and calcium Sensitive studies of the calcium/parathyroid hormone axis (using citrate and calcium infusions) have shown a shift to the right of parathyroid hormone set point and increased serum calcium concentrations in seven patients taking lithium for an average of 5 years who had normal baseline total calcium and parathyroid hormone concentrations (37[c]). Two patients who had taken lithium for 17 and 19 years had hyperparathyroidism and reduced bone mineral density (38[c]). The abnormal findings persisted despite withdrawal of lithium in both cases, but did remit in one after two parathyroid adenomas had been resected. A 51-year-old man who had taken lithium for more than 10 years had hypercalcemia (3.08 mmol/l) and raised parathyroid hormone concentrations, which persisted despite stopping lithium (39[c]). After an oxyphilic parathyroid adenoma had been excised, both values normalized. Another patient, who had taken lithium for 19 years, developed hyperparathyroidism associated with hypertension and a bradydysrhythmia (bone mineral density was not altered), which persisted after lithium was withdrawn. After surgery for parathyroid hyperplasia, there was improvement in his parathyroid hormone and lithium concentrations, blood pressure, and the dysrhythmia (40[c]). A retrospective chart review comparing patients on lithium who had persistent hypercalcemia ($n = 12$) with normocalcemic lithium patients ($n = 40$) and normocalcemic bipolar patients taking anticonvulsant mood stabilizers ($n = 20$) showed a higher frequency of cardiac conduction disturbances in the hypercalcemic lithium group (41[C]). An interaction between lithium and hypercalcemia was postulated to play a pathogenic role in the conduction disturbances.

Hyperglycemia A reversible case of hyperosmolar non-ketotic hyperglycemia occurred in a 45-year-old man after 2 weeks of severe polyuria (he had taken lithium for 10 years with mild polyuria for the previous 5 years); he had no history of diabetes mellitus (42[c]). The syndrome resolved after withdrawal of lithium and supportive treatment, and the urine volume fell from 4–5 to 1.7 l/day.

Weight gain In an open study of eight women who had gained a mean of 17 kg while taking tricyclic antidepressants and lithium, treatment with the opiate antagonist naltrexone for 8 weeks was associated with a small but significant weight loss (43[c]). The role of naltrexone in treating lithium-associated weight gain remains unclear.

Urinary system Despite many years of study and debate, the long-term impact of lithium on the kidneys continues to arouse controversy. A brief review of *lithium-induced renal disease* has concluded that, "... a small number of patients treated with lithium developed progressive renal damage associated with chronic interstitial nephritis" (44[R]). While I find this a reasonable statement, others may disagree. In a study of 107 patients treated with lithium for 1–15 years (mean 54 months) compared with 29 psychiatric controls, those taking lithium had significantly higher 24-h urine volumes and urinary excretion of β_2-microglobulin and glycosaminoglycan (indicators of renal damage) but no differences in plasma creatinine and 24-h creatinine clearance (45[C]).

The conclusion of a report of three patients with end-stage renal disease was that lithium was the most likely cause (46[c]). The first patient stopped taking lithium in 1984 after 12 years of treatment when the serum creatinine was 160 μmol/l. Despite only a brief exposure to lithium after that, renal insufficiency was progressive and dialysis was initiated in 1992. The second had taken lithium for 11 years when the serum creatinine was 141 μmol/l. Despite lithium withdrawal, the renal disease progressed and hemodialysis was started 8 years later. In the third patient, lithium was stopped after 8 years of treatment, when an episode of lithium toxicity was associated with a serum creatinine of 239 μmol/l. Over the course of 10 years and two intervening pregnancies, renal function deteriorated further and hemodialysis was begun. A search for causes other than lithium was unrewarding in all three patients and two had renal biopsies consistent with, but not diagnostic of, lithium-induced nephrotoxicity (interstitial fibrosis). While a causal relation between lithium and renal insufficiency could not be firmly established, it could also not be excluded. The progressive nature of the conditions in the absence of lithium suggests an unrelated process, although concern remains that lithium could have initiated the irreversibility.

The fact that lithium-induced *nephrogenic diabetes insipidus* is sometimes irreversible has been illustrated by a patient who developed severe polyuria after 11 years of lithium treatment (47[c]). The polyuria was still present 10 years after withdrawal of lithium, when he was hospitalized with marked hypernatremia (serum sodium 181 mmol/l) and a 24-h urine volume of 8 l. Indomethacin was useful for the polyuria as it was in two other patients.

An 82-year-old man who had been taking lithium for 31 years developed neurotoxic symptoms (serum lithium 0.7 mmol/l) associated with dehydration, impaired renal function and hypernatremia (serum sodium 172 mmol/l). Lithium-induced nephrogenic diabetes insipidus was diagnosed and treated effectively with indomethacin 25 mg tds, later supplemented with hydrochlorothiazide 25 mg daily (48[c]).

A similar prompt reduction in urine volume from indomethacin, 150 mg/day, occurred in a 47-year-old neurotoxic woman dehydrated secondary to fluid restriction and lithium-induced polyuria (serum lithium 1.1 mmol/l, serum sodium 170 mmol/l, urine volume as high as 24 l/day) after desmopressin, amiloride, and hydrochlorothiazide had failed to control output (49[cR]).

These reports illustrate the ever-present risk of dehydration in the presence of lithium-induced polyuria and the beneficial effects of indomethacin in controlling excessive urine output.

Another case of lithium-associated *nephrotic syndrome* and a review of 19 cases in the literature has served as a reminder of this rare adverse effect (50[cR]). While the onset of nephrotic syndrome in the 40-year-old woman after 20 years on lithium suggests a relationship more likely to be coincidental than causal, the syndrome remitted fully within 6 weeks of stopping lithium. Renal biopsy showed minimal-change disease. One further case with similar biopsy findings involved a lithium toxic (serum concentration 2.9 mmol/l) 59-year-old man with a 24-h urine protein concentration of 12.08 g (51[c]).

Skin and appendages The cutaneous effects of lithium have been reviewed and examples of *exacerbation of psoriasis* by lithium provided (52[cR]), (53[c]). Worsening of psoriasis by lithium was first reported in 1972, but a recent report of a similar reaction from drinking 'holy water' was unusual (54[c]). A 19-year-old's psoriasis was exacerbated after drinking spring water containing lithium 6.9 mmol/l (her serum lithium concentration was 0.3 mmol/l), subsided after stopping the water, and recurred after consumption resumed.

Two patients developed *pityriasis versicolor* while taking lithium, although a causal relation was not formally established (55[c]).

Hidradenitis suppurativa was associated with lithium in a 47-year-old woman, but whether it was caused by lithium was not clear (56[c]).

In contrast, an ointment of lithium succinate was more effective than placebo in a double-blind study of 12 HIV-positive patients with seborrheic dermatitis (57[C]).

Special senses Controversy continues over the long-term effects of lithium on vision. In 24 patients who had taken lithium for a mean of 7.3 years, there were no differences compared with 21 aged-matched controls using electro-oculography and electroretinography (58[C]). In contrast, 50 patients who took lithium for 1 week to 23 years had "subtle but significant" reductions in sensitivity to light compared with aged-matched controls; these effects did not correlate with duration of treatment (59[C]).

Second-generation effects Several reviews have addressed the use of lithium during and after pregnancy (60[R])–(62[R]) and have placed the risks (often overstated previously) in proper perspective with regard to the benefits (often underappreciated), and have also provided guidelines for the management of women with bipolar disorder during pregnancy and lactation. The low, but nevertheless increased, risk of *teratogenesis* with first trimester exposure to lithium must be balanced against the risk of affective recurrence if lithium is discontinued—a risk that is increased if lithium is discontinued too rapidly (which has often been the case in pregnancy) (63[C]).

A woman with an increased serum lithium concentration (2.6 mmol/l) just before delivery gave birth to an infant who had a serum concentration of 2.1 mmol/l (64[c]). *Lethargy* and *poor suck–swallow coordination* was present initially but resolved gradually over a week.

Whether women taking lithium should breast-feed remains controversial. The American Academy of Pediatrics considers it contraindicated; some experts agree (65[R]) but others are more open to a risk/benefit analysis case by case (61[R]), (62[R]), (66[R]).

Interactions *Angiotensin-converting enzyme (ACE) inhibitors* There have been sporadic reports of lithium toxicity associated with ACE inhibitors. Six weeks after starting lisinopril, verapamil, and aspirin, a 55-year-old woman who had taken lithium for 17 years without toxicity was hospitalized with confusion, slurred speech, and a serum lithium concentration of 4.9 mmol/l (67[c]). The authors proposed a complex interaction, in which aspirin had increased the lisinopril concentration, lisinopril had increased the lithium concentration, and verapamil had contributed to the neurotoxic symptoms. However, this sequence was not substantiated.

Angiotensin II receptor antagonists A 77-year-old woman developed symptoms of lithium toxicity and a serum lithium concentration of 2.0 mmol/l (previously 0.63) 5 weeks after starting to take losartan, an angiotensin II (type AT_1) receptor antagonist (68[c]). Losartan did not alter renal lithium excretion in rats (69[c]), but this case report suggests the possibility of an interaction in humans.

Antibiotics The authors of a review of the neuropsychiatric effects and interactions of antibiotics have briefly and incompletely summarized the literature on lithium/antibiotic interactions (70[R]). A case report suggested that doxycycline 100 mg bd was responsible for neurological symptoms and a trough lithium concentration of 1.5 mmol/l in a 68-year-old woman whose serum concentration was usually between 0.8 and 1.1 mmol/l (71[c]). Her symptoms began 1 day after she started to take doxycycline and resolved 1 day after stopping it. Reports of lithium/antibiotic interactions have been restricted to a few cases, from which generalizations are not possible.

Calcium antagonists Nifedipine 40–80 mg/day for 12 weeks caused a 30% reduction in renal lithium clearance, used as a measure of proximal tubular renal function, in 14 hypertensive patients (72[C]). Consistent with this effect, a subsequent report described a 30-year-old man who shortly after starting to take nifedipine 60 mg/day required a lithium carbonate dosage reduction from 1500 to 900 mg/day to maintain his serum concentration within the therapeutic range (73[c]).

Idebenone In 12 healthy subjects, idebenone, a memory enhancer, did not alter lithium pharmacokinetics after single or multiple doses (74[C]).

Neuroleptic drugs Since the 1974 report of neurotoxicity associated with lithium and haloperidol, the relative risk of combining lithium with antipsychotic drugs has been debated. The authors of a brief review reached no firm conclusions, but suggested that caution be exercised, especially if lithium is combined with high dosages of high-potency neuroleptic drugs (75[R]).

A 44-year-old woman with therapeutic lithium concentrations developed an acute encephalopathy consistent with neuroleptic malignant syndrome 2 days after starting to take haloperidol 6 mg/day

(76[c]). The syndrome worsened when haloperidol was reintroduced several days later, and despite withdrawal of both drugs, she was left with a permanent cerebellar syndrome.

The possibility of adverse interactions between lithium and the atypical neuroleptic, clozapine, has been summarized in a description of 10 reported cases of variable substantiation, including neurotoxicity ($n = 4$), seizures ($n = 2$), agranulocytosis ($n = 1$), organic psychosis ($n = 1$, following clozapine withdrawal when lithium concentrations increased), neuroleptic malignant syndrome ($n = 1$), and diabetic ketoacidosis ($n = 1$, 5 weeks after clozapine had been added) (77[R]). A report in abstract form indicated that the addition of an unspecified dose of quetiapine to lithium for 14 days in an unspecified number of patients did not increase extrapyramidal adverse effects (78[c]).

Non-steroidal anti-inflammatory drugs (NSAIDs) Reports continue to emerge associating the use of NSAIDs with increased serum lithium concentrations and possible lithium toxicity. In a single-blind, crossover study in 11 women with bipolar disorder, flurbiprofen 100 mg every 12 h for a week significantly increased trough lithium concentrations and AUC (79[C]). Four subjects had a clinically significant increase in trough concentration, defined by an increase of greater than 25% or more than 0.2 mmol/l. Similarly, ketorolac 10 mg qds caused a 24% increase in lithium AUC in five male volunteers, associated with moderate adverse effects (such as ataxia, tremors, difficulty concentrating, and sedation) (80[C]).

In contrast, over-the-counter dosages of naproxen (220 mg tds) or acetaminophen (650 mg qds) in 12 young healthy male volunteers produced no significant change in plasma lithium concentrations (81[C]). Nevertheless, caution should be exercised when any NSAID is combined with lithium, since dosage, age, renal function, and other factors can predispose certain individuals to problems.

Serotonin syndrome Several reports have suggested that the use of lithium in combination with drugs that enhance serotonin-mediated functions (such as monoamine reuptake inhibitors, the serotonin receptor agonist sumatriptan, MAO inhibitors, and the serotonin precursor tryptophan) is associated with the serotonin syndrome. Further reports of the serotonin syndrome in patients taking reuptake inhibitors have supported that suggestion.

A 59-year-old woman whose serum paroxetine concentrations were six times higher than customary developed shivering, tremor, flushing, agitation, and mildly impaired mental focusing 6 days after lithium was started (serum lithium concentration 0.63 mmol/l). Although she continued to take lithium, her symptoms resolved when the paroxetine dosage was reduced (82[c]).

A 77-year-old woman who took paroxetine and lithium for several days (serum lithium 1.2 mmol/l) developed a fever (39.5°C), confusion, hypertonicity, hyper-reflexia, and ataxia (83[c]). With discontinuation of the drugs and supportive care, the syndrome resolved in 4 days.

While taking venlafaxine and lithium, a 50-year-old woman became restless with "hyper-reflexia of arms and legs, spontaneous tossing of arms, muscular rigor, discrete myoclonia and moderate tachycardia" (84[c]). Her symptoms resolved when both drugs were stopped, but did not recur when both were restarted.

On the other hand, despite concerns about the use of *sumatriptan*, a $5HT_{1a}$ receptor agonist, in patients taking lithium, the authors of a review have concluded that the few reports of adverse reactions to lithium and sumatriptan could not be clearly defined as cases of the serotonin syndrome (85[r]).

While it is possible that combining lithium with serotonergic drugs may increase the risk of the serotonin syndrome, this is far from well established and should not deter the use of such combinations for overcoming otherwise treatment-resistant depression (86[C]).

Overdosage and toxicity Prompt and efficient treatment of lithium intoxication should reduce the risk of death or permanent damage (neurological, renal, and other). A comprehensive review based on literature from 1984 to 1996 has discussed reducing absorption with whole bowel irrigation and sodium polystyrene sulfonate resin and enhancing elimination by forced saline diuresis (of questionable efficacy), low-dose dopamine infusion (a single case report), theophylline (of limited value), continuous arteriovenous or venovenous hemodiafiltration (promising), and hemodialysis (the acknowledged treatment of choice for severe intoxication) (87[R]). Two patients with chronic lithium toxicity who were studied pharmacokinetically during and after hemodialysis demonstrated both the efficiency with which dialysis removes lithium from the body and the tendency for a rebound increase in serum lithium concentration after termination of treatment (88[c]).

The possibility of neurotoxic manifestations of lithium despite therapeutic concentrations has once again been illustrated by the case of a 56-year-old woman who developed "disorientation, aphasia, ideatoric apraxia, parkinsonism, restlessness, and severe sleep disorder" in the absence of toxic lithium concentrations (89[c]). Symptoms reappeared with re-exposure to therapeutic lithium and resolved fully when it was discontinued—a reminder that while serum lithium concentrations are often helpful in assessing lithium neurotoxicity, they should never replace sound clinical judgement.

Interference with diagnostic routines It has been suggested that inaccurate serum lithium concentrations might be related to 'ageing' of ion-selective electrodes (90[c]). A lithium concentration of 0.4 mmol/l was reported in a patient not taking lithium, and higher than expected concentrations were noted in 13 patients taking the drug. When five samples were also analyzed by atomic absorption spectrophototometry, the results averaged 0.3 mmol/l lower. A similar false-positive result with an ion-selective electrode led to incrimination of either the silicone surfactant or silica clot activator in the Becton-Dickinson Vacutainer Plus Tube used to collect the blood (91[c]). Whether these or similar tubes were used in the first study is not known.

REFERENCES

1. Schou M. Forty years of lithium treatment. Arch Gen Psychiatry 1997;54:9–13.
2. Cookson J. Lithium: balancing risks and benefits. Br J Psychiatry 1997;171:120–4.
3. Jefferson JW. Lithium. Still effective despite its detractors. Br Med J 1998;316:1330–1.
4. Moncrieff J. Lithium: evidence reconsidered. Br J Psychiatry 1997;171:113–19.
5. Solomon DA, Keitner GI, Miller IW, Shea MT, Keller MB. Course of illness and maintenance treatments for patients with bipolar disorder. J Clin Psychiatry 1995;56:5–13.
6. Gershon S, Soares JC. Current therapeutic profile of lithium. Arch Gen Psychiatry 1997;54:16–20.
7. Sharma V, Yatham LN, Haslam DRS, Silverstone PH, Parikh SV, Matte R, Kutcher SP, Kusumakar V. Continuation and prophylactic treatment of bipolar disorder. Can J Psychiatry 1997;42:92S–100S.
8. Greil W, Ludwig-Mayerhofer W, Erazo N, Schöhlin C, Schmidt S, Engel RR, Czernik A, Giedke H, Müller-Oerlinghausen B, Osterheider M, Rudolf GAE, Sauer H, Tegeler J, Wetterling T. Lithium versus carbamazepine in the maintenance treatment of bipolar disorders—a randomised study. J Affect Disord 1997;43:151–61.
9. Denicoff KD, Smith-Jackson EE, Disney ER, Ali SO, Leverich GS, Post RM. Comparative prophylactic efficacy of lithium, carbamazepine, and the combination in bipolar disorder. J Clin Psychiatry 1997;58:470–8.
10. Maj M, Pirozzi R, Magliano L, Bartoli L. Long-term outcome of lithium prophylaxis in bipolar disorder: a 5-year prospective study of 402 patients at a lithium clinic. Am J Psychiatry 1998;155:30–5.
11. Tondo L, Baldessarini RJ, Hennen J, Floris G. Lithium maintenance treatment of depression and mania in bipolar I and bipolar II disorders. Am J Psychiatry 1998;155:638–45.
12. Tondo L, Baldessarini RJ, Hennen J, Floris G, Silvetti F, Tohen M. Lithium treatment and risk of suicidal behavior in bipolar disorder patients. J Clin Psychiatry 1998;59:405–14.
13. Baldessarini RJ, Tondo L, Faedda GL, Suppes TR, Floris G, Rudas N. Effects of the rate of discontinuing lithium maintenance treatment in bipolar disorders. J Clin Psychiatry 1996;57:441–8.
14. Baldessarini RJ, Tondo L, Floris G, Rudas N. Reduced morbidity after gradual discontinuation of lithium treatment for bipolar I and II disorders: a replication study. Am J Psychiatry 1997;154:551–3.
15. Baldessarini RJ, Tondo L. Recurrence risk in bipolar manic-depressive disorders after discontinuing lithium maintenance treatment: an overview. Clin Drug Invest 1998;15:337–51.
16. Post RM, Leverich GS, Altshuler L, Mikalauskas K. Lithium-discontinuation-induced refractoriness: preliminary observations. Am J Psychiatry 1992;149:1727–9.
17. Maj M, Pirozzi R, Magliano L. Nonresponse to reinstituted lithium prophylaxis in previously responsive bipolar patients: prevalence and predictors. Am J Psychiatry 1995;152:1810–11.
18. Tondo L, Baldessarini RJ, Floris G, Rudas N. Effectiveness of restarting lithium treatment after its discontinuation in bipolar I and bipolar II disorders. Am J Psychiatry 1997;154:548–50.

19. Coryell W, Solomon D, Leon AC, Akiskal HS, Keller MB, Scheftner WA, Mueller T. Lithium discontinuation and subsequent effectiveness. Am J Psychiatry 1998;155:895–8.
20. Greil W, Ludwig-Mayerhofer W, Erazo N, Engel RR, Czernik A, Giedke H, Müller-Oerlinghausen B, Osterheider M, Rudolf GAE, Sauer H, Tegeler J, Wetterling T. Lithium versus carbamazepine in the maintenance treatment of schizoaffective disorder—a randomised study. Eur Arch Psychiatry Clin Neurosci 1997;247:42–50.
21. Hussain KMA, Kostandy G, Kurz L, Pachter BR. Hemodynamic, electrocardiographic, metabolic, and hematologic abnormalities resulting from lithium intoxication. A case report. Angiology 1997;48:351–4.
22. Joseph M, Vieweg V. Electrocardiographic changes of sinus bradycardia and sinus node dysfunction among patients with therapeutic levels of lithium. Depression 1994/1995;2:226–31.
23. Terao T, Abe H, Abe K. Irreversible sinus node dysfunction induced by resumption of lithium therapy. Acta Psychiatr Scand 1996;93:407–8.
24. Kores B, Lader MH. Irreversible lithium neurotoxicity: an overview. Clin Neuropharmacol 1997;20:283–99.
25. Mangano WE, Montine TJ, Hulette CM. Pathologic assessment of cerebellar atrophy following acute lithium intoxication. Clin Neuropathol 1997;16:30–3.
26. Meyer-Lindenberg A, Krausnick B. Tardive dyskinesia in a neuroleptic-naive patient with bipolar-I disorder: persistent exacerbation after lithium intoxication. Mov Disord 1997;12:1108–9.
27. Khan AU, Chang F-L, Howsepian A. Central pontine myelinolysis related to lithium toxicity. Gen Hosp Psychiatry 1997;19:150–2.
28. Higes-Pascual F, de Arriba de la Fuente G, de Pedro-Esteban F. Coreoatetosis, una manifestación infrecuente de intoxicación por litio. Rev Neurol 1998;26:841.
29. Gordon PH, Hirsch LJ, Balmaceda C. Transient aphasia associated with lithium intoxication. J Clin Psychopharmacol 1997;17:55–6.
30. Jiménez-Jiménez FJ, Garcia-Ruiz PJ, Molina JA. Drug-induced movement disorders. Drug Saf 1997;16:180–204.
31. Bschor T, Bauer M. Schilddrüsenfunktoin bei lithiumbehandlung. Nervenarzt 1998;69:189- 95.
32. Leutgeb U. Lithiumwirkungen auf die schilddrüse. Nervenheilkunde 1998;17:114–9.
33. Lazarus JH. Effect of lithium on the thyroid gland. In: Weetman AP, Grossman A, editors. Pharmacotherapeutics of the Thyroid Gland. Handb Exp Pharmacol 1997;128:207–23.
34. Loviselli A, Bocchetta A, Mossa P, Velluzzi F, Bernardi F, del Zompo M, Mariotti S. Value of thyroid echography in the long-term follow-up of lithium-treated patients. Neuropsychobiology 1997;36:37–41.
35. Shimizu M, Hirokawa M, Manabe T, Shimozuma K, Sonoo H, Harada T. Lithium associated autoimmune thyroiditis. J Clin Pathol 1997; 50:172–4.
36. Dickstein G, Shechner C, Adawi F, Kaplan J, Baron E, Ish-Shalom S. Lithium treatment in amiodarone-induced thyrotoxicosis. Am J Med 1997;102:454–8.
37. Haden ST, Stoll AL, McCormick S, Scott J, El-Hajj Fuleihan G. Alterations in parathyroid dynamics in lithium-treated subjects. J Clin Endocrinol Metab 1997;82:2844–8.
38. Laroche M, Lamboley V, Amigues J-M, Cantagrel A, Mazières B. Hyperparathyroidism during lithium therapy. Two new cases. Rev Rhum Engl Ed 1997;64:132–4.
39. de Celis G, Fiter M, Latorre X, Llebaria C. Oxyphilic parathyroid adenoma and lithium therapy. Lancet 1998;352:1070.
40. Wolf ME, Moffat M, Mosnaim J, Dempsey S. Lithium therapy, hypercalcemia, and hyperparathyroidism. Am J Ther 1997;4:323–5.
41. Tsai S-J, Chen Y-S. Lithium, hypercalcemia, and arrhythmia. J Clin Psychopharmacol 1998; 18:420–3.
42. Azam H, Newton RW, Morris AD, Thompson CJ. Hyperosmolar nonketotic coma precipitated by lithium-induced nephrogenic diabetes insipidus. Postgrad Med J 1998;74:39–41.
43. Zimmermann U, Rechlin T, Plaskacewicz GJ, Barocka A, Wildt L, Kaschka WP. Effect of naltrexone on weight gain and food craving induced by tricyclic antidepressants and lithium: an open study. Biol Psychiatry 1997;41:747–9.
44. Braden GL. Lithium-induced renal disease. In: Greenberg A, ed. Primer on Kidney Diseases. Academic Press: San Diego, CA, 1998:332–4.
45. Coskunol H, Vahip S, Dorhout-Mees E, BasCCi A, Bayindir O, Tuglular I. Renal side-effects of long-term lithium treatment. J Affect Disord 1997;43:5–10.
46. Chugh S, Yager H. End-stage renal disease after treatment with lithium. J Clin Psychopharmacol 1997;17:495–7.
47. Thompson CJ, France AJ, Baylis PH. Persistent nephrogenic diabetes insipidus following lithium therapy. Scott Med J 1997;42:16–17.
48. Meinardi JR, Donders SHJ. Nephrogenic diabetes insipidus in a lethargic lithium-treated patient. Neth J Med 1997;50:105–9.
49. Lam SS, Kjellstrand C. Emergency treatment of lithium-induced diabetes insipidus with nonsteroidal anti-inflammatory drugs. Renal Failure 1997;19:183–8.
50. Bosquet S, Descombes E, Gauthier T, Fellay G, Regamey C. Nephrotic syndrome during lithium therapy. Nephrol Dial Transplant 1997; 12:2728–31.
51. Gill DS, Chhetri M, Milne JR. Nephrotic syndrome associated with lithium therapy. Am J Psychiatry 1997;154:1318–19.
52. Mantelet S, Féline A. Effets cutanés du lithium: revue de la littérature à propos d'un cas. Ann Med Psychol 1997;155:664–8.
53. Herrero Ambrosio A, Ruano Encinar M, Hernández-Cano N, Gutiérrez Ramos R, Jiménez

Caballero E. Exacerbación de psoriasis por litio. Farm Hosp 1997;21:175–7.
54. Hanada K, Sawamura D, Sone K, Hashimoto I. Can lithium in spring water provoke psoriasis? Lancet 1997;350:1522.
55. Fearfield LA, Bunker CB. Pityriasis versicolor associated with oral lithium therapy. Clin Exp Dermatol 1997;22:57–9.
56. Marinella MA. Lithium therapy associated with hidradenitis suppurativa. Acta Dermatol Venereol 1997;77:483.
57. Langtry JAA, Rowland Payne CME, Staughton RCD, Stewart JCM Horrobin DF. Topical lithium succinate ointment (Efalith) in the treatment of AIDS-related seborrhoeic dermatitis. Clin Exp Dermatol 1997;22:216–19.
58. Lam RW, Allain S, Sullivan K, Beattie CW, Remick RA, Zis AP. Effects of chronic lithium treatment on retinal electrophysiologic function. Biol Psychiatry 1997;41:737–42.
59. Wirz-Justice A, Remé C, Prünte A, Heinen U, Graw P, Urner U. Lithium decreases retinal sensitivity, but this is not cumulative with years of treatment. Biol Psychiatry 1997;41:743–6.
60. Yonkers KA, Little BB, March D. Lithium during pregnancy. Drug effects and their therapeutic implications. CNS Drugs 1998;9:261–9.
61. Schou M. Treating recurrent affective disorders during and after pregnancy. What can be taken safely? Drug Saf 1998;18:143–52.
62. Llewellyn A, Stowe ZN, Strader JR. The use of lithium and management of women with bipolar disorder during pregnancy and lactation. J Clin Psychiatry 1998;59 Suppl 6:57–64.
63. Viguera A, Nonacs R, Cohen LS, Tondo L, Murray A, Baldessarini RJ. Risk of discontinuing lithium maintenance in pregnant vs. nonpregnant women with type I or II bipolar disorder. New Clinical Drug Evaluation Unit Program. Presented at the NCDEU 38th Annual Meeting, Boca Raton, FL, June 10–13, 1998, Poster No. 28.
64. Flaherty B, Krenzelok EP. Neonatal lithium toxicity as a result of maternal toxicity. Vet Hum Toxicol 1997;39:92–3.
65. Chisholm CA, Kuller JA. A guide to the safety of CNS-active agents during breastfeeding. Drug Saf 1997;17:127–42.
66. Spigset O, Hägg S. Excretion of psychotropic drugs into breast milk. Pharmacokinetic overview and therapeutic implications. CNS Drugs 1998; 9:111–34.
67. Chandragiri SS, Pasol E, Gallagher RM. Lithium, ACE inhibitors, NSAIDs, and verapamil. A possible fatal combination. Psychosomatics 1998;39:281–2.
68. Blanche P, Raynaud E, Kerob D, Galezowski N. Lithium intoxication in an elderly patient after combined treatment with losartan. Eur J Clin Pharmacol 1997;52:501.
69. Imbs J-L, Barthelmebs M, Danion J-M, Singer L. Mécanisme des interactions médicamenteuses avec l'élimination rénale du lithium. Bull Acad Natl Med 1997;181:685–97.
70. Sternbach H, State R. Antibiotics: neuropsychiatric effects and psychotropic interactions. Harv Rev Psychiatry 1997;5:214–26.
71. Miller SC. Doxycycline-induced lithium toxicity. J Clin Psychopharmacol 1997;17:54–5.
72. Bruun NE, Ibsen H, Skøtt P, Toftdahl D, Giese J, Holstein-Rathlou NH. Lithium clearance and renal tubular sodium handling during acute and long-term nifedipine treatment in essential hypertension. Clin Sci 1988;75:609–13.
73. Pinkofsky HB, Sabu R, Reeves RR. A nifedipine-induced inhibition of lithium clearance. Psychosomatics 1997;38:400–1.
74. Rost KL, Wierich W, Hadler D, Stark M, Müller-Oerlinghausen B, Herrmann WM. Idebenone does not significantly change the pharmacokinetics of amitriptyline, fluvoxamine, and lithium. NS Arch Pharmacol 1997;355:R120.
75. ZumBrunnen TL, Jann MW. Drug interactions with antipsychotic agents. Incidence and therapeutic implications. CNS Drugs 1998;9:381–401.
76. Gill M, Ghariani S, Piéret F, Delbecq J, Depré A, Saussu F, de Barsy T. Encéphalomyopathie aiguë et syndrome cérébelleux persistant après intoxication par sel de lithium et halopéridol. Rev Neurol 1997;153:268–70.
77. Edge SC, Markowitz JS, DeVane CL. Clozapine drug-drug interactions: a review of the literature. Hum Psychopharmacol 1997;12:5–20.
78. Kalali AH, Franklin D, Carreon D, Potkin SG. Adding seroquel to lithium does not increase extrapyramidal effects. Biol Psychiatry 1997; 41:95S.
79. Hughes BM, Small RE, Brink D, McKenzie ND. The effect of flurbiprofen on steady-state plasma lithium levels. Pharmacotherapy 1997; 17:113–20.
80. Cold JA, ZumBrunnen TL, Simpson A, Augustin BG, Awad E, Jann MW. Increased lithium serum and red blood cell concentrations during ketorolac coadministration. J Clin Psychopharmacol 1998;18:33–7.
81. Levin GM, Grum C, Eisele G. Effect of over-the-counter dosages of naproxen sodium and acetaminophen on plasma lithium concentrations in normal volunteers. J Clin Psychopharmacol 1998;18:237–40.
82. Sobanski T, Bagli M, Laux G, Rao ML. Serotonin syndrome after lithium add-on medication to paroxetine. Pharmacopsychiatry 1997;30:106–7.
83. Onen F Courpron PH. Le syndrome sérotoninergique: une iatropathogénie à connaître. Rev Geriatr 1997;22:213–4.
84. Mekler G, Woggon B. A case of serotonin syndrome caused by venlafaxine and lithium. Pharmacopsychiatry 1997;30:272–3.
85. Anonymous. Sumatriptan and serotonin syndrome. Psychiatry Drug Alerts 1998;12:19–20.
86. Baumann P, Nil R, Souche A, Montaldi S, Baettig D, Lambert S, Uehlinger C, Kasas A, Amey M, Jonzier-Perey M. A double-blind, placebo-controlled study of citalopram with and

without lithium in the treatment of therapy-resistant depressive patients: a clinical, pharmacokinetic, and pharmacogenetic investigation. J Clin Psychopharmacol 1996;16:307–14.
87. Scharman EJ. Methods used to decrease lithium absorption or enhance elimination. Clin Toxicol 1997;35:601–8.
88. Bosinski T, Bailie GR, Eisele G. Massive and extended rebound of serum lithium concentrations following hemodialysis in two chronic overdose cases. Am J Emerg Med 1998;16:98–100.
89. Fallgatter AJ, Strik WK. Reversible neuropsychiatrische nebenwirkungen von lithium bei normalen serumspiegeln. Eine fallbeschreibung. Nervenarzt 1997;68:586–90.
90. Lovell RW, Bunker WW. Lithium assay errors. Am J Psychiatry 1997;154:1477.
91. Sampson M, Ruddel M, Albright S, Elin RJ. Positive interference in lithium determinations from clot activator in collection container. Clin Chem 1997;43:675–9.

Eileen J. Wong, Jayendra K. Patel and Alan I. Green

4 Drugs of abuse

AMPHETAMINES

Methylenedioxymethamphetamine (MDMA)

MDMA (also referred to as Ecstasy, XTC, MDM, 'E', or Adam) is a popular drug of abuse world wide, often used during 'rave' parties with dancing, the adverse effects of which have been reviewed in previous years (SEDA-19, 24; SEDA-20, 19; SEDA-21, 22).

Psychiatric Neuropsychiatric complications have been reported (1[cr]).

A 17-year-old man, previously healthy. He took one tablet of MDMA and had an acute sense of impending doom, extreme discomfort in his lower back, and sympathomimetic symptoms (including tachycardia and pupillary dilatation). Two months later he sought medical help for incapacitating symptoms: trance-like states, memory lapses, and sporadic episodes of depersonalization. Other symptoms included depression, paranoia, derealization, deja vu, panic, and suicidal ideation. Occasionally, he had episodes of uncontrolled anger, sudden bursts of energy, and photophobia. He also had chronic headaches, blurred vision, and visceral sensations. A brain electrical activity mapping (BEAM) test showed abnormal electrical discharges arising from within the posterior temporal region, particularly during evoked potential analysis.

The authors suggested that MDMA may have affected the serotonergic system and also considered a possible diagnosis of *temporal lobe epilepsy* precipitated by MDMA.

Current drug users recruited from non-clinical settings in the UK have been interviewed to study the adverse psychological effects of MDMA, cocaine, and amphetamine (2[CR]). The 158 subjects were mostly white unemployed men and all had used one or more of these drugs in the previous month. Amphetamines were associated with the most adverse effects, and they were more severe than the effects of MDMA or cocaine. More than one-third of the amphetamine users described severe *sleep disturbances*, and 10–20% reported severe problems with *paranoia*, *depression*, *anxiety*, and *irritability*. Users of cocaine powder reported few adverse effects.

Endocrine, metabolic A case of profound acute *hypoglycemia* after MDMA abuse has been reported (3[cr]).

A 25-year-old woman took three tablets of MDMA, collapsed 4 h later, and had a generalized tonic–clonic seizure. She became agitated, tachycardic, and febrile (41.9°C), with a blood glucose of 7.2 mmol/l. Six hours after the initial presentation her blood glucose fell to 0.6 mmol/l and responded to 50% dextrose intravenously. She was subsequently treated for progressive coagulopathy and rhabdomyolysis.

Mineral and fluid balance Three new cases of *hyponatremia* after the use of MDMA have been reported.

A 20-year-old woman, who occasionally took MDMA, was found comatose and vomiting 2 days after taking MDMA while dancing vigorously (4[cr]). Her plasma sodium concentration was 119 mmol/l and she had a metabolic acidosis but normal renal function. Her presentation was consistent with the syndrome of inappropriate antidiuretic hormone secretion (SIADH). She responded well to treatment and within 48 h was able to communicate.

A 15-year-old healthy girl took MDMA at a dance, consumed large amounts of water (as recommended by the UK Health Education Authority to counteract the hyperthermic effects of MDMA), and 5 h later started to vomit; 5 h after that she became drowsy and confused, and had a respiratory arrest (5[cr]). She was intubated, but had bilateral papilledema and hypotension, a serum sodium concentration of 125 mmol/l, and cerebral edema on a CT scan. She died within 3 days.

The authors felt that the cause of death had been hypoxic encephalopathy secondary to respiratory arrest, which had itself resulted from acute water intoxication. They further sug-

Side Effects of Drugs, Annual 22
J.K. Aronson, ed.

gested that young people using MDMA should be told to drink moderate amounts of fluids and immediately to seek attention for non-resolving symptoms; this opinion was shared by others (6[r]).

A 24-year-old woman took MDMA and was admitted stuporose, with brief periods of agitation (7[cr]). She had SIADH, with a serum sodium concentration of 113 mmol/l. She rapidly improved with fluid restriction, regaining consciousness within 16 h.

The authors noted that this and other reported cases had involved premenopausal women and suggested that premenopausal women who abuse MDMA and drink excess water may be at particular risk of SIADH. Furthermore, arginine vasopressin may play an important role in the pathology. Rapid changes in osmolarity may underlie the significant morbidity and mortality associated with this condition.

Hematological Severe *aplastic anemia* with multiple complications after MDMA has been described (8[cr]).

A 19-year-old man presented with a 3-day history of rash, sore throat, hemoptysis, and vomiting after taking MDMA for the first time 2 weeks before. He had fever, widespread petechiae, and pustular tonsillitis. His leukocyte count was 1.0×10^9/l (no neutrophils) and his platelet count was 7×10^9/l. A bone marrow aspirate and biopsy showed an almost completely acellular marrow; a specimen assessed for progenitor content showed no evidence of hemopoietic activity. He eventually recovered after a peripheral blood progenitor cell transplant with rapid neutrophil engraftment.

Although it is difficult to know for sure whether MDMA caused aplastic anemia in this case, all other causes were ruled out. The authors suggested that the aplastic anemia could have been an idiosyncratic reaction to MDMA or possibly related to contaminants.

Liver Acute reversible *liver failure* has been attributed to MDMA (9[cr]).

An 18-year-old man who had been consuming MDMA one to two tablets/week for 8 months developed right upper abdominal pain, weight loss, vomiting, yellow discoloration of the skin, and abnormal liver function tests. The diagnosis was acute liver failure secondary to MDMA abuse, and 15 days later he developed hepatic encephalopathy and required liver transplantation. Later his own liver regenerated and the transplant atrophied and was removed because of an abscess.

Musculoskeletal Reports of *rhabdomyolysis* with raised creatine kinase activity after MDMA continue to appear (10[cr]).

A 33-year-old man developed generalized muscle aches and diarrhea 7 h after taking MDMA at a dance. His muscle pains worsened and his urine turned dark brown 3 days later. His creatine kinase activity peaked at 112 000 IU/l within 24 h and fell to near normal 30 days later.

A 25-year-old woman collapsed at a party after taking one MDMA tablet with alcohol. She had a generalized tonic–clonic seizure and became febrile, hypoglycemic, and unconscious. Her platelet count fell below 45×10^9/l without coagulopathy. Her creatine kinase activity peaked at 99 700 IU/l within 1 day and gradually returned to normal within 2 weeks.

In neither case was renal function impaired. The authors concluded that creatine kinase activity can remain high for much longer than has previously been recognized after the ingestion of MDMA. Furthermore, creatine kinase activity may not reliably predict the extent of muscle damage and the risk of acute renal failure.

However, others have used isoforms of creatine kinase as qualitative indicators of rhabdomyolysis (11[cr]).

A healthy 21-year-old man collapsed at a dance 5 h after taking alcohol, seven tablets of MDMA, and 2 g of amphetamine. He was unconscious and febrile (42°C) and was sweating profusely. He had muscle rigidity, dilated pupils, hypotension, tachycardia, and tachypnea. His creatine kinase activity was extremely high and he subsequently developed myoglobinuria, disseminated intravascular coagulation, and pulmonary edema. He recovered with aggressive medical treatment.

The peak creatine kinase activity of 122 341 U/l is the highest ever recorded value in a case of MDMA toxicity. The high activity of the MM_3 isoform relative to the ratio of MM_2 to MM_1 confirmed continuous progressive rhabdomyolysis. He also had a high activity of the MB isoform with a high ratio of MB_2 to MB_1, indicating myocardial injury.

Miscellaneous A 19-year-old white man had a history of *excessive thirst and tiredness* on the first 3 days of each week for a year (12[cr]). There was no underlying basis for these symptoms, except that he habitually used MDMA while attending weekend raves. The authors thought that these effects may have been due to changes in brain serotonin activity.

Overdosage A 31-year-old previously healthy man was found dead at home, and postmortem and toxicological analysis confirmed the presence of MDEA (3,4-MDMA); he may have taken up to six tablets (14[cR]).

Methamphetamine

Hematological *Methemoglobinemia* has been reported in a woman who took methamphetamine (13[cr]).

A 31-year-old woman became cyanotic a day after taking methamphetamine. She was alert and awake, but dyspneic, with pulse oximetry of 88% on room air. With a 100% oxygen non-rebreather mask, her readings continued to fall. Her methemoglobin concentration was 51% and her oxygen saturation 52%. She responded well to methylene blue.

The author postulated that an adulterant, benzocaine, cut into the methamphetamine, may have caused the methemoglobinemia.

COCAINE

Cardiovascular Cocaine use and *myocardial infarction* have been reviewed extensively before (SEDA-18, 36). Myocardial infarction can occur after illicit or therapeutic cocaine exposure. A new case with serial angiography has been reported (15[cr]).

A 29-year-old man, a non-smoker with no cardiac risk factors, underwent nasal septoplasty, with 12.5% cocaine hydrochloride for topical anesthesia, and 6 h later became sweaty and had chest pain radiating to the left arm and jaw. The electrocardiogram showed the changes of an acute inferior myocardial infarction. Coronary angiography showed that the posterior descending and posterolateral branches of the right coronary arteries were occluded; 3 months later they were patent.

Based on the findings of repeated angiography, the authors suggested that a mechanism such as thrombosis with or without vasospasm may underlie cocaine-related coronary occlusion.

Aortic dissection can occur after cocaine use (SEDA-18, 36; SEDA-19, 26; SEDA-21, 29). A case of a rare type of thoracic aortic dissection has been reported (16[cr]).

A 33-year-old man with no significant medical history complained of dull chest pain, shortness of breath, and blood-tinged sputum 3 days after an all-night crack binge. He had a new cardiac murmur, a harsh triphasic pericardial friction rub, and a blood pressure difference of 30 mmHg between the right and left arms. He had a Type A aortic dissection, with aortic insufficiency and a pericardial effusion. He underwent surgery with interposition grafting of the proximal aorta and resuspension of the aortic valve and made a full recovery.

The authors discussed how cocaine can contribute to conditions that cause shearing in the thoracic aorta. With raised arterial blood pressure and increased afterload secondary to peripheral vasoconstriction, stress in the wall of the aorta can undergo a steep rise, predisposing to dissection.

Peripheral vascular occlusive disease associated with cocaine has been reported for the first time (17[cr]).

A 37-year-old man developed severe pain and numbness of his feet after using cocaine. His distal legs and feet were cool, with reduced sensation and peripheral pulses. Arteriography showed bilateral occlusions of the superficial femoral, popliteal, and trifurcation arteries.

A 22-year-old woman had burning pain and numbness in both feet within an hour of smoking crack cocaine. Her feet were cold with reduced peripheral pulses. Arteriography showed diffuse vasospasm extending from the iliac arteries distally in both lower extremities; it responded to an infusion of glyceryl trinitrate.

The authors suggested that cocaine may have caused peripheral vascular occlusion through vasoconstriction, increased platelet aggregation, and possibly atherogenesis.

Respiratory Cocaine can cause lung damage, including edema, hemorrhage, alveolar damage, interstitial inflammation, and fibrosis. To investigate the possibility that cocaine-induced immunological effects might contribute to acute lung injury, 24 crack users received cocaine (i.v. or by inhalation) or placebo after abstaining for at least 8 h (18[CR]). Cocaine caused activation of circulating neutrophil-mediated antibacterial and antitumor activity. The production of interleukin 8, a potent neutrophil mediator in acute and chronic lung injury, was also increased. Based on these findings, the authors concluded that bursts of anti-inflammatory activity from repeated short-term use of crack may contribute to chronic lung injury.

Crack cocaine can be smoked as particles rolled into a cigarette or as crystals in a pipe. In a novel technique, shotgunning, a second person forcibly blows the crack vapors through a special pipe into the smoker's mouth. This method delivers a greater amount of drug more rapidly than inhalation alone. *Retropharyngeal emphysema* after shotgunning has been reported (19[cr]).

A 47-year-old woman, a daily crack smoker who also engaged in shotgunning on a weekly basis, developed a sore throat, progressive neck swelling, and an inability to swallow. She had a bulging posterior pharyngeal wall with reddened mucosa and there was air in the retropharyngeal space. She later developed an abscess.

The authors suggested that shotgunning crack may have traumatically introduced air into the retropharyngeal space. Microperforation of the pharyngeal mucosa may have allowed the entry of air and bacteria.

Pneumothorax, *pneumomediastinum*, and *pneumoperitoneum* are rare consequences of cocaine use (20[Cr]).

A 17-year-old girl attempted suicide by smoking crack cocaine. She developed midsternal chest pain, shortness of breath, a sore throat, and pressure in the neck. She was tachycardic, tachypneic and wheezy. There was subcutaneous emphysema in her face, neck, and anterior chest. Chest and abdominal X-rays showed small bilateral pneumothoraces, pneumomediastinum, and pneumoperitoneum. She responded to oxygen.

Nervous system Long-term neuroleptic drug treatment causes dopamine receptor blockade, resulting in functional dopamine deficiency. Chronic abuse of cocaine also leads to central dopamine deficiency. This raises the question of whether chronic cocaine use is a risk factor for *parkinsonism* in subjects taking long-term neuroleptic drugs. Male chronic schizophrenics, including 19 cocaine users on long-term depot neuroleptic drugs and 24 non-cocaine users on long-term depot neuroleptic drugs as controls were examined using the United Parkinson's Disease Scale (21[CR]). There were no significant differences, suggesting that chronic cocaine use does not aggravate or increase the signs of parkinsonism in patients taking long-term neuroleptic drugs.

Acute dystonic reactions after crack cocaine use have been described (SEDA-18, 36) and a new case report has appeared (22[cR]).

A 34-year-old woman presented with acute facial dystonia, with jaw tightness and left-sided facial droop, after a crack binge the previous night. She had four further episodes of dystonia, each lasting 10–40 min, during the next 12 h.

The authors also reviewed three published cases. In all cases the dystonic reactions had involved the muscles of the head and neck and had occurred 12–18 h after crack exposure.

Stroke in young adult cocaine users has been documented (SEDA-20, 26; SEDA-20, 21). The medical records of patients aged 20–39 years admitted to an inner city hospital during 1990–4 have been reviewed and 66 of 144 young crack users admitted with stroke were compared with 99 of 147 young crack users admitted with other diagnoses (23[CR]). There was no association between stroke or cerebral infarction and either acute crack use (within 48 h of admission) or crack use at any time. It was commented that the use of a different control group (i.e. age-matched cocaine users in the general population) might have led to a different conclusion (24[r]), but the original authors disputed this point (24[r]).

The first case of pupillary-sparing *third cranial nerve palsy* after the use of crack cocaine has been reported (25[cr]).

A 29-year-old man with no significant medical history, except intermittent cocaine use, developed drooping of the right eyelid, double vision, and headache. He had motor impairment of the third cranial nerve with normal vision and pupillary function. A cerebral arteriogram and MRI scan were normal. His symptoms resolved gradually.

Neuropsychological development Several new studies of second-generation neurodevelopmental effects associated with in utero cocaine exposure have been published. In one longitudinal study, *early language development* was investigated in children of low socioeconomic status (26[cr]). Children with prenatal cocaine exposure ($n = 76$) and children with no exposure ($n = 81$) were assessed using the Preschool Language Scale. Performance scores in areas of expressive, receptive, or total language were similar at age 2.5 years in both groups.

The possible effect of prenatal cocaine exposure on the development of *visual attention abilities* has been investigated in 31 children aged 8–40 months, 14 who had been exposed and 17 who had not (27[CR]). Cocaine-exposed children were consistently slower to orient to targets in the right visual field than controls. They were also more likely to orient to the left when given the choice to look to the left or right. The authors discussed how the visual attention system, mediated by dopaminergic pathways, when disrupted by prenatal cocaine exposure, could impair visual attention. Dopamine is distributed asymmetrically, and cocaine exposure might cause lateralized deficits.

Psychiatric Residual behavioral changes associated with repeated cocaine smoking have been studied in nine crack cocaine users, who were allowed to self-administer up to six doses of crack cocaine 25 mg during 2 or 3 days (28[CR]). They reported greater cocaine craving and subtle mood changes (*anxiety*, *confusion*, *feeling high*, *less friendly*) on the day after three binges than on the day after two binges. The reported behavioral changes were related to the amount of drug they took and inversely related to the time since the last exposure.

Impairment of concentration, *memory*, *problem solving*, and *abstraction* have been described in 36 active and abstinent cocaine abusers (SEDA-17, 37). In a recent study, neuropsychological functioning during the 48 h after cocaine withdrawal has been assessed (29[CR]). The latency of the P300 cognitive event-related potential, a measure of rate of information processing, was more reduced among intravenous users than smokers and was not affected in nasal users. The authors suggested that the pattern of cocaine use may in part determine the risks of its cognitive effects.

Gastrointestinal Gastric perforation after cocaine use has previously been reported (SEDA-17, 37; SEDA-20, 23; SEDA-21, 29). In a 6-year retrospective study of 78 surgical cases of peptic ulcer disease (24 confirmed crack cocaine users and 54 non-users), the patients who had used crack were younger and had perforations primarily in the duodenum (30[CR]).

Ischemia in the small bowel and colon is a rare complication of cocaine use. A new case of *ischemic colitis* has been reported (31[cR]).

A 36-year-old woman complained of 2 days of vomiting, abdominal pain, and no bowel movements or flatus, followed by two episodes of coffee-ground vomiting after a 2-day crack binge. At surgery an infarcted transverse colon and an inflamed gall-bladder were removed. Microscopic examination showed multiple small-vessel thrombi.

Urinary system Pathological investigation of cocaine-induced renal damage is a new area of inquiry. In one study, renal vascular alterations in 40 autopsy specimens from individuals who had cocaine-related deaths were compared with 40 kidney specimens from road accident victims (32[CR]). In the cocaine-exposed specimens there was a greater degree of *hyalinosis of the glomeruli*, *interstitial cellular infiltration*, and *glomerulosclerosis*. The authors commented that there was advanced hyperplastic damage in a surprisingly high percentage (75%) of cocaine cases.

Skin and appendages Rapid *gingival recession with dental erosion*, diagnosed and treated as necrotizing ulcerative periodontitis, was in fact secondary to contact with cocaine (33[cr]). After several years of treatment, the patient divulged that she had regularly applied cocaine to the affected gums.

Special senses The rewards and reinforcing effects of cocaine abuse involve the brain's dopaminergic system. Dopamine, which is present in high concentrations in the retina, also has an important role in color vision. The possible adverse effects of cocaine use on the visual system have been investigated.

In one study, 31 former cocaine users who had recently stopped using the drug were compared with matched controls; the cocaine users showed some *blue-yellow color vision loss* (34[CR]). In a second study, the effect of cocaine on blue cone retinal function was examined (35[Cr]). Eight cocaine users in withdrawal abstinence (range 3–62 days) had significantly reduced blue cone b-wave amplitudes (i.e. a reduced retinal response to flashes of blue light) on electroretinogram. In the same patients repeat electroretinography showed no significant changes over the course of 8 weeks, and the authors concluded that the dysregulation of blue cone functioning found in the initial phase of cocaine withdrawal remained stable over this period (36[CR]).

The neurophysiological sequelae associated with cocaine use are under investigation. Two previous studies of smooth pursuit eye movement (SPEM) functioning among cocaine users in early abstinence produced contrary results (SEDA-18, 38). Now a new study of 35 recently abstinent cocaine users has reproduced the earlier findings of *enhanced SPEM tracking* (37[CR]). SPEM tracking was more accurate in patients without a paternal history of alcoholism, while those with a paternal history of alcoholism had subnormal performance. The authors suggest that SPEM functioning in recently abstinent cocaine users may be influenced by this familial factor as well as by cocaine.

Immunological and hypersensitivity reactions A case of *Goodpasture's syndrome* after crack cocaine has been reported (38[cR]).

A 32-year-old man who smoked two packets of cigarettes a day and who smoked crack over 3 weeks, developed acute respiratory distress, diffuse pulmonary hemorrhage, and progressive renal failure. Goodpasture's syndrome without linear IgG deposits was confirmed by renal biopsy and antibody titers. Plasmapheresis and immunosuppressive therapy led to prompt recovery of respiratory status but not renal function.

The authors thought that a causative role of cocaine in this case was unclear.

Use in pregnancy Cocaine use during pregnancy is associated with an *increased risk of sexually transmitted diseases*, and the possibility that cocaine alters immunological functioning during pregnancy is being studied. The effect of cocaine on induced lymphocyte proliferation has been investigated in peripheral blood mononuclear cells obtained from 39 pregnant women and non-pregnant controls (39[CR]). Cocaine added to cell cultures stimulated with the mitogen concanavalin A did not suppress lymphocyte proliferation in either group. The authors proposed that other factors associated with cocaine use, such as poor nutrition, poor medical and prenatal care, and multiple partners, may contribute to altered immune function during pregnancy.

Obstetric complications are associated with cocaine use (SEDA-19, 29). In one case-control analysis of 40 cases of confirmed *placenta previa* at delivery, cocaine use increased the risk of placenta previa more than 4-fold (40[CR]). Cocaine users were more likely to have had a cesarean section, a risk factor for placenta previa.

Autopsy in an infant who died at 3 months showed *congenital heart disease* and slight *pericardial petechiae* (41[cr]). Although there was no evidence of abuse, nail clippings tested positive for cocaine, indicating prenatal drug exposure, particularly during early gestation. The death of this infant was not thought to be connected to prenatal cocaine exposure. However, the authors suggested that nail clippings can provide vital clues to drug exposure during the prenatal period.

Tumor-inducing effects The use of tobacco, alcohol, and 10 specific recreational drugs as possible risk factors for the development of *non-Hodgkin's lymphoma* has been investigated in a case–control study (42[Cr]). In 378 HIV-negative participants, previous use of cocaine, amphetamines, Quaalude, and lysergic acid diethylamide were each associated with an increased risk of non-Hodgkin's lymphoma in men. More frequent substance use was correlated with a higher risk, as was multiple drug use. Cocaine use had the greatest effect.

Interactions The combined use of cocaine with *alcohol* increases plasma concentrations of cocaine and norcocaine, reduces plasma benzoylecgonine concentrations, and induces cocaethylene conversion. Adverse outcomes associated with the combination of cocaine with alcohol have been described previously (SEDA-19, 65). Eight healthy participants who engaged in recreational cocaine and alcohol use were given intranasal cocaine 100 mg and alcohol (vodka) 0.8 g/kg in a double-blind, double-dummy, controlled study (43[CR]). The combination produced greater increases in heart rate, rate-pressure product (systolic blood pressure times heart rate), and pleasurable feelings. Plasma cortisol concentrations rose more with the combination than with cocaine alone.

Overdosage Body stuffers swallow the evidence to avoid arrest or prosecution while in possession of drugs. However, packets are typically not prepared for ingestion and are often not suitably wrapped. Cocaine is the drug most commonly involved. A retrospective case series study of emergency room visits to a California county hospital identified 98 body stuffers during 28 months (44[Cr]). Symptoms of mild cocaine intoxication, such as *tachycardia*, *hypertension*, and *agitation* were common. All cases of *seizure* (4%) occurred within 4 h of ingestion. However, the study was limited by the fact that self-reporting was used in lieu of toxicological screening to confirm drug exposure (45[r]).

OPIATES

Nervous system *Progressive spongiform leukoencephalopathy* can occur secondary to a practice known as 'chasing the dragon', wherein the user inhales heated heroin vapor (46[c]).

A 21-year-old woman with a 6-month history of inhaling heroin vapor, developed progressive bradykinesia, ataxia, and slurred speech over 2 weeks. She had abulia and a decorticate posture, with normal reflexes. Over the next 2 weeks she became mute, spastic, and nearly quadriplegic. Heroin, cocaine, and methadone were found in her blood. An MRI scan showed diffuse symmetrical areas of hyperintensity in white matter of the cerebellum, posterior cerebrum, corticospinal tracts, and lemniscal pathways. A brain biopsy showed spongiform degeneration of white matter with relative sparing of subcortical fibers.

Her friend, a 40-year-old man with a 6-month history of intranasal use of cocaine and heroin, had inhaled heroin vapor with her daily for 2 weeks. He developed dysarthria, scanning speech, and saccadic eye movements with ocular dysmetria. His arm movements were ataxic with dysdiadochokinesis and rebound. An MRI scan showed diffuse symmetrical areas of white matter hyperintensity, most prominently in the cerebellum, but also involving the posterior cerebrum, the splenium of the corpus callosum, and the posterior limbs of the internal capsule. He improved after treatment with ubiquinone.

Two cases of *ballistic movements* due to ischemic infarcts after intravenous heroin abuse have been reported (47[cr]).

A 34-year-old man became semi-comatose after injecting heroin intravenously. He responded to naloxone, but later developed continuous ballistic movements of all four limbs. An MRI scan showed bilateral ischemic lesions of the globus pallidus, suggesting generalized cerebral hypoxia during coma.

A 19-year-old man, who had been an intravenous heroin addict for a year, was found unconscious 12 h after using heroin. He recovered promptly with naloxone but developed ballistic limb movements with moderate distal weakness of the left limbs. An MRI scan showed ischemic infarcts in the territories of the right lenticulostriate vessels and the inferior branch of the right middle cerebral artery, suggesting recent embolism.

Overdosage This year several reports have focused on severe morbidity and mortality from heroin use. A survey of heroin users in the UK showed that over half had had accidental overdoses. It has been recommended that to prevent heroin-related deaths, emergency resuscitation kits be given to addicts and their contacts (48[r]). It was also proposed that naloxone, an opioid receptor antagonist, should be available in a nasal spray as a preventive measure.

Accidental overdosage is the largest contributor to the excess mortality associated with the use of heroin. There were 44 heroin-related deaths in south-western Sydney in Australia in 1995, an increase of 120% compared with 1992 (49[Cr]). Those who died were significantly older and were more likely to be men. Multiple drug use was very frequent.

The contribution of methadone and heroin overdosage to deaths due to accidental and intentional self-poisoning has been investigated (50[CR]). In England and Wales there were 43 231 self-poisoning deaths between 1974 and 1992. The number fell by 32% from 8958 (in 1974–7) to 6125 (in 1990–2). In contrast, lethal self-poisonings involving heroin alone and methadone with or without heroin, rose from seven to 90 and from 26 to 240, respectively. The proportion of poisoning deaths involving methadone alone or in combination with heroin rose by 80% per 3-year period. The authors concluded that the impact of opiate addiction on rates of death by poisoning is rising rapidly. Poisoning deaths due to methadone had risen faster than those due to heroin in this period.

A death from oral overdosage of heroin has been reported (51[cr]).

A 40-year-old man with a long history of heroin abuse in a detention center for drug trafficking submitted to daily body searches for drugs. One evening, he hid a sachet of heroin by swallowing it. He was found dead the next day. Heroin and its metabolites were found in high concentrations.

Body packers or smugglers who swallow packets of illicit drugs or insert them into body cavities for transport occasionally die due to absorption of the contents. Nine fatal cases in the southern US have been described (52[CR]). The prodromal symptoms were those of intoxication with a depressant drug. The authors pointed out that pulmonary edema is often prominent in heroin cases, and may help differentiate heroin- from cocaine-related deaths in body packers.

Interactions In another study, blood toxicology results from 39 heroin overdose fatalities were compared with those of 100 active heroin users who had injected within the preceding 24 h (53[CR]). Heroin-related deaths had a higher median concentration of morphine than active heroin users (0.35 vs 0.09 mg/l). However, the blood morphine concentrations in the two groups had substantial overlap in the range 0.08–1.45 mg/l. One-third of current users had morphine concentrations more than twice the designated toxic concentrations. Alcohol was detected in 51% of fatal cases but in only 1% of current users. The authors questioned the roles of heroin and alcohol separately and in combination in contributing to the outcomes. Specifically, they suggested that in the presence of alcohol, tolerance to heroin is lower and that death occurs with smaller amounts.

REFERENCES

1. Cohen RS, Cocores J. Neuropsychiatric manifestations following the use of 3,4-methylenedioxymethamphetamine (MDMA; 'Ecstasy'). Prog Neuro-Psychopharmacol Biol Psychiatry 1997;21:727–34.
2. Williamson S, Gossop M, Powis B, Griffiths P, Fountain J, Strang J. Adverse effects of stimulant drugs in a community sample of drug users. Drug Alcohol Depend 1997;44:87–94.
3. Montgomery H, Myerson S. 3,4-Methylenedioxymethamphetamine (MDMA or 'Ecstasy') and associated hypoglycemia. Am J Emerg Med 1997;15:218.
4. Nuvials X, Masclans JR, Peracaula R, De Latorre FJ. Hyponatraemic coma after ecstasy ingestion. Intensive Care Med 1997;23:480.
5. Parr MJA, Low HM, Botterill P. Hyponatraemia and death after 'Ecstasy' ingestion. Med J Aust 1997;166:136–7.
6. Hall AP. Hyponatraemia, water intoxication and 'Ecstasy'. Intensive Care Med 1997;23:1289.
7. Watson ID, Serlin M, Moncur P, Tames F. Acute hyponatraemia. Postgrad Med J 1997; 73:443–4.
8. Clark AD, Butt N. Ecstasy-induced very severe aplastic anaemia complicated by invasive mucormycosis treated with allogenic peripheral blood progenitor cell. Clin Lab Haematol 1997;19:279–81.
9. Hellinger A, Rauen U, De Groot H, Erhard J. Auxiliare Lebertransplantation bei akutem Leberversagen nach Einnahme von 3,4-Methoxylendioxymethamphetamin ('Ecstasy'). Dtsch Med Wochenschr 1997;122:716–20.
10. Williams A, Unwin R. Prolonged elevation of serum creatine kinase (CK) without renal failure after ingestion of ecstasy. Nephrol Dial Transplant 1997;12:361–2.
11. Murthy BV, Wilkes RG, Roberts NB. Creatine kinase isoform changes following Ecstasy overdose. Anaesth Intensive Care 1997;25:156–9.
12. Sturrock NDC, Morris R. Monday to Wednesday tiredness and thirst. Br J Hosp Med 1997;58:454.
13. Verzosa JD. Methemoglobinemia: cyanosis and street methamphetamine. J Am Board Fam Pract 1997;10:137–40.
14. Tsatsakis AM, Michalodimitrakis MN, Patsalis AN. MDEA related death in Crete: a case report and literature review. Vet Hum Toxicol 1997;39:241–4.
15. Williams JA, Stewart RA. Serial angiography in cocaine-induced myocardial infarction. Chest 1997;111:822–4.
16. Perron AD, Gibbs M. Thoracic aortic dissection to crack cocaine ingestion. Am J Emerg Med 1997;15:507–9.
17. Gutierrez A, England JD, Krupski WC. Co-

caine-induced peripheral vascular occlusive disease. Angiology 1998;49:221–4.
18. Baldwin GC, Buckley DM, Roth MD, Kleerup EC, Tashkin DP. Acute activation of circulating polymorphonuclear neutrophils following in vivo administration of cocaine. A potential etiology for pulmonary injury. Chest 1997;111:698–705.
19. Nadel DM, Lyons KM. 'Shotgunning' crack cocaine as a potential cause of retropharyngeal abscess. Ear Nose Throat J 1997;77:47–50.
20. Uva JL. Spontaneous pneumothoraces, pneumomediastinum, and pneumoperitoneum: consequences of smoking crack cocaine. Pediatr Emerg Care 1997;13:24–6.
21. Dhopesh V, Macfadden A, Maany I, Gamble G. Absence of parkinsonism among patients in long-term neuroleptic therapy who abuse cocaine. Psychiatr Serv 1997;48:95–7.
22. Catalano G, Catalano M, Rodriguez R. Dystonia associated with crack cocaine use. South Med J 1997;90:1050–2.
23. Qureshi AI, Akbar MS, Czander E, Safdar K, Janssen RS, Frankel MR. Crack cocaine use and stroke in young patients. Neurology 1997;48:341–5.
24. Riggs JE, Gutmann L. Crack cocaine use and stroke in young patients. Neurology 1997; 49:1473–4.
25. Migita DS, Devereaux MW, Tomsak RL. Cocaine and pupillary-sparing oculomotor nerve paresis. Neurology 1997;49:1466–7.
26. Hurt H, Malmud E, Betancourt L, Brodsky NL, Giannetta J. A prospective evaluation of early language development in children with in utero cocaine exposure and in control subjects. J Pediatr 1997;130:310–12.
27. Heffelfinger A, Craft S, Shyken J. Visual attention in children with prenatal cocaine exposure. J Int Neuropsychol Soc 1997;3:237–45.
28. Foltin RW, Fischman MW. Residual effects of repeated cocaine smoking in humans. Drug Alcohol Depend 1997;47:117–24.
29. Noldy NE, Carlen PL. Event-related potential changes in cocaine withdrawal: evidence for long-term cognitive effects. Neuropsychobiology 1997;36:53–6.
30. Sharma R, Organ CH, Hirvela ER, Henderson VJ. Clinical observation of the temporal association between crack cocaine and duodenal ulcer perforation. Am J Surg 1997;174:629–33.
31. Boutros HH, Pautler S, Chakrabarti S. Cocaine-induced ischemic colitis with small-vessel thrombosis of colon and gallbladder. J Clin Gastroenterol 1997;24:49–53.
32. DiPaolo N, Fineschi V, Di Paolo M, Wetly CV, Garosi G, Del Vecchio MT, Bianciardi G. Kidney vascular damage and cocaine. Clin Nephrol 1997;47:298–303.
33. Kapila YL, Kashani H. Cocaine-associated rapid gingival recession and dental erosion. A case report. J Periodontol 1997;68:485–8.
34. Desai P, Roy M, Roy A, Brown S, Smelson D. Impaired color vision in cocaine-withdrawn patients. Arch Gen Psychiatry 1997;54:696–9.
35. Roy M, Smelson D, Roy A. Longitudinal study of blue cone retinal function in cocaine-withdrawn patients. Soc Biol Psychiatry 1997;41:252–3.
36. Roy M, Roy A, Williams J, Weinberger L, Smelson D. Reduced blue cone electroretinogram in cocaine-withdrawn patients. Arch Gen Psychiatry 1997;54:153–6.
37. Bauer L. Smooth pursuit eye movement dysfunction in abstinent cocaine abusers: effects of a paternal history of alcoholism. Alcohol Clin Exp Res 1997;21:910–15.
38. Garcia-Rostan y Perez GM, Bragado FG, Puras Gil AM. Pulmonary hemorrhage and antiglomerular basement membrane antibody-mediated glomerulonephritis after exposure to smoked cocaine (crack): a case report and review of the literature. Pathol Int 1997;47:692–7.
39. Hedstrom SA, Monga M, Bishop K, Blanco JD. The effect of cocaine on mitogen-induced lymphocyte proliferation in pregnant women. Am J Perinatol 1997;14:583–6.
40. Macones GA, Sehdev HM, Parry S, Morgan MA, Berlin JA. The association between maternal cocaine use and placenta previa. Am J Obstet Gynecol 1997;177:1097–100.
41. Skopp G. Potsch L. A case report on drug screening of nail clippings to detect prenatal drug exposure. Ther Drug Monit 1997;19:386–9.
42. Nelson RA, Levine AM, Marks G, Bernstein L. Alcohol, tobacco and recreational drug use and the risk of non-Hodgkin's lymphoma. Br J Cancer 1997;76:1532–7.
43. Farre M, De La Toffe R, Gonzalez ML, Teran M, Roset PN, Menoyo E, Cami J. Cocaine and alcohol interactions in humans: neuroendocrine effects and cocaethylene metabolism. J Pharmacol Exp Ther 1997;283:164–76.
44. Sporer KA, Firestone J. Clinical course of crack cocaine body stuffers. Ann Emerg Med 1997;29:596–601.
45. Nordt SP, Fuchs MA. Clinical course of crack cocaine body stuffers. Ann Emerg Med 1997;30:714.
46. Kriegstein AR, Armitage BA, Kim PY. Heroin inhalation and progressive spongiform leukoencephalopathy. New Engl J Med. 1997;336:589–90.
47. Vila N, Chamorro A. Ballistic movements due to ischemic infarcts after iv heroin overdose: report of two cases. Clin Neurol Neruosurg 1997;99:259–62.
48. Abbasi K. Deaths from overdose are preventable. Br Med J 1997;316:331.
49. Darke SG, Zador DA, Sunjic SD. Heroin-related deaths in South-western Sydney. Med J Aust 1997;167:107.
50. Neeleman J, Farrell M. Fatal methadone and heroin overdoses: time trends in England and Wales. J Epidemiol Community Health 1997;51:435–7.

51. Rop PP, Fornaris M, Salmon T, Burle J, Bresson M. Concentrations of heroin, 06-monoacetylmorphine, and morphine in a lethal case following an oral heroin overdose. J Anal Toxicol 1997;21:232–5.
52. Wetli CV, Rao A, Rao VJ. Fatal heroin body packing. Am J Forensic Med Pathol 1997;18:312–18.
53. Darke SG, Sunjic SD, Zador DA, Prolov T. A comparison of blood toxicology of heroin-related deaths and current heroin users in Sydney, Australia. Drug Alcohol Depend 1997;47:45–53.

Stephen Curran and Sukhjeet Lally

5 Hypnotics and sedatives

GENERAL

Insomnia can be defined as nocturnal disturbance of the normal sleep cycle. When this occurs there will be adverse daytime consequences, such as fatigue, irritability, and reduced performance. The causes of insomnia are complex; they include: (1) physiological (e.g. jet lag); (2) physical (e.g. various types of physical illness); (3) psychological (e.g. examination stress); (4) psychiatric (e.g. depression).

Insomnia due to these factors should generally not be treated with hypnotic drugs. The underlying difficulty needs to be identified and managed, and this requires a fairly detailed assessment of the patient. In addition, non-pharmacological approaches should also be tried (so-called sleep hygiene). Hypnotics are not usually indicated for insomnia that is transient (lasting 1 or 2 days) or chronic (lasting more than a month). When they are used, they should be reserved for short-term insomnia (usually up to 1 month) that has no underlying cause and that has failed to respond to non-pharmacological approaches. In addition, hypnotics should not be used on a continuous basis for more than about 1 month. If they need to be given for longer, treatment should be intermittent (e.g. on 1 or 2 days a week).

AZASPIRONES *(SED-13, 112; SEDA-19, 36; SEDA-21, 39)*

Buspirone

Nervous system In a placebo-controlled trial of buspirone 30 mg/day for 9 weeks in social phobia adverse effects included *nausea*, *abdominal distress*, *restlessness*, *insomnia*, *vivid dreams*, *depression*, and *sexual disturbances* (1^C).

In a randomized, double-blind, placebo-controlled trial of buspirone 20–60 mg/day for 4 months in 10 patients with cerebellar cortical atrophy, adverse effects included *headache*, *dizziness*, *hypersomnia*, *insomnia*, *diarrhea*, and '*mental discomfort*' (2^C). Two patients were unable to tolerate doses greater than 20 mg/day.

Interactions Studies in rats have suggested that buspirone increases *fluoxetine* concentrations, and the authors speculated that buspirone may enhance antidepressant activity by this mechanism (3).

The effects of *erythromycin* 1.5 g/day, *itraconazole* 200 mg/day, or placebo on a single 10 mg dose of buspirone after 4 days of treatment have been studied (4^c). Erythromycin and itraconazole, respectively, increased the AUC of buspirone 6- and 19-fold and the peak concentration 5- and 13-fold. The mechanism was inhibition of the first-pass metabolism of buspirone via CYP3A4.

An interaction of buspirone with *clozapine* has been described (5^c).

A 33-year-old schizophrenic man, who had been previously medically well and had been taking clozapine 600 mg/day for over 1 year, took buspirone 15 mg/day for 4 weeks, and then increased the dosage to 20 mg/day. At various times before he had temporarily taken lorazepam, clonazepam, and β-blockers without ill effects. He had a major hematemesis and severe diabetic ketoacidosis, requiring temporary treatment with insulin. Both drugs were withdrawn and he was re-started on clozapine without ill effect.

These adverse effects are known with clozapine and it may be that clozapine concentrations are increased by the addition of buspirone, although there is no evidence for this.

Side Effects of Drugs, Annual 22
J.K. Aronson, ed.

BARBITURATES

Nervous system High rates of *agitation* and *respiratory depression* have been reported with pentobarbital in sedation during emergency pediatric radiology (6[R]).

Of 11 epileptic children aged 7–14 years, both on and off medication with phenobarbital and mephobarbital, six were *irritable* and *overactive* whilst on medication (7[C]). However, there were no effects on the EEG and little effect on a battery of neuropsychological tests.

BENZODIAZEPINES *(SED-13, 104; SEDA-19, 33; SEDA-20, 31; SEDA-21, 37)*

Abecarnil

In a comparison of the effects of single doses of abecarnil (2.5 and 5 mg) with lorazepam 2 mg and placebo, the 5-mg dose produced the same adverse effects as lorazepam on the Digit Symbol Substitution memory test, keypad reaction time, a tracking test, a test for ataxia, and a test of peripheral vision (8[C]). The effects were significant with the 2.5-mg dose. Adverse effects were significantly worse than with placebo and included *drowsiness*, *poor concentration*, *visual disturbance*, *fatigue*, *dizziness*, *loss of equilibrium*, and *euphoria*.

A multicenter, randomized, double-blind, placebo-controlled study of abecarnil (3–9 mg/day) and alprazolam (1.5–4.5 mg/day) has been conducted in 180 out-patients with generalized anxiety disorder, with flexible dosing for 4 weeks followed by up to a 2-week tapering off period (9[C]). There were no significant differences in drop-out rates (70–80% completion) or in adverse effects. Adverse effects in the 67 patients treated with abecarnil included *back pain* (three), *headache* (four), and *depression* (three). During withdrawal, significantly more suffered *nausea*, *dysphoric mood*, and *anxiety* compared with placebo. There were also strong trends for *appetite loss* and *poor coordination*.

In a trial of similar design and patients a high-dosage group took 7.5–22.5 mg/day of abecarnil and a low-dosage group took 3–9 mg/day for 6–24 weeks (10[C]). In the high-dosage group there was a significantly greater attrition rate because of adverse events, including *drowsiness*, *lack of concentration* (both also significant with the low dosage), *dizziness*, *fatigue*, *confusion*, *difficulty in coordination*, and *ataxia*. Patients treated for more than 12 weeks had significantly more *withdrawal symptoms* after abrupt withdrawal. However, these effects were not replicated in a separate placebo-controlled study in patients with anxiety, aged 68 years, who took abecarnil 7.5–17.5 mg/day or 3–7 mg/day or for 6 weeks (11[C]). After abrupt withdrawal the patients were followed for a further 2 weeks. Discontinuation owing to adverse events was much more frequent in the high-dosage group (44%) compared with placebo (12%). The adverse effects that were especially more common than with placebo were *drowsiness*, *insomnia*, and *nausea*. After withdrawal the symptoms were significantly worse in the high-dosage group and included *insomnia*, *difficulty in concentrating*, *tremor*, *headache*, *agitation*, *anxiety*, *loss of appetite*, *flu-like symptoms*, *poor coordination*, *confusion*, and *depersonalisation*. *Insomnia*, *difficulty in concentrating*, and *tremor* were also significantly more common in the low-dosage group compared with placebo.

Alprazolam

In a placebo-controlled study of alprazolam in panic disorder, alprazolam produced significantly greater *sedation*, *ataxia*, *slurred speech*, *fatigue*, *constipation*, *amnesia*, and *reduction in libido* (12[C]). Other adverse effects that led to withdrawal of treatment were *mania*, *depression*, and *hepatitis*.

Nervous system In a double-blind placebo-controlled trial of alprazolam 0.5–4 mg/day in patients with anxiety disorder, patients taking alprazolam had significantly greater *sedation* and *drowsiness* (13[C]). There were also trends for *increased forgetfulness* and *impairment of cognitive function*.

Gastrointestinal A 7% incidence of *gastric*

irritation and vomiting has been reported (6[R]).

Withdrawal In a study in which patients were treated with a mean dose of alprazolam of 5.5 mg/day for 8 months, despite discontinuation over a 4-week period, one-third of the patients had withdrawal symptoms; these included *anxiety*, *insomnia*, *dizziness*, *hyperacusis*, *enhanced sense of smell*, *tremor*, *poor concentration*, *depersonalization*, *sweating*, *headache*, *reduced appetite*, *nausea*, and *restlessness* (cited in Ref. (12[C])).

Diazepam

Hematological In an in vitro study (14[C]) diazepam and clonazepam both inhibited the activity of natural killer cells, but further work is needed to clarify this phenomenon and to examine its implications for therapeutic use.

Gastrointestinal In rats diazepam increased gastric secretions (15). The implications of these findings for humans needs to be investigated.

Interactions In a randomized, double-blind, placebo-controlled trial, 20 male volunteers took *sertraline* up to 200 mg/day (16[C]). After 3 weeks they were given a single 10-mg intravenous dose of diazepam. There was a 13% increased clearance of diazepam, but this was not significant, probably because the study was small.

A 51-year-old man taking diazepam 20 mg/day had *clozapine* 25 mg/day added to his treatment; he suffered severe cardiorespiratory collapse (17[c]). Similar complications occurred in a 36-year-old man treated with diazepam and flurazepam when only 12.5 mg of clozapine was given. The authors reviewed other cases; typical symptoms were delirium, unconsciousness, severe hypotension, and respiratory arrest.

Lorazepam

A 15-year-old boy being given a continuous infusion of lorazepam (2–25 mg/h) for 42 days while being ventilated developed *hyperosmolality*, *hypotension*, *an increased requirement for red blood cell transfusions*, and *bilateral knee effusions* (18[c]). These symptoms are consistent with the toxic effects of propylene glycol, which was present as an additive in the lorazepam formulation. The symptoms resolved when midazolam was used instead.

Gastrointestinal A 57-year-old lady who had been taking lorazepam 2 mg/day for 2 years presented with a 2-week history of severe *dysphagia* (19[c]). Radiology showed that half the contrast was retained in the pharynx. Two weeks after withdrawal of lorazepam her dysphagia resolved both clinically and radiologically. She was asymptomatic 1 year later.

Interactions The importance of considering interactions with drugs not traditionally considered as psychoactive has been illustrated in a recent study in 48 healthy volunteers, in which the impairment of attentional tasks by the centrally acting antihypertensive drug *moxonidine* was compounded when it was co-administered with lorazepam (20[C]).

Midazolam

Cardiorespiratory The many cases of *fatal respiratory depression and cardiac arrest* that have occurred with midazolam have been reviewed (21[R]). These are particularly likely in elderly people and children, especially midazolam with opioids (e.g. fentanyl). Instances of *ventricular bigeminy*, *trigeminy*, and *tachycardia* after premedication with midazolam have also been reported; all were self-limiting.

Nervous system Reports of *athetoid movements* after premedication with midazolam have been reviewed (21[R]). *Hiccups* also appear to be relatively common. Prolonged infusions have been associated with acute *withdrawal symptoms including seizures*.

Gastrointestinal The rate of *vomiting* with midazolam in pediatric radiology has been reported to be 10% (6[R]).

Immunological and hypersensitivity reactions There have been two reports of *anaphylaxis with bronchospasm* (21[R]).

Interactions A 32-year-old man with advanced HIV disease taking the protease inhibitor *saquinavir* had prolonged sedation requiring flumazenil when he was given midazolam 5 mg intravenously for bronchoscopy; before saquinavir treatment he had received the same dose of midazolam without problems (22[c]). This effect could have been due to competition for metabolism by CYP3A4.

In 10 individuals, 5 days of treatment with *rifampicin* 15 mg/day caused 94 and 96% respective reductions in C_{max} and AUC for a 15-mg oral dose of midazolam (23[R]). The likely mechanism was induction of cytochrome P450.

In rabbits midazolam had a synergistic effect with *fentanyl* on the phrenic nerve and therefore on ventilation (24). This interaction has been examined in a randomized, double-blind, placebo-controlled study of intravenous fentanyl 200 g and midazolam 0.2 mg/kg in 15 patients undergoing orthopedic surgery (25[C]). Fentanyl caused a 30% reduction in the clearance of midazolam and a 50% increase in its elimination half-life, probably because of competitive inhibition via cytochrome P450.

There was a 2- to 3-fold increase in midazolam half-life, AUC, and peak concentration after prior administration of *fluconazole* in nine healthy volunteers (26[C]). The effect was greater for oral than for intravenous administration.

Triazolam

Nervous system Triazolam produced dose-dependent *impairment of learning*, *recall*, and *performance* for at least 6 h after a single dose in seven healthy volunteers (27[c]).

Interactions In a randomized placebo-controlled study in eight healthy volunteers *rifampicin* reduced concentrations of triazolam by over 80% (28[C]). There was a corresponding effect on psychomotor test performance. The mechanism of this interaction is probably induction of CYP3A4.

Overdosage A 71-year-old patient committed suicide by taking triazolam and amitriptyline; the respective plasma concentrations were 46 and 521 ng/g of whole blood (29[c]). This report suggests that triazolam may enhance the toxicity of amitriptyline when both are taken in overdose.

CHLORAL HYDRATE *(SED-13, 112; SEDA-21, 39)*

Nervous system A 2-year-old boy with no previous history of seizures who received an oral dose of chloral hydrate (70 mg/kg) before echocardiography had a *seizure* 1 h later, followed by a second 30 min later; at this point his Glasgow Coma Scale was 8/15 but he made a full recovery (30[c]).

CYCLOPYRROLONES *(SED-13, 111; SEDA-19, 37; SEDA-20, 33; SEDA-21, 40)*

Zolpidem

In a recent randomized double-blind placebo-controlled study of the effect of zolpidem 10–15 mg for 31 days in chronic insomnia, seven of the 75 patients who took zolpidem had to be withdrawn owing to adverse effects (none in the placebo group) (31[C]). These effects included *dry mouth*, *confusion*, *headache*, *light-headedness*, *anxiety*, and *panic attacks*. Adverse effects that were significantly more common than with placebo included drowsiness, lethargy, dizziness, pharyngitis, and rhinitis.

Nervous system In a comparison of zolpidem with triazolam the authors concluded that the two drugs cause similar *reductions in cognitive performance and memory function*, and *rebound insomnia* in therapeutic doses (32[R]).

Interactions In a randomized placebo-controlled study in eight healthy volunteers *rifampicin* reduced plasma concentrations of zolpidem by 58% (33[C]). There was a corresponding effect on psychomotor test performance. The mechanism of this interaction is probably induction of CYP3A4.

Zopiclone

Interactions In a randomized placebo-controlled study in eight healthy volunteers, *rifampicin* reduced plasma concentrations of zopiclone by over 80% (34[C]). There was a corresponding effect on psychomotor test performance. The mechanism of this interaction is believed to be induction of CYP3A4.

REFERENCES

1. Vliet IM, Den Boer JA, Westenberg HGM, Pian KLH. Clinical effects of buspirone in social phobia: a double blind placebo controlled study. J Clin Psychiatry 1997;58:164–8.
2. Trouillas P, Xie J, Adeleine P, Michel D Vighetto A, Honnorat J, Dumas R, Nighoghossian N, Laurant B. Buspirone, a 5HT agonist, is active in cerebellar ataxia. Arch Neurol 1997;54:749–52.
3. Gobert A, Rivet JM, Cistarelli L, Millan MJ. Buspirone enhances duloxetine and fluoxetine induced increases in dialysate levels of dopamine and noradrenaline, but not serotonin, in frontal cortex of freely moving rats. J Neurochem 1997;68:1326–9.
4. Kivisto KT, Lamberg TS, Kantola T, Neuvonen PJ. Plasma buspirone concentrations are greatly increased by erythromycin and itraconazole. Clin Pharmacol Ther 1997;62:348–54.
5. Good MI. Lethal interaction of clozapine and buspirone? Am J Psychiatry 1997;154:1472–3.
6. Frush DP, Bisset GS. Sedation of children for emergency imaging. Radiol Clin North Am 1997;35:789–97.
7. Willis J, Nelson A, Black SW, Borges A, An A, Rice J. Barbiturate anticonvulsants; a neuropsychological and quantitative electroencephalographic study. J Child Neurol 1997;12:169–71.
8. Hege SG, Ellinwood EH, Wilson WH, Helligers CAM, Graham SM. Psychomotor effects of the anxiolytic abecarnil: a comparison with lorazepam. Psychopharmacology 1997;131:101–7.
9. Lydiard RB, Ballenger JC, Rickels K. A double-blind evaluation of the safety and efficacy of abecarnil, alprazolam and placebo in out-patients with generalised anxiety disorder. J Clin Psychiatry 1997;58 (Suppl 11):11–18.
10. Pollack MH, Worthington JJ, Manfro GG, Otto MW, Zucker B. Abecarnil for the treatment of generalised anxiety disorder: a placebo-controlled comparison of two dose ranges of abecarnil and buspirone. J Clin Psychiatry 1997;58 (Suppl 11):19–23.
11. Small GW, Bystritsky A. Double-blind, placebo-controlled trial of two doses of abecarnil for geriatric anxiety. J Clin Psychiatry 1997;58 (Suppl 11):24–9.
12. Davidson JRT, Barlow DH, Rosenbaum JF, Shear MK. The use of benzodiazepines in panic disorder. J Clin Psychiatry 1997;58 (Suppl 2):26–8.
13. Roache JD, Stanley MA, Creson DR, Shah NN, Meisch RA. Alprazolam reinforced medication use in out-patients with anxiety. Drug Alcohol Depend 1997;45:143–55.
14. Bessler H, Caspi B, Gavish M, Rehavi M, Hart J, Weisman R. Peripheral type benzodiazepine receptor ligands modulate human natural killer cell activity. Int J Immunopharmacol 1997;19:249–54.
15. Lin W-C. Stimulatory effect of diazepam on gastric acid secretion in the continuously perfused stomach in rats under anaesthesia. Res Commun Mol Pathol Pharmacol 1997;95:157–68.
16. Gardner MJ, Baris BA, Wiliner KD, Preskom SH. Effect of sertraline on the pharmacokinetics and protien binding of diazepam in healthy volunteers. Clin Pharmacokin 1997;32 (Suppl 1):43–9.
17. Faisal I, Lindenniayer JP, Taintor Z, Cancro R. Clozapine-benzodiazepine interactions. J Clin Psychiatry 1997;58:547–8.
18. Seay RE, Graves EJ, Wiliin MK. Comment: Possible toxicity from propylene glycol in lorazepam infusion. Ann Pharmacother 1997;31:647–8.
19. Dantas RO, Souza MAN. Dysphagia induced by chronic ingestion of benzodiazepine. Am J Gastroenterol 1997;92:1194–6.
20. Wesnes K, Simpson PM, Jansson B, Grahnen A, Weiman HJ, Kuppers H. Moxonidine and cognitive function: interactions with moclobemide and lorazepam. Eur J Clin Pharmacol 1997; 52:351–8.
21. Nordt SP, Clark RF. Midazolam: a review of therapeutic uses and toxicity. J Emerg Med 1997;15:357–65.
22. Merry C, Mulcahy F, Barry M, Gibbons S, Back D. Saquinavir interaction with midazolam: pharmacokinetic considerations when prescribing protease inhibitors for patients with HIV disease. AIDS 1997;11:268–9.
23. Strayhorn VA, Baciewzcz AM, Self TH. Update on rifampicin drug interactions, III. Arch Intern Med 1997;157:2453–8.

24. Ma D, Sapsed-Byrne SM, Chakrabarti MK, Whitwam JG. Synergistic effect of fentanyl and midazolam on phrenic nerve activity in rabbits. Br J Anaesth 1997;79:686–7.
25. Hase I, Oda Y, Tanaka K, Mizutani K, Nakamoto T, Asada A. Intravenous fentanyl decreases the clearance of midazolam. Br J Anaesth 1997;79:740–3.
26. Ahonen J, Olkkola KT, Neuvonen PJ. Effect of route of administration of flucanozole on the interaction between flucanozole and midazolam. Eur J Clin Pharmacol 1997;51:415–19.
27. Rush CR, Madakasira S, Hayes CA, Johnson CA, Goldman NH, Pazzaglia PJ. Trazodone and triazolam: acute subject-rated and performance-impairing effects in healthy volunteers. Psychopharmacology 1997;131:9–18.
28. Villikka K, Kivisto KT, Backman JT, Olkkola KT, Neuvonen PJ. Triazolam is ineffective in patients taking rifampicin. Clin Pharmacol Ther 1997;61:8–14.
29. Kudo K, Imamura T, Jitsufuchi N, Zhang XX, Tokunaga H, Nagata T. Death attributed to the toxic interaction of triazolam, amitriptyline and other psychotropic drugs. Forensic Sci Int 1997;86:35–41.
30. Munoz M, Gomez A, Soult JA, Marquez C, Lopez-Castilla JD, Cervera A, Cano M. Seizures caused by chloral-hydrate sedative doses. J Paediatr 1997;131:787–8.
31. Lahmeyer H, Wilcox CS, Kann J, Leppik I. Subjective efficacy of zolpidem in outpatients with chronic insomnia: a double-blind comparison with placebo. Clin Drug Invest 1997;13:134–44.
32. Lobo BL, Greene WL. Zolpidem: distinct from triazolam? Ann Pharmacother 1997;31:625–32.
33. Villikka K, Kivisto KT, Luurila H, Neuvonen PJ. Rifampicin reduces plasma concentrations and effects of zolpidem. Clin Pharmacol Ther 1997;62:629–34.
34. Villikka K, Kivisto KT, Lamberg TS, Kantola T, Neuvonen PJ. Concentrations and effects of zopiclone are greatly reduced by rifampicin. Br J Clin Pharmacol 1997;43:471–4.

Alfonso Carvajal and Luis H. Martín Arias

6 Antipsychotic drugs

GENERAL

Pharmacological profiles of typical and atypical neuroleptic drugs have been compared, and especial emphasis has been devoted to adverse effects (1[R]). Moreover, a general review on neuroleptic drugs has been published (2[R]).

Concern has been expressed about patients who do not obtain the therapeutic benefits of antipsychotic drugs because of neuroleptic drug intolerance (3[R]).

Incidence Of 10 994 psychiatric admissions, 29 patients were transferred to a General Hospital because of adverse drug reactions (4[C]). Antipsychotic drugs were implicated in 48% of the cases. There were no fatalities and only eight patients required hospitalization. Since no figures were available about antipsychotic drug exposure, it is not possible to know the real risk of being transferred to an emergency room owing to an adverse drug reaction.

Dose-dependency Although several published studies have suggested that there is little benefit from increasing dosages of conventional antipsychotic drugs above 500–800 mg/day chlorpromazine equivalents, institutionalized patients with schizophrenia often receive larger doses. Equations and graphs that describe dose-associated likelihood of treatment response, adverse effects, and benefit:risk ratios have been developed (5[C]). These predict that if each of 1000 psychotic schizophrenic patients receives 200 mg/day chlorpromazine equivalents, 773 will respond and 55 will develop serious neuroleptic drug-associated adverse effects within a maintenance period of 6 months. Doubling the dose gives figures of 940 responders and 105 with serious adverse effects.

Side Effects of Drugs, Annual 22
J.K. Aronson, ed.

Cardiovascular Recommendations for the avoidance of cardiovascular risks of neuroleptic drugs have been published (6[R]): (1) avoidance of the low-potency phenothiazines, such as thioridazine and chlorpromazine in cardiac patients; (2) monitoring of cardiac status after starting treatment; (3) obtaining an electrocardiogram before starting the drug and again 1 month later to look for QT interval prolongation.

Conduction disturbances are a matter of concern, as they may be life-threatening (SEDA-21, 43). Recently, published reports from 1966 to 1996 have been reviewed to identify conduction disturbances associated with the butyrophenones in critically ill patients (7[R]). There were 11 reports describing 18 patients with conduction disturbances associated with therapeutic dosages of droperidol or haloperidol, of whom 13 patients had a history of cardiovascular disease. Using a reference range for the QT_c interval of 463–503 ms, 11 of 14 patients had prolongation of the QT_c interval and eight of them developed torsade de pointes. Another case has been reported (8[c]).

A 66-year-old woman developed torsade de pointes after taking a second dose of haloperidol (4 mg total) for controlling her psychosis. Her QT interval before treatment had been 360 ms and she had had T wave inversion in the lateral chest leads, consistent with myocardial ischemia, but no other known cardiac risk factors; her serum potassium concentration was 4.6 mmol/l.

This was claimed to be the first case associated with such a low dose.

Hypotension, syncope, and sudden death might be a continuum of events caused by antipsychotic drugs in some predisposed patients. From a database of spontaneously reported adverse drug effects, 55 cases of *orthostatic hypotension* were identified among 4154 reported in 1990–4 to the Midi-Pyrenees Regional Pharmacovigilance Center (9[C]). Two cases were associated with carpipramine or flupenthixol.

Syncope is frequent in elderly people, and its consequences account for substantial mortality, morbidity, and disability. The risk of syncope in elderly people has been assessed in a multicenter case–control study (588 cases and 1807 controls) according to drug consumption within the 3 days before (10[C]). After adjustment for age, sex, and cardiovascular disease, neuroleptic drugs were associated with syncope (OR 1.7; 95% CI 1.2, 2.4). Aceprometazine (2.0; 1.5, 2.5) and haloperidol (2.8; 2.0, 3.6) had the highest risks.

A case of *unexplained sudden death* in a young psychiatric patient has been reported (11[c]). The authors discussed the contribution of both medication and physical restraint to the death.

Respiratory Antipsychotic drugs and sedatives are contraindicated during acute attacks of asthma because sedation hampers respiratory drive (12[R]). The risk of asthma death and hospital readmission is increased among users of psychotropic drugs (SEDA-21, 51).

Nervous system Drug-induced *stuttering* in 22 published cases has been reviewed; in three cases neuroleptic drugs were involved (13[R])

In 27 women with chronic schizophrenia receiving neuroleptic drugs tested for right or left turning behavior there was no substantial right or left asymmetry (14[C]).

Extrapyramidal signs Acute extrapyramidal symptoms have been studied in patients who had been treated for at least 3 months with similar chlorpromazine equivalent doses of clozapine ($n = 41$), risperidone ($n = 23$), and conventional antipsychotic drugs ($n = 42$) (15[C]). The point-prevalences of *akathisia* were 7.3, 13, and 24%, respectively. The point-prevalences for rigidity and cogwheeling were 4.9 and 2.4%, 17 and 17%, and 36 and 26%. However, since there was no random allocation, these results must be questioned.

Pimozide and haloperidol have been compared in a double-blind, 24-week, placebo-controlled double crossover study in 22 children and adolescents with Tourette's syndrome (16[C]). In equivalent dosages, pimozide was superior to haloperidol for controlling symptoms of Tourette's syndrome. The number of extrapyramidal symptoms in the haloperidol group (dose range 1–8 mg/day) was higher than with placebo or pimozide (dose range 1–6 mg/day). Most of the adverse events with haloperidol were attributable to extrapyramidal symptoms and included akathisia ($n = 2$) and akinesia ($n = 2$). Two pimozide-treated patients experienced weight gain, and one had treatment emergent anxiety.

Low dose fluspirilene (1.5 mg/week) is occasionally used to treat generalized anxiety disorders. In an open-label study ($n = 205$) over 6 weeks 49 patients (16%) developed adverse effects, the most common being fatigue (5.9%), weight gain (4.4%), and mild Parkinson-like symptoms (2%) (17[C]).

Are the new antipsychotic drugs associated with a reduced risk of extrapyramidal syndromes and tardive dyskinesia? This question has been responded to in the affirmative (18[R]). In fact, many patients may benefit with the so-called 'atypical' antipsychotic drugs, and this is why, increasingly, many other patients are being switched from conventional antipsychotic drugs to these emerging atypical drugs. All aspects of changing antipsychotic drugs have been extensively reviewed (19[R]). Adverse effects, such as persistent extrapyramidal symptoms, tardive dyskinesia, and hyperprolactinemia, are indications for switching. Crossover techniques for avoiding antipsychotic and anticholinergic withdrawal drug effects are fully described. In two extensive reviews, focused on neuroleptic drug-induced movement disorders, the possible coexistence of two or more types of these disorders in the same patient has been pointed out (20[R]), (21[R]).

Different risk factors have been considered in published studies. Cocaine blocks dopamine reuptake, resulting in potentiation of neurotransmission. However, chronic use of cocaine eventually causes depletion of dopamine. Thus, it is reasonable to expect aggravation of, or an increase in, parkinsonian signs among patients receiving long-term neuroleptic drugs who abuse cocaine. Of 43 schizophrenic patients with a history of long-term psychiatric hospitalizations, 19 had a history of cocaine abuse (22[C]). Mean scores on the

14-item, 70-point United Parkinson's Disease Scale were not affected by cocaine abuse.

A pre-existing movement disorder is a predictor of an underlying organic disturbance originating in the basal ganglia (SEDA-20, 38). Of 35 neuroleptic drug-naive schizophrenic patients, 13 developed parkinsonism within 1 year of follow-up; 67% of those who had rigidity before treatment ($n = 13$) developed parkinsonism, compared with 22% of the non-rigid patients ($n = 22$) (23[C]). Advanced age, but not psychopathology, neuroleptic dosage, or prophylactic use of anticholinergic drugs, was also a predictor.

An association between depressive symptoms and extrapyramidal adverse effects has also been described (SED-13, 122). In 125 schizophrenic patients there was a positive association between extrapyramidal adverse effects and depressive symptoms (24[C]). Extrapyramidal adverse effects may cause subjective dysphoria in some patients and so contribute to depressive symptoms.

Low dosages of neuroleptic drugs are currently used to manage behavioral and psychiatric disturbances in Alzheimer's disease. Predictive factors of extrapyramidal adverse effects in these patients have been explored in 24 patients (25[C]). Several independent variables were chosen as potential predictors of neuroleptic drug-induced parkinsonism: the existence at baseline of clinical parkinsonian signs, such as bradykinesia, rigidity, and tremor; the dosage of the neuroleptic drug (haloperidol or thioridazine); the potency of the drug; age; and cognitive status. Nine patients had mild-to-moderate parkinsonian signs before treatment and this figure increased to 16 at some time during the 9-month follow-up period. Only pretreatment instrument-measured bradykinesia reached statistical significance as an independent predictor of neuroleptic drug-induced parkinsonism at 3 months and drug potency at 9 months.

Correlation of antipsychotic drug plasma concentrations with extrapyramidal signs is being paid much attention (SED-13, 117; SEDA-19, 41; SEDA-20, 45). There was no correlation between extrapyramidal signs and biperiden or haloperidol plasma concentrations in 29 chronically ill schizophrenic patients receiving both drugs (26[C]). In another study in 53 Chinese schizophrenic patients treated with a fixed dose of haloperidol for 2 weeks haloperidol concentrations did not correlate with extrapyramidal signs, although the concentrations of reduced haloperidol, a weak or non-active metabolite, did (27[C]).

In 31 schizophrenic out-patients negative symptoms were not correlated with either dosage in chlorpromazine equivalents or neuroleptic drug plasma concentrations, and neither were parkinsonism or akathisia (28[C]). There was, however, a significant correlation between dosage or plasma concentrations and positive symptoms and also with tardive dyskinesia as assessed using the Abnormal Involuntary Movement Scale (AIMS). In a multiple regression analysis of the contribution of age, sex, duration of illness, and dosage to the AIMS score, only dose contributed significantly.

Elderly and critically ill patients are often exposed to neuroleptic drugs. What happens in the elderly during acute haloperidol treatment with regard to adverse effects has been addressed in a study in 19 schizophrenic patients, aged 55–83 years (29[C]). Baseline scores on the Positive and Negative Syndrome Scale correlated with baseline scores and changes in scores on the Simpson–Angus Scale for extrapyramidal symptoms. Age was positively associated with baseline and second extrapyramidal scores.

The existence of tardive tremor as a distinct entity that, according to the authors, is worthy of recognition because of its satisfactory response to tetrabenazine has been supported by the case of a 63-year-old schizophrenic woman who developed tremor in the few years after the diagnosis had been made and neuroleptic treatment had been started (30[c]).

Different strategies have been proposed to counteract neuroleptic drug-induced parkinsonism (SEDA-18, 48), including dopamine agonists (SEDA-21, 44). Pramipexole, a dopamine D_2/D_3 receptor agonist, in dosages up to 10.25 mg/day, has been added in an open-label, non-randomized study to the haloperidol currently being taken by 15 schizophrenic patients (31[C]). Pramipexole is supposed to exert its activity by stimulation of presynaptic D_2 receptors, inhibiting the synthesis and release of dopamine. The Positive and Negative Syndrome Scale score fell by 16% after 4 weeks of treatment. The most frequent non-serious adverse events were insomnia (four patients), euphoria and schizophrenic exacerbation (three each). Reported as severe were insomnia (two), euphoria (three), schizophrenic exacerbation (three), auditory hallucinations (one), depression (one), a paranoid reaction (one), and tiredness (one). Three patients dropped out prematurely owing to adverse effects.

Akathisia occurred in 22% of 73 in-patients receiving antipsychotic drugs in a 4-week prospective study (32[C]). Dosage increase was identified as a risk factor.

A new scale (Akathisia Rating of Movement Scale, ARMS) intended to assess akathisia in mentally retarded patients has been used to study three groups of subjects: (a) neuroleptic drug-free subjects ($n = 20$); (b) subjects who had received neuroleptic drugs for at least 3 years, without changes in the previous 6 months ($n = 66$); (c) subjects who after long periods of neuroleptic treatment underwent a period of neuroleptic dosage reduction ($n = 8$) (33[C]). The respective prevalence rates for akathisia were 5, 17, and 25%.

The question of whether there is increased susceptibility to extrapyramidal adverse effects in patients with adrenocortical hormone dysfunction has been raised by the case of a 64-year-old woman with acute persistent akathisia and early-onset tardive dyskinesia after 6 weeks of neuroleptic drug treatment (34[c]). She had had symptoms of Cushing's syndrome for 18 months, but diagnosed only a month before she started to take flupenthixol.

Many schizophrenic patients smoke tobacco (more than in the general population; SEDA-20, 44) and it has been supposed that nicotine has some beneficial neuropharmacological effect. In a single-blind study of whether nicotine reduces neuroleptic drug-induced akathisia nicotine patches 14 mg were administered to 16 patients with akathisia due to antipsychotic drugs (35[C]). On the nicotine day, 15 of the subjects had lower akathisia scores compared with baseline, and 12 had lower values than on the control day when no patch was administered. However, although the rater was blind, the patients were aware of the day on which they wore the patch and may have been vulnerable to the effects of suggestion.

It has been suggested that dopamine/serotonin imbalance, with relative enhancement of serotonergic activity, might be one of the pathophysiological mechanisms underlying neuroleptic drug-induced akathisia. In the light of this hypothesis, buspirone, a partial 5-HT_{1A} receptor agonist in divided doses of up to 30 mg/day was given for 4 days to 10 patients with acute neuroleptic drug-induced akathisia (36[C]). There were no significant changes during treatment as rated using the Barnes Akathisia Scale. In contrast, mianserin a $5\text{-HT}_{2A/2C}$ receptor antagonist did improve akathisia in the same patients.

Bruxism resulting from antipsychotic drug treatment has been described as an adverse effect of chronic drug exposure and treated as a form of tardive dyskinesia. Two cases of nocturnal bruxism have been reported as an early adverse effect of antipsychotic drug treatment (37[cr]). Both were associated with neuroleptic drug-induced parkinsonism and akathisia and responded to a combination of anticholinergic drugs and β-blockers.

Dyskinesia There is some evidence that the prevalence of tardive dyskinesia differs in different ethnic groups. Nevertheless, the currently available surveys have not provided conclusive evidence of such ethnic differences (38[R]). However, prevalence rates may be misleading, as they vary depending on the number of years of exposure.

The possible involvement of oxygen radicals in the pathophysiology of tardive dyskinesia has been discussed previously (SED-13, 123). A recent study in 30 schizophrenic patients has addressed the possible relation between the activity of superoxide dismutase (SOD) and tardive dyskinesia (39[C]). The patients had received typical neuroleptic drugs for more than 10 years and were classified according to their AIMS score as having definite ($n = 10$), questionable ($n = 12$), or no tardive dyskinesia ($n = 8$). Erythrocyte Cu,Zn-SOD activity was significantly lower in those with tardive dyskinesia compared with no or questionable tardive dyskinesia.

The frequency and risk factors of severe tardive dyskinesia in older psychiatric out-patients ($n = 378$) has been studied (40[C]) in an extension of previously reported studies involving smaller numbers of patients (SEDA-21, 45). The cumulative proportion of all enrolled patients who developed severe tardive dyskinesia was 2.5% (0.5–4.5%) after 1 year, 12% (6.7–18%) after 2 years, and 23% (15–31%) after 3 years. Cox regression analysis showed that cumulative life-time neuroleptic drug dosage was a significant predictor of severe tardive dyskinesia. A higher neuroleptic dosage in mg/day chlorpromazine equivalents at study entry and an increased severity of negative symptoms from baseline to the last visit, were also predictors. None of the demographic, clinical, or neuropsychological variables, including those that had previously been found to be predictors of at least mild tardive dyskinesia (e.g. a history of alcohol misuse or dependence), predicted the development of severe tardive dyskinesia. Nevertheless, not every patient treated with neuroleptic drugs for long periods develops tardive dyskinesia, suggesting that individual characteristics may be important.

The possibility that molecular variants of a dopamine D_2 receptor gene may confer different susceptibility to tardive dyskinesia has been explored in 93 patients with tardive dyskinesia and 84 non-tardive dyskinesia patients matched for age, chronicity of disease, and dosage of neuroleptic drugs (41[C]). There were significant differences of genotype (TaqI A) and allele frequencies, but only in women with tardive dyskinesia. Genetic variation of the dopamine D_3 receptor gene has also been studied as a putative risk factor for tardive dyskinesia in schizophrenic patients receiving long-term antipsychotic drugs (42[C]). There was a high frequency (22–24%) of homozygosity for the Ser9Gly variant of the dopamine D_3 receptor gene in subjects with tardive dyskinesia compared with relative under-representation (4–6%) in patients with no or fluctuating tardive dyskinesia. Potential artefacts affecting the genetic association have been reviewed (43[R]).

In a 4-year follow-up study of young patients with recent-onset psychoses (n = 125; mean age at baseline 26 years), older age and male sex were risk factors for tardive dyskinesia (44[C]). The duration of previous exposure to antipsychotic drugs, alcohol, and/or drug misuse and negative symptoms at follow-up were also independently associated with tardive dyskinesia.

In another study tardive dyskinesia was also associated with age and the number of years of treatment with neuroleptic drugs (45[C]). Since aged patients are likely to take neuroleptic drugs for longer than young patients, age might be a confounder.

A history of alcohol abuse or dependence increase the incidence of tardive dyskinesia (SEDA-20, 38). In a retrospective analysis of 1027 patients with schizophrenia, schizoaffective disorder, or schizophreniform disorder, a history of substance abuse correlated positively with tardive dyskinesia, as were age and years of neuroleptic exposure (46[C]). However, the analysis of variance used in this study cannot independently have considered age and years of exposure. The type of substance abused was not specified, although based on epidemiological literature it is assumed that the majority of patients were alcohol abusers.

The poor metabolizer genotype might be associated with neuroleptic drug-induced dyskinesia (SEDA-20, 39; (47[C])). This has been further investigated in two new studies (48[C]), (49[C]), data from which are summarized in Table 1. Neither showed a significant association between poor metabolizer genotype and tardive dyskinesia.

The Curaçao Extrapyramidal Syndromes Studies have addressed different topics with regard to neuroleptic drug-induced neurological adverse effects: inter-relations of tardive dyskinesia, parkinsonism, akathisia, and tardive dystonia (n = 194; mean age, 53.1 years) (50[C]); intermittent neuroleptic drug treatment and risk of tardive dyskinesia (51[C]). In the first of these the prevalences of combinations of extrapyramidal syndrome were: tardive dyskinesia and parkinsonism 13%; tardive dyskinesia and tardive dystonia 9.8%; tardive dyskinesia and akathisia 5.2%; parkinsonism and tardive dystonia 4.6%; parkinsonism and akathisia 2.6%; and akathisia and tardive dystonia 1.0%. Having tardive dyskinesia increased the probability of akathisia six-fold (OR 6.2, 95% CI 1.6, 24) and of tardive dystonia 9-fold (8.7, 2.3, 32), but had no effect on parkinsonism (0.6, 0.3, 1.3). The cross-sectional design of this study does not allow one to distinguish between factors that affect the development of extrapyramidal symptom and factors that affect the course of these symptoms once they have occurred. In the

Table 1. *Distribution of poor metabolizer genotype in schizophrenic patients with and without tardive dyskinesia*

Number of poor metabolizers				
With tardive dyskinesia†	Without tardive dyskinesia	Odds ratio*	95% CI*	Reference
1/13	7/100‡	1.11	0.13, 9.79	(47[C])
5/51	5/49	0.96	0.26, 3.53	(48[C]) (cross-sectional)
5/25	3/50	3.92	0.85, 18.0	(48[C]) (longitudinal)
4/35	1/41	5.16	0.55, 48.5	(49[C])

*Not given in the studies.
†In (49[C]) tardive dyskinesia and/or parkinsonism.
‡Frequency in population of healthy white Swedish volunteers.

other study three life-time medication variables (cumulative dose of neuroleptic drugs, number of interruptions in neuroleptic drug treatment, cumulative dose of anticholinergic drugs) were assessed in relation to the occurrence and severity of tardive dyskinesia. This retrospective study included 133 Afro-Caribbean psychiatric patients from Curaçao who had received neuroleptic drugs for at least 3 months. The prevalence of tardive dyskinesia was 36%. Only the number of neuroleptic drug interruptions was significantly related both to the occurrence (two versus more than two interruptions: OR 3.29, 95% CI 1.27, 8.49) and to the severity of tardive dyskinesia. According to the authors, this finding supports the use of long-term low-dose neuroleptic drug treatment for schizophrenia, rather than targeted or intermittent neuroleptic drug treatment.

A buccolinguomasticatory dyskinesia, similar to tardive dyskinesia, occurred after 10 days of treatment with a neuroleptic and an anticholinergic drug in a 22-year-old woman (52[c]). It lasted 6 days and subsided on withdrawal.

A report of tardive diaphragmatic flutter in a 68-year-old man who had taken prochlorperazine 15–30 mg/day for 7 years has further extended the range of tardive involuntary movements (53[c]). He also had parkinsonism and orofacial stereotypies. After unsuccessful treatment with an anticholinergic drug, trihexyphenidyl, he was given a putative acetylcholine precursor, deanol 100 mg/day. Within 2 weeks, there was an improvement that was sustained for at least 2 years.

Extrapyramidal adverse effects of long-term low-dose neuroleptic drugs have been studied in non-psychiatric, anxious-depressive patients treated with either low-dose neuroleptic drugs ($n = 106$) or with antidepressants and benzodiazepines ($n = 37$) (54[C]). Tardive dyskinesia occurred in six patients, all of whom had been treated with neuroleptic drugs (chlorpromazine equivalents 47 mg/day); in contrast, other extrapyramidal adverse effects, such as pseudoparkinsonism, occurred in 28 of those treated and in six of those not treated with neuroleptic drugs.

The risk of dyskinesias has been studied in 118 autistic children aged 2–8 years in a long-term prospective study (55[C]). Children received haloperidol mean dose 1.75 mg/day for 6 months followed by placebo for 4 weeks, this sequence being repeated if required (range of treatment period 25–3610 days). Drug-related dyskinesias developed in 40, mostly during the first placebo period (18). There were no differences between children in whom dyskinesias developed and those in whom they did not.

There have been two reports of severe neuroleptic withdrawal dyskinesia (56[c]). The condition did not improve until concomitant stimulant therapy with methylphenidate was withdrawn.

Acetazolamide is often the treatment of choice for a number of diseases characterized by movement disorders, such as periodic paralysis and some forms of epileptic seizures. In combination with thiamine it has been examined in the treatment of tardive dyskinesia and other extrapyramidal symptoms in 33 patients with chronic treatment-resistant psychoses; all had been receiving maintenance doses of various neuroleptic drugs for at least 1 year before the start of the study (57[C]).

Parkinsonian effects decreased by about 40% as did symptoms of tardive dyskinesia. There was complete relapse within a week of withdrawal.

The successful use of posteroventral pallidotomy has been described in a 31-year-old man with tardive dyskinesia of the buccolinguomasticatory type rapidly progressing to severe tardive dystonia (58[c]).

Neuroleptic drugs can cause extrapyramidal symptoms that can affect swallowing (SEDA-19, 44; SEDA-21, 44). Three new cases of severe neuroleptic drug-induced dysphagia have been reported (59[c]).

A 79-year-old man with Alzheimer's disease was taking loxapine 5 mg/day orally or intramuscularly for aggressive behavior. About 1 week after the dose had been increased gradually to 5 mg bd he started choking on his medication and liquid dosage forms were required. Videofluoroscopy showed moderate-to-severe oropharyngeal dysphagia, which improved after loxapine was withdrawn and chlorpromazine, 10 mg every 8 h, was given.

A 61-year-old woman with atypical psychosis continuously treated with neuroleptic drugs for 13 years developed dysphagia, and was unable to eat or drink. She had been taking daily oral chlorpromazine 25 mg, levomepromazine 25 mg, and trihexyphenidyl 4 mg. Her medication was changed to daily sulpiride 500 mg, diazepam 15 mg, and biperiden 3 mg, given via a stomach tube. Her dysphagia gradually disappeared but the tardive dyskinesia involving her tongue and upper extremities did not completely resolve.

A 53-year-old schizophrenic woman who had received various neuroleptic drugs for 18 years developed tardive dyskinesia. She could drink but could no longer eat solid food. Her medication was changed from daily propericiazine 50 mg to oxypertine 60 mg, chlorpromazine 25 mg, and clonazepam 2 mg. Polygraphic studies were compatible with rabbit syndrome. Oxypertine was changed to thioridazine 100 mg and trihexyphenidyl 4 mg was added. After 1 week her tremors had completely resolved along with her dysphagia.

Dystonia Cocaine is a risk factor for neuroleptic drug-induced dystonia. This is the conclusion of a prospective study of 29 patients who developed dystonia within 7 days after starting to take a neuroleptic drug for the first time (60[C]). More cocaine users developed dystonia (six of nine) than did non-users (three of 20; RR = 4.4; 95% CI 1.4, 14).

On two different occasions, dystonia appeared after neuroleptic drug withdrawal (61[c]) in a 52-year-old man, who could not close his mouth after withdrawal of haloperidol and on another occasion after withdrawal of sulpiride.

Bilateral ulnar paralysis has also been reported as a complication of neuroleptic drug-induced extrapyramidal rigidity (62[c]). Treatment consisted of anticholinergic medication and physiotherapy. The patient recovered over 8 months.

Dystonic reactions may sometimes present as Bell's palsy (63[c]).

An 11-year-old boy developed acute left-sided facial paralysis. He had been treated with amoxicillin for left-sided otitis media and with oral prochlorperazine 10 mg every 6 h for nausea and vomiting. A diagnosis of Bell's palsy, presumably caused by otitis, was made. At the time of discharge he was unable to maintain an upright position while standing. After the recognition of a possible dystonic reaction, intravenous diphenhydramine 50 mg was given and within 5 min he was able to stand erect and walk normally. His facial palsy also completely resolved.

Laryngeal dystonia can mimic anaphylaxis (64[c]).

A 24-year-old man with a provisional diagnosis of schizophrenia received haloperidol 1.5 mg at night; after 2 weeks, the dosage was increased to 1.5 mg bd. Four days later, within 90 min of taking haloperidol, he developed a hoarse almost inaudible voice associated with tachypnea and a sensation of tongue swelling. A provisional diagnosis of acute anaphylaxis of unknown cause was made and he was given intravenous adrenaline, hydrocortisone, metoclopramide, and ranitidine, and an oral antihistamine and diazepam. Two days later, his symptoms recurred more severely, with dyspnea and respiratory distress. He began to shake violently after the administration of adrenaline and developed unilateral temporomandibular joint dislocation. Intravenous diazepam, given to treat the jaw dislocation, unexpectedly caused dramatic improvement in his respiratory symptoms as well as resolution of the dislocation. Since a neuroleptic drug-induced dystonia was strongly suspected, haloperidol was withdrawn and risperidone begun. Skin tests using small quantities of the patient's own haloperidol showed no evidence of hypersensitivity.

Some investigators believe that tardive dystonia is related to tardive dyskinesia. Consequently, vitamin E, which has been used to treat tardive dyskinesia (SED-13, 123; SEDA-21, 47), has now been used to treat tardive dystonia (65[c]).

A 21-year-old psychotic man who had taken neuroleptic drugs and lithium for 5 years developed involuntary dystonic movements of the trunk and limbs. Five months later the treatment was discontinued and replaced by carbamazepine as a sole agent, without any relief of dystonic movements. He had symptoms of tardive dystonia, with slow persistent movements of overextension and overflexion of the hands, a sideways deviation of one foot at a time, a retro-or-side flexion of the head and neck, and slow torsion of the trunk. He could not eat, drink, walk, or button his clothes. Treatment with vitamin E was begun and after 4 weeks his functional capacity had improved and he was able to eat, walk, swim, and button his clothes. The treatment was maintained and no exacerbation occurred during the 15-month follow-up after his discharge.

Botulinum toxin type A is used in patients with dystonia and spasticity (SEDA-19, 45). Severity scores in six of seven patients with tardive cervical dystonia improved during 5 years of treatment with Botulinum toxin injections (66[c]). The number of treatments was four to 17, and the average number of days between injections was 82–276 days.

A custom-made mechanical device that delivers a sensory stimulus to the head and shoulders has been successfully used to treat six patients with severe axial tardive dystonia with retrocollis and back arching (67[c]). The authors suggested that a device that delivers pressure to the occiput and shoulders may improve sitting, standing, and walking in patients who suffer a combination of severe retrocollis and back arching.

Neuroleptic malignant syndrome A retrospective case–control study (68[C]) and several case reports (69[cR]), (70[c]) have added further information on the neuroleptic malignant syndrome (SEDA-20, 41). In 25 patients with neuroleptic malignant syndrome matched with 50 patients also treated with neuroleptic drugs, neuroleptic malignant syndrome was more likely to occur in a patient who was agitated (OR 4.3) or dehydrated (OR 3.5), who receives large doses of a neuroleptic drug within 24 h of admission to the hospital (<600 vs >600 mg chlorpromazine equivalents, OR 3.33), or who continues to receive high doses over the next few days (maximum neuroleptic drug dose 600 vs >600 mg chlorpromazine equivalents, OR 4.30). A past history of ECT also emerged as a risk factor (OR 5.89). Lithium, medical or neurological illness, and mental retardation were not risk factors.

The neuroleptic malignant syndrome has been described in patients with AIDS (SEDA-19, 47). In the light of a new case, the subject has been reviewed and the main features of the nine reported cases discussed (69[cR]).

Cases of isolated thrombocytopenia associated with neuroleptic drugs have previously been described (SED-11, 51; SEDA-19, 48). A case of neuroleptic malignant syndrome with acute thrombocytopenia has been claimed to be the first report of this type (70[c]).

A 32-year-old woman had neuroleptic malignant syndrome and a severe hemorrhagic thrombocytopenia after treatment with perphenazine 4 mg tds and haloperidol 5 mg qds. Detailed investigations for thrombocytopenia were negative and it resolved after withdrawal of the neuroleptic drugs, along with her fever, obtundation, autonomic instability, and oculogyric crisis.

Psychiatric *Mood* Dysphoria has deserved recent attention, although it is not a newly discovered adverse effect of neuroleptic drugs (SED-13, 121; SEDA-21, 46; (71[r])). Eight men with developmental stuttering participated in a study to assess the effect of 6 weeks of pimozide treatment on speech fluency and mood (72[C]). Four of seven who were compliant developed marked depression.

Cognitive function Neuroleptic drugs are often used to treat behavioral problems in patients with dementia, but they can cause more rapid impairment of cognitive function. This has been observed in a 2-year longitudinal non-randomized study in 71 patients with dementia (73[C]). The fall in the mean score for the expanded examination in the patients who took neuroleptic drugs ($n = 16$) was twice that in patients who did not. Three commentaries (74[Cr]), (75[cr]), (76[cr]), plus the authors' reply (77[r]) have underlined the interest aroused by this topic.

Based on a follow-up of 135 subjects from the Camberwell (UK) dementia case register, the association between neuroleptic drug exposure and cognitive decline has been further emphasized (74[Cr]). During 1 year, subjects who took neuroleptic drugs ($n = 23$) had a greater fall in Minimental State Examination than those who did not (21 vs 9.3 points). There was a higher proportion of cognitive decline in carriers of the apolipoprotein E4 allele. An anticholinergic mechanism has been suggested to explain cognitive decline, since differences in anticholinergic potency may account for differences in cognitive impairment (75[cr]). Alternatively, it has been suggested that patients who were already on a steeper trajectory of cognitive decline were more likely to be given neuroleptic drugs (76[cr]). In contrast, some other studies have shown no impairment in cognitive function, although differences in the outcome variables, and particularly in the follow-up periods, might have explained such discrepancies.

Attentional dysfunction, as assessed by continuous performance tests, did not change in drug-naive ($n = 24$) or drug-withdrawn ($n = 20$) schizophrenic patients during, or on average 6 months after, treatment with neuroleptic drugs and after a significant reduction in symptom severity (78[C]).

Memory The effect of haloperidol withdrawal on memory performance has been studied in 21 schizophrenic patients (79[C]). Recent memory was slightly impaired in patients who underwent haloperidol withdrawal, whereas access to old, remote memory increased slightly. It had previously been shown that haloperidol did not appreciably affect the structure of the attentional system (80[C]).

Endocrine, metabolic Drug-related *hyperprolactinemia* has been reviewed (81[R]). Antipsychotic agents remain a frequent cause, but the newer neuroleptic drugs have a smaller effect on prolactin concentrations (82[cr]).

Gynecomastia is associated with antipsychotic drugs (SED-13, 125; SEDA-20, 43; SEDA-21, 50). There has been discussion of the prevalence of gynecomastia during puberty, and the mechanisms involved in the light of the case of a 13-year-old boy who developed bilateral gynecomastia after taking lithium carbonate 1500 mg/day and perphenazine 12 mg/day and then switching to risperidone 3 mg bd (83[cr]).

Hematological The reported incidence of *agranulocytosis* associated with antipsychotic drugs is variable, ranging from 1:3000–4000 to 1:250 000 (SED-13, 126). Reported cases have further illustrated some of the features of the condition (SEDA-18, 51; SEDA-19, 48).

A 67-year-old man treated for mania with chlorpromazine 50–150 mg/day and lithium developed severe granulocytopenia (0.7×10^9/l) (84[c]). After withdrawal of chlorpromazine he recovered and his white cell count was in the reference range by 11 days.

Although It is not uncommon for patients receiving phenothiazines to develop leukopenia, only very few develop severe granulocytopenia below 1.0×10^9/l.

Gastrointestinal Yohimbine caused *increased salivary flow* in 10 patients treated with either antidepressants or neuroleptic drugs (85[C]). This was observed in a randomized, double-blind, cross-over comparison of yohimbine with anetholtithione. There were no adverse effects in the 5 days of treatment.

In a multicenter, double-blind, randomized study, the efficacy and safety of tiapride was compared with that of melperone in patients with dementia ($n = 176$) (86[C]). After 4 weeks, adverse events did not significantly differ between the two groups. Two patients in the tiapride group withdrew because of *duodenal ulceration*, which was considered serious.

Urinary tract *Urinary retention and incontinence* have been reported in relation to neuroleptic drugs (SED-13, 127) and there have been two further reports (87[c]), (88[c]).

A 75-year-old man developed acute urinary retention. He had been treated for psychotic depression with haloperidol 1 mg/day, alprazolam 0.5 mg/day, and venlafaxine 37.5 mg/day for 1 week. The retention resolved spontaneously in a few days after withdrawal of all drugs.

A 32-year-old woman had an exacerbation of her psychosis. Two days later her haloperidol and diazepam were withdrawn in order to simplify her treatment, and chlorpromazine was increased to 500 and then to 700 mg/day. She also received depot fluphenazine decanoate 25 mg after 3 days. After 4 days of increased chlorpromazine and 5 days after the depot, she developed urinary incontinence. Chlorpromazine was withdrawn and the reaction resolved within 24 h.

Special senses Episodes of *perceptual alteration*, mainly of vision and/or hearing occurred in three schizophrenic patients on long-term maintenance neuroleptic drugs (89[c]). Although these episodes seemed like relapse of schizophrenia, oral anticholinergic drugs and dosage reduction of the neuroleptic drugs reduced their frequency.

Sexual function *Priapism* has been occasionally been related to neuroleptic drugs (SED-13, 125; SEDA-20, 43; SEDA-21, 50). A 53-year-old man with a history of untreated hypertension developed priapism a few days after starting treatment with the phenothiazine prothipendylhydrochloride 40 mg tds (90[c]). Decompression by a caverno-spongious fistula was successfully performed. An 11-year-old boy developed priapism while being treated with thioridazine; it resolved with direct instillation of phenylephrine into the corpus cavernosum (91[c]). Since a hematoma developed at the needle site, others recommended that this be prevented by directing the needle through the glans into the corpus cavernosum (92[r]).

Withdrawal effects Neuroleptic drug withdrawal in schizophrenic patients has been previously reviewed in these Annuals (SEDA-20; 44). The hypothesis of the authors of a recent meta-analysis on how to achieve neuroleptic drug withdrawal was that slow withdrawal would delay and perhaps even reduce the risk of relapses (93[CR]). However, there were no significant differences in the resulting survival functions for those who discontinued treatment abruptly ($n = 1006$) versus gradually ($n = 104$). The risk of relapse after 12 months of abrupt withdrawal of oral neuroleptic drugs was 54% (95% CI 51, 58).

Neuroleptic drugs are commonly used in patients with dementia who are physically aggressive. There has now been a randomized, double-blind, baseline neuroleptic drug-controlled trial of the effects of short-term (3 weeks) neuroleptic drug withdrawal on aggression (94[C]). Based on the observed instances of physically aggressive behavior in 20 patients from the withdrawn group, excluding two who needed remedication, and all 14 from the not-withdrawn group, there were no significant differences. Thus, withdrawal of neuroleptic drugs in some patients reduces the probability of adverse events.

Use in pregnancy It is not clear whether neuroleptic drugs cause fetal malformations (SED-13, 128). In a recent review devoted to the use of antipsychotic drugs in pregnancy, the possible risks have been discussed (95[R]). Four prospective studies have focused on the *teratogenicity* of low-potency antipsychotic drugs, giving information about 45 687 exposed and unexposed children. Only one of the studies showed significantly more malformations in the infants of women who had taken phenothiazines during the first 3 months of pregnancy than in those whose mothers had not. There is less information on high-potency antipsychotic drugs; one in four studies showed a minimal increase in the risk of malformations. There are no data on atypical antipsychotic drugs.

There have been a few case reports of neonatal toxicity or perinatal syndromes; no differences have been observed in behavioral and intellectual functioning between exposed or unexposed children. Although there are no clearly established guidelines for the use of antipsychotic drugs in the acutely psychotic pregnant woman, non-pharmacological therapy, such as individual psychotherapy, therapy for the patient's partner and family, social casework, and hospitalization in a supportive structured milieu, should usually be attempted before drug therapy. But, if necessary, the use of the lowest possible dosage for the shortest possible time is wise to minimize fetal exposure.

Interactions Pharmacokinetic interactions of psychotropic drugs have been identified by using information from a therapeutic drug monitoring database (96[C]). Patients who had been exposed to one of five agents known for their capacity to induce (*phenytoin*, *phenobarbital*, and *carbamazepine*) or to inhibit (*thioridazine* and *levomepromazine*) the metabolism of psychotropic drugs ($n = 105$) were matched by age, sex, and psychotropic medication with 105 patients randomly selected from a pool of subjects who had not been exposed to target co-medication. Co-medication with a phenothiazine (thioridazine or levomepromazine) led to significantly higher concentrations of demethylated metabolites of *clomipramine*, *imipramine*, *amitriptyline*, and *mianserin*. Concentrations of *moclobemide* were also increased.

Carbamazepine reduced concentrations of haloperidol, clopenthixol, and flupenthixol. Plasma concentrations of bromperidol fell in 13 patients to whom *carbamazepine* was given (97[C]). Conversely, they rose in 26 schizophrenic patients to whom levomepromazine was given, although this effect was not observed with thioridazine (98[C]) or with trihexyphenidyl or biperiden (99[C]).

Various antipsychotic drugs inhibit the metabolism of *tricyclic antidepressants* (SED-13, 129; SEDA-20, 45; SEDA-21, 51). Perphenazine increases plasma concentrations of *nortriptyline* by inhibiting CYP2D6 (100[C]).

Selective serotonin reuptake inhibitors (SSRIs) inhibit CYP2D6 (SEDA-20, 50; SEDA-21, 51). After pretreatment of eight healthy extensive CYP2D6 metabolizers with paroxetine 20 mg/day for 10 days, perphenazine peak plasma concentrations increased from 2- to 13-fold, in association with a significant increase in central nervous system adverse effects, including oversedation, extrapyramidal symptoms, and impairment of psychomotor performance and memory (101[C]).

When compared with the high neuroleptic dosages typically used to treat psychiatric disorders, the low dosages used in Tourette's syndrome uncommonly cause drug-induced parkinsonism; however, three cases of acute, severe, drug-induced parkinsonism have been reported (102[c]). The adverse effect was observed in three of 14 adult patients treated with neuroleptic drugs and SSRIs for Tourette's syndrome, but in none of the 75 children treated. Dosages of fluphenazine, the neuroleptic used in the three cases, did not exceed 4 mg/day. Since SSRIs inhibit cytochrome P450 isoenzymes, plasma concentrations of concomitant neuroleptic drugs could increase. The combination of a neuroleptic and a tricyclic antidepressant does not appear to be associated with the same risk.

A system of strategies in France (Opposable Medical References), forming part of a panoply of measures aimed at controlling prescription, has been implemented in relation to the use of antiparkinsonian drugs in patients taking neuroleptic drugs; clearly, one should avoid using them altogether.

Monitoring therapy Since CYP2D6 is involved in the metabolism of both haloperidol and dextromethorphan, the relation between baseline dextromethorphan metabolic ratios (dextromethorphan to dextrophan) and steady-state plasma haloperidol concentrations and reduced haloperidol/haloperidol ratios could be of interest. In a recent study in 18 Chinese schizophrenic patients, there were significant correlations between dextromethorphan/dextrorphan ratios and haloperidol concentrations, reduced haloperidol concentrations, and reduced haloperidol/haloperidol ratios (103[C]). Ten patients who had extrapyramidal symptoms had significantly higher reduced haloperidol/haloperidol ratios than the other eight patients. The authors suggested that phenotyping for dextromethorphan metabolism might predict extrapyramidal symptoms in some patients.

INDIVIDUAL DRUGS

Amisulpiride

Amisulpiride is a substituted benzamide with high selectivity for dopamine D_2 and D_3 receptors, preferentially in the limbic system rather than the striatum, it especially blocks presynaptic dopamine autoreceptors. It has no affinity for other receptors. In a multicenter, randomized, double-blind study (n = 141), amisulpiride 100 mg/day for 6 months was more effective than placebo in the treatment of schizophrenic patients (104[C]). There was at least one adverse event in 41 patients in the amisulpiride group (n = 69) and 33 in the placebo group (n = 72). With amisulpiride the most common events were *sleep disorders* (eight), *increased weight* (six), *anxiety* (four), *nervousness* (four), and *amenorrhea* (four of the 23 women). Five patients (one taking placebo and four taking amisulpiride) developed *parkinsonism* requiring treatment.

Amisulpiride 800 mg/day was at least as effective as haloperidol 20 mg/day in the treatment of acute exacerbations of schizophrenia whilst causing less parkinsonism: this was the conclusion of a multicenter, double-blind trial in which patients were randomly allocated to amisulpiride ($n = 95$) or haloperidol ($n = 96$) for 6 weeks (105[C]). Adverse events were reported in 54 amisulpiride-treated patients and in 72 haloperidol-treated patients; *neurological adverse events* using spontaneous reporting were almost twice as frequent in the haloperidol group ($n = 59$) than in the amisulpiride group ($n = 34$) with a tendency to be more severe in patients receiving haloperidol. One patient taking haloperidol committed *suicide* 2 days after starting active treatment. Since some data suggest that there is no further improvement with doses over 10 mg/day, the haloperidol dose used in this study may have led to bias in favor of amisulpiride.

Amisulpiride has been compared with either haloperidol or flupenthixol in three double-blind randomized trials (106[R]). Amisulpiride was as effective as the reference drugs in acute exacerbations of schizophrenia and caused fewer extrapyramidal adverse effects.

Chlorpromazine

Immunological and hypersensitivity reactions Neuroleptic drugs have been associated with *lupus-like syndrome* (SED-13, 127; SEDA-21, 50). Since anti-phospholipid antibodies may occur in drug-induced lupus-like syndrome, its relation with the major histocompatibility complex markers has been studied in 93 psychiatric patients chronically treated with chlorpromazine (107[C]). In 41 patients there were positive results for antibodies and there were significantly increased frequencies of HLA-B44 and HLA-DRZ antigens. This suggests that major histocompatibility antigens could play some role in chlorpromazine-induced lupus-like syndrome.

Clozapine *(SED-13, 118; SEDA-19, 51; SEDA-20, 46; SEDA-21, 52)*

Clozapine 100–900 mg ($n = 205$) has been compared with haloperidol 5–30 mg ($n = 218$) in a randomized double-blind trial in patients with refractory schizophrenia (108[C]). Compliance was 55% in the patients taking clozapine compared with 28% for haloperidol. In an intent-to-treat analysis, Positive and Negative Syndrome Scale scores were significantly better with clozapine. Patients assigned to clozapine had less tardive dyskinesia and akathisia and fewer extrapyramidal adverse effects. There was *leukopenia* in four patients taking clozapine and in two patients taking haloperidol; there was *neutropenia* in eight patients taking clozapine and nine patients taking haloperidol. *Agranulocytosis* developed in only three patients taking clozapine, all of whom recovered fully after withdrawal. Clozapine is more expensive, but patients taking it spent 24 fewer days at the hospital in 1 year than those taking haloperidol.

The long-term outcome of clozapine treatment in chronic treatment-resistant schizophrenic patients has been studied in 122 patients (109[C]). At follow-up, 74 were still taking clozapine, and of the remaining 48 only 11 had discontinued treatment owing to adverse effects (five *blood dyscrasias* and six other events).

Clozapine has also been studied in 40 Chinese schizophrenic patients in a 12-week, double-blind comparison with chlorpromazine (110[C]). Two clozapine-treated patients were withdrawn, one because of *leukopenia and nausea* and the other because of *vomiting and hypotension*. Chlorpromazine was prematurely withdrawn in two patients, because of *jaundice and oversedation* in one, and because of *severe weight loss* (9 kg) in the other. The rate of moderate-to-severe *hypersalivation* was high in clozapine-treated patients (29%). Two clozapine-treated patients and two chlorpromazine-treated patients had significant improvements in previously existing tardive dyskinesia and one chlorpromazine-treated patient had worsened tardive dyskinesia.

In a prospective 10-year open study in 80 schizophrenic patients considered refractory, 60% of the patients improved significantly after treatment with clozapine (111[C]). Adverse effects were mild and well tolerated, with no cases of hematological disturbances and only five withdrawals because of adverse reactions. There was mild *somnolence* in 57 patients, *hypersalivation* in 39, *hypotension* in 20, *gastrointestinal symptoms* in 20, *weight gain* in 11, *increased sweating* in 11, *seizures* in three, and *myoclonus* in three. Similarly, in an open 1-year follow-up study, schizophrenic patients with ($n = 41$) and without ($n = 19$) bipolar features were treated with clozapine (75–600 mg/day) (112[C]). The main adverse effects were: *drowsiness* or *sedation*, 40%; *hypersalivation*, 35%; *tachycardia*, 18%; over 10% *weight gain*, 18%; *hypotension*, 10%; and *leukopenia*, 3%. There were four withdrawals owing to adverse effects. *Tachycardia* only occurred in the patients with bipolar features.

Sociodemographic, behavioral, and clinical predictors of tardive dyskinesia are said to be useful in identifying a subset of schizophrenic individuals who benefit from treatment with clozapine (113[R]); this favorable motor adverse effect profile of clozapine contributes to improve patient outcomes by reducing noncompliance, substance abuse, and suicide.

Cardiovascular *Tachycardia* (25%) is the most common cardiovascular adverse effect of clozapine, hypotension being the second (114[R]). Hypotension may be caused by both typical and atypical neuroleptic drugs and two cases of hypertension associated with clozapine (SEDA-19, 51; SEDA-21, 52) have been considered as 'paradoxical hypertension'. However, two new cases of hypertension have been reported (115[c]), (116[c]). Like previous cases, the patients were young men and their blood pressure before treatment had been normal (see Table 2).

Nervous system There is increasing evidence that seizures associated with clozapine are dose-dependent (SED-13, 121; SEDA-21, 53). Specific EEG changes during clozapine therapy have been prospectively studied in 50 patients who were randomly assigned to one of three non-overlapping clozapine serum concentration ranges (50–150, 200–300, and 350–450 ng/ml) (119[C]). EEGs were obtained before and after 10 weeks of treatment. There were EEG changes in 53% of the patients and three seizures, one in a patient taking clozapine 900 mg (serum concentration 320 ng/ml), and two in patients with lower serum concentrations (200–300 ng/ml) who had prior histories of seizures and inadequate valproate coverage.

Treatment of psychosis related to Parkinson's disease deserves particular attention, and some studies devoted to this topic have recently been published (120[C])–(122[C]). The severity of *parkinsonian motor disability and dyskinesias* was evaluated in seven levodopa-responsive patients with Parkinson's disease after an acute challenge with the mixed dopamine agonist apomorphine, before and after low-dose clozapine (50 mg/day) for 18 days (120[C]). There was improvement in apomorphine-induced dyskinesias without aggravation of parkinsonian motor signs after clozapine treatment. On the other hand, since levodopa-induced psychosis can complicate the treatment of Parkinson's disease, a retrospective uncontrolled study (121[C]) has addressed the efficacy and safety of treatment with clozapine in 27 such patients; most had rapid improvement from baseline within 1 month, but there were adverse effects in 21 patients and five withdrew owing to adverse effects (two with confusion/agitation, one with severe orthostatic hypotension, one with seizures, and one with sedation). There has also been a double-blind crossover comparison of low-dose clozapine with benztropine in the treatment of tremor in Parkinson's disease (122[C]). Twenty-two subjects were enrolled and 19 completed the study; there were significant adverse events with each drug, but leukopenia was not encountered.

A dose-related *tic-like syndrome* associated with clozapine has been reported (SEDA-20, 47). This disturbance, which affected speech, was described as a grunting or 'hiccuping' motor tic. In addition, a case of *orolaryngeal myoclonus* with speech disturbance in a 40-year-old man has been reported (123[c]). The problem was also related to dose and reduction of the dosage of clozapine to 350 mg/day was accompanied by partial remission; cloza-

Table 2. *Some recently published cases of hypertension associated with clozapine*

Age (years)	Dosage of clozapine (mg/day)	Blood pressure (mmHg)	References
34	62.5	160/108	(117[c])
19	175	170/115	(115[c])
32	200–400	164/116	(118[c])
27	300	146/106	(116[c])

pine was further reduced to 250 mg/day and the speech disturbance completely resolved.

Neuroleptic malignant syndrome has been rarely associated with clozapine (SEDA-19, 53), and it is questionable whether published cases fulfil the criteria for neuroleptic malignant syndromes (SEDA-21, 54). Although there is consensus about diagnosis of the fully developed syndrome, there is controversy about mild, early, and atypical cases (124[r]). In contrast, some authors (125[r]) have claimed that some of the classical signs and symptoms of neuroleptic malignant syndrome are not reported with clozapine, and that their absence might be explained by the emergence of a different 'atypical' neuroleptic malignant syndrome. Meanwhile, new cases have been described (126[c]), (127[c]).

A 45-year-old man developed neuroleptic malignant syndrome 16 days after starting clozapine therapy, with rigidity, fever, and an increase in creatinine kinase activity (i.e. at least three major manifestations). Moreover, he developed a raised creatinine kinase activity 2 days after a clozapine rechallenge.

A 67-year-old woman developed neuroleptic malignant syndrome after taking clozapine (300 mg/day) for 38 days; she had fever, sweating, tachycardia, confusion, and an increased creatinine kinase activity.

A case of clozapine withdrawal catatonia and neuroleptic malignant syndrome in a 30-year-old man has also been reported (128[c]). The authors suggested that neuroleptic malignant syndrome may be regarded as a neuroleptic drug-induced retarded (stuporous) subtype of malignant catatonia, clinically indistinguishable from non-neuroleptic retarded malignant catatonia but different from the excited form.

Delirium associated with clozapine, an uncommon adverse effect, probably due to its anticholinergic properties, has been reported (129[c]).

A 48-year-old woman with a schizoaffective disorder was treated with clozapine therapy, initially 12.5 mg bd. On day 10 of treatment, after 3 days at a dose of 50 mg in the morning and 100 mg at bedtime, she became disoriented, was ataxic, and had slurred speech and visual hallucinations. Clozapine was withdrawn and her delirium resolved within 3 days. Subsequently she responded well to clozapine rechallenge at a much lower dosage of 37.5 mg at bedtime.

Neurogenic *stuttering*, which is an infrequent adverse effect of psychoactive drugs, has been reported in a 28-year-old woman treated with clozapine (130[c]). Stuttering occurred during the second month of clozapine therapy and ceased when the clozapine dose was at or below 700 mg/day.

Endocrine, metabolic *Diabetic ketoacidosis and insulin-dependent hyperglycemia* associated with clozapine have previously been described (SEDA-19, 53; SEDA-21, 54). There has since been published a four-case series in which clozapine therapy was associated with either de novo onset (two patients) or severe exacerbation of pre-existing diabetes mellitus (two patients) (131[c]). Two men aged 32 and 44 years, with no prior history or laboratory evidence of diabetes mellitus developed hyperglycemia after taking clozapine for 5 weeks. Two other 51-year-old men with a history of type 2 diabetes mellitus, well controlled, had worse glycemic control. In addition, ketoacidosis occurred in a 50-year-old man after 6 days of clozapine treatment (132[c]).

Hematological In a review of published reports of blood dyscrasias other than agranulocytosis, associated with clozapine, 20 cases were discussed (133[R]). Eosinophilia was the most frequent abnormality. The reported incidence of eosinophilia is very variable, from 0.2–1.0%, an underestimated incidence based on spontaneous adverse event reporting, up to a considerably higher incidence of 46 or 62% in other studies (134[r]). In a recent study it was identified in 13% of 160 patients who had begun to take clozapine within a 3.5-year period (135[C]). All cases developed within 4 weeks of the first dose of clozapine. In one case, clozapine was withdrawn and in all other cases the eosinophilia resolved without intervention. Because it can resolve spontaneously, withdrawal of clozapine may be unjustified in patients with eosinophilia (136[c]).

A 22-year-old man with recurrent suicidal ideas was given clozapine after failed treatment with thiothixene, haloperidol, and risperidone. On day 27, his leukocyte count was 9.1×10^9/l with 23% eosinophils (2.1×10^9/l) and 46% neutrophils (4.1×10^9/l). Clozapine was withdrawn and 6 months later he died from suicide while taking a combination of loxapine and risperidone.

Eosinophilia does not predict agranulocytosis, but in one 37-year-old man eosinophilia and agranulocytosis co-existed (137[c]). In another case lupus anticoagulant and an abnormal activated partial thromboplastin time were detected in a 38-year-old man taking clozapine (138[c]).

R *Agranulocytosis and clozapine*

Incidence *Although premarketing data suggested an incidence of agranulocytosis of 1–2%, the actual incidence based on data from The Clozaril National Registry in the US was 0.38%: 382 cases in 99 502 exposed patients in 1990–4; 12 patients died (0.012%) (139[C]). A patient monitoring system in the UK and Ireland during the same period found fatal agranulocytosis in 0.03% of patients. Among individuals at risk, the critical period of developing agranulocytosis is within the first 6 months after the start of therapy. The FDA advisory committee therefore recommended in July 1997 that mandatory weekly blood monitoring should be reduced in frequency (e.g. every 2 weeks) after 6 months. However, incidence figures from data collected by Sandoz in New Zealand are higher (140[CR]). Between April 1988 and June 1995, there were eight cases of agranulocytosis among 693 patients exposed to clozapine (1.15%), none fatal. There were also 14 cases of neutropenia (2.02%).*

Course *The New Zealand experience with clozapine-induced neutropenia or agranulocytosis suggests that there are two responses: (i) transient neutropenia of usually short duration (2–5 days); the neutrophil count typically falls just below 1.5×10^9/l and then recovers spontaneously after clozapine withdrawal; (ii) frank agranulocytosis of longer duration (8–22 days); patients often become ill, for example with sore throat and fever; the neutrophil count falls steadily or in a few cases sharply from low normal to zero or near zero; neutrophil recovery after withdrawal can take 14–22 days, but deaths can occur.*

A 37-year-old man who developed agranulocytosis after 11 weeks of clozapine monotherapy deteriorated rapidly and developed extreme hyperglycemia, severe lactic acidosis, recurrent cardiac arrest, cardiogenic shock, and coma (141[c]). He died 36 h later.

Diagnosis *Blood dyscrasias constitute a reason for withdrawing clozapine, although rechallenge in patients who developed agranulocytosis has been discussed. Negative rechallenge in a patient with previous agranulocytosis has been reported (SEDA-20, 54) and further cases have appeared (142[c]).*

A 29-year-old man developed an increasingly severe neutropenia that necessitated withdrawal of clozapine. After 3 weeks of treatment with lithium clozapine was restarted. One year later, while he was taking clozapine, his granulocyte count was within the reference range.

However, positive rechallenge has also been reported (143[c]).

A 53-year-old man's weekly white blood cell count fell to 3.8×10^9/l and clozapine had to be withdrawn. When it was restarted his leukocyte count was 8200×10^9/l; after 7 weeks the leukocyte count fell to 3900×10^9/l and clozapine had to be withdrawn again.

Liver The rate of liver dysfunction associated with clozapine has been estimated at 1%, and *hepatitis* and *raised liver enzymes* have been reported (SEDA-20, 49). Hepatotoxicity in 238 patients treated with either haloperidol or clozapine has been investigated as part of a prospective drug monitoring program (144[C]). The most commonly abnormal liver function test was a raised AlT with both drugs. Clozapine-treated patients had an increase in AlT (to above twice the upper limit of the reference range) significantly more often than patients treated with haloperidol (37 vs 17%). Higher clozapine plasma concentrations were associated with an increase in AlT; men were at a higher risk. At least 60% of the increases in the different enzymes resolved within the first 13 weeks of treatment despite continued administration. Two cases of marked rises in liver enzyme with clozapine have been reported, in 27- and 49-year-old men, which had several characteristics in common (145[c]).

Fatal *acute fulminant liver failure* due to clozapine has been reported in a 39-year-old man, 8 weeks after starting clozapine (350 mg/day) (146[c]).

Gastrointestinal *Hypersalivation* is a common and well-known adverse effect of clozapine (SEDA-20, 49). It has been suggested that it reflects an imbalance between M_3 muscarinic receptor blockade, leading to a reduction in salivation, and M_4 receptor stimulation, leading to an increase in salivation (147[r]). Trihexyphenidyl, an anticholinergic drug, has been proposed for the treatment of clozapine-induced hypersalivation (148[C]). Trihexyphenidyl 5–15 mg/day was given for 15 days to 14 patients with hypersalivation due to clozapine; there was a 44% reduction in hypersalivation.

Of 36 patients treated with clozapine, four developed *reflux esophagitis* within 6 weeks of starting clozapine (149[C]). Subsequent endoscopy showed moderately severe erosive esophagitis in three; one had taken treatment for a peptic ulcer in the past but the other two had no previous history of any upper gastrointestinal disorder. The authors suggested that the anticholinergic effect of clozapine predisposes towards reflux of stomach contents and may account for this adverse effect.

Constipation is an adverse effect that often has been associated with clozapine; it may be serious and even fatal (SEDA-20, 50). In 100 patients treated with clozapine, constipation was a major problem in four cases (all men); two patients refused to continue taking the drug, one (aged 60 years) had two general hospital admissions, and one (aged 49 years) died suddenly and unexpectedly (150[C]).

Necrotizing colitis is an adverse effect that rarely has been linked to neuroleptic drugs. The first case of this condition associated with clozapine has been reported (151[c]).

A 36-year-old man was given clozapine and the dosage was gradually increased to 600 mg/day, which he took for about 4 months. He then complained of feeling unwell and had abdominal discomfort. An emergency laparotomy showed marked dilatation of the colon. Death occurred within several hours, and autopsy showed a focal area with hemorrhagic adhesions of serosa in the distal ileum.

The authors suspected that clozapine, with its marked anticholinergic properties, had precipitated the colitis, and that the concomitant use of benztropine may have played a contributory role.

Urinary system *Enuresis* has been associated with clozapine (SEDA-19, 54; SEDA-20, 50; SEDA-21, 54). In 71 patients with clozapine therapy, there were seven cases of urinary incontinence (152[C]). Six cases arose de novo after the start of therapy, and one case represented an exacerbation of pre-existing stress urinary incontinence. In all cases the incontinence resolved with treatment, five with oxybutynin and two with intranasal desmopressin.

Immunological and hypersensitivity reactions A case of *polyserositis* that included concurrent pericarditis, pericardial effusion, and pleural effusion has been associated with clozapine treatment (153[c]).

A 21-year-old man had been given clozapine for 8 weeks for schizophrenia before developing tachypnea, tachycardia, and fever. He had pericardial and pleural effusions and constrictive pericarditis was suspected. He was treated after discharge with clozapine 200 mg bd and presented 9 days after discharge with tachycardia and congestive heart failure. Clozapine was withdrawn in favor of risperidone. Two months later he had no further cardiorespiratory problems.

Unilateral pleural effusion and cellulitis with eosinophilia but no pericarditis was associated with clozapine therapy in a 37-year-old man and recurred on rechallenge (154[c]).

Spiking *fevers* have been reported in three patients during the first 3 weeks of clozapine therapy (155[c]). The mechanisms are unknown, but an immunological reaction has been suggested, since recent studies have shown that clozapine increases the plasma concentrations of soluble interleukin-2 receptors, reaching a peak after 2 weeks (156[c]).

Risk factors *Children* Clozapine therapy in children and adolescents has previously been studied (SEDA-21, 53). In a recent study, 11 neuroleptic drug-resistant children, aged 9–13 years, with a diagnosis of schizophrenia were treated with clozapine and monitored for 16 weeks (157[C]). The adverse effects were *drowsiness* (90%), *hypersalivation* (90%), *non-*

specific excitatory EEG changes (2%), transient *psychomotor agitation* (27%), and transient *eosinophilia* (18%). There were no cases of agranulocytosis and extrapyramidal symptoms during this short time. The mean dosage at week 16 was 230 mg/day.

It is said that patients with organic brain disease are more prone to adverse effects of clozapine; thus, special care should be taken in this group. This has been observed in a double-blind randomized trial in 33 patients with Huntington's chorea (158[C]). They were given clozapine (a maximum of 150 mg/day) or placebo for a period of 31 days and all those treated with clozapine ($n = 17$) had some adverse effects, severe in some cases: six patients were unable to complete the trial because of adverse effects and a reduction in clozapine dose was necessary in eight patients. The adverse effects most often reported were *drowsiness* (14 patients), *dizziness* (six), *walking difficulties* (six), *fatigue* (four), and *hypersalivation* (four). In seven patients there was an *increase in liver enzymes*.

Genetic susceptibility The effect of genetic variation in the serotonin 5-HT_{2C} receptor in the response to clozapine ($n = 152$) has been studied (159[C]). There was no consistent association between genetic variation of the 5-HT_{2C} receptor and the observed adverse effects, but there was a positive association between electrocardiographic changes (including moderate to severe disturbance of background activity) and the 5-HT_{2C} variant (Ser23) in men who had taken clozapine for at least 56 days.

Clozapine-induced agranulocytosis has been associated with different HLA types and HSP70 variants, suggesting that a gene within the MHC region is associated with agranulocytosis. In a recent study common genetic markers for this disorder were compared in 33 schizophrenic patients (12 Jewish and 21 non-Jewish) who had agranulocytosis during treatment with clozapine with a control group of 33 genetically unrelated schizophrenic patients (18 Jewish and 15 non-Jewish) who had taken clozapine for at least 52 weeks but had not developed agranulocytosis (160[C]). Tumor necrosis factor microsatellites d3 and b4 were found in higher frequencies in both the Jewish and non-Jewish patients with agranulocytosis: 51 of 66 (77%) and 48 of 66 (57%), respectively. Comparisons of these frequencies with those of the controls (28 of 66 (42%) and 18 of 66 (27%)) were statistically significant. Tumor necrosis factor microsatellite b5 was under-represented in the patients with agranulocytosis (nine of 66 (14%)) compared with the control subjects (43 of 66 (65%)) and this was probably related to protection from clozapine-induced agranulocytosis.

Of 43 patients who were serotyped for human leukocyte antigens (HLA-A, HLA-B, HLA-C, and HLA-DQ antigens) three developed agranulocytosis (161[C]). One of those had a combination of both 'high-risk' haplotypes (HLA-B16(38,39), DR4, DQ3 and HLA-DR2, DQ1); another had HLA-DR2, DQ1; the last had a totally different haplotype. Of patients without agranulocytosis, one was found to carry the HLA-B16(38,39), DR4, DQ3 haplotype and 14 (of 40) had the HLA-DR2, DQ1 haplotype.

In a recent review of 58 patients taking clozapine, its metabolite, *N*-desmethylclozapine, was not a marker for impending clozapine-induced granulocytopenia and agranulocytosis (162[C]).

Withdrawal effects A case of *catatonia and neuroleptic malignant syndrome* in a 30-year-old man associated with clozapine withdrawal has been published (128[c]). Psychosis and/or delirium have also been previously associated with clozapine withdrawal (SED-13, 128; SEDA-20, 55). Three new case reports of clozapine withdrawal resulting in delirium with psychosis have been reported (163[c]); symptoms resolved rapidly and completely upon resumption of low doses of clozapine. The authors suggest that symptoms were perhaps the result of central cholinergic rebound. Other explanations involved serotonergic receptor alterations (164[r]).

Interactions The metabolism of clozapine appears to be largely controlled by CYP1A2 (165[r]). Compounds that induce CYP1A2 activity (*carbamazepine*, *tobacco*) can reduce plasma clozapine concentrations. Inhibitors of CYP1A2 (*caffeine*, *erythromycin*) have the opposite effect, but drugs that inhibit CYP2D6 have also been reported to increase plasma clozapine, although the mechanism of this interaction is unclear.

Serious symptoms due to dangerous interactions with *benzodiazepines* in patients treated with clozapine have been reported before (SEDA-19, 55; SEDA-20, 50). In a recent review of the published cases (166[R]), the authors stated that in a study in 189 patients exposed to the clozapine–benzodiazepine combination, 2.1% had severe drug interactions. However, according to unpublished data of the Novartis Pharmaceutical Corporation the risk was lower: 15 311 patients were treated with clozapine during the first 18 months of its reintroduction into the US and about 11% of these patients received concomitant benzodiazepine therapy. There were only six cases of respiratory depression/arrest, representing 0.31% of the clozapine–benzodiazepine group.

Potentially lethal gastrointestinal bleeding and marked hyperglycemia occurred in a 33-year-old man after *buspirone* had been added to clozapine (167[c]). The authors suggested that the addition of buspirone may have increased the serum concentration of clozapine, but the clozapine concentration was not determined.

Selective serotonin reuptake inhibitors can increase clozapine plasma concentrations (SEDA-19, 55; SEDA-20, 50; SEDA-21, 55).

Fluvoxamine caused worsening of their psychoses in two women aged 26 and 24 years (168[c]). Plasma clozapine concentrations were increased in correspondence to the worsening of their psychoses. In another case very high blood clozapine concentrations occurred during concomitant use of fluvoxamine (169[c]). The patient developed dizziness and mild hypotension while taking clozapine 200 mg/day. The blood clozapine concentration was 2040 ng/ml and fluvoxamine was withdrawn; 5 days later the clozapine concentration was 175 mg/ml.

The dose-dependence of the interaction between selective serotonin reuptake inhibitors and clozapine has been emphasized (170[c]).

A 53-year-old man taking clozapine 400 mg/day was given paroxetine 20 mg qds for depression. The clozapine plasma concentration was 1161 ng/ml (target range 100–800 ng/ml); 19 days later he developed an anticholinergic syndrome. At a later date, when he was taking paroxetine 20 mg qds and clozapine 200 mg/day (clozapine plasma concentrations 325–339 ng/ml), he did not have any anticholinergic symptoms.

There have been two reports of leukopenia associated with the combination of paroxetine with clozapine, after the patients had taken clozapine for 6–12 months without adverse effects (171[c]). Although clozapine might have caused the neutropenia itself, the time-course of the effect and the fact that paroxetine increases plasma clozapine concentrations suggested an interaction.

The combination of clozapine with the fluoroquinolone *ciprofloxacin* in a 72-year-old man led to a significant increase in plasma clozapine concentration (172[c]). Inhibition of CYP1A2 by ciprofloxacin may explain this.

A beneficial interaction of clozapine with *sulpiride* has been proposed in 28 patients, who were only partially responsive to clozapine and who were given additional sulpiride 600 mg/day or placebo double-blind for 10 weeks (173[C]). The addition of sulpiride produced substantially greater and significant improvements in psychotic symptoms. The major adverse effect was a 4- to 7-fold increase in serum prolactin. The authors suggested that the mechanism of action was synergistic enhancement of D_2 blockade, although pharmacokinetic interactions could not be ruled out, since both clozapine and sulpiride are metabolized by the cytochrome isozymes.

Monitoring therapy Clozapine plasma concentration measurement is not routinely used in clinical practice; clozapine fulfils a number of criteria that make it a candidate for therapeutic monitoring: an identifiable target range, an unpredictable dose–concentration relation between patients, a potential for clinically relevant pharmacokinetic interactions with other drugs, and a high probability of patient non-compliance. The therapeutic threshold plasma concentration is about 400 μg/l, and concentrations above 1000 μg/l increase the risk of adverse effects on the central nervous system (confusion, delirium, and generalized seizures) (174[r]). There is no evidence linking increased concentrations of clozapine or its metabolite to agranulocytosis.

Droperidol *(SEDA-19, 55; SEDA-20, 50; SEDA-21, 55)*

In an open-label study, 35 patients with migraine were treated with intravenous droperidol 2.5 mg every 30 min until either three doses had been given or the patient was completely or almost headache-free (175[C]). Four patients had an asymptomatic *fall in systolic blood pressure* of 20 mmHg or more. Most (34 of 35) were *sedated*. Five patients developed akathisia and one developed dystonia.

In a study of the analgesic efficacy and adverse effects of tramadol ($n = 18$) versus tramadol plus droperidol ($n = 16$) for post-operative patient-controlled analgesia over 48 h (176[C]) there were no major complications. The combination provided similar analgesia with less nausea and vomiting and without increased sedation.

In contrast, an anesthesiologist has recounted anecdotal experience of patients who have experienced unpleasant sensations subsequent to their previous anaesthetics, suspected of being induced by droperidol for postoperative nausea and vomiting (177[r]). The experiences were described as *agitation*, *'feeling trapped'*, *an inability to relax*, and *sleep disturbances coupled with nightmares*.

Flupenthixol

Skin and appendages Diagnosis of *photosensitivity* to flupenthixol has been made by photoprick testing (178[c]).

A 38-year-old psychotic man developed an erythematous eruption that first appeared on light-exposed skin. The lesions appeared and worsened after regular injections of flupenthixol. Whereas conventional photopatch testing was negative, photoprick gave a reaction to flupenthixol.

Haloperidol

Nervous system A possible *toxic encephalopathy* has been reported after high-dose intravenous haloperidol in a 54-year-old African-American man who had received 270 mg intravenously over the course of a day to control agitation (179[c]).

Intravenous haloperidol is commonly used to control delirium in critically ill patients and may cause *extrapyramidal symptoms* (180[c]).

A 55-year-old woman with respiratory distress syndrome was given haloperidol and over 3 weeks received a total of 910 mg of haloperidol intravenously and 108 mg intramuscularly. She developed masked facies, bradykinesia, cogwheel rigidity of her upper extremities, and a pill-rolling tremor of her hands. Haloperidol was withdrawn and she recovered over the next 8 days.

Differentiating between generalized psychotic agitation and akathisia that manifests as violence is clinically important in order to avoid a vicious cycle of violence in patients taking antipsychotic drugs. Violence has been attributed to haloperidol (181[c]).

A 47-year-old man was taken to the emergency room because he was screaming in the streets and was given haloperidol qds and benzotropine 1 mg every morning. Within 24 h he started pacing about, became restless, agitated, and violent, and attacked a staff member. On day 17 haloperidol was withdrawn and he became calmer and did not require further room restrictions. After 5 days haloperidol was restarted and again he became violent and required room restriction. Haloperidol was finally withdrawn and his agitation and violence resolved; a week later he was discharged.

Risk factors Two patients developed severe extrapyramidal adverse effects after discontinuing *clozapine* and starting haloperidol (182[c]). The authors therefore wondered whether clozapine had somehow changed receptor sensitivity, increasing vulnerability to the extrapyramidal adverse effects of haloperidol.

Withdrawal effects Another five cases of *movement disorders* associated with haloperidol withdrawal while in an intensive care unit have been reported (183[c]). Dosages were always above 240 mg/day, the duration of treatment was 14–23 days, and dyskinesia lasted 4–13 days. These five patients represented only 2% of patients in the unit who had received haloperidol.

Nemonapride

Nemonapride is a novel neuroleptic drug that has recently been marketed in Japan. It has been given in daily doses of 3–50 mg to 19 schizophrenic patients in an 8-week open-label trial (184[C]). The major adverse effects were *drowsiness* and *akathisia*, but there were no severe extrapyramidal symptoms.

Olanzapine *(SEDA-21, 56)*

Olanzapine, a thienobenzodiazepine with a receptor affinity profile similar to that of clozapine and a serotonin/dopamine receptor antagonist, became available in the US for the treatment of schizophrenia and other psychotic disorders in 1996.

Adverse effects from high dosages of olanzapine (30–40 mg/day) in patients with treatment-refractory schizophrenia have been described (185[c]). The current guidelines for using olanzapine in schizophrenia patients suggest a maximum dosage of 20 mg/day, and the safety of higher dosages has not yet been evaluated; however, many patients continue to have substantial psychopathology after several weeks of treatment.

Olanzapine has been compared with haloperidol and placebo, and according to a recent review (186[R]) olanzapine had been studied in over 2500 schizophrenic patients at the time of submission for regulatory approval in the US. The main conclusions were presented in last year's Annual (SEDA-21, 56). In a review of further published studies and abstracts of unpublished Phase III clinical trials provided by the manufacturer it was concluded that in general olanzapine was well tolerated with significantly fewer extrapyramidal adverse effects than haloperidol (187[R]). There were no significant hematological abnormalities nor increased prolactin. In contrast, there was a dose-related *increase in hepatic transaminases* in patients treated with olanzapine, and two anticholinergic adverse effects, *constipation* and *dry mouth*, occurred more often with olanzapine than with haloperidol. Significant *weight gain* occurred more often with olanzapine than with haloperidol.

In a more recent double-blind randomized comparison of olanzapine and haloperidol 335 in-patients with schizophrenia were given placebo (n = 68), low-dose olanzapine (n = 65), medium-dose olanzapine (n = 64), high-dose olanzapine (n = 69), or haloperidol (n = 69) for 52 weeks (188[C]). The mean modal maintenance doses of olanzapine for patients with at least 3 weeks of therapy were 6.6, 11.6, and 16.3 mg/day; the dose of haloperidol was 16.4 mg/day. There was significantly greater improvement with high-dose olanzapine than with placebo or haloperidol. The most common treatment-related adverse events across all five treatment groups were psychomotor slowing (*somnolence*, *weakness*) and psychomotor activation (*agitation*, *nervousness*, *insomnia*, *anxiety*). Only somnolence was significantly related to olanzapine dosage. Use of the Simpson–Angus scale for extrapyramidal adverse effects and the Barnes Akathisia Scale showed that mean scores from baseline to endpoint were not affected by olanzapine but were altered by haloperidol.

However, despite these comparisons, the exact place of olanzapine in the therapy of psychotic patients remains unclear (189[r]).

Less is known about how olanzapine compares with atypical neuroleptic drugs, such as clozapine. Such comparisons would be desirable, particularly for patients who are refractory to conventional neuroleptic drugs who have subsequently responded to clozapine (190[r]). However, olanzapine has been compared with risperidone in an international, multicenter, double-blind, parallel-group, 28-week prospective study in 339 patients who met DSM-IV criteria for schizophrenia, schizophreniform disorder, or schizoaffective disorder (olanzapine, n = 172; risperidone, n = 167) (191[C]). Both olanzapine (starting dosage 15 mg/day) and risperidone (starting dosage 1 mg bd) were effective in the management of psychotic symptoms. However, olanzapine had significantly greater efficacy in negative symptoms, as well as overall response rate, and a statistically significantly greater proportion of the olanzapine-treated than risperidone-treated patients maintained their response after 28 weeks. The most commonly observed adverse events were *somnolence*, *headache*, *insomnia*, *rhinitis*, *depression*, and *nausea*. *Weight gain* was reported significantly more often with olanzapine, whereas *nausea*, *amblyopia*, *extrapyramidal syndrome*, *increased salivation*, *attempted suicide*, *abnormal ejaculation*, *back pain*, *increased creatine phosphokinase*, and *urinary tract infection* were reported statistically significantly more often with risperidone. A significantly greater proportion of patients taking olanzapine had raised AlT activity at any time than those taking risperidone. Similarly, significantly more patients taking olanzapine had *low neutrophil counts* at any time (olanzapine 4.3%, risperidone 0.6%).

Nervous system Data from three multicenter, double-blind, randomized comparisons of olanzapine and haloperidol (SEDA-21, 56) have been reviewed and reanalysed by investigators from Eli Lilly, the manufacturers, with a focus on *extrapyramidal adverse effects* (192[C]) and *tardive dyskinesia* (193[CR]). Olanzapine had a better profile.

Four patients had improvement in preexisting tardive dyskinesia after olanzapine (194[c]). All required a maximum dosage of olanzapine (20 mg) for persistent psychotic symptoms, and the most significant reduction in AIMS scores occurred after 2 months of therapy, with a continuing but lesser reduction during the next 4 months.

Psychiatric In a study of treatment-refractory schizophrenic patients ($n = 25$) who received olanzapine 15–25 mg/day, one patient discontinued treatment because of depression, and the most common adverse effects were *anxiety* (in 36% of patients), *hallucinations* (20%), *delusions* (16%), and *insomnia*, *personality disorders*, and *schizophrenic reactions* (each in 12% of the patients) (195[C]).

Endocrine, metabolic Data from a trial (SEDA-21, 56) have been reanalysed in order to compare the effects of olanzapine and haloperidol on *serum prolactin concentrations* (196[CR]). Olanzapine increased the concentrations less than haloperidol (about one-half to one-third) and the rises were more transient.

Hematological Olanzapine is relatively free of hematological adverse effects, but three consecutive patients who were switched to olanzapine when they had reduced granulocyte counts associated with clozapine, had prolonged *granulocyte depression* (197[c]). The authors warned that until further evidence is available, it would be prudent to avoid starting olanzapine in patients with clozapine-induced granulocyte depression until the leukocyte count has normalized.

Withdrawal effects *Koro* is a Malay term that describes the intense fear that one's genitals are shrinking into the body and may recede into the abdomen, possibly causing death. This psychiatric disorder has been observed in ethnic Chinese, in association with organic mental illness, depression, anxiety, psychosis, and phobic disorder. A 19-year-old white man developed koro when he abruptly stopped taking olanzapine and recovered when olanzapine was subsequently restarted (198[c]).

Interactions An open-label, three-way randomized crossover study of olanzapine (5 mg) and *imipramine* (75 mg) alone and together has been carried out in nine healthy men, aged 32–54 years (199[C]). Sedation, postural hypotension, and minor alterations in vital signs occurred with all treatments. Olanzapine alone and in combination reduced motor-speed tasks (finger tapping and visual-arm random reach) compared with baseline or imipramine. Olanzapine concentrations were 19% greater when it was given with imipramine, but this difference was not significant. The authors concluded that olanzapine did not inhibit CYP2D6.

Quetiapine

In a 6-week, double-blind, randomized, multicenter, parallel-group comparison of quetiapine ($n = 101$) and chlorpromazine ($n = 100$) in hospitalized schizophrenics, the treatments were equally effective (200[C]). The most frequent adverse events with quetiapine were *somnolence* (14%) and *insomnia* (10%), but no other event was reported with an incidence over 10%. Severe adverse events with quetiapine included *anxiety* ($n = 4$), *agitation* ($n = 3$), and *hostility* ($n = 3$). Four patients withdrew owing to adverse events, including *generalized tonic–clonic seizures* and *increased alkaline phosphatase*, *AlT*, *AsT*, and *γ-glutamyltransferase*. In addition, one patient taking quetiapine withdrew on day 14, having developed mild *leukopenia* on day 7. There was a statistically significant difference in *akathisia* between treatment groups at the end of the study, and fewer patients in the quetiapine group had become 'worse' (5 vs 14%). Quetiapine was not associated with a sustained increase in serum prolactin. In contrast, there was clinically significant *weight gain* in a slightly higher proportion of patients taking quetiapine (27%) than chorpromazine (18%).

In another study 361 patients who completed a single-blind, placebo-washout phase were randomized double-blind to quetiapine (75, 150, 300, 600, or 750 mg/day), haloperidol (12 mg/day), or placebo, and were evaluated weekly for 6 weeks (201[C]). Quetiapine was no different from placebo across the dosage range studied regarding extrapyramidal symptoms and changes in prolactin concentrations. Three adverse events occurred at an incidence rate twice that of placebo, but none led to withdrawal: *headache*, *constipation*, and *dyspepsia*. *Agitation* and *insomnia* were reported in all the groups. *Postural hypotension*, in one patient, was the only adverse effect of quetiapine that led to withdrawal. There were significant *increases in AlT* in 17 patients taking quetiapine. Quetiapine was associated with a dose-dependent *fall in total* T_4 *and free* T_4 *concentrations*.

In a multicenter, double-blind, placebo-controlled trial, 286 hospitalized schizophrenic patients were randomized to 6 weeks of treatment with high-dose quetiapine (750 mg/day, $n = 96$), low-dose quetiapine (250 mg/day, $n = 94$), or placebo ($n = 96$) (202[C]). Of 280 patients in whom efficacy was evaluated, 159 (42% of those taking high-dose treatment, 57% of those taking low-dose treatment, and 59% of those taking placebo) withdrew before the end of the trial, primarily because of treatment failure. *Agitation* was the most frequently reported adverse event in each group, and *somnolence* occurred with quetiapine (25% in the high-dose group and 19% in the low-dose group) as well as with placebo (15%). Motor system adverse events were limited, and quetiapine had no clinically important effects on hematological measurements. Hepatic transaminase activities, particularly AlT, were significantly raised (three times the upper limit of the reference range) in 14 patients (five with high-dose quetiapine, eight with low-dose quetiapine, and one with placebo. At the end, differences among treatment groups were significant for mean changes from baseline in total triiodothyronine (T_3) and total thyroxine (T_4); for total T_4 the mean change from baseline in the low-dose group was also significantly greater than the mean change in the placebo group, suggesting dose-responsiveness. Treatment with quetiapine was associated with clinically significant *weight gain* in 25% of the patients in the high-dose group compared with 16% in the low-dose group and 5% in the placebo group.

Striatal D_2 receptor occupancy has been investigated with SPECT using [^{123}I]iodobenzamide in patients treated with quetiapine (n = 4), clozapine ($n = 6$), and haloperidol (n = 8), and in eight healthy controls (203[C]). There was significantly lower striatal D_2 occupancy with quetiapine and clozapine than with haloperidol, and there were no extrapyramidal motor adverse effects with quetiapine and clozapine. These data support the view that quetiapine is an atypical antipsychotic drug.

Risperidone *(SED-13, 118; SEDA-19, 55; SEDA-20, 52; SEDA-21, 57)*

Since the introduction in 1993 of the novel serotonin/dopamine receptor antagonist risperidone, over 12 million patient-months of exposure have accumulated, and it has been suggested to be more effective on negative symptoms of schizophrenia (204[R]). However, this suggested superiority of risperidone on negative symptoms may be artifactual, since standard neuroleptic drugs, supposedly because of extrapyramidal adverse effects, can mimic or exacerbate negative symptoms (205[R]).

In a open study 25 patients were assessed at baseline and after taking risperidone for 4 weeks (206[C]). All were selected because of prominence of negative symptoms, which improved with risperidone. The authors suggested that negative symptoms and cognitive deficit have a common underlying substrate, which is targeted by risperidone, and that certain cognitive deficits depend on negative symptoms.

Data from in two double-blind trials have

been reanalysed in a study supported by Janssen, the manufacturers (207[CR]). In these so-called North American trials, 513 patients were randomly assigned to receive placebo, fixed doses of risperidone (2, 6, 10, or 16 mg/day), or haloperidol 20 mg/day for 8 weeks. Risperidone was significantly better than haloperidol in reducing negative symptoms, even at the lowest dose (2 mg/day). Haloperidol was associated with substantially more severe *parkinsonism* than placebo or risperidone. The severity of parkinsonism tended to be higher at higher doses of risperidone, although at week 8 it was similar in patients taking placebo and risperidone 2–10 mg/day. If extrapyramidal symptoms produce or aggravate negative symptoms, as has been proposed, patients who took 10 or 16 mg/day, which produced more extrapyramidal symptoms than 6 mg/day, would have been expected to have lower improvement rates of negative symptoms than patients who took 6 mg/day of risperidone, and that was not the case, despite significantly greater improvements with 6 mg/day than 10 or 16 mg/day in three of the factors analysed.

Risperidone has been compared with conventional neuroleptic drugs in a recent meta-analysis of 11 randomized, double-blind, controlled trials (208[CR]). Slightly more patients taking risperidone improved (57 vs 52%; OR 1.04–1.56). Concomitant medications for extrapyramidal adverse effects were used significantly less often with risperidone than, for example, haloperidol (23 vs 38%; OR 0.51, 95% CI 0.41, 0.63). The drop-out rate was lower with risperidone (29 vs 34%; OR 0.75, 95% CI 0.61, 0.94). *Weight gain* and *tachycardia* were more common with risperidone.

In an open-label, multicenter phase IV study of the use of risperidone in 945 schizophrenic patients, 558 completed the 10-week trial (209[C]). The primary reason for premature discontinuation was an adverse event in 107 (11% of the total): *extrapyramidal adverse effects* (n = 22) and *nausea/vomiting* (22) were the main reasons. Information on adverse events was available for 842 patients, of whom 361 (43%) had at least one. The most frequent adverse effects were *insomnia* (5.9%), *nausea* (5.6%), *dizziness* (4.4%), *excessive sedation* (3.3%), and *headache* (3.2%). Severe adverse event occurred in 47 patients (5.6%), the most frequent being *agitation* (1.1%), *insomnia* (0.7%), and *dizziness* (0.7%). *Extrapyramidal adverse effects* were reported by 17 patients and akathisia by 16. However, the open design of this study makes it difficult to rely on the results.

Information on comparability with clozapine has recently come from a controlled double-blind, multicenter study in 86 in-patients randomly assigned to risperidone (n = 43) or clozapine (n = 43) for 8 weeks after a 7-day washout period (210[C]). After a 1-week dose-titration phase, dosages were fixed at 6 mg/day of risperidone and 300 mg/day of clozapine for 1 week and then adjusted according to response. The final mean doses were 6.4 mg/day of risperidone and 291 mg/day of clozapine. The drugs had similar efficacy. *Extrapyramidal symptoms* were few in the two groups and only three in each group needed antiparkinsonian drugs. Adverse events reported by 5% or more of patients were: *weakness*, *sedation*, *weight gain*, *failing memory*, *concentration difficulties*, *sleep disorders*, *nausea*, *dizziness*, and *reduced sexual drive*. There were no significant differences between the groups, except for weakness, which was reported by more patients taking clozapine than those taking risperidone. One patient in the risperidone group had *neutropenia* on days 7–9 of treatment.

As the number of novel antipsychotic drugs increases, switching among these agents becomes more probable. Clinical guidelines for these exchanges remain to be established. Of 28 patients who were taking risperidone and clozapine, 10 had taken both simultaneously and treatment was changed in other 18: six from clozapine to risperidone and 12 from risperidone to clozapine (211[C]). No patient who switched from risperidone to clozapine deteriorated, but two of the six patients who stopped clozapine had rapid worsening of psychotic symptoms. Overall, 50% of adverse effects occurred with clozapine alone, 29% with risperidone alone, and 21% during concurrent use. The rate of adverse effects was lowest with combined treatment (when monitoring would be intensified), and significantly lower than with clozapine alone. No adverse effects were unexpected or serious, regardless of the change in therapy. Cautious co-administration of therapeutic doses of risperidone and clozapine during gradual overlapping transition was well tolerated.

Cardiovascular *Fatal cardiac arrest* has been associated with risperidone (212[cr]).

A 34-year-old woman with no previous history of cardiac disease developed postural hypotension and her risperidone dosage was held at 2 mg bd; however, on day 5 of therapy she had a cardiac arrest and electromechanical dissociation. Her electrocardiogram showed a prolonged QRS complex (160 ms) and an abnormal QT_c interval (480 ms).

Nervous system *Extrapyramidal signs* In an open-label uncontrolled study, 22 patients with a first episode of schizophrenia were examined before any treatment and during and after treatment with risperidone (213[C]). The mean duration of treatment was 7.1 weeks and the endpoint was discharge from hospital. There were no clinically significant extrapyramidal adverse effects with risperidone 2–4 mg/day; however, with 5–8 mg/day 32% developed mild akathisia or parkinsonism, both of which diminished with dosage reduction.

D_2 receptor occupancy has been studied by [^{123}I]iodobenzamide SPECT in subjects treated with risperidone ($n = 12$) or haloperidol ($n = 7$) (214[C]). There was no significant difference. There was drug-induced parkinsonism in subjects treated with risperidone (42%) and haloperidol (29%) and it occurred at occupancies above 60%. The authors concluded that 5-HT_2 blockade with risperidone at D_2 occupancy rates of 60% and above does not protect against extrapyramidal adverse effects.

Severe extrapyramidal adverse effects occurred in a 55-year-old man with neurofibromatosis taking risperidone 4 mg/day (215[c]). The authors suggested that patients with frontal lobe damage may be at higher risk of complete occupancy of D_2 receptors, which in turn would negate the 5-HT_2-mediated protection against extrapyramidal symptoms.

Tardive dyskinesia Tardive dyskinesia associated with risperidone has been previously reported (SEDA-20, 53; SEDA-21, 59), although causality has been questioned (216[r]). However, new cases continue to be reported (217[c])–(219[c]). Patients with a history of psychiatric diseases had been exposed to risperidone for longer than 4 months.

Data from seven 1-year trials of risperidone in over 1100 patients, 503 of whom had taken this drug for at least 1 year, indicate that the annual incidence of tardive dyskinesia in patients taking risperidone (7.6–9.4 mg/day) is 0.3%, lower than 5–10% of conventional neuroleptic drugs. This is stated in a recent review carried out by investigators from the manufacturer, Janssen (204[R]).

Neuroleptic malignant syndrome New cases of neuroleptic malignant syndrome have been reported (220[c]), (221[c]). One occurred in a 73-year-old woman after monotherapy with risperidone and reversed after drug withdrawal and treatment with dantrolene and bromocriptine; the other was in a 75-year-old man who, after 3 weeks of risperidone, developed fever, mental changes, tremor, rigidity, increased serum creatine phosphokinase, hypernatremia, and metabolic acidosis. A 51-year-old man developed neuroleptic malignant syndrome without rigidity (222[cr]). The authors considered this syndrome to be atypical and pointed out that in seven published cases of neuroleptic malignant syndrome associated with risperidone, none occurred without rigidity.

Seizures Seizures occurred in an elderly woman treated with risperidone (223[c]).

A 64-year-old Chinese schizophrenic woman without seizures or a history of substance abuse was treated with risperidone, co-trimoxazole for a mild urinary tract infection, and astemizole. After 2 days, 9 h after taking the first four doses of risperidone, she had a single generalized tonic–clonic seizure lasting 1 min, with 5 min of postictal confusion. Risperidone and astemizole were withdrawn, while co-trimoxazole was continued for 7 days. Risperidone was restarted 15 days later in a lower dosage and she was free of seizures for 4 months.

The authors pointed out that seizures occurred in 0.3% (9/2607) of risperidone-treated patients during premarketing testing and that no postmarketing risperidone-associated seizure had been previously reported. They suggested that a drug interaction and age had been possible contributory elements.

Psychiatric Although it has been suggested

that risperidone has acute antimanic effects in some patients (224[c]), several cases of *behavioral stimulation*, *hypomania*, and *mania* have been reported (SEDA-20, 53; SEDA-21, 59). Two new cases in which risperidone was the only drug being taken (225[cr]) have suggested that this is probably a dose-related phenomenon. The emergence of mania was within 6 weeks in the first case and 3 weeks in the second. In the 13 previously reported cases, most patients developed mania within the first week and only one at 6 weeks. Two other cases of mania associated with risperidone have been reported in patients taking therapeutic dosages of lithium and valproate (226[c]).

Data from an open study that suggested efficacy of risperidone in patients with obsessive–compulsive symptoms have previously been published (SEDA-21, 57). However, two cases of risperidone-associated *obsessive–compulsive symptoms* have also been reported.

A 38-year-old woman with chronic paranoid schizophrenia developed obsessive–compulsive symptoms after she started to take risperidone (227[c]). This subsequently responded to clomipramine.

A 46-year-old man reported obsessive–compulsive symptoms after starting to take risperidone (228[c]). The severity of the symptoms was related to increasing doses of risperidone. As the obsessive–compulsive symptoms remained severe, he was given sertraline and improved.

A 21-year-old woman taking risperidone 0.5 mg bd had feelings of *generalized anxiety*, *visual distortions*, and *panic attacks*; her symptoms resolved on withdrawal of risperidone (229[c]).

Weight gain and *bulimia nervosa* has been reported in a 12-year-old girl (230[c]).

Endocrine, metabolic *Weight gain* is a relatively common adverse effect of risperidone (SEDA-21, 57). In a randomized, double-blind comparison of risperidone and clozapine, weight gain occurred in 23 and 37% of cases, respectively, after 2 months (210[C]). In a meta-analysis the incidence was 31% in subjects taking risperidone and 23% in controls, mainly taking haloperidol (208[C]). However, in a recent review of the reports collected by the manufacturers from postmarketing surveillance, it was suggested that weight gain over 13.6 kg occurs in less than 0.003% (231[R]). Children seem to be more prone to weight gain, and a recent study has suggested an association between long-term risperidone therapy, weight gain, and hepatotoxicity in children (232[C]).

Hyperprolactinemia and galactorrhea (SEDA-20, 53) occurred after 3 weeks of treatment with a low dose of risperidone in a 42-year-old premenstrual woman (233[c]).

Mineral and fluid balance *Hyponatremia* associated with risperidone has been reported, purportedly for the first time (234[c]).

A 48-year-old man without endocrine disease or polydipsia, not taking diuretics, and with no renal disease, started to take risperidone 6 mg/day. Seven days later, he developed hyponatremia, generalized seizures, and possible aspiration pneumonia.

It was assumed that the mechanism of hyponatremia was similar to that of other psychotropic medications, in that it was secondary to the syndrome of inappropriate antidiuretic hormone secretion.

Hematological Risperidone has rarely been associated with blood dyscrasias, such as leukopenia (SEDA-21, 59). Recently risperidone-induced *leukopenia and neutropenia* has been reported in a 63-year-old man (235[c]). He had previously developed a blood dyscrasia with clozapine.

Liver *Hepatotoxicity* has been reported with risperidone (SEDA-21, 59), and a new study has focused on this (232[C]). Hepatic adverse effects were sought in the medical records of 13 psychotic children taking risperidone (10 girls, three boys). Two boys who presented with obesity, liver enzyme abnormalities, and confirmatory evidence of fatty liver were identified, and in each case liver damage was reversed after withdrawal of risperidone.

It has been suggested that long-term risperidone therapy is probably associated with hepatotoxicity in boys. However, a causal relation has been questioned by investigators from Janssen, who have stated that raised liver function tests have a rate of two per

100 000 risperidone-treated children the US (236[r]).

Pancreas *Pancreatitis* associated with risperidone has been reported, purportedly for the first time (237[c]).

A 32-year-old man with schizophrenia, hypertension, and hypercholesterolemia, and with no history of hepatitis or HIV, was treated with risperidone, doxepin, benztropine mesylate, and nifedipine. Full dosage of risperidone (6 mg/day) was achieved after 2 weeks and 1 week later acute pancreatitis was diagnosed. Clinical and laboratory symptoms abated after withdrawal of risperidone without further intervention or consequence.

Urinary system Several cases of *enuresis* have previously been described in patients taking risperidone and a selective serotonin reuptake inhibitor (SSRI); the package insert of risperidone lists this adverse effect in up to 1% of patients (SEDA-21, 59). In the light of the case of a 33-year-old man who developed enuresis after risperidone monotherapy, it has been suggested that the frequency of enuresis may range from 1 to 10% in patients treated with combined risperidone and SSRIs (238[c]).

Special senses Effects on eye movement activity have been compared between risperidone and haloperidol in 20 patients (10 taking risperidone and 10 haloperidol) and 10 matched healthy subjects (239[C]). Risperidone, but not haloperidol, was associated with *prolonged latency and reduced peak velocity and accuracy of saccadic eye movements* 4 weeks after the start of treatment. The authors suggested that the adverse effects of risperidone may be due to the lack of development of acute tolerance to its powerful 5-HT_{2A} receptor antagonism, which could be responsible for disruption of brainstem physiology in regions that control saccadic eye movements.

Immunological and hypersensitivity reactions *Allergic reactions* are not common with risperidone.

A 67-year-old Japanese man had a severe allergic reaction to risperidone, resulting in edema, rash, and stridor (240[c]). The edema occurred 31 days after the start of therapy and lasted for 26 days, while the rash and stridor began after 43 and 46 days and lasted for 20 and 17 days, respectively.

It is not clear whether risperidone itself or the other components in the tablet contributed to this allergic reaction, and it is thus noteworthy that the Japanese version of the risperidone tablet includes wax in place of the pigment found in the US tablet.

Risk factors Several studies have addressed the efficacy and safety of risperidone in special groups of patients (SEDA-21, 57), and there have since been further studies.

Age Of 122 geriatric patients (age range 65–95 years) newly treated with risperidone, 18% were withdrawn because of intolerability (11%) or inefficacy (7%) (241[C]). There were adverse events in 32% of the patients (36% of those who withdrew); these included *hypotension* (29% of total adverse events), *symptomatic orthostatic hypotension* (10%), *cardiac arrest* (1.6%) with *death* (0.8%), *extrapyramidal adverse effects* (11%), and *delirium* (1.6%).

Schizophrenia has been recognized in childhood, although there has not been much experience with neuroleptic drugs in children. Risperidone has been used in an 8-year-old boy (242[c]). Adverse effects included *drowsiness* and a 21% *weight gain* (6.3 kg) during treatment with 2 mg/day for 4 months.

In an open study, six autistic children (aged 5–9 years) were treated with risperidone (mean dosage 1.1 mg/day) (243[C]). After 8 weeks the most common adverse effect was *weight gain* (range 0.5–3.1 kg). *Sedation* occurred in two.

In another study, 11 men (mean age, 18 years) with explosive aggressive autism improved with risperidone 0.5–1.5 mg/day (244[C]). *Weight gain* was a prominent adverse effect (average increase 0.47 kg/week).

Withdrawal effects An association between risperidone and withdrawal-emergent *dyskinesia* has been previously reported (SEDA-21, 60). A case of a Tourette-like syndrome has now been published, as an episode of withdrawal dyskinesia in a 12-year-old child when risperidone was discontinued (245[c]).

Protracted *akathisia* occurred in a 69-year-old woman and persisted for 8 weeks after risperidone withdrawal (246[c]).

Overdosage Two cases of overdosage have been reported (247[c]), (248[c]).

A 15-year-old girl took an acute overdose of risperidone 40 mg and 1.5 h later developed prolonged hypotension and orthostasis.

A 35-year-old woman took 228 mg of risperidone and was unaffected, except for akathisia; the only abnormal laboratory result was a mildly raised lactic dehydrogenase.

Interactions Severe extrapyramidal adverse effects and possible laryngospasm occurred in a 26-year-old man taking low-dose risperidone and *fluoxetine*, and a pharmacokinetic interaction was suggested (249[c]). However, it is also possible that fluoxetine interacted pharmacodynamically with risperidone, since fluoxetine has caused a variety of acute extrapyramidal adverse effects even when used as monotherapy (250[r]).

Carbamazepine caused a greater than 2-fold reduction in the plasma risperidone concentration in a 22-year-old extensive metabolizer (251[c]). Since carbamazepine induces CYP3A, this isozyme may participate in the metabolism of risperidone. There may thus be interactions with other drugs that affect CYP3A. This is of particular interest, since risperidone is known to be metabolized by CYP2D6.

Sertindole

Sertindole is a novel antipsychotic medication that was approved in several countries in 1997. It is a phenylindole derivative with high potency as a D_2 dopamine receptor antagonist and also has affinity for $5HT_2$ receptors.

The manufacturers, Abbot Laboratories (USA) and H. Lunbeck (Denmark), recently voluntarily suspended sertindole in the UK and other European countries. This followed concerns about reports of *cardiac dysrhythmias and sudden cardiac death* associated with sertindole (252[r]). Different studies had identified cardiac abnormalities that had not been considered worrisome. For instance, in a multicenter, double-blind, placebo-controlled study of sertindole (12, 20, and 24 mg/day), haloperidol (4, 8, and 16 mg/day), and placebo in treating psychotic symptoms in 497 patients with schizophrenia, both drugs were effective (253[C]). Analysis of more than 2700 electrocardiograms showed that the QT and QT_c intervals were significantly prolonged in all three sertindole groups. Although there were significant differences in mean changes from baseline, there were no statistically significant differences between any sertindole group and placebo in the percentages of patients who had a QT or QT_c interval 500 ms or longer at any time during the study. In addition, no electrocardiographic changes were related to clinical signs or symptoms (e.g. syncope) and there were no dysrhythmias (e.g. torsade de pointes) in any of the sertindole groups. For all extrapyramidal symptoms, sertindole was indistinguishable from placebo, changes in hematological and clinical chemistry measures were insignificant, and there was no evidence of agranulocytosis or liver dysfunction. Only 5.6% of patients discontinued sertindole because of adverse events, while 9.1% discontinued haloperidol. Nasal congestion and reduced ejaculatory volume occurred more often with sertindole. Body weight increased by 2.2–3.3 kg with haloperidol 8 mg and with all three dosages of sertindole; these increases were significantly greater than with placebo.

Four clinical trials have been reviewed on behalf of the manufacturers, not surprisingly supporting the claim that sertindole 12–24 mg/day is a potent antipsychotic drug (254[R]). Its most distinctive characteristic is a reduction in motor adverse effects, compared with traditional antipsychotic drugs. It's two most noteworthy adverse effects are *QT interval prolongation* and *reduced ejaculatory volume*, reversible on withdrawal in the 20% of patients in whom it occurs. Three studies have provided data about the lengthening of the QT interval with sertindole: 22–26, 11–21, and 19 ms on average. In one of them, 3% of the patients had a QT_c interval longer than 500 ms.

In five patients with schizophrenia and more than 30 patient-months of exposure, sertindole was associated with slight increases in QT_c that were not considered clinically significant, and abnormal ejaculation, which was one patient's reason for withdrawing from the study (255[c]).

Interaction In a 30-year-old man sertindole significantly worsened the symptoms of *paroxetine* withdrawal (256[c]). The authors noted the possible increased risk of a serotonergic withdrawal syndrome with paroxetine in patients being treated with sertindole.

Sulpiride

Nervous system Levosulpiride has been associated with *parkinsonism and dyskinesia* (257[c]).

A 60-year-old woman, who for 2 years had taken levosulpiride 100 mg/day, clomipramine 75 mg/day, and diazepam 10 mg/day for a depressive disorder, developed resting tremor, rigidity, and bradykinesia. Levosulpiride and clomipramine were withdrawn, and her parkinsonism improved. A few weeks after withdrawal she developed a severe tongue-jaw-lip dyskinesia, which persisted until the last follow-up visit 6 months later.

Endocrine, metabolic Neuroleptic drug-induced endocrine imbalance presumed to be involved in the development of *obesity* has been studied in young women who were randomized to sulpiride (n = 17) or placebo (n = 17) (258[C]). Although the women treated with sulpiride gained more body weight, the difference was not statistically significant. Prolactin concentrations were significantly increased by sulpiride and 17β-estradiol concentrations fell. The latter is said to affect the ratio of estradiol to testosterone, increasing androgenic activity, as observed in women with well-established obesity. The authors concluded that this effect, along with genetic predisposition, increased appetite, hypoactivity, and ignorance of proper dietary habits, may explain the excessive weight gain and obesity observed in women during chronic treatment with sulpiride or other antipsychotic agents.

Interaction A beneficial interaction of sulpiride with *clozapine* is discussed above under clozapine (173[C]).

Veralipride

Respiratory dyskinesia occurred in a 52-year-old woman taking veralipride (259[c]). After 4 months she started to have buccolingual movements and marked dyspnea, which caused difficult irregular breathing and severe thoracic discomfort. After drug withdrawal there was a progressive improvement and then resolution of her symptoms. Respiratory dyskinesia is seldom described, probably because it is only detected when it is severe enough to cause functional effects.

Zotepine

Plasma concentrations of zotepine and prolactin and adverse effects were monitored for 36 h after the administration of a single oral dose of zotepine 25 mg to 14 healthy men (260[C]). *Changes in prolactin concentrations* and adverse effect scores were correlated with drug concentrations. There was *sleepiness* and *difficulty in concentrating* in all the subjects. Other frequent adverse effects were *reduced salivation* (n = 9), *weakness* (n = 7), and *orthostatic dizziness* (n = 4).

Two cases of *acute deep vein thrombosis* after the administration of a combination of paroxetine and zotepine have been reported (261[c]).

REFERENCES

1. Casey DE. The relationship of pharmacology to side effects. J Clin Psychiatry 1997;58 (Suppl 10):55–62.
2. Lachaux B, Sechter D, Morasz L, Adouard D. Une nouvelle lecture des effets secondaires en matière de prescription des neuroleptiques. Encèphale 1997;23 (Special Issue II):25–34.
3. Hansen TE, Casey DE, Hoffman WF. Neuroleptic intolerance. Schizophr Bull 1997;23:567–82.
4. Popli AP, Hegarty JD, Siegel AJ, Kando JC, Tohen M. Transfer of psychiatric inpatients to a general hospital due to adverse drug reactions. Psychosomatics 1997;38:35–7.
5. Mossman D. A decision analysis approach to neuroleptic dosing: insights from a mathematical model. J Clin Psychiatry 1997;58:66–73.
6. Burggraf GW. Are psychotropic drugs at therapeutic levels a concern for cardiologists? Can J Cardiol 1997;13:75–80.
7. Lawrence KR, Nasraway SA. Conduction disturbances associated with administration of butyrophenone antipsychotics in the critically ill: a review of the literature. Pharmacotherapy 1997; 17:531–7.
8. Jackson T, Ditmanson L, Phibbs B. Torsade de pointes and low-dose oral haloperidol. Arch Intern Med 1997;157:2013–15.
9. Montastruc JL, Laborie I, Bagheri H, Senard JM. Drug-induced orthostatic hypotension. A five-year experience in a regional pharmacovigilance centre in France. Clin Drug Invest 1997;14:61–5.
10. Cherin P, Colvez A, Deville de Periere G, Sereni D. Risk of syncope in the elderly and consumption of drugs: a case-control study. J Clin Epidemiol 1997;50:313–20.
11. Kumar A. Sudden unexplained death in a psychiatric patient—a case report: the role of phenothiazines and physical restraint. Med Sci Law 1997;37:170–5.
12. Joseph KS. Asthma mortality and antipsychotic or sedative use. What is the link? Drug Saf 1997;16:351–4.
13. Brady JP. Drug-induced stuttering: a review of the literature. J Clin Psychopharmacol 1998; 18:50–4.
14. Levine J, Martine T, Feraro R, Kimhi R, Bracha HS. Medicated chronic schizophrenic patients do not demonstrate left turning asymmetry. Neuropsychobiology 1997;36:22–4.
15. Miller CH, Mohr F, Umbricht D, Woerner M, Fleischhacker WW, Lieberman JA. The prevalence of acute extrapyramidal signs and symptoms in patients treated with clozapine, risperidone, and conventional antipsychotics. J Clin Psychiatry 1998;59:69–75.
16. Sallee FR, Nesbitt L, Jackson C, Sine L, Sethuraman G. Relative efficacy of haloperidol and pimozide in children and adolescents with Tourette's disorder. Am J Psychiatry 1997;154:1057–62.
17. Wurthmann C, Klieser E, Lehmann E. Side effects of low dose neuroleptics and their impact on clinical outcome in generalized anxiety disorder. Prog Neuropsychopharmacol Biol Psychiatry 1997;21:601–9.
18. Casey DE. Will the new antipsychotics bring hope of reducing the risk of developing extrapyramidal syndromes and tardive dyskinesia? Int Clin Psychopharmacol 1997;12 (Suppl 1):S19–27.
19. Weiden PJ, Aquila R, Dalheim L, Standard JM. Switching antipsychotic medications. J Clin Psychiatry 1997;58 (Suppl 10):63–72.
20. Holloman LC, Marder SR. Management of acute extrapyramidal effects induced by antipsychotic drugs. Am J Health-Syst Pharm 1997; 54:2461–77.
21. Jiménez-Jiménez FJ, García-Ruíz PJ, Molina JA. Drug-induced movement disorders. Drug Saf 1997;16:180–204.
22. Dhopesh V, Macfadden A, Maany I, Gamble G. Absence of parkinsonism among patients in long-term neuroleptic therapy who abuse cocaine. Psychiatr Serv 1997;48:95–7.
23. Caligiuri MP, Lohr JB. Instrumental motor predictors of neuroleptic-induced parkinsonism in newly medicated schizophrenia patients. J Neuropsychiatry Clin Neurosci 1997;9:562–7.
24. Krakowski M, Czobor P, Volavka J. Effect of neuroleptic treatment on depressive symptoms in acute schizophrenic episodes. Psychiatr Res 1997;71:19–26.
25. Caligiuri MP, Rockwell E, Jeste DV. Extrapyramidal side effects in patients with Alzheimer's disease treated with low-dose neuroleptic medication. Am J Geriatr Psychiatry 1998;6:75–82.
26. Meszaros K, Lenzinger E, Hornik K, Schönbeck G, Hatzinger R, Langer G, Sieghart W, Aschauer HN. Biperiden and haloperidol plasma levels and extrapyramidal side effects in schizophrenic patients. Neuropsychobiology 1997; 36:69–72.
27. Lane H-Y, Lin H-N, Hu OY-P, Chen C-C, Jann MW, Chang W-H. Blood levels of reduced haloperidol versus clinical efficacy and extrapyramidal side effects of haloperidol. Prog Neuro-Psychopharmacol Biol Psychiatry 1997;21:299–311.
28. Tugg LA, Desai D, Prendergast P, Remington G, Reed K, Zipursky RB. Relationship between negative symptoms in chronic schizophrenia and neuroleptic dose, plasma levels and side effects. Schizophr Res 1997;25:71–8.
29. Weisbard JJ, Pardo M, Pollack S. Symptom change and extrapyramidal side effects during acute haloperidol treatment in chronic geriatric schizophrenics. Psychopharmacol Bull 1997; 33:119–22.
30. Storey E, Lloyd J. Tardive tremor. Mov Disord 1997;12:808–10.
31. Kasper S, Barnas C, Heiden A, Volz HP, Laakmann G, Zeit H, Pfolz H. Pramipexole as adjunct to haloperidol in schizophrenia. Safety

and efficacy. Eur Neuropsychopharmacol 1997; 7:65–70.

32. Miller CH, Hummer M, Oberbauer H, Kurzthaler I, DeCol C, Fleischhacker WW. Risk factors for the development of neuroleptic induced akathisia. Eur Neuropsychopharmacol 1997;7:51–5.
33. Bodfish JW, Newell KM, Sprague RL, Harper VN, Lewis MH. Akathisia in adults with mental retardation: development of the akathisia ratings of movement scale (ARMS). Am J Ment Retard 1997;101:413–23.
34. Brüne M, Schröder SG. Neuroleptic-induced akathisia and early onset tardive dyskinesia in affective disorder due to Cushing's syndrome. Gen Hosp Psychiatry 1997;19:445–7.
35. Anfang MK, Pope HG. Treatment of neuroleptic-induced akathisia with nicotine patches. Psychopharmacology 1997;134:153–6.
36. Poyurovsky M, Weizman A. Serotonergic agents in the treatment of acute neuroleptic-induced akathisia: open-label study of buspirone and mianserin. Int Clin Psychopharmacol 1997; 12:263–8.
37. Amir I, Hermesh H, Gavish A. Bruxism secondary to antipsychotic drug exposure: a positive response to propranolol. Clin Neuropharmacol 1997;20:86–9.
38. Swartz JR, Burgoyne K, Smith M, Gadasally R, Ananth J, Ananth K. Tardive dyskinesia and ethnicity: review of the literature. Ann Clin Psychiatry 1997;9:53–9.
39. Yamada K, Kanba S, Anamizu S, Ohnishi K, Ashikari I, Yagi G, Asai M. Low superoxide dismutase activity in schizophrenic patients with tardive dyskinesia. Psychol Med 1997;27:1223–5.
40. Caligiuri MP, Lacro JP, Rockwell ER, McAdams LA, Jeste DV. Incidence and risk factors for severe tardive dyskinesia in older patients. Br J Psychiatry 1997;171:148–53.
41. Chen C-H, Wei F-C, Koong F-J, Hsiao K-J. Association of TaqI a polymorphism of dopamine D_2 receptor gene and tardive dyskinesia in schizophrenia. Biol Psychiatry 1997;41:827–9.
42. Steen VM, Lovlie R, MacEwan T, McCreadie RG. Dopamine D_3-receptor gene variant and susceptibility to tardive dyskinesia in schizophrenic patients. Mol Psychiatry 1997;2:139–45.
43. Jeste DV, Kelsoe JR. Schizophrenia, tardive dyskinesia, and a D_3 receptor gene variant: a new twist on dyskinesias? Mol Psychiatry 1997;2:86–8.
44. Van Os J, Fahy T, Jones P, Harvey I, Toone B, Murray R. Tardive dyskinesia: who is at risk? Acta Psychiatr Scand 1997;96:206–16.
45. Labbate LA, Lande RG, Jones F, Oleshansky MA. Tardive dyskinesia in older out-patients: a follow-up study. Acta Psychiatr Scand 1997; 96:195–8.
46. Bailey L, Maxwell S, Brandabur MM. Substance abuse as a risk factor for tardive dyskinesia: a retrospective analysis of 1,027 patients. Psychopharmacol Bull 1997;33:177–81.
47. Arthur H, Dahl M-L, Siwers B, Sjöqvist F. Polymorphic drug metabolism in schizophrenic patients with tardive dyskinesia. J Clin Psychopharmacol 1995;15:211–16.
48. Andreassen OA, MacEwan T, Gulbrandsen AK, McCreadie RG, Steen VM. Non-functional CYP2D6 alleles and risk for neuroleptic-induced movement disorders in schizophrenic patients. Psychopharmacology 1997;131:174–9.
49. Armstrong M, Daly AK, Blennerhassett R, Ferrier N, Idle JR. Antipsychotic drug-induced movement disorders in schizophrenics in relation to CYP2D6 genotype. Br J Psychiatry 1997; 170:23–6.
50. Van Harter PN, Hoek HW, Matroos GE, Koeter M, Kahn RS. The inter-relationships of tardive dyskinesia, parkinsonism, akathisia and tardive dystonia: the Curaçao extrapyramidal syndromes study II. Schizophr Res 1997;26:235–42.
51. Van Harter PN, Hoek HW, Matroos GE, Koeter M, Kahn RS. Intermittent neuroleptic treatment and risk for tardive dyskinesia: Curaçao extrapyramidal syndromes study III. Am J Psychiatry 1998;155:565–7.
52. Tawara Y, Nishikawa T, Koga I, Uchida Y, Yamawaki S. Transient and intermittent oral dyskinesia appearing in a young woman ten days after neuroleptic treatment. Clin Neuropharmacol 1997;20:175–8.
53. Burn DJ, Coulthard A, Connolly S, Cartlidge NEF. Tardive diaphragmatic flutter. Mov Disord 1998;13:190–2.
54. Fritze J, Spreda I. Tolerability of low dose neuroleptics: a case control study of flupenthixol. Eur Neuropsychopharmacol 1997;7:261–6.
55. Campbell M, Armenteros JL, Malone RP, Adams PB, Eisenberg ZW, Overall JE. Neuroleptic-related dyskinesias in autistic children: a prospective, longitudinal study. J Am Acad Child Adolesc Psychiatry 1997;36:835–43.
56. Connor DF. Stimulants and neuroleptic withdrawal dyskinesia. J Am Acad Child Adolesc Psychiatry 1998;37:247–8.
57. Cowen MA, Green M, Bertollo DN, Abbott K. A treatment for tardive dyskinesia and some other extrapyramidal symptoms. J Clin Psychopharmacol 1997;17:190–3.
58. Weetman J, Anderson IM, Gregory RP, Gill SS. Bilateral posteroventral pallidotomy for severe antipsychotic induced tardive dyskinesia and dystonia. J Neurol Neurosurg Psychiatry 1997; 63:554–6.
59. Sokoloff LG, Pavlakovic R. Neuroleptic-induced dysphagia. Dysphagia 1997;12:177–9.
60. Van Harten PN, Van Trier JC, Horwitz EH, Matroos GE, Hoek HW. Cocaine as a risk factor for neuroleptic-induced acute dystonia. J Clin Psychiatry 1998;59:128–30.
61. Modrego Pardo P, Pérez-Trullen JM. Distonía aguda recurrente secundaria a la supresión de neurolépticos. Rev Clin Esp 1997;197:211–12.
62. Sampath G, Pandurangi AK. Bilateral ulnar nerve paralysis: an unreported complication of drug-induced extrapyramidal rigidity. Aust NZ J Psychiatry 1997;31:427–8.

63. Bhopale S, Seidel JS. Dystonic reaction to a phenothiazine presenting as Bell's palsy. Ann Emerg Med 1997;30:234–6.
64. Ilchef R. Neuroleptic-induced laryngeal dystonia can mimic anaphylaxis. Aust NZ J Psychiatry 1997;31:877–9.
65. Dannon PN, Grunhaus L, Iancu I, Braf A, Lepkifker E. Vitamin E treatment in tardive dystonia. Clin Neuropharmacol 1997;20:434–7.
66. Brashear A, Ambrosius WT, Eckert GJ, Siemers ER. Comparison of treatment of tardive dystonia and idiopathic cervical dystonia with botulinum toxin type A. Mov Disord 1998;13:158–61.
67. Krack P, Schneider S, Deuschl G. Geste device in tardive dystonia with retrocollis and opisthotonic posturing. Mov Disord 1998;13:155–7.
68. Sachdev P, Mason C, Hadzi-Pavlovic D. Case-control study of neuroleptic malignant syndrome. Am J Psychiatry 1997;154:1156–8.
69. Hernández JL, Palacios-Araus L, Echevarría S, Herran A, Campo JF, Riancho JA. Neuroleptic malignant syndrome in the acquired immunodeficiency syndrome. Postgrad Med J 1997;73:779–84.
70. Ray JG. Neuroleptic malignant syndrome associated with severe thrombocytopenia. J Intern Med 1997;241:245–7.
71. Hollister LE. Antipsychotic drug-induced dysphoria. Br J Psychiatry 1997;170:387–90.
72. Bloch M, Stager S, Braun A, Calis KA, Turcasso NM, Grothe DR, Rubinow DR. Pimozide-induced depression in men who stutter. J Clin Psychiatry 1997;58:433–6.
73. McShane R, Keene J, Gedling K, Fairburn C, Jacoby R, Hope T. Do neuroleptic drugs hasten cognitive decline in dementia? Prospective study with necropsy follow up. Br Med J 1997;314:266–70.
74. Holmes C, Fortenza O, Powell J, Lovestone S. Do neuroleptic drugs hasten cognitive decline in dementia? Carriers of apolipoprotein E e4 allele seem particularly susceptible to their effect. Br Med J 1997;314:1411.
75. Tobiansky R, Blanchard M. Do neuroleptic drugs hasten cognitive decline in dementia? Trials must determine which neuroleptics are best in dementia. Br Med J 1997;314:1411
76. Bentham PW, Goh SE, Gregg EM, Madeley P, Patel AR, Taylor AP. Do neuroleptic drugs hasten cognitive decline in dementia? Authors have not proved their argument. Br Med J 1997;314:1412.
77. McShane R, Hope T, Jacoby R, Keene J. Do neuroleptic drugs hasten cognitive decline in dementia? Authors' reply. Br Med J 1997; 314:1412.
78. Finkelstein JRJ, Cannon TD, Gur RE, Gur RC, Moberg P. Attentional dysfunctions in neuroleptic-naive and neuroleptic-withdrawn schizophrenic patients and their siblings. J Abnorm Psychol 1997;106:203–12.
79. Gilbertson MW, Van Kammen DP. Recent and remote memory dissociation: medication effects and hippocampal function in schizophrenia. Biol Psychiatry 1997;42:585–95.
80. Allen DN, Gilbertson MW, Van Kammen DP, Kelley ME, Gurklis JA, Barry EJ. Chronic haloperidol treatment does not affect structure of attention in schizophrenia. Schizophr Res 1997;25:53–61.
81. Davies PH. Drug-related hyperprolactinaemia. Adverse Drug React Toxicol Rev 1997; 16:83–94.
82. Al-Adwani A. Neuroleptics and bone mineral density. Am J Psychiatry 1997;154:1173.
83. Storch DD. Gynecomastia with antipsychotics. J Am Acad Child Adolesc Psychiatry 1997;36:161.
84. Yen C-F, Chong M-Y, Kuo M-C, Chang C-S. Severe granulocytopenia secondary to chlorpromazine despite concurrent lithium treatment: a case report. Kaohsiung J Med Sci 1997;13:635–8.
85. Bagheri H, Schmitt L, Berlan M, Montastruc JL. A comparative study of the effects of yohimbine and anetholtrithione on salivary secretion in depressed patients treated with psychotropic drugs. Eur J Clin Pharmacol 1997;52:339–42.
86. Gutzmann H, Kühl K-P, Kanowski S, Khan-Boluki J. Measuring the efficacy of psychopharmacological treatment of psychomotoric restlessness in dementia: clinical evaluation of tiapride. Pharmacopsychiatry 1997;30:6–11.
87. Benazzi F. Urinary retention with venlafaxine-haloperidol combination. Pharmacopsychiatry 1997;30:27.
88. Alvi T, Reza H. Neuroleptic induced incontinence: case report. J Pak Med Assoc 1997;47:195–6.
89. Higuchi H, Shimizu T, Hishikawa Y. Recurrent paroxysmal episodes characterized by perceptual alteration in three schizophrenic patients on neuroleptic medication. Psychiatry Clin Neurosci 1997;51:99–101.
90. Michielsen D, Lamberts G, De Boe V, Braeckman J, Keuppens F. Prothipendylhydrochloride-induced priapism: case report. Acta Urol Belg 1997;65:43–4.
91. Siegel JF, Reda E. Intracorporeal phenylephrine reduces thioridazine (Mellaril) induced priapism in a child. J Urol 1997;157:648.
92. Hatch DA. Re: intracorporeal phenylephrine reduces thioridazine (Mellaril) induced priapism in a child. J Urol 1997;158:888–9.
93. Viguera AC, Baldessarini RJ, Hegarty JD, Van Kammen DP, Tohen M. Clinical risk following abrupt and gradual withdrawal of maintenance neuroleptic treatment. Arch Gen Psychiatry 1997;54:49–55.
94. Bridges-Parlet S, Knopman D, Steffes S. Withdrawal of neuroleptic medications from institutionalized dementia patients: results of a double-blind, baseline-treatment-controlled pilot study. J Geriatr Psychiatry Neurol 1997;10:119–26.
95. Trixler M, Tényi T. Antipsychotic use in pregnancy. Drug Saf 1997;16:403–10.
96. Gex-Fabry M, Balant-Gorgia AE, Balant LP. Therapeutic drug monitoring databases for postmarketing surveillance of drug-drug interactions:

evaluation of a paired approach for psychotropic medication. Ther Drug Monit 1997;19:1–10.
97. Otani K, Ishida M, Yasui N, Kondo T, Mihara K, Suzuki A, Furukori H, Kaneko S, Inoue Y. Interaction between carbamazepine and bromperidol. Eur J Clin Pharmacol 1997;52:219–22.
98. Suzuki A, Otani K, Ishida M, Yasui N, Kondo T, Mihara K, Kaneko S, Inoue Y, Shibata M, Ikeda K. Increased plasma concentrations of bromperidol and its reduced metabolite with levomepromazine, but not with thioridazine. Ther Drug Monit 1997;19:261–4.
99. Otani K, Ishida M, Yasui N, Kondo T, Mihara K, Suzuki A, Kaneko S, Inoue Y, Shibata M, Ikeda K. No effect of the anticholinergic drugs trihexyphenidyl and biperiden on the plasma concentrations of bromperidol and its reduced metabolite. Ther Drug Monit 1997;19:165–8.
100. Mulsant BH, Foglia JP, Sweet RA, Rosen J, Lo KH, Pollock BG. The effects of perphenazine on the concentration of nortriptyline and its hydroxymetabolites in older patients. J Clin Psychopharmacol 1997;17:318–21.
101. Ozdemir V, Naranjo CA, Herrmann N, Reed K, Sellers EM, Kalow W. Paroxetine potentiates the central nervous system side effects of perphenazine: contribution of cytochrome P4502D6 inhibition in vivo. Clin Pharmacol Ther 1997;62:334–47.
102. Kurlan R. Acute parkinsonism induced by the combination of a serotonin reuptake inhibitor and a neuroleptic in adults with Tourette's syndrome. Mov Disord 1998;13:178–9.
103. Lane H-Y, Hu OY-P, Jann MW, Deng H-C, Lin H-N, Chang W-H. Dextromethorphan phenotyping and haloperidol disposition in schizophrenic patients. Psychiatry Res 1997;69:105–11.
104. Loo H, Poirier-Littre MF, Theron M, Rein W, Fleurot O. Amisulpride versus placebo in the medium-term treatment of the negative symptoms of schizophrenia. Br J Psychiatry 1997;170:18–22.
105. Möller HJ, Boyer P, Fleurot O, Rein W. Improvement of acute exacerbations of schizophrenia with amisulpride: a comparison with haloperidol. Psychopharmacology 1997;132:396–401.
106. Freeman HL. Amisulpride compared with standard neuroleptics in acute exacerbations of schizophrenia: three efficacy studies. Int Clin Psychopharmacol 1997;12 (Suppl 2):S11–17.
107. Vargas-Alarcón G, Yamamoto-Furusho JK, Zuòiga J, Canoso R, Granados J. HLA-DR7 in association with chlorpromazine-induced lupus anticoagulant (LA). J Autoimmun 1997;10:579–83.
108. Rosenheck R, Cramer J, Xu W, Thomas J, Henderson W, Frisman L, Fye C, Charney D. A comparison of clozapine and haloperidol in hospitalized patients with refractory schizophrenia. New Engl J Med 1997;337:809–15.
109. Lindström LH, Lundberg T. Long-term effect on outcome of clozapine in chronic therapy-resistant schizophrenic patients. Eur Psychiatry 1997;12 (Suppl 5):353s-5s.
110. Hong CJ, Chen JY, Chiu HJ, Sim CB. A double-blind comparative study of clozapine versus chlorpromazine on Chinese patients with treatment-refractory schizophrenia. Int Clin Psychopharmacol 1997;12:123–30.
111. Alvarez E, Barón F, Perez-Blanco J, Soriano DPJ, Masip C, Pérez-Solá V. Ten years' experience with clozapine in treatment-resistant schizophrenic patients: factors indicating the therapeutic response. Eur Psychiatry 1997;12 (Suppl 5):343s-6s.
112. Cassano GB, Ciapparelli A, Villa M. Clozapine as a treatment tool: only in resistant schizophrenic patients? Eur Psychiatry 1997;12 (Suppl 5):347s-51s.
113. Casey DE. Effects of clozapine therapy in schizophrenic individuals at risk for tardive dyskinesia. J Clin Psychiatry 1998;59 (Suppl 3):31–7.
114. Lieberman JA. Maximizing clozapine therapy: managing side effects. J Clin Psychiatry 1998;59 (Suppl 3):38–43.
115. Ennis LM, Parker RM. Paradoxical hypertension associated with clozapine. Med J Aust 1997;166:278
116. Li JKY, Yeung VTF, Leung CM, Chow CC, Ko GTC, So WY, Cockram CS. Clozapine: a mimicry of phaeochromocytoma. Aust NZ J Psychiatry 1997;31:889–91.
117. Gupta S. Paradoxical hypertension associated with clozapine. Am J Psychiatry 1994;151:148.
118. George TP, Winther LC. Hypertension after initiation of clozapine. Am J Psychiatry 1996;153:1363–9.
119. Freudenreich O, Weiner RD, McEvoy JP. Clozapine-induced electroencephalogram changes as a function of clozapine serum levels. Biol Psychiatry 1997;42:132–7.
120. Durif F, Vidailhet M, Assal F, Roche C, Bonnet AM, Agid Y. Low-dose clozapine improves dyskinesias in Parkinson's disease. Neurology 1997;48:658–62.
121. Widman LP, Burke WJ, Pfeiffer RF, McArthur-Campbell D. Use of clozapine to treat levodopa-induced psychosis in Parkinson's disease: retrospective review. J Geriatr Psychiatry Neurol 1997;10:63–6.
122. Friedman JH, Koller WC, Lannon MC, Busenbark K, Swanson-Hyland E, Smith D. Benztropine versus clozapine for the treatment of tremor in Parkinson's disease. Neurology 1997; 48:1077–81.
123. Knoll JL. Clozapine-related speech disturbance. J Clin Psychiatry 1997;58:219.
124. Lee JW. Comment on neuroleptic malignant syndrome and clozapine monotherapy. Aust NZ J Psychiatry 1997;31:435.
125. Chatterton R, Cardy S, Schramm MT. Response to Lee's comment on neuroleptic malignant syndrome and clozapine monotherapy. Aust NZ J Psychiatry 1997;31:435–6.
126. Dalkilic A, Grosch WN. Neuroleptic malignant syndrome following initiation of clozapine therapy. Am J Psychiatry 1997;153:881–2.
127. Amore M, Zazzeri N, Berardi D. Atypical

drawal catatonia and neuroleptic malignant syndrome: a case report. Ann Clin Psychiatry 1997;9:165–9.
129. Wilkins-Ho M, Hollander Y. Toxic delirium with low-dose clozapine. Can J Psychiatry 1997;42:429–30.
130. Ebeling TA, Compton AD, Albright DW. Clozapine-induced stuttering. Am J Psychiatry 1997;154:1473.
131. Popli AP, Konicki PE, Jurjus GJ, Fuller MA, Jaskiw GE. Clozapine and associated diabetes mellitus. J Clin Psychiatry 1997;58:108–11.
132. Pierides M. Clozapine monotherapy and ketoacidosis. Br J Psychiatry 1997;171:90–1.
133. Barbui C, Campomori A, Bonati M. Clozapine and blood dyscrasias different from agranulocytosis. Can J Psychiatry 1997;42:981–2.
134. Bailey P. Clozapine treatment, eosinophilia and agranulocytosis. Br J Psychiatry 1997;171:90.
135. Chatterton R. Eosinophilia after commencement of clozapine treatment. Aust NZ J Psychiatry 1997;31:874–6.
136. Adityanjee MD, Jampala VC, Mohan MS. Eosinophilia, agranulocytosis and clozapine. Br J Psychiatry 1997;171:485–6.
137. Amital D, Gross R, Amital H, Zohar J. Coexistence of eosinophilia and agranulocytosis in a clozapine-treated patient. Br J Psychiatry 1997; 170:194.
138. Kanjolia A, Valigorsky JM, Joson-Pasion ML. Clozaril-induced lupus anticoagulant. Am J Hematol 1997;54:345–6.
139. Honigfeld G, Arellano F, Sethi J, Bianchini A, Schein J. Reducing clozapine-related morbidity and mortality: 5 years of experience with the Clozaril National Registry. J Clin Psychiatry 1998;59 (Suppl 3):3–7.
140. Miller PR, Cutten AEC. Haematological side effects of clozapine: patient characteristics. NZ Med J 1997;110:125–7.
141. Koren W, Kreis Y, Duchowiczny K, Prince T, Sancovici S, Sidi Y, Gur H. Lactic acidosis and fatal myocardial failure due to clozapine. Ann Pharmacother 1997;31:168–70.
142. Silverstone PH. Prevention of clozapine-induced neutropenia by pretreatment with lithium. J Clin Psychopharmacol 1998;18:86–8.
143. Szarek BL, Goethe JW, Pentz PG. Unsuccessful reexposure to clozapine. J Clin Psychopharmacol 1997;17:71–3.
144. Hummer M, Kurz M, Kurzthaler I, Oberbauer H, Miller C, Fleischhacker WW. Hepatotoxicity of clozapine. J Clin Psychopharmacol 1997;17:314–7.
145. Markowitz JS, Grinberg R, Jackson C. Marked liver enzyme elevations with clozapine. J Clin Psychopharmacol 1997;17:70–1.
146. Macfarlane B, Davies S, Mannan K, Sarsam R, Pariente D, Dooley J. Fatal acute fulminant liver failure due to clozapine: a case report and review of clozapine-induced hepatotoxicity. Gastroenterology 1997;112:1707–9.
147. Szabadi E. Clozapine-induced hypersalivation. Br J Psychiatry 1997;171:89.
148. Spivak B, Adlersberg S, Rosen L, Gonen N, Mester R, Weizman A. Trihexyphenidyl treatment of clozapine-induced hypersalivation. Int Clin Psychopharmacol 1997;12:213–5.
149. Laker MK, Cookson JC. Reflux oesophagitis and clozapine. Int Clin Psychopharmacol 1997; 12:37–9.
150. Drew L, Herdson P. Clozapine and constipation: a serious issue. Aust NZ J Psychiatry 1997;31:149–50.
151. Shammi CM, Remington G. Clozapine-induced necrotizing colitis. J Clin Psychopharmacol 1997;17:230–2.
152. Lurie SN, Hosmer C. Oxybutynin and intranasal desmopressin for clozapine-induced urinary incontinence. J Clin Psychiatry 1997;58:404.
153. Catalano G, Catalano MC, Wetter RLF. Clozapine induced polyserositis. Clin Neuropharmacol 1997;20:352–6.
154. Chatterjee A, Safferman AZ. Cellulitis, eosinophilia, and unilateral pleural effusion associated with clozapine treatment. J Clin Psychopharmacol 1997;17:232–3.
155. Trémeau F, Clark SC, Printz D, Kegeles LS, Malaspina D. Spiking fevers with clozapine treatment. Clin Neuropharmacol 1997;20:168–70.
156. Pollmacher T, Hinze-Selch D, Mullington J, Holsboer F. Clozapine-induced increase in plasma levels of soluble interleukin-2 receptors. Arch Gen Psychiatry 1995;52:877–8.
157. Turetz M, Mozes T, Toren P, Chernauzan N, Yoran-Hegesh R, Mester R, Wittenberg N, Tyano S, Weizman A. An open trial of clozapine in neuroleptic-resistant childhood-onset schizophrenia. Br J Psychiatry 1997;170:507–10.
158. Van Vugt JPP, Siesling S, Vergeer M, Van der Velde EA, Roos RAC. Clozapine versus placebo in Huntington's disease: a double blind randomized comparative study. J Neurol Neurosurg Psychiatry 1997;63:35–9.
159. Rietschel M, Naber D, Fimmers R, Möller HJ, Propping P, Nöthen MM. Efficacy and side-effects of clozapine not associated with variation in the 5-HT_{2C} receptor. Neuroreport 1997; 8:1999–2003.
160. Turbay BD, Lieberman J, Alper CA, Delgado JC, Corzo D, Yunis JJ, Yunis EJ. Tumor necrosis factor-constellation polymorphism and clozapine-induced agranulocytosis in two different ethnic groups. Blood 1997;89:4167–74.
161. Theodoropoulou ST, Pappa H, Lykouras L, Papageorgiou G, Papasteriades C, Sakalis G. Human Leukocyte antigen system in clozapine-induced agranulocytosis. Neuropsychobiology 1997;36:5–7.
162. Combs MD, Perry PJ, Bever KA. N-Desmethylclozapine, an insensitive marker of clozapine-induced agranulocytosis and granulocytopenia. Pharmacotherapy 1997;17:1300–4.
163. Stanilla JK, De Leon J, Simpson GM. Clozapine withdrawal resulting in delirium with psychosis: a report of three cases. J Clin Psychiatry 1997;58:252–5.
164. Meltzer HY. Clozapine withdrawal: sero-

tonergic or dopaminergic mechanism? Arch Gen Psychiatry 1997;54:760–3.
165. Taylor D. Pharmacokinetic interactions involving clozapine. Br J Psychiatry 1997;171:109–12.
166. Faisal I, Lindenmayer JP, Taintor Z, Cancro R. Clozapine-benzodiazepine interactions. J Clin Psychiatry 1997;58:547–8.
167. Good MI. Lethal interaction of clozapine and buspirone? Am J Psychiatry 1997;154:1472–3.
168. Chong SA, Tan CH, Lee HS. Worsening of psychosis with clozapine and selective serotonin reuptake inhibitor combination: two case reports. J Clin Psychopharmacol 1997;17:68–9.
169. Armstrong SC, Stephans JR. Blood clozapine levels elevated by fluvoxamine: potential for side effects and lower clozapine dosage. J Clin Psychiatry 1997;58:499.
170. Joos AA, König F, Frank UG, Kaschka WP, Mörike KE, Ewald R. Dose-dependent pharmacokinetic interaction of clozapine and paroxetine in an extensive metabolizer. Pharmacopsychiatry 1997;30:266–70.
171. George TP, Innamorato L, Sernyak MJ, Baldessarini RJ, Centorrino F. Leukopenia associated with addition of paroxetine to clozapine. J Clin Psychiatry 1998;59:31.
172. Markowitz JS, Gill HS, Devane CL, Mintzer JE. Fluoroquinolone inhibition of clozapine metabolism. Am J Psychiatry 1997;153:881.
173. Shiloh R, Zemishlany Z, Aizenberg D, Radwan M, Schwartz B, Dorfman-Etrog P, Modai I, Khaikin M, Weizman A. Sulpiride augmentation in people with schizophrenia partially responsive to clozapine. Br J Psychiatry 1997;171:569–73.
174. Freeman DJ, Oyewumi LK. Will routine therapeutic drug monitoring have a place in clozapine therapy? Clin Pharmacokinet 1997;32:93–100.
175. Wang SJ, Silberstein SD, Young WB. Droperidol treatment of status migrainosus and refractory migraine. Headache 1997;37:377–82.
176. Ng KF, Tsui SL, Yang JC, Ho ET. Comparison of tramadol and tramadol/droperidol mixture for patient-controlled analgesia. Can J Anaesth 1997;44:810–15.
177. Marsland AR. Droperidol and dysphoria. Anaesth Intensive Care 1997;25:726–7.
178. Bourrain JL, Paillet C, Woodward C, Beani JC, Amblard P. Diagnosis of photosensitivity to flupenthixol by photoprick testing. Photodermatol Photoimmunol Photomed 1997;13:159–61.
179. Maxa JL, Taleghani AM, Ogu CC, Tanzi M. Possible toxic encephalopathy following high-dose intravenous haloperidol. Ann Pharmacother 1997;31:736–7.
180. Blitzstein SM, Brandt GT. Extrapyramidal symptoms from intravenous haloperidol in the treatment of delirium. Am J Psychiatry 1997; 154:1474–5.
181. Galynker II, Nazarian D. Akathisia as violence. J Clin Psychiatry 1997;58:31–2.
182. Bobba R, Carr A. Severe extrapyramidal side effects when discontinuing clozapine and starting haloperidol. Can J Psychiatry 1997; 42:530.
183. Riker RR, Fraser GL, Richen P. Movement disorders associated with withdrawal from high-dose intravenous haloperidol therapy in delirious ICU patients. Chest 1997;111:1778–81.
184. Satoh K, Someya T, Shibasaki M. Nemonapride for the treatment of schizophrenia. Am J Psychiatry 1997;154:292.
185. Sheitman BB, Lindgren JC, Early J, Sved M. High-dose olanzapine for treatment-refractory schizophrenia. Am J Psychiatry 1997;154:1626.
186. Beasley CM Jr, Tollesfson GD, Tran PV. Safety of olanzapine. J Clin Psychiatry 1997;58 (Suppl 10):13–17.
187. Kando JC, Shepski JC, Satterlee W, Patel JK, Reams SG, Green AI. Olanzapine: a new antipsychotic agent with efficacy in the management of schizophrenia. Ann Pharmacother 1997;31:1325–34.
188. Tollefson GD, Sanger TM. Negative symptoms: a path analytic approach to a double-blind, placebo- and haloperidol-controlled clinical trial with olanzapine. Am J Psychiatry 1997;154:466–74.
189. Olanzapine for schizophrenia. Med Lett Drugs Ther 1997;39:5–6.
190. Reus VI. Olanzapine: a novel atypical neuroleptic agent. Lancet 1997;349:1264–5.
191. Tran PV, Hamilton SH, Kuntz AJ, Potvin JH, Andersen SW, Beasley C, Tollefson GD. Double-blind comparison of olanzapine versus risperidone in the treatment of schizophrenia and other psychotic disorders. J Clin Psychopharmacol 1997;17:407–18.
192. Tran PV, Dellva MA, Tollefson GD, Beasley CM, Potvin JH, Kiesler GM. Extrapyramidal symptoms and tolerability of olanzapine versus haloperidol in the acute treatment of schizophrenia. J Clin Psychiatry 1997;58:205–11.
193. Tollefson GD, Beasley CM, Tamura RN, Tran PV, Potvin JH. Blind, controlled, long-term study of the comparative incidence of treatment-emergent tardive dyskinesia with olanzapine or haloperidol. Am J Psychiatry 1997;154:1248–54.
194. Littrell KH, Johnson CG, Littrell S, Peabody CD. Marked reduction of tardive dyskinesia with olanzapine. Arch Gen Psychiatry 1998;55:279–80.
195. Martìn J, Gómez JC, García-Bernardo E, Cuesta M, Alvarez E, Gurpegui M. Olanzapine in treatment-refractory schizophrenia: results of an open-label study. J Clin Psychiatry 1997; 58:479–83.
196. Crawford AMK, Beasley CM, Tollefson GD. The acute and long-term effect of olanzapine compared with placebo and haloperidol on serum prolactin concentrations. Schizophr Res 1997;26:41–54.
197. Flynn SW, Altman S, MacEwan GW, Black LL, Greenidge LL, Honer WG. Prolongation of clozapine-induced granulocytopenia associated with olanzapine. J Clin Psychopharmacol 1997; 17:494–5.
198. Ramos RH, Budman CL. Emergence of koro

after abrupt cessation of olanzapine. J Clin Psychiatry 1998;59:86–7.
199. Callaghan JT, Cerimele BJ, Kassahun KJ, Nyhart EH, Hoyes-Beehler PJ, Kondraske GV. Olanzapine: interaction study with imipramine. J Clin Pharmacol 1997;37:971–8.
200. Peuskens J, Link CG. A comparison of quetiapine and chlorpromazine in the treatment of schizophrenia. Acta Psychiatr Scand 1997;96:265–73.
201. Arvanitis LA, Miller BG, Borison RL, Pitts WM, Sharif ZA, Hammer MB, et al (30 authors). Multiple fixed doses of Seroquel (quetiapine) in patients with acute exacerbation of schizophrenia: a comparison with haloperidol and placebo. Biol Psychiatry 1997;42:233–46.
202. Small JG, Hirsch SR, Arvanitis LA, Miller BG, Link CG. Quetiapine in patients with schizophrenia. Arch Gen Psychiatry 1997;54:549–57.
203. KHfferle B, Tauscher J, Asenbaum S, Vesely C, Podreka I, Brücke T, Kasper S. IBZM SPECT imaging of striatal dopamine-2 receptors in psychotic patients treated with the novel antipsychotic substance quetiapine in comparison to clozapine and haloperidol. Psychopharmacology 1997;133: 323–8.
204. Gutierrez-Esteinou R, Grebb JA. Risperidone: an analysis of the first three years in general use. Int Clin Psychopharmacol 1997;12 (Suppl 4):S3–10.
205. Mattes JA. Risperidone: how good is the evidence for efficacy? Schizophr Bull 1997;23:155–61.
206. Rossi A, Mancini F, Stratta P, Mattei P, Gismondi R, Pozzi F, Casacchia M. Risperidone, negative symptoms and cognitive deficit in schizophrenia: an open study. Acta Psychiatr Scand 1997;95:40–3.
207. Marder SR, Davis JM, Chouinard G. The effects of risperidone on the five dimensions of schizophrenia derived by factor analysis: combined results of the North American trials. J Clin Psychiatry 1997;58:538–46.
208. Song F. Risperidone in the treatment of schizophrenia: a meta-analysis of randomized controlled trials. J Psychopharmacol 1997;11:65–71.
209. Jeste DV, Klausner M, Brecher M, Clyde C, Jones R. A clinical evaluation of risperidone in the treatment of schizophrenia: a 10-week, open-label, multicenter trial. Psychopharmacology 1997;131:239–47.
210. Bondolfi G, Dufour H, Patris M, May JP, Billeter U, Eap CB. Risperidone versus clozapine in treatment-resistant chronic schizophrenia: a randomized double-blind study. Am J Psychiatry 1998;155:499–504.
211. Gardner DM, Baldessarini RJ, Benzo J, Zarate CA, Tohen M. Switching between clozapine and risperidone treatment. Can J Psychiatry 1997;42:430–1.
212. Ravin DS, Levenson JW. Fatal cardiac event following initiation of risperidone therapy. Ann Pharmacother 1997;31:867–70.
213. Kopala LC, Good KP, Honer WG. Extrapyramidal signs and clinical symptoms in first-episode schizophrenia: response to low-dose risperidone. J Clin Psychopharmacol 1997;17:308–13.
214. Knable MB, Heinz A, Raedler T, Weinberger DR. Extrapyramidal side effects with risperidone and haloperidol at comparable D_2 receptor occupancy levels. Psychiatr Res Neuroimaging 1997;75:91–101.
215. De León OA, Jobe TH, Furmaga KM, Gaviria M. Severe extrapyramidal reaction due to risperidone in a case of neurofibromatosis. J Clin Psychiatry 1997;58:323.
216. Edleman RJ. TD From risperidone? J Am Acad Child Adolesc Psychiaty 1997;36:867.
217. Haberfellner EM. Tardive dyskinesia during treatment with risperidone. Pharmacopsychiatry 1997;30:271.
218. Saran BM. Risperidone-induced tardive dyskinesia. J Clin Psychiatry 1998;59:29–30.
219. Gwinn KA, Caviness JN. Risperidone-induced tardive dyskinesia and parkinsonism. Mov Disord 1997;12:119–21.
220. Gleason PP, Conigliaro RL. Neuroleptic malignant syndrome with risperidone. Pharmacotherapy 1997;17:617–21.
221. Bajjoka I, Patel T, O'Sullivan T. Risperidone-induced neuroleptic malignant syndrome. Ann Emerg Med 1997;30:698–700.
222. Newman M, Adityanjee, Jampala C. Atypical neuroleptic malignant syndrome associated with risperidone treatment. Am J Psychiatry 1997;154:1475.
223. Lane H-Y, Chang W-H, Chou JC-Y. Seizure during risperidone treatment in an elderly woman treated with concomitant medications. J Clin Psychiatry 1998;59:81–2.
224. McIntyre R, Young LT, Hasey G, Patelis-Siotis I, Jones BD. Risperidone treatment of bipolar disorder. Can J Psychiatry 1997:42:88–90.
225. Lane H-Y, Lin Y-C, Chang W-H. Mania induced by risperidone: dose related? J Clin Psychiatry 1998;59:85–6.
226. Barkin JS, Pais VN, Gaffney MF. Induction of mania by risperidone resistant to mood stabilizers. J Clin Psychopharmacol 1997;17:57–8.
227. Alzaid K, Jones BD. A case report of risperidone-induced obsessive-compulsive symptoms. J Clin Psychopharmacol 1997;17:58–9.
228. Dodt JE, Byerly MJ, Cuadros C, Christensen RC. Treatment of risperidone-induced obsessive-compulsive symptoms with sertraline. Am J Psychiatry 1997;154:582.
229. Morehead DB. Exacerbation of hallucinogen-persisting perception disorder with risperidone. J Clin Psychopharmacol 1997;17:327–8.
230. Crockford DN, Fisher G, Barker P. Risperidone, weight gain, and bulimia nervosa. Can J Psychiatry 1997;42:326–7.
231. Brecher M, Geller W. Weight gain with risperidone. J Clin Psychopharmacol 1997;17:435–6.
232. Kumra S, Herion D, Jacobsen LK, Briguglia C, Grothe D. Case study: risperidone-induced

hepatotoxicity in pediatric patients. J Am Acad Child Adolesc Psychiatry 1997;36:701–5.
233. Schreiber S, Segman RH. Risperidone-induced galactorrhea. Psychopharmacology 1997;130:300–1.
234. Whitten JR, Ruehter VL. Risperidone and hyponatremia: a case report. Ann Clin Psychiatry 1997;9:181–3.
235. Dernovsek Z, Tavcar R. Risperidone-induced leucopenia and neutropenia. Br J Psychiatry 1997;171:393–4.
236. Gueller WK, Zuiderwijk PB. Risperidone-induced hepatotoxicity? J Am Acad Child Adolesc Psychiatry 1998;37:246–7.
237. Berent I, Carabeth J, Cordero MM, Cordero R, Sugerman B, Robinson D. Pancreatitis associated with risperidone treatment? Am J Psychiatry 1997;154:130–1.
238. Poyurovsky M, Weizman A. Risperidone-induced nocturnal enuresis. Isr J Psychiatry Relat Sci 1997;34:247–8.
239. Sweeney JA, Bauer KS, Keshavan MS, Haas GL, Schooler NR, Kroboth PD. Adverse effects of risperidone on eye movement activity: a comparison of risperidone and haloperidol in antipsychotic-naive schizophrenic patients. Neuropsychopharmacology 1997;16:217–28.
240. Terao T, Kojima H, Eto A. Risperidone and allergic reactions. J Clin Psychiatry 1998;59:82–3.
241. Zarate CA, Baldessarini RJ, Siegel AJ, Nakamura A, McDonald J, Muir-Hutchinson LA, Cherkerzian T, Tohen M. Risperidone in the elderly: a pharmacoepidemiologic study. J Clin Psychiatry 58:311–17.
242. Sourander A. Risperidone for treatment of childhood schizophrenia. Am J Psychiatry 1997; 154:1476.
243. Findling RL, Maxwell K, Wiznitzer M. An open clinical trial of risperidone monotherapy in young children with autistic disorder. Psychopharmacol Bull 1997;33:155–9.
244. Horrigan JP, Barnhill LJ. Risperidone and explosive aggressive autism. J Autism Dev Disord 1997;27:313–23.
245. Rowan AB, Malone RP. Tics with risperidone withdrawal. J Am Acad Adolesc Psychiatry 1997;36:162–3.
246. Rosebush PI, Kennedy K, Dalton B, Mazurek MF. Protracted akathisia after risperidone withdrawal. Am J Psychiatry 1997;154:437–8.
247. Himstreet JE, Daya M. Hypotension and orthostasis following a risperidone overdose. Ann Pharmacother 1998;32:267.
248. Moore NC, Shukla P. Risperidone overdose. Am J Psychiatry 1997;154:289–90.
249. Brown ES. Extrapyramidal side effects with low-dose risperidone. Can J Psychiatry 1997; 42:325–6.
250. Pies R. Re: extrapyramidal side effects with low-dose risperidone. Can J Psychiatry 1997; 42:881.
251. De Leon J, Bork J. Risperidone and cytochrome P450 3A. J Clin Psychiatry 1997;58:450.
252. Rawlins M. Suspension of availability of Serdolect (sertindole). Media Release 1998;2:3–7.
253. Zimbroff DL, Kane JM, Tamminga CA, Daniel DG, Mack RJ, Wozniak PJ, Sebree TB, Wallin BA, Kashkin KB. Controlled, dose-response study of sertindole and haloperidol in the treatment of schizophrenia. Am J Psychiatry 1997;154:782–91.
254. Tamminga CA, Mack RJ, Granneman GR, Silber CJ, Kashkin KB. Sertindole in the treatmente of psychosis in schizophrenia: efficacy and safety. Int Clin Psychopharmacol 1997;12 (Suppl 1):S29–35.
255. Brown GR, Radford JM. Sertindole hydrochloride: a novel antipsychotic medication with a favorable side effect profile. South Med J 1997;90:691–3.
256. Walker-Kinnear M, McNaughton S. Paroxetine discontinuation syndrome in association with sertindole therapy. Br J Psychiatry 1997;170:389.
257. Benazzi F. Side-effects of benzamide derivatives. Int J Geriatr Psychiatry 1997;12:132.
258. Baptista T, Molina MG, Martinez JL, De Quijada M, Calanche de Cuesta I, Acosta A, Páez X, Martinez JM, Hernández L. Effects of the antipsychotic drug sulpiride on reproductive hormones in healthy premenopausal women: relationship with body weight regulation. Pharmacopsychiatry 1997;30:256–62.
259. Marta-Moreno E, Gracia-Naya M, Marzo-Sola ME. Discinesia respiratoria inducida por veralipride. Rev Neurol 1997;25:245–7.
260. Tanaka O, Kondo T, Otani K, Yasui N, Tokinaga N, Kaneko S. Single oral dose kinetics of zotepine and its relationship to prolactin response and side effects. Ther Drug Monit 1998;20:117–19.
261. Pantel J, Schröder J, Eysenbach K, Mundt CH. Two cases of deep vein thrombosis associated with a combined paroxetine and zotepine therapy. Pharmacopsychiatry 1997;30:109–11.

Emilio Perucca

7 Antiepileptic drugs

GENERAL TOPICS *(SED-13, 136; SEDA-19, 61; SEDA-20, 58; SEDA-21, 66)*

Cardiovascular *Cardiac dysrhythmias* caused by antiepileptic drugs in therapeutic dosages have been reviewed (1[R]). Dysrhythmias induced by antiepileptic drugs are rare and occur mainly in patient populations different from those known to be at high risk for sudden unexpected death. Phenytoin has been rarely associated with bradydysrhythmias, almost exclusively after intravenous dosing, and some of these have been fatal. Carbamazepine can depress the cardiac conduction system, mostly in elderly or otherwise predisposed patients. There have been no reports of dysrhythmias induced by other antiepileptic drugs.

Endocrine, metabolic *(SEDA-20, 58)* Assessment of serum electrolyte concentrations in 1086 patients with epilepsy taking various anticonvulsants has shown an association between oxcarbazepine or carbamazepine treatment and reduction in serum sodium (2[c]). The proportions of patients taking oxcarbazepine or carbamazepine who presented with *subnormal sodium concentrations* were 44 and 30%, respectively, for those on monotherapy compared with 69 and 42% for those on polytherapy. Hyponatremia correlated with serum concentrations of the monohydroxy metabolite of oxcarbazepine and with the use of diuretics. Although the association of hyponatremia with oxcarbazepine and carbamazepine is well known, the proportion of hyponatremic patients, particularly among those treated with carbamazepine, was higher in this study than in other reports. Hyponatremic patients had a higher frequency of seizures than those with normal sodium concentrations, possibly due to a facilitating effect of hyponatremia on seizure susceptibility. However, since drug dosages were not specified, it could not be excluded that patients with more severe epilepsy were taking higher dosages than the other patients.

Nervous system An assessment of published data has suggested that in patients taking polytherapy the *neurotoxic effects* of antiepileptic drugs relate more to total drug load than to the actual number of drugs taken (3[C]). Drug load was expressed as the sum of ratios between the actual prescribed daily dose and the average defined daily dose for each drug, or as the sum of ratios between the observed serum concentration and the average toxic concentration. These data suggested that polytherapy is not by itself necessarily associated with more frequent adverse effects: the dosage and serum concentrations of each drug are obviously important. The authors suggested that this should lead to a re-assessment of the potential merits of polytherapy, at least in patients who do not respond to a well-tolerated dose of a single drug.

Three patients, aged 16, 19, and 65 years, developed *epileptic negative myoclonus status* (almost continuous lapses in muscle tone associated with epileptiform discharges and interference with postural control and motor coordination) 48–72 h after rapid withdrawal of clobazam or valproate (6 days or less), taken in combination with other anticonvulsants (4[C]). All the patients had a long history of partial epilepsy and none had had negative myoclonus in the past. The condition was diagnosed by polygraphic recordings, and it might have been misinterpreted as a recrudescence of partial seizures, which were also more frequent in these patients. Clonazepam 1 mg intravenously terminated the status, which did not recur in the ensuing 9–36 months. This appears to be the first report of de novo appearance of epileptic negative

Side Effects of Drugs, Annual 22
J.K. Aronson, ed.

myoclonus triggered by withdrawal of antiepileptic drugs.

R

Adverse psychiatric effects of anticonvulsants

The adverse psychiatric effects of antiepileptic drugs have been reviewed (5[R]). Although epilepsy is itself associated with an increased risk of psychiatric disturbances, antiepileptic drugs can contribute to worsening behavior and mood.

Individual drugs *Phenobarbital-induced behavioral disturbances, especially hyperactivity, are especially common in children: the incidence is 20–50% and drug withdrawal is required in 20–30% of cases. Owing to a paucity of systematic studies, it is unclear whether and to what extent phenobarbital causes adverse psychiatric effects in adults.*

Phenytoin has also been implicated in the pathogenesis of psychiatric adverse effects with or without other signs of toxicity, and at serum concentrations above or below the upper limit of the optimal range, but the actual incidence of these reactions is unknown.

Compared with phenobarbital and phenytoin, benzodiazepines may be less likely to cause psychiatric disturbances; however, paradoxical excitatory effects of benzodiazepines may be observed, particularly in children and in anxious patients, and several other psychiatric symptoms can complicate the syndrome of benzodiazepine withdrawal.

Psychiatric/behavioral disorders have been reported with ethosuximide, but the lack of systematic studies prevents assessment of their incidence and cause–effect relation.

Among older drugs, valproic acid and carbamazepine are least likely to cause adverse psychiatric effects. Valproate can rarely cause an encephalopathy and reversible pseudodementia.

Among newer drugs, vigabatrin has been implicated most commonly in psychiatric adverse effects. Psychotic/behavioral reactions associated with vigabatrin are sometimes but not always related to forced normalization (a condition in which disappearance of EEG abnormalities and/or seizures leads to psychosis) and may be dose-related (see SEDA-18, 71). The overall incidence of vigabatrin-associated psychotic/behavioral disorders is probably around 1% or less, but it may increase up to 6% in patients with severe refractory epilepsy. Several reports suggest that vigabatrin may also cause depression, though evidence for this is inconsistent.

Gabapentin has rarely been associated with psychiatric disturbances, although preliminary evidence suggests that aggressiveness and/or hyperactivity can occur when it is given to adults and children with previous behavioral problems or learning disability.

Adverse psychiatric reactions to lamotrigine are uncommon (but see 'Lamotrigine' below), whereas with topiramate, felbamate, and other new drugs the data are too sparse for meaningful evaluation.

Avoidance *Overall, the problem of drug-induced psychiatric disorders can be minimized by avoiding unnecessarily large dosages and drug combinations and by careful monitoring of the clinical response. In patients with a previous history of psychiatric disorders, carbamazepine and valproate are the first-line drugs that are least likely to cause behavioral disturbances.*

Management *The ideal management of a drug-induced psychiatric reaction is discontinuation of the offending agent. When continuation of treatment is necessary for seizure control, the disorder may be managed with psychosocial intervention and psychotropic medication.*

Hematological Compared with 74 age-matched controls, patients taking monotherapy with phenobarbital ($n = 33$) or carbamazepine ($n = 36$) had significantly *reduced serum folate* concentrations (6[Cr]). Serum folate was not reduced in patients taking valproate ($n = 41$) and zonisamide ($n = 25$), which are not known to induce hepatic enzymes. These results are consistent with the hypothesis that enzyme induction plays a role in the pathogenesis of folate deficiency.

Skin and appendages The risks of *serious cutaneous reactions* requiring hospitalization within 60 days of starting therapy with phenytoin, carbamazepine, or sodium valproate have been assessed in a record linkage study (7[Cr]). There were eight confirmed reactions (including two probable and two possible cases of hypersensitivity syndrome) among 8888 new phenytoin users, six (including one probable and four possible cases of hypersensitivity syndrome) among 9738 new carbamazepine users, and none among 1504 new valproate users.

In another study, the risk of cross-sensitivity of skin rashes with antiepileptic drugs was assessed retrospectively (8[Cr]). Among 633 patients who had 1875 exposures to 14 anticonvulsants, 14 had rashes from two or more drugs, involving predominantly phenytoin and carbamazepine. Of 17 patients who had a rash from phenytoin, 10 (58%) also had a rash from carbamazepine. Ten of 25 patients (40%) who had a rash from carbamazepine also had a rash from phenytoin. Four of five patients with a phenobarbital-associated rash also developed a rash with phenytoin or carbamazepine. Valproate or clobazam were safer alternatives in patients who had had a rash from aromatic anticonvulsants. However, in a 41-year-old man a fixed drug eruption that occurred after separate exposure to phenytoin and carbamazepine also occurred after challenge with sodium valproate (9[cr]).

Special senses Epileptic patients taking phenytoin or carbamazepine monotherapy had blue-yellow *color vision disturbances* which correlated significantly with signs of neurotoxicity (10[Cr]). There were no color vision disturbances in patients taking valproate or no drugs. The authors suggested that color vision testing may provide a sensitive method for early detection of clinical neurotoxicity caused by phenytoin and carbamazepine.

Immunological and hypersensitivity reactions Although carbamazepine-induced *systemic lupus erythematosus* usually develops within months of treatment, a case report has suggested that it may occur after as late as 8 years (11[cr]). Rash, enlarged lymph nodes, joint involvement, myalgia, fever, leukopenia, and positive antinuclear antibodies were among the manifestations found in a 34-year-old man who had been taking carbamazepine (1200–1600 mg/day) for 8 years. Complete recovery occurred when carbamazepine was substituted with valproate and anti-inflammatory agents were given for 2 months. There was no relapse after 18 months.

Interactions Interactions of clobazam with other anticonvulsants have been assessed in 74 children with intractable seizures (12[Cr]). Clobazam had no discernible effect on serum concentrations of other anticonvulsants, except for *valproic acid* and *primidone*, whose concentrations were increased. Since the interaction affecting valproate was considered to be particularly significant, monitoring of valproic acid concentrations was recommended. Serum clobazam concentrations were reduced by phenobarbital and serum concentrations of *N*-desmethylclobazam were increased by phenytoin or carbamazepine, but these interactions are likely to have modest clinical significance.

Evidence on the effect of *ethosuximide* on serum *valproic acid* concentrations is controversial. In nine children with epilepsy, valproic acid concentrations increased by an average of 37% after withdrawal of ethosuximide (13[Cr]). Conversely, the addition of ethosuximide to valproate resulted in a 28% fall in valproic acid concentrations in four children. The mechanism of this possible interaction is unclear.

A Japanese study based on non-linear mixed effects modelling of plasma concentration data suggested that co-medication with *carbamazepine* reduced the apparent oral clearance of *phenobarbital* by 17% (14[C]). The reduction was largest (54%) in early childhood, and there were minimal changes in adults. Although a slight reduction in phenobarbital clearance after adding carbamazepine has been described before, its age-dependency and its greater magnitude in children, as found in this study, are surprising, and the possibility of assessment bias cannot be excluded.

There have been several reports of potential interactions involving lamotrigine and other anticonvulsants. In patients co-medicated with *oxcarbazepine*, serum *lamotrigine* concentration/dose ratios were about 30% lower than in patients taking lamotrigine monotherapy and about 30% higher than in patients taking carbamazepine co-medication (15[c]). These data suggest that oxcarbazepine induces the metabolism of lamotrigine, though less than carbamazepine. *Methsuximide* can also reduce serum *lamotrigine* concentrations (15[c]), (16[cr]). In 10 patients, serum lamotrigine concentrations averaged 11.9 (SD 3.1) mg/l off methsuximide compared with 5.5 (2.2) mg/l when methsuximide was given concurrently (16[cr]). Methsuximide would therefore be expected to reduce the clinical response to lamotrigine, whereas signs of lamotrigine intoxication may be anticipated when methsuximide is withdrawn. The finding of unusually high serum primidone/phenobarbital ratios (1:1 to 2:1) in three patients comedicated with lamotrigine led to the suggestion that *lamotrigine* may impair the conversion of *primidone* to phenobarbital (17[C]). However, the information provided was insufficient to assess the probability of an interaction, and a rise in primidone/phenobarbital ratio may be caused by other factors, including poor compliance. Finally, several studies have shown that the addition of *lamotrigine* to *carbamazepine* often produces clinical signs suggestive of carbamazepine toxicity. Careful monitoring of serum concentrations of carbamazepine and carbamazepine-10,11-epoxide in these patients did not show any changes, leading to the conclusion that this interaction is pharmacodynamic (18[Cr]).

In a retrospective survey, the apparent oral clearance of *felbamate* was lower in 10 patients co-medicated with *gabapentin* compared with 41 patients taking felbamate alone (0.42 vs 0.67 l/kg per day) (19[c]). It was speculated that gabapentin reduces the renal clearance of felbamate, but within-patient studies are required to confirm this interaction.

℞ *Overdosage with antiepileptic drugs*

Carbamazepine *After large overdoses of carbamazepine, absorption may be delayed and peak serum concentrations may not be reached until as late as 72 h (20[R]). Manifestations are dominated by neurological features and may include nystagmus, dysarthria, ataxia, tremor, seizures (including status epilepticus), dizziness, mydriasis, convergent strabismus, external ophthalmoplegia, fixed dilated pupils, and altered reflexes and posture. Cardiovascular signs include tachycardia or bradycardia, sinoatrial or atrioventricular block, QRS prolongation, loss of P wave, and hypotension or hypertension. In severe cases, coma (sometimes cyclic) and respiratory depression may be observed. Management consists of supportive measures; gastric lavage is indicated within 1 h of a massive overdosage, provided airways can be protected. Activated charcoal in repeated oral doses enhances carbamazepine elimination, as does charcoal hemoperfusion. Hemodialysis and peritoneal dialysis are not effective because carbamazepine is highly protein bound and has a high volume of distribution. Adults have survived the ingestion of doses as high as 640 mg/kg. Death can result from cardiac dysrhythmias, aspiration pneumonitis, hepatitis, or status epilepticus.*

An unusual manifestation of overdosage has been described in a 36-year-old woman who attempted suicide by ingesting 60 tablets of carbamazepine 200 mg (21[cr]). At admission after 5 h she was unconscious and she was treated with gastric aspiration and hemodialysis. Within 48 h she developed respiratory failure, and a diagnosis of acute interstitial pneumonia or diffuse alveolar damage was made 13 days later, based on extensive investigations, including bronchoalveolar lavage and lung tissue biopsy. A similar presentation recurred after a second overdose 15 months later.

Ethosuximide *Intoxication with ethosuximide can cause lethargy, headache, dizziness, ataxia, fatigue, nausea, vomiting, euphoria, and in more severe cases respiratory depression (20[R]). Supportive measures are required. Gastric lavage and activated charcoal may be considered within 1 h, though their value is unproven.*

Phenytoin *Phenytoin overdose can be associated with slow gastrointestinal absorption (20[R]). Clinical features include nausea, vomiting, sedation, cerebellar signs, seizures, and altered reflexes, tone, and ocular motility. Hyperkinesias and dyskinesias, including choreoathetosis, are less common. Coma and respiratory depression are unusual. Alterations in heart rhythm and blood pressure are more common with parenteral overdose, but they have also been seen after massive oral over-*

dose, especially when there was pre-existing cardiac disease. Hypoglycemia, hyperglycemia, and hypernatremic coma have been reported. Management is primarily supportive. Gastric lavage and multiple-dose activated charcoal may be considered within 1 h of overdose. Multiple-dose charcoal also increases phenytoin clearance, but the associated benefits are unclear. Forced diuresis, peritoneal dialysis, exchange transfusion, and hemodialysis are of little or no value, and charcoal hemoperfusion is of questionable benefit. Plasmapheresis has been suggested for young children with features of cardiotoxicity.

Valproate *Valproate overdosage causes sedation, apathy, stupor, and confusion (20[R]). Coma may occur with doses in excess of 20 mg/kg and may be related to hyperammonemia. Other features include cerebral edema, asterixis, seizures, hypotension, nausea, vomiting, diarrhea, hypernatremia, hypoglycemia, hypocalcemia, hypophosphatemia, and metabolic acidosis. Bone marrow suppression, leukopenia, thrombocytopenia, pancreatitis and, rarely, hepatotoxicity have been reported. Unlike other antiepileptic drug toxicity, dysarthria, nystagmus, and ataxia are not features of valproate poisoning. Management is supportive. Gastric lavage may be useful within 1 h of the overdose. Continuous activated charcoal by nasogastric tube increases valproic acid elimination, but its benefits are unclear. Naloxone has been beneficial in some cases, but its therapeutic role and dose–response relation have not been defined.*

Hemodialysis and hemoperfusion should be considered, but their potential value has not been adequately assessed. However, there has been a report of the usefulness of hemoperfusion (22[cr]).

A 19-year-old woman was hospitalized 6 h after ingesting 18 g of valproate. Her plasma valproic acid concentration was 800 mg/l and she presented with coma and lactic acidosis. Metabolic studies suggested that coma could be related to inhibition of β-oxidation of fatty acids. She was hemoperfused with activated charcoal, which shortened the half-life of valproic acid to 1.8 h (compared with 4.4 h before hemoperfusion). Over a period of about 6 h, her valproic acid concentration fell from 471 to 45 mg/l, at which point she became alert.

Lamotrigine *Lamotrigine overdose causes sedation, ataxia, diplopia, nausea, vomiting, hypertonia, nystagmus, and a prolonged QRS interval (20[R]). Gastric lavage has been proposed within 1–2 h of overdose, and cardiac rhythm should be monitored. Activated charcoal has been recommended but its value is unproven.*

Vigabatrin *Doses of vigabatrin of up to 10 g have been ingested without serious effects. Large overdose causes vertigo, tremor, sedation, coma, myoclonic jerks, and psychosis. Gastric lavage within 1–2 h is recommended after doses in excess of 12 g in adults and 2 g in children. Activated charcoal is recommended after vigabatrin overdose, but its value is unproven.*

A 33-year-old woman with complex partial seizures treated with vigabatrin (dose unspecified) accidentally ingested 20 g and was comatose for several hours (23[c]). Vigabatrin was withdrawn, and 6 days later she developed discontinuous partial complex status epilepticus for 3 days. It was suggested that abrupt withdrawal after the overdose had activated a pre-existing focal epileptogenic area.

INDIVIDUAL DRUGS

Carbamazepine *(SED-13, 145; SEDA-19, 64; SEDA-20, 60; SEDA-21, 69)*

Nervous system Carbamazepine worsens absence and myoclonic seizures, but aggravation of other generalized seizure types is less common. A 23-year-old man with a history of drug-refractory West syndrome had about 50 *tonic seizures* per month for 15 years while taking a combination of primidone and carbamazepine (24[c]). Withdrawal of carbamazepine resulted in dramatic and long-lasting reduction of seizure frequency, down to a maximum of three seizures per month. Aggravation of tonic seizures by carbamazepine was confirmed at rechallenge.

Gastrointestinal A 5-year-old boy developed watery diarrhea about 3 weeks after starting carbamazepine (dosage unspecified) (25[c]). Extensive investigations over the years led eventually to a diagnosis of *lymphocytic colitis*, a possibly autoimmune disorder characterized by increased numbers of mucosal surface lymphocytes. The condition persisted for 4 years and then disappeared over a 2-month period when the child was weaned from carbamazepine. The temporal relation suggested that carbamazepine may have triggered the condition.

Immunological and hypersensitivity reactions A 13-year-old boy developed rash, fever, conjunctivitis, facial edema, chest pain, tachycardia, hepatomegaly, and eosinophilia about 4 weeks after starting carbamazepine in a maintenance dosage of 800 mg/day (26[c]). He died within 2 days from uncontrollable cardiac dysrhythmias. Post-mortem investigation showed *eosinophilic myocarditis*, a serious complication of carbamazepine hypersensitivity.

Interactions *Dextropropoxyphene* inhibits carbamazepine metabolism. In a study of the relevance of this interaction, 59 of 7263 mostly elderly patients in a drug-dispensing program from pharmacies in Sweden were taking a combination of these two drugs (27[Cr]). A questionnaire on 30 symptoms of well-being was distributed to four groups of 21 patients taking carbamazepine and dextropropoxyphene in combination, only carbamazepine or dextropropoxyphene, or neither of the two. In patients taking the combination, serum carbamazepine concentrations were significantly higher and carbamazepine-10,11-epoxide concentrations were significantly lower compared with patients taking only carbamazepine, despite the fact that carbamazepine dosage was higher in the latter. The average number of symptoms was significantly higher in patients taking the combination than in the other groups. Dizziness and a readiness to cry were more common with the combination compared with carbamazepine alone. The authors concluded that in elderly people the combination of carbamazepine with dextropropoxyphene increases the risk of carbamazepine adverse effects. However, the number of concomitant drugs was also higher in patients taking the combination, and it is not possible to exclude the possibility that symptoms were related to underlying ailments or other comedication.

In eight patients stabilized on carbamazepine, the addition of *ketoconazole* (200 mg/day for 10 days) resulted in a rise in serum carbamazepine concentrations by about 30%, presumably due to inhibition of CYP3A-mediated oxidation (28[C]). Although signs of toxicity were not observed, all the patients had low serum carbamazepine concentrations at baseline. Monitoring for serum carbamazepine concentrations and potential adverse effects is recommended whenever patients are given this combination.

In 12 patients taking anticonvulsant therapy (principally carbamazepine), the systemic availability of a single 20-mg oral dose of conventional-release *nifedipine* was only 22% of that in 12 healthy controls, presumably due to induction of first-pass metabolism (29[C]). Similar interactions have been previously reported with felodipine (30[C]), nisoldipine (31[C]), and nimodipine (32[C]). Patients taking enzyme-inducing anticonvulsants are unlikely to have an adequate response to usual dosages of dihydropyridine drugs.

A single case report in a 24-year-old man has suggested that carbamazepine dose-dependently reduces the anticoagulant effect of *phenprocoumon* (33[cr]). This interaction is probably caused by enzyme induction.

Felbamate *(SED-13, 153; SEDA-19, 67; SEDA-20, 61; SEDA-21, 70)*

Aplastic anemia and felbamate

The use of felbamate has been curtailed because of its association with aplastic anemia and hepatotoxicity. Two recent reviews have concluded that these problems should not be underestimated, but that felbamate remains a valuable alternative in difficult-to-treat epilepsies (particularly the Lennox–Gastaut syndrome) unresponsive to safer agents (34[R]), (35[R]).

Risk factors *To date, a total of 34 cases of felbamate-associated aplastic anemia have been reported. Of these 20 occurred in combination with other compounds implicated as a possible cause of aplastic anemia and five occurred concurrently with viral infections (34[R]). Although five patients were taking felbamate monotherapy, 13 of the 34 suffered from auto-*

immune diseases, and one was taking cytostatic therapy. The mean age of the 34 patients was 41 (range 13–75) years, with a mean time of felbamate exposure of 154 days. There had been previous allergic or toxic reactions to other antiepileptic drugs in 65% of the patients; blood dyscrasias were reported in 45%, while 32% had serological evidence of an immune disorder in the past. Eight of nine patients tested had experienced at least one episode of aplastic anemia-associated HLA antigens. While risk factors have not been identified with certainty, it would be wise at this stage to avoid felbamate in patients with previous blood dyscrasias or autoimmune disorders, especially lupus erythematosus.

Incidence *In an attempt to define incidence rates better, the first 31 reported cases of aplastic anemia associated with felbamate have been re-evaluated (35[Cr]). According to the criteria of the International Agranulocytosis and Aplastic Anemia Study, 23 cases (15 women and eight men, median age 40 years) were confirmed as aplastic anemia. Of these, seven had died and two had been lost to follow-up; the median length of follow-up among the remaining 14 survivors was 29 (range 24–34) months. Felbamate was considered the only plausible cause in three cases and the most likely cause in 11; in the remaining nine cases, there was at least one other plausible cause in addition to felbamate. With an estimated exposure rate of 110 000 patients (based on sales data), the incidence of felbamate-induced aplastic anemia was estimated to be 27–209 per million (with a 'most probable' estimate of 127 per million), compared with a risk of aplastic anemia of 2–2.5 per million in the general population.*

Mechanism *Superoxide dismutase activity in erythrocytes and glutathione peroxidase activity in plasma and erythrocytes from seven patients with a history of felbamate-associated aplastic anemia were significantly reduced compared with matched healthy controls and patients without idiosyncratic reactions to felbamate (36[c]). These data suggest that a deficiency in free radical scavenging activity may play a role in felbamate-induced aplastic anemia.*

Avoidance *Before starting felbamate, patients should be fully informed of the potential risks and educated about symptoms that might herald bone marrow toxicity. Hematological tests should be performed at baseline and during treatment, and dose escalations should be made slowly.*

Liver and pancreas Twenty-three cases of *hepatic failure* have been reported in patients on felbamate, but only 10 (including five patients who died) were probably related to the drug (34[R]). There have been also 20 cases of *hepatitis* in which no deaths occurred, and in five of these a relation with felbamate was considered unlikely. Overall, the incidence of fatal liver toxicity caused by felbamate is estimated at one per 26 000–34 000. A careful history, asking about previous hepatic damage with other drugs, and the routine measurement of liver function tests are recommended before starting felbamate. Patients should be seen regularly to monitor hepatic function, and alerted about signs and symptoms of possible hepatotoxicity.

Gabapentin *(SED-13, 153; SEDA-19, 70; SEDA-20, 61; SEDA-21, 71)*

Nervous system A 58-year-old woman developed *stuttering* after she had started to take gabapentin in an unspecified dosage (37[c]). Although the symptom disappeared after withdrawal, a cause–effect relation remains speculative.

Endocrine, metabolic Evidence is emerging that *weight gain* is a significant adverse effect of gabapentin. Of 44 adults with epilepsy treated with high-dosage gabapentin (mean 3520 mg/day) for at least 12 months, 10 gained more than 10% and 15 gained between 5 and 10% of their baseline weight (38[C]). Gain in weight started after 2–3 months and tended to stabilize after 6–9 months. Among 45 patients who had been taking high-dose gabapentin monotherapy (mean 3900 mg/day) for a mean of 252 days, body weight increased by an average of 3.5 kg (5% of total body weight) compared with baseline (39[c]). This was considered an adverse effect in four patients whose average weight gain was 11 kg (7–20 kg) or 14% of their initial body weight.

Hematological Among 275 patients who took part in a comparison of three dosages of gabapentin (600, 1200, and 3600 mg/day), the only serious adverse event leading to withdrawal was *granulocytopenia* in one patient, who was also taking carbamazepine and valproate (40[c]). Granulocytopenia was present at pretreatment, worsened with gabapentin (600 mg/day), and resolved after withdrawal. No other details were given, and the potential cause–effect relation is open to speculation.

Liver A 26-year-old man developed *raised liver enzymes* (increase in AsT from 25 to 855 U/l and AlT from 35 to 1670 U/l) 12 weeks after gabapentin had been added to phenytoin and primidone (41[c]). Serological tests for hepatitis A, B, and C were negative, and recovery occurred after withdrawal of gabapentin. Gabapentin is rarely involved in idiosyncratic reactions, and insufficient details were given to assess its possible role in this case.

Skin and appendages Diffuse *alopecia* developed in a 15-year-old girl after she had taken gabapentin (1800 mg/day) for about 1 month, and regressed within 1 month of withdrawal (42[c]). This observation suggests that gabapentin may be added to the list of anticonvulsants (phenytoin, carbamazepine, vigabatrin, and especially valproate) capable of causing alopecia.

Urinary system *Urinary incontinence* after the administration of gabapentin has been reported previously (43[c]), and has again been described in a 43-year-old man, a 34-year-old woman, and a 12-year-old boy, who took 600–1800 mg/day (44[c]). In all cases the symptom disappeared after withdrawal.

Lamotrigine *(SED-13, 153; SEDA-19, 70; SEDA-20, 62; SEDA-21, 72)*

The long-term tolerability of lamotrigine has been evaluated in 11 316 patients included in a non-interventional cohort study carried out in the context of the UK Prescription Event Monitoring System (45[C]). A follow-up study provided data on the first 3994 patients who took lamotrigine for 6 months or more. Rash was the most common non-epileptic event (19.7/1000 patient months) in the first month of treatment and led to withdrawal in 2% of patients; it was more common in children aged 2–12 years (29.4/1000 patient months). The most common events leading to withdrawal were *rash* ($n = 210$), *drowsiness* ($n = 74$), *nausea* ($n = 66$), *dizziness* ($n = 63$), *headache* ($n = 61$), *vomiting* ($n = 33$), *ataxia* ($n = 32$), *malaise* ($n = 29$), and *aggression* ($n = 26$). Rare serious adverse events included *Stevens–Johnson syndrome* ($n = 12$), *neutropenia* ($n = 4$), *thrombocytopenia* ($n = 3$), *disseminated intravascular coagulation* ($n = 2$), *leukopenia* ($n = 1$), *meningitic reaction* ($n = 1$), *acute renal failure* ($n = 1$), *hepatotoxicity* ($n = 1$), and a *lupus-like reaction* ($n = 1$). For Stevens–Johnson syndrome, the risk in the first month of therapy was 0.8/1000 patients. Sixty-nine women took lamotrigine in the first trimester of pregnancy and six later in pregnancy; there were two terminations for spina bifida in mothers co-medicated with valproate. Among the 55 live births from these pregnancies, there were three with major *congenital malformations*, but other drugs had been taken concurrently and a specific role of lamotrigine could not be established.

Cardiovascular Isolated cases of *multiorgan dysfunction* and *disseminated intravascular coagulation* were observed during early clinical studies, but at least some of these were ascribed to underlying disorders rather than lamotrigine itself. The condition has again been observed in two children aged 3.5 and 11 years, 9 days after lamotrigine had been added to their antiepileptic therapy, which included valproic acid (46[cr]). The presentation included fever, rash, hepatic and renal dysfunction, hypoalbuminemia, disseminated intravascular coagulation, and changes in alertness. Since no other causative factor was detected, lamotrigine was probably responsible. One of the children had rhabdomyolysis during the episodes, suggesting that the reaction may involve muscular tissue.

Nervous system Among 19 intellectually handicapped adults with epilepsy given add-on lamotrigine, 10 developed *aggressive behaviour* (47[cr]). Five required drug withdrawal after 7–47 days (drug dosage 25–200 mg/day), two were withdrawn from treatment but required lamotrigine reintroduction complemented with psychiatric assistance, one responded to a decrease in dosage, one continued treatment with psychiatric assistance, and one had aggression unrelated to treatment. Four other patients had behavioral problems besides aggression. Irritability and other manifestations of disturbed behavior have also been described in three mentally retarded adults given add-on lamotrigine (0.7–4.5 mg/kg/day), but there were also three patients whose behavior improved on lamotrigine (48[C]). These data suggest that lamotrigine may carry some risk of inducing irritability and aggressive or violent behaviour in mentally retarded patients.

Downbeat nystagmus can occur at high serum concentrations of lamotrigine (49[c]).

Three patients taking lamotrigine (300–400 mg/day, serum concentrations 17–24 mg/l) in combination with valproate (1500–2500 mg/day) developed downbeat nystagmus in primary position with exacerbation on oblique and downward gaze and no nystagmus on extreme upward gaze. Nausea, vomiting and truncal ataxia were also present. The symptoms resolved after lamotrigine concentrations had been reduced to below 10 mg/l.

Hematological *Anemia* associated with increased platelet counts has been described in two men aged 17 and 35 years after they had taken lamotrigine for about 2 months (50[cr]). Although the condition reversed after lamotrigine withdrawal, other drugs were also administered and a cause–effect relation cannot be ascertained.

Skin and appendages Lamotrigine-induced severe *skin rashes*, including *toxic epidermal necrolysis* and *Stevens–Johnson syndrome*, have an estimated frequency of 1:50 to 1:300 in children compared with 1:1000 in adults (SEDA-20, 72). In trials sponsored by the manufacturer, 11 of 3499 adults (0.3%) developed a rash leading to hospitalization; four of these were reported as possible Stevens–Johnson syndrome (51[c]). Eleven of 966 children (1%) developed a rash associated with hospitalization, with possible Stevens–Johnson syndrome in five (0.5%). Usually the rash occurs during the first 8 weeks. Risk factors include exceeding the recommended dose escalation rate and co-administration of valproate.

In a retrospective survey, minor *skin rashes* were observed in 20 (15%) of 130 epileptic children (mean age 8 years) (52[c]). The rashes developed within 1 day to 5 months (median 17 days) after starting lamotrigine and were usually urticarial or maculopapular. There were no cases of Stevens–Johnson syndrome. Contrary to previous reports, the rash was not more common when valproate was co-administered. The incidence of rash fell from 25% (14/57) before 1996 to 8% (6/73) thereafter, probably as a consequence of the more conservative dosage escalation regimens used recently. In two children, aged 2 and 13 years, who developed a macular or maculopapular rash 27 and 16 days after starting lamotrigine, the rash was associated with a marked increase in the percentage of activated T helper and T suppressor lymphocytes, a smaller increase in the percentage of B lymphocytes, and a larger increase in serum IgE (53[C]). This confirms that the condition is immune mediated. An immune-mediated reaction was also suggested by a positive lymphocyte transformation test to lamotrigine in a 30-year-old man who developed Stevens–Johnson syndrome 5 weeks after lamotrigine had been added to valproate (54[c]).

When six patients who developed a skin rash while taking lamotrigine were switched to phenobarbital ($n = 5$) or phenytoin ($n = 1$), a similar rash reappeared (55[c]). One patient was then exposed to felbamate and the rash recurred. Since lamotrigine is structurally unrelated to aromatic anticonvulsants, such cross-allergy is intriguing. A general predisposition to immunologically mediated reactions might be an explanation.

Immunological and hypersensitivity reactions A 24-year-old man developed erythematous and hemorrhagic papules 1 week after he started to take lamotrigine, 400 mg/day (56[c]). The condition worsened during the next 2–3 weeks, when he developed a fever, leukocytosis, and laboratory evidence of liver and kidney dysfunction. Lamotrigine withdrawal and high-dosage steroid therapy resulted in complete recovery after 1 week. The condition was considered to resemble phenytoin hypersensitivity syndrome, and its precipitation may have been facilitated by an inappropriately large initial dosage, although surprisingly this was not commented on.

Interactions Preliminary data suggest that *sertraline* may increase serum lamotrigine concentrations (57[c]). In one patient, the addition of sertraline (25 mg/day) was associated with a doubling of lamotrigine concentrations and symptoms of toxicity, while in another a reduction in sertraline dosage (by 25 mg/day) resulted in halving of serum lamotrigine concentrations, despite a 33% increase in lamotrigine dosage. No other details were given.

Phenytoin *(SED-13, 141; SEDA-19, 72; SEDA-20, 64; SEDA-21, 73)*

Cardiovascular The *purple-glove syndrome*, defined as the progressive development of edema, discoloration, and pain in the limb, is a recognized complication of intravenous phenytoin. Its sequelae include soft-tissue necrosis and limb ischemia. Retrospective analysis of data from 140 patients treated with intravenous phenytoin identified eight (5.7%) who developed purple-glove syndrome; they had received a higher median initial dose of phenytoin (700 vs 362 mg) and a higher total dose (900 vs 500 mg) than those without the complication, and they were older (70 vs 49 years) (58[c]). One patient required surgical therapy while the others resolved within 3 weeks with conservative management.

Skin and appendages A 19-year-old girl developed *acromelanosis* (hyperpigmentation of all fingers and toes) after she had taken phenytoin for 7 years (59[c]). The condition regressed partially when phenytoin was withdrawn for 1 year, but recurred within 3 months of restarting treatment. This adverse effect does not appear to have been reported before.

Immunological and hypersensitivity reactions Phenytoin is rarely implicated in hypersensitivity reactions with pulmonary involvement. The first case of histopathologically documented *bronchiolitis obliterans organizing pneumonia* diagnosed by open-lung biopsy has been described in a 40-year-old man with severe phenytoin hypersensitivity syndrome (60[c]). Cold agglutinin disease was also documented, together with hemodynamic changes mimicking sepsis. The patient improved rapidly on high-dosage steroid therapy.

Interactions The addition of *ticlopidine* (250 mg bd) to phenytoin (350 mg/day) in a 44-year-old man resulted in a rise in serum phenytoin concentrations from 15–20 to 46.5 mg/l within 25 days, with signs of phenytoin toxicity (61[cr]). Although this interaction has been described before, in this study the mechanism was investigated using human liver microsomes and was found to involve inhibition of CYP2C19.

In a 69-year-old man, serum concentrations of intravenous phenytoin fell markedly after the addition of *ciprofloxacin* (800 mg/day intravenously for 1 week) and increased again when the ciprofloxacin was withdrawn (62[cr]). This seems to be the fourth patient to have shown a fall in serum phenytoin after the addition of ciprofloxacin (63[r]). The mechanism is unknown. The time course is not consistent with enzyme induction, and a change in phenytoin serum protein binding is also unlikely because ciprofloxacin is not highly bound to plasma proteins. Monitoring serum phenytoin concentrations and clinical response is recommended whenever ciprofloxacin is added or withdrawn.

In an 8-year-old girl treated with phenytoin and *ifofosfamide*, the plasma concentration of the *R*- and *S*-enantiomers of ifofosfamide were much lower than in children not co-medicated with phenytoin, whereas the concentrations of some ifofosfamide dechloroethyl metabolites were increased (64[c]). The data were interpreted as evidence that phenytoin induces CYP2B6- and CYP3A4-mediated ifofosfamide metabolism. The child's acute lymphoblastic leukemia responded well to ifofosfamide.

Tiagabine *(SEDA-19; 73; SEDA-20, 65; SEDA-21, 74)*

In a placebo-controlled add-on comparison of tiagabine 16 mg bd with tiagabine 8 mg qds in 318 patients with refractory partial seizures, adverse events that occurred significantly more often with active treatment were *nervousness*, *vomiting*, *abdominal and other pain*, *emotional lability*, and *amnesia* (65[c]). None of these events affected more than 10% of patients. Although the incidence of adverse events did not vary with dosing frequency, there was a trend for patients taking a twice-daily schedule to have more adverse events.

Nervous system Of 123 patients with refractory epilepsy in a randomized trial, those who could be converted successfully to tiagabine monotherapy (6 or 36 mg) showed some improvement in mood and adjustment (low-dose group) or in motor speed, concentration and verbal fluency measures (high-dose group) (66[C]). However, the subgroup of 18 patients in the high-dose group who could not achieve monotherapy had a deterioration in measures in *mood and adjustment*. The effect was ascribed to an excessively fast titration rate (12 mg/week).

The possibility that tiagabine can cause *non-convulsive status epilepticus* was discussed in SEDA-21 (p. 74). In another report, two of nine patients included in an open add-on tiagabine trial developed non-convulsive status with electroclinical features consistent with atypical absence seizures (67[C]). Both were women with partial epilepsy, and one had never had atypical absences before. The dosage of tiagabine when status developed was 30 mg/day, and in both patients drug withdrawal was followed by sustained electroclinical remission. GABAergic drugs aggravate absence seizures, but de novo appearance of absences in patients with partial epilepsy is unusual.

Topiramate *(SEDA-20; 66; SEDA-21, 75)*

Nervous system In a retrospective survey, five of 80 patients who started to take topiramate developed *psychotic symptoms* within 2–46 days; these included paranoid delusions in four, auditory hallucinations in three, suicidal thoughts in two, aggressive thoughts or actions in two, and mood swings and depersonalization in one (68[c]). The dosage of topiramate at the onset of symptoms was 50–400 mg/day. The condition resolved after withdrawal in three cases, a dosage reduction from 300 to 200 mg/day in one, and neuroleptic treatment in one patient who had become seizure-free. Three patients had no significant psychiatric history. Although a cause–effect relation cannot be ascertained, the possibility of a drug-induced reaction should be considered in patients developing psychotic symptoms on topiramate.

Dose-dependent *impairment in attention* (assessed by weekly digit span) was reported in four of nine patients who took topiramate in dosages of 100–700 mg/day over a 3-month period (69[C]). Because of the small number of patients, the uncontrolled design, and the lack of comprehensive evaluation, these data cannot be regarded as conclusive.

Valproate sodium *(SED-13, 149; SEDA-19, 73; SEDA-20, 67; SEDA-21, 76)*

In a double-blind trial (70[c]), 143 patients with poorly controlled partial seizures were switched to divalproex sodium monotherapy and randomized to serum valproic acid concentrations in a low range (25–50 mg/l) or a high range (80–150 mg/l). Adverse effects were more common in the high-range group, and included *tremor* (64 vs 6%), *thrombocytopenia* (31 vs 0%), *alopecia* (28 vs 4%), *weakness* (17 vs 0%), *diarrhea* (21 vs 4%), *vomiting* (17 vs 0%), and *anorexia* (15 vs 0%). Valproate was discontinued because of adverse events in 32% of patients in the high-range group compared with 2% in the low-range group. To meet regulatory requirements, the study aimed to show a difference in efficacy between the groups, which explains the allocation to concentration ranges outside the normally quoted optimal range of 50–100 mg/l. Seizure control was better in the high-range group, but many patients tolerated high concentrations poorly.

Endocrine, metabolic Muscle biopsies in seven children treated with valproate showed *accumulation of microvesicular lipid* droplets between myofibrils adjacent to mitochondria (71[c]). There were ultrastructural abnormalities in the mitochondria, and it was suggested that lipid deposits were a result of impaired mitochondrial fatty acid oxidation. Lipid accumulation and mitochondrial changes were also seen in the muscle of rats given 100 mg/kg valproate intraperitoneally for 14 days.

Hematological In a controlled trial, 36 (27%) of 131 patients with epilepsy randomized to high plasma concentrations of valproic acid (80–150 mg/l) had at least one platelet count below 75×10^9/l, compared with only one patient in the group randomized to low valproic acid concentrations (25–50 mg/l) (72[c]). Logistic regression analysis showed that the probability of valproate-induced *thrombocytopenia* increases when trough unbound and total valproic acid concentrations exceed 30 and 135 mg/l, respectively, in men and 20 and 110 mg/l, respectively, in women.

An unusual case report has suggested that hematological complications may occur following exposure to valproate in breast milk (73[c]). *Thrombocytopenic purpura*, *anemia*, and *reticulocytosis* were observed in a 3-month-old breast-fed infant whose mother was taking valproic acid at a dosage of 1200 mg/day. The serum valproic acid concentration in the infant was 6.6 mg/l. Recovery occurred when breast feeding was stopped.

Liver and pancreas A boy with delayed psychomotor development, attention deficit disorder, and epilepsy died of *liver failure* after taking valproate for 4 months (74[Cr]). Postmortem investigations with cultured fibroblasts suggested medium chain acyl-CoA dehydrogenase deficiency, an unexpected finding, because the boy had not shown the typical manifestations of this disease. This metabolic disorder is considered to predispose to valproate hepatotoxicity.

Pancreatitis developed in a 14-year-old girl and a 12-year-old boy after they had taken valproate for 2 years (75[Cr]). The girl also had manifestations of hepatotoxicity and died. Both children had end-stage renal failure, raising the possibility that this might predispose to valproate-associated pancreatitis.

Interactions A 43-year-old woman with partial seizures stabilized on valproic acid (750 mg tds) developed *status epilepticus* 12 days after starting to take *clomipramine*, 75 mg/day for depression (76[c]). The status was ascribed to clomipramine toxicity and the serum clomipramine concentration was high (342 ng/ml), in spite of the low dosage. The authors speculated that valproic acid inhibited the metabolism of clomipramine, a suggestion consistent with evidence that valproic acid can increase the serum concentrations of amitriptyline and nortriptyline.

Vigabatrin *(SED-13, 155; SEDA-19, 76; SEDA-20, 70; SEDA-21, 77)*

Special senses Following initial reports in 1997 of a possible association between vigabatrin and *visual field defects* (SEDA-21, 78), this issue has been a hot topic among physicians treating epilepsy. While prospective studies providing conclusive evidence for a cause–effect relation have not been completed, the bulk of evidence suggests that vigabatrin-treated patients have an increased risk of developing possibly irreversible constriction of the visual fields.

The incidence of the visual field defects is still uncertain, partly because recognition is difficult without careful ophthalmological testing. Among 38 patients treated with vigabatrin, two complained of constricted visual field and two had blurred vision after 2–40 months of therapy at dosages of 2–4.5 g/day (77[C]). Electroretinography showed bilateral retinal dysfunction consistent with reduced inner retinal cone response in all four patients. Oscillatory potentials were lost. Two of the patients had normal visual-evoked responses and minimal abnormalities at clinical ophthalmological examination. Impairment of cone function was ascribed to selective vulnerability of the retina of affected patients to the GABAergic effects of vigabatrin. Another study involving ophthalmological assessment was carried out in a group of patients in a randomized comparative monotherapy trial of vigabatrin and carbamazepine in newly diagnosed epilepsy (78[c]), (79[c]). Of 32 patients still taking vigabatrin after 3–9 years, 13 (42%) had constricted visual fields, and the defects were rated as severe in two patients. Of seven patients with field defects, five had reduced oscillatory potentials and two also had abnormal a and b waves in rod and cone electroretinograms. By contrast, none of the 20 patients taking carbamazepine had abnormal visual fields.

A total of 23 additional cases of vigabatrin-associated visual field defects were reported in abstract form at the European Epilepsy Congress in May 1998 (80[c])–(82[c]). The only case described in detail was that of a 17-year-old boy who developed symptomatic bilateral constriction of the peripheral visual field 18 months after starting to take vigabatrin 4 g/day, in addition to valproate 2400 mg/day (82[c]). Electro-oculography and visual evoked responses were normal, but Gantzfeld electroretinography showed reduced oscillatory potentials, suggesting damage to the outer retina rather than the optic nerve.

As mentioned above, visual field defects may not be recognized easily. In fact, even patients with relatively severe constriction can partly compensate for the defect by adjustments in eye movements. Owing to the slow development of the disorder, these patients may be unaware of their condition, even though their visual impairment may place them at risk in special situations, for example when driving a car. Visual field defects are also difficult to detect by simple clinical examination, even in patients who have severe constriction at perimetric assessment.

Pending further information, the manufacturers have recommended visual field testing before treatment and at regular intervals during treatment. Patients should also be questioned about visual disturbances and should be referred to an ophthalmologist if symptoms suggestive of a field defect are recognized.

Zonisamide *(SED-13, 156; SEDA-19, 76; SEDA-21, 80)*

Assessment of tolerability data in 197 patients in seven clinical trials has suggested that the adverse effects of zonisamide are related to the rate of dose escalation (83[c]). In particular, adverse events in the first 4 weeks of therapy occurred in 90% of 25 patients started at 400 mg/day, compared with 49% when the same dosage was reached over a 4-week escalation period. No details were given about the type of adverse events recorded.

Interactions In vitro studies have suggested that zonisamide should not inhibit the oxidative metabolism of drugs metabolized by CYP1A2, CYP2D6, or CYP3A4 (84[c]). However, it may have a minor inhibitory effect on the clearance of drugs metabolized by CYP2A6, CYP2C9, CYP2C19, and CYP2E1. Zonisamide itself is partly metabolized by CYP3A4 and to a lesser extent CYP2C19 and CYP3A5. In vitro studies have also predicted that the CYP3A4 inhibitors ketoconazole, cyclosporin, and miconazole should reduce zonisamide clearance by 31, 23, and 17%, respectively (85[C]). No clinically significant inhibition of zonisamide metabolism is expected from therapeutic dosages of carbamazepine, fluconazole, itraconazole, dihydroergotamine, or triazolam.

REFERENCES

1. Tomson T, Kenneback G. Arrhythmia, heart rate variability, and antiepileptic drugs. Epilepsia 1997;38 (Suppl 11):S48–51.
2. Huuskonen UEJ, Isojarvi JIT. Antiepileptic drugs and serum sodium. Epilepsia 1997;38 (Suppl 8):89–90.
3. Deckers CLP, Hekster YA, Keyser A, Meinardi H, Renier WO. Reappraisal of polytherapy in epilepsy: a critical review of drug load and adverse effects. Epilepsia 1997;38:570–5.
4. Gambardella A, Aguglia U, Oliveri RL, Russo C, Zappia M, Quattrone A. Negative myoclonus status due to antiepileptic drug tapering: report of three cases. Epilepsia 1997;38:819–23.
5. Wong ICK, Tavernor SJ, Tavernor RME. Psychiatric adverse effects of anticonvulsant drugs: incidence and therapeutic implications. CNS Drugs 1997;8:492–509.
6. Kishi T, Fujita N, Eguchi T, Ueda K. Mechanism of reduction of serum folate by antiepileptic drugs during prolonged therapy. J Neurol Sci 1997;145:109–12.

7. Tennis P, Stern RS. Risk of serious cutaneous disorders after initiation of use of phenytoin, carbamazepine, or sodium valpoate: a record linkage study. Neurology 1997;49:542–6.
8. Hyson C, Sadler M. Cross sensitivity of skin rashes with antiepileptic drugs. Can J Neurol Sci 1997;24:245–9.
9. Chan JL, Tan KC. Fixed drug eruption to three anticonvulsant drugs: an unusual case of polysensitivity. J Am Acad Dermatol 1997; 36:259.
10. Bayer AU, Thiel HJ, Zrenner E, Dichgans J, Kuehn M, Paulus W, Ried S, Schmidt D. Color vision tests for early detection of antiepileptic drug toxicity. Neurology 1997;48:1394–7.
11. Toepfer M, Sitter T, Lechmuller H, Pontgraz LD, Muller-Felber W. Drug-induced systemic lupus erythematosus after 8 years of treatment with carbamazepine. Eur J Clin Pharmacol 1998;54:193–4.
12. Theis JG, Koren G, Daneman R, Sherwin AL, Menzano E, Cortez M, Hwang P. Interactions of clobazam with conventional antiepileptics in children. J Child Neurol 1997;12:208–13.
13. Salke-Kellerman RAT, Boenigk HE. Influence of ethosuximide on valproic acid serum concentrations. Epilepsy Res 1997;26:345–9.
14. Yukawa E, To H, Ohdo S, Higuchi S, Aoyama T. Detection of a drug-drug interaction on population-based phenobarbitone clearance using nonlinear mixed-effects modeling. Eur J Clin Pharmacol 1998;54:69–74.
15. May TW, Rambeck B. Influence of oxcarbazepine and methsuximide on lamotrigine concentrations. Epilepsia 1998;39 (Suppl 2):25.
16. Besag FMC, Berry DJ, Pool F. Methsuximide lowers lamotrigine blood levels: a pharmacokinetic antiepileptic drug interaction. Epilepsia 1998;39 (Suppl 2):25.
17. Collins M, McKee S, Beinlich B, Gidal B. Potential interaction between lamotrigine and primidone. Epilepsia 1997;38 (Suppl 8):101.
18. Besag FMC, Berry DJ, Pool F, Newbery JE, Subel B. Carbamazepine toxicity with lamotrigine: pharmacokinetic or pharmacodynamic interaction? Epilepsia 1998;39:183–7.
19. Troupin AS, Montouris G, Hussein G. Felbamate: therapeutic range and other kinetic information. J Epilepsy 1997;10:26–31.
20. Jones AL, Proudfoot AT. Features and management of poisoning with modern drugs used to treat epilepsy. Q J Med 1998;91:325–32.
21. Wilschut FA, Cobben NAM, Thunnissen FBJM, Lamer RJS, Wouters EFM, Drent M. Recurrent respiratory distress associated with carbamazepine overdose. Eur Resp J 1997;10:2163–5.
22. Matsumoto J, Ogawa H, Maeyama R, Okudaira K, Shinka T, Kuhara T, Matsumoto I. Successful treatment by direct hemoperfusion of coma possibly resulting from mitochondrial dysfunction in acute valproate intoxication. Epilepsia 1997;38:950–3.
23. Wu HM, Tsai JJ. Bilateral periodic epileptiform discharges as postictal change in a case with vigabatrin withdrawal discontinuous complex partial status epilepticus seizure. Epilepsia 1998;39 (Suppl 2):95.
24. Kramer G, Mothersill IW, Ried S. Carbamazepine-induced tonic seizures. Epilepsia 1998;39 (Suppl 2):108.
25. Mahajan L, Wyllie R, Goldblum J. Lymphocytic colitis in a pediatric patient: a possible adverse reaction to carbamazepine. Am J Gastroenterol 1997;92:2126–7.
26. Salzman MB, Valderrama E, Sood SK. Carbamazepine and fatal eosinophilic myocarditis. New Engl J Med 1997;336:878–9.
27. Bergendal L, Friberg A, Schaffrath AM, Holmdahl M, Landahl S. The clinical relevance of the interaction between carbamazepine and dextropropoxyphene in elderly patients in Gothenburg, Sweden. Eur J Clin Pharmacol 1997;53:203–6.
28. Spina E, Arena D, Scordo MG, Fazio A, Pisani F, Perucca E. Elevation of plasma carbamazepine concentrations by ketoconazole in patients with epilepsy. Ther Drug Monit 1997;19:535–8.
29. Routledge PA, Soryal I, Eve MD, Williams J, Richens A, Hall R. Reduced bioavailability of nifedipine in patients with epilepsy receiving anticonvulsants. Br J Clin Pharmacol 1998; 45:196P.
30. Capewell S, Freestone S, Critchley JAJH, Pottage A, Prescott. Reduced felodipine bioavailability in patients taking anticonvulsants. Lancet 1988;31:68–74.
31. Tartara A, Galimberti CA, Manni R, Parietti L, Zucca C, Baasch H, Caresia L, Muck W, Barzaghi N, Gatti G, Perucca E. Differential effects of valproic acid and enzyme inducing anticonvulsants on nimodipine bioavailability in epileptic patients. Br J Clin Pharmacol 1991;32:335–40.
32. Michelucci R, Cipolla G, Passarelli D, Gatti G, Ochan M, Heinig R, Tassinari CA, Perucca E. Reduced plasma nisoldipine concentrations in phenytoin-treated patients with epilepsy. Epilepsia 1996;37:1107–10.
33. Bottcher T, Buchmann J, Zettl UK, Benecke R. Carbamazepine-phenprocoumon interaction. Eur Neurol 1997;38:132–3.
34. Pellock JM, Brodie MJ. Felbamate: 1997 update. Epilepsia 1997;38:1261–4.
35. Kaufman DW, Kelly JP, Anderson T, Harmon DC, Shapiro S. Evaluation of case reports of aplastic anemia among patients treated with felbamate. Epilepsia 1997;38:1265–9.
36. Glauser TA, Titanic MK, Armstrong D, Pippenger CE. Abnormalities in free radical scavenging enzyme activity in patients with felbamate-associated aplastic anemia. Epilepsia 1998;39 (Suppl 2):40.
37. Nissani M, Sanchz EA. Stuttering caused by gabapentin. Ann Intern Med 1997;126:410–11.
38. DeToledo JC, Toledo C, DeCerce J, Ramsay RE. Changes in body weight with chronic, high-dose gabapentin therapy. Ther Drug Monit 1997;19:394–6.
39. Beydoun A, Fakhoury T, Nasreddine W,

Abou-Khalil B. Conversion to high-dose gabapentin monotherapy in patients with medically refractory partial epilepsy. Epilepsia 1998;39:188–93.
40. Beydoun A, Fisher J, Labar DR, Harden C, Cantrell D, Uthman BM, Sackellares JC, Abou-Khalil B, Ramsay RE, Hayes A, Greiner M, Garofalo E, Pierce M, and the US Gabapentin Study Group 82/83. Gabapentin monotherapy: II. A 26-week, double-blind, dose-controlled, multicenter study of conversion from polytherapy in outpatients with refractory complex partial or secondarily generalized seizures. Neurology 1997; 47:746–52.
41. Singh BK, White-Scott S. Side effects of add-on gabapentin in individuals with epilepsy, mental retardation, and developmental disabilities. Epilepsia 1997;38 (Suppl 8):180.
42. Picard C, Jonville-Bera AP, Billard C, Autret E. Alopecia associated with gabapentin: first case. Ann Pharmacother 1997;31:1260.
43. Doherty KP, Gates JR, Penovich PE, Moriarty MD. Gabapentin in a medically refractory epilepsy population: seizure response and unusual side effects. Epilepsia 1995;36 (Suppl 4):71.
44. Gil-Nagel A, Gapany S, Blesi K, Villanueva N, Bergen D. Incontinence during treatment with gabapentin. Neurology 1997;48:1467–8.
45. Mackay FJ, Wilton LV, Pearce GL, Freemantle SN, Mann RD. Safety of long-term lamotrigine in epilepsy. Epilepsia 1997;38:881–6.
46. Chattergoon DS, McGuigan MA, Koren G, Hwang P, Ito S. Multiorgan dysfunction and disseminated intravascular coagulation in children receiving lamotrigine and valproic acid. Neurology 1997;49:1442–4.
47. Beran RG, Gibson RJ. Aggressive behaviour in intellectually challenged patients with epilepsy treated with lamotrigine. Epilepsia 1998;39:280–2.
48. Ettinger AB, Weisbrot DM, Saracco J, Dhoon A, Kanner A, Devinsky O. Positive and negative psychotropic effects of lamotrigine in patients with epilepsy and mental retardation. Epilepsia 1998; 39:874–7.
49. Tasch E, Bernasconi A, Kirkham T, Sherwin A, Andermann F. Reversible downbeat nystagmus: a new sign of lamotrigine toxicity. Epilepsia 1997;38 (Suppl 8):103.
50. Esfahani FE, Dasheiff RM. Anemia associated with lamotrigine. Neurology 1997;49:306–7.
51. Giorgi L, Messenhemer J, Risner M. Safety overview of Lamictal in adult and pediatric clinical trials. Epilepsia 1998;39 (Suppl 2):61.
52. Hahn JS, Humberg-Roether S, Crowley T, Low C. Incidence of rash in children treated with lamotrigine. Epilepsia 1997;38 (Suppl 8):193.
53. Iannetti P, Raucci U, Zuccaro PG, Pacifici R. Lamotrigine hypersensitivity in childhood epilepsy. Epilepsia 1998;39:502–7.
54. Sachs B, Ronnau AC, Von Schmiedebrg S, Ruzicka T, Gleichmann EE, Schuppe HC. Lamotrigine-induced Stevens-Johnson syndrome: demonstration of specific lymphocyte reactivity in vitro. Dermatology 1997;195:60–4.
55. Gudin M, Galindo PA, Garrido JA, Del Real MA, Ibanez R, Diaz Obregon MC. Lamotrigine and aromatic skin rash. Epilepsia 1997;38 (Suppl 8):100.
56. Jones D, Chhiap V, Resor S, Appel G, Grossman ME. Phenytoin-like hypersensitivity associated with lamotrigine. J Am Acad Dermatol 1997;36:1016–18.
57. Kaufman KR, Gerner R. Lamotrigine toxicity secondary to sertraline. Epilepsia 1997;38 (Suppl 8):100–1.
58. O'Brien TJ, Cascino GD, So EL, Hanna DR. Incidence and clinical consequences of the purple-glove syndrome in patients receiving intravenous phenytoin. Epilepsia 1997;38 (Suppl 8):90–1.
59. Kanwar AJ, Jaswal R, Thami GP, Bedi GK. Acquired acromelanosis due to phenytoin. Dermatology 1997;194:373–4.
60. Angle P, Thomas P, Chiu B, Freedman J. Bronchiolitis obliterans with organizing pneumonia and cold agglutinin disease associated with phenytoin hypersensitivity syndrome. Chest 1997;112:1697–9.
61. Donahue SR, Flockhart DA, Abernethy DR, Ko JW. Ticlopidine inhibition of phenytoin metabolism mediated by potent inhibition of CYP2C19. Clin Pharmacol Ther 1997;62:572–7.
62. Brouwers PJ, De Boer LE, Guchelaar HJ. Ciprofloxacin-phenytoin interaction. Ann Pharmacother 1997;31:498.
63. Pollack PT, Slayter KL. Comment: ciprofloxacin-phenytoin interaction. Ann Pharmacother 1997;31:1549–50.
64. Ducharme MP, Bernstein ML, Granvil CP, Gehrcke B, Wainer IW. Phenytoin-induced alteration in the N-dechloroethylation of ifosfamide stereoisomers. Cancer Chemother Pharmacol 1997;40:531–3.
65. Sachdeo RC, Leroy RF, Krauss GL, Drake ME, Green PM, Leppik IE, Shu VS, Ringham GL, Sommerville KW, for the Tiagabine Study Group. Tiagabine therapy for complex partial seizures. A dose-frequency study. Arch Neurol 1997;54:595–601.
66. Dodrill CB, Arnett JL, Shu V, Pixton GC, Lenz GT, Sommerville KW. Effects of tiagabine monotherapy on abilities, adjustment, and mood. Epilepsia 1998;39:33–42.
67. Eckardt KM, Steinhoff BJ. Nonconvulsive status epilepticus in two patients receiving tiagabine treatment. Epilepsia 1998;39:671–4.
68. Khan A, Faught E, Kuzniecki R, Gilliam F, Laich E. Acute psychotic symptoms induced by topiramate. Epilepsia 1997;38 (Suppl 8):97.
69. Burton LA, Harden C. Effect of topiramate on attention. Epilepsy Res 1997;27:29–32.
70. Beydoun A, Sackellares JC, Shu V, and the Depakote Monotherapy for Partial Seizures Study Group. Safety and efficacy of divalproex sodium monotherapy in partial epilepsy: a double-blind, concentration response design clinical trial. Neurology 1997;48:182–8.

71. Melegh B, Trombitas K. Valproate treatment induces lipid globule accumulation with ultrastructural abnormalities of mitochondria in skeletal muscle. Neuropediatrics 1997;28:257–61.
72. Carney P, Nasreddine W, Drury I, Varma N, Payne T, Shu V, Beydoun A. Relation between thrombocytopenia and valproate dose. Epilepsia 1997;38 (Suppl 8):102.
73. Stah MMS, Neiderud J, Vinge E. Thrombocytopenic purpura and anemia in a breast-fed infant whose mother was treated with valproic acid. J Pediatr 1997;130:1001–3.
74. Njolstad PR, Skjeldal OH, Agsteribbe E, Huckriede A, Wannag E, Sovik O, Waaler PE. Medium chain acyl CoA dehydrogenase deficiency and fatal valproate toxicity. Pediatr Neurol 1997;16:160–2.
75. Levin TL, Berdon WE, Seigle RR, Nash MA. Valproic acid-associated pancreatitis and hepatic toxicity in children with endstage renal disease. Pediatr Neurol 1997;27:192–3.
76. DeToledo JC, Haddad H, Ramsay RE. Status epilepticus associated with the combination of valproic acid and clomipramine. Ther Drug Monit 1997;19:71–3.
77. Krauss GL, Johnson MA, Miller NR. Vigabatrin-associated retinal cone system dysfunction: electroretinogram and ophthalmologic findings. Neurology 1998;50:614–18.
78. Kalviainen R, Nousianen I, Nikoskelainen E, Partanen J, Partanen K, Mantyjarvi M, Riekkinen PJ. Visual field defects associated with initial vigabatrin monotherapy as compared with initial carbamazepine monotherapy. Epilepsia 1998;39 (Suppl 2):5.
79. Kalviainen R, Nousianen I, Mantyjarvi M, Riekkinen PJ. Initial vigabatrin monotherapy is associated with increased risk of visual field constriction. A comparative follow-up study with patients on initial carbamazepine monotherapy and healthy controls. Epilepsia 1998;39 (Suppl 6):72.
80. Beran RG, Currie J, Sandbach J, Plunkett M. Visual field restriction with new antiepileptic medication. Epilepsia 1998;39 (Suppl 2):6.
81. Black AB. Vigabatrin and visual field loss. Epilepsia 1998;39 (Suppl 2):5–6.
82. Pung T, Ruether K, Schmitz B, Grosse P. Visual field constriction during treatment with vigabatrin. Epilepsia 1998;39 (Suppl 2):40–1.
83. Wilder BJ, French JA, Ramsey RE, Bergen C, Padgett CS. Zonisamide introduction and tolerance. Epilepsia 1997;38 (Suppl 8):108.
84. Mather GG, Carlson S, Trager WF, Buchanan RA, Levy RH. Prediction of zonisamide interactions based on metabolic isozymes. Epilepsia 1997;38 (Suppl 8):108.
85. Nakasa H, Nakamura H, Ono S, Tsutsui M, Kiuchi M, Ohmori S, Kitada M. Prediction of drug-drug interactions of zonisamide metabolism in humans from in vitro data. Eur J Clin Pharmacol 1998;54:177–83.

A.H. Ghodse and R.E. Edwards

8 Opioid analgesics and narcotic antagonists

GENERAL

The common adverse effects of opioids are *respiratory depression*, *nausea*, *vomiting*, *sedation*, and *constipation*. These, in addition to a more comprehensive list of adverse effects encountered during long-term opioid therapy, have been listed in a review of management of chronic pain (1[R]). Those mentioned are *dry mouth*, *urinary retention*, *pruritus*, *myoclonus*, *altered cognitive function*, *sleep disturbance*, *dysphoria*, *euphoria*, *sexual dysfunction*, *inappropriate ADH secretion*, *physiological dependence*, and *tolerance*.

Nervous system The evidence that opioids can cause *seizures or seizure-like activity* has been reviewed, including the mechanisms by which opioids are neuroexcitatory and, although there is no evidence that opioids should be withheld in non-epileptic patients, the authors suggested that caution is necessary in patients with a documented history of epilepsy (2[R]).

Routes of administration The effects of conventional epidural analgesia during labor have been compared with those of a combined epidural spinal technique in a large prospective randomized trial, in which 775 women were encouraged or discouraged to ambulate (3[C]). The aim of the study was to test the hypothesis that the combined technique with ambulation encouraged is associated with a lower incidence of dystocia. The women were randomly assigned to one of three groups: one group received conventional epidural analgesia with 6 ml of 0.25% bupivacaine plus fentanyl 50 μg, followed by an infusion of 0.125% bupivacaine and fentanyl 20 μg/h; the other two groups received sufentanil 10 μg in 2 ml of isotonic saline via the subarachnoid space with a continuous infusion of 0.0625% bupivacaine and fentanyl 24 μg/h via the epidural catheter. Of the two groups receiving combined epidural/spinal analgesia, one was encouraged to walk. There were no differences in the incidence of adverse effects between the groups, although the incidence of pruritus in the group receiving conventional epidural analgesia was significantly less than in the other two groups (8 vs 47 and 46%). There were no significant differences in the incidences of sedation, nausea, fetal heart rate changes, hypotension or headache between the groups. Furthermore, the combination of spinal and epidural analgesia did not result in a lower incidence of cesarean section.

OPIOID AGONISTS

Alfentanil *(SED-13, 173; SEDA-19, 82; SEDA-20, 76; SEDA-21, 86)*

Intravenous opioids produce their effects by activation of opioid receptors in the periphery, brain and spinal cord. However, the end results of this activation can be mediated by activation of other receptor types. Noradrenaline and acetylcholine are released in the spinal cord by systemically administered opioids, and the release of acetylcholine into the cerebrospinal fluid is enhanced by intrathecal neostigmine. It has been suggested that spinally released noradrenaline and acetylcholine contribute to the analgesia produced by intravenous opioids. A study has been performed in 40 healthy volunteers to determine whether intravenous alfentanil increased CSF

Side Effects of Drugs, Annual 22
J.K. Aronson, ed.

concentrations of acetylcholine, and whether intrathecal neostigmine enhanced this effect and the analgesic effects of alfentanil (4[C]). Evidence of enhancement of the adverse effects of the drugs when used concurrently was also sought. The subjects were randomized to receive isotonic saline or neostigmine 50, 100, or 200 μg intrathecally in 2 ml of 5% dextrose. Pain measurements and visual analog scales for nausea, weakness and sedation were taken after 60 min. Alfentanil was then given by computer-controlled intravenous infusion to produce a pre-set plasma alfentanil concentration. Less alfentanil was administered if the volunteers were being given intrathecal neostigmine. Neostigmine produced more analgesia in the foot than the hand, whereas alfentanil produced equivalent analgesia. With regard to adverse effects, neostigmine did not enhance respiratory depression associated with alfentanil (determined by end tidal CO_2 and pulse oximetry), but did enhance alfentanil induced *sedation* and *nausea* synergistically; this may limit the usefulness of the combination. Neostigmine, but not alfentanil, produced *weakness* and this was synergistically enhanced by alfentanil. Alfentanil was detected in the CSF in all volunteers and it increased CSF acetylcholine concentrations, an effect that was independent of plasma alfentanil concentration; intrathecal neostigmine produced a dose-dependent increase in this effect of alfentanil.

Codeine *(SED-13, 173; SEDA-19, 82; SEDA-21, 86)*

Codeine is *O*-demethylated to morphine by CYP2D6. There are two major phenotypes (extensive and poor metabolizers) and a new phenotype of ultrarapid metabolizers has been identified, with very high CYP2D6 activity.

An ultrarapid codeine metabolizer has been described: a 33-year-old woman who experienced *severe epigastric pain*, *euphoria* and *dizziness* within 30 min of taking codeine 60 mg (5[c]). Following further ingestion of 30 mg codeine her symptoms recurred but were less severe than before. She was phenotyped and genotyped as an ultrarapid metabolizer and the cause of her pain was presumed to have been due to rapid formation of morphine by the liver, a high concentration in the biliary tracts causing biliary spasm.

Risk factors Last year's review included a message of caution with regard to the use of over-the-counter cough suppressants. A statement by the American Academy of Pediatrics Committee on Drugs has emphasized that the efficacy of codeine and dextromethorphan as cough suppressants has not been demonstrated in children (6[R]). Hepatic metabolism of the drugs contained in antitussive medications is reduced in infants, enhancing the risk of adverse effects. Doses of codeine of 3–5 mg/kg per day have produced *somnolence*, *ataxia*, *miosis*, *vomiting*, *rash*, *facial swelling* and *pruritus*. *Respiratory depression* occurred in 3% of children receiving in excess of 5 mg/kg per day, with two deaths. The authors suggested that cough suppression in children may be contraindicated and that acute viral airway infection should be managed with fluids and humidity. Parents should be educated with regard to the lack of proven effects of antitussives in children and the potential risk of their administration.

Fentanyl *(SED-13, 174; SEDA-19, 82; SEDA-20, 77; SEDA-21, 88)*

The addition of epidural fentanyl 100 μg to morphine 2 or 4 mg produced superior analgesia without an increase in the incidence of adverse effects, compared with morphine alone, in 122 patients undergoing gastrectomy (7[C]). Visual analog scale scores were significantly lower in the first 6 h after surgery in those who received morphine 4 mg with fentanyl, although 10% of patients still required supplemental analgesia in the first 4 h after surgery. Not surprisingly, in the later postoperative phase, those who received morphine 4 mg, with or without fentanyl, had significantly lower visual analog scale scores than those who received morphine 2 mg. No patient who received morphine 4 mg/fentanyl 100 μg had clinically significant respiratory depression and, although the incidence of *pruritus* was high in this group (30%), this was not significantly higher than in patients who received other combinations of epidural opioids.

Fentanyl is often added to extradural bupivacaine during labor to improve on the onset, quality and duration of analgesia produced by the local anesthetic alone. In a study designed to determine the bupivacaine sparing effect of various concentrations of fentanyl in women in labor, the incidence of pruritus was significantly higher (23%) at a concentration of 4 μg/ml, although this was the concentration that was associated with the greatest bupivacaine sparing effect (8[C]). The optimum concentration was therefore suggested to be 3 μg/ml.

In 20 primigravidae, in whom epidural analgesia was contraindicated in labor, intravenous patient-controlled fentanyl was used as an analgesic; fentanyl is short acting and may be less sedating than morphine (9[C]). Three of 10 women randomized to intravenous fentanyl were withdrawn because of inadequate analgesia and were given epidural block. Adverse effects were greater in those given fentanyl, and *dizziness* and *tiredness* reached statistical significance. Other adverse effects included *nausea and vomiting*. There was no effect on the cardiotocogram or neonatal outcome. Patient-controlled fentanyl may have a place in women in whom epidural analgesia is contraindicated and in multiparous women with shorter labors.

The effects of different patient-controlled management practices on outcomes, including adverse effects, have been evaluated (10[C]) in 40 patients who received patient-controlled analgesia and were managed by primary service physicians (usually surgeons), compared with a retrospective group matched for age, sex and type of surgery and who were treated by acute pain service physicians. Nausea, vomiting, sedation, respiratory depression and mental state changes were documented every 4 h. The patients managed by the primary service physicians had a significantly higher incidence of adverse effects than the patients who were managed by acute pain service physicians. *Nausea* and *urinary retention* were significantly higher, whilst the incidence of *pruritus* was comparable. No patient had respiratory depression. The pain service physicians avoided morphine if the patient reported previous bad experiences with the drug, but the primary service physicians did not. Not unexpectedly, regular and repeated visits by experienced physicians concentrating on quality of analgesia and adverse effects resulted in superior management. As the authors pointed out, improved education of primary service staff may lead to improved analgesia in postoperative patients.

Nervous system The *amnesic effects* of equisedative doses of intravenous fentanyl with ondansetron pretreatment, midazolam, propofol and thiopental have been compared in 67 healthy volunteers in a randomized double-blind study (11[CR]). The drugs were administered by computer-controlled infusion to achieve three target concentrations at increasing levels of sedation followed by two decreasing sedative concentrations. Fentanyl had no amnesic effects, in contrast to the other non-opioids used. In a previous study the authors found that fentanyl, at the same maximum serum concentrations as in this study, did have an effect on memory impairment and they discussed the possible antagonism by ondansetron of mild impairment by fentanyl in relation to effects on serotonergic neurones, which have a role in memory. A possible explanation for this effect may be that the presence of nausea in subjects in the previous study reduced their level of sedation and thus improved their memory performance.

Gastrointestinal Although *dysphagia* has been reported with intrathecal sufentanil, dysphagia after intrathecal fentanyl has been reported for the first time in two women receiving combined epidural-spinal analgesia during labor (12[c]). One woman was given 20 μg, the other 25 μg. One hour after the fentanyl, the first woman had difficulty swallowing and an inability to clear her throat. The second had dysphagia, generalized itching and tingling in her lips and fingers after 20 min. Both cases resolved spontaneously. The authors proposed cephalad spread of the opioid as a cause of these symptoms, with cranial nerve involvement.

Musculoskeletal Opioid-induced *rigidity* is well described with large doses of opioids.

Severe muscle rigidity has now also been described after a small dose of fentanyl (13[c]).

A 21-year-old pregnant woman, an in-patient in a psychiatric unit, was taking haloperidol and paroxetine for major depression. She received fentanyl 50 μg intravenously to facilitate vaginal examination, followed 30 min later by a second dose of 100 μg. Severe muscle rigidity and apnea ensued and manual ventilation was impossible. With naloxone spontaneous ventilation returned and she regained consciousness.

The authors suggested that reduced anesthetic requirements in pregnancy and the concurrent administration of butyrophenones had played a significant role in this complication.

Morphine *(SED-13, 176; SEDA-19, 83; SEDA-20, 79; SEDA-21, 89)*

Intrathecal morphine has been evaluated in 40 patients undergoing coronary artery bypass grafting to determine its effects on the timing of extubation and postoperative analgesic requirements (14[C]). The patients were randomly allocated to either intrathecal morphine 10 μg/kg or placebo (isotonic saline) before induction of anesthesia. After extubation they received intravenous PCA morphine. They were directly questioned about the presence of pruritus, nausea and vomiting postoperatively. The mean time from arrival in ICU and extubation was significantly longer in the patients who received intrathecal morphine. Three of 19 patients who received intrathecal morphine had extubation delayed because of *respiratory depression*. The authors pointed out that large doses of intravenous fentanyl, which would have had an additive effect with morphine, had been used (20 μg/kg), and that the ideal dose of intrathecal morphine required to produce optimal analgesia with minimal respiratory depression remains to be evaluated.

The effects of intravenous morphine or fentanyl given postoperatively on adequacy of analgesia, incidence of adverse effects and readiness for discharge postoperatively have been studied in 58 patients undergoing ambulatory day-case surgery in a randomized double-blind comparison (15[C]). The drugs were titrated postoperatively according to pain scores on a visual analog scale until the patient had a score of less than 40 mm or to a maximum of 20 mg morphine or 250 μg fentanyl. The incidence of *nausea and vomiting* was not significantly different in the two groups before discharge but was significantly higher with morphine after discharge. There were no significant differences in sedation or dizziness. Not unexpectedly, owing to its longer duration of action, morphine produced sustained analgesia with less requirement for postoperative analgesia, although both opioids produced similar analgesia in the first 20 min. The authors did not comment on the high male to female ratio in the fentanyl group compared with the morphine group (15:14 vs 21:8), a factor that may have influenced differences in postoperative nausea and vomiting.

In a study designed to evaluate the effects of pre-emptive analgesia with epidural morphine, 30 patients undergoing lumbar laminectomy were randomly assigned to a control group (epidural placebo 60 min before start of surgery followed by epidural morphine 3 mg at the end of surgery) or a study group (morphine 3 mg at the start of surgery and epidural placebo at the end of surgery) (16[C]). The mean visual analog scale scores in the study group were significantly less than the control group at 8, 12, and 24 h after surgery. There was a statistically significant higher incidence of *sedation* and *nausea and vomiting* in the control group, although the number of patients who had nausea and vomiting was not stated. This can be explained by the greater need for supplementary intravenous morphine (mean dose 31 mg/day in controls vs 9.5 mg/day in the study group). There were, however, no other significant adverse effects.

Gastrointestinal Morphine increases lower esophageal sphincter pressure during esophageal relaxation induced by swallowing. This effect has been evaluated in eight patients with reflux disease and healthy volunteers to establish whether morphine could reduce the incidence of reflux (17[C]). Although morphine, as expected, reduced reflux by this mechanism, the impact on the amount of reflux was minimal, as swallowing-induced relaxation of the lower esophageal sphincter is not the major mechanism of reflux in these patients. An unexpected observation was that morphine reduced the rate of transient lower esophageal sphincter relaxations in the patients, thus reducing the number of episodes of reflux. This did not happen in the healthy subjects, possibly because of the small number of episodes of transient lower esophageal sphincter relaxation in this group and the short observation time. The mechanism of this effect is uncertain. The effect was reversed by naloxone, suggesting the involvement of μ-opioid receptors. The site postulated was the afferent pathway, since lower esophageal sphincter relaxation pressure and duration were unaffected, making the efferent pathway unlikely.

Risk factors The pharmacokinetics of morphine are altered in patients with liver disease, and different types of disease affect drug kinetics in different ways. A study of the pharmacokinetics of modified-release morphine in patients with cirrhosis after hepatitis showed that clearance was reduced in the patients with cirrhosis compared with controls (18[c]). The reduction in liver cell mass led to a 3-fold increase in peak plasma concentrations due to reduction in first-pass metabolism. The patients were more sedated than controls and there was a higher incidence of opioid-related adverse effects. The authors therefore recommended reduced doses and longer intervals between doses in patients with cirrhosis receiving oral opioids, such as morphine.

A similar study of intravenous oxycodone in patients with end-stage cirrhosis requiring transplantation showed reduced drug clearance (19[c]), prompting the recommendation that dosage intervals of oxycodone be reduced in these patients.

Remifentanil

Remifentanil is a new opioid with a very short duration of action; it is metabolized by non-specific esterases in tissue and plasma.

Remifentanil has been used for maintenance of anesthesia in 62 children undergoing surgery for strabismus in a comparison with propofol, isoflurane and alfentanil (20[C]). There was no difference in recovery time between the groups, nor any significant difference in the incidence of adverse effects, with the exception of a greater incidence of hypoxia in those given alfentanil. However, the incidence of *vomiting* in those given remifentanil was high (31%) and similar to the incidence in the other groups (alfentanil 26%, isoflurane 32%, propofol 30%). The dose of remifentanil used in the study was twice the ED_{50} of adults and may have been much larger than required.

Remifentanil has also been compared with alfentanil in a multicenter study of 201 patients scheduled for day-case surgery (21[C]). Patients who received remifentanil had significantly fewer responses to surgical stimulation and had better psychomotor and psychometric function during the recovery period, although there was no significant difference in time to recovery room or hospital discharge. There was a higher incidence of *hypotension* during anesthesia in those given remifentanil, presumably related to the concurrent use of a relatively high dose of isoflurane, which was probably unnecessary. There was no statistically significant difference in the incidence of adverse effects between the two groups.

Sufentanil *(SED-13, 178; SEDA-19, 85; SEDA-20, 81; SEDA-21, 89)*

Serious consequences related to the use of intrathecal sufentanil in parturients have been described in a series of case reports.

A 17-year-old primigravida had a respiratory arrest requiring intubation 4 min after intrathecal sufentanil 10 mg (22[c]). This prompted the authors to review all parturients who had received intrathecal or epidural analgesia between 1990 and 1996. Of the 4870 patients who had received intrathecal sufentanil, in most cases 10 mg, the case described was the only one of respiratory arrest, giving a risk of 0.021% (95% CI 0–0.061%).

Severe maternal hypotension and fetal bradycardia occurred 4 min after sufentanil 7.5 mg and bupivacaine 2.5 mg intrathecally (23[c]). There was no motor blockade, making a significant contribution from bupivacaine unlikely.

A case of maternal hypotension (requiring brief external cardiac massage) and respiratory arrest and one of respiratory arrest have been described after intrathecal sufentanil 10 mg and bupivacaine 2.5 mg (24[c]). Both women had received intravenous fentanyl before regional anesthesia, in one case 90 min and in the other 120 min before. Both patients responded readily to intravenous naloxone.

It may well be that prior narcotics and the concurrent use of intrathecal or even epidural bupivacaine may contribute to serious adverse effects, and these reports should caution anesthesiologists to the potential for serious adverse effects with these techniques.

The dose–response relation and adverse effects of intrathecal sufentanil have been analysed in 18 healthy women (25[C]) in a random double-blind study of intrathecal sufentanil 12.5, 25 or 50 mg. Analgesia was assessed by pressure algometry at the tibia. Respiratory rate, pulse oximetry, arterial blood gas analysis, ventilatory response to CO_2 and a respiratory intervention score (designed to standardize detection and treatment of hypoxemia in this study) provided thorough assessment of respiratory depression, and a nausea and pruritus scoring system were used. P_aCO_2 rose significantly in all groups for 10 h after drug administration, although the changes were not dramatic (maximum 12.4 mmHg, 1.65 kPa). There were 29 episodes of *hypoxemia*, defined as pulse oximetry readings of less than 85% for 5 s, which we would describe as severe hypoxemia. Supplementary oxygen at 2 l/min restored the saturation to over 90%, although this still constitutes significant hypoxia. Increasing doses of sufentanil produced a higher incidence of *nausea*. The incidence of *pruritus* was high (15/20), but there was no dose–response relation. Respiratory rate and sedation did not significantly change in any subject. In summary, therefore, there was no analgesic advantage in increasing the dose of intrathecal sufentanil to above 12.5 mg in this group, and increasing doses led to more respiratory depression and nausea and vomiting.

The effect of adding dextrose to alter the baricity of intrathecal sufentanil has been examined in two studies of women in labor, and therefore the spread of the solution and possibly the incidence of adverse effects (26[CR]), (27[C]). In one study (26[CR]) intrathecal sufentanil 10 mg was diluted with saline or dextrose 10% and the needle aperture was directed either up or down, to attempt to influence the extent of spread. In the other study sufentanil was diluted with saline or dextrose 7.5% and injected in either the lateral decubitus or sitting position, again to influence the spread of the solution (27[C]). In both studies the duration of analgesia with intrathecal sufentanil was reduced when the spread of the solution was limited, and in one (26[CR]) there was less analgesic effect with the hypobaric solution. Limiting spread also significantly reduced the incidence of pruritus. Needle orientation had no effect on the spread of the solution.

Epidural sufentanil and fentanyl have been compared in 80 women after cesarean section (28[C]). When they complained of postoperative pain they were randomly allocated to one of eight groups: fentanyl 25, 50, 100 or 200 mg, or sufentanil 5, 10, 20 or 30 mg. Intraoperative analgesia was provided by epidural lidocaine with adrenaline. The ED_{95} for fentanyl was 92 mg and for sufentanil 17.5 mg, giving an analgesic potency ratio of 1:5. There was no difference between the groups in the incidence of adverse effects. In all, 45% of the patients had at least one adverse effect, *pruritus* being the most common (41%). Only four patients complained of *nausea* and none had a respiratory rate below 10/min, although more sensitive indices of respiratory depression were not evaluated. The incidence of adverse effects did not increase with increasing dose. As the authors discussed, there was probably a contribution from residual blockade due to the epidural local anesthetic administered for the operation, although this was likely to have been consistent in all the groups.

Large doses of intravenous opioids, commonly administered on induction of anesthesia for cardiac surgery, cause *difficulty in ventilation* and *muscular rigidity*. The contribution of closure of the vocal cords to difficulty in ventilation has been assessed in 30 patients undergoing cardiac surgery (29[C]). Each received intravenous sufentanil 3 mg/kg and photographs were taken via a fiberoptic bronchoscope positioned above the glottis under local anesthesia. Pulmonary compliance was severely impaired in 28 of the patients and all had closed vocal cords. The mechanism for this effect is not understood; however, the authors commented that animal experiments have suggested an increase in efferent motor impulses, causing muscle contraction and rigidity due to central μ_1 receptor stimulation.

Tramadol *(SED-13, 176; SEDA-20, 81; SEDA-21, 90)*

The use of caudal tramadol has been studied in 90 boys aged 13–53 months undergoing hypospadias surgery who received either bupivacaine 2 mg/kg, tramadol 2 mg/kg or both (30[C]). The group who received tramadol alone had significantly greater requirements for additional analgesia within 1 h of surgery compared with the other two groups. Additional analgesia was administered when the pain score was greater than 3/10. In the other patients there was no significant difference in the time to next analgesic request between the three groups. There was no significant difference in the incidence of adverse effects between the groups.

Nervous system A single dose of 100 mg tramadol produced *ataxia*, *pupillary dilatation and visual disturbance*, *numbness of the arms and legs*, *tremulousness* and *dysphoria* in a healthy 32-year-old man (31[c]). This patient was an ultrarapid CYP2D6 metabolizer and so the effects may have been due to the O-desmethyl metabolite of tramadol.

Psychiatric A 27-year-old woman with bipolar disorder developed marked *insomnia* and other *manic symptoms* 4 days after taking tramadol 200 mg/day (32[c]). She had had one previous episode of mania whilst taking steroids. She had been treated with valproic acid, carbamazepine and haloperidol, all of which had been discontinued for 5 months before the accident that led to the use of tramadol prescription. This may have been a natural recurrence of her mania although, as tramadol is a noradrenaline and serotonin reuptake inhibitor and also stimulates serotonin release, it may exacerbate mania in a similar manner to antidepressants.

Interactions An interaction between tramadol and *phenprocoumon*, leading to an increase in INR, has been described in two patients (33[c]), (34[c]). This was probably due to either potentiation of the effect of phenprocoumon on vitamin K epoxide reductase or inhibition of phenprocoumon metabolism by tramadol. An interaction of *warfarin* with tramadol has also been reported (35[c]).

A possible interaction of *sertraline* with tramadol, leading to a 'serotonin syndrome', has been described (36[c]). Tramadol inhibits serotonin reuptake and stimulates its release. Several possible factors may have been involved in this case, including inhibition of CYP2D6 by sertraline and tramadol accumulation, but there are many unanswered questions.

PARTIAL OPIOID AGONISTS

Buprenorphine *(SED-13, 180; SEDA-19, 89; SEDA-20, 82; SEDA-21, 91)*

Buprenorphine is a synthetic opioid which is a partial agonist and, it is claimed that although *respiratory depression* occurs, there is a ceiling effect, with no further respiratory depression at higher doses. It is metabolized to buprenorphine glucuronide and *N*-dealkylated to norbuprenorphine. Norbuprenorphine is a weak analgesic, but no research into its respiratory effects has previously been undertaken. Now, the respiratory depressant effects of both buprenorphine and norbuprenorphine have been evaluated in rats (37). There was no respiratory depression with buprenorphine at doses of 0.008–3 mg/kg. There was a dose-dependent depression of respiration with norbuprenorphine, reaching a peak effect after 15 min; the effect was 10 times more potent than that of buprenorphine. The respiratory depressant effect of norbuprenorphine was far less after intra-arterial injection than intravenous injection, and lung concentrations were four times higher after intravenous injection, suggesting that the effect may be via opioid receptors in the lung rather than the brain. Further evaluation of norbuprenorphine with various opioid receptor antagonists suggested that its effects are mediated via μ receptors and that norbuprenorphine has a higher affinity for the μ_2 receptor subtype, which is involved mainly in respiratory depressant effects, than buprenorphine.

Nalbuphine *(SED-13, 182)*

Nalbuphine is a mixed opioid agonist-antagonist which is thought to have efficacy at both μ and κ receptors, and which has a ceiling effect for both its analgesic and respiratory depressant effects. It has been studied in healthy volunteers to determine its psychological, physiological and subjective effects and to compare it with equianalgesic doses of morphine in 15 subjects (38[CR]). Psychomotor performance and subjective effects were dose related. There was no effect on delayed recall, only on immediate recall. There were significant effects on heart rate, oxygen saturation, respiratory rate, and pupillary size, although only miosis was dose related. There was no effect on blood pressure. The subjective effects included increased scores on the Pentobarbital-Chlorpromazine-Alcohol Group scale (sensitive to sedation effects) and the Lysergic Acid Diethylamide scale (sensitive to somatic and dysphoric changes) of the Addiction Research Centre Inventory rating scales. There were also increased adjective checklist ratings, for example, 'numb' and 'sweating', increased visual analog scale ratings of, for example, 'high' and 'sleepy', and increased drug-liking ratings. The authors pointed out that, although the study showed that nalbuphine 10 mg was comparable with morphine 10 mg, they had not compared other doses.

OPIOID ANTAGONISTS

Nalmefene

Nalmefene is an opioid antagonist with a longer duration of action than naloxone. *Pulmonary edema* after naloxone is well known. A 21-year-old man, previously fit and healthy, developed pulmonary edema 15 min after being given nalmefene 75 mg in 25-mg increments over 10 min after an exploratory laparotomy (39[c]).

Naltrexone *(SED-13, 180; SEDA-20, 83; SEDA-21, 92)*

Pruritus associated with cholestasis may be mediated via enkephalins, and the opioid antagonists naloxone and nalmefene have successfully used in its treatment. In 16 patients with pruritus due to cholestasis randomized to receive naltrexone 50 mg/day or placebo for 4 weeks, naltrexone produced a significant reduction in pruritus (40[C]). The adverse effects comprised *malaise* initially in four patients, *dizziness* (two), *drowsiness* (two), *headache* (one), *nightmares* (one) and *tremor* (one). The symptoms improved after 3 days. One patient required a reduction in dosage to 25 mg/day after 1 week; although his symptoms persisted he completed the study. Other adverse effects reported with naltrexone were *abdominal cramps* (five), *dry mouth* (two), *night sweats* and *peripheral edema*. One patient withdrew after 2 weeks of naltrexone, as the itching increased. There was no deterioration in liver function.

REFERENCES

1. Garcia J, Altman RD. Chronic pain states: pathophysiology and medical therapy. Semin Arthritis Rheum 1997;27:1–16.
2. Manninen PH. Opioids and seizures. Can J Anaesth 1997;44:463–6.
3. Nageotte MP, Larson D, Rumney PJ, Sidhu M, Hollenbach K. Epidural analgesia compared with combined spinal-epidural analgesia during labor in nulliparous women. New Engl J Med 1997;337:1715–19.
4. Hood DD, Mallak KA, James RL, Tuttle R, Eisenach JC. Enhancement of analgesia from systemic opioid in humans by spinal cholinesterase inhibition. J Pharmacol Exp Ther 1997;282:86–92.
5. Dalen P, Frengell C, Dahl M-L, Sjoqvist F. Quick onset of severe abdominal pain after codeine in an ultrarapid metabolizer of debrisoquine. Ther Drug Monit 1997;19:543–4.
6. Berlin CM Jr, McCarver-May DG, Notterman DA, Ward RM, Weismann DN, Wilson GS, Wilson TJ, March J, Bennett DR, Hoskins IA, Mulinare J, Kaufman P, Mithani S, MacLeod SM, Troendle G, Yaffe SJ, Cote CJ, Szefler SJ. Use of

codeine- and dextromethorphan-containing cough remedies in children. Pediatrics 1997;996:918–20.
7. Tanaka M, Watanabe S, Matsumiya N, Okada M, Kondo T, Takahashi S. Enhanced pain management for post-gastrectomy patients with combined epidural morphine and fentanyl. Can J Anaesth 1997;44:1047–52.
8. Lyons G, Columb M, Hawthorne L, Dresner M. Extradural pain relief in labour: bupivacaine sparing by extradural fentanyl is dose dependent. Br J Anaesth 1997;78:493–7.
9. Nikkola EM, Ekblad UU, Kero PO, Alihanka JJM, Salonen MAO. Intravenous fentanyl PCA during labour. Can J Anaesth 1997;44:1248–55.
10. Stacey BR, Rudy TE, Nellhaus D. Management of patient-controlled analgesia: a comparison of primary surgeons and a dedicated pain service. Anesth Analg 1997;85:130–4.
11. Veselis RA, Reinsel RA, Feschenko VA, Wronski M. The comparative amnestic effects of midazolam, propofol, thiopental, and fentanyl at equisedative concentrations. Anesthesiology 1997;87:749–64.
12. Currier DS, Levin KR, Campbell C. Dysphagia with intrathecal fentanyl. Anesthesiology 1997;87:1570–1.
13. Viscomi CM, Bailey PL. Opioid-induced rigidity after intravenous fentanyl. Obstet Gynecol 1997;89 (Suppl II):822–4.
14. Chaney MA, Furry PA, Fluder EM, Slogoff S. Intrathecal morphine for coronary artery bypass grafting and early extubation. Anesth Analg 1997;84:241–8.
15. Claxton AR, McGuire G, Chung F, Cruise C. Evaluation of morphine versus fentanyl for postoperative analgesia after ambulatory surgical procedures. Anesth Analg 1997;84:509–14.
16. Kundra P, Gurnani A, Bhattacharya A. Preemptive epidural morphine for postoperative pain relief after lumbar laminectomy. Anesth Analg 1997;85:135–8.
17. Penagini R, Bianchi PA. Effect of morphine on gastroesophageal reflux and transient lower esophageal sphincter relaxation. Gastroenterology 1997;113:409–14.
18. Kotb HIM, El-Kabsh MY, Emara SES, Fouad EA. Pharmacokinetics of controlled release morphine (MST) in patients with liver cirrhosis. Br J Anaesth 1997;79:804–6.
19. Tallgren M, Olkkola KT, Seppala T, Hockerstedt K, Lindgreen L. Pharmacokinetics and ventilatory effects of oxycodone before and after liver transplantation. Clin Pharmacol Ther 1997; 61:655–61.
20. Davis PJ, Lerman J, Suresh S, McGowan FX, Cote CJ, Landsman I, Henson LG. A randomized multicenter study of remifentanil compared with alfentanil, isoflurane, or propofol in anesthetized pediatric patients undergoing elective strabismus surgery. Anesth Analg 1997;85:982–9.
21. Cartwright DP, Kvalsvik O, Cassuto J, Jansen J-P, Wall C, Remy B, Knape JTA, Noronha D, Upadhyaya BK. A randomized, blind comparison of remifentanil and alfentanil during anesthesia for outpatient surgery. Anesth Analg 1997; 95:1014–19.
22. Ferouz F, Norris MC, Leighton BL. Risk of respiratory arrest after intrathecal sufentanil. Anesth Analg 1997;85:1088–90.
23. D'Angelo R, Eisenach JC. Severe maternal hypotension and fetal bradycardia after a combined spinal epidural anesthetic. Anesthesiology 1997;87:166–8.
24. Lu JK, Manullang TR, Staples MH, Kern SE, Bailey PL. Maternal respiratory arrests, severe hypotension, and fetal distress after administration of intrathecal, sufentanil, and bupivacaine after intravenous fentanyl. Anesthesiology 1997; 87:170–2.
25. Lu JK, Schafer PG, Gardner TL, Pace NL, Zhang J, Niu S, Stanley TH, Bailey PL. The dose-response pharmacology of intrathecal sufentanil in female volunteers. Anesth Analg 1997;85:372–9.
26. Ferouz F, Norris MC, Arkoosh VA, Leighton BL, Boxer LM, Corba RJ. Baricity, needle direction and intrathecal sufentanil labor analgesia. Anesthesiology 1997;86:592–8.
27. Gage JC, D'Angelo R, Miller R, Eisenach JC. Does dextrose affect analgesia or the side effects of intrathecal sufentanil? Anesth Analg 1997; 85:826–30.
28. Grass JA, Sakima NT, Schmidt R, Michitsch R, Zuckerman RL, Harris AP. A randomized, double-blind, dose-response comparison of epidural fentanyl versus sufentanil analgesia after cesarean section. Anesth Analg 1997;85:365–71.
29. Bennett JA, Abrams JT, Van Riper DF, Horrow JC. Difficult or impossible ventilation after sufentanil-induced anesthesia is caused primarily by vocal cord closure. Anesthesiology 1997; 87:1070–4.
30. Prosser DP, Davis A, Booker PD, Murray A. Caudal tramadol for postoperative analgesia in paediatric hypospadias surgery. Br J Anaesth 1997;79:293–6.
31. Gleason PP, Frye RF, O'Toole T. Debilitating reaction following the initial dose of tramadol. Ann Pharmacother 1997;31:1150–2.
32. Watts BV, Grady TA. Tramadol-induced mania. Am J Psychiatry 1997;154:1624.
33. Madsen H, Moller Rasmussen J, Brosen K. Interaction between tramadol and phenprocoumon. Lancet 1997;350:637.
34. Boeijinga JK, Van Meegen E, Van den Ende R, Schook CE, Cohen AF, Madsen H, Rasmussen JM, Brosen K. Is there interaction between tramadol and phenprocoumon? (multiple letters). Lancet 1997;350:1552–3.
35. Scher ML, Huntington NH, Vitillo JA. Potential interaction between tramadol and warfarin. Ann Pharmacother 1997;31:646–7.
36. Mason BJ, Blackburn KH. Possible serotonin syndrome associated with tramadol and sertraline coadministration. Ann Pharmacother 1997;31: 175–7.

37. Ohtani M, Kotaki H, Nishitateno K, Sawada Y, Iga T. Kinetics of respiratory depression in rats induced by buprenorphine a metabolite, norbuprenorphine. J Pharmacol Exp Ther 1997; 281:428–33.
38. Zacny JP, Conley K, Marks S. Comparing the subjective, psychomotor and physiological effects of intravenous nalbuphine and morphine in healthy volunteers. J Pharmacol Exp Ther 1997; 280:1159–69.
39. Henderson CA, Reynolds JE. Acute pulmonary edema in a young male after intravenous nalmefene. Anesth Analg 1997;84:218–9.
40. Wolfhagen FHJ, Sternieri E, Hop WCJ, Vitale G, Bertolotti M, Van Buuren HR. Oral naltrexone treatment for cholestatic pruritus: a double-blind, placebo-controlled study. Gastroenterology 1997;113:1264–9.

A. Del Favero

9 Anti-inflammatory and antipyretic analgesics and drugs used in gout

NON-STEROIDAL ANTI-INFLAMMATORY DRUGS (NSAIDs)

Cardiovascular There is evidence that NSAIDs can adversely affect cardiovascular function in many ways. They can cause *edema*, induce or aggravate *hypertension* or *congestive heart failure*, and interact negatively with the effects of *antihypertensive drugs and diuretics* (SEDA-11, 85; SEDA-20, 89; (1[R]), (2[R]), (3[C])).

The mechanisms involved in these clinically important adverse effects of NSAIDs are complex and controversial, and may include, among others, reduced renal blood flow, a reduction in the filtered load of sodium, an increase in tubular reabsorption of sodium, and a reduction in PGE_1 synthesis, which may be associated with raised blood viscosity and increased peripheral vascular resistance due to increased renal synthesis of endothelin-1 (SEDA-11, 85; (3[C])).

However, only a minority of patients using NSAIDs develop the above-mentioned adverse effects. The reason for that is not clear, but it is probably related to the fact that extracellular volume and sodium homeostasis are very closely regulated by other control systems, or it may be that a combination of NSAIDs with other risk factors (such as advanced age) is necessary. It is therefore important to quantify the actual risk of developing such adverse effects.

Reliable data are available for hypertension in the elderly (2[CR]): recent users of NSAIDs have a 1.7-fold increase in the risk of initiating antihypertensive therapy compared with non-users, and the use of NSAIDs significantly predicts the presence of hypertension (OR 1.4; 95% CI 1.1–1.7). Much less is known about the risk of developing congestive heart failure. In a recent study (4[C]) the rate of hospitalization for congestive heart failure in more than 10 000 patients over 55 years of age during exposure to both diuretics and NSAIDs was compared with the rate in those exposed to diuretics only. The patients were followed up for an average of 4.7 years, a total observation time of 49 512 person-years. There was an overall increased risk of hospitalization for congestive heart failure during periods of concomitant use of diuretics and NSAIDs compared with diuretics alone (relative risk 1.8; 95% CI 1.4–2.4). Most hospitalizations occurred during the first month of concomitant treatment. The risk was even greater in patients with a pre-existing diagnosis of congestive heart failure (RR 2.4; 95% CI 1.7–3.4). There were no significant differences in the risk of hospitalization for congestive heart failure among the various NSAIDs used.

Nervous system After reviewing 120 spontaneous reports the Australian Drug Reaction Advisory Committee recently reported that *paresthesia* is a class effect of NSAIDs, although it is rare and reversible (5[c]).

Side Effects of Drugs, Annual 22
J.K. Aronson, ed.

Rx Gastrointestinal problems with NSAIDs

Despite a wider appreciation among physicians that NSAIDs cause a significant number of gastrointestinal disorders, NSAID-induced gastrointestinal complications remain a problem (6[R]), (7[C]), (8[C]).

This topic has been previously reviewed in these volumes (SEDA-17, 102; SEDA-18, 99), but some recently published data deserve attention.

Does the risk of upper gastrointestinal toxicity persist during continuous treatment with NSAIDs and after their withdrawal? *Several studies have suggested that upper gastrointestinal toxicity shortly after exposure does not persist (9[C])–(12[C]). This may be either because there is adaptation to NSAID-induced mucosal damage or because in these studies susceptible patients were selected.*

However, contrasting findings have recently been published. A population-based cohort study has provided evidence that upper gastrointestinal toxicity is constant during exposure to NSAIDs and continues for some time after treatment stops (8[C]). The study included 52 293 patients aged over 50 years who had received one or more prescriptions for NSAIDs in 1989–91, and 73 792 controls who had not. The increased risks of admission to hospital for both complications (bleeding or perforation) and any upper gastrointestinal event associated with exposure to NSAIDs were constant during continuous exposure. Moreover, despite the fact that the increased risk of gastrointestinal toxicity in NSAID users falls with increasing time since the last exposure, some excess risks seemed to persist for at least a year after the last exposure. This last finding might be explained by the fact that intermittent self-treatment with left-over drug, combined with the use of non-prescription drugs (such as aspirin), may occur in general practice more often than is usually anticipated.

Can educational interventions reduce NSAID-related problems? *NSAIDs are among the most frequently used analgesics, and their use may be accompanied by serious problems, in particular upper gastrointestinal bleeding and perforation (13[C]), (14[C]). Our knowledge of the epidemiology, pathogenic mechanisms, and predisposing risk factors of NSAID-related gastrointestinal toxicity has greatly improved in the last decade. It is now clear that avoidance of unnecessary prescribing, use of the lowest efficacious dose of the safer NSAIDs, and careful monitoring of patients, especially those with known risk factors for gastrointestinal damage, are all key factors in achieving a reduction in the incidence of such severe adverse effects. However, to attain this objective it is necessary that doctors prescribe these analgesics wisely and that patients become better acquainted with them. Unfortunately, recent reports have shown that both these requirements are far from being fulfilled (13[C])–(15[C]). In a study of hospital admissions of elderly patients in Scotland (13[C]) 5.3% of admissions were probably or definitely caused by drugs; NSAIDs were most frequently implicated (28% of the cases). Most importantly, more than 66% of hospitalizations due to NSAID-related adverse events were considered to have been definitely preventable by more judicious prescription. Moreover, two independent surveys in the US have shown that many patients using NSAIDs are unaware of the severe adverse effects that they can cause (14[C]), (15[C]), and that low awareness may put patients (mainly elderly patients) at unnecessary increased risks of severe reactions (16[C]).*

The first survey showed that 37% of elderly patients had not been warned by their doctors about possible adverse effects of analgesics, and 48% had not been advised against potential interactions associated with them (14[C]). The second survey (15[C]) gave similar results, showing that 30% of individuals using prescription NSAIDs had not been informed about potential adverse effects by their pharmacist, compared with 68% of those using over-the-counter NSAIDs. Elderly patients, a high-risk group, had the poorest information about analgesics.

The relevance of patient information in the prevention of adverse effects of NSAIDs has been nicely illustrated in a study of 50 consecutive patients who were admitted to the hospital with acute gastrointestinal bleed and who had taken NSAIDs 3 days before admission, compared with 100 matched control patients who had not bled (16[C]). All the patients were visited at home to assess their knowledge of their therapy. In particular they were asked if they had received any information about possible adverse effects of NSAIDs, and if so what they had been advised to do if adverse effects developed. Not only did the patients who suffered gastrointestinal bleeding know less about the adverse effects of NSAIDs or what to do when they occurred than the controls, but they also adhered more closely to the prescribed dosage of NSAIDs. In fact 18 patients (36%) who bled had had epigastric pain before the bleed and all but two had continued to take the NSAID, whereas only 15 (15%) of the controls had had epigastric discomfort, of whom 10 had reduced their analgesic intake. Despite the potential limitations of the study (17[r]), it looks as if ignorance of adverse effects can lead to failure in recognizing warning symptoms and to inappropriate compliance. In fact, if the patients who bled had reduced their intake of NSAIDs to the same extent as the apparently better informed control patients in response to epigastric pain, it is possible that some episodes of acute gastrointestinal bleeding would have been avoided.

On the basis of these data we should consider educational interventions as one of the main preventive strategies against NSAID-related toxicity. Initiatives to fill gaps in patients' knowledge about the adverse effects of NSAIDs have been taken in the US by the FDA, which requires special labelling information on the geriatric use of NSAIDs (18[C]), and by the American Gastroenterology Association and Searle (an NSAID manufacturer), who have launched an educational campaign called Risk Education to Decrease Ulcer Complications and their Effects from NSAIDs (REDUCE) (15[C]).

Unfortunately experience of educational initiatives to improve the safe prescribing of NSAIDs is at best scanty (13[C]), (19[C]). Some of the intervention strategies were not demonstrably effective (13[C]), while others were able to modify prescribing habits only in the short term (19[C]).

To maintain long-term benefits a continuous educational program for prescribers may be necessary.

Selective cyclo-oxygenase (COX)-2 inhibitors: are they the answer to NSAID gastropathy?

This topic has previously been reviewed in these volumes (SEDA-19, 96), but it deserves further attention, as new data from experimental studies have raised questions regarding the premises on which the development of highly selective inhibitors of COX-2 as gastrointestinal-sparing anti-inflammatory agents is based. Selective inhibitors of COX-2 are being developed, based on the premise that this inducible isoform is solely responsible for prostaglandin synthesis at sites of inflammation, whereas constitutively produced COX-1 produces prostaglandins important for the maintenance of mucosal integrity. Therefore, a drug that specifically inhibits COX-2 without affecting COX-1 would theoretically reduce inflammation without causing gastrointestinal damage. Despite some experimental evidence in healthy animals and humans that selective COX-2 inhibitors have both anti-inflammatory and gastrointestinal sparing properties (20[R]), recent studies have provided important notes of caution. In an ex vivo study in 16 healthy volunteers, the range of COX-1 inhibition varied at least 1000-fold among the 25 NSAIDs studied, and all drugs also inhibited COX-2 activity in the blood, with a potency varying almost 4000-fold. All of the NSAIDs tested, even the COX-2 'selective' inhibitors, had sufficient COX-1 inhibitory activity to cause potent inhibitory effects on gastric prostaglandin E_2 synthesis at therapeutic concentrations achieved in vivo (21[C]), showing that COX-2 selectivity does not guarantee less gastric toxicity. Very interesting data came from an animal study of the relation between suppression of inflammation by COX-2 'selective' inhibitors and their effects on gastric prostaglandin synthesis. There were significant anti-inflammatory effects only at doses that also inhibited COX-1. At these doses, the drugs also significantly suppressed gastric prostaglandin synthesis and caused gastric mucosal damage. The degree of suppression of prostaglandin synthesis at the site of inflammation correlated significantly with inhibition of COX-1 but not COX-2. Therefore, COX-1 inhibition may make an important contribution to the anti-inflammatory activity of NSAIDs. To achieve desirable therapeutic effects COX-2 'selective' inhibitors need to be given in dosages at which selectivity is lost, leading to suppression of gastric prostaglandin synthesis and to mucosal *damage. Thus, the hope that the anti-inflammatory and gastrotoxic effects of NSAIDs can eventually be dissociated may not be realistic. Moreover, evidence is emerging that COX-2 activity may actually be beneficial in resolving inflammation, and in the stomach this isoenzyme has been implicated in mucosal healing and protective processes (22[C]).*

How do these experimental findings mesh with the few clinical data on the efficacy and tolerability of available COX-2 'selective' NSAIDs? Only the results of large, long-term clinical studies, incorporating careful evaluation of both the efficacy and safety of these new compounds can provide an answer.

Strategies for managing ulcers associated with the use of NSAIDs *NSAIDs can cause gastrointestinal mucosal damage by several mechanisms that may impair mucosal defence and repair capability (SEDA-17, 104). There are several lines of evidence that gastric acidity can play an important role in favoring NSAID-related upper gastrointestinal toxicity. In fact, the direct toxic action on the gastric and duodenal mucosa of some NSAIDs is exacerbated by acidity, since a low pH promotes the absorption of NSAIDs in their non-ionized form, and when mucosal cells have been damaged by other mechanisms (e.g. by loss of prostaglandin-dependent mucosal protective mechanisms) luminal acidity may increase the damage. It is not therefore surprising that increasing the gastric pH with a potent acid-inhibiting drug, such as omeprazole, has been studied as a promising option for both the treatment and prophylaxis of ulcers in patients taking NSAIDs continuously (23[R]), (24[C])–(30[C]). Four such studies deserve attention.*

The purpose of the Scandinavian Collaborative Ulcer Recurrence (SCUR) study (27[C]) was to investigate whether the empirical use of omeprazole, without any endoscopic screening, could reduce the incidence of upper gastrointestinal adverse effects with respect to placebo in 175 patients with a history of peptic ulcer disease or dyspepsia starting NSAID therapy. Treatment failure was defined as the presence after 1 or 3 months of treatment of moderate to severe dyspepsia or of endoscopic peptic ulceration or more than 10 erosions. Among omeprazole-treated patients 24% experienced treatment failure compared with 50% of those taking placebo, providing evidence that omeprazole 20 mg od provides effective prophylactic therapy in patients at risk of developing NSAID-associated ulcers, erosions, or dyspeptic symptoms.

The Omeprazole versus Placebo as Prophylaxis of Ulcers and Erosions from NSAID Treatment (OPPULENT) study (28[C]) enrolled 169 patients free of gastric or duodenal ulcers and with fewer than 10 gastric or duodenal erosions and only mild dyspepsia, a group of patients who are at low risk of developing NSAID-induced gastrotoxicity. They were endoscoped at 1, 3, and 6 months. The probability of remaining free from gastroduodenal toxicity (ulcers, multiple erosions, and moderate or severe dyspepsia) with continuous NSAID therapy for 6 months was 78% with omeprazole (20 mg od) and 53% with placebo.

In both of these prophylactic studies fewer patients taking omeprazole developed peptic ulcers and a large proportion of this overall reduction of ulcer occurrence was attributed to duodenal ulcer.

The other two studies, the Acid Suppression Trial: Ranitidine versus Omeprazole for NSAID-Associated Ulcer Treatment (ASTRONAUT) study (29[C]) and the Omeprazole versus Misoprostol for NSAID-Induced Ulcer Management (OMNIUM) trial (30[C]), had similar designs. They were large, randomized, double-blind, multicenter, controlled comparisons and both had an initial healing (therapeutic) phase followed by a prophylactic phase. A total of 1476 patients, 541 in ASTRONAUT and 935 in OMNIUM, were studied, to evaluate whether omeprazole and ranitidine (ASTRONAUT study) or omeprazole and misoprostol (OMNIUM study) were comparable in healing and maintaining remission in patients with gastroduodenal ulcers (over 3 mm in diameter) or gastroduodenal erosions (over 10) who required continuous treatment with NSAIDs.

Patients in the therapeutic phase were randomly assigned to omeprazole (20 or 40 mg od) in both studies and to ranitidine (150 mg bd), in ASTRONAUT and to misoprostol (200 mg qds), in OMNIUM. Success in this healing phase was defined as the achievement, at either 4- or 8-week endoscopy, of complete healing of any ulcer, less than five erosions in the stomach or duodenum, and only dyspeptic symptoms. In ASTRONAUT, healing rates at 8 weeks were 80 and 79% in the low- and high-dose omeprazole groups, respectively, and 63% with ranitidine. In contrast, in OMNIUM treatment success at 8 weeks was similar in all groups: 76 and 75% for low- and high-dose omeprazole, and 71% in the misoprostol-treated patients. Patients in whom treatment was successful were then randomized again, this time to maintenance treatment (prophylactic phase). In ASTRONAUT, 432 patients were randomly assigned to either omeprazole 20 mg od or ranitidine 150 mg bd for 6 months. In OMNIUM, 732 patients were randomized to maintenance therapy for 6 months with omeprazole 20 mg od, misoprostol 200 mg bd, or placebo. In both studies patients taking omeprazole remained in remission at 6 months at a higher rate than patients taking ranitidine (72 vs 59%) or misoprostol (61 vs 48%).

In conclusion, these studies have provided good overall evidence that in patients with ulcers or multiple erosions in the stomach or duodenum who require continuous NSAID treatment, therapy with omeprazole gives greater benefit than ranitidine but not misoprostol. However, misoprostol may be less effective in healing duodenal ulcers and is not as well tolerated as omeprazole. A daily dose of omeprazole over 20 mg does not confer any clinical advantage. As far as maintenance therapy is concerned, these studies have shown that in patients taking NSAIDs omeprazole 20 mg od prevents gastroduodenal damage more effectively than ranitidine or misoprostol.

Some limitations of the prophylactic studies are worthy of note:

(1) none was designed to investigate the severe upper gastrointestinal complications of NSAIDs (bleeding, perforation), and we are therefore left with doubts about whether the low rate of gastrointestinal ulcers translates into fewer complications;

(2) the relevance of preventing endoscopic lesions such as erosions may be doubtful, since there is contrasting evidence on whether erosions are an important prognostic factor for gastroduodenal ulceration (SEDA-20, 86);

(3) failure during the maintenance phase of the OMNIUM study was defined not only as recurrence of an ulcer or multiple erosions, but also as the occurrence of moderate symptoms of dyspepsia; since the correlation between symptoms and mucosal damage is poor, this definition may introduce bias in favor of omeprazole, which is particularly effective in controlling symptoms such as epigastric pain and heartburn; this bias may be relevant, as the difference in the relapse rates between misoprostol and omeprazole is mainly due to differences in the recurrence of dyspeptic symptoms, since the rates of recurrence of ulcers, erosions, or both were the same in the two groups (28%) (31[C]).

What is therefore the clinical relevance of these studies? The initial message is that with omeprazole we now have a better choice for therapy of NSAID-related gastroduodenal ulcers and possibly maintenance of remission in patients who take these drugs continuously. However, taking into account the limitations of these studies, these results should not lead to uncritical prescription of proton pump inhibitors for primary prophylaxis in NSAID-treated patients.

As previously mentioned (SEDA-19, 96), prophylactic therapy may be justified only in high-risk patients, such as the elderly, patients with history of peptic ulcer, gastrointestinal bleeding, or concomitant cardiovascular disease, or patients who are concurrently taking warfarin or high-dosage glucocorticoids.

An appropriate pharmacoeconomic evaluation of this approach would also be welcome (32[C])–(34[C]).

No association between NSAIDs and acute appendicitis *A case–control study has shown no association between appendicectomy for acute appendicitis and the use of NSAIDs (35[C]).*

Urinary system Several groups of patients are highly susceptible to functional *renal insufficiency* caused by NSAIDs (SEDA-11, 85). However the level of risk associated with community use of these drugs is unknown.

A case–control study of the relation between recent use of NSAIDs and the presence of functional renal impairment at the time of hospitalization has shown that there is a weak association between the use of NSAIDs (including non-prophylactic aspirin) and renal dysfunction (36[C]). The odds ratio for reversible renal dysfunction was 1.5 (95% CI 0.80–2.9) for patients who had used an NSAID in the previous week and 1.8 (95% CI 0.97–3.4) for the previous month. Patients at higher risk were subjects with a previous history of renal disease (OR 6.6; 95% CI 0.75–57.8) and those with a history of gout and hyperuricemia (OR 7.2; 95% CI 1.3–40.2). While NSAID dosage showed only a weak positive relation with renal impairment, there was a statistically significant difference between compounds with half-lives shorter or longer than 4 h: the OR increased from 1.2 (95% CI 0.61–2.4) to 4.8 (CI 1.5–15.8) for compounds with a half-life of over 12 h.

Long half-life drugs should be avoided in subjects at risk of renal impairment.

Infections Sporadic case reports of a possible association between NSAIDs and *necrotizing fasciitis* have been published (SEDA-12, 79; (37[R])) and continue to be reported (38[C]), but a causal link between this severe infection and NSAIDs is far from proven. A retrospective review of the cases reported to the FDA's Spontaneous Reporting System, has shown that necrotizing soft tissue infections are only rarely associated with NSAIDs (33 cases) and are unlikely to occur without other risk factors. The most frequently implicated NSAIDs were diclofenac (16 cases) and ibuprofen (11 cases), probably reflecting their more widespread use compared with other NSAIDs. The organisms cultured were compatible with the range of bacteria typically associated with necrotizing fasciitis (39[CR]).

NSAIDs are often prescribed to treat the symptom complex of fever and pain, but when these symptoms are due to an infection their use may mask signs of infection and delay appropriate treatment. On the other hand, there are several lines of evidence that NSAIDs can impair host defence mechanism against infection and can modulate the acute inflammatory response in such a way as to alter the course of infection, predisposing the patient to bacteremia, shock, and multiorgan failure (40[R]), (41[C]). Until appropriate studies have better defined the potential relation between NSAIDs and severe soft tissue infections, it would be wise to avoid using them, if possible, until the cause of the fever is known.

Use in pregnancy As inhibitors of cyclo-oxygenase, NSAIDs given during pregnancy have the potential to cause adverse maternal and fetal effects (SEDA-11, 88; (42[C])). However, little is know about the possible long-term effects of NSAIDs on the physical and mental development of the offspring of patients with inflammatory rheumatic diseases treated with NSAIDs during pregnancy (SEDA-21, 107). A cohort of 88 pregnant patients with rheumatic disease, 45 of whom were treated and 43 not treated with NSAIDs during pregnancy, has been studied. The mean duration of exposure to standard doses of NSAIDs was 15 weeks. A comparison of pregnancies that had or had not been exposed to NSAIDs showed no differences in pregnancy outcome, duration of labor, complications at delivery, neonatal health, and the health or development of the offspring at follow-up. Unfortunately, this study was too small to allow firm conclusions. NSAIDs should not be used in the third trimester of pregnancy, as they can alter fetal physiology and prolong gestation and labor (43[C]).

Tumor-preventing effects Evidence that aspirin and NSAIDs reduce the risk of colorectal cancer has prompted an interest in their ability to prevent other cancers. A case–control comparison of the use of over-the-counter analgesics in 503 women with epithelial ovarian cancer and 523 women from the general population has shown a statistically significant inverse association between paracetamol and the risk of ovarian cancer (44[C]). There was also a modest non-significant inverse association with aspirin use and ovarian cancer but no association with ibuprofen.

ACETYLSALICYLIC ACID AND RELATED COMPOUNDS *(SED-13, 170; SEDA-19, 97; SEDA-20, 90; SEDA-21, 100)*

Hematological Aspirin is currently recommended as an antithrombotic agent for patients with essential thrombocythemia. However, it is also associated with increased risk of *bleeding* in these patients, compared with the risk of bleeding in other patients treated with aspirin. The reason for this has been clarified by a study showing that aspirin prolonged the bleeding time in 82% of the patients with essential thrombocythemia but only in 27% of healthy volunteers (45[C]).

Gastrointestinal *Diaphragm-like strictures* in the small bowel have been related to the chronic use of non-aspirin NSAIDs (SEDA-17, 102). A recent report from Canada has described two cases of strictures in the small bowel caused by chronic use of acetylsalicylic acid (46[c]).

Immunological and hypersensitivity reactions Aspirin intolerance manifested as bronchospasm or urticaria/angio-edema is well known (SED-13, 170). *Unilateral periorbital angio-edema* is an unusual manifestation of aspirin intolerance (47[c]).

Use in pregnancy Aspirin is used for the prevention of complications in pregnancy and, in association with heparin, in the treatment of infertility. Pregnant women are at greater risk of bleeding with anticoagulation therapy than the general population and have other hemorrhagic risks, such as placental bleeding. However, few studies have provided data on maternal or neonatal hemorrhagic complications during anticoagulation or antiplatelet drug treatment. A meta-analysis of 11 trials of low-dose aspirin in pregnancy has shown that aspirin is not associated with most hemorrhagic complications, although it does appear to be associated with a small increase in the risk of maternal blood transfusion (48[C]). A report of pregnancy-related death associated with heparin and aspirin treatment for infertility has also been published, but the patient died from a cerebral hemorrhage associated with a congenital arteriovenous malformation. Because there is a potential for bleeding with heparin and aspirin, the risks and the benefits of such therapy for infertility require rigorous research before they can be accepted in routine practice (49[CR]).

Aspirin poisoning during pregnancy is rare. A recent report has shown that the fetus is at greater risk than the mother of serious injury by salicylate poisoning (50[c]).

Preoperative withdrawal of low-dose aspirin As the number of proven indications for low-dosage aspirin continues to increase, so does the population exposed to it. As no conventional prophylactic aspirin regimen is free from a risk of hemorrhagic complications (SEDA-21, 100), the benefit:risk ratio of aspirin prophylaxis needs to be reassessed carefully in patients at risk of such complications, for example those undergoing major surgery (51[C]), (52[C]). Unfortunately, evidence-based guidelines on how the problem should be managed are lacking. It is not, therefore, surprising that a questionnaire-based survey in the UK has shown that only one-third of 116 neuroanesthetists had a policy, either personal or departmental, regarding the discontinuation of low-dose aspirin before intracranial surgery (51[C]). When they were asked to express their opinions and working practices with regard to patients taking low-dose aspirin who present for elective intracranial surgery, 44% felt that these patients were at an increased risk of perioperative hemorrhage and 12% had personal experience of patients with such problems who had required another operation. The anesthetists who recommended discontinuation of aspirin before surgery had varying policies, ranging from 1 to 42 days (mean 11.3). Furthermore, about 50% advocated the use of platelet infusions, either alone or in combination with other blood products or hemostatic agents, if hemorrhagic complications occurred.

ANILINE DERIVATIVES

Paracetamol *(SED-13, 199; SEDA-20, 96; SEDA-21, 103)*

Liver In addition to the well-known dose-related toxic liver damage that paracetamol can cause, it can also rarely cause non-dose-related severe prolonged *cholestasis* or *granulomatous hepatitis* with cirrhosis, according to a survey of all the liver reactions to paracetamol reported to the Swedish Adverse Drug Reactions Advisory Committee from 1973 to 1993 (53[C]).

Immunological and hypersensitivity reactions Selective allergy to paracetamol without concomitant intolerance of aspirin or NSAIDs is uncommon. A report of five patients who developed hypersensitivity reactions (*angioedema, urticaria*) to paracetamol, but who tolerated aspirin, has been published (54[C]).

Overdosage A retrospective study in the US has shown that patients who take an accidental overdose of paracetamol while using the drug for pain relief have higher rates of morbidity and mortality than those who attempt suicide by paracetamol overdose (55[C]). The study included 50 patients who attempted suicide (median dose 20 g) and 21 who had taken an accidental overdose (median dose 12 g). In the accidental overdose group peak serum transaminase activities were 19–34 720 (median 3490) and were significantly higher than those in the suicidal group (11–15 890, median 31), despite the lower dose. The same difference was found for peak serum creatinine (median 1.3 mg/dl, 115 μmol/l, in the accidental overdose group versus 0.9 mg/dl, 80 μmol/l, in the suicidal group). Hepatic coma occurred in 33% of the patients in the accidental overdose group and in 6% in the suicide group, despite the fact that acetylcysteine was given to the same percentage of patients (80%). Four in the accidental group (20%) and one in the suicide group (2%) died, despite the fact that four of the five had received acetylcysteine. The results of this study may also be relevant to paracetamol overdosage in children, as dosing errors by parents are not infrequent (56[C]).

Paracetamol overdosage is common in many parts of the world, and despite the availability of acetylcysteine as an effective specific treatment, overdosage is characterized by severe liver damage and even death. Therefore, pressure is growing to define preventive measures (SEDA-21, 103). Among these measures, adding the antidote methionine to paracetamol tablets is one possibility (57[CR]). Paracetamol toxicity in overdosage is due to excessive production of *N*-acetyl-*para*-benzoquinoneimine, a toxic metabolite of paracetamol, which depletes hepatic glutathione, leading to covalent binding and necrosis of hepatic cells. Methionine protects against this damage by promoting synthesis of glutathione. In order to convert methionine to cysteine, for the synthesis of glutathione, hepatocytes must be intact, and it is therefore necessary to administer methionine within 10 h of paracetamol overdose.

The question of whether methionine should be added to all paracetamol formulations to reduce the incidence and severity of liver damage in cases of overdosage has prompted contrasting opinions (57[C])–(60[C]). The main objection to this strategy stems from the lack of convincing data on the efficacy and safety of long-term methionine. Paracetamol and methionine combination formulations are not currently available in the US or Europe, with the exception of the UK, where Paradote® (paracetamol 500 mg and methionine 100 mg) can be purchased. It is unlikely that more proprietary combinations will become available in the future.

Propacetamol *(SEDA-21, 103)*

New cases of occupational *contact dermatitis* caused by propacetamol have been reported (61[C]). Careful allergological investigation showed no evidence of sensitization to paracetamol or diethylglycine, leaving the allergen unknown.

ARYLALKANOIC ACID DERIVATIVES *(SED-13, 227; SEDA-20, 91; SEDA-21, 103)*

Bromfenac *(SEDA-21, 104)*

Bromfenac received FDA approval in July 1997 for short-term (less than 10 days) management of acute pain, and its safety profile appeared to be similar to that of other NSAIDs (SEDA-21, 104). However, the manufacturer recently sent a 'Dear Doctor' letter to US doctors warning them about hepatotoxicity associated with bromfenac. Severe hepatitis and liver failure were associated with treatment longer than 10 days. The FDA initially asked the manufacture to strengthen the warning on the labelling about duration of therapy and the risk of hepatotoxicity, but in June 1998 the manufacturers announced the voluntary withdrawal of the compound because of postmarketing reports of *severe hepatic failure* resulting in four deaths and eight liver transplants. It is noteworthy that 11 of 12 patients who died or required liver transplantation had used bromfenac for more than 10 days and the other had pre-existing liver disease (62[C]).

Diclofenac *(SED-13, 232; SEDA-19, 98; SEDA-20, 91; SEDA-21, 104)*

Hematological Immune hemolytic anemia is an uncommon adverse reaction to diclofenac (SEDA 20, 91).

A 75-year-old woman developed acute Coombs' positive *hemolytic anemia* complicated by *renal failure* during treatment with diclofenac (63[c]). She had been taking diclofenac intermittently for 2 years for osteoarthritis. She had taken two tablets of diclofenac 75 mg about 2 weeks before hospital admission and one tablet 24 h before the onset of her symptoms. Complete recovery occurred within 1 month. Hemolytic anemia was caused by sensitivity to a diclofenac metabolite, the 4-hydroxylated glucuronide ester of diclofenac.

Skin and appendages Pemphigus and pemphigoid are uncommon manifestation of NSAID toxicity (SEDA-13, 72). The possible involvement of diclofenac in triggering *pemphigus vulgaris* has been described in a 79-year-old woman who was using it rectally and topically (64[C]).

Diclofenac can be added to the list of NSAIDs that can cause *photosensitivity* after topical application (65[c]).

Treatment of toxic effects Many cases of hepatic injury attributed to diclofenac have been reported (SEDA-20, 91). In the large majority of patients early discontinuation of the drug accompanied recovery of normal liver function. However, hepatic failure leading to death has been reported. Successful treatment of diclofenac-induced fulminant *hepatic failure* by liver transplantation has been described (66[c]).

Etodolac *(SED-13, 238)*

Gastrointestinal De novo *colitis* has been described, albeit rarely, with the use of many different NSAIDs (SEDA-15, 92), but has never been reported with the use of etodolac. Two patients, aged 67 and 62 years, developed bloody diarrhea and abdominal pain after taking etodolac for arthritis (67[c]). In the first patient symptoms began few days after starting the NSAID; in the second, symptoms developed after 3 months of therapy. In both patients endoscopy showed *acute colitis*. The gastrointestinal symptoms and diarrhea resolved on discontinuation of etodolac. Rechallenge with etodolac, carried out in the second patient, led to similar symptoms as before.

Etodolac can be added to the list of NSAIDs (SEDA-15, 92) that can cause *colonic strictures* (68[CR]).

Fenbufen *(SED-13, 235)*

Immunological and hypersensitivity reactions Severe skin reactions and laboratory evidence of hepatotoxicity have been reported with fenbufen (69[c]).

A 61-year-old man developed *toxic epidermal necrolysis*, *raised serum liver enzymes* and *interstitial nephritis* 5 days after starting fenbufen for lower back pain. After withdrawal he made an uneventful complete recovery within 8 weeks.

Interaction Fenbufen interacts with the fluoroquinolone *enoxacin*, causing convulsions (SEDA-15, 100). It would therefore be wise to avoid concomitant use of any NSAID with fluoroquinolones that are known to have a proconvulsant activity. However, when the potential effect of concurrent administration of fenbufen and *ciprofloxacin*, a widely prescribed fluoroquinolone, on central nervous system activity in healthy young volunteers was investigated by electroencephalography, none of the EEG or clinical parameters were significantly different from those measured when the drugs were given alone (70[C]).

Ibuprofen *(SED-13, 228; SEDA-19, 98; SEDA-20, 93; SEDA-21, 105)*

Skin and appendages NSAIDs have been blamed for increasing the risk of severe infections (see above). The possible association between ibuprofen and *dermatological superinfection* in children with recent *varicella* infection has been investigated in a retrospective cohort study (71[C]). Among 7013 cases of *varicella*, 89 superinfections developed and the 30-day risk of superinfection was calculated comparing users and non-user of ibuprofen. There was no statistically significant difference between the two groups of children.

Immunological and hypersensitivity reactions Anaphylaxis to NSAIDs is thought to depend on cyclo-oxygenase inhibition coupled with upregulation of 5-lipoxygenase-dependent pathways. The administration of leukotriene receptor antagonists should therefore provide some protection against aspirin-induced anaphylaxis. However, there has been a report of a patient with moderately severe asthma who had an episode of *anaphylaxis* after taking ibuprofen 400 mg while also taking cafirlukast (72[c]). Patients sensitive to aspirin should avoid all NSAIDs even while taking leukotriene receptor antagonists.

Overdosage *Renal involvement* in cases of overdose may be more common than previously thought (73[C])–(75[C]). *Acute papillary necrosis* (76[C]) has also been described.

Interaction High-dosage ibuprofen can slow the progression of lung disease in patients with cystic fibrosis and appears to be free of serious toxicity (SEDA-20, 93). *Aminoglycosides* are often given to these patients to treat pulmonary infections and are nephrotoxic. There has been a report of four children with cystic fibrosis who had transient renal failure during exacerbations of their lung disease, probably due to the combination of an intravenous aminoglycoside and oral ibuprofen (77[C]). This adverse effect was not observed when ibuprofen was given alone or in combination with nebulized aminoglycoside. Ibuprofen should probably be withdrawn during intravenous aminoglycoside therapy.

Ketoprofen *(SED-13, 229; SEDA-20, 93; SEDA-21, 105)*

Gastrointestinal In some epidemiological studies, ketoprofen at prescription doses has been found to be more gastrotoxic than other NSAIDs (SEDA-18, 99). However, very few data are available on the gastrointestinal effects of over-the-counter doses of ketoprofen (78[C]). Ketoprofen (75 mg/day) and paracetamol (4 g/day) have been compared in an endoscopic short-term (7 days) randomized, placebo-controlled, crossover study in healthy subjects (79[C]). Ketoprofen was associated with significant gastrointestinal toxicity, including *gastric ulceration*. However, the results of endoscopic studies must be interpreted with caution (SEDA-14, 79). Despite the relevant difference in endoscopic tolerability there were no significant differences between treatment groups with respect to subjective symptoms of gastric discomfort or adverse events.

Another endoscopic study (80[C]) has shown that the *R*-enantiomer of ketoprofen has less gastrointestinal toxicity than the racemic mixture or the *S*-enantiomer, while retaining good analgesic activity (81[c]).

Skin and appendages A series of reports has shown that topical ketoprofen can cause *pho-*

todermatitis (65[C]), (82[C]), (83[C]). One of these reports has shown that patients who develop photosensitization with ketoprofen may also have cross-reactivity to fenofibrate and some benzophenones, because of their structural similarities (83[C]).

Ketorolac *(SED-13, 240; SEDA-19, 95; SEDA-20, 93; SEDA-21, 105)*

Cardiovascular Rapid intravenous administration of ketorolac during or after surgery can result in reversible *bradycardia* in children (84[C]), (85[C]).

Pancreas *Acute pancreatitis* occurred in a 44-year-old woman after intramuscular treatment with ketorolac 30 mg for chest pain (86[c]). This association requires confirmation before ketorolac is included in the list of drugs believed to cause pancreatitis.

Gastrointestinal Further evidence on the unfavorable benefit:risk profile of ketorolac compared with other NSAIDs has come from a case–control study on hospitalization for upper *gastrointestinal tract bleeding* and/or *perforation*. Ketorolac was five times more gastrotoxic than all other NSAIDs (RR 25, 95% CI 9.6–63.5 vs RR 5.5, 95% CI 2.1–14.4). The relative risk with intramuscular ketorolac was higher than that associated with oral ketorolac (87[C]).

Urinary system The debate on the assessment of the potential of ketorolac to cause postoperative *nephrotoxicity* continues (88[C]), (89[C]).

Interaction Case reports of an interaction of ketorolac with *lithium*, resulting in *lithium toxicity* have been published (90[c])–(92[c]). Interactions of lithium with many NSAIDs have been reported (SED-13, 213).

Loxoprofen *(SED-13, 240)*

Immunological and hypersensitivity reactions Two cases of a type I hypersensitivity reaction, characterized by a generalized *urticarial rash* and *dyspnea*, have been described (SEDA-15, 101). Another report has now been published in a 27-year-old woman (93[c]).

Nabumetone *(SED-13, 239; SEDA-20, 93)*

Skin and appendages *Pseudoporphyria* has been reported with nabumetone (SEDA-16, 111). A new case report has been published and additional reports have been received by the UK's Committee on Safety of Medicines (94[C]).

Naproxen *(SED-13, 231; SEDA-19, 99; SEDA-20, 93; SEDA-21, 106)*

Gastrointestinal Esophageal damage is a rare adverse reaction to NSAIDs. The published evidence comprises a small number of case-reports and few specific studies (SEDA-15, 92).

A recent report from the FDA's Spontaneous Reporting System in the US has described a case series involving predominantly young healthy people who developed *esophageal problems* after taking over-the-counter naproxen sodium (95[Cr]).

Naproxen sodium was approved for over-the-counter marketing in January 1994. By December 1995 the FDA had received 81 reports of esophageal symptoms; tablets (as opposed to capsules) were implicated in 77% of cases. In 42 cases the patients reported that the tablet had stuck in their throat; nine required either barium swallow testing or upper endoscopy for evaluation of symptoms, and seven had *esophageal ulcerations*. No hemorrhages were reported.

The mechanism of esophageal injury was not clear. In 15 reports it was specifically noted that the patients had not taken the tablets with fluids or had lain down after taking the drug. Most of the patients had no history of esophageal problems and were not taking concomitant medications. While further information on the use of over-the-counter medication would be helpful to identify factors contributing to esophageal injury, it seems wise to reiterate the suggestion that patients taking

NSAIDs must swallow their pills with large amounts of water in the upright position, at least 1 h before retiring (SEDA-15, 92).

Additional data on the gastrointestinal safety of over-the-counter naproxen sodium has come from a comparative case–cohort study on the risk of *gastrointestinal tract bleeding* requiring hospitalization associated with naproxen sodium or ibuprofen, using a prescribing database to approximate over-the-counter dosing (96[C]). The use of naproxen sodium versus ibuprofen was associated with an adjusted relative risk of upper gastrointestinal tract bleeding of 2.0 (95% CI 1.1–3.8). Among patients with multiple prescriptions, the crude relative risk for those receiving therapy in a dose typical of over-the-counter use was 4.1 (95% CI 1.2–13.8). So, although the incidence of upper gastrointestinal tract bleeding was low with both drugs, the use of low-dose naproxen compared with low-dose ibuprofen appears to put patients at increased risk of *gastrointestinal bleeding*. This difference between the two compounds may be of particular relevance in patients with an increased baseline risk of bleeding.

Oxaprozin *(SED-13, 238; SEDA-20, 93; SEDA-21, 106)*

Immunological and hypersensitivity reactions A life-threatening reaction (*respiratory distress requiring intubation*, *facial edema*, *lethargy*) developed in a 53-year-old woman after a single dose oxaprozin 600 mg (97[c]). This was a not unexpected reaction in a woman with a history of severe asthma and aspirin allergy.

INDOMETHACIN AND RELATED COMPOUNDS

Indomethacin *(SED-13, 225; SEDA-21, 107)*

Interactions Behavioral changes have been described in elderly patients taking indomethacin (SED-13, 225; (98[C])) albeit rarely. An increased risk of *encephalopathic* or *psychotic features* has been reported in patients receiving concomitant treatment with muromonab CD_3 (OKT_3) monoclonal antibody (99[Cr]).

Renal failure and severe *metabolic acidosis* developed in a patient with type 2 diabetes mellitus on long-term metformin therapy after recent treatment with indomethacin (100[C]). NSAIDs can reduce glomerular filtration rate, with subsequent impairment of renal function, and metformin can accumulate in the presence of acute renal insufficiency, contributing to the development of lactic acidosis.

Sulindac *(SED-13, 225; SEDA-20, 94; SEDA-21, 107)*

Use in pregnancy A prospective comparison of oral sulindac with intravenous indomethacin for closure of patent ductus arteriosus has shown that sulindac can promote ductal constriction without compromising renal function in preterm infants, but its use was accompanied by *severe gastrointestinal complications* (101[C]).

OXICAM DERIVATIVES *(SED-13, 244; SEDA-20, 95)*

Ampiroxicam

Ampiroxicam is a monoacid ether carbonate prodrug of piroxicam. In humans it is completely converted to piroxicam after oral administration. In clinical doses there was no detectable portal or systemic exposure to ampiroxicam, indicating that conversion to piroxicam was complete during the absorption process. The pharmacokinetics of piroxicam from ampiroxicam were the same as those for piroxicam (102[c]), (103[c]).

The adverse effects profile of this prodrug is still unknown, but it can be expected to be similar to that of piroxicam.

Skin and appendages A few reports of ampiroxicam-induced *photosensitivity* have been published (104[C])–(106[C]).

PYRAZOLONE DERIVATIVES
(SED-13, 220)

Dipyrone can induce or exacerbate *pemphigus vulgaris* according to a recent report (107[cr]). An active amide group might be responsible for disease induction (108[C]).

MISCELLANEOUS COMPOUNDS

Diacerein *(SEDA-14, 96; SEDA-15, 103)*

Acute hepatitis has been associated with diacerein (109[c]).

Glucosamine sulfate

This compound is claimed to have a chondroprotective activity in patients with osteoarthritis and comparative efficacy but better tolerability with respect to NSAIDs (110[C]). However, adequate studies documenting both its efficacy and long-term safety are lacking (111[R]).

Hyaluronan *(SEDA-15, 103)*

Intra-articular injection of hyaluronan may have some short-term benefit in patients with osteoarthritis (112[R]). However, its adverse effects include *joint pain*, *effusion*, and *swelling*, and septic arthritis. *Acute pseudogout* and *anaphylaxis* following intra-articular injection have also been reported (113[c]), (114[c]).

Nimesulide *(SED-13, 248)*

Urinary system *Acute oliguric renal failure* followed the ingestion of one tablet of nimesulide 100 mg to relieve myalgia in a 68-year-old woman with diffuse arteriosclerosis but normal renal function. A renal biopsy showed interstitial nephritis. Recovery of renal function was complete (115[C]).

Skin and appendages Nimesulide can be added to the list of NSAIDs that can cause *toxic epidermal necrolysis* (116[C]).

DRUGS USED IN THE TREATMENT OF GOUT

Colchicine *(SED-13, 252; SEDA-19, 101; SEDA-21, 109)*

Interaction Reports documenting the potential adverse effects of continued use of colchicine with *cyclosporin* have appeared (SEDA-19, 101). The concomitant use of these drugs caused acute *myopathy* with or without *neuropathy* in two young renal transplant recipients. All patients taking concomitant cyclosporin and colchicine must be monitored closely (117[CR]), (118[C]).

REFERENCES

1. Feenstra J, Grobbee DE, Mosterd A, Stricker BH. Adverse cardiovascular effects of NSAIDs in patients with congestive heart failure. Drug Saf 1997;17:166–80.
2. Johnson AG. NSAIDs and blood pressure. Clinical importance for older patients. Drugs Aging 1998;12:17–27.
3. Johnson AG, Nguyen TV, Owe-Young R, Williamson DJ, Day RO. Potential mechanisms by which nonsteroidal anti-inflammatory drugs elevate blood pressure: the role of endothelin-1. J Hum Hypertens 1996;10:257–61.
4. Heerdink ER, Leufkens HG, Herings RMC, Ottervanger JP, Striker BHC, Bakker A. NSAIDs associated with increased risk of congestive heart failure in elderly patients taking diuretics. Arch Intern Med 1998;158:1108–12.
5. Anonymous. Paraesthesia with NSAIDs. Aust Adv Drug React Bull. 1997;16:7 May.
6. Griffin MR. Epidemiology of nonsteroidal anti-inflammatory drug-associated gastrointestinal injury. Am J Med 1998;104:23S–29S.
7. Blower AL, Brooks A, Fenn GC, Hill A, Pearce MY, Morant S, Bardhan KD. Emergency admissions for upper gastrointestinal disease and their relation to NSAID use. Aliment Pharmacol Ther 1997;11:283–91.
8. MacDonald TM, Morant SV, Robinson GC,

Shield MJ, McGilchrist MM, Murray FE, McDevitt DG. Association of upper gastrointestinal toxicity of non-steroidal anti-inflammatory drugs with continued exposure: cohort study. Br Med J 1997;315:1333–7.
9. Langman MJS, Weil J, Wainwright P, Lawson DH, Rawlins MD, Logan RF, Murphy M, Vessey MP, Colin-Jones DG. Risks of bleeding peptic ulcer associated with individual non-steroidal anti-inflammatory drugs. Lancet 1994;343:1075–8.
10. Henry D, Dobson A, Turner C. Variability in the risk of major gastrointestinal complications from nonaspirin nonsteroidal anti-inflammatory drugs. Gastroenterology 1993;105:1078–88.
11. Griffin MR, Piper JM, Daugherty JR, Snowden M, Ray WA. Nonsteroidal anti-inflammatory drug use and increased risk for peptic ulcer disease in elderly persons. Ann Intern Med 1991;114:257–63.
12. Griffin MR, Ray WA, Schaffner W. Nonsteroidal anti-inflammatory drug use and death from peptic ulcer in elderly persons. Ann Intern Med 1998;109:359–63.
13. Cunningham G, Dodd TRP, Grant DJ, McMurdo MET, Richards RM-E. Drug-related problems in elderly patients admitted to Tayside hospitals, methods for prevention and subsequent reassessment. Age Ageing 1997;26:375–82.
14. Anonymous. Low awareness of analgesic adverse effects in elderly Americans. Reactions 1997;656:3.
15. Anonymous. Many patients unaware of ADRs associated with NSAID use. Reactions 1998; 694:2.
16. Wynne HA, Long A. Patient awareness of adverse effects of non-steroidal anti-inflammatory drugs (NSAIDs). Br J Clin Pharmacol 1996; 42:253–6.
17. Herxheimer A. Many NSAID users who bleed don't know when to stop. Br Med J 1998;316:492.
18. Anonymous. Labelling information on geriatric use of drugs will be required. Reactions 1997;667:3.
19. Sutters C, Keat A, Lant A. Improving prescribing of non-steroidal anti-inflammatory drugs in hospital: an educational approach. Br J Rheumatol 1993;32:618–22.
20. Yeomans ND, Cook GA, Giraud AS. Selective COX-2 inhibitors: are they safe for the stomach? Gastroenterology 1998;115:227–9.
21. Cryer B, Feldman M. Cyclooxygenase-1 and cyclooxygenase-2 selectivity of widely used nonsteroidal anti-inflammatory drugs. Am J Med 1998;104:413–21.
22. Wallace JL, Bak A, McKnight W, Asfaha S, Sharkey KA, MacNaughton WK. Cyclooxygenase 1 contributes to inflammatory responses in rats and mice: implications for gastrointestinal toxicity. Gastroenterology 1998;115:101–9.
23. Dent J. Why proton pump inhibition should heal and protect against nonsteroidal anti-inflammatory drug ulcers. Am J Med 1998;104:52S–55S.
24. Daneshmend TK, Stein AG, Bhaskar NK, Hawkey CJ. Abolition by omeprazole of aspirin induced gastric mucosal injury in man. Gut 1990;31:514–17.
25. Scheiman JM, Behler EM, Loeffler KM, Elta GH. Omeprazole ameliorates aspirin-induced gastroduodenal injury. Dig Dis Sci 1994;39:97–103.
26. Walan A, Bader J-P, Classen M, Lamers CB, Piper DW, Rutgersson K, Eriksson S. Effect of omeprazole and ranitidine on ulcer healing and relapse rates in patients with benign gastric ulcer. New Engl J Med 1989;320:69–75.
27. Ekstrom P, Carling L, Wetterhus S, Wingren PE, Anker-Hansen O, Lundegardh G, Thorhallsson E, Unge P. Prevention of peptic ulcer and dyspeptic symptoms with omeprazole in patients receiving continuous non-steroidal anti-inflammatory drug therapy. A Nordic multicentre study. Scand J Gastroenterol 1996;31:753–8.
28. Cullen D, Bardhan KD, Eisner M, Kogut DG, Peacock RA, Thomson JM, Hawkey CJ. Primary gastroduodenal prophylaxis with omeprazole for non-steroidal anti-inflammatory drug users. Aliment Pharmacol Ther 1998;12:135–40.
29. Yeomans ND, Tulassay Z, Juhasz L, Racz I, Howard JM, van Rensburg CJ, Swannell AJ, Hawkey CJ. A comparison of omeprazole with ranitidine for ulcers associated with nonsteroidal antinflammatory drugs. Acid Suppression Trial: Ranitidine versus Omeprazole for NSAID-associated Ulcer Treatment (ASTRONAUT) Study Group. New Engl J Med 1998;338:719–26.
30. Hawkey CJ, Karrasch JA, Szczepanski L, Walker DG, Barkun A, Swannell AJ, Yeomans ND. Omeprazole compared with misoprostol for ulcers associated with nonsteroidal antiinflammatory drugs. Omeprazole versus Misoprostol for NSAID-induced Ulcer Management (OMNIUM) Study Group. New Engl J Med 1998;338:727–34.
31. Guslandi M. Therapies for ulcers associated with nonsteroidal antiinflammatory drugs. New Engl J Med 1998;339:350.
32. Stucki G, Johannesson M, Liang MH. Is misoprostol cost-effective in the prevention of nonsteroidal anti-inflammatory drug-induced gastropathy in patients with chronic arthritis? A review of conflicting economic evaluations. Arch Intern Med 1994;145:2020–5.
33. Maetzel A, Ferraz MB, Bombardier C. The cost-effectiveness of misoprostol in preventing serious gastrointestinal events associated with the use of nonsteroidal antiinflammatory drugs. Arthritis Rheum 1998;41:16–25.
34. Johnson RE, Hornbrook MC, Hooker RS, Woodson GT, Shneidman R. Analysis of the costs of NSAID associated gastropathy: experience in a US health maintenance organisation. PharmacoEconomics 1997;12:76–88.
35. Evans JMM, Macgregor AM, Murray FE, Vaidya K, Morris AD, MacDonald TM. No association between non-steroidal anti-inflammatory drugs and acute appendicitis in a case-control study. Br J Surg 1997;84:372–4.
36. Henry D, Page J, Whyte I, Nanra R, Hall C.

Consumption of non-steroidal anti-inflammatory drugs and the development of functional renal impairment in elderly subjects. Results of a case-control study. Br J Clin Pharmacol 1997;44:85–90.
37. Holder EP, Moore PT, Browne BA. Nonsteroidal anti-inflammatory drugs and necrotising fasciitis. An update. Drug Saf 1997;17:369–73.
38. Rivey MP, Allington DR, Dubham ALH. Necrotizing fasciitis associated with nonsteroidal antiinflammatory drug use. J Pharm Technol 1998;14:58–62.
39. Kahn LH, Styrt BA. Necrotizing soft tissue infections reported with nonsteroidal anti-inflammatory drugs. Ann Pharmacother 1997; 31:1034–9.
40. Stevens DL. Could nonsteroidal antiinflammatory drugs (NSAIDs) enhance the progression of bacterial infections to toxic shock syndrome? Clin Infect Dis 1995;21:977–80.
41. Barnham M, Anderson AW. Non-steroidal anti-inflammatory drugs (NSAIDs). A predisposing factor for streptococcal bacteraemia? Adv Exp Med Biol 1997;418:145–7.
42. Vermillion ST, Scardo JA, Lashus AG, Wiles HB. The effect of indomethacin tocolysis on fetal ductus arterious constriction with advancing gestational age. Am J Obstet Gynecol 1997;177:256–9.
43. Ostensen M, Ostensen H. Safety of nonsteroidal antinflammatory drugs in pregnant patients with rheumatic disease. J Rheumatol 1996; 23:1045–9.
44. Cramer DW, Harlow BL, Titus-Ernstoff L, Bohlke K, Welch WR, Greenberg ER. Over the counter analgesics and risk of ovarian cancer. Lancet 1998;351:104–7.
45. Cortelazzo S, Marchetti M, Orlando E, Falanga A, Barbui T, Buchanan MR. Aspirin increases the bleeding side effects in essential thrombocythemia independent of the cyclooxygenase pathway: role of the lipoxygenase pathway. Am J Hematol 1998;57:277–82.
46. Zalev AH, Gardiner GW, Warren RE. NSAID injury to the small intestine. Abdom Imag 1998;23:40–4.
47. Price KS, Thomson DMP. Localized unilateral periorbital edema induced by aspirin. Ann Allergy Asthma Immunol 1997;79:420–2.
48. Macones GA, Regan C, Stamilio D, Parry S, Morgan MA. Maternal and neonatal safety of low dose aspirin in pregnancy: a meta-analysis. Am J Obstet Gynecol 1998;178:126S.
49. Center for Disease Control and Prevention. Pregnancy-related death associated with heparin and aspirin treatment for infertility, 1996. J Am Med Assoc 1998;279:1860–1.
50. Palatnick W, Tenenbein M. Aspirin poisoning during pregnancy: increased fetal sensitivity. Am J Perinatol 1998;15:39–41.
51. James DN, Fernandes JR, Calder I, Smith M. Low-dose aspirin and intracranial surgery. A survey of the opinions of consultant neuroanaesthetists in the UK. Anaesthesia 1997;52:169–72.
52. Wierod FS, Frandsen NJ, Jacobsen JD, Hartvigsen A, Olsen PR. Risk of haemorrage from transurethral prostatectomy in acetylsalicylic acid and NSAID-treated patients. Scand J Urol Nephrol 1998;32:120–2.
53. Lindgren A, Aldenborg F, Norkrans G, Olaison L, Olsson R. Paracetamol-induced cholestatic and granulomatous liver injuries. J Intern Med GBR 1997;241:435–9.
54. Mendizabal SL, Gòmez MLD. Paracetamol sensitivity without aspirin intolerance. Allergy Eur J Allergy Clin Immunol 1998;53:457–8.
55. Schiodt FV, Rochling FA, Casey DL, Lee WM. Acetaminophen toxicity in an urban county hospital. New Engl J Med 1997;337:1112–17.
56. Rivera-PeneraT, Gugig R, Davis J, McDiarmid S, Vargas J, Rosenthal P, Berquist W, Heyman MB, Ament ME. Outcome of acetaminophen overdose in pediatric patients and factors contributing to hepatotoxicity. J Pediatr 1997; 130:300–4.
57. Jones AL, Hayes PC, Proudfoot AT, Vale JA, Prescott LF. Controversies in management: should methionine be added to every paracetamol tablet? No: the risks are not well enough known. Br Med J 1997;315:301–3.
58. Krenzelok EP. Controversies in management: should methionine be added to every paracetamol tablet? Yes: But perhaps only in developing countries. Br Med J 1997;315:303–4.
59. Saha SK, Kale R. Adding methionine to every paracetamol tablet. Br Med J 1998;316:473–4.
60. Chada N. Drugs as important as paracetamol in developing counries should not be tainted. Br Med J 1998;316:474.
61. Barbaud A, Reichert-Penetrat S, Trechot P, Cuny JF, Weber M, Schmuts J-L. Occupational contact dermatitis to propacetamol. Allergological and chemical investigations in two new cases. Dermatology 1997;195:329–31.
62. Bradburg J. And another drug is with drawn from the market. Lancet 1998;351:1937.
63. Bougie D, Johnson ST, Weitekamp LA, Aster RH. Sensitivity to a metabolite of diclofenac as a cause of acute immune hemolytic anemia. Blood 1997;90:407–13.
64. Matz H, Bialy-Golan A, Brenner S. Diclofenac: a new trigger of pemphigus vulgaris? Dermatology 1997;195:48–9.
65. Adamski H, Benkalfate L, Delaval Y, Olliver I, Le Jean S, Toubel G, le Hir-Garreau I, Chevrant-Breton J. Photodermatitis from non-steroidal anti-inflammatory drugs. Contact Dermatitis 1998;38:171–4.
66. Jones AL, Latham T, Shallcross TM, Simpson KJ. Fulminant hepatic failure due to diclofenac treated succesfully by orthotopic liver transplantation. Transplant Proc 1998;30:192–4.
67. Wilcox GM, Porensky RS. Acute colitis associated with etodolac. J Clin Gastroenterol 1997;25:367–8.
68. Eis MJ, Watkins BM, Philip A, Welling RE. Nonsteroidal-induced benign strictures of the colon: a case report and review of the literature. Am J Gastroenterol 1998;93:120–1.

69. Krivoy N, Azzam Z, Oren I, Ben-Itzhak O, Alroy G. Interstitial nephritis, toxic epidermal necrolysis and liver dysfunction associated to fenbufen. Clin Rheumatol 1997;16:489–90.
70. Kamali F, Ashton CH, Marsh VR, Cox J. Assessment to the effects of combination therapy with ciprofloxacim and fenbufen on the central nervous system of healthy volunteers by quantitative electroencephalography. Antimicrob Agents Chemother 1998;42:1256–8.
71. Choo P-W, Donahue JG, Platt R. Ibuprofen and skin and soft tissue superinfections in children with varicella. Ann Epidemiol 1997;7:440–5.
72. Menendez R, Venzor J, Ortiz G. Failure of zafirlukast to prevent ibuprofen-induced anaphylaxis. Ann Allergy Asthma Immunol 1998;80:225–6.
73. Kim J, Gazarian M, Verjee Z, Johnson D. Acute renal insufficiency in ibuprofen overdose. Pediatr Emerg Care 1995;11:107–8.
74. Le HT, Bosse GM, Tsai Y. Ibuprofen overdose complicated by renal failure, adult respiratory distress syndrome, and metabolic acidosis. J Toxicol Clin Toxicol 1994;32:315–20.
75. Al-Harbi NN, Domrongkitchaiporn S, Lirenman DS. Hypocalcemia and hypomagnesemia after ibuprofen overdose. Ann Pharmacother 1997;31:432–4.
76. Atta MG, Whelton A. Acute renal papillary necrosis induced by ibuprofen. Am J Ther 1997;4:55–60.
77. Kovesi TA, Swartz R, MacDonald N. Transient renal failure due to simultaneous ibuprofen and aminoglycoside therapy in children with cystic fibrosis. New Engl J Med 1998;338:65–6.
78. Moore N, Vuillemin N, Abiteboul M, Boudignat O, Paliwoda A, Robins J-L, Jacobs L-D. Large scale safety study of ketoprofen 25 mg (Toprec) in febrile and painful conditions. Pharmacoepidemiol Drug Saf 1996;5:295–302.
79. Lanza FL, Codispoti JR, Nelson EB. An endoscopic comparison of gastroduodenal injury with over-the-counter doses of ketoprofen and acetaminophen. Am J Gastroenterol 1998;93: 1051–4.
80. Jerussi TP, Caubet JF, McCray JE, Handley DA. Clinical endoscopic evaluation of the gastroduodenal tolerance to (R)-ketoprofen, (R)-flurbiprofen, racemic ketoprofen, and paracetamol: a randomized, sigle-blind, placebo-controlled trial. J Clin Pharmacol 1998;38 (Suppl):19S–24S.
81. Cooper SA, Reynolds DC, Reynolds B, Hersh EV. Analgesic efficacy and safety of (R)-ketoprofen in postoperative dental pain. J Clin Pharmacol 1998;38 (Suppl):11S–18S.
82. Mirande-Romero A, Gonzales-Lopez A, Esquivias JI, Bajo C, Garcia-Munoz M. Ketoprofen-induced connubial photodermatitis. Contact Dermatitis 1997;375:242.
83. Leroy D, Dompmartin A, Szczurko C, Michel M, Louvet S. Photodermatitis from ketoprofen with cross-reactivity to fenofibrate and benzophenones. Photodermatol Photoimmunol Photomed 1997;13:93–7.
84. Foster PN, Williams JG. Bradycardia following intravenous ketorolac in children. Eur J Anaesthesiol 1997;14:307–9.
85. Chiaretti A, Simeone E, Langer A, Butera G, Piastra M, Tortorolo L, Polidori G. Comparison of ketorolac and fentanyl for pain relief in pediatric intensive care. Pediatr Med Chir 1997; 19:419–24.
86. Goyal SB, Goyal RS. Ketorolac tromethamine-induced acute pancreatitis. Arch Intern Med 1998;158:411.
87. Garcia Rodriguez LA, Cattaruzzi MG, Troncon MG, Agostinis L. Risk of hospitalization for upper gastrointestinal tract bleeding associated with ketorolac, other nonsteroidal anti-inflammatory drugs, calcium antagonists, and other antihypertensive drugs. Arch Intern Med 1998;158:33–9.
88. Myles PS, Power I. Does ketorolac cause postoperative renal failure: how do we assess the evidence? Br J Anaesth 1998;80:420–1.
89. Buller GK, Perazella MA. Acute renal failure and ketorolac. Ann Intern Med 1997;127:493–4.
90. Langlois R, Paquette D. Increased serum lithium due to ketorolac therapy. Can Med Assoc J 1994;150:1455–6.
91. Iyer V. Ketorolac (Toradol) induced lithium toxicity. Headache 1994;34:442–4.
92. Cold JA, ZumBrunnen TL, Simpson MA, Augustin BG, Awad E, Jann MW. Increased lithium serum and red blood cell concentrations during ketorolac coadministration. J Clin Psychopharmacol 1998;18:33–7.
93. Kimura M, Kawada A, Hiruma M, Ishibashi A. A case of urticarial drug eruption from loxoprofen sodium. Clin Exp Dermatol 1997;22:303–4.
94. Varma S, Lanigan SW. Pseudoporphyria caused by nabumetone. Br J Dermatol 1998; 138:549–50.
95. Kahn LH, Chen Min MS, Eaton R. Over-the-counter naproxen sodium and esophageal injury. Ann Intern Med 1997;126:1006.
96. Strom BL, Schinnar R, Bilker WB, Feldman H, Farrar JT, Carson JL. Gastrointestinal tract bleeding associated with naproxen sodium vs ibuprofen. Arch Intern Med 1997;157:2626–31.
97. Hailemeskel B, Namanny MD, Metzger SD. Severe asthmatic reaction to contraindicated anti-inflammatory drug. Am J Health-Syst Pharm 1997;54:199–200.
98. Mallet L, Kuyumjian J. Indomethacin-induced behavioral changes in an elderly patient with dementia. Ann Pharmacother 1998;32:201–3.
99. Mignat C. Clinically significant drug interactions with new immunosuppressive agents. Drug Saf 1997;16:267–78.
100. Chan NN, Fauvel NJ, Feher MD. Non-steroidal anti-inflammatory drugs and metformin: a cause for concern? Lancet 1998;352:201.
101. Ng PC, So KW, Fok TF, Yam MC, Wong MY, Wong W. Comparing sulindac with indomethacin for closure of ductus arteriosus in preterm infants. J Pediatr Child Health 1997;33:324–8.

102. Carty TJ, Marfat A, Moore PF, Falkner FC, Twomey TM, Weissman A. Ampiroxicam, an anti-inflammatory agent which is a prodrug of piroxicam. Agents Actions 1993;39:157–65.
103. Falkner FC, Twomey TM, Borgers AP, Garg D, Weidler D, Gerber N, Browder IW. Disposition of ampiroxicam, a prodrug of piroxicam, in man. Xenobiotica 1990;20:645–52.
104. Chishiki M, Kawada A, Fujioka A, Hiruma M, Ishibashi A, Banba H. Photosensitivity due to ampiroxicam. Dermatology 1997;195:409–10.
105. Toyohara A, Chen K-R, Miyakawa S-I, Inada M, Ishiko A. Ampiroxicam-induced photosensitivity. Contact Dermatitis 1996;34:101–2.
106. Kurumaji Y. Ampiroxicam-induced photosensitivity. Contact Dermatitis 1996;34:298–9.
107. Brenner S, Bialy-Golan A, Crost N. Dipyrone in the induction of pemphigus. J Am Acad Dermatol 1997;36:488–90.
108. Wolf R, Brenner S. An active amide group in the molecule of drugs that induce pemphigus: a casual or causal relationship. Dermatology 1994;189:1–4.
109. Vial T, Mille R, Bory RM, Evreux JC. Acute hepatitis associated with ingestion of diacerein. Gastroenterol Clin Biol 1997;21:795–6.
110. Gui-Xing-Qiu, Shu-Neng-Gao, Giacovelli G, Rovati L, Setnikar I. Efficacy and safety of glucosamine sulfate versus ibuprofen in patients with knee osteoarthritis. Arzneim Forsch Drug Res 1998;48:469–74.
111. Da Camara CC, Dowless GV. Glucosamine sulfate for osteoarthritis. Ann Pharmacother 1998;32:580–7.
112. Anonymous. Hyaluronan injections for osteoarthrosis of the knee. Med Lett Drugs Ther 1998;40:69–70.
113. Maillefert JF, Hirschhorn P, Pascaud F, Piroth C, Tavernier C. Acute attack of chondrocalcinosis after an intraarticular injection of hyaluronan. Rev Rhum Engl Ed 1997:64;593–4.
114. Luzar MJ, Altawil B. Pseudogout following intra-articular injection of sodium hylauronate. Arthritis Rheum 1998;41:939–40.
115. Apostolou T, Sotsiou F, Yfanti G, Andreadis E, Nikolopoulou N, Diamantopoulos E, Billis A. Acute renal failure induced by nimesulide in a patient suffering from temporal arteritis. Nephrol Dial Transplant 1997;12:1493–6.
116. Senna GE, Governa M, Dama AR, Crivellaro MA, Lombardi C. Toxic epidermal necrolysis due to nimesulide. Allergy 1997;52 (Suppl 37):133.
117. Lee BI, Shin SJ, Yoon SN, Choi YJ, Yang CW, Bang BK. Acute myopathy induced by colchicine in a cyclosporine-treated renal transplant recipient: a case report and review of the literature. J Korean Med Sci 1997;12:160–1.
118. Jagose JT, Bailey RR. Muscle weakness due to colchicine in a renal transplant recipient. NZ Med J 1997;110:343.

T.G. Short and M.A. Faigan

10 General anesthetics and therapeutic gases

GENERAL TOPICS

There have been several recent comparisons of the efficacy and safety of various anesthetic agents during monitored anesthesia care. The short-acting hypnotic propofol has been compared with the ultra-short acting opioid remifentanil in 44 patients undergoing breast biopsy under local anesthesia (1[c]). These agents both have the advantage of allowing easy titration of the level of sedation, as well as a rapid recovery. All patients received intravenous midazolam 2 mg and then either propofol 75 μg/kg per min or remifentanil 0.1 μg/kg per min. The infusions were titrated to maintain optimal patient comfort without respiratory depression. Of those who were given remifentanil, 22% fewer patients required supplemental local anesthetics, and none of this group required rescue fentanyl for analgesia. Rescue fentanyl was required by 18% of the patients who were given propofol. Propofol resulted in significantly higher median sedation scores, but was associated with less respiratory depression and more rapid recovery.

Immunological and hypersensitivity reactions The pathogenesis of allergic reactions to anesthetic drugs has been reviewed (2[R]). In a survey of *allergic reactions* during anesthesia in 1750 patients, 58% were due to IgE-mediated anaphylaxis, confirmed by a raised serum tryptase in the 2 h after the reaction. Identification of the drug responsible for the adverse reaction was by skin testing and detection of specific IgE using radiolabeled anti-IgE antibody.

Some patients develop *severe hypotension* after the use of propofol and a muscle relaxant, perhaps because of histamine release, since the combination of propofol and a muscle relaxant potentiates the release of histamine in vitro.

Risk factors Past studies of chronic occupational exposure to trace concentrations of inhalational agents have shown possible neurological, psychomotor, hematological, and reproductive adverse effects. However, the methods used in many of those studies have been criticized and the findings have often been inconclusive or contradictory. Despite the inconclusive evidence, threshold values for exposure to nitrous oxide and volatile agents have been recommended by national Occupational Safety and Health Organizations. In a recent study these concentrations were measured accurately using a photoacoustic infrared spectrometer during 20 pediatric anesthetics (3[C]). Pediatric anesthesia predisposes to high concentrations of waste gases, because of the frequent use of inhalational inductions, uncuffed tracheal tubes, and high fresh gas flow rates. High concentrations of nitrous oxide and volatile anesthetics were detected in the operating theatre during inhalational induction for several minutes in some patients, but after tracheal intubation trace concentrations of gases fell to concentrations that were mostly within the recommended limits. In a review of this topic other common causes of pollution in operating theatres were identified: leaks from ill-fitting face-masks, loose connections in breathing systems, and leaks from laryngeal masks at the end of surgery (4[R]). Testing for leaks, using infrared analysers, has been recommended as an important aid in the identification of hidden sources of pollution.

Side Effects of Drugs, Annual 22
J.K. Aronson, ed.

ANESTHETIC VAPORS *(SED-13, 265; SEDA-19, 104; SEDA-20, 106; SEDA-21, 116)*

Tumor-inducing effects Recent evidence suggests that exposure to anesthetic drugs can adversely affect the immune response. When mice were exposed to equipotent concentrations of isoflurane or halothane without surgical intervention, there were equal increases in the incidences of pulmonary metastases of melanoma (5). Previous findings of in vitro inhibition of natural killer cell cytotoxicity following exposure to volatile agents and nitrous oxide were confirmed.

Desflurane

The use of desflurane and sevoflurane in neuroanesthesia has been criticized in a recent review (6[R]). Their rapid recovery characteristics allow faster awakening at the end of anesthesia and therefore the advantage of earlier neurological evaluation. However, as with other volatile anesthetics, they are cerebral vasodilators, and can cause *increased intracranial pressure*; they also cause metabolic uncoupling, resulting in *increased cerebral blood flow and reduced cerebral metabolic oxygen consumption*. Although both sevoflurane and desflurane preserve carbon dioxide reactivity, they do so less than isoflurane. Desflurane has anticonvulsant properties, but there are reports that sevoflurane may have a proconvulsant effect. Both agents cause *depression of the EEG*, which may interfere with its use for diagnosis and monitoring. Desflurane is an airway irritant, which can trigger a sympathetic response, with *hypertension* and *tachycardia* on sudden exposure.

Halothane

Respiratory General anesthesia with halothane can cause *pulmonary microvascular injury* (7[C]). In 30 patients undergoing spinal surgery, randomized to receive either halothane or isoflurane, there were no significant differences between the groups on pulmonary function testing preoperatively or postoperatively. However, radionuclide lung clearance was significantly impaired on the third postoperative day in the halothane group, with gradual improvement to preoperative values by the tenth postoperative day. In order to demonstrate acute-phase changes under general anesthesia and to perform pathological examinations, a complementary animal study was performed. Rabbits had pulmonary radionuclide imaging studies before and after anesthesia using the same agents, and then underwent lung biopsy. There was abnormal radionucleotide lung clearance in the rabbits who had been exposed to halothane, and pathological examination showed endothelial damage. The mechanism of this pulmonary microvascular injury after exposure to a volatile anesthetic is not clear.

Liver The immunotoxicology of the liver has been reviewed (8[R]). The immunoallergic basis of *halothane hepatitis*, which results from a reaction of the oxidative metabolite trifluoroacetate with proteins to form a neoantigen that causes antibody formation, has been well described. However many points still remain unclear, including the precise mechanism of the adverse immune response, the very rare occurrence of the disease, and the risk factors involved. There is some evidence that a genetically determined susceptibility may predispose to halothane hepatitis.

An ‘in vitro cytotoxicity assay’ to identify genetically determined susceptibility of cells to destruction by reactive metabolites, as well as assessing the efficiency of systems of detoxification, has been developed (9[c]). The assay uses as target cells lymphocytes, which are exposed to the reactive metabolites of the tested drug. The susceptibility to halothane hepatitis was studied using this test in the presence of phenytoin and a compound that inhibits the enzyme epoxide hydrolase, which is involved in the detoxification of reactive metabolites of some drugs by the liver. Lymphocyte destruction was markedly higher in the patients with halothane hepatitis than in controls. Family studies showed increased lymphocyte cytotoxicity in half of the relatives of patients with halothane hepatitis.

Interactions Volatile anesthetics augment the effects of *neuromuscular blocking drugs*. Halothane has the weakest effect of all the commonly used volatile agents, and previous studies of the interaction between halothane and mivacurium have been contradictory. In 60 adults anesthetized with thiopental, fentanyl, and *mivacurium* for intubation, a computer-controlled closed-loop infusion of mivacurium was used to maintain neuromuscular block at 95% (10[C]). The patients received fentanyl and nitrous oxide, or halothane at various end-tidal concentrations. There was a linear relation between plasma cholinesterase activity and mivacurium requirements in all the patients. Halothane anesthesia reduced mivacurium infusion requirements by 15–25% compared with nitrous oxide–fentanyl anesthesia; however, the individual differences in the extent of this interaction were large.

Isoflurane

Liver Fatal *hepatic necrosis* occurred after isoflurane-based anesthesia in a 36-year-old woman without previous liver disease (11[C]). Although acute hepatotoxicity has been reported after exposure to isoflurane, under 10 cases of liver failure have been reported.

A previously healthy woman had taken no drugs before undergoing uneventful anesthesia with isoflurane for a gynecological procedure. She had previously been exposed to enflurane. Other drugs given perioperatively included clorazepate, thiopental, alfentanil, suxamethonium, alcuronium, nitrous oxide, atropine, neostigmine, naloxone, flumazenil, and piritramide. She developed fatal hepatic necrosis within 12 days of anesthesia, and no other cause could be found. No anti-trifluoroacetyl antibodies were detected in her serum, but the absence of those antibodies does not rule out the possibility of isoflurane toxicity.

Many factors thought to be associated with hepatitis after exposure to volatile anesthetics were present in this case, and it is possible that there may have been cross-sensitization between enflurane and isoflurane.

Interactions Volatile anesthetics prolong the effects of *non-depolarizing muscle relaxants*. The duration of anesthesia with isoflurane also influences the degree of potentiation seen with the muscle relaxant *mivacurium*, as has been shown in a study of 45 children who received 0.2 mg/kg mivacurium during anesthesia with 1.5 MAC isoflurane for either 10 or 30 min (12[c]). Those who received isoflurane for 30 min had recovery times of mivacurium prolonged by 55–58% and the onset time of neuromuscular blockade was significantly shorter than in patients who received isoflurane for 10 min. Thus, the potentiation of neuromuscular blockade by volatile anesthetics may be both a time- and concentration-dependent phenomenon.

In a study of 50 patients the MAC of isoflurane, postoperative analgesic requirements, and the hemodynamic response to tracheal intubation and extubation were reduced by *dexmeditomidine* (13[c]). However, hypotension and bradycardia were more frequent in 49 patients treated with dexmeditomidine (14[c]).

Sevoflurane

The recovery characteristics of anesthesia based on sevoflurane and propofol have been compared in a multicenter study of 169 outpatients of ASA grades I and II undergoing knee arthroscopy (15[c]). In previous comparisons of sevoflurane and propofol for outpatient anesthesia mixed populations with different surgical procedures have been studied. The patients received diclofenac 100 mg before induction of anesthesia with fentanyl 1.0–1.5 μg/kg and propofol 2.0–2.5 mg/kg. Maintenance of anesthesia was with 60% nitrous oxide via a laryngeal mask and continuous administration of either sevoflurane or propofol. In agreement with previous studies, the patients who were given sevoflurane emerged more rapidly from anesthesia but had a higher incidence of *nausea*, *vomiting*, and *dizziness* compared with the patients who received propofol. There was a higher incidence of cardiovascular adverse events, such as *bradycardia*, in the patients who received sevoflurane (19 vs 4%). None of the adverse effects resulted in a delay in recovery room discharge time or time to discharge. One of the patients given sevoflurane had *myoclonic seizures* after initial emergence from anesthesia and again 27 h later. Epileptiform movements have previously been reported during sevoflurane induction of anesthesia in children. However, in this case the seizures occurred during recovery, when end-tidal concentration of sevoflurane was low. Another possible explanation may have been the use of propofol for induction. The EEG was normal and a neurologist regarded the case as 'functional'. It is not possible to draw any firm conclusions about this reported adverse effect.

Cardiovascular The hemodynamic responses to surgical stimulation during sevoflurane and isoflurane anesthesia (1.5 MAC) with and without nitrous oxide have been compared in 24 patients undergoing gastrectomy (16[C]). During steady-state surgical stimulation the patients were randomized to continue receiving either 1.5 MAC of the designated anesthetic or an equipotent mixture of volatile anesthetic plus nitrous oxide. Neither sevoflurane nor isoflurane prevented the hemodynamic responses to surgical incision and the responses were similar. Sevoflurane plus nitrous oxide was associated with *higher central venous and pulmonary capillary wedge pressures* than sevoflurane alone, while no such effect was seen with isoflurane.

Dose-related *depression of left ventricular function and cardiac output* with sevoflurane has been reported in adults and children, but not infants (17[C]). The hemodynamic effects of sevoflurane and halothane were compared in 30 healthy infants undergoing elective surgery, who were anesthetized with either sevoflurane or halothane. Heart rate, blood pressure, and echocardiographic data were recorded at 1 and 1.5 MAC. Halothane, but not sevoflurane, caused a *fall in heart rate and cardiac index* compared with awake values. Halothane caused a greater fall in blood pressure than sevoflurane at all concentrations, and both agents significantly reduced systemic vascular resistance at all concentrations. There was a *reduction in myocardial contractility* in both groups, but in those given sevoflurane it was mild and was compensated for by a greater fall in systemic vascular resistance and maintenance of heart rate. Sevoflurane therefore reduced cardiac output less than halothane. Avoiding bradycardia was found to be crucial to maintaining normal cardiac output in infants. A larger study is needed to determine whether sevoflurane is safer than halothane for induction of anesthesia in infants.

Nervous system There was a higher incidence of *delirium* during recovery from sevoflurane anesthesia compared with halothane anesthesia in 63 preschool boys compared with 53 school-aged boys who underwent minor urological surgery with sevoflurane or isoflurane (18[C]). As well as general anesthesia, all the boys received caudal local anesthesia with bupivacaine and topical infiltration with lidocaine. There was quicker emergence and earlier recovery in those given sevoflurane, but a significantly higher incidence of delirium during recovery in the preschool group that had received sevoflurane. In the past, postoperative delirium was common after cyclopropane anesthesia, and it has recently been reported to be more frequent with desflurane. It may therefore be a problem associated with a rapid return to consciousness in an unfamiliar environment, although it has not been observed after the use of remifentanil in children.

Hematological Halothane *suppresses platelet function and prolongs bleeding time*. Sevoflurane has previously been shown to have a greater suppressive effect on platelet aggregation in vitro than halothane, possibly by suppression of thromboxane A2. To study the effect clinically, 38 elective surgical patients were randomly divided to receive either sevoflurane or isoflurane anesthesia (19[C]). Anesthesia was induced with thiopental and maintained with the volatile agent and nitrous oxide. Blood was collected before induction of anesthesia and then again 5 and 10 min after tracheal intubation, but before the start of surgery, and again when end-tidal concentration of volatile agent had reached 1–1.5 MAC. Platelet aggregation was induced by adenosine diphosphate and epinephrine. In all samples obtained during sevoflurane anesthesia, primary but not secondary platelet aggregation could be induced. In contrast, secondary platelet aggregation was only abolished in one of the 15 patients given isoflurane. Despite these findings, few investigators have confirmed any increased blood loss during general anesthesia compared with regional anesthesia. This may be partly because the neuroendocrine response to surgical stress induces a hypercoagulable state, and the anti-aggregatory effects of anesthetics may be overcome by increased catecholamines induced by the stress response. The suppressive effect on platelet function caused by volatile anesthetics may be either beneficial or harmful depending on clinical circumstances (20[c]).

Urinary system The safety of low-flow sevoflurane anesthesia in humans has been questioned, because it is degraded by strong bases in carbon dioxide absorbers to 'compound A', which causes dose-dependent nephrotoxicity in rats at concentrations above 50 ppm.

The effects of low-flow sevoflurane anesthesia on renal function have been compared with those of isoflurane in a detailed study of 73 patients (21[C]). Total fresh gas flow through the anesthetic breathing circuit was 1 l/min, with recirculation through a barium hydroxide lime absorber to remove carbon dioxide. The duration of anesthesia averaged 3.8 h. Maximum inspired compound A concentrations averaged 27 (range 10–67) ppm. There were no significant differences between sevoflurane and isoflurane. There was no evidence of renal damage attributable to compound A using the biochemical markers, serum blood urea nitrogen and creatinine, urinary excretion of protein, glucose, *N*-acetyl-β-D-glucosamine and α- or π-glutathione-*S*-transferase or postoperative alanine and aspartate aminotransferase concentrations.

In another study the renal effects of high (6–10 l/min) and low (1 l/min) flow sevoflurane were compared with the effects of low-flow isoflurane anesthesia in operations that lasted a mean of 6 h in 48 patients (22[C]). There was increased formation of compound A in the low-flow sevoflurane group (mean 20 ppm), but no evidence of renal damage or differences in renal function attributable to compound A. Tests of renal function included serum blood urea nitrogen and creatinine, creatinine clearance, and urinary *N*-acetyl-β-D-glucosaminidase and alanine aminopeptidase. In each group 33% of the patients had values after anesthesia above the upper limit of the reference range. The significance of these changes in the surgical setting remains unknown.

This subject has also been reviewed (23[CR]).

It was concluded that sevoflurane is as safe as isoflurane when it is used at low flow rates. However, until more is known it has been recommended that sevoflurane be avoided in patients with impaired kidney function.

Musculoskeletal Sevoflurane can trigger *malignant hyperthermia*. Prolonged skeletal muscle weakness has been reported in a 27-year-old man recovering from malignant hyperthermia resulting from sevoflurane anesthesia (24[C]). Neither the patient nor his family had a prior history of neuromuscular disease, and during anesthesia for tonsillectomy no other known triggering agents for malignant hyperthermia were given. A typical malignant hyperthermia reaction occurred 25 min after induction of anesthesia, and was successfully treated with dantrolene 100 mg. The day after this reaction he complained of severe muscle weakness in the arms and legs, most severe in the distal rather than proximal muscles, which took 3 months to resolve completely. Histology of muscle specimens obtained from patients recovering from malignant hyperthermia has shown various degrees of muscle destruction, so although it has not been previously reported, it was not surprising that subsequent muscle weakness occurred.

GASES

Nitrous oxide *(SED-13, 274; SEDA-19, 109; SEDA-20, 111; SEDA-21, 121)*

Nervous system Three episodes of *seizures* have been reported in a 7-month-old child exposed to nitrous oxide (25[c]).

An otherwise healthy 7-month-old girl, weight 10 kg, was admitted for reduction of hip dysplasia. On induction of anesthesia with nitrous oxide in oxygen she developed generalized tonic–clonic seizures. Inspired oxygen was immediately increased to 100%. The blood glucose was 2–4 mmol/l. Surgery was cancelled and a 16-channel EEG recorded on the same day was normal. A week later she was given dextrose in water until 2 h before induction of anesthesia for the same procedure. Anesthesia was induced with nitrous oxide and 1.5% halothane in oxygen, via a face-mask. During induction generalized seizures occurred again, but resolved quickly with discontinuation of nitrous oxide. Her blood glucose concentration was again normal. When she returned for a scheduled change of plaster the next month, continuous 10-lead EEG monitoring was performed perioperatively. Nitrous oxide in oxygen was started at 20% and increased stepwise. Two minutes after the inspired concentration of nitrous oxide had been increased to 70%, the EEG showed seizure activity, her arms hyperextended, and her eyes rolled upwards. The nitrous oxide was immediately discontinued and 100% oxygen plus 1.2% halothane were given by face-mask. The EEG showed continued seizure activity, maximum over both anterior regions and both temporal regions, and becoming diffuse after 10 s. She then developed generalized clonic movements for about 60 s. Spontaneous breathing was assisted and there was no hypoxia.

Despite evidence of cerebral excitatory actions and increased motor activity associated with its use, there has been no previous documentation of seizure activity after the administration of nitrous oxide.

Special senses Nitrous oxide can rapidly enter enclosed air containing spaces, increasing the pressure within them. It has therefore been suggested that nitrous oxide should be avoided in middle ear surgery, because of the potential risk of displacement of tympanic membrane grafts or ossicular prostheses. However, studies in this area have cited equivocal results. Of 97 patients randomized to receive halothane with or without nitrous oxide those who received nitrous oxide had significantly greater *fluctuations in middle ear pressure* than those who received halothane alone, but there was no difference in surgical outcome (26[c]). The Eustachian tube functions as a pressure-release mechanism, and fluctuations in pressure in the middle ear occur in both normal and some abnormal ears. The question of risk associated with the use of nitrous oxide anesthesia in middle ear surgery was not answered.

Interactions Both *methotrexate* and nitrous oxide affect folate-dependent processes. In an in vitro study pretreatment with methotrexate prevented irreversible inactivation of methionine synthase by nitrous oxide (27). Toxicity using this drug combination may depend on the sequence of administration.

INTRAVENOUS AGENTS

BARBITURATES *(SED-13, 275; SEDA-19, 119; SEDA-20, 112; SEDA-21, 122)*

Thiopental sodium

Use in pregnancy In 70 pregnant women at 7–13 weeks gestation the dose of thiopental for hypnosis was 17% less, and that for anesthesia 18% less, than in non-pregnant women (28[c]). Previous human and animal studies have also shown that pregnancy increases sensitivity to inhalational anesthetics. The changes in sensitivity to anesthetics in the later stages of pregnancy are unknown.

MISCELLANEOUS NON-BARBITURATE ANESTHETICS

Benzodiazepines *(SED-13, 277; SEDA-19, 112; SEDA-20, 112; SEDA-21, 122)*

Immunological and hypersensitivity reactions In vitro studies of benzodiazepines have shown evidence of an *immunosuppressive action* by natural killer T cell inhibition (29[c]). The clinical implications of these findings are unknown.

Midazolam

The therapeutic use and toxicity of midazolam have been reviewed (30[R]).

Data on 19 112 patients from 14 hospitals have been analyzed retrospectively to investigate whether there is an association between the use of midazolam and serious cardiorespiratory events or death. The study included patients admitted to hospital between March 1986 and October 1987 who received either injectable diazepam or midazolam on the same day as they had medical interventions, including endoscopy, general anesthesia, or conscious sedative procedures. After adjustment for confounding factors, the death rate was significantly lower in patients who received midazolam than in those who received diazepam. The study had major limitations in the reliability and completeness of information on confounding factors. It was not certain that serious cardiorespiratory adverse events could be reliably identified. Doses of the study drugs were also not controlled for (31[C]).

Interactions The pharmacokinetics of midazolam are altered by drugs that are metabolized by the CYP3A or that affect CYP3A activity. These include *macrolide antibiotics*, *antimycotics*, *calcium antagonists*, and *cimetidine*. CYP3A also metabolizes midazolam at extrahepatic sites, particularly in the gut wall, and inhibitors and inducers of CYP3A interfere with the metabolism of midazolam at these sites (32[r]), (33[c]).

Grapefruit juice inhibits the presystemic metabolism of benzodiazepines by inhibition of CYP3A in the small intestine (34[r]).

Saquinavir, a protease inhibitor used in HIV disease, may potentiate the effects of midazolam, probably via CYP3A inhibition (35[r]).

Combined use of midazolam with *opioid analgesics* has a supra-additive hypnotic effect and causes respiratory depression. The clearance of midazolam was reduced by fentanyl in 30 patients, probably as a result of competitive inhibition of the activity of the isoenzyme CYP3A (36[C]). In a recent study of 150 patients undergoing endoscopy, low-dose midazolam (35 μg/kg) was not associated with more frequent oxygen desaturation when it was used in combination with an opioid (37[c]). However, the combination of midazolam with pethidine did not improve patient tolerance or pain scores compared with either drug given alone. The benzodiazepine antagonist flumazenil enhanced the analgesic effect of morphine in 71 postoperative patients who had received diazepam preoperatively. Benzodiazepines antagonize opioid analgesia in animals, probably by activation of GABA receptors and it has been suggested that benzodiazepines may also have this effect in humans (38).

Ketamine *(SED-13, 277; SEDA-19, 114; SEDA-20, 113; SEDA-21, 124)*

Ketamine is often favored for pediatric sedation, because it lacks the respiratory depressant effects of other anesthetic agents, and maintains upper airway patency and reflexes. In 30 children who received intravenous ketamine 1–2 mg/kg for painful procedures in the emergency department, 1.5 mg/kg produced optimal sedation within 2 min (39[C]). The median time to fulfil discharge criteria was 25 min. The most common adverse effect reported was *ataxia*, which occurred in nine patients and persisted for 0.5–2 h. *Vomiting*, *agitation*, *hallucinations*, and *nightmares* were occasionally reported. The findings were in agreement with those of previous reports. Ketamine appears to be safe for sedation of children, because it rarely causes airway complications such as laryngospasm or aspiration. Transient respiratory depression has been reported when ketamine was injected intravenously over a period of under 10 s. The authors recommended that intravenous ketamine should be given over 30–60 s.

Propofol *(SED-13, 278; SEDA-19, 115; SEDA-20, 114; SEDA-21, 125)*

A meta-analysis of 84 randomized controlled studies in 6069 patients of the effect of propofol compared with other anesthetics on *postoperative nausea and vomiting* has been performed (40[R]). In a high-risk setting, in which the incidence of postoperative nausea and vomiting is 20–60% without prophylaxis, propofol can produce a short-term 20% reduction when it is given as a maintenance regimen. In other circumstances, including the use of propofol for induction only, late postoperative nausea and vomiting, and settings in which the risk of postoperative nausea and vomiting is low, the authors concluded that, while the effect of propofol may be statistically significant, it is clinically unimportant.

Data from three meta-analyses have been used to study the antiemetic efficacy of propofol anesthesia compared with another anesthetic; anesthesia using the same agents with or without nitrous oxide; and propofol anesthesia without nitrous oxide compared with anesthesia with another anesthetic with nitrous oxide (41[R]). Either propofol maintenance of anesthesia, or omitting nitrous oxide in general anesthesia had similar effects on both early (0–6 h) or late (0–24 h) postoperative vomiting, and the NNT was 6. Propofol reduced the incidence of early nausea to the same extent as early vomiting, whereas omitting nitrous oxide had no effect on early nausea.

The induction characteristics of 2% propofol in 45 children of ASA grade I have been evaluated in a prospective randomized study (42[c]). At a dose of 3 mg/kg there was a 90% incidence of *spontaneous movements*. A dose of 5 mg/kg was associated with a high incidence of *coughing* (90%), which interfered with manual ventilation. A dose of 4 mg/kg allowed rapid and smooth induction, with few adverse effects and excellent conditions for manual ventilation. Hemodynamic stability and pain on injection were the same as with the 1% formulation. The 2% formulation had the advantages of reducing the volume of drug required and the time taken for injection. Propofol has previously been reported to inhibit cytochrome P450 CYP3A4, but current evidence suggests that it does not inhibit the metabolism of midazolam at clinically important concentrations (43[c]).

Nervous system *Abnormal movements and seizures* have been widely reported after propofol. A healthy 24-year-old woman who developed seizures over the 24 h after the use of propofol differed from previous patients in that she had been previously exposed to propofol without any complications (44[c]).

A survey of the incidence and content of *dreams* intraoperatively and of emotional status on recovery has been conducted in 112 patients undergoing surgery for varicose veins (45[C]). They were anesthetized with propofol total intravenous anesthesia, propofol induction followed by a volatile anesthesia including nitrous oxide, or thiopental induction followed by volatile anesthesia including nitrous oxide. As in previous studies the patients who received propofol had more dreams than those who were anesthetized with thiopental. The incidence of recall of dreams was also higher. However, contrary to previous reports there was no difference in the sexual content of the dreams. Postoperative nausea and vomiting were less in those who received propofol groups, and they reported feeling happier than those who received thiopental.

Risk factors The issue of the use of propofol sedation in pediatric intensive care has been reviewed and investigated (46[R]), (47[R]). Its use has been contentious since a 1992 report of five deaths in children who had received high infusion rates (exceeding 6 mg/kg per h) and all of whom had evidence of respiratory tract infection. Several possible mechanisms for these deaths have been suggested, including hypertriglyceridemia in the presence of impaired lipid metabolism, extrinsic bacterial contamination of propofol, or an idiosyncratic syndrome of propofol-associated metabolic acidosis. Nine children ventilated in intensive care after cardiac surgery were prospectively studied and received propofol 1–4 mg/kg per h and fentanyl 1–5 μg/kg per h for 48 h (46[R]). The children had no evidence of respiratory infections and did not receive parenteral nutrition containing additional intralipid. There was no evidence of metabolic acidosis or any other metabolic or biochemical alterations, and the children were cardiovascularly stable. The authors recommended that until more information is available, propofol should not be given to children with an acute infective process, especially an upper respiratory tract infection. The rate of infusion should not exceed 5 mg/kg per h and it should not be used as the sole sedative agent. Its continued use should be reviewed daily. Larger studies are needed before criteria for the safe use of propofol in pediatric intensive care can be defined.

It has been suggested that the 2% formulation may be a useful alternative in order to reduce the lipid load in patients who require high doses of propofol over long periods of time (48[r]), (49[c]).

Interactions Recent studies have suggested that propofol may alter its own distribution and elimination (50[r]). Accurate performance of a target-controlled infusion device may fall with increasing blood propofol concentration, and this may be due to a reduction in cardiac output and liver blood flow, reducing the redistribution and clearance of propofol.

Opioid analgesics and propofol also interact synergistically. Opioids reduce the redistribution and elimination of propofol, and propofol inhibits the metabolism of some opioids.

A randomized double-blind study of the anesthetic induction requirements in 60 healthy patients showed a 24% reduction in dose after an intravenous dose of *metoclopramide* 0.15 mg/kg (51[c]).

REFERENCES

1. Smith I, Avramov MN, White PF. A comparison of propofol and remifentanil during monitored anesthesia care. J Clin Anesth 1997;9:148–54.
2. Aimone-Gastin I, Gueant JL, Laxenaire MC, Moneret-Vautrin DA. Pathogenesis of allergic reactions to anaesthetic drugs. Int J Immunopathol Pharmacol 1997;10:193–6.
3. Hoerauf K, Funk W, Harth M, Hobbhahn J. Occupational exposure to sevoflurane, halothane and nitrous oxide during paediatric anaesthesia. Anaesthesia 1997;52:215–19.
4. Barker JP, Abdelatti MO. Anaesthetic pollution: potential sources, their identification and control. Anaesthesia 1997;52:1077–83.
5. Moudgil GC, Singal DP. Halothane and isoflurane enhance melanoma tumour metastasis in mice. Can J Anaesth 1997;44:90–4.
6. Templehoff R. The new inhalational anesthetics desflurane and sevoflurane are valuable additions to the practice of neuroanesthesia. J Neurosurg Anesthiol 1997;9:69–71.
7. Gunaydin B, Karadenizli Y, Babacan A, Kaya K, Unlu M, Inanir S, Mahki A, Akcabay M, Yardim S. Pulmonary microvascular injury following general anesthesia with volatile anaesthetics—halothane and isoflurane: a comparative clinical and experimental study. Respir Med 1997;91:351–60.
8. Beaune PH, Lecoeur S. Immunotoxicology of the liver: adverse reactions to drugs. J Hepatol Suppl 1997;26:37–42.
9. Larrey D, Pageaux GP. Genetic predisposition to drug-induced hepatotoxicity. J Hepatol Suppl 1997;26:12–21.
10. Kansanaho M, Olkkola KT. The effect of halothane on mivacurium infusion requirements in adult surgical patients. Acta Anaesthesiol Scand 1997;47:754–9.
11. Weitz J, Kienle P, Bohrer H, Hofmann, Theilmann L, Otto G. Fatal hepatic necrosis after isoflurane anaesthesia. Anaesthesia 1997;52:884–95.
12. Jalkanen L, Meretoja OA. The influence of the duration of isoflurane anaesthesia on neuromuscular effects of mivacurium. Acta Anaesthesiol Scand 1997;41:248–51.
13. Lawrence CJ, De Lange S. Effects of a single pre-operative dexmedetomidine dose on isoflurane requirements and peri-operative haemodynamic stability. Anaesthesia 1997;52:736–44.
14. Aantaa R, Jaakola M-J, Kallio A, Kanto J. Reduction of the minimum alveolar concentration of isoflurane by dexmedetomidine. Anesthesiology 1997;86:1055–60.
15. Raeder J, Gupta A, Pedersen FM. Recovery characteristics of sevoflurane or propofol based anaesthesia for day-care surgery. Acta Anaesthesiol Scand 1997;41:988–94.
16. Inada T, Inada K, Kawachi S, Takubo K, Tai M, Yasugi H. Haemodynamic comparison of sevoflurane and isoflurane anaesthesia in surgical patients. Can J Anaesth 1997;44:140–5.
17. Wodey E, Pladys P, Copin C, Lucas MM, Chaumont A, Carre P, Lelong B, Azzis O, Ecoffey C. Comparative hemodynamic depression of sevoflurane versus halothane in infants. Anesthesiology 1997;87:795–800.
18. Aono J, Ueda W, Mamiya K, Takimoto K, Manabe M. Greater incidence of delirium during recovery from sevoflurane anaesthesia in preschool boys. Anesthesiology 1997;87:1298–300.
19. Hirikata H, Nakamura K, Sai S, Okuda H, Hatano Y, Urabe N, Mori K. Platelet aggregation is impaired during anaesthesia with sevoflurane but not with isoflurane. Can J Anaesth 1997;44:1157–61.
20. Aoki H, Mizobe TH. Platelet aggregation inhibited by sevoflurane, or by ethanol? Anesthesiology 1997;87:1016.
21. Karasch ED, Frink EJ, Zager R, Bowdle TA, Artu A, Nogami WM. Assessment of low-flow sevoflurane and isoflurane effects on renal function using sensitive markers of tubular toxicity. Anesthesiology 1997;86:1238–53.
22. Bito H, Ikeuchi Y, Ikeda K. Effects of low-flow sevoflurane anesthesia on renal function. Anesthesiology 1997;86:1231–7.
23. Mazze RI, Jamison RL. Low-flow (1 l/min) sevoflurane. Is it safe? Anesthesiology 1997;86:1225–7.
24. Maeda H, Iranami H, Hatano Y. Delayed recovery from muscle weakness due to malignant hyperthermia during sevoflurane anesthesia. Anesthesiology 1997;87:425–6.
25. Lannes M, Desparmet JF, Zifkin BJ. Generalised seizures associated with nitrous oxide in an infant. Anesthesiology 1997;87:705–8.
26. Chinn K, Brown OE, Manning SC, Crandell CC. Middle ear pressure variation: effect of nitrous oxide. Laryngoscope 1997;107:357–63.

27. Fiskerstrand T, Ueland PM, Refsum H. Folate depletion induced by methotrexate affects methionine synthase activity and its susceptibility to inactivation by nitrous oxide. J Pharmacol Exp Ther 1997;282:1305–11.
28. Gin T, Mainland P, Chan MTV, Short TG. Decreased thiopental requirements in early pregnancy. Anesthesiology 1997;86:73–8.
29. Bessler H, Caspi B, Gavish M, Rehavi M, Hart J, Weizman R. Peripheral-type benzodiazepine receptor ligands modulate human natural killer cell activity. Int J Immunopharmacol 1997;19:249–54.
30. Nordt SP, Clark RF. Midazolam: a review of therapeutic uses and toxicity. J Emerg Med 1997;15:357–65.
31. Dai WS, Xue S, Yoo K, Jones JK, Labraico J. An investigation of the safety of midazolam use in hospital. Pharmacoepidemiol Drug Saf 1997;6:79–87.
32. Strayhorn VA, Baciewicz AM, Self TH. Update on rifampin drug interactions, III. Arch Intern Med 1997;157:2453–8.
33. Ahonen J, Olkola KT, Neuvonen PJ. Effect of route of administration of fluconazole and midazolam. Eur J Clin Pharmacol 1997;51:415–19.
34. Ameer B, Weintraub RA. Drug interactions with grapefruit juice. Clin Pharmacokinet 1997; 33:103–21.
35. Merry C, Mulcahy F, Barry M, Gibbons S, Back D. Saquinavir interaction with midazolam: pharmacokinetic considerations when prescribing protease inhibitors for patients with HIV disease. AIDS 1997;11:268–9.
36. Hase I, Oda Y, Tanaka K, Mizutani K, Nakamoto T, Asada A. I.v. fentanyl decreases the clearances of midazolam. Br J Anaesth 1997; 79:740–3.
37. Froehlich F, Thorens J, Shwizer W, Preisig M, Kohler M, Hays RD, Fiedd M, Gonvers J-J. Sedation and analgesia for colonoscopy: patient tolerance, pain and cardiorespiratory parameters. Gastrointest Endosc 1997;45:1–9.
38. Gear RW, Miaskowski C, Heller PH, Paul SM, Gordon MC, Levine JD. Benzodiazepine mediated antagonism of opioid analgesia. Pain 1997;71:25–9.
39. Dachs RJ, Innes GM. Intravenous ketamine sedation of pediatric patients in the emergency department. Ann Emerg Med 1997;29:146–50.
40. Tramer M, Moore A, McQuay H. Propofol anaesthesia and postoperative nausea and vomiting: quantitative systematic review of randomised controlled studies. Br J Anaesth 1997;78:247–55.
41. Tramer M, Moore A, McQuay H. Meta-analytic comparison of prophylactic antiemetic efficacy for postoperative nausea and vomiting: propofol anaesthesia vs omitting nitrous oxide vs total i.v. anaesthesia with propofol. Br J Anaesth 1997;78:256–9.
42. Borgeat A, Fuchs T, Tassonyi E. Induction characteristics of 2% propofol in children. Br J Anaesth 1997;78:433–5.
43. Leung B, Millar E, Park G. The effect of propofol on midazolam metabolism in human liver microsome suspension. Anaesthesia 1997; 52:945–8.
44. Harrigan PWJ, Browne SM, Quail AW. Multiple seizures following re-exposure to propofol. Anaesth Intensive Care 1996;24:261–4.
45. Brandner B, Blagrove M, McCallum G, Bromley LM. Dreams, images and emotions associated with propofol anaesthesia. Anaesthesia 1997;52:750–5.
46. Martin PH, Murphy BVS, Petros AJ. Metabolic, biochemical and haemodynamic effects of infusion of propofol for long-term sedation of children under going intensive care. Br J Anaesth 1997;79:276–9.
47. Hatch DJ. Propofol in paediatric care. Br J Anaesth 1997;79:274–5.
48. Mateu de Antonio J, Barrachina F. Propofol infusion and nutritional support. Am J Health-Syst Pharm 1997;54:2515–16.
49. Servin FS, Desmonts JM, Melloni C, Martinelli G.A. Comparison of 2% and 1% formulations of propofol for the induction and maintenance of anaesthesia in surgery of moderate duration. Anaesthesia 1997;52:1216–21.
50. Vuyk J. Pharmacokinetic and pharmcodynamic interactions between opioids and propofol. J Clin Anaesth 1997;9 (Suppl):23–6S.
51. Page VJ, Chhipa JH. Metoclopramide reduces the induction dose of propofol. Acta Anaesthesiol Scand 1997;41:256–9.

Stephan A. Schug and Joanne E. Ritchie

11 Local anesthetics

Immunological and hypersensitivity reactions *Type I reactions* Pruritus and generalized urticaria occurred 20 min after administration of an amide local anesthetic in a 30-year-old woman (1[c]). Skin prick tests were negative for all local anesthetic drugs tested. However, intradermal tests were positive for lidocaine, mepivacaine, and bupivacaine, as were placebo-controlled, double-blind, subcutaneous challenges with lidocaine and mepivacaine. The authors were unable to detect specific IgE antibodies to these local anesthetics. Even so, they concluded that the characteristics of the reaction and the positive skin tests and challenge tests pointed to a type 1 hypersensitivity reaction.

An urticarial reaction and possible type I hypersensitivity occurred in a 35-year-old woman after the administration of articaine for a dental procedure (2[c]). Again skin prick tests were negative, but intradermal tests with lidocaine, prilocaine, and bupivacaine were all positive, demonstrating possible cross-reactivity between the amide local anesthetic drugs.

A similar case of probable type I reactions to lidocaine and mepivacaine, with cross-reactivity to articaine has been reported in a 54-year-old woman with asthma and eczema (3[c]). The report was unusual insofar as this patient had previously experienced four possible allergic reactions to amide local anaesthetics: an initial minor reaction to topical lidocaine (possibly sensitizing her); an episode of respiratory distress and loss of consciousness after intra-articular lidocaine; a life-threatening reaction to lidocaine via a peripheral nerve block, with severe hypotension and bradycardia requiring adrenaline; and finally another similar episode after mepivacaine for dental anaesthesia.

Delayed reactions Over a 20-year period 208 patients with a history of local anesthetic allergy were referred to an anesthetics allergy clinic (4[C]). These patients were tested with progressive intradermal challenges and 198 patients had negative tests for local anesthetics; 36 reacted to an additive (two with anaphylaxis), either methylparaben or metabisulfite, and 193 subsequently received preservative-free local anesthetics without problems. Two patients had an immediate reaction to the local anesthetic and four had delayed hypersensitivity. One patient had a delayed systemic reaction to four different local anesthetics and an alternative drug had yet to be found. Other diagnoses included: vasovagal attacks, other psychological causes, and reactions to other drugs and intravascular adrenaline.

A delayed reaction to prilocaine has been reported (5[c]). The patient developed local itching, redness, and edema 3 days after infiltration anesthesia with prilocaine plus adrenaline for removal of a lipoma. This responded to topical corticosteroids. Patch tests showed reactions to prilocaine, EMLA and articaine, but not to the disinfectant or dressings used, or to lidocaine, or to a number of other ester or amide local anesthetics. This patient had had previous exposure to prilocaine, and it seemed that this caused cross-reactivity with articaine.

EFFECTS RELATED TO DIFFERENT MODES OF USE

Brachial plexus anesthesia *(SED-13, 287; SEDA-19, 127; SEDA-20, 122)*

Plasma concentrations of mepivacaine after radiographically guided injection of 50 ml of 1.5% solution into the axillary sheath in six patients have been compared with those after

Side Effects of Drugs, Annual 22
J.K. Aronson, ed.

extra-sheath injection in another six (6[C]). Extra-sheath injections caused higher plasma concentrations than intra-sheath injection, which exceeded minimum toxic plasma concentrations for mepivacaine (mean 8 μg/ml). However, only two patients in this study developed mild central nervous system toxicity within 30 min of injection.

Dental anesthesia *(SEDA-13, 288; SEDA-19, 127; SEDA-20, 124; SEDA-21, 131)*

In a survey of the local anesthetic techniques of 1600 German dentists in 2731 patients there was a 4.5% incidence of complications (7[C]). These included: *dizziness*, *tachycardia*, *agitation*, *nausea*, *tremor*, *syncope*, *seizures* (one patient), and *bronchospasm* (one patient). This complication rate increased to 5.7% if risk factors were present, such as cardiovascular disease, allergies, and pregnancy. Cardiovascular disease was associated with a higher incidence of tachycardia, but not angina, myocardial infarction, dysrhythmias, or cardiac arrest. Premedication at home also increased the incidence of complications to 9.1%. Articaine (the drug most frequently used) with 1:200 000 adrenaline and lidocaine were associated with the least frequent complications (3.1 and 0%, respectively). Mepivacaine and articaine with 1:100 000 adrenaline were associated with the most frequent complications (7.2 and 6.1%, respectively). The authors suggested that an adequate medical history should be taken, that safe dosages need to be calculated by weight before use, that low concentrations of adrenaline should be used, and that dentists should match drug and technique to the procedure and the individual patient.

Special senses Ocular and visual symptoms occurred in two patients after block for a dental procedure (8[c]). The first followed an injection of lidocaine with adrenaline for a mandibular block. Within minutes the patient complained of *dizziness and double vision*, accompanied by *partial blindness*. He also had *blanching of the forehead and upper eyelid*, with *left eye adduction*. This lasted for about 20 min, with no anesthesia of the mandible. The authors postulated that these symptoms result directly from entry of the local anesthetic into the ophthalmic artery via the middle meningeal artery, thereby affecting the portion of the sixth cranial nerve, which innervates the lateral rectus muscle. This would have resulted in blanching of the skin, partial amaurosis, and ophthalmoplegia.

The second case followed a posterior superior alveolar injection of lidocaine with adrenaline. This resulted in a good block for the dental procedure. But on standing the patient complained of *dizziness and diplopia*, with accompanying *numbness of the eyebrow and lids* and some *loss of motor function*. This lasted about 3 h and resolved as the local anesthesia subsided. In this patient, the positional and delayed presentation may have been due to an arteriovenous shunt or anastomosis between the superior ophthalmic vein and the ophthalmic artery, causing reflux into the artery from the valveless vein when the patient became upright.

Epidural anesthesia *(SED-13, 290; SEDA-19, 127; SEDA-20, 124; SEDA-21, 131)*

Epidural analgesia (bupivacaine 0.0625% and fentanyl 3.3 μg/ml) has been compared with patient-controlled analgesia (intravenous morphine) in 111 women (9[C]). There was a similar incidence of *vomiting* in the two groups (33% in the epidural group) and a higher incidence of *pruritus* (32%) and *leg weakness* (18%) in the epidural group. The epidural technique provided better-quality analgesia.

In a comparison of bolus epidural morphine with epidural infusion of 0.1% bupivacaine plus fentanyl in postoperative analgesia in 31 children, the bupivacaine/fentanyl infusion was significantly better with fewer adverse effects (10[C]). All had some degree of *sedation*. In the bupivacaine/fentanyl group 13% had *pruritus* and 60% *vomited*. One in this group had *hypotension* with subsequent headache, possibly secondary to the hypotension, which resolved with intravenous fluids and discontinuation of the epidural. Another child was severely sedated and so the epidural was discontinued. Two had their infusion doses reduced, one because of asymptomatic *bradycardia* and the other because of *paresthesia of the legs*. There were no episodes of respiratory depression or motor blockade in either group.

In a comparison of bupivacaine alone with bupivacaine plus sufentanil in 100 postoperative patients using patient-controlled epidural analgesia, bupivacaine plus sufentanil produced better analgesia but more *sedation* (11[C]). There were three cases of early *respiratory depression* (one in the bupivacaine group), three of postoperative *disorientation* (two in the bupivacaine group), and one of *hallucinations* (in the bupivacaine plus sufentanil group).

Of 2000 consecutive patients receiving postoperative epidural analgesia with bupivacaine 0.25% plus morphine, three had episodes of *respiratory depression* requiring naloxone and discontinuation of the epidural infusion, and another 31 had respiratory rates of 6–7 per min but did not require treatment (12[C]). Four had *hypotension* (systolic blood pressures under 80 mmHg), and required vasopressors. Only 0.05% had *paralysis of the legs*, while 12% had some degree of *motor block*. *Nausea* occurred in 36%, 14% *vomited*, and 4.6% had severe nausea without vomiting. The authors also reported two trauma patients who developed *epidural abscesses* after 3 weeks of treatment, causing permanent paralysis. They felt that in these cases there had been a late response to early warning signs.

Epidural analgesia masked a neurological deficit in a 34-year-old man with type 1 diabetes mellitus (13[c]). He received postoperative epidural analgesia of 0.125% bupivacaine plus fentanyl 5 μg/ml after a 4-h procedure, during which he was in the lithotomy position. Postoperatively he complained of heaviness in his legs, which was attributed to the epidural infusion until discontinuation of his epidural 3 days postoperatively, when his leg heaviness continued. Three months later, EMG studies showed peripheral lesions at the right femoral nerve and the left lateral femoral cutaneous nerve of the thigh. It is likely that this was due to the lengthy intraoperative lithotomy position, masked by the epidural infusion.

Two further cases of postoperative problems masked by epidural analgesia occurred during orthopedic surgery in two children, in whom postoperative epidural bupivacaine and fentanyl analgesia were used and compartment syndrome developed (14[c]). The authors thought that the use of postoperative epidural analgesia with bupivacaine had masked the symptoms of excessive pressure from the splints, but not the pain of the subsequent compartment syndrome. They suggested that the addition of bupivacaine to fentanyl for orthopedic postoperative epidurals is unnecessary and increases the risk of pressure-related problems. However, they largely ignored the fact that poor pressure area care and inadequate positioning are other causative factors in this previously described problem.

In 600 obstetric patients who received slow epidural injection of local anesthetic (by gravity flow) or by bolus injection, gravity flow was associated with a reduced incidence of hypotension, nausea, sedation, and an *increased heart rate* (15[C]). Four of the 300 patients who received a local anesthetic as a bolus had mild symptoms of local anesthetic toxicity compared with none of those who received the anesthetic by gravity flow.

A comparison of epidural single end-holed catheters and multi-holed catheters in 364 obstetric patients showed that a multi-orifice catheter may be more efficacious when used for continuous infusion of low-concentration local anesthetic solutions, owing to a lower risk of unilateral block (16[c]). However, there was a higher rate of blood in the multi-holed than the single-holed catheters, and the authors proposed that this was probably related to detection of vascular trauma at insertion rather than intravascular placement. Three patients in each group developed early local anesthetic toxicity from the test dose.

Cardiovascular A 71-year-old woman had a *cardiopulmonary arrest* 1 h after an epidural injection of 18 ml of 0.5% bupivacaine for a total knee joint replacement (17[c]). She required full cardiopulmonary resuscitation, including intubation and ventilation. However, she made a full recovery 6 h later. A CT scan showed air in the subarachnoid space, indicating a dural puncture at the time of location of the epidural space. The authors thought that the delay in presentation might have been due to a slow leak of local anesthetic solution into the subarachnoid space, causing a high spinal block.

Respiratory In 2000 consecutive patients using postoperative epidural analgesia with morphine plus bupivacaine 0.25% one catheter was placed in the subarachnoid space and the patient had a episode of late *severe respiratory depression* requiring treatment with naloxone (12[C]).

Nervous system An episode of *polymyoclonus* has been reported after epidural steroid injection (18[c]).

A 56-year-old man with chronic back pain and neurological symptoms was given an injection of 13 ml of 1% lidocaine and 120 mg of triamcinolone, and 20 min later became sedated and hypotensive and developed a high patchy sensory and motor block and a myoclonus in his upper extremities, which then developed into generalized myoclonus, with brief, jerky, involuntary, asymmetrical, asynchronous movements of his extremities every 15–45 s. This was treated with intravenous midazolam and resolved over 30 min, but was followed by anxiety and restless legs for about 1 h.

The authors postulated that a subdural injection had occurred, because of negative aspiration of blood or CSF at the time of injection, resulting, because of the narrow subdural space and trabeculae within, in a high level of sensory, motor, and autonomic block of patchy distribution, with delayed onset. The myoclonus might have been due to an effect of the injectate on the cerebellum, a drug-induced spinal seizure, or hypotension-induced cerebral hypoperfusion.

Two episodes of *severe leg pain* occurred after epidural labor analgesia in a patient who had had one previous uncomplicated epidural catheter for labor analgesia (19[c]).

During a second epidural for cesarean section with 3 ml of bupivacaine 0.25% plus 15 ml of lidocaine 2%, a woman developed bilateral cramping pain in the anterior thighs, which resolved as the epidural block wore off. After a third epidural catheter insertion and administration of 20 ml of bupivacaine 0.25% followed by 20 ml of lidocaine 2% plus 2 ml of 8.4% sodium bicarbonate, she developed severe pain in her lower limbs, anterior abdomen, and anterior thighs; this resolved as the sensory block regressed.

The authors concluded that this could have been due to a neurotoxic effect of 2% lidocaine and transient radicular irritation. However, using recent definitions of transient radicular irritation, namely pain or dysesthesia that occurs within 24 h of the resolution of a block, this is unlikely to have been a true case. Otherwise, this would have been the second case of neurological irritation after the epidural use of 2% lidocaine.

Urinary system In 3364 obstetric deliveries over a 10-month period there were 30 cases of *urinary retention* requiring catheterization (20[C]). Epidural analgesia increased the risk of urinary retention: 27 of the 30 cases occurred after epidural analgesia, which was only used in 1000 cases (30%). There was no significant difference in the incidence of urinary retention between the two epidural solutions used (bupivacaine 0.25% or bupivacaine 0.125% plus sufentanil), despite the assumption that lowering the local anesthetic dose may reduce the incidence of urinary retention. The authors therefore concluded that adding sufentanil counteracts the effects of reducing the dose of bupivacaine.

Intrathecal (spinal) anesthesia

(SED-13, 290; SEDA-19, 127; SEDA-20, 124; SEDA-21, 131)

In 55 obstetric patients given intrathecal morphine and bupivacaine 2.5 mg, the first and second stages of labor were longer than in a control group given systemic analgesia (mean 318 vs 176 min and 74 vs 37 min, respectively) and instrument-assisted delivery was more common (31 vs 14%) (21[C]). There were no differences in the rate of cesarean section or neonatal Apgar scores. However, in those who received intrathecal analgesia there was a high incidence of mild adverse events, such as *pruritus* (48%), *nausea* (40%), *vomiting* (37%), *somnolence* (27%), *shivering* (27%), *urinary retention* (21%), *hypotension* (15%), and *bradycardia* (13%). Respiratory depression and spinal headache were not reported.

Respiratory arrest, *severe hypotension*, and *fetal distress* occurred in two women who received intravenous fentanyl followed by intrathecal sufentanil and bupivacaine (22[c]). Soon after the intrathecal injection, each became unresponsive, bradycardic, hypotensive, and apneic, and there was fetal bradycardia. These episodes required circulatory and ventilatory support, including naloxone, but they later delivered healthy babies without further incident. The authors suggested that an interaction between the intravenous and intrathecal opioids had been mainly responsible for this, as only mild respiratory depression has previously been reported with sufentanil alone.

Cardiovascular Sufentanil and low-dose bupivacaine caused marked *hypotension* in a parturient (23[c]). This was associated with a high sensory block, but no motor block. In view of the lack of motor block, this was possibly due to the sympatholytic effects of sufentanil in combination with the local anesthetic.

Hypotension (a 15% reduction in baseline systolic blood pressure) also occurred in 13 of 14 patients who received 10 mg of hyperbaric tetracaine as spinal anesthesia in a randomized comparison of the effects of treatment of hypotension with either adrenaline or phenylephrine (24[C]).

In a further comparison of single-dose and continuous spinal analgesia, the latter significantly reduced the incidence of hypotension and bradycardia (25[c]).

Nervous system After spinal anesthesia with 80 mg of lidocaine 5% and 20 μg of fentanyl, a 45-year-old man developed sudden *bradycardia*, *unresponsiveness*, *apnea*, and *cyanosis* (26[c]). At this time he had a sensory block height of T5–6. He was initially treated with atropine, with some improvement, but required naloxone to re-establish respiration on three further occasions. This was probably due to cephalad spread of the opioid, but again there may also have been a contribution from high spinal local anesthesia.

A 57-year-old woman, who underwent knee arthroscopy under spinal anesthesia with 0.5% tetracaine, developed *rhythmic clonic movements* of her pelvis, legs, and ankles postoperatively (27[c]). She had residual sensory block to T12, with absent ankle jerks, and made a full recovery after 1 h. The authors postulated that this was partially due to a sensory abnormality caused by the local anesthesia at the spinal cord level, and a more central action by inhibition of inhibitory pathways causing transient excitation of the central nervous system.

Mepivacaine has been implicated in two cases of *transient radicular irritation*. In both cases 4% hyperbaric mepivacaine was used for spinal anesthesia during a short procedure in the lithotomy position (28[c]). The first patient complained of buttock pain radiating to the posterior thighs 3 h after the spinal anesthetic and lasting 12 h. The second complained of severe pain in the lower back radiating to the thighs and calves 4 h after the spinal anesthesia and lasting 24 h.

In a comparison of 4% mepivacaine with 0.5% bupivacaine in spinal anesthesia in 100 patients each, 30 had transient radicular irritation with mepivacaine and three with bupivacaine (29[C]). The duration of symptoms was less with bupivacaine (up to 12 h) than mepivacaine (12–120 h). In addition, all patients in the bupivacaine group were satisfied with their treatment, whereas 20% of those in the mepivacaine group were not. Three patients in the mepivacaine group had had previous problems; one after hyperbaric 5% lidocaine and two after 4% mepivacaine. Two patients in the bupivacaine group also described transient hearing deterioration. However, all of these problems were transient and the overall conclusion was that 0.5% bupivacaine can be used safely in patients undergoing minor procedures of relatively short duration, with greater patient satisfaction than with mepivacaine.

In a study of the spinal administration of 0.5% tetracaine with differing concentrations of glucose and with or without phenylephrine in 160 patients undergoing elective lower limb surgery, there was a higher incidence of transient radicular irritation in those given phenylephrine, but no difference between each concentration of glucose (30[C]). The authors therefore postulated that the same mechanism that increases duration of block via reduced vascular uptake and increased exposure of spinal nerves to local anesthetic may also increase neurotoxicity. Vasoconstriction and local ischemia were discussed as possible indirect factors. Hyperesthesia was associated with pain in one patient; this has not previously been reported, and it is possible that it was due to an independent mechanism.

Four other cases of transient radicular irritation after spinal anesthesia with high-concentration lidocaine have been reported; one with plain 2% lidocaine (31[c]), another with hyperbaric 2% lidocaine (32[c]), and two with hyperbaric 5% lidocaine (33[c]). All of these involved procedures in the lithotomy position.

Two cases of *cauda equina syndrome* after intrathecal bupivacaine have been reported (34[c]).

A 63-year-old man received 3.6 ml of hyperbaric 0.5% bupivacaine for spinal anesthesia. This produced inadequate sensory block for the operative procedure, and he was therefore given a general anesthetic. Postoperatively he had signs and symptoms of cauda equina syndrome. Electromyography showed neurological damage to the sacral roots and MRI showed a lumbar spinal stenosis. Two years later there was very little recovery.

A 70-year-old woman undergoing combined spinal-epidural anesthesia for knee arthroplasty received 3.5 ml of bupivacaine 0.5% intrathecally preoperatively and an epidural infusion for 42 h postoperatively. After stopping the epidural infusion, she also had signs and symptoms of cauda equina syndrome. However, MRI failed to show compression.

In the first case the authors thought that the spinal stenosis had caused poor spread of the local anesthetic and therefore poor sensory block and neurotoxicity. In the second case, the possible causes were catheter or needle trauma or contamination of the ampoule or the bupivacaine epidural infusion (if not causing, then certainly masking the symptoms of cauda equina syndrome).

In 603 continuous spinal anesthetics (127 via a 28-gauge microcatheter) the incidence of neurological sequelae has been retrospectively surveyed (35[C]). Three patients reported postoperative *paresthesia* (one in the microcatheter group). Two of these resolved in 4 days; one was discharged 8 days later with residual foot pain. Only one patient had sensory cauda equina syndrome after continuous spinal anesthesia. Microcatheters have previously been held responsible for this problem. However, in this case, a 20-gauge macrocatheter was used with 5% lidocaine, which again suggests that 5% lidocaine should not be used intrathecally.

Intravenous regional anesthesia

A comparison of 0.5% lidocaine, articaine, and prilocaine used for intravenous regional anesthesia in 30 patients showed no signs or symptoms of toxicity, even though lidocaine plasma concentrations peaked at a mean of 8.5 μg/ml (articaine 1.85 μg/ml, prilocaine 4.4 μg/ml) (36[C]).

Ocular anesthesia *(SED-13, 1420; SEDA-19, 129; SEDA-20, 126; SEDA-21, 133)*

Postoperative hypotropia, causing *vertical diplopia*, occurred in 31 of 2143 patients who underwent retrobulbar block with either 50:50 bupivacaine 0.75% and lidocaine 4% or with bupivacaine 0.5% alone (37[C]). This was due to misdirection of the needle and probable injection of the local anesthetic into the inferior rectus muscle. The authors postulated that the muscle was either directly damaged by myotoxicity of the local anesthetic solution or that the volume used caused tissue pressure and subsequent ischemia.

Two other cases of local anesthetic myotoxicity from direct injection of local anesthetic agent into muscle during retrobulbar anesthesia have been reported (38[c]). Both patients developed postoperative *strabismus* from contracture of the extraocular lateral rectus and superior rectus muscles.

A 62-year-old woman who underwent strabismus surgery developed *retrobulbar hemorrhage* after episcleral (sub-Tenon) block with 3 ml of lidocaine 2% (39[c]). This caused raised intraocular pressure (68 mmHg), which was treated with lateral canthotomy. This is probably the first reported case after this usually very safe block, and the authors postulated that this could have been caused by rupture of a sclerotic vessel by the high volume of fluid.

Complete loss of light perception occurred in a 40-year-old man who underwent repair of a dehisced corneal graft, after topical anesthesia (4% lidocaine) and intracameral local anesthesia (1% lidocaine 0.5 ml) (40[c]). His vision returned within hours. The authors speculated about the possibility of local anesthetic toxicity on the retina and optic nerve, but concluded that this was probably total anesthesia of the retinal nerve fiber layer at or near the optic nerve, with resolution when the anesthetic wore off. In this case, the normal barrier of the lens capsule, the zonules, and the vitreous humor had virtually been lost, allowing local anesthetic access to the posterior chamber.

A 29-year-old man suffered *ocular pain*, *reduced visual acuity*, *edema*, *delayed healing*, and *corneal stromal ring infiltrates* after photorefractive keratectomy (41[c]). After a number of pharmacological and surgical therapies, it was found that for 6 months he had intermittently been using proparacaine eyedrops. Discontinuation of this and patching led to resolution of all but the stromal infiltrates, and he was left with permanent visual impairment.

Four other cases of topical local anesthetic abuse have been reported; these presented as a *ring keratitis* resembling a parasitic infectious keratitis (42[c]). All the patients had self-medicated with local anesthetic drops (tetracaine or proparacaine) to treat pain after minor eye irritation or injury. After a protracted course, a diagnosis was finally made and the local anesthetic drops were withdrawn, with improvement. However, three of the four were left with long-term visual impairment. The authors discussed the development of 'dependence': increasing pain occurs as the local anesthetic causes further tissue and nerve damage, thus requiring further analgesia. Theories on the mechanism of the damage range from direct toxicity to immunological causes and preservative toxicity. These cases come as a warning that local anesthetic abuse can cause persistent keratitis.

Local anesthetic toxicity has been shown in a study in which injection of 0.2 ml of one of four local anesthetic solutions (bupivacaine 0.75%, lidocaine 4%, proparacaine 0.5%, and tetracaine 0.5%) into the anterior chamber in rabbits produced *corneal thickening and opacification* via endothelial damage (43). Proparacaine caused the worst reaction, while tetracaine was no more toxic than the saline solution that was used as a placebo. Dilutions of 1:10 also produced mild but statistically insignificant changes, which resolved completely.

Stellate ganglion anesthesia *(SED-13, 292; SEDA-19, 130; SEDA-21, 134)*

High central neural block after stellate ganglion blockade occurred in a 19-year-old patient after injection of 8 ml of bupivacaine 0.25% (44[c]). The patient complained of nausea and 'sensations' in the arm before becoming apneic and losing consciousness. After 2 h of ventilation the patient made a full recovery. Ultrasonography showed a local anesthetic depot at the root of C6, and the authors recommended that ultrasound be used to guide stellate blockade, to look for the development of a local anesthetic depot, and possibly to prevent intravascular injection by direct visualization of the great vessels.

Topical anesthesia *(SEDA-19, 131; SEDA-20, 127; SEDA-21, 135)*

The incidence of perioperative adverse effects was significantly increased after the use of lidocaine gel as a lubricant for insertion of laryngeal mask airway in a comparison of this with saline in 126 patients (45[C]). There was no difference in the incidence of *sore throats*, and the use of lidocaine gel was associated with significantly more intraoperative *hiccups* and postoperative *hoarseness* (four patients), *paresthesia of the tongue* (one patient), *nausea* (three patients), and *vomiting* (one patient). The authors concluded that there is no advantage to the use of lidocaine gel over saline for lubrication of laryngeal mask airways; because of the increase in adverse effects, it is not recommended for this purpose.

EMLA was used for analgesia in 68 healthy neonates undergoing circumcision in a randomized, controlled, double-blind study (46[C]). The pain of the procedure was attenuated by the EMLA, and there was no detectable increase in methemoglobin. However, there was mild localized *pallor*, one neonate developed mild *edema*, and one developed *a local infection* treated with a topical antibiotic.

Respiratory Lidocaine 10% spray used for upper airway anesthesia before fiberoptic intubation caused *acute airway obstruction* in a grossly obese woman with a large goiter (47[c]). Intubation was impossible, but it was possible to ventilate her via a laryngeal mask airway, when she was anesthetized with intravenous propofol. Repeated attempts to waken her resulted in airway obstruction. A definitive airway was eventually provided when percutaneous tracheostomy was performed with difficulty. The authors postulated that this had been due to a combination of laryngospasm and loss of upper airway muscle tone caused by the local anesthetic. An alternative suggested mechanism (48[r]) was inhibition of laryngeal receptors, removing reflexes involved with airway maintenance.

Hematological High-dose EMLA has been responsible for at least two cases of neonatal *methemoglobinemia* (49[c]), (50[c]).

A 2-day-old baby had a 60-min application of EMLA 3.5 g for circumcision. He was cyanotic, with pulse oximetry of 91% and a methemoglobin concentration of 16%. Treatment was with 100% oxygen only.

Symptomatic methemoglobinemia developed when EMLA was used in a 6-week-old baby with a large hemangioma on the buttock and perianal region requiring laser treatment. About 4 h after application, the child was noted to be lethargic and pale, with lip cyanosis. Instead of the recommended 2 g of cream, five tubes of 5 g had been applied, giving a huge dose of 625 mg of lidocaine and 625 mg of prilocaine.

The second case not only highlights the problems of using EMLA in neonates, but also those of patient/parent misunderstanding of instructions and the quality of those instructions.

Skin and appendages Five patients developed localized *purpura* within 1 h of application of EMLA, four of these after only 30 min of exposure to EMLA for removal of molluscum contagiosum (these patients also had contact dermatitis) and one after a lip biopsy (51[c]). Patch tests were negative for EMLA itself, all of the other individual ingredients of EMLA, placebo, and tegaderm. The reduced barrier function of the skin in patients with contact dermatitis, especially around areas of molluscum contagiosum, as well as application to the lip, would be associated with increased absorption of local anesthetic. So, with negative patch testing, this could possibly have been a toxic effect on capillary endothelium after increased absorption.

EMLA caused *blanching or transient local erythema* in seven low-birth-weight infants randomized to receive 1–1.25 g of either EMLA or placebo 1 h before insertion of a percutaneous central venous line. There was no significant difference in methemoglobinemia between the two groups, and there were no problems with local anesthetic toxicity (52[C]).

INDIVIDUAL COMPOUNDS

Benzocaine *(SED-13, 293; SEDA-19, 131; SEDA-21, 135)*

Three cases of benzocaine-induced *methemoglobinemia* requiring treatment with methylene blue have been reported (53[c])–(55[c]).

After the insertion of an orogastric tube a terminally ill patient became cyanotic and tachypneic with methemoglobinemia of up to 40% requiring treatment with methylene blue. A cause was not initially found until, after a second orogastric tube insertion with similar symptoms, it was realised that benzocaine had been used before both episodes.

Another patient with syncope and methemoglobinemia of 46% had taken analgesia for a toothache; this included an entire bottle of a solution containing 6.3% benzocaine.

A third patient who underwent ERCP developed marked cyanosis and pulse oximetry saturation of 75% after being given a 1-s spray of 20% benzocaine to the back of throat. A blood sample was chocolate brown in colour, and the methemoglobin concentration was 40%. After treatment the methemoglobin concentration fell to 0.8% by the following morning.

Bupivacaine *(SED-13, 293; SEDA-19, 131; SEDA-20, 128; SEDA-21, 135)*

The use of bupivacaine as a preincisional intra-articular injection before arthroscopy has been highlighted as causing potential problems with toxicity. There has been at least one fatal result from bupivacaine used in this manner (56[r]).

Cardiovascular A severe *dysrhythmia* occurred in a patient with late-onset isovaleric acidemia (an autosomal recessive disorder of leucine catabolism causing episodes of acidosis during catabolic stress), who underwent liposuction (57[c]).

Under general anesthesia a 16-year-old woman was given subcutaneous bupivacaine 22 mg in 300 ml with 300 μg of adrenaline. She soon developed a junctional bradycardia, then idioventricular rhythm with associated hypotension. This was treated with ephedrine and she then developed ventricular tachycardia requiring lidocaine and adrenaline, with reversion to sinus tachycardia. When she woke her electrocardiogram showed QT prolongation, and echocardiography showed mild left ventricular dysfunction. One week later, her electrocardiogram was normal.

The authors postulated that carnitine deficiency and other aspects of isovaleric acidemia could lower the threshold for bupivacaine-induced dysrhythmias.

2-Chloroprocaine

Formulations of 2-chloroprocaine containing EDTA can cause *severe burning back pain* in epidural anesthesia. In a randomized double-blind study, 30 patients for out-patient knee arthroscopy were divided into two groups to receive either 30 ml of epidural Nesacaine CE 3% (2-chloroprocaine with calcium disodium edetate and sodium bisulfite) or lidocaine 1.33% (58[C]). In the first 24 h, 10 patients given 2-chloroprocaine had pain (mainly mild and in the region of the injection) compared with seven of those given lidocaine. Only one patient described more diffuse pain of mild intensity in the perilumbar region. The author of an accompanying editorial suggested that the mechanism of pain caused by EDTA-containing solutions is chelation of calcium ions by the EDTA (59[R]). Injection into the epidural space of large volumes of solution causes leakage into the paravertebral space, which may result in hypocalcemic tetany of the surrounding muscles. However, the mild localized pain described in the above study is much more likely to have been related to the needle puncture itself.

Cocaine *(SED-13, 294; SEDA-19, 132; SEDA-20, 128; SEDA-21, 135)*

Cardiovascular A fit 29-year-old patient developed *myocardial ischemia* after the topical application of 12.5% cocaine for nasal surgery (60[c]). Angiography showed occlusion of the posterior descending and posterolateral branches of the right coronary artery, which was unrelieved by either intravenous glyceryl trinitrate or intracoronary verapamil. This is consistent with the systemic effects of cocaine, which causes coronary vasoconstriction and platelet activation. In this case there were no other cocaine-induced adrenergic signs and the occlusion was not relieved by vasodilators, suggesting that thrombosis had played a part.

Lidocaine *(SED-13, 292; SEDA-19, 132; SEDA-20, 128; SEDA-21, 136)*

Nervous system A *tonic–clonic seizure* occurred in a 40-year-old patient after the injection of 400 mg of lidocaine 2% jelly into the ureter for manipulation of a ureteric stone. It is probable that rapid absorption of high-dose lidocaine occurred via a previously traumatized mucosa, causing central nervous system toxicity (61[c]).

Prilocaine *(SED-13, 294; SEDA-20, 128)*

There have been two reports of *methemoglobinemia* from the use of prilocaine for penile block for circumcision in neonates. One of the children developed severe symptomatic methemoglobinemia after 15 mg of prilocaine (62[c]). It is probable that there was increased absorption of prilocaine from the very vascular penis, in addition to immature methemoglobin reductase systems and residual fetal hemoglobin in the neonate, increasing the risk of symptomatic methemoglobinemia.

Ropivacaine *(SED-13, 295; SEDA-20, 129)*

The efficacy and pharmacokinetics of a 72-h infusion of epidural ropivacaine have been assessed in 11 patients (63[c]). One patient, with previous liver disease, had an increase in alkaline phosphatase and γ-glutamyltransferase activities; this patient also had the highest plasma concentrations. Two patients developed postoperative hypotension treatable with fluids, nine developed a pyrexia during treatment, seven developed urinary retention requiring catheterization, and three had pulse oximetry readings below 94% on more than two occasions.

Hypotension was the most frequent adverse event found during a randomized comparison of epidural bupivacaine 0.25% with ropivacaine 0.25% as analgesia during labor in 75 patients (64[C]). *Motor block* occurred in 74% of patients in the ropivacaine group, 14% with degree 3 on the modified Bromage scale. There was motor block in 53% of the patients given bupivacaine, but this difference was not statistically significant. There was also a high incidence of augmented and instrumental deliveries in both groups. The authors concluded that the two drugs produced very similar block, with high maternal and fetal tolerance; however, ropivacaine has greater cardiac safety and would be the preferred drug.

Cardiovascular Bupivacaine and ropivacaine infusions have been compared in 12 healthy volunteers in a cross-over study (65[C]). Higher doses of ropivacaine than bupivacaine were tolerated (mean of 115 vs 103 mg) by more subjects (9/12), with a more rapid recovery of symptoms. The maximum tolerated unbound plasma concentration of ropivacaine was double that of bupivacaine (0.6 vs 0.3 mg/l). Cardiovascular effects were more pronounced with bupivacaine than ropivacaine at the maximum tolerated doses. Bupivacaine caused *QRS prolongation* and *reduced left ventricular systolic and diastolic function*, whereas ropivacaine only reduced systolic function.

Nervous system In a crossover study of the pharmacokinetics and effects of intravenous infusions of three doses of ropivacaine in nine subjects, there was one episode of *numbness of the lower lip* after an infusion of 80 mg (the highest dose); this correlated with an extrapolated total plasma concentration of 1.7 mg/l and an unbound plasma concentration of 0.08 mg/l (66[C]).

A previously healthy 66-year-old woman developed *seizures* shortly after the injection of 20 ml of ropivacaine 0.75% (2.3 mg/kg) for an interscalene block (67[c]). This required treatment with thiopental and muscle relaxation with suxamethonium. There were no cardiac manifestations and she made a full recovery with no memory of events but also no indication of a brachial plexus block. Despite negative aspiration, it was felt that ropivacaine had probably been injected intra-arterially, causing direct central nervous system toxicity.

REFERENCES

1. Cuesta-Herranz J, Heras M, Fernandez M, Lluch M, Figueredo E, Umpierrez A, Lahoz C. Allergic reaction caused by local anesthetic agents belonging to the amide group. J Allergy Clin Immunol 1997;99:427–8.
2. Warrington RJ, McPhillips S. Allergic reaction to local anesthetic agents of the amide group. J Allergy Clin Immunol 1997;100:855.
3. Bourezane Y, Adessi B, Didier JM, Vuitton DA, Laurent R. Allergic immediate aux anesthesiques du groupe amide. Gastroenterol Clin Biol 1997;21:344–5.
4. Fisher MM, Bowey CJ. Alleged allergy to local anaesthetics. Anaesth Intensive Care 1997; 25:611.
5. Suhonen R, Kanerva L. Contact allergy and cross-reactions caused by prilocaine. Am J Contact Dermatitis 1997;8:231–5.
6. Yamamoto K, Nomura T, Shibata K, Ohmura S. Failed axillary brachial plexus block techniques result in high plasma concentrations of mepivacaine. Reg Anesth 1997;22:557–61.
7. Daublander M, Muller R, Lipp MD. The incidence of complications associated with local anesthesia in dentistry. Anesth Prog 1997;44:132–41.
8. Goldenberg AS. Transient diplopia as a result of block injections. Mandibular and posterior superior alveolar. NY State Dent J 1997;63:29–31.
9. Tsui SL, Lee DK, Ng KF, Chan TY, Chan

WS, Lo JW. Epidural infusion of bupivacaine 0.0625% plus fentanyl 3.3 μg/ml provides better postoperative analgesia than patient-controlled analgesia with intravenous morphine after gynaecological laparotomy. Anaesth Intensive Care 1997;25:476–81.

10. Kart T, Walther-Larsen S, Svejborg TF, Feilberg V, Eriksen K, Rasmussen M. Comparison of continuous epidural infusion of fentanyl and bupivacaine with intermittent epidural administration of morphine for postoperative pain management in children. Acta Anaesthesiol Scand 1997;41:461–5.

11. Wiebalck A, Brodner G, Van Aken H. The effects of adding sufentanil to bupivacaine for postoperative patient-controlled analgesia. Anesth Analg 1997;85:124–9.

12. Rygnestad T, Borchgrevink PC, Eide E. Postoperative epidural infusion of morphine and bupivacaine is safe on surgical wards. Organisation of the treatment, effects and side-effects in 2000 consecutive patients. Acta Anaesthesiol Scand 1997;41:868–76.

13. Kahn L. Neuropathies masquerading as an epidural complication. Can J Anaesth 1997; 44:313–16.

14. Dunwoody JM, Reichert CC, Brown KL. Compartment syndrome associated with bupivacaine and fentanyl epidural analgesia in pediatric orthopaedics. J Pediatr Orthop 1997;17:285–8.

15. Cohen S, Amar D. Epidural block for obstetrics: comparison of bolus injection of local anesthetic with gravity flow technique. J Clin Anesth 1997;9:623–38.

16. Dickson MA, Moores C, McClure JH. Comparison of single, end-holed and multi-orifice extradural catheters when used for continuous infusion of local anaesthetic during labour. Br J Anaesth 1997;79:297–300.

17. Jerez A, Molina JA, Benito-Leon J. Epidural anesthesia. Neurology 1997;48:294–5.

18. Dreskin S, Bajwa ZH, Lehmann L, Warfield CA. Polymyoclonus resulting from possible accidental subsural injection of local anesthetic. Anesth Analg 1997;84:692–3.

19. Clarke JP, Buchanan CCR. Pain associated with 2% lignocaine epidural anaesthesia. Anaesth Intensive Care 1997;25:435–6.

20. Olofsson CI, Ekblom AO, Ekman-Ordeberg GE, Irestedt LE. Post-partum urinary retention: a comparison between two methods of epidural analgesia. Eur J Obstet Gynecol Reprod Biol 1997;71:31–4.

21. Wu JL, Hsu MS, Hsu TC, Chen LH, Yang WJ, Tsai YC. The efficacy of intrathecal coadministration of morphine and bupivacaine for labor analgesia. Acta Anaesthesiol Sin 1997; 35:209–16.

22. Lu JK, Manullang TR, Staples MH, Kem SE, Balley PL. Maternal respiratory arrests, severe hypotension, and fetal distress after administration of intrathecal, sufentanil, and bupivacaine after intravenous fentanyl. Anesthesiology 1997; 87:170–2.

23. D'Angelo R, Eisenach JC. Severe maternal hypotension and fetal bradycardia after a combined spinal epidural anesthetic. Anesthesiology 1997;87:166–8.

24. Brooker RF, Butterworth JF, Kitzman DW, Berman JM, Kashtan HI, McKinley A. Treatment of hypotension after hyperbaric tetracaine spinal anesthesia. A randomised, double-blind, cross-over comparison of phenylephrine and epinephrine. Anesthesiology 1997;86:797–805.

25. Holst D, Mollmann M, Karmann S, Wendt M. Kreislaufverhalten unter Spinalanästhesie. Kathetertechnik versus Single-dose-Verfahren. Anesthetist 1997;46:38–42.

26. Cornish PB. Respiratory arrest after spinal anesthesia with lidocaine and fentanyl. Anesth Analg 1997;84:1387–8.

27. Lee MS, Lyoo CH, Kim WC, Kang HJ. Periodic bursts of rhythmic dyskinesia associated with spinal anesthesia. Mov Disord 1997;12:816–17.

28. Lynch J, Zur Nieden M, Kasper S, Radbruch L. Transient radicular irritation after spinal anesthesia with hyperbaric 4% mepivacaine. Anesth Analg 1997;85:872–3.

29. Hiller A, Rosenberg P. Transient neurological symptoms after spinal anaesthesia with 4% mepivacaine and 0.5% bupivacaine. Br J Anaesth 1997;79:301–5.

30. Sakura S, Sumi M, Sakaguchi Y, Saito Y, Kosaka Y, Drasner K. The addition of phenylephrine contributes to the development of transient neurologic symptoms after spinal anesthesia with 0.5% tetracaine. Anesthesiology 1997; 87:771–8.

31. Ramasamy D, Eadie R. Transient radicular irritation after spinal anaesthesia with 2% isobaric lignocaine. Br J Anaesth 1997;79:394–5.

32. Grange C, Bright S, Douglas J. Radicular irritation with 2% lignocaine spinal. Anaesth Intensive Care 1997;25:89–90.

33. Newman L, Iyer N, Tuman K. Transient radicular irritation after hyperbaric lidocaine spinal anesthesia in parturients. Int J Obstet Anesth 1997;6:132–4.

34. Kubina P, Gupta A, Oscarsson A, Axelsson K, Bengtsson M. Two cases of cauda equina syndrome following spinal-epidural anesthesia. Reg Anesth 1997;22:447–50.

35. Horlocker T, McGregor D, Matsushige D, Chantigian R, Schroeder D, Besse J. Neurologic complications of 603 consecutive continuous spinal anesthetics using macrocatheter and microcatheter techniques. Anesth Analg 1997;84:1063–70.

36. Simon MA, Gieen MJ, Alberink N, Vree TB, Van Egmond J. Intravenous regional anesthesia with 0.5% articaine, 0.5% lidocaine or 0.5% prilocaine. A double-blind randomised clinical study. Reg Anesth 1997;22:29–34.

37. Corboy J, Jiang X. Postanesthetic hypotropia: a unique syndrome in left eyes. J Cataract Refract Surg 1997;23:1394–8.

38. Ando K, Oohira A, Takao M. Restrictive stra-

bismus after retrobulbar anesthesia. Jpn J Ophthalmol 1997;41:23–6.
39. Olitsky SE, Juneja RG. Orbital hemorrhage after the administration of sub-Tenon's infusion anesthesia. Ophthalmic Surg Lasers 1997;28:145–6.
40. Hoffman RS, Fine IH. Transient no light perception visual acuity after intracameral lidocaine injection. J Cataract Refract Surg 1997;23:957–8.
41. Kim JY, Choi YS, Lee JH. Keratitis from corneal anesthetic abuse after photorefractive keratectomy. J Cataract Refract Surg 1997; 23:447–9.
42. Varga JH, Rubinfeld RS, Wolf TC, Stutzman RD, Peele KA, Kimberly MAJ, Clifford WS, Madigan W. Topical anesthetic abuse ring keratitis: report of four cases. Cornea 1997;16:424–9.
43. Judge AJ, Najafi K, Lee DA, Miller KM. Corneal endothelial toxicity of topical anesthesia. Ophthalmology 1997;104:1373–9.
44. Kapral S, Krafft P, Gosch M, Fridrich P, Weinstabl C. Subdurale, extraarachnoidale Blockade als Komplikation des Ganglion-Stellatum-Blocks: Dokumentation mittels Sonographie. Anaesthesiol Intensivmed Notfallmed Schmerzther 1997;32:638–40.
45. Keller C, Sparr HJ, Brimacombe JR. Laryngeal mask lubrication. A comparative study of saline versus 2% lignocaine gel with pressure cuff control. Anaesthesia 1997;52:592–6.
46. Taddio A, Stevens B, Craig K, Rastogi P, Ben-David S, Shennan A, Mulligan P, Koren G. Efficacy and safety of lidocaine-prilocaine cream for pain during circumcision. New Engl J Med 1997;336:1197–201.
47. Shaw IC, Welchew EA, Harrison BJ, Michael S. Complete airway obstruction during awake fibreoptic intubation. Anaesthesia 1997;52:582–5.
48. Moscuzza E. Complete airway obstruction during awake fibreoptic intubation. Anaesthesia 1997;52:1024–5.
49. Kumar AR, Dunn N, Naqvi M. Methemoglobinemia associated with a prilocaine-lidocaine cream. Clin Pediatr Phil 1997;36:239–40.
50. Elsner P, Dummer R. Signs of methaemoglobinaemia after topical application of EMLA cream in an infant with haemangioma. Dermatology 1997;195:153–4.
51. De Waard Van Der Spek FB, Oranje AP. Purpura caused by EMLA is of toxic origin. Contact Dermatitis 1997;36:11–13.
52. Garcia OC, Reichberg S, Brion LP, Schulman M. Topical anesthesia for line insertion in very low birthweight infants. J Perinatol 1997;17:477–80.
53. Cooper HA. Methemoglobinemia caused by benzocaine topical spray. South Med J 1997; 90:946–8.
54. Gilman CS, Veser FH, Randall D. Methemoglobinemia from a topical oral anesthetic. Acad Emerg Med 1997;4:1011–13.
55. Guerriero SE. Methemoglobinemia caused by topical benzocaine. Pharmacotherapy 1997; 17:1038–40.
56. Abbott PJ, Sullivan G. Cardiovascular toxicity following preincisional intra-articular injection of bupivacaine. Arthroscopy 1997;13:282.
57. Weinberg GL, Laurito CE, Geldner P, Pygon BH, Burton BK. Malignant ventricular dysrhythmias in a patient with isovaleric acidemia receiving general and local anesthesia for suction lipectomy. J Clin Anesth 1997;9:668–70.
58. Drolet P, Veillette Y. Back pain following epidural anesthesia with 2-chloroprocaine (EDTA-free) or lidocaine. Reg Anesth. 1997; 22:303–7.
59. Stevens RA. Back pain following epidural anesthesia with 2-chloroprocaine. Reg Anesth 1997;22:299–302.
60. Williams M, Stewart R. Serial angiography in cocaine-induced myocardial infarction. Chest 1997;111:822–4.
61. Pantuck AJ, Goldsmith JW, Kuriyan JB, Weiss RE. Seizures after ureteral stone manipulation with lidocaine. J Urol 1997;157:2248.
62. Prineas S, Wilkins BH, Halliday RJ. Circumcision blues. Med J Aust 1997;166:615.
63. Scott DA, Emanuelsson BM, Mooney PH, Cook RJ, Junestrand C. Pharmacokinetics and efficacy of long-term epidural ropivacaine infusion for postoperative analgesia. Anesth Analg 1997;85:1322–30.
64. Gaiser RR, Venkateswaren P, Cheek TG, Persiley E, Buxbaum J, Hedge J. Comparison of 0.25% ropivacaine and bupivacaine for epidural analgesia for labor and vaginal delivery. J Clin Anesth 1997;9:564–8.
65. Knudsen K, Beckman-Suurkula S, Blomberg S, Sjovall J, Edvardsson N. Central nervous and cardiovascular effects of iv infusions of ropivacaine, bupivacaine and placebo in volunteers. Br J Anaesth 1997;78:507–14.
66. Emanuelsson BM, Persson J, Sandin S, Alm C, Gustafsson LL. Intraindividual and interindividual variability in the disposition of the local anesthetic ropivacaine in healthy subjects. Ther Drug Monit 1997;19.126–31.
67. Korman B, Riley RH. Convulsions induced by ropivacaine during interscalene brachial plexus block. Anesth Analg 1997;85:1128–9.

O. Zuzan and M. Leuwer

12 Neuromuscular blocking agents and skeletal muscle relaxants

GENERAL TOPICS

Nervous system Many reports of *persistent paralysis* after long-term administration of neuromuscular blocking agents to critically ill patients in intensive care units have been published. As most of these reports have featured the steroidal agents vecuronium and pancuronium, some authors have recommended the use of benzylisoquinolone relaxants instead of steroidal relaxants for long-term administration. However, several cases of *persistent paralysis* after long-term administration of atracurium have been reported during the last few years. Cisatracurium, one of the stereoisomers of atracurium, might have some advantages in intensive care patients, as it is associated with less release of laudanosine than atracurium (1[C]). However, recently, persistent paralysis has also been observed after long-term administration of cisatracurium (2[c]).

A 45-year-old woman developed aspiration pneumonitis and acute respiratory distress after bilateral total knee replacement. In order to facilitate inverse ratio ventilation, a cisatracurium infusion was started and continued for 13 days. Throughout the period of relaxant administration, one to four responses to train-of-four stimulation of a peripheral nerve were detected. Methylprednisolone was given over several days to attenuate the fibroproliferative sequelae of adult respiratory distress syndrome. After withdrawal of the relaxant she could not move nor be weaned from the ventilator. After 11 days she could move her fingertips and another 6 days later was weaned from ventilation. Extensive rehabilitation measures were required for several months.

Several authors have suggested that neuromuscular transmission monitoring, by helping to avoid overdosing of neuromuscular blocking agents, might prevent persistent paralysis. However, this case illustrates that neuromuscular disturbances can occur in spite of such monitoring. Indeed, prolonged neuromuscular blockade due to accumulation of cisatracurium was probably avoided, as suggested by the results of train-of-four stimulation. This alone should be reason enough to use neuromuscular transmission monitoring routinely during long-term administration of muscle relaxants. However, myopathic changes or changes at the neuromuscular junction not caused by muscle relaxants will not be reliably detected by such monitoring.

One important risk factor for persistent paralysis in this case was the combination of high-dosage glucocorticoid therapy and long-term administration of a muscle relaxant. Glucocorticoids have been linked to acute quadriplegic myopathy and severe muscle weakness in patients who were also receiving neuromuscular blocking agents (SEDA-19, 141; (3[c]), (4[c]), (5[C]), (6[C]), but it is not known how these factors combine to produce persistent paralysis (7[cr]). Electromyographic testing would have helped to classify the neuromuscular disturbances in this case. As the authors conceded, other reasons for failure to wean and muscle weakness, such as critical illness polyneuropathy, should also be taken into account. An exact diagnosis cannot be made by clinical assessment alone.

Musculoskeletal system Several authors have described *heterotopic ossification* or *myositis ossificans* after long-term administration of neuromuscular blocking agents to patients in

Side Effects of Drugs, Annual 22
J.K. Aronson, ed.

intensive care units (SEDA-20, 136; SEDA-19, 141; (8[c])–(10[c]). However, recently, the causative role of muscle relaxants has been questioned (11[c]), in the light of the observation that heterotopic ossification occurred in critically ill patients not treated with such agents (12[c]). It was suggested that prolonged immobilization is important in the pathogenesis of heterotopic ossification and that both deep sedation and neuromuscular blockade, by producing complete immobilization, might contribute to the pathophysiology of this severe complication in critical illness.

Immunological and hypersensitivity reactions Current knowledge about the pathogenesis of *allergic reactions* to muscle relaxants has been reviewed (13[R]). The key statements are:

(1) allergic reactions result in a massive release of cell mediators, such as histamine, tryptase, serotonin, kinins, prostaglandins, and leukotrienes;
(2) this release is usually triggered by the bridging of IgE receptor complexes with allergens;
(3) activation of mast cells and basophil leukocytes can occur independent of the binding of drugs to IgE (in these cases, histamine release is probably dose-dependent);
(4) tertiary and quaternary ammonium ions are important elements at the allergenic site of muscle relaxants, which may explain cross-reactivity among muscle relaxants;
(5) there is no correlation between plasma concentrations of histamine, tryptase, or serotonin and the severity of anaphylaxis;
(6) plasma tryptase concentration is a sensitive and relatively specific marker of anaphylaxis.

Laudanosine toxicity One of the breakdown products of atracurium is laudanosine. When atracurium is given over long periods there is a possibility of laudanosine accumulation. In animals, high plasma concentrations of laudanosine provoke seizure activity, hypotension, and bradycardia (14). So far, no toxic effects of laudanosine have been reported in humans. Higher concentrations of laudanosine can occur in patients with severely impaired renal function (SED-13, 324). A recent example has illustrated the effect of atracurium infusion for several weeks on laudanosine plasma concentrations and EEG activity (15[c]).

A 23-year-old woman had a sickle cell crisis, and developed hepatic and renal insufficiency and progressive respiratory distress requiring endotracheal intubation and ventilatory support, for which she was given atracurium 0.3–0.96 mg/kg per h for 38 days. The speed of infusion was adjusted according to her response to stimuli such as suctioning. The laudanosine plasma concentration was 3.7 μg/ml before withdrawal of atracurium and had fallen to 0.8 μg/ml 24 h later. The elimination half-life of laudanosine was 10.3 h. An EEG recorded 3 days before withdrawal was interpreted as normal without epileptiform activity. Several days later she died from respiratory failure.

As in previous reports, plasma laudanosine concentrations were high during long-term infusion in a critically ill patient without evidence of cerebral adverse effects. The highest reported laudanosine plasma concentration in an intensive care patient was 8.7 μg/ml. However, a lack of adverse effects of long-term infusion of atracurium does not justify the conclusion that this may be regarded as a safe technique. First, there is a risk of persistent paralysis after long-term infusion of any neuromuscular blocking agent. Secondly, there is no information available on other than cerebral adverse effects of laudanosine accumulation. Furthermore, it may be difficult to diagnose laudanosine adverse effects accurately in patients in intensive care units, because they have depressed consciousness and hemodynamic fluctuations produced by the underlying disease.

DEPOLARIZING NEUROMUSCULAR BLOCKING AGENTS *(SED-13, 301; SEDA-19, 136; SEDA-20, 137; SEDA-21, 141)*

Succinylcholine

Cardiovascular Not every cardiac arrest after succinylcholine is due to hyperkalemia. A case of massive *pulmonary embolism* coincident with the administration of succinylcholine has been reported (16[c]).

A 71-year-old woman had intense fasciculations after being given ketamine 70 mg plus succinylcholine 100 mg. After intubation, manual ventilation required a peak airway pressure of more than 40 cmH_2O and there was bilateral wheezing. Within 1–2 min after induction, her systolic blood pressure fell from 190 to 40 mmHg and her end-tidal carbon dioxide to 12 mmHg. Adrenaline and a short period of chest compression returned the blood pressure to baseline, but it fell again 10 min later. Prolonged resuscitative efforts were unsuccessful. Postmortem examination showed occlusive pulmonary emboli in the right and left main pulmonary arteries and an occlusive thrombus in the left popliteal vein.

Intraoperative massive pulmonary embolism is rare. Here it occurred shortly after the administration of succinylcholine, which led the authors to speculate on a causative role. Referring to the fact that some cases have occurred after manipulations of the lower limbs, they thought that succinylcholine-induced fasciculations might have resulted in the propagation of a deep vein thrombus. Such a mechanism cannot be definitely excluded, but this premature speculation should not prompt us to regard massive pulmonary embolism as an adverse effect of succinylcholine. Other factors that might have facilitated the dislocation of a deep vein thrombus during induction of anesthesia should be considered, for example drastic changes in intrathoracic pressure associated with bronchospasm after intubation.

Mineral and fluid balance *Hyperkalemia* is a life-threatening complication of succinylcholine administration. One major risk factor is the presence of large masses of denervated muscle, such as in patients with paraplegia. Even functional denervation associated with prolonged immobility can produce alterations at the neuromuscular junction, resulting in hyperkalemic cardiac arrest if succinylcholine is given, but it is not known how long the patient must be immobilized to be regarded as being at risk. In a recent case, fatal hyperkalemia occurred after succinylcholine had been given to a previously healthy young woman after 5 days of immobilization (17[c]).

A 23-year-old woman with bacterial meningitis required intubation for respiratory failure due to aspiration of gastric contents 4 days after diagnosis. A few seconds after the administration of succinylcholine she developed a wide-complex bradycardia and cardiac arrest which was not reversed by adrenaline and calcium chloride. After 60 min resuscitative efforts were stopped. A blood sample taken 10 min after cardiac arrest contained potassium in a concentration of 8.4 mmol/l. There were no risk factors for hyperkalemia other than immobilization.

This is the shortest period of immobilization that has been reported to increase the risk of succinylcholine-induced hyperkalemia. While undetected muscle disease cannot be ruled out, the danger of succinylcholine-induced hyperkalemia militates against the use of succinylcholine in patients immobilized for more than a few days. This is especially true in critically ill patients treated in intensive care units. Further examples of hyperkalemic cardiac arrest in patients in intensive care units have appeared (18[c]), (19[c]).

Among other risk factors for succinylcholine-induced hyperkalemia are spinal cord lesions. It is generally agreed that succinylcholine can be given during the first few days after an injury without risking hyperkalemic complications. It is not known, however, whether the pathophysiological changes on the muscle cell surface resolve sufficiently with time to allow the safe administration of succinylcholine after the period of risk has passed. A recent review on anesthesia in patients with spinal cord lesions has caused some controversy (20[R]). The authors stated that succinylcholine could be used safely if the onset of the condition dated back more than 9 months. Furthermore, referring to their observation that all patients with spinal cord lesions who had succinylcholine-induced hyperkalemic cardiac arrest had been resuscitated successfully, they regarded the use of succinylcholine as justified if there was a strong indication. Unfortunately, they failed to list examples of such indications. Indeed, one wonders if there is such an indication in the face of an increased risk of cardiac arrest. In response, it was suggested that succinylcholine should be regarded inappropriate in patients with upper motor neurone lesions, such as spinal cord injuries, if the onset of the lesion dated back more than a few days (21[r]).

Special senses Succinylcholine can cause *increased intraocular pressure*, the clinical impact of which has been the subject of debate for decades (SEDA-21, 145). In the case of penetrating eye injuries the prevention of factors that increase intraocular pressure is an important element of anesthetic management. Several drugs, including non-depolarizing muscle relaxants, have been suggested for pretreatment before injecting succinylcholine, but no single drug has hitherto completely blocked the rise in intraocular pressure. Recently, the effect of mivacurium pretreatment has been studied in 40 patients randomized to either mivacurium 0.02 mg/kg or saline 3 min before a rapid sequence induction of anesthesia with propofol 2 mg/kg, alfentanil 20 μg/kg, and succinylcholine 1.5 mg/kg (22[C]). The mean increase in intraocular pressure was 0.4 mmHg after mivacurium compared with 3.5 mmHg after saline. There was no information on the intraocular pressure response in individual patients, but the mean increase of 0.4 mmHg, although small, suggests that some patients given mivacurium may have had a considerable increase in intraocular pressure after succinylcholine.

In a previous study (23[C]) the intraocular pressure response to succinylcholine and endotracheal intubation was completely blocked without non-depolarizer pretreatment when propofol 2 mg/kg plus alfentanil 40 μg/kg was used for rapid sequence induction of anesthesia, the only apparent difference to the above study being the higher dose of alfentanil. Therefore, a deep level of anesthesia and the suppression of sympathoadrenal responses seem to be prerequisite for avoiding increases in intraocular pressure during induction of anesthesia in patients with penetrating eye injuries. Pretreatment with a small dose of a non-depolarizing muscle relaxant might have an additional beneficial effect.

Musculoskeletal system *Masseter muscle rigidity* due to succinylcholine can prevent successful airway management. While severe rigidity is comparatively rare, smaller increases in jaw tension often occur. Three different techniques of induction of anesthesia have been compared (24[C]) in 60 patients randomized to thiopental 5 mg/kg, thiopental 5 mg/kg plus atracurium 0.05 mg/kg, or propofol 2.5 mg/kg for induction of anesthesia, followed in each case by succinylcholine 1.5 mg/kg. Jaw tension was recorded using a force transducer between the upper and lower incisors. After succinylcholine the mean increase in jaw tension was significantly less with thiopental/atracurium (6.4 N) and propofol group (5.0 N) than with thiopental (12.4 N). The authors concluded that the increase in masseter muscle tone after succinylcholine was affected by the choice of induction agent and that pretreatment with atracurium attenuated the increase.

NON-DEPOLARIZING NEUROMUSCULAR BLOCKING AGENTS *(SED-13, 310; SEDA-19, 140; SEDA-20, 138; SEDA-21, 144)*

Cardiovascular The antinicotinic and antimuscarinic actions of non-depolarizing muscle relaxants and associated adverse effects, such as *hypotension* and *tachycardia*, have been reviewed (25[R]).

Rocuronium

There have been several reports of *pain during injection* of rocuronium (26[c]), (27[c]). Eight of 10 patients complained of severe pain, one complained of moderate pain, and another reported an unpleasant sensation (26[c]). This suggests that rocuronium will almost invariably cause pain. The mechanism of this phenomenon is not clear, but there appear to be some similarities to propofol injection pain. Several authors have suggested that rocuronium should not be given to conscious patients (26[c]), (27[c]). On the other hand, small doses of rocuronium have been used, with some success, to prevent fasciculations and myalgia after succinylcholine (28[C])–(31[C]).

SKELETAL MUSCLE RELAXANTS *(SED-13, 328; SEDA-17, 143; SEDA-20, 133; SEDA-21, 140)*

Baclofen *(SED-13, 328; SEDA-17, 156; SEDA-19, 144; SEDA-20, 140)*

Sexual function In a systematic study of the effects of intrathecal baclofen on sexual function, nine men on continuous treatment via an implantable pump for severe and disabling spasticity were interviewed by questionnaire (32[C]). There was no effect on libido or the ability to obtain psychogenic or reflexive erections. Eight reported *a reduction in erection rigidity and duration*. When ejaculation was possible before the start of baclofen treatment it disappeared or was more difficult to obtain during treatment. These effects resolved after withdrawal of baclofen.

Risk factors Baclofen is 70% excreted unchanged in the urine (33[R]), and a review of 16 individual patients, most of whom were on hemodialysis, has highlighted the problem of the adverse effects of baclofen in patients with *severe renal insufficiency* (34[C]). These patients typically presented with altered consciousness after very small doses of baclofen. Seizures and respiratory depression were rare, but abdominal pain was common. Patients who received hemodialysis shortly after baclofen improved thereafter and had a shorter recovery time than a patient who received only supportive care.

Overdosage While major adverse effects are rare with proper administration, overdosage of baclofen results in *progressively impaired consciousness and coma* (SEDA-20, 140). Unfortunately, it is used illicitly as a so-called 'date-rape' drug. The first report of mass exposure to baclofen in adolescents seeking intoxication has recently been published (35[c]). A group of adolescents became symptomatic after ingesting 3–30 tablets of baclofen 20 mg during a party. Because several children were very lethargic, their chaperones suspected drug abuse. A poisons control center identified the white tablets found at the party as baclofen. Of 14 patients who were taken to hospital, nine required endotracheal intubation and ventilatory support. The most common findings within 1–2 h after ingestion were *coma*, *hypothermia*, *bradycardia*, *hypertension*, and *hyporeflexia*. Three had *unifocal premature ventricular contractions* and two had *tonic–clonic seizures*. The mean duration of mechanical ventilation was 40 h. Serial serum baclofen concentrations ranged from 0.049 to 6.0 μg/ml in intubated patients, target concentrations being 0.08–0.4 μg/ml. Concentrations 14 h after ingestion correlated with the duration of mechanical ventilation. All the patients recovered and were discharged home within 5 days.

The authors recommended that baclofen overdosage be treated with a single dose of activated charcoal, atropine for symptomatic bradycardia, nitroprusside for hypertension, and meticulous supportive care. None of the patients required physostigmine.

Chlorzoxazone *(SED-13, 331; SEDA-21, 148)*

Two episodes of chlorzoxazone overdosage have been described in the same patient (36[c]).

A 57-year-old man became *somnolent*, with *slurred speech* after he had taken oral chlorzoxazone 3.5 mg. He had a history of chronic alcohol abuse, chronic back pain, seizures, depression, and chronic obstructive pulmonary disease. He rapidly became comatose and required endotracheal intubation and ventilatory support for 24 h. A month later he was again found unconscious. On this occasion, however, intubation was averted and his symptoms were reversed by intravenous flumazenil up to a total of 0.35 mg.

This experience led the authors to think that chlorzoxazone, although not classified as a benzodiazepine, might interact with benzodiazepine receptors, making flumazenil potentially useful in cases of chlorzoxazone overdose.

Tizanidine *(SED-13, 149; SEDA-21, 149)*

The central α_2-adrenoceptor agonist tizanidine, an imidazole derivative, has similar effects to baclofen. Its pharmacology, efficacy, and tolerability in the management of spasticity have been reviewed, with emphasis on its favorable tolerability profile (37[R]). Its adverse effects are *drowsiness*, *dry mouth*, *mild muscle weakness*, and rarely *liver damage* (SEDA-21, 149).

Botulinum toxin *(SED-13, 330; SEDA-17, 156; SEDA-19, 144; SEDA-20, 141; SEDA-21, 147)*

Nervous system Botulinum toxin 50 μl (50 IE/ml) either intrafascicularly, extrafascicularly, or extraneurally, has been compared with 10% phenol 50 μl in rats (38). Nerves injected intraneurally with phenol were badly damaged, whereas nerves treated with botulinum toxin retained their normal architecture without cellular infiltration or demyelination.

During recent years some cases of ipsilateral *brachial plexus neuropathy* have been reported after the use of botulinum toxin to treat cervical or arm dystonia (39[c]), (40[c]). Contralateral brachial plexus neuropathy has been reported after botulinum toxin treatment of rotational torticollis and laterocollis (41[c]).

Ten days after injection of botulinum toxin into the right splenius capitis (90 units), the right levator scapulae (40 units), and the right sternomastoid (30 units), a 55-year-old man became unable to lift the left arm for several days. There were signs of denervation electromyographically. Within 7 months full strength had returned and the patient received four subsequent injections of botulinum toxin without recurrence of left arm weakness.

There is some evidence that brachial plexus neuropathy may be immune mediated, and is associated with mononuclear inflammatory T lymphocyte infiltrates surrounding epineural and endoneural vessels (42[c]). As this patient did not have recurrence of brachial plexus neuropathy, despite four subsequent exposures to botulinum toxin, a causal relation remains unclear. Hitherto, five patients with brachial plexus neuropathy after botulinum toxin have been reported. The estimated incidence is 1.64/100 000 person-years (43[C]). Coincidence is a possible explanation in these cases.

Infections *Necrotizing fasciitis* has been reported after treatment with botulinum toxin (44[c]).

An 80-year-old woman with blepharospasm and chronic myeloid leukemia developed necrotizing fasciitis around her right eye 3 days after subcutaneous injection of botulinum toxin. Both eyes had been treated at the same time, but only one was affected. A hemolytic streptococcus was found in specimens taken at the time of emergency debridement. Despite proper antibiotic therapy and additional extensive debridement the course was complicated, and finally a rectus abdominis flap and split skin graft were required.

In this case there was no evidence to suggest that the fasciitis had been caused by anything other than contamination from the patient's own skin, and the streptococci may have been introduced directly into the muscle. Thus, a specific contribution of botulinum toxin remains doubtful.

Interactions Botulinum toxin inhibits acetylcholine release, and can interfere with *neuromuscular blocking agents*. An example has been described (45[c]).

A 68-year-old man underwent general anesthesia twice during treatment with botulinum toxin for blepharospasm. Neuromuscular block produced by vecuronium 0.05 mg/kg was monitored electromyographically at the abductor digiti minimi, using 2-Hz train-of-four stimulation every 20 s. Compared with that seen in 24 individuals without neuromuscular disease his sensitivity to vecuronium was low 90 days after the seventh treatment with botulinum toxin and normal 8 days after the ninth treatment.

Anticipating increased sensitivity, the authors had originally given a reduced dose of vecuronium. To explain the surprising results they suggested that repeat treatment with botulinum toxin could have caused remodelling of neuromuscular synapses. They speculated that each dose of botulinum toxin may have two effects: first, a direct increase in sensitivity to neuromuscular blocking agents; secondly, compensatory remodelling resulting in reduced sensitivity. Even if this hypothesis is tentatively accepted, the effects of neuromuscular blocking agents on neuromuscular transmission in patients receiving botulinum toxin cannot be predicted.

REFERENCES

1. Boyd AH, Eastwood NB, Parker CJ, Hunter JM. Comparison of the pharmacodynamics and pharmacokinetics of an infusion of cis-atracurium (51W89) or atracurium in critically ill patients undergoing mechanical ventilation in an intensive therapy unit. Br J Anaesth 1996;76:382–8.
2. Davis NA, Rodgers JE, Gonzalez ER, Fowler AA. Prolonged weakness after cisatracurium infusion: a case report. Crit Care Med 1998; 26:1290–2.
3. Barohn RJ, Jackson CE, Rogers SJ, Ridings LW, McVey AL. Prolonged paralysis due to nondepolarizing neuromuscular blocking agents and corticosteroids. Muscle Nerve 1994;17:647–54.
4. Hirano M, Ott BR, Raps EC, Minetti C, Lennihan L, Libbey NP, Bonilla E, Hays AP. Acute quadriplegic myopathy: a complication of treatment with steroids, nondepolarizing blocking agents, or both. Neurology 1992;42:2082–7.
5. Leatherman JW, Fluegel WL, David WS, Davies SF, Iber C. Muscle weakness in mechanically ventilated patients with severe asthma. Am J Respir Crit Care Med 1996;153:1686–90.
6. Subramony SH, Carpenter DE, Raju S, Pride M, Evans OB. Myopathy and prolonged neuromuscular blockade after lung transplant. Crit Care Med 1991;19:1580–2.
7. Ruff RL. Why do ICU patients become paralyzed? Ann Neurol 1998;43:154–5.
8. Ackman JB, Rosenthal DI. Generalized periarticular myositis ossificans as a complication of pharmacologically induced paralysis. Skelet Radiol 1995;24:395–7.
9. Goodman TA, Merkel PA, Perlmutter G, Kelleher Doyle M, Krane SM, Polisson RP. Heterotopic ossification in the setting of neuromuscular blockade. Arthritis Rheum 1997;40:1619–27.
10. Ray TD, Lowe WD, Anderson LD, Muller AL, Brogdon BG. Periarticular heterotopic ossification following pharmacologically induced paralysis. Skelet Radiol 1995;24:609–12.
11. Dellestable F, Gaucher A, Voltz C. Heterotopic ossification in critically ill patients: comment on the article by Goodman et al. Arthritis Rheum 1998;41:1329–30.
12. Dellestable F, Voltz C, Mariot J, Perrier JF, Gaucher A. Heterotopic ossification complicating long-term sedation. Br J Rheumatol 1996;35:700–1.
13. Aimone-Gastin I, Gueant JL, Laxenaire MC, Moneret-Vautrin DA. Pathogenesis of allergic reactions to anaesthetic drugs. Int J Immunopathol Pharmacol 1997;10:193–6.
14. Chapple DJ, Miller AA, Ward JB, Wheatley PL. Cardiovascular and neurological effect of laudanosine. Br J Anaesth 1987;59:218–25.
15. Grigore AM, Brusco L, Kuroda M, Koorn R. Laudanosine and atracurium concentrations in a patient receiving long-term atracurium infusion. Crit Care Med 1998;26:180–3.
16. Greilich PE, Randle DW, Froelich EG, Yee LL. Massive intraoperative pulmonary embolism coincident with the administration of succinylcholine. Anesth Analg 1998;87:491–3.
17. Hansen D. Suxamethonium-induced cardiac arrest and death following 5 days of immobilization. Eur J Anaesthesiol 1998;15:240–1.
18. Berkahn JM, Sleigh JW. Hyperkalaemic cardiac arrest following succinylcholine in a longterm intensive care patient. Anaesth Intensive Care 1997;25:588–9.
19. Lee YM, Fountain SW. Suxamethonium and cardiac arrest. Singapore Med J 1997;38:300–1.
20. Hambly PR, Martin B. Anaesthesia for chronic spinal cord lesions. Anaesthesia 1998; 53:273–89.
21. Gronert GA. Use of suxamethonium in cord patients—whether and when. Anaesthesia 1998; 53:1035–6.
22. Chiu CL, Lang CC, Wong PK, Delilkan AE, Wang CY. The effect of mivacurium pretreatment on intra-ocular pressure changes induced by suxamethonium. Anaesthesia 1998;53:501–5.
23. Zimmerman AA, Funk KJ, Tidwell JL. Propofol and alfentanil prevent the increase in intraocular pressure caused by succinylcholine and endotracheal intubation during a rapid sequence induction of anesthesia. Anesth Analg 1996; 83:814–17.
24. Ummenhofer WC, Kindler C, Tschaler G, Hampl KF, Drewe J, Urwyler A. Propofol reduces succinylcholine induced increase of masseter muscle tone. Can J Anaesth 1998;45:417–23.
25. Vizi ES, Lendvai B. Side effects of nondepolarizing muscle relaxants: relationship to their antinicotinic and antimuscarinic actions. Pharmacol Ther 1997;73:75–89.
26. Borgeat A, Kwiatkowski D. Spontaneous movements associated with rocuronium: is pain on injection the cause? Br J Anaesth 1997;79:382–3.
27. Steegers M, Robertson E. Pain on injection of rocuronium bromide. Anesth Analg 1996;83:203.
28. Demers-Pelletier J, Drolet P, Girard M, Donati F. Comparison of rocuronium and d-tubocura-

rine for prevention of succinylcholine-induced fasciculations and myalgia. Can J Anaesth 1997; 44:1144–7.
29. Findlay GP, Spittal MJ. Rocuronium pretreatment reduces suxamethonium-induced myalgia: comparison with vecuronium. Br J Anaesth 1996;76:526–9.
30. Motamed C, Choquette R, Donati F. Rocuronium prevents succinylcholine-induced fasciculations. Can J Anaesth 1997;44:1262–8.
31. Tsui BC, Reid S, Gupta S, Kearney R, Mayson T, Finucane B. A rapid precurarization technique using rocuronium. Can J Anaesth 1998; 45:397–401.
32. Denys P, Mane M, Azouvi P, Chartier Kastler E, Thiebaut JB, Bussel B. Side effects of chronic intrathecal baclofen on erection and ejaculation in patients with spinal cord lesions. Arch Phys Med Rehabil 1998;79:494–6.
33. Faigle JW, Keberle H, Degen PH. Chemistry and pharmacokinetics of baclofen. In: Feldman RG, Young RR, Koella WP, editors. Spasticity: Disordered Motor Control. Chicago: Year Book, 1980:461–75.
34. Chen KS, Bullard MJ, Chien YY, Lee SY. Baclofen toxicity in patients with severely impaired renal function. Ann Pharmacother 1997; 31:1315–20.
35. Perry HE, Wright RO, Shannon MW, Woolf AD. Baclofen overdose: drug experimentation in a group of adolescents. Pediatrics 1998;101:1045–8.
36. Roberge RJ, Atchley B, Ryan K, Krenzelok EP. Two chlorzoxazone (Parafon forte) overdoses and coma in one patient: reversal with flumazenil. Am J Emerg Med 1998;16:393–5.
37. Wagstaff AJ, Bryson HM. Tizanidine. A review of its pharmacology, clinical efficacy and tolerability in the management of spasticity associated with cerebral and spinal disorders. Drugs 1997;53:435–52.
38. Lu L, Atchabahian A, Mackinnon SE, Hunter DA. Nerve injection injury with botulinum toxin. Plast Reconstr Surg 1998;101:1875–80.
39. Glanzman RL, Gelb DJ, Drury I, Bromberg MB, Truong DD. Brachial plexopathy after botulinum toxin injection. Neurology 1990;40:1143.
40. Sampaio C, Castro-Caldas A, Sales-Luis ML, Alves M, Pinto L, Apolinario P. Brachial plexopathy after botulinum toxin administration for cervical dystonia. J Neurol Neurosurg Psychiatry 1993;56:220.
41. Tarsy D. Brachial plexus neuropathy after botulinum toxin injection. Neurology 1997;49: 1176–7.
42. Suarez GA, Giannini C, Bosch EP, Barohn RJ, Wodak J, Ebeling P, Anderson R, McKeever PE, Bromberg MB, Dyck PJ. Immune brachial plexus neuropathy: suggestive evidence for an inflammatory-immune pathogenesis. Neurology 1996;46:559–61.
43. Beghi E, Kurland LT, Mulder DW, Nicolosi A. Brachial plexus neuropathy in the population of Rochester, Minnesota, 1970–1981. Ann Neurol 1985;18:320–3.
44. Latimer PR, Hodgkins PR, Vakalis AN, Butler RE, Evans AR, Zaki GA. Necrotising fasciitis as a complication of botulinum toxin injection. Eye 1998;12:51–3.
45. Fiacchino F, Grandi L, Soliveri P, Carella F, Bricchi M. Sensitivity to vecuronium after botulinum toxin administration. J Neurosurg Anesthesiol 1997;9:149–53.

Michael Schachter

13 Drugs affecting autonomic functions or the extrapyramidal system

Many of the reports included in this chapter emphasize the possibility of new reactions to old drugs. Readers should note that the inhaled β_2-adrenoceptor agonists are discussed in Chapter 16.

DRUGS STIMULATING BOTH α- AND β-ADRENOCEPTORS *(SED-13, 153; SEDA-19, 147; SEDA-20, 145; SEDA-21, 153)*

There is very extensive non-prescribed use of this class of agent, so it is not surprising that adverse effects continue to be reported.

Endocrine, metabolic Epinephrine and norepinephrine are used in some patients after cardiopulmonary bypass, as part of the management of hypotension. In a study designed to determine whether either drug contributes to the *lactic acidosis* that sometimes occurs in these patients, 17 patients were randomized to receive norepinephrine and 19 to receive epinephrine (1[C]). Six patients developed lactic acidosis, all of them in the epinephrine group. The authors concluded that there was no evidence of confounding factors to account for this difference and that the epinephrine was acting via β_2-adrenoceptors to increase blood flow in the legs, which were the principal source of the lactate. The outcome was not unfavorable in these patients, since the acidosis resolved after the end of the epinephrine infusion. The authors therefore suggested that lactate concentrations may not be a good marker of clinical status in these patients.

Skin and appendages Ephedrine and pseudoephedrine have been reported to cause a *fixed drug rash* in an 18-year-old woman (2[c]). Both drugs produced an identical rash on challenge. Although such reactions have been described before, they appear to be rare.

Interactions An interaction between ephedrine and *cocaine* has been reported (3[c]).

A 42-year-old man developed coronary artery spasm and ventricular tachycardia after having been given intravenous ephedrine to increase his blood pressure during spinal anesthesia. He was a regular cocaine user, most recently about 4 days before surgery. Coronary arteriography showed very minor atheromatous lesions.

Previous reports have suggested that chronic cocaine use sensitizes coronary arterial α-adrenoceptors to agonists (4[C]).

DRUGS PREDOMINANTLY STIMULATING α-ADRENOCEPTORS *(SEDA-21, 153)*

These drugs are now mainly used topically, as nasal decongestants. Systemic effects nevertheless occur.

Cardiovascular *Cardiac dysrhythmias* have been reported with oxymetazoline (5[c]).

A 43-year-old man had several episodes of ventricular tachycardia associated with the use of oxymetazoline nasal spray. He proved to have an intra-

Side Effects of Drugs, Annual 22
J.K. Aronson, ed.

mural calcified cardiac fibroma near both fascicles of the bundle of His. It was thought that this was an ectopic focus that had been stimulated by the oxymetazoline. The patient was advised to avoid the spray and the dysrhythmia resolved.

A reminder that dopamine has significant α-agonist properties at high doses comes from a report of two cases of symmetrical *peripheral gangrene* in patients who had been treated with dopamine (20 μg/kg per min) for septic shock (6[c]). One patient died and the other required amputation of both hands and both feet. Although both patients had received epinephrine as well as dopamine, and one had also been given phenylephrine, these cases demonstrate the potential dangers of using dopamine in infusion rates over 10 μg/kg per min.

Nervous system The possibility that phenylephrine (added to a local anesthetic) may be a factor in the transient neurological symptoms associated with spinal anesthesia has been investigated in Japan (7[C]). Of 80 patients given phenylephrine, 10 developed transient symptoms such as *dysesthesia*. By contrast, this occurred in only one of the 80 patients who did not receive phenylephrine. An accompanying editorial suggested that the problem may have arisen from the combination of phenylephrine with the local anesthetic (tetracaine), although tetracaine may nevertheless be the anesthetic of first choice in this procedure (8[r]).

Gastrointestinal *Enterocolitis* has been described with phenylephrine (9[c]).

A 47-year-old man took a cold medication containing phenylephrine at the same time as amoxicillin/clavulanic acid (co-amoxiclav). After 5 days of medication he developed a hemorrhagic enterocolitis around the hepatic flexure. After the drugs had been withdrawn he made a full recovery within days.

Clearly the precise cause was difficult to ascertain under these conditions, but the authors postulated that this may have been ischemic colitis related to vasoconstriction.

Tolerance *Rebound nasal congestion* is a well recognised adverse effect of the chronic use of nasal decongestant sprays: they should therefore not be used for more than 3–5 days. However, it has been suggested that this problem can be avoided, at least with oxymetazoline, provided it is used only once nightly in a low dose (10[C]). Under these conditions the spray retained its efficacy for up to 8 weeks in 10 volunteers. It is not entirely clear how far this can be extrapolated to patients with rhinitis, as the authors themselves pointed out.

DRUGS PREDOMINANTLY STIMULATING β_1-ADRENOCEPTORS *(SED-13, 354; SEDA-19, 147; SEDA-20, 145; SEDA-21, 154)*

Dobutamine

Because of its widespread use in stress echocardiography there is continued interest in the adverse effects of dobutamine. Obviously its use is not often necessary in children, but a report on 46 patients from Cincinnati Children's Hospital has confirmed its safety. The mean age of the patients was about 10 (range 1–22) years. *Ventricular extra beats* and *hypertension* necessitated termination of the procedure in one patient; fewer severe cardiac adverse effects were seen in 9% of patients; and non-cardiac adverse effects, such as *nausea* and *headache*, occurred in 19% (11[C]).

Dobutamine has also been compared with adenosine in exercise radionuclide ventriculography (12[Cr]). Both drugs were well-tolerated: dobutamine caused less *flushing*, *headache*, and *nausea* but more *ventricular extra beats* (20% of 41 patients).

The safety and adverse effects of over 3000 dobutamine echocardiography studies carried out over 5 years have been surveyed (13[C]). More intensive test protocols have evolved over this period but have not been associated with increased risks. No deaths occurred in this series of patients, although there was one *myocardial infarction* and five cases of *sustained ventricular tachycardia*. The protocols were stopped prematurely in 7.6% of patients, mostly because of *hypotension* (3.8%) or *dysrhythmias* (1.6%).

In a small study from Japan the hypothesis

that intravenous estrogen administration could diminish dobutamine-induced ischemia in eight post-menopausal women has been tested. This proved to be so, with dose-dependent improvements in symptoms, electrocardiographic changes, and left ventricular function (14[c]).

DRUGS PREDOMINANTLY STIMULATING β_2-ADRENOCEPTORS *(SEDA-19, 147; SEDA-20, 145; SEDA-21, 154)*

Interference with diagnostic tests β_2-Adrenoceptor agonists are still widely used (though on rather weak grounds) to suppress premature labor. In a series of 140 women in Japan, ritodrine caused *increased plasma amylase activity* in 43%, while ephedrine had a similar effect in 54 of 160 women: the two drugs had additive effects when given together (15[C]). However, the amylase was entirely of the salivary type and there was no pancreatic dysfunction. This should be borne in mind to avoid spurious diagnoses of acute pancreatitis.

LEVODOPA AND DRUGS STIMULATING DOPAMINE RECEPTORS *(SED-13, 354, 355; SEDA-19, 148; SEDA-20, 146; SEDA-21, 155)*

Nervous system The difficulties associated with levodopa therapy in Parkinson's disease are well-recognised and remain largely intractable. Motor and neuropsychiatric problems have been reviewed, with emphasis on the former (16[R]). Nevertheless, the author pointed out that after 30 years levodopa still remains the most effective treatment. One approach to minimizing motor fluctuations is essentially pharmacokinetic, by prolonging the half-life of levodopa. This has been done with the selective monoamine oxidase inhibitor selegiline (17[R]) and more recently with inhibitors of catechol-O-methyltransferase, such as entacapone. In a placebo-controlled double-blind randomized trial of 205 patients entacapone increased 'on' time by about 1 h/day and reduced levodopa requirements by 100 mg/day (18[c]). However, there was some increase in dyskinesia and nausea, though this did not lead to withdrawals. (Another drug of the same class, tolcapone, has recently been withdrawn throughout the world following reports of severe hepatotoxicity, in some cases fatal.)

Respiratory Since the early 1980s there have been several reports of *pleural fibrosis* associated with bromocriptine, as well as other dopamine-agonist ergolines (19[cR]). In 15 patients from Sweden and Australia it was noted that treatment with bromocriptine had been preceded years earlier by exposure to asbestos (20[C]). There was significant clinical improvement after drug withdrawal, but fibrosis usually persisted. The authors suggested that asbestos may potentiate the fibrogenic effects of bromocriptine. This was discussed further in an accompanying editorial, in which it was concluded that the interaction remains to be proved but merits further attention and investigation (21[R]). Pleural fibrosis due to bromocriptine and other ergot derivatives is usually reversible, unlike the cases described above.

AGENTS WITH ANTICHOLINERGIC EFFECTS *(SED-13, 369; SEDA-19, 148; SEDA-20, 147)*

Atropine

Atropine is often used in patients with bradycardia when increased vagal tone is present or suspected. An unexpected adverse reaction has been reported in three out of 23 male heart transplant recipients given intravenous atropine: *second- or third-degree heart block* (22[c]). The mechanism is unknown but it appears that particular caution is needed when atropine is used in this group of patients.

Benzatropine

The use of anticholinergic drugs in treating patients with Parkinson's disease has long been associated with neuropsychiatric adverse effects. This can be aggravated by drug interactions, as has been reported with *paroxetine* (23[c]).

A 17-year-old boy taking haloperidol and benztropine was given paroxetine, a selective serotonin reuptake inhibitor, which also inhibits CYP2D6. After 8 days he became delirious and had a serum benzatropine concentration 40% higher than that considered to be toxic. He recovered within 2 days after all medication had been discontinued and there were no problems when haloperidol was reintroduced.

Oxybutynin

In recent years anticholinergic drugs have been used increasingly in the treatment of bladder detrusor instability. Unfortunately, their effects are not confined to the urinary tract, especially since they can cross the blood–brain barrier. *Confusional states* and *hallucinations* have been described in four elderly men (aged 79–85 years) with Parkinson's disease, whose urinary symptoms were treated with oxybutynin (24[c]). The mental changes subsided rapidly on withdrawal.

A 42-year-old woman with multiple sclerosis developed not only a dry mouth and blurred vision but also *drowsiness* when treated with oral oxybutynin (25[c]). A year later she was given the drug intravesically and this caused *numbness in the distribution of the sacral dermatomes*. This did not disappear completely when oxybutynin was withdrawn and there was no evidence that her disease had relapsed at this point. The authors pointed out that this reaction was not observed in patients who were given oxybutynin after spinal injury.

Scopolamine (hyoscine)

Scopolamine is widely used during a variety of anesthetic procedures. Attention has been drawn to potentially confusing clinical signs associated with the drug (26[c]).

Hyoscine was given by transdermal patch as an antiemetic to a 38-year-old woman who had undergone combined epidural and general anesthesia for a hysterectomy; the patch was placed behind the right ear. She developed a right fixed dilated pupil and became uncooperative. She recovered dramatically after intravenous physostigmine. A high level of suspicion in this case averted the need for unnecessary investigations.

Tolterodine

It has been asserted that tolterodine, an antimuscarinic drug used in the treatment of the hyperactive bladder, has significantly fewer systemic adverse effects than oxybutynin at equi-effective doses (particularly dry mouth), although the reason for this difference was not explained (27[C]). This needs to be confirmed.

Trihexyphenidyl (benzhexol)

Anticholinergic withdrawal can precipitate *encephalopathy* (28[c]).

A 61-year-old woman with mild Parkinson's disease took trihexyphenidyl 6 mg/day for 1 year. When it was withdrawn her conscious level fell and she became comatose after 2 days, with extreme miosis and decerebrate posturing in response to painful stimuli. She recovered after the drug had been re-administered by nasogastric tube. Drug withdrawal led to similar effects.

The authors concluded that the patient's clinical state had been due to central cholinergic overactivity.

REFERENCES

1. Totaro RJ, Raper RF. Epinephrine-induced lactic acidosis following cardiopulmonary bypass. Crit Care Med 1997;25:1693–9.
2. Garcia Ortiz JC, Terron M, Bellido J. Nonpigmenting fixed exanthema from ephedrine and pseudoephedrine. Allergy Eur J Allergy Clin Immunol 1997;52:229–30.
3. Lustik SJ, Chhibber AK, van Vliet M, Pomerantz RM. Ephedrine-induced coronary artery vasospasm in a patient with prior cocaine use. Anesth Analg 1997;84:931–3.
4. Lange RA, Cigarroa RG, Yancy CW, Willard JE, Popma JJ, Sills MN, McBride W, Kim AS, Hillis LD. Cocaine-induced coronary artery vasoconstriction. New Engl J Med 1989;321:1157–62.
5. Khan A, Dewhurst N. Use of a sympathomimetic nasal spray in association with cardiac fibroma: an unusual cause of ventricular tachycardia. Br J Clin Pract 1997;51:192–3.
6. Park JY. Dopamine-associated symmetric peripheral gangrene. Arch Dermatol 1997; 133:247–8.
7. Sakura S, Sumi M, Sakaguchi Y, Saito Y, Kosaka Y, Drasner K. The addition of phenylephrine contributes to the development of transient neurologic symptoms after spinal anesthesia with 0.5% tetracaine. Anesthesiology 1997; 87:771–8.
8. Rowlingson JC. Tranisent neurologic symptoms: now, with phenylephrine? Anesthesiology 1997;87:737–8.
9. Pérez-Castrillon JL, Duenas A, Goyeneche MA, Martin-Escudero JC, Herreros V. Hemorrhagic colitis due to amoxicillin/clavulanate and nasal decongestants? J Clin Gastroenterol 1997; 25:701.
10. Yoo JK, Seikaly H, Calhoun KH. Extended use of topical nasal decongestants. Laryngoscope 1997;107:40–3.
11. Kimball TR, Witt SA, Daniels SR. Dobutamine stress echocardiography in the assessment of suspected myocardial ischemia in children and young adults. Am J Cardiol 1997;79:380–4.
12. Nagaoka H, Isobe N, Kubota S, Iizuka T, Imai S, Suzuki T, Nagai R. Comaprison of adenosine, dobutamine, and exercise radionuclide ventriculography in the detection of coronary artery disease. Cardiology 1997;88:180–8.
13. Secknus M-A, Marwick TH. Evolution of dobutamine echocardiography protocols and indications: safety and side-effects in 3,011 studies over 5 years. J Am Coll Cardiol 1997;29:1234–40.
14. Alpaslan M, Shimokawa H, Kuroiwa-Matsumoto M, Harasawa Y, Tekeshita A. Short-term estrogen administration ameliorates dobutamine-induced myocardial ischemia in post-menopausal women with coronary artery disease. J Am Coll Cardiol 1997;30:1466–71.
15. Takahashi T, Minamaki H, Tamada T, Sato I. Hypeamyalasemia in response to ritodrine or ephedrine administered to pregnant women. J Am Coll Surg 1997;184:31–6.
16. Hurtig HI. Problems with current pharmacologic treatment of Parkinson's disease. Exp Neurol 1997;144:10–16.
17. Golbe LI, Langston JW, Shoulson I. Selegiline and Parkinson's disease. Protective and symptomatic considerations. Drugs 1990;39:646–51.
18. Parkinson Study Group. Entacapone improves motor fluctuations in levodopa-treated Parkinson's disease patients. Ann Neurol 1997; 42:747–55.
19. Bhatt MH, Keenan SP, Fleetham JA, Calne DB. Pleuropulmonary disease associated with dopamine agonist therapy. Ann Neurol 1991; 30:613–16.
20. Hillerdal G, Lee J, Blomkvist A, Rask-Andersen A, Uddenfeldt M, Koyi H, Rasmussen E. Pleural disease during treatment with bromocriptine in patients previously exposed to asbestos. Eur Respir J 1997;10:2711–15.
21. De Vuyst P, Pfitzenmeyer P, Camus P. Asbestos, ergot drugs and the pleura. Eur Respir J 1997;10:2695–8.
22. Brunner–La Rocca HP, Kiowski W, Bracht C, Weilenmann D, Follath F. Atrioventricular block after administration of atropine in patients following cardiac transplantation. Transplantation 1997; 63:1838–9.
23. Armstrong SC, Schweitzer SM. Delirium associated with paroxetine and benztropine combination. Am J Psychiatry 1997;154:581–2.
24. Donnellan CA, Fook L, McDonald P, Playfer JR. Oxybutynin and cognitive dysfunction. Br Med J 1997;315:1363–4.
25. Vaidyanathan S, Krishnan KR, Soni BM, Fraser MH. Exaggerated neurological side-effects of oral and intravesical oxybutynin in a patient with multiple sclerosis. Spinal Cord 1997;35:190–1.
26. Elias MAY, Abouleish E. Scopolamine patch can be confusing to the patient and anesthesiologist: a case report. Anesthesiology 1997;86:743–4.
27. Appell RA, Norton PA, Kawabe K, Wein AJ, Malone Lee J. Clinical efficacy and safety of tolterodine in the treatment of overactive bladder: a pooled analysis. Urology 1997;50 (Suppl 6A): 90–9.
28. Johkura K, Matsumoto S, Hasegawa O, Kuroiwa Y. Trihexyphenidyl withdrawal encephalopathy. Ann Neurol 1997;41:133–4.

Anton C. de Groot

14 Dermatological drugs, topical agents, and cosmetics

R ## *Ingredient labeling of cosmetic products: new opportunities, new problems*

(Note: This Special Review has been adapted from (1[R]) with the kind permission of the Editor (Dr RJG Rycroft) and the Publisher (Munksgaard) of the journal Contact Dermatitis.)

Opportunities *On 1 January 1997 the Sixth Amendment to the EU Cosmetics Directive (76/768) came into force. This Directive requires, inter alia, that all cosmetic products marketed in the European Union should display their ingredients on the outer package or, in certain cases, on an accompanying leaflet, label, tape, or tag (2[R]). The primary purpose of ingredient labeling is to allow dermatologists to identify specific ingredients that cause allergic responses in their patients and to enable such patients to avoid cosmetic products containing the substances to which they are allergic by checking their labels (3[R]), (4[R]). It is expected that labeling will also boost scientific research in the field of cosmetic dermatitis and that new cosmetic allergens will be identified much sooner, which will help the cosmetics industry to create safer cosmetic products (3[R]).*

Labeling rules *The nomenclature used throughout the European Union for labeling is the INCI (International Nomenclature Cosmetic Ingredient), based on the American CTFA (Cosmetic, Toiletry and Fragrance Association) nomenclature. Most CTFA terms have been retained unchanged. However, all colorants are listed as color index (CI) numbers, except hair dyes, which have INCI names. For botanicals (cosmetic ingredients directly derived from plants) the INCI nomenclature is based on the Linnean system, in which the Latin genus and species names of the plant are used. 'Trivial names' is the term used for the names of ingredients that should be well known to consumers. The INCI names for such ingredients are based on those used in the European Pharmacopoeia.*

Although all ingredients have to be declared, certain materials are not considered as ingredients and therefore do not need to be labeled: (1) impurities in the raw materials used; (2) subsidiary technical materials used in the preparation but not present in the final product; (3) materials used in strictly necessary quantities as solvents or as carriers for perfume and aromatic compositions.

Confidential substances are listed under a unique seven-digit code.

Labeling always starts with the word: INGREDIENTS. Then follows a list of ingredients in descending order of concentration. Ingredients in concentrations of less than 1% may be listed in any order after those in concentrations of more than 1%. Coloring agents may be listed in any order after the other ingredients. Perfume ingredients are not listed individually, but their presence is indicated by the word 'Perfume'. Flavoring ingredients (as in mouthwashes or toothpaste) are denoted as 'Aroma'.

The words 'May contain' or '+/−' sometimes precede a number or colorants. These are colorants that are used in a particular brand of decorative cosmetic products marketed in several color shades. Which of these colors is present in any particular product remains unknown to the consumer.

Problems *The source of information on ingredients is the European Inventory, published in all official EU languages. The information*

Side Effects of Drugs, Annual 22
J.K. Aronson, ed.

includes the INCI names (in alphabetical order), CAS-number, EINECS-ELINCS numbers, chemical/IUPAC names, and functions. Unfortunately, the Inventory has several disadvantages.

The major problem is the 'translation' of plant products and colors from the CTFA nomenclature to the INCI. Lists of synonyms are not provided. Only those who have access to botanical literature and specific literature on colors can find relevant names. Apart from the fact that dermatologists will have to get used to some very exotic names, who would be able to find Myroxylon pereirae for balsam of Peru, Eugenia caryophyllus for clove oil, or 'CI 77000' for aluminum?

The order of listing is sometimes illogical: for p-*aminophenol, look under 'Pa . . .' instead of 'Am . . .'. Benzophenone-11 comes before Benzophenone-2 (because 11 begins with 1, ergo before 2).*

It is stated that fragrances have not been included in the INCI, as they need not to be declared. However, I have found many fragrance names (e.g. geraniol, *hydroxycitronellal, cinnamal, cinnamyl alcohol), described as 'additives'. Additives are defined as 'Substances which, often in fairly small amounts, are added to cosmetic products to create or improve desired properties or minimize or suppress undesired properties'. In this context one may think of 'masking perfumes', the classic example of which is ethylene brassylate (indeed mentioned in the inventory). However, I do not know whether producers of cosmetics will actually declare such fragrances on the label. In addition, dermatologists will have to check the inventory, whether or not a specific fragrance is included, before advising patients allergic to these individual fragrance compounds.*

In spite of the fact that fragrances do not need to be declared, Part II of the Inventory lists some 2500 fragrances (including plant extracts) and aroma chemicals. In itself this could be very useful; however, the chemicals are not listed in alphabetical order, but in ascending order of EINECS/ELINCS numbers, and therefore impossible for almost all dermatologists to trace.

Clearly, patients who are allergic to certain cosmetics ingredients should be supplied with the INCI names of their allergens. They will seek in vain for well-known names, such as Kathon CG, oxybenzone, balsam of Peru, Amerchol L 101, dibromodicyanobutane, or orange oil. Dermatologists should therefore be familiar with INCI names.

From the above it is clear that the relevant names are sometimes very hard or impossible to find. To overcome this problem, a list has been made of substances that can be present in cosmetics and have been described as allergens ((5[R]), (6[R]), and see also recent issues of the journal 'Contact Dermatitis'), in which their names (CTFA, Merck Index, names provided by the producers of commercially available allergens, 'common names', commonly used trade names) have been compared with INCI. Chemicals whose INCI names are different are summarized in Table 1. Not included are chemicals whose names are virtually identical or contain a common part of the name (rose oil = rosa; propolis = propolis cera) and can therefore easily be recognized by patients, and ingredients that are prohibited in the EU (e.g. captan, sodium omadine, pyrogallol) (4[R]). This list should enable dermatologists to adequately instruct those of their patients who are allergic to cosmetics ingredients. I could not find the INCI names for 11 reported allergens, eight of which are essential oils. It may be that these substances are not used in cosmetic products in the EU or are outdated, and were therefore not included in the INCI. Alternatively, I may not have searched hard enough for their INCI counterparts.

I suggest that: (1) Trolab and Chemotechnique (the providers of test allergens) should in future include INCI names in their lists of synonyms (and preferably use INCI names as first entry); (2) the Liaison Committee on Cosmetic Nomenclature and/or Colipa should provide alphabetical lists of all chemicals whose INCI names differ from CTFA or other commonly used names; (3) Part II of the Inventory should be supplemented with an alphabetical listing of fragrance and aroma chemicals.

ORAL PHOTOCHEMOTHERAPY (PUVA) *(SED-13, 380; SEDA-19, 154; SEDA-20, 153; SEDA-21, 160)*

Several review articles on the efficacy and toxicity of photochemotherapy in psoriasis

Table 1. *Conversion list to INCI names*

Commonly used name CTFA name common trade name names used by Trolab Chemotechnique	INCI name
Abitol®	Hydroabietyl alcohol
Acid red 18	CI 16255
Acid red 27	CI 16185
Acid red 87	CI 45380
Acid yellow 3	CI 47005
Acid yellow 23	CI 19140
Ale oil	INNF*
Aluminum	CI 77000
Amaranth	CI 16185
Amerchol® L 101	Lanolin alcohol and paraffinum liquidum
p-Aminobenzoic acid	PABA
p-Aminodiphenylamine	*N*-Phenyl-*p*-phenylenediamine sulfate
Angelica root oil	Angelica acutiloba/polymorpha
Anise oil	*Pimpinella anisum*
Arlacel Æ 83	Sorbitan sesquioleate
Atlas® G-1441	PEG-40 sorbitan lanolate
Avocado oil	*Persea gratissima*
Balsam of Peru	*Myroxylon pereirae*
Balsam of Pine	*Pinus*
Balsam of Tolu	*Myroxylon toluiferum*
Basil oil	*Ocimum basilicum*
Bay oil	*Pimenta acris*
Beech tar	*Fagus sylvatica*
Benzoin resinoid	Styrax benzoin
Benzyl-4-hydroxybenzoate	Benzylparaben
Bergamot oil	*Citrus bergamia*
Birch tar	*Betula alba*
Bismuth oxychloride	CI 77163
Bitter almond oil	*Prunus amara*
Bitter orange oil	*Citrus amara*
Brilliant lake red R	CI 15800
Bronopol	2-Bromo-2-nitropropane-1,3-diol
2,6-ditert-Butyl-4-cresol	BHT
Butyl hydroxyanisole	BHA
Butyl-4-hydroxybenzoate	Butylparaben
Butyl hydroxytoluene	BHT
4-*tert*-Butyl-4′-methoxydibenzoylmethane	Butyl methoxydibenzoylmethane
2-*tert*-Butyl-4-methoxyphenol	BHA
Calamus oil	*Acorus calamus*
Cananga oil	*Cananga odorata*
Carboxyvinyl polymer	Carbomer
Cassia oil	*Cinnamonum cassia*
Castor oil	*Ricinus communis*
Cedarwood oil	*Cedrus atlantica*
Cetylsteraryl alcohol	Cetyl alcohol, stearyl alcohol
Chamomilla Romana	*Anthemis nobilis*
Cherry pit oil	*Prunus avium*
1-(3-Chloroallyl)-3,5,7-triaza-1-azonia-adamantane chloride	Quaternium-15
Chlorocresol	*p*-Chloro-*m*-cresol
4-Chloro-3-cresol	*p*-Chloro-*m*-cresol
4-Chloro-3-xylenol	Chloroxylenol
Chromium hydroxide	CI 77289
Citronella oil	*Cymbopogon nardus*
Clary sage oil	*Salvia sclarea*
Cl+Me-isothiazolinone	Methylisothiazolinone, methylchloroiso-thiazolinone
Clove oil	*Eugenia caryophyllus*
Coal tar	Pix ex carbone
Cochenille red A	CI 16255

Table 1. *Continued*

Commonly used name CTFA name common trade name names used by Trolab Chemotechnique	INCI name
Coconut diethanolamide	Cocamide DEA
Colocynth	*Citrullus colocynthis*
Copaiba oil	*Copaifera officinalis*
Coriander oil	*Coriandrum sativum*
Costus oil	INNF*
Cypress oil	*Cupressus sempervirens*
Dandelion	*Taraxacum officinale*
DC blue 6	CI 73000
DC blue 9	CI 69825
DC red 10	CI 15630
DC red 17	CI 26100
DC red 19	CI 45170
DC red 21	CI 45380
DC red 30	CI 73360
DC red 31	CI 15800
DC red 36	CI 12085
DC yellow 10	CI 47005
DC yellow 11	CI 47000
2,5-Diaminotoluene sulfate	Toluene-2,5-diamine sulfate
Dibromodicyanobutane	Methyldibromoglutaronitrile
Dichlorodifluoromethane	INNF*
Dihydroabietyl alcohol	Hydroabietyl alcohol
Diisopropanolamine	DIPA (not present as such)
Dowicil® 200	Quaternium-15
Eosin	CI 45380
Escalol® 507	Octyl dimethyl PABA
Escalol® 557	Octyl methoxycinnamate
Escalol® 567	Benzophenone-3
Ethyl chloride	INNF
Ethylenediamine tetraacetic acid disodium	Disodium EDTA dihydrate
2-Ethylhexyl-*p*-dimethylaminobenzoate	Octyl dimethyl PABA
2-Ethylhexyl-*p*-methoxycinnamate	Octyl methoxycinnamate
Ethyl-4-hydroxybenzoate	Ethylparaben
Eucalyptus oil	*Eucalyptus globulus*
Eusolex® 4360	Benzophenone-3
Eusolex® 6007	Octyl dimethyl PABA
Eusolex® 6300	4-Methylbenzylidene camphor
Eusolex® 8020	Isopropyl dibenzoylmethane
Euxyl® K 100	Methylisothiazolinone, methylchloroisothiazolinone
Euxyl® K 400	Methyldibromo glutaronitrile, phenoxyethanol
Ext DC orange 4	CI 12120
FDC red 2	CI 16185
FDC yellow 3	CI 15985
FDC yellow 5	CI 19140
Feverfew	*Chrysanthemum parthenium*
Food orange 4	CI 16230
Food red 7	CI 16255
Food red 9	CI 16185
Food yellow 4	CI 19140
Food yellow 6	CI 15985
Frankincense oil	*Boswellia carterii*
Germall® 115	Imidazolidinyl urea
Germall® II	Diazolidinyl urea
Glutaraldehyde	Glutaral
Glutardialdehyde	Glutaral
Glyceryl-3(glyceroxy)-anthranilate	INNF*
Glyceryl monothioglycolate	Glyceryl thioglycolate
Greengrass oil	INNF*

Table 1. *Continued*

Commonly used name CTFA name common trade name names used by Trolab Chemotechnique	INCI name
Guanine	CI 75170
Guiac wood oil	*Guaiacum officinale*
Helindone pink	CI 73360
Hexamethylenetetramine	Methenamine
Hexamine	Methenamine
Horsechestnut extract	*Aesculus hippocastanum*
2-Hydroxy-4-methoxybenzophenone	Benzophenone-3
2-Hydroxy-4-methoxy-4′-methylbenzophenone	Benzophenone-10
2(2-Hydroxy-5-methylphenyl)benzotriazole	Drometrizole
1-(4-Isopropylphenyl)-3-phenyl-1,3-	Isopropyl dibenzoylmethane-propanedione
Jojoba oil	*Buxus chinensis*
Juniper (berry) oil	*Juniperus communis/oxycedris*
Karaya gum	*Sterculia urens*
Kathon® CG	Methylisothiazolinone, methylchloroisothiazolinone
Laurel oil	*Laurus nobilis*
Lavandin oil	*Lavandula hybrida*
Lavender oil/absolute	*Lavandula angustifolia*
Lemongrass oil	Cymbopogon
Lemon oil	*Citrus limonum*
Lithol red	CI 15630
Litsea cubeba oil	INNF*
Lovage oil	*Levisticum officinale*
Marjoram oil	*Origanum majorana*
Merthiolate	Thimerosal
Methyl-4-hydroxybenzoate	Methylparaben
Mexenone	Benzophenone-10
Microcrystalline wax	Cera microcrystallina
Mineral oil	Paraffinum liquidum
Myrrh oil	*Commiphora myrrha*
Narcissus oil	*Narcissus pseudonarcissus*
Natural white 1	CI 75170
Neroli oil (= orange flower oil)	*Citrus aurantium dulcis*
Niaouli oil	INNF*
Nigella sativa black seed oil	INNF*
Olive oil	*Olea europaea*
Orange oil	*Citrus dulcis*
Oxybenzone	Benzophenone-3
Parabens	Benzylparaben
	Butylparaben
	Ethylparaben
	Methylparaben
	Propylparaben
Parsol® 1789	Butyl methoxydibenzoylmethane
Parsol® MCX	Octyl methoxycinnamate
Patchouli oil	*Pogostemon cablin*
Peppermint oil	*Mentha piperita*
Petitgrain bigarade oil	*Citrus amara*
4-Phenylenediamine base	*p*-Phenylenediamine
2-Phenyl-5-methyl benzoxazole	INNF*
Pigment blue 15	CI 74160
Pigment red 3	CI 12120
Pigment red 4	CI 12085
Pigment red 7	CI 12420
Pigment red 48:4	CI 15865
Pigment red 49	CI 15630
Pigment red 64	CI 15800
Pigment yellow 1	CI 11680
Pine tar	*Pinus*

Table 1. *Continued*

Commonly used name CTFA name common trade name names used by Trolab Chemotechnique	INCI name
Pix betulae	*Betula alba*
Pix fagi	*Fagus sylvatica*
Pix liquida	*Pinus*
Pix oxycedri	Juniper tar
Polyethyleneglycol ointment	PEG-. . . (number)
Polyoxyethylene sorbitan lanolate	PEG-40 sorbitan lanolate
Polyoxyethylene sorbitan monopalmitate	Polysorbate 40
Polyoxyethylene sorbitan oleate	Polysorbate 80
Pomerance flower oil	INNF*
Propyl-4-hydroxybenzoate	Propylparaben
Quinoline yellow	CI 47005
Rosin	*Colophonium*
Sage oil	*Salvia officinalis*
Sandalwood oil	*Santalum album*
Sesame oil	*Sesamum indicum*
Solvent red 1	CI 12150
Solvent red 3	CI 12010
Solvent red 23	CI 26100
Solvent yellow 33	CI 47000
Sorbitan monooleate	Sorbitan oleate
Span® 80	Sorbitan oleate
Spearmint oil	*Mentha viridis*
Spike oil	*Lavandula angustifolia*
Spruce oil	*Picea excelsa*
Storax	Styrax benzoin
Sudan III	CI 26100
Sunset yellow	CI 15985
Tannin, synthetic	Tannic acid
Tansy extract	*Tanacetum vulgare*
Tartrazine	CI 19140
Tea tree oil	*Melaleuca alternifolia*
Thuja essential oil	*Thuya occidentalis*
Thyme oil	*Thymus vulgaris*
Tinuvin® P	Drometrizole
Toluenesulfonamide/formaldehyde resin	Tosylamide/formaldehyde resin
Toluidine red	CI 12120
Toney red	CI 26100
3,4,4′-Trichlorcarbanilide	Triclocarban
Trolamine	Triethanolamine
Tween® 80	Polysorbate 80
Vat blue 1	CI 73000
Vat blue 6	CI 69825
Vat red 1	CI 73360
Vetiver oil	INNF*
Witch hazel	*Hamamelis virginiana*
Wool alcohols	Lanolin alcohol
Yarrow	*Achillea millefolium*
Ylang-ylang oil	*Cananga odorata*
Zinc oxide	CI 77947

*INNF = INCI name not found.

(7^R), (8^R) and vitiligo (9^R) have recently been published.

Skin and appendages *Phototoxicity* The most significant short-term adverse effect of PUVA is phototoxicity. Apart from the initial reports of multicenter studies that evaluated efficacy (SEDA-7, 166), there has been little study of this adverse effect. The incidence and possible causes of phototoxicity of sufficient degree (painful erythema) to cause interruption of treatment for at least one subsequent session, have been determined in a retrospective study of 16 506 PUVA treatments given to 414 patients (10[Cr]). Phototoxicity occurred in 51 patients (11%) and was an adverse effect in 0.3% of treatments. The most common cause was suspected to be a defect in the treatment protocol, notably the administration of a dose of UVA radiation that exceeded the patient's threshold for phototoxicity (n = 18). The second most common problem appeared to be high absorption of methoxsalen, as indicated by nausea or other evidence of gastrointestinal discomfort ($n = 6$) (these symptoms are triggered by high serum concentrations of methoxsalen). Treatment on consecutive days, the addition of UVB radiation to the treatment, and shifting the treatment time from evening to morning were less common problems with the treatment protocol. Concurrent use of phototoxic medications (methotrexate, doxycycline) was considered to be the cause of phototoxic erythema in three patients. Patients forgetting to wear protective clothing, excessive exposure to sunlight, and erratic attendance were examples of poor compliance leading to erythema. Technical errors in UV administration were responsible for two cases of phototoxicity. Finally, in 14% of instances of erythema there was no apparent cause.

Ingestion of psoralen-containing vegetables, such as celery, fennel, parsnip, parsley, dill, cumin, and other members of the *Umbellifera* family, in significant amounts before PUVA sessions might, in some patients, account for unexpected variations in phototoxic responses (11[c]).

Vitiligo during PUVA Pigmentary changes during PUVA therapy usually manifest as PUVA lentigines (SEDA-9, 130). Vitiligo-like depigmentation during PUVA has been observed in one patient treated for vitiligo and two for mycosis fungoides. The depigmentation was not confined to clinically involved areas, nor was it associated with obvious phototoxicity (SEDA-9, 130). Now vitiligo has also been observed during treatment for psoriasis (12[cr]).

A 19-year-old Caucasian man, who presumably had suffered from a vitiligo patch at age 5, received topical PUVA with 0.1% trimethoxsalen cream for 3 months for psoriasis. UVA light was applied at 0.1 J/cm^2 with an increment of 0.1 J/cm^2 at each session, as tolerated. At the 10th session, depigmented lesions were noted around the margins of the regressing psoriatic plaques. This progressed until the vitiligo-like lesions completely replaced the resolved psoriatic plaques in exactly the same configuration. In a biopsy melanocytes were absent (as in vitiligo).

PUVA kills melanocytes in experimental animals. However, this reaction could not be attributed to this effect only, as the vitiligo did not conform to the trimethoxsalen application sites, but rather was solely confined to areas involving the psoriatic plaques and did not extend beyond those margins. Thus, the authors hypothesized that topical PUVA activated an immunological reaction, and that this reaction was clinically relevant only in inflammatory (psoriatic) skin lesions.

Tumor-inducing effects *(SED-13, 380; SEDA-18, 166)* *Non-cutaneous cancers* Although many years ago, some clinicians hypothesized that psoriasis may protect against cancer, several subsequent population-based studies have suggested that the risk of some types of non-cutaneous cancers may be increased in people with psoriasis (13[Cr]). Psoralen and ultraviolet A radiation are mutagenic and may have immunosuppressive effects (SEDA-13, 119). Long-term PUVA treatment increases the risk of squamous cell cancer (14[R]). Because of these observations, there is concern that an increased risk of non-cutaneous cancers, especially *lymphoreticular malignancy* (SEDA-10, 125; SEDA-14, 124) might be a long-term adverse effect of PUVA (15[Cr]).

To test this hypothesis, the members of the PUVA Follow-up Study have prospectively followed 1380 patients who first began PUVA treatment for psoriasis in 1975–6. The risk of non-cutaneous cancers in this cohort was compared with that expected based on general population incidence rates. The overall risk of non-cutaneous cancers was nearly identical to that expected in the general population. However, for three separate sites, significant increases were noted: thyroid cancer (RR 3.57; 95% CI 1.16–8.34), breast cancer (RR

1.81; 95% CI 1.19–2.64), and central nervous system neoplasms (RR 2.80; 95% CI 1.13–5.57). Since 1987, however, the risk of central nervous system neoplasms has not increased and the relative risk of breast cancer was lower than in the prior decade and not statistically significant. There was no association between higher degrees of exposure to PUVA and the risk of any of these cancers. The was no significant increase in the risk of lymphomas or leukemia. Thus, this study did not support the hypothesis that long-term PUVA treatment increases the risk of non-cutaneous cancers.

℞ Does long-term PUVA therapy increase the risk of malignant melanoma?

Is an increased risk to be expected? *Photochemotherapy using the psoralen methoxsalen and ultraviolet A radiation (PUVA) is highly effective in moderate to severe psoriasis. However, long-term therapy increases the risk of squamous cell carcinoma of the skin (SED-13, 380; SEDA-18, 166; SEDA-19, 156).*

In many patients who receive PUVA therapy, irregular pigmented macules (PUVA lentigines) develop and persist long after therapy is stopped. Histologically these lesions are proliferations of large cytologically atypical melanocytes. PUVA induces melanocytic tumors in mice (16), and it stimulates the growth of melanoma cells in vivo (17). Moreover, experiments in animals suggest that exposure to ultraviolet A radiation may contribute to the induction and progression of malignant melanoma. Thus, although the relation between cumulative exposure to sunlight and the risk of melanoma is controversial, and no definite melanoma risk of UVA-emitting tanning lamps has been established (18[R]), there has always been concern that PUVA increases the risk of malignant melanoma.

Except in anecdotal reports, malignant melanoma has so far not been observed in patients with psoriasis who have received long-term treatment with PUVA, and this has been comforting. However, a recent report from the PUVA Follow-up Study has suggested that there is indeed a modest but significant increased risk of malignant melanoma in PUVA-treated patients, which begins about 15 years after the first treatment and is observed especially in patients who have received 250 treatments or more (19[Cr]).

Results of the PUVA Follow-up Study *The PUVA Follow-up Study prospectively evaluated 1380 patients who began PUVA treatment for psoriasis at 16 university centers in 1975 and 1976 (19[Cr]). Of the 1380 patients, 984 were still alive on 29 February 1996. At the time of enrolment, the average age of the patients was 44 years. The mean interval from the first treatment to the most recent follow-up interview was 19 years. A total of 11 melanomas were found in nine patients. Overall, the risk of melanoma was significantly higher in the study patients than in persons of similar age, sex, and ethnicity in the US population (RR 2.3; 95% CI 1.1–4.1). From enrolment to the end of 1990, four malignant melanomas were detected in four patients, an incidence nearly identical to that expected on the basis of the incidence data of the Surveillance, Epidemiology, and End Results program of the National Cancer Institute (RR 1.1; 95% CI 0.3–2.9). However, from the beginning of 1991 to February 1996, a total of seven melanomas were detected in six patients (RR 5.4; 95% CI 2.2–11.1). The patients who received 250 treatments or more had the greatest increased risk (incidence-rate ratio 4.1; 95% CI 1.3–13.4). Using the time from the first treatment as an independent predictor, there was a significant increase beginning in 1991 compared with the earlier period of surveillance, from 1975 to 1990 (incidence rate ratio 4.7; 95% CI 1.4–16.1). In five other patients, not included in the analysis, other melanocytic tumors developed: four melanomas in situ and one melanoma of the ocular choroid. Two of the nine patients with malignant melanoma died from metastatic disease.*

Should PUVA be abandoned? *This study raises the strong suspicion that PUVA increases the risk of malignant melanoma. High degrees of exposure to PUVA, a period of at least 15 years from the time of the first exposure, or both are required before the risk* *of melanoma increases substantially. Does this mean that PUVA should be abandoned (20)?*

Clearly these data are alarming, because malignant melanoma is fatal if left untreated. Even more alarming is the fact that melanomas appeared only after a long latency period, which suggests that more patients treated with PUVA in the past may have melanomas in the future, and that the risk persists after the end of treatment. However, it should be realized that the study lacks certain important data. For instance, the total phototoxic dose delivered was not mentioned, nor was it clear whether other potentially carcinogenic or co-carcinogenic factors were found in the melanoma patients. Most importantly, it is unknown whether the melanoma patients were at greater risk of melanoma in the first place—specifically, whether they had atypical nevocellular nevi or a family history of melanoma. One of the nine patients had three primary melanomas; if one assumes that he had familial melanoma or the dysplastic nevus syndrome and excludes him from the cohort, the statistics of the study look less frightening.

Before abandoning PUVA as a treatment for psoriasis, we should also ask what other options there are for dealing with the severe forms of this disease. Topical treatments, including ultraviolet B irradiation, corticosteroids, and calcipotriol, are not sufficiently effective in severe psoriasis. Systemic treatments, such as methotrexate or cyclosporin, are highly effective, but they pose the risk of immunosuppression and systemic toxicity; the latter is also true of the retinoids. None of these treatments has been as carefully studied for long-term side-effects as PUVA has.

After more than 20 years' experience, it has become clear that PUVA offers many patients the chance to resume a normal life. Taking this into account, considering the questions raised here, and weighing the risks and benefits of the other options for treating severe psoriasis, PUVA need not and cannot be abandoned now (20). Nevertheless, the results of the PUVA Follow-up Study (19[Cr]) should not be taken lightly. It has clearly shown that the guidelines for treating psoriasis with PUVA should be rigidly observed ((21[R]); SEDA-19, 154), that patients receiving long-term treatment with PUVA should be carefully followed throughout their lives, and most important, that those who are at increased risk from melanoma should not be given this treatment. Meanwhile, cohorts of patients treated in other multicenter studies should be carefully re-evaluated to determine whether the observations of the PUVA Follow-up Study can be validated (20).

RETINOIDS *(SED-13, 382; SEDA-19, 156; SEDA-20, 154; SEDA-21, 162)*

A useful review article on the clinical efficacy and toxicity of retinoids has recently been published (22[R]).

Indications for treatment with isotretinoin When isotretinoin was first introduced in the early 1980s, its use was restricted predominantly to patients with severe nodulocystic acne. With increasing clinical experience; however, many physicians have expanded its use to include patients with less severe disease. An international expert panel now advises that "acne patients should, where appropriate, be prescribed isotretinoin sooner rather than later" (23[R]).

The criteria for prescribing isotretinoin in patients with mild or moderate acne include acne that improves less than 50% after 6 months of conventional oral antibiotic and topical combination therapy, acne that scars, acne that produces psychological distress, and acne that relapses significantly either during or soon after conventional therapy. Treatment can be initiated with daily doses of 0.5–1.0 mg/kg to achieve a total cumulative dose of 120–150 mg/kg. There are significant cost savings in treating acne with oral isotretinoin compared with other types of treatment (23[R]).

Urinary system *Renal impairment* is not a classical complication of retinoid treatment. Only two such cases caused by etretinate have been previously documented (24[cr]), (25[cr]). Now there has been a report of a similar case of renal impairment possibly caused by isotretinoin (26[cr]).

A 34-year-old man had taken isotretinoin 40 mg/day for 2 months for severe acne. He presented with severe bilateral lumbar pain suggestive of renal colic. His blood pressure was normal, he was apyrexial, and he had normal urinary output. The serum creatinine was 259 μmol/l and there was microscopic hematuria and proteinuria (0.8 g/l). There was evidence of inflammation (ESR 30 mm/h, C reactive protein 77 g/l), but there was no evidence of infection and immunological test results were normal (autoantibodies, complement, immunoglobulins). Urinary analysis did not show inversion of the Na/K ratio. There was no eosinophilia. A renal ultrasound scan showed kidneys of normal size. An intravenous pyelogram was normal. An abdominal CAT scan showed no renal infarction and investigations of abdominal pain only showed an elongated colon. When isotretinoin was withdrawn and intravenous hydration given, the creatinine returned to normal in 7 days and the proteinuria, hematuria, and inflammatory markers disappeared after 3 days.

Another case of renal impairment caused by *polyarteritis nodosa* manifesting as multiple small aneurysms detected by selective renal arteriography has been attributed to isotretinoin (27[cr]). Vasculitis due to retinoids is rare (SEDA-13, 123; SEDA-15, 142).

Skin and appendages *Epidermal stripping of the skin by wax epilation* Isotretinoin and etretinate can cause severe dryness of the skin and epidermal fragility (SEDA-11, 137; SEDA-15, 142). As a result of the fragility of the skin, wax depilatory treatment of the legs and face may not only remove the hair but also large areas of the epidermis of women taking isotretinoin. It has been recommended that young women taking isotretinoin should be advised to avoid wax epilation while taking isotretinoin and for up to 2 months afterwards (28[Cr]).

Drug–disease and drug–drug interactions Since oral isotretinoin is the only therapy that addresses all major causes of acne, it remains the most effective antiacne therapy available. Its adverse effects are predictable and can be managed easily; severe adverse effects are rare. Acne patients with serious concomitant systemic diseases, such as insulin-dependent diabetes mellitus, epilepsy, or spina bifida, transplant patients, patients with renal failure, patients with multiple sclerosis, motor neuron disease, and others can also safely be treated with a standard cumulative dose of 120 mg/kg per treatment course (29[R]). Experience has shown, however, that dosage adjustments may be advisable (30[R]), as shown in Table 2.

Possible drug–drug interactions are of particular concern in patients with concurrent systemic diseases.

In epileptics, no increase in seizure susceptibility was noted in a number of patients taking retinoids and phenytoin, sodium valproate, or carbamazepine; however, the authors recommended measuring *carbamazepine* concentrations during retinoid therapy, since plasma concentrations of carbamazepine and its main metabolite can fall, which can be attributed to either reduced absorption or increased clearance (29[R]).

The insulin requirements of diabetics do not appear to be affected by courses of isotretinoin (29[R]). Although no changes in lipid metabolism were seen compared to the non-diabetic patients, blood sugar and lipid concentrations should be monitored regularly in diabetics treated with isotretinoin.

The reliability of oral contraceptives is not influenced by isotretinoin (29[R]).

Concurrent use of *tetracycline* has been considered contraindicated in patients taking isotretinoin, because of the risk of benign intracranial hypertension (29[R]). Either compound alone can provoke this rare effect, but there is no evidence of any additive effect.

CONTACT ALLERGY *(SED-13, 385; SEDA-19, 158; SEDA-20, 156; SEDA-21, 164)*

An issue of the *Clinics in Dermatology* entirely devoted to the subject of *contact dermatitis* contains useful reviews of recent developments in contact dermatitis from cosmetics (31[R]), preservatives (32[R]), fragrances ((33[R]); SEDA-20, 149), topical medicaments (34[R]), and corticosteroids ((35[R]); SEDA-21, 158). Pigmented contact dermatitis (36[R]) and contact urticaria (37[R]), (38[R]) have also been reviewed.

Other articles focused on contact dermatitis from cinnamic aldehyde (cinnamal) (39[R]) and hydroquinone (40[R]). Cinnamic aldehyde is a potent skin sensitizer. Up to 2% of patients with dermatitis are allergic to this fragrance

Table 2. *Dosage adjustments for retinoid therapy in acne in patients with other diseases*

Concomitant disease	Regimen
Diabetes mellitus Epilepsy Crohn's disease Ulcerative colitis	Protocol A: standard dose regimen
Chronic renal failure Immunosuppression (transplant patients) Neurological diseases	Protocol B: half the standard dose regimen initially, with gradual increase to standard dose
Behçet's disease Leukemia Liver transplantation Retinitis pigmentosa	Protocol C: once a week regimen with gradual dosage increase

material, particularly users of cosmetic products. Its occupational importance is low and it may only play a role in dental staff or people in the food industry (39[R]). Hydroquinone, commonly encountered in the chemicals industry, is extensively used as a hypopigmenting or lightening agent for melasma therapy, as a photographic developer, and as a stabilizing agent. Standard dermatological textbooks imply that hydroquinone may be a common allergen. However, when the literature is critically reviewed using criteria such as appropriate controls and clinical relevance and ruling out excited skin syndrome, the current data imply that, although hydroquinone allergic contact dermatitis occurs, its frequency is low rather than high (40[R]).

Bufexamac Although their efficacy remains controversial, ointments and creams containing bufexamac (a topical non-steroidal anti-inflammatory drug) are widely used by patients with eczematous disorders as an alternative to topical corticosteroids (41[CR]). As early as 1973, the first cases of contact allergy to a cream containing 5% bufexamac were reported (42[C]). Many reports followed (SEDA-18, 163), and more recently erythema multiforme-like eruptions from contact allergy to bufexamac have been observed (43[Cr]) (SEDA-16, 155; SEDA-17, 188). To evaluate the prevalence of use of bufexamac and the rate of sensitization in a patch-test population of Austrian dermatitis patients, 504 consecutive patients were tested with bufexamac 5% pet and Parfenac® ointment, the only commercial bufexamac product in Austria. The packaging of the commercial product was shown to the entire study population, to decide whether or not they had ever used this product. A total of 30 patients (6%) agreed that they had definitely used bufexamac, and five others had probably used it. In 20 (57%) of these 35 patients there were positive and relevant patch-test reactions to bufexamac, as well as the bufexamac-containing ointment, and sensitization occurred even after short-term application. This study has shown that bufexamac has a very high sensitization rate. With a frequency of 4% of positive reactions in an unselected population of dermatitis patients, bufexamac should, according to the authors, be added to the standard series in countries with a high usage of bufexamac-containing products (41[R]).

Contact vasculitis due to topical non-steroidal anti-inflammatory drugs In recent decades, many non-steroidal anti-inflammatory drugs (NSAIDs) have been introduced as topical formulations for the treatment of acute soft tissue trauma, inflammatory and degenerative musculoskeletal disorders, and some inflammatory skin diseases. These include benzydamine, bufexamac (see above), diclofenac, etofenamic acid, ibuprofen, ibuproxam, indomethacin, ketoprofen, piroxicam, and tiaprofenic acid. Formulations containing oxyphenbutazone, phenylbutazone, and suprofen have previously been withdrawn from the market in some countries. Topical NSAIDs can cause allergic contact dermatitis (including erythema multiforme-like reactions), and also phototoxicity, photoallergic contact dermatitis, and immediate contact reactions (contact urticaria) (SEDA-18, 163).

Apparently, such formulations can also cause contact vasculitis, and seven such cases have been reported from France (44[Cr]). The mean age of the patients (four women, three men) was 39 years. The topical NSAIDs used were ketoprofen ($n = 3$), phenylbutazone ($n = 2$), and mephenesin ($n = 2$). Cutaneous lesions occurred after a mean duration of 4 days. Histological examination of skin biopsy specimens showed a leukocytoclastic vasculitis in two cases, a lymphocytic vasculitis in two cases, and a mixed vasculitis in three cases. Previous sensitization to the drug was noted in five patients, three of whom had had drug rashes from oral use. Patch tests with the drugs were positive in all cases, indicating that the reaction had been caused by contact allergy. The authors warned that there is a risk of systemic reactions when sensitized patients take the culprit drug orally.

Other contact allergens Each year 'new' allergens (i.e. chemicals that have not previously been known to cause contact allergy) are described. These allergens and updated information on chemicals already known to be sensitizers in topical drugs and cosmetics are presented in Table 3.

PHOTOSENSITIVITY *(SED-13, 393; SEDA-15, 145; SEDA-17, 187; SEDA-19, 161)*

The British Photodermatology Group has provided a concise and up-to-date summary of the methods and clinical use of photopatch testing. They recommended the following standard series of potential photoallergens: PABA, butyl methoxydibenzoylmethane, 2-ethylhexyl-*p*-methoxycinnamate, benzophenone-3, musk ambrette, and octyl dimethyl PABA. Patients' own products, diluted appropriately, should of course always be tested as well (64[r]).

Cross-reactivity of the photosensitizer ketoprofen *(SEDA-17, 187; SEDA-18, 163)* The incidence of allergic, photoallergic, and phototoxic contact dermatitis to non-steroidal anti-inflammatory drugs is increasing, due in part to the dramatic expansion in the marketing of NSAIDs. Among propionic acid derivatives, ketoprofen is one that often causes photoallergic contact dermatitis. Cross-photosensitization has been reported with ketoprofen and other topical NSAIDs and also with fenofibrate. The cross-photoreaction with fenofibrate may be due to a common benzoylketone structure, and for this reason it was suspected that ketoprofen may also photocross-react with benzophenones, UV filters that have structural similarity. To test this hypothesis, seven patients with photodermatitis from ketoprofen underwent photopatch tests with ketoprofen, fenofibrate, benzophenone-3, benzophenone-4, benzophenone-10, and personal products (65[Cr]). All had positive photopatch test reactions to ketoprofen and fenofibrate, four had positive UVA photopatch tests to benzophenone-3, and two to benzophenone-10. It was concluded that patients with photosensitization to ketoprofen may also have cross-reactivity to fenofibrate and some benzophenones, notably benzophenone-3.

Some patients may become photosensitized to ketoprofen used by their partner ('connubial' or 'consort' photodermatitis) (66[Cr]).

Contact and photocontact sensitivity to sunscreens *(SEDA-18, 174)* The 15-year experience with sunscreen allergy and photoallergy in the Department of Dermatology at the University of Göttingen has been reported and the pertinent literature reviewed (67[CR]). From 1981 to 1996, 402 patients with suspected clinical photosensitivity were patch and photopatch tested with the commercial sunscreens and the facial cosmetics that they had used, and with chemical UV absorbers, fragrance allergens, preservatives, and emollients. In all, 80 patients (20%) (28 men, 52 women), had allergic and/or photoallergic contact dermatitis to one or more UV absorber. In 47 patients with photodermatoses or photoaggravated dermatoses and in 33 subjects with normal photosensitivity, there were 91 allergic and 84 photoallergic reactions to UV filters. Over the years, sunscreens were added to the test series, which since 1989 has comprised 10 UV absorbers which induced (photo)allergic reactions (Table 4). 47 patients reacted to fragrance materials, 11 to

Table 3. *Contact allergy to ingredients of topical drugs and cosmetics*

Ingredient	Use	Conc and vehicle	No.	Comments	Ref
1,3-Butylene glycol	Moisturizer	5% water	1	No cross-reactivity to propylene glycol	(45[cr])
Chlorphenesin	Antimicrobial	1% pet	1	Uncommonly used in cosmetics	(46[cr])
Colophony	Fixative for pigments in lipstick	30% pet	1	First report of contact allergy to colophony in lipsticks	(47[cr])
Crotamiton	Antipruritic	1% and 10% pet	1	Rare contact allergen (see SEDA-15, 146)	(48[cr])
Dexpanthenol	Vitamin B5 derivative	5% pet	1	Worsening of dermatitis by oral provocation with calcium-D-pantothenate and by nutritional vitamin B5 (see SEDA-20, 158)	(49[cr])
Diethyl sebacate	Penetration enhancer; adds viscosity (see SEDA-15, 146; SEDA-16, 155: under di-isopropyl sebacate)	30% alcohol	1	30 control patients were negative	(50[cr])
2,7-Dihydroxy-naphthalene	Hair dye	0.1% water	1	First report of contact sensitization. Adequate controls performed	(51[cr])
Eumulgin® L	Emulsifier	10% pet and water	1	Eumulgin L is cetylstearyl alcohol with two added molecules of propylene oxide and nine of ethylene oxide. First report of contact allergy. Adequate controls performed	(52[cr])
Gentian violet (pyoctanin, crystal violet)	Topical antiseptic dye	0.05–0.25% water	2	Rare contact allergen	(53[cr])
Henna	Vegetable hair dye	10% pet	1	Rare allergen	(54[cr])
6β-Methyl-prednisolone	Corticosteroid	1% alcohol	1	Cross-reaction from hydroacetonate cortisone-17-butyrate. First report of contact allergy. No controls performed, but report reliable (see SEDA-21, 158)	(55[cr])
Metronidazole	Antibiotic for treatment of rosacea	1% pet	1	No cross-reactions to other imidazoles	(56[cr])
Neticonazole	Antimycotic	1% and 10% pet	1	First report of contact allergy. No controls performed, but report is reliable. Possible cross-reactions to econazole and sulconazole (see SEDA-20, 156; SEDA-21, 164)	(57[cr])
Nitrocellulose	Film former in nail lacquer	10% isopropyl alcohol	1	First well-documented case of contact allergy	(58[cr])
Octyldodecanol	Solvent	5–10% liquid paraffin	1	Rare contact allergen	(59[cr])
Oleth-3-phosphate	Opacifier, surfactant	1% pet	1	First report of contact allergy. Adequate controls performed. The patient was also allergic to the related oleth-5 (1% pet) present in the product (hair wax)	(60[cr])

Table 3. *Continued*

Ingredient	Use	Conc and vehicle	No.	Comments	Ref
Oleth-5	See under Oleth-3-phosphate				(60[cr])
Oleyl alcohol	Emulsifier, emollient	10% pet	1	Possible cross-reactions to ricinoleic acid and lanolin (see SEDA-19, 162)	(61[cr])
Propyl gallate	Antioxidant	1% pet	1		(62[cr])
Tea tree oil	Essential oil in wart paint	1% water	1	See SEDA-18, 170	(63[cr])

Table 4. *UV absorbers eliciting (photo)allergic reactions during 1981–96 (65[CR])*

Sunscreen	Contact allergy (number)	Photocontact allergy (number)
Benzophenone-3	3	9
Benzophenone-4	–	–
Butyl methoxydibenzoyl-methane	15	13
Isoamyl *p*-methoxycinnamate	4	10
Isopropyl dibenzoylmethane	30	32
4-Methylbenzylidene camphor	32	5
Octyl dimethyl PABA	1	2
Octyl methoxycinnamate	3	4
PABA	2	2
Phenylbenzimidazole sulfonic acid	1	7

preservatives, and two to lanolin alcohol. Frequent (photo)sensitization to isopropyl dibenzoylmethane was the reason that its production was discontinued in 1993. The authors concluded that clinicians should consider contact and photocontact allergy to sunscreens, especially in patients with photodermatoses and photo-aggravated dermatoses, and that they should perform photopatch testing.

MISCELLANEOUS ADVERSE REACTIONS

Calcipotriol *(SED-13, 396; SEDA-20, 157)*

Topical treatment of psoriasis with the vitamin D_3 analogues calcipotriol and the newer tacalcitol and their adverse effects have been reviewed (68[R]). With the use of doses larger than the recommended maximum of 100 g/week, a few reports have documented *hypercalcemia* and *hypercalciuria* (SED-13, 396; SEDA-8, 176).

Calcipotriol exerts its effects on systemic calcium homeostasis by increasing intestinal absorption of calcium and probably phosphate. This results in suppression of parathyroid hormone and 1,25-dihydroxycholecalciferol (69[Cr]).

Tacalcitol is currently under investigation in the treatment of psoriasis. No reliable information on the possible induction of changes in the calcium homeostasis or other adverse events is yet available (68[R]).

Nitrogen mustard

Immunological and hypersensitivity reactions Topical nitrogen mustard (mechlorethamine) is effective in the early stages of mycosis fungoides. The most common adverse reaction is an *allergic contact dermatitis* at the site of application in 30–60% of patients (70[CR]). A *local bullous reaction* has also been reported. Less commonly, *immediate urticarial or anaphylactoid reactions* have occurred. In addition, topical nitrogen mustard can act as a carcinogen or tumor promoter, as evidenced by the increased incidence of *cutaneous malignancies*; these include basal cell carcinomas, squamous cell carcinomas, and keratoacanthomas. Other adverse effects include *hyperpigmentation*, *xerosis*, and *superficial dermatophyte infections*.

Another patient developed *Stevens–Johnson syndrome* while being treated with nitrogen mustard for mycosis fungoides (70[CR]). Other possible causes were excluded. The patient may have become allergic to the topical medication. Erythema multiforme-like eruptions are sometimes caused by contact allergic reactions (SEDA-15, 145; see also under bufexamac, p. 169). Unfortunately, the authors did not perform patch tests for fear of inducing another systemic reaction.

Selenium sulfide

Hair discoloration can occur secondary to underlying diseases, drugs, or exposure to exogenous chemicals. Selenium sulfide lotion can now be added to this list (71[cr]).

A 4-year-old black girl presented with a 6-week history of generalized flaking of her scalp in association with patchy hair loss and pruritus. Potassium hydroxide examination and culture were consistent with a dermatophyte infection (*Tinea tonsurans*), and treatment with oral griseofulvin was started. Her mother was asked to shampoo her daughter's scalp with selenium sulfide 2.5% lotion three times a week to alleviate the scaling and the pruritus. Two weeks later, the girl returned with a complaint of prominent green hair discoloration. No other products had been applied to the hair or scalp, and there was no history of swimming pool exposure. Selenium sulfide lotion was discontinued, and treatment with ketoconazole 2% shampoo started. Oral griseofulvin was continued. One week later the girl's hair had returned to normal.

The mechanism of hair discoloration from selenium sulfide is unknown. Product information states that selenium sulfide lotion can cause hair discoloration, but data to substantiate this were previously unavailable.

Tar

The main drawbacks of tar are its *messiness*, *staining*, and *odor*; however, these complaints lessen with the use of modified tar formulations. The other adverse effects can be classified as *allergic*, (*photo*)*toxic*, and non-specific reactions, such as *folliculitis* and *bronchoconstriction*. Of greater concern is the possibility that tar, which contains some potent carcinogens (polycyclic aromatic hydrocarbons in crude coal tar such as benzo(*a*)pyrene, benz(*a*)anthracene and dibenz(*a*,*h*)anthracene), may be *carcinogenic*. Another concern is its potential *teratogenicity*, as has been seen in animal studies.

Topical therapy of psoriasis and other skin disorders such as atopic dermatitis with tar and its adverse effects have been reviewed (72[R]), with the following conclusions and recommendations.

(1) Coal tar is important in the treatment of (atopic) dermatitis and psoriasis. It has been extensively used for centuries and appears to be safe.

(2) However, in view of the fact that coal tar may pose a potential carcinogenic effect, as has been observed in vitro and in animals, and by the proven induction of squamous cell carcinoma in workmen chronically and extensively exposed to industrial tar, some restriction seems to be appropriate.

(3) Long-term treatment with pix lithantracis in a concentration over 5% is undesirable and not recommended.

(4) Because of its possible teratogenic effects, coal tar should be restricted to intermittent use in a low concentration on a relatively small percentage of body surface in the second and third trimesters of pregnancy only.

Obviously, these are the personal opinions of the author of this review. Many dermatologists in France, Germany, and Switzerland feel that coal tar is safe (73). Nevertheless, in certain countries (e.g. Holland, Germany, and Switzerland) health authorities have banned the use of coal tar in consumer products, notably shampoos that were until recently available over the counter.

REFERENCES

1. De Groot AC, Weijland JW. Conversion of common names of cosmetic allergens to the INCI nomenclature. Contact Dermatitis 1997; 37: 145–50.
2. Dillarstone A. Letter to the Editor. Contact Dermatitis 1996;35:64–5.
3. De Groot AC. Labeling cosmetics with their ingredients. Br Med J 1990;300:1636–8.
4. De Groot AC, White IR. Cosmetic ingredient labeling in the European Community. Contact Dermatitis 1991;25:273–5.
5. De Groot AC, Weijland JW, Nater JP. Unwanted Effects of Cosmetics and Drugs Used in Dermatology, 3rd ed. Amsterdam: Elsevier, 1994.
6. De Groot AC, Frosch PJ. Adverse reactions to fragrances: a clinical review. Contact Dermatitis 1997;36:57–86.
7. Lowe NJ, Chizhevsky V, Gabriel H. Photo-(chemo)therapy: general principles. Clin Dermatol 1997;15:745–52.
8. Laurahanta J. Photochemotherapy. Clin Dermatol 1997;15:769–80.
9. Grimes PE. Psoralen photochemotherapy for vitiligo. Clin Dermatol 1997;15:921–6.
10. Morison WL, Marwaha S, Beck L. PUVA-induced phototoxicity: incidence and causes. J Am Acad Dermatol 1997;36:183–5.
11. Puig L. Pharmacodynamic interaction with phototoxic plants during PUVA therapy. Br J Dermatol 1997;136:973–4.
12. Halcin C, Hann S-K, Kauh YC. Vitiligo following the resolution of psoriatic plaques during PUVA therapy. Int J Dermatol 1997;36:534–6.
13. Olsen JH, Moller H, Frentz G. Malignant tumors in patients with psoriasis. J Am Acad Dermatol 1992;27:716–22.
14. Stern RS, Laird N, members of the Photochemotherapy Follow-up Study. The carcinogenic risk of treatments for severe psoriasis. Cancer 1994;73:2759–64.
15. Stern RS, Vakeva LH, and the PUVA Follow-up Study. Noncutaneous malignant tumors in the PUVA follow-up study: 1975–1996. J Invest Dermatol 1997;108:897–900.
16. Alcalay J, Bucana C, Kripke ML. Cutaneous pigmented melanocytic tumor in a mouse treated with psoralen plus ultraviolet A radiation. Photodermatol Photoimmunol Photomed 1990;7:28–31.
17. Aubin F, Donawho CK, Kripke ML. Effect of psoralen plus ultraviolet A radiation on in vivo growth of melanoma cells. Cancer Res 1991; 51:5893–7.
18. Swerdlow AJ, Weinstock MA. Do tanning lamps cause melanoma? An epidemiological assessment. J Am Acad Dermatol 1998;38:89–98.
19. Stern RS, Nichols KT, Vakeva LH, for the PUVA Follow-up Study. Malignant melanoma in patients treated for psoriasis with methoxsalen (psoralen) and ultraviolet A radiation (PUVA). New Engl J Med 1997;336:1041–5.
20. Wolff K. Should PUVA be abandoned? New Engl J Med 1997;336:1090–1.
21. Morison WL, Baughman RD, Day RM, Forbes PD, Hoenigsmann H, Krueger GG, Lebwohl M, Lew R, Naldi L, Parrish JA, Piepkorn M, Stern RS, Weinstein GD, Whitmore SE. Consensus workshop on the toxic effects of long-term PUVA therapy. Arch Dermatol 1998;134:595–8.
22. Gollnick HPM, Dummler U. Retinoids. Clin Dermatol 1997;15:799–810.
23. Cunliffe WJ, van de Kerkhof PCM, Caputo R, Cavicchini S, Cooper A, Fyrand OL, Gollnick H, Layton AM, Leyden JJ, Mascaró J-M, Ortonne J-P, Shalita A. Roaccutane treatment guidelines: results of an international survey. Dermatology 1997;194:351–7.
24. Horber FF, Zimmermann A, Frey FJ. Impaired renal function and hypercalcaemia associated with etretinate. Lancet 1984;i:1093.
25. Cribier B, Welsch M, Heid E. Renal impairment probably induced by etretinate. Dermatology 1992;185:266–8.
26. Pavese P, Kuentz F, Belleville C, Rougé P-E, Elsener M. Renal impairment induced by isotretinoin. Nephrol Dial Transplant 1997;12:1299.
27. Chochrad D, Langhendries J-P, Stolear J-C, Godin J. Isotretinoin-induced vasculitis imitating polyarteritis nodosa, with perinuclear antineutrophil cytoplasmic antibody in titers correlated with clinical symptoms. Rev Rhum Engl Ed 1997; 64:129–31.
28. Woollons A, Price ML. Roaccutane and wax epilation: a cautionary tale. Br J Dermatol 1997;137:839–40.
29. Meigel WN. How safe is oral isotretinoin? Dermatology 1997;195 (Suppl 1):22–8.
30. Cunliffe WJ, Stables A. Optimum use of isotretinoin. J Cutaneous Med Surg 1996;1 (Suppl):2–20.
31. De Groot AC. Cosmetic dermatitis. Clin Dermatol 1997;15:485–92.
32. Gruvberger B, Bruze M. Preservatives. Clin Dermatol 1997;15:493–8.
33. Nethercott JR, Larsen WG. Fragrances. Clin Dermatol 1997;15:499–504.
34. Guin JD, Kincannon J. Medication-induced contact reactions. Clin Dermatol 1997;15:511–26.
35. Isaksson M, Dooms-Goossens A. Corticosteroids. Clin Dermatol 1997;15:527–32.
36. Ebihara T, Nakayama H. Pigmented contact dermatitis. Clin Dermatol 1997;15:593–600.
37. Hannuksela M. Mechanisms in contact urticaria. Clin Dermatol 1997;15:619–22.
38. Warner MR, Taylor JS, Leow Y-H. Agents causing contact urticaria. Clin Dermatol 1997; 15:623–36.
39. Schnuch A. Zimtaldehyd. Dermatosen Beruf Umwelt 1997;45:281–3.
40. Dalloo D, Makar S, Maibach HI. Hydroquinone as a contact allergen. Dermatosen Beruf Umwelt 1997;45:208–10.

41. Kranke B, Szolar-Platzer C, Komericki P, Derhaschnig J, Aberer W. Epidemiological significance of bufexamac as a frequent and relevant contact sensitizer. Contact Dermatitis 1997; 36:212–15.
42. Achten G, Bourlond A, Haven E, Lapière CM, Piérard J, Reynaers H. Étude du bufexamac crème et du bufexamac onguent dans le traitement de diverse dermatoses. Dermatologica 1973; 146:1–7.
43. Koch P, Bahmer FA. Erythema multiforme-like, urticarial papular and plaque eruptions from bufexamax: report of 4 cases. Contact Dermatitis 1994;31:97–101.
44. Delbarre M, Joly P, Balguerie X, Thomine E, Lauret Ph. Vasculites de contact aux topiques contenant des anti-inflammatoires non steroidiens ou des antalgiques. Ann Dermatol Venereol 1997;124:841–4.
45. Sugiura M, Hayakawa R. Contact dermatitis due to 1,3-butylene glycol. Contact Dermatitis 1997;37:90.
46. Wakelin SH, White IR. Dermatitis from chlorphenesin in a facial cosmetic. Contact Dermatitis 1997;37:138–9.
47. Batta K, Bourke JF, Foulds IS. Allergic contact dermatitis from colophony in lipsticks. Contact Dermatitis 1997;36:171–2.
48. Kawada A, Hiruma M, Fujioka A, Tajima S, Akiyama M, Ishibashi A. Simultaneous contact sensitivity due to lidocaine and crotamiton. Contact Dermatitis 1997;37:45.
49. Hemmer W, Bracun R, Wolf-Abdolvahab S, Focke M, Gotz M, Jarisch R. Maitenance of hand eczema by oral panthotenic acid in a patient sensitized to dexpanthenol. Contact Dermatitis 1997; 37:51.
50. Sasaki E, Hata M, Aramaki J, Honda M. Allergic contact dermatitis due to diethyl sebacate. Contact Dermatitis 1997;36:172.
51. Eskelinen A, Molitor C, Kanerva L. Allergic contact dermatitis from 2,7-dihydroxynaphthalene in hair dye. Contact Dermatitis 1997; 36:312–13.
52. Corazza M, Lombardi AR, Virgili A. Non-eczematous urticarioid allergic contact dermatitis due to Eumulgin® in a deodorant. Contact Dermatitis 1997;36:159–60.
53. Schoppelrey H-P, Mily H, Agathos M, Breit R. Allergic contact dermatitis from pyoctanin. Contact Dermatitis 1997;36:221–4.
54. Garcia Ortez JC, Terron M, Bellido J. Contact allergy to henna. Int Arch Allergy Immunol 1997;114:298–9.
55. Balato N, Patruno C, Lembo G, Cuccurullo FM, Ayala F. Contact sensitization to 6 alpha-methylprednisolone aceponate. Am J Contact Dermatitis 1997;8:24–5.
56. Voncenzi C, Lucente P, Ricci C, Tosti A. Facial contact dermatitis due to metronidazole. Contact Dermatitis 1997;36:116–17.
57. Kawada A, Hiruma M, Fujioka A, Tajima S, Ishibashi A, Kawada I. Contact dermatitis from netilconazole. Contact Dermatitis 1997;36:106–7.
58. Castelain M, Veyrat S, Laine G, Montastier C. Contact dermatitis from nitrocellulose in a nail varnish. Contact Dermatitis 1997;36:266–7.
59. Dharmagunawardena B, Charles-Holmes R. Contact dermatitis due to octyldodecanol in clotrimazole cream. Contact Dermatitis 1997;36:231.
60. Abdullah A, Walker S, Tan CY, Foulds IS. Sensitization to oleth-3-phosphate and oleth-5 in a hair wax. Contact Dermatitis 1997;37:188.
61. Tan BB, Noble AL, Roberts ME, Lear JT, English JSC. Allergic contact dermatitis from oleyl alcohol in lipstick cross-reacting with ricinoleic acid in castor oil and lanolin. Contact Dermatitis 1997;37:41–2.
62. Hernandez N, Assier-Bonnet H, Terki N, Revuz J. Allergic contact dermatitis from propyl gallate in desonide cream (Locapred®). Contact Dermatitis 1997;36:111.
63. Bhushan M, Beck MH. Allergic contact dermatitis from tea tree oil in a wart paint. Contact Dermatitis 1997;36:117–18.
64. British Photodermatology Group. Workshop report. Photopatch testing: methods and indications. Br J Dermatol 1997;136:371–6.
65. Leroy D, Dompmartin A, Szczurko C, Michel M, Louvet S. Photodermatitis from ketoprofen with cross-reactivity to fenofibrate and benzophenones. Photodermatol Photoimmunol Photomed 1997;13:93–7.
66. Mirande-Romero A, Gonzalez-Lopez A, Esquivias JI, Bajo C, García-Munoz M. Ketoprofen-induced connubial photodermatitis. Contact Dermatitis 1997;37:242.
67. Schauder S, Ippen H. Contact and photocontact sensitivity to sunscreens. Review of a 15-year experience and of the literature. Contact Dermatitis 1997;37:221–32.
68. Fogh K, Kragballe K. Vitamin D3 analogues. Clin Dermatol 1997;15:705–13.
69. Bourke JF, Mumford R, Whittaker P, Iqbal SJ, Le Van LW, Trevellyan A, Hutchinson PE. The effect of topical calcipotriol on systemic calcium homeostasis in patients with chronic plaque psoriasis. J Am Acad Dermatol 1997;37:929–34.
70. Newman JM, Rindler JM, Bergfeld WF, Bryan IK. Stevens-Johnson syndrome associated with topical nitrogen mustard. J Am Acad Dermatol 1997;36:112–4.
71. Fitzgerald EA, Purcell SM, Goldman HM. Green hair discoloration due to selenium sulfide. Int J Dermatol 1997;36:238–9.
72. Arnold WP. Tar. Clin Dermatol 1997;15:739–44.
73. Plantin P. Should coal tar be forbidden? Ann Dermatol Venereol 1997;124:205–7.

Anthony N. Nicholson

15 Antihistamines

R *Antihistamines and cardiac dysrhythmias*

For many years it was accepted that antihistamines were among the safest drugs in the world, and their enviable reputation was further enhanced by the development of drugs free of adverse effects on vigilance and performance, and free of anticholinergic activity. However, cardiotoxicity has become a prominent issue with antihistamines that have been introduced in the past few years. Intentional overdoses of terfenadine or astemizole have led to prolongation of the QT_c interval with ventricular dysrhythmias similar to those seen with quinidine. There is no correlation between antihistaminic potency, and there is little, if any, possibility that cardiotoxicity may in some circumstances or with some compounds be due to blockade of H_1 receptors.

Mechanism *The cellular event leading to dysrhythmias is blockade of the delayed rectifier potassium current, although the involvement of other channels cannot be excluded. Certainly, terfenadine is a potent blocker of the myocardial potassium channels that control the QT_c interval, and patients with dysrhythmias associated with terfenadine have high plasma concentrations of the parent compound, because of overdosage, inhibition of metabolism, or hepatic insufficiency.*

Risk factors *Inhibition of metabolism is a particularly important issue (1[R]), and some individuals may even be poor metabolizers. Terfenadine is normally rapidly metabolized by the P450 enzyme CYP3A4 to fexofenadine, which has negligible cardiac effects, while astemizole is similarly metabolized to desmethylastemizole and norastemizole, though these metabolites may not be free of the potential to prolong the QT_c interval. Inhibitors of CYP3A4 include the antifungals, ketoconazole, itraconazole, and terbinafine, the macrolide antibiotics erythromycin, clarithromycin, and troleandomycin, the azalide antibiotic azithromycin, 6,7-dihydroxybergamottin (an active principle of the flavonoids of grapefruit juice), and ethinylestradiol. Many antidepressants, particularly serotonin reuptake inhibitors (SSRIs), have affinity for CYP3A4 and should therefore be used with caution. Cimetidine and ranitidine also inhibit CYP3A4. Caution must be exercised with any drug that inhibits CYP3A4 and raises the plasma concentration of the parent antihistamine or its metabolite, even if clinical trials, inevitably of limited prognostic value, do not reveal cardiac effects.*

Caution must also be exercised in the use of antihistamines in patients with congenital prolongation of the QT_c interval, bradycardia, ischemic heart disease, congestive cardiac failure, electrolyte changes (especially hypokalemia), and drugs that prolong the QT_c interval, such as quinidine. Essentially, all potential H_1-antihistamines must be screened for cardiotoxicity, as some patients may be susceptible to plasma concentrations near to the therapeutic target range. Furthermore, it is in patients who may be peculiarly susceptible to antihistamines that raised plasma concentrations can be particularly relevant.

Interactions *Antifungal imidazoles A 36-year-old woman who took terfenadine 120 mg/day for hay fever and itraconazole 100 mg bd for mycosis had several episodes of syncope with a prolonged QT_c interval (2[C]).*

Plasma concentrations of astemizole and desmethylastemizole and the QT_c interval were measured after ingestion of 10 mg astemizole in male volunteers taking itraconazole 200 mg bd for 11 days (3[C]). Astemizole clearance was reduced, and hypokalaemia was observed in

Side Effects of Drugs, Annual 22
J.K. Aronson, ed.

one volunteer. The QT_c interval was not altered by itraconazole or within 24 h of the addition of astemizole. There was no evidence of cardiotoxicity in these studies, but the reduction in astemizole clearance and hypokalemia in one volunteer suggest a cautious approach to the use of itraconazole with astemizole.

QT_c intervals were measured after 7 days of ketoconazole (200 mg bd) either alone or after azelastine (4.4 mg bd for 14 days) (4[C]). There were no changes in QT_c interval. This suggests that there is no pharmacokinetic interaction between azelastine and ketoconazole, and that azelastine can be given with CYP3A4 inhibitors. However, it is essential to confirm the absence of a pharmacokinetic interaction, as raised plasma concentrations, even in the absence of evidence of cardiac effects in a clinical trial, would suggest a cautious approach.

Macrolide antibiotics *Erythromycin inhibits the metabolism of the newer antihistamines, although dirythromycin, a metabolite of erythromycin, may be less of a problem. Astemizole 30 mg was given to healthy young adults who had taken dirythromycin 500 mg/day for 4 days (5[C]). The half-life of astemizole was prolonged but the clearance of desmethylastemizole was unchanged. There was no evidence of an adverse change in QT_c intervals during dirythromycin administration for up to 12 h after astemizole. However, there were substantial between-subject differences in the pharmacokinetic data, and this observation, together with reduced clearance of the parent compound, suggest that caution should be exercised in the co-administration of astemizole with dirythromycin. On the other hand, dirythromycin appears to have no significant effects on the pharmacokinetics of terfenadine (6[C]).*

Use in pregnancy Antihistamines are generally contraindicated during pregnancy, essentially because of lack of relevant data. However, they are used and not infrequently. An important question is the preferred antihistamine for pregnancy, and opinions differ. Many years of clinical use and reassuring animal studies have suggested that chlorpheniramine, introduced in the 1940s, is safe during pregnancy. Certainly, caution should be exercised with the second-generation, non-sedating compounds.

In a prospective controlled study (7[C]) 120 women were studied after exposure to either hydroxyzine ($n = 53$) or to cetirizine, its active carboxylic acid metabolite ($n = 39$), during the first trimester of pregnancy. There were no significant differences in the rates of live births, spontaneous or therapeutic abortions, or stillbirths between women who had taken hydroxyzine or cetirizine and a control group of pregnant women (matched for age, smoking, and alcohol consumption) who had been exposed to non-teratogenic drugs. There were also no differences in the rate of anomalies, mean birth rates, mode of delivery, gestational ages or neonatal distress. The authors concluded that neither hydroxyzine nor cetirizine increases the risk of major malformations, even when used during the period of organogenesis, and that pregnant women with significant allergic symptoms should probably not be denied these drugs.

In another prospective study (8[r]) similar end-points were used in 114 women taking astemizole (10 mg/day) during pregnancy. There were more pregnancies with astemizole than in the matched control group, but there was no evidence of an increase in the rate of major malformations, which remained well within the expected rate for the population. The authors concluded that although further investigation was necessary to determine the absolute risk to the fetus, the results suggested that astemizole was safe during pregnancy.

However, in both studies the samples may not have been large enough to provide adequate statistical power or to establish the true incidence of individual malformations. Indeed, the author of an editorial comment on the study of hydroxyzine and cetirizine (9[R]) was unable to accept the recommendations and concluded that brompheniramine and hydroxyzine had some risk, and that chlorpheniramine was the preferred antihistamine for use during pregnancy. It could be added that if there is some risk with hydroxyzine, caution should also be exercised with cetirizine, its metabolite. Although there is the advantage of lack of sedation with the second-generation antihistamines, the editorial still preferred chlorpheniramine, as there is much less clinical experience in the use of second-generation antihistamines during pregnancy.

INDIVIDUAL H_1-ANTIHISTAMINES

Astemizole *(SED-13, 417; SEDA-18, 183; SEDA-19, 170; SEDA-20, 162)*

A woman who had taken astemizole 10 mg/day for 10 months developed syncope 60 min after taking quinine sulfate 260 mg (10[c]). Quinine is a substrate of CYP3A4 (11), and although the case was complicated by the fact that she was also taking alprazolam (a substrate of CYP3A4) and fluoxetine (an inhibitor of CYP3A4), clearly a combination of the known effects of quinine on the QTc interval (12[C]) and inhibition of the clearance of astemizole could have caused this effect.

Azelastine *(SED-13, 417; SEDA-20, 162; SEDA-21, 172)*

Azelastine is an antihistamine that also inhibits histamine release from mast cells and the action or release of leukotrienes. It is given as an intranasal spray for perennial rhinitis, to alleviate symptoms in the nose, eyes, and throat. Its most common adverse effects are *pharyngitis*, *cough*, and *bronchitis*. In a patient with bronchial asthma and epilepsy an *epileptic seizure* was attributed to a single dose of azelastine (4 mg) (13[c]).

Cetirizine *(SEDA-21, 172)*

Skin reactions have been reported with cetirizine (14[C]) and a probable interaction with *acenocoumarol*, with increased anticoagulant activity (15[c]). There is no evidence that cetirizine prolongs the QT_c interval or causes cardiac dysrhythmias, and there is no evidence of an interaction with erythromycin.

Cinnarizine and flunarizine *(SED-13, 417, 537; SEDA-20, 191; see also Chapter 19)*

Drug-induced *parkinsonism* occurs mainly in psychotic patients after exposure to neuroleptics, but it can also be caused by cinnarizine and flunarizine. The natural course of drug-induced parkinsonism was followed in elderly patients exposed to one or other of these drugs for an average of 7 months (16[C]). Clinical assessments were carried out for 7 years after withdrawal and none of the patients had full recovery of extrapyramidal signs.

Blepharospasm has been attributed to flunarizine in an elderly woman (17[c]). *Insomnia* has also been reported in association with flunarizine (18[c]).

Diphenhydramine *(SEDA-21, 174)*

Central effects of diphenhydramine (19[C]) include *agitation* on intravenous injection (20[C]), *cognitive impairment* in the elderly (21[C]) and *psychosis* (22[c]).

Hydroxyzine *(SEDA-17, 201)*

Skin reactions have been recorded with hydroxyzine. Four children with restlessness who were treated with hydroxyzine hydrochloride developed *fixed drug eruptions of the penis*; drug withdrawal was followed by complete resolution (23[C]). In three patients with urticaria and atopic dermatitis, hydroxyzine caused *generalized maculopapular eruptions* associated with positive patch tests but no evidence of cross-allergy to ethylenediamine, piperazine, or other antihistamines (24[C]). In another case *contact dermatitis* occurred with hydroxyzine in a patient who was patch tested positive to ethylenediamine (25[c]).

Loratadine *(SEDA-19, 174)*

The performance of male subjects on various tasks considered to be relevant to air-crew were studied after the administration of loratadine 10 mg in a hypobaric environment (simulated altitude of 8000 ft) with arterial saturations of 89–93% (26[C]). The study included an active control (triprolidine 5 mg) and placebo. There were no significant effects of loratadine on performance compared with placebo, but triprolidine had detrimental effects on both subjective and objective measures.

Mequitazine *(SED-13, 417)*

Syncopal attacks due to *cardiac dysrhythmias* in a 21-year-old woman with congenital prolongation of the QT_c interval have been attributed to the simultaneous ingestion of mequitazine and spiramycin over 48 h (27[c]).

Terfenadine *(SED-13, 417; SEDA-19, 176; SEDA 20, 163; SEDA-21, 177)*

Skin and appendages Adverse drug reactions reported to the Norwegian Medicine Control Authority from 1970 to 1994 included five cases of *photosensitivity* related to terfenadine (28[r]).

Interactions Healthy volunteers took terfenadine 120 mg 30 min after drinking 300 ml of freshly squeezed *grapefruit juice* (29[C]). The AUC and C_{max} of terfenadine were increased by the concomitant administration of grapefruit juice, but there was no change in the QT_c interval. Although the increase in the systemic availability of terfenadine did not lead to evidence of cardiotoxicity in these healthy subjects, it is not possible to exclude a cardiotoxic effect of the concomitant administration of terfenadine and grapefruit juice in individuals with risk factors, and it is therefore prudent to avoid such a combination.

Zileuton is a 5-lipoxygenase inhibitor, and inhibition of the production of leukotrienes has potential therapeutic benefits in asthma. Healthy volunteers took terfenadine 60 mg bd on days 1–7 and zileuton 600 mg 6-hourly on days 1–10 (30[C]). Co-administration resulted in a small increase in the AUC and C_{max} of terfenadine and of carboxyterfenadine, suggesting some inhibitory effect on metabolism, but there were no changes in the QT_c interval. These results suggest a minimal interaction.

Healthy men were given two single doses of terfenadine (60 mg) after an eighth dose of *fluoxetine* 60 mg/day (31[C]). There was no evidence that fluoxetine inhibited the metabolism of terfenadine. Fluoxetine is an inhibitor of CYP3A4, but it appears that a clinically relevant drug–drug interaction is unlikely. This conclusion is also likely to hold for astemizole.

REFERENCES

1. Zhang M-Q. Chemistry underlying the cardiotoxicity of antihistamines. Curr Med Chem 1997;4:171–84.
2. Romkes JH, Froger CL, Wever EFD, Westerhof PW. Wegrakingen tijdens simultaan gebruik van terfenadine en itraconazol. [Syncope during simultaneous use of terfenedine and itraconazole.] Ned Tijdschr Geneeskd 1997;141:950–3.
3. Lefebvre RA, Van Peer A Woestenborghs R. Influence of itraconazole on the pharmacokinetics and electrocardiographic effects of astemizole. Br J Clin Pharmacol 1997;43:319–22.
4. Morganroth J, Lyness WH, Perhach JL, Mather GG, Harr JE, Trager WF, Levy RH. Rosenberg A. Lack of effect of azelastine and ketoconazole co-administration on electrocardiographic parameters in healthy volunteers. J Clin Pharmacol 1997;37:1065–72.
5. Bachmann K, Sullivan TJ, Reese JH, Jauregui L, Miller K, Scott M, Stotka J, Harris J. A study of the interaction between dirythromycin and astemizole in healthy adults. Am J Ther 1997;4:73–9.
6. Watkins VS, Polk RE, Stotka JL. Drug interactions of macrolides: emphasis on dirythromycin. Ann Pharmacother 1997;31:349–56.
7. Einarson A, Bailey B, Jung G, Spizzirri D, Baillie M, Koren G. Prospective controlled study of hydroxyzine and cetirizine in pregnancy. Ann Allergy Asthma Immunol 1997;78:183–6.
8. Mazzotta P, Koren G. Non sedating antihistamines in pregnancy: considering astemizole. Can Fam Phys 1997;43:1509–11.
9. Schatz M, Pettiti D. Antihistamines and pregnancy. Ann Allergy Asthma Immunol 1997; 78:157–9.
10. Martin ES, Rogalski K, Black JN. Quinine may trigger torsades de pointes during astemizole therapy. PACE 1997;20:2024–5.
11. Zhao XJ, Ishizaki T. The in vitro hepatic met-

abolism of quinine in mice, rats and dogs: comparison with human liver microsomes. J Pharmacol Exp Ther 1997;283:1168–76.
12. Karbwang J, Davis TM, Looareesuwan S, Molunto P, Bunnag D, White NJ. A comparison of the pharmacokinetic and pharmacodynamic properties of quinine and quinidine in healthy Thai males. Br J Clin Pharmacol 1993;35:265–71.
13. Watanabe H, Imai M, Ling M, Sugihara N, Ohtami S, Hayakawa, Miura H, Kawai S, Kobayashi H. Epileptic seizure most probably caused by azelastine treatment in a patient with bronchial asthma and genuine epilepsy [original in Japanese]. Jpn J Allergol 1997;46:605–8.
14. Stingeni L, Caraffini S, Agostinelli D, Ricci F, Lisi P. Maculopapular and urticarial eruption from cetirizine. Contact Dermatitis 1997;37:249–50.
15. Berod T, Mathiot I. Probable interaction between cetirizine and acenocoumarol. Ann Pharmacother 1997;31:122.
16. Negrotti A, Calzetti S. A long-term follow-up study of cinnarizine- and flunarizine-induced parkinsonism. Mov Disod 1997;12:107–10.
17. Koukoulis A, Herrero JS, Gomez-Alonso J. Blepharospasm induced by flunarizine. J Neurol Neurosurg Psychiatry 1997;63:412–13.
18. Pradalier A, Vincent D. Insomnia induced by flunarizine. Thérapie 1997;52:81–2.
19. Kay GG, Berman B, Mockoviak SH, Morris CE, Reeves D, Starbuck V, Sukenik E, Harris AG. Initial and steady-state effects of diphenyhydramine and loratadine on sedation, cognition, mood, and psychomotor performance. Arch Intern Med 1997;157:2350–6.
20. Cheng KL, Dwyer PN, Amsden GW. Paradoxic excitation with diphenhydramine in an adult. Pharmacotherapy 1997;17:1311–14.
21. Sands L, Katz IR, DiFilippo S, D'Angelo, K, Boyce A, Cooper T. Identification of drug-related cognitive impairment in older individuals. Am J Geriatr Psychiatry 1997;5:156–66.
22. Sexton JD, Pronchik DJ. Diphenhydramine-induced psychosis with therapeutic doses. Am J Emerg Med 1997;15:548–9.
23. Cohen HA, Barzilai A, Matalon A, Harel L, Gross S. Fixed drug eruption of the penis due to hydroxyzine hydrochloride. Ann Pharmacother 1997;31:327–9.
24. Michel M, Dompmartin A, Louvet S, Szczurko C, Castel B, Leroy D. Skin reactions to hydroxyzine. Contact Dermatitis 1997;36:147–9.
25. Ash S, Scheman AJ. Systemic contact dermatitis to hydroxyzine. Am J Contact Dermatitis 1997;8:2–5.
26. Valk PJL, Simons RM, Stryvenberg PA, Kruit H, van Berge MT. Effects of a single dose of loratadine on flying ability under conditions of simulated cabin pressure. Am J Rhinol 1997; 11:27–33.
27. Verdun F, Mansourati J, Jobic Y, Bouquin V, Munier S, Guillo P, Pagès Y, Boschat J, Blanc J-J. Torsades de pointes sous traitement par spiramycine et méquitazine. A propos d'un cas. Arch Mal Coeur Vass 1997;90:103–6.
28. Selvaag E. Clinical drug photosensitivity. A retrospective analysis of reports to the Norwegian Adverse Drug Reactions Committee from the years 1970–1994. Photodermatol Photoimmunol Photomed 1997;13:21–3.
29. Clifford CP, Adams DA, Murray S, Taylor GW, Wilkins MR, Boobis AR, Davies DS. The cardiac effects of terfenedine after inhibition of its metabolism by grapefruit juice. Eur J Clin Pharmacol 1997;52:311–15.
30. Awni WM, Cavanagh JH, Leese P, Kasier J, Coa G, Locke CS, Dube LM. The pharmacokinetic and pharmacodynamic interaction between zileuton and terfenedine. Eur J Clin Pharmacol 1997;52:49–54.
31. Bergstrom RF, Goldberg MJ, Cerimele BJ, Hatcher BL. Assessment of the potential for a pharmacokinetic interaction between fluoxetine and terfenadine. Clin Pharmacol Ther 1997; 62:643–51.

J.W. Paterson and K.M. Lulich

16 Drugs acting on the respiratory tract

INHALER PROPELLANTS

We have previously discussed the phasing out of chlorofluorocarbon (CFC) gases as propellants for pressurized multidose aerosols (SED-13, 427). Ventolin® contains the propellants CFC 11 and CFC 12. Proventil-HFA® contains instead the hydrofluorocarbon propellant HFA-134a. The efficacy and safety of HFA-134a has been confirmed in 565 patients, aged 18–65 years, studied for 12 weeks in 33 centers across the USA (1[C]), (2[C]). The subjects were randomly allocated to salbutamol (Proventil-HFA; $n = 193$), salbutamol (Ventolin Rotacaps with Rotahaler; $n = 186$), or placebo (HFA-134a alone; $n = 186$). Randomization was stratified so that half the patients in each group were taking inhaled corticosteroids. They all had at least a 12-month history of asthma requiring inhaled β_2-agonists for symptom relief. Asthma had been stable for 1 month before the study. Inhaled bronchodilators were withheld for 8 h and theophylline for 24 h before lung function testing. Baseline FEV_1 was 40–80% of predicted and increased by at least 15% within 30 min of inhaling 200 μg of Ventolin. At weeks 0, 4, 8, and 12 spirometry was performed before and serially over 6 h after dosing.

There were no significant differences between Proventil-HFA and Ventolin for FEV_1 at any time; the average peak changes in FEV_1 were 32 and 33%, respectively. Proventil-HFA had a similar safety profile to Ventolin during regular use. A dosage of 16 puffs (4 puffs qds) of the propellant HFA-134a was well tolerated. Regular use of either Proventil-HFA or Ventolin did not cause asthma to deteriorate.

Mean changes in heart rate over 6 h after dosing were between −1.6 and +0.5 beats/min on any test day. When all test days were examined, only 12 (6%), eight (4%), and 23 (12%) of the patients had a greater than 20 beats/min increase in heart rate at any time over the 6 h after dosing with Proventil-HFA, Ventolin, and HFA-134a placebo, respectively. Mean changes in systolic blood pressure over 6 h after dosing were between −2.0 and +0.9 mmHg. When all test days were examined, there were only 42 patients who had a greater than 20 mmHg increase over the 6 h after dosing with Proventil-HFA (15), Ventolin (13), and HFA-134a placebo (14), respectively. Similar trends were found for diastolic blood pressure. Full blood counts, serum biochemistry, and urine analysis were carried out at the start and end of the study and were unchanged.

All adverse events reported by patients at twice-weekly visits were recorded. Adverse events were reported by 172 (89%) patients who took Proventil-HFA, 160 (86%) in those who took Ventolin, and 153 (82%) in those who used HFA-134a placebo. The most frequent events were *headache* (163 patients), *an acute attack of asthma* (133), *upper respiratory tract infection* (111), *increased asthma symptoms* (98), and *rhinitis* (97). However, similar numbers of adverse events were attributed to the study drug in each treatment group; Proventil-HFA 71 (37%), Ventolin 68 (37%), and HFA-134a alone 63 (34%).

Proventil-HFA has been compared with Proventil and Ventolin in a randomized, single-blind, placebo-controlled, four-period, crossover study in 20 men with documented exercise-induced bronchoconstriction (3[C]). On each occasion two puffs of the aerosol were self-administered 30 min before exer-

Side Effects of Drugs, Annual 22
J.K. Aronson, ed.

cise. The Proventil-HFA provided protection against exercise-induced bronchoconstriction comparable to Ventolin and Proventil and superior to placebo. Changes in heart rate, blood pressure, and QT interval were similar with the three active treatments.

DRUGS USED IN ASTHMA

INHALED CORTICOSTEROIDS

(SED-13, 428; SEDA-19, 181; SEDA-20, 169; SEDA-21, 187)

The type of delivery device for inhaled corticosteroids can alter the delivered dose. Large-volume spacers enhance lung delivery and reduce oropharyngeal deposition; hence, the dose of inhaled steroid may be lowered.

Beclomethasone dipropionate is dispensed from a pressurized multidose inhaler (MDI). A new multidose powder inhaler, MDPI (Easyhaler Orion, Pharma Finland), which delivers 500 μg per puff, has recently been compared with a beclomethasone pressurized MDI with a large-volume spacer (4[C]). Asthmatics ($n = 148$) taking 800–1000 μg of inhaled steroid were recruited for the 12-week study; 74 used the MDPI and 74 the pressurized MDI and spacer. The dose of beclomethasone was 500 μg bd. Correct inhalation technique was taught and checked at each visit. After inhalation the mouth was thoroughly rinsed with water.

There was no difference between the two delivery systems in therapeutic efficacy, as judged by the scoring of symptoms, home PEFR measurements, clinic spirometry, rescue medication with inhaled β_2-agonists, or the need for oral corticosteroids. *Hoarseness* was reported by 17 of the patients who used the MDPI and nine of the patients who used the pressurized MDI plus spacer; *sore throat* occurred in seven (9%) and three (4%), respectively. The mean morning serum cortisol concentration did not differ between the two groups. Visually detected *thrush* occurred in three of those who used the MDPI and three of those who used the pressurized MDI. Mouth rinsing reduces local effects, such as *Candida* infection, which was uncommon in this study. It also reduces systemic absorption and protects against systemic adverse effects. The multidose powder inhaler of beclomethasone dipropionate is clearly as effective and well tolerated as the pressurized multidose aerosol.

Adverse effects of corticosteroids on bone R

Studies of the effects of inhaled corticosteroids on bone density and metabolism have been reviewed (5[R]).

Investigative techniques *Biochemical markers of bone metabolism have often been measured as potential indicators of changes in bone resorption and formation. In population studies, hydroxyproline, calcium, and pyridinyline cross-links are markers of bone resorption, and osteocalcin, alkaline phosphatase, and procollagen peptides are markers of bone formation. These markers may have a role in indicating short-term changes in bone metabolism when they are measured sequentially. There is considerable interindividual variation in each marker, and so in population studies they have been poor predictors of the risk of osteoporosis. In long-term studies there appear to be compensatory mechanisms, and the clinical implications of short-term changes are unclear. Osteocalcin is a 49-amino acid protein produced by osteoblasts, and 10–30% of it enters the circulation. In the past, assays have proved difficult, with poor comparability between centers. Two other potentially important markers are PICP (procollagen type 1 carboxy-terminal propeptide), and ICTP (type 1 collagen carboxy-terminal telopeptide). PICP is formed during the conversion of procollagen to collagen and is a measure of bone formation. ICTP is a breakdown product of collagen and is a measure of bone resorption.*

Several techniques are used to measure bone density. Cortical bone can be assessed in peripheral sites by single-photon absorptiometry (SPA), and a combination of cortical and trabecular bone in central sites by dual X-ray absorptiometry (DXA). Trabecular bone can be assessed by quantitative computer tomography scanning of the lumbar spine. Since SPA and DXA give a negligible dose of radiation, they are useful both for population screening and for providing data on the fracture risk in an individual patient. However, these two techniques are not sensitive enough to show subtle changes in bone density over a shorter and more easily assessable time-frame. Quantitative computer tomography (QCT) gives a significant dose of radiation (of the order of one-tenth of a lateral X-ray of the spine) but can focus on trabecular bone, which has a 10-fold increase in turnover compared with cortical bone. QCT is more sensitive to changing bone density over time.

Effects on bone density *Oral corticosteroids can adversely affect bone density in several ways. Available calcium is reduced by a reduction in calcium absorption and an increase in urinary excretion. Osteoblast activity is reduced and osteoclast activity increased, so that resorption exceeds formation. Corticosteroids also prevent the bone-sparing effect of calcitonin.*

Corticosteroids accelerate bone loss; the risk of fracture doubles in patients taking over 7.5 mg/day of prednisolone. Because of the rapid turnover of trabecular bone, typical fracture sites are in the vertebrae, ribs, and pelvis (6[R]).

Initially, short-term studies raised concerns about an effect of inhaled corticosteroids on bone metabolism. Beclomethasone 2 mg/day, in eight healthy volunteers reduced serum osteocalcin concentrations at 1 and 2 weeks, but these returned to normal at 1 and 2 weeks after withdrawal (7[C]). The effects of inhaled corticosteroids on markers of bone resorption/formation were considerably less than those seen with oral corticosteroids.

The adverse effects profile of nebulized budesonide (2 mg bd) has been compared with that of oral prednisolone (30 mg/day) in a 5-day randomized parallel-group study of 19 adults with severe airway obstruction (8[C]). Budesonide produced an increase in FEV_1 that was not significantly different to that seen with oral prednisolone. Serum osteocalcin was significantly higher 2.3 (95% CI 0.9, 3.7) ng/ml with budesonide compared with 0.6 (0–1.2) ng/ml with prednisolone. The 24-h urinary calcium to creatinine ratios were significantly lower with budesonide. The authors concluded that biochemical markers associated with steroid adverse effects improve in patients treated with nebulized corticosteroids compared with patients treated with oral corticosteroids.

The transient nature of the effect of inhaled corticosteroids on serum osteocalcin has been confirmed in patients with asthma. In 15 steroid-naïve asthmatics who took budesonide 800 μg/day or beclomethasone dipropionate 800 μg/day for 4 weeks, there were significant but paradoxical changes in osteocalcin and PICP (which are both markers of bone formation) (9[C]). Osteocalcin concentrations fell but PICP concentrations rose. In the same study, 70 patients taking beclomethasone dipropionate 800 μg/day were followed for 30 months. There were no change in markers of resorption (ICTP) or formation (PICP) compared with a group taking β_2-agonists only.

Studies in which markers of bone turnover are measured for 1–2 months have little relevance, except as a way of comparing the potential effects of two different corticosteroids. The effect on bone metabolism of fluticasone propionate 750 μg/day for 6 weeks has been compared with that of beclomethasone dipropionate 1500 μg/day in a crossover study in 21 patients with asthma (10[C]). Beclomethasone dipropionate significantly reduced markers of bone formation (osteocalcin and PICP concentrations), whereas fluticasone propionate had no effect. Neither drug affected markers of bone resorption.

A study in older women with asthma, who have an increased risk of osteoporosis, showed no significant change in bone mineral density over a 1-year period (11[C]). Asthmatic patients (n = 19, mean age 53 years, range 43–67) were treated with beclomethasone dipropionate 1000 μg/day and compared with a group of healthy women (n = 19, mean age 53 years, range 43–67). Bone mineral density was measured with DXA in both groups at baseline and after 6 and 12 months.

Because high doses of inhaled corticosteroids reduce serum osteocalcin concentrations, the effects of inhaled steroids on bone density (measured using DXA of the spine and hip) and biochemical parameters have been documented over 18 months in 37 adult asthmatic patients who took 800 μg/day or more of either beclomethasone or budesonide for comparison with a control group of 37 asthmatics who used little or no inhaled steroids (less than 500 μg/day) (12[C]). Mean serum osteocalcin concentrations were significantly lower in the high-dose group and mean urinary phosphorus was significantly higher. However, bone mineral densities of the lumbar spine and hip were similar in the two groups. In another study the effect of inhaled steroids on bone density was investigated in growing children (13[C]). Bone mineral density was measured (using DXA) over 7–16 months in 21 asthmatic children over the age of 5, of whom 19 used regular inhaled steroids, and over 13–60 months in 14 healthy children. As there was no difference in bone density between the asthmatic and normal children it was concluded that advancement of bone density proceeded normally in asthmatic children taking inhaled steroids.

These studies are reassuring, but they did not use the most sensitive techniques for assessing bone mineral density and were relatively short compared with a patient's potential lifetime use of inhaled corticosteroids.

Three prospective comparative studies of patients taking inhaled fluticasone propionate showed no adverse effects on bone mineral density (14[C])–(16[C]). In a 12-month multicenter crossover comparison of asthmatic patients taking fluticasone propionate 250–500 μg/day or beclomethasone dipropionate 500–1000 μg/day, the two drugs had equal therapeutic effects but fluticasone propionate was associated with a higher bone mineral density (assessed at the hip) and higher serum osteocalcin concentrations (16[C]).

In a prospective randomized comparison of the effects of fluticasone propionate 1000 μg/day and budesonide 1600 μg/day over 1 year, bone mineral density measured in the spine was normal at the start of the study and increased slightly with time in both groups, as did serum osteocalcin concentration (15[C]).

In a prospective comparison of fluticasone propionate 1000 μg/day and beclomethasone dipropionate 2000 μg/day over 2 years, there was no change in markers of bone metabolism (14[C]). Bone mineral density, measured by DXA or SPA, showed no consistent changes. However, when bone mineral density was measured using QCT of the lumbar spine, beclomethasone dipropionate was associated with a small fall in bone mineral density, which stabilized by 24 months. Fluticasone propionate had no effect on QCT bone density measurements.

The author of the review concluded that low- and medium-dose inhaled corticosteroids are remarkably safe and have little or no effect on bone density and metabolism, particularly compared with oral corticosteroids, which they often replace (5[R]).

Prevention and management The prophylaxis of osteoporosis caused by long-term treatment with oral corticosteroids has been documented in a randomized study of the effect of intermittent intravenous administration of disodium pamidronate in 27 patients about to start long-term, high-dose corticosteroid treatment, in most cases for inflammatory rheumatic disease (17[C]). Simultaneously with the start of steroid therapy one group received an intravenous infusion of pamidronate (Aredia®, Ciba-Geigy, Basel, Switzerland), 90 mg in 500 ml 0.9% saline over 4 h and then every 3 months 30 mg in 250 ml 0.9% saline over 30 min, for as long as steroid treatment continued. Both groups took 800 mg/day of elemental calcium as calcium carbonate. BMD was measured every 3 months in the lumbar spine and hip (total and subregions) using dual energy X-ray absorptiometry. In the pamidronate group BMD increased significantly: lumbar spine +3.6%, femoral neck +2.2%. In contrast the controls had a reduction in BMD: lumbar spine −5.3%, femoral neck −5.3%. Differences between the groups were significant at all sites measured. The authors concluded that intermittent intravenous pamidronate achieves primary prevention of steroid-induced osteoporosis as assessed by BMD measurements over 1 year.

The management of corticosteroid-induced osteoporosis has been reviewed (18[R]). Most physicians are aware that osteoporosis is a major complication of corticosteroid therapy. However only a minority simultaneously prescribe medication to prevent it. In a survey of 65 000 people in the UK, 303 (0.5%) had taken oral corticosteroids for at least 3 months. The mean dose was 8 mg/day of prednisolone and the medium duration of treatment was 3 years. In the course of 4 years, only 41 (14%) of the patients had received medication to prevent osteoporosis.

This is in clear contrast with the Osteoporo-

sis Guidelines published by the American College Rheumatology Task Force. These recommend that patients starting long-term corticosteroid treatment should have bone mineral density (BMD) measurements performed. Patients with a BMD 1 standard deviation or more below the peak bone mass (T score below −1) are considered to have a low BMD and those with a BMD 2.5 standard deviations below (T score below −2.5) are considered to have osteoporosis. The BMD measurement determines the patient's risk for osteoporotic fractures.

All patients should be educated about steroid-induced bone loss and lifestyle modifications (mainly smoking, alcohol, and exercise) should be discussed. Calcium and vitamin D supplementation should be started. Further treatment depends on the BMD measurement. In a woman with a T score below −1 hormone replacement therapy should be started. If there are contraindications to hormone replacement therapy, a bisphosphonate or calcitonin should be prescribed. BMD measurement should be repeated 6–12 months after starting corticosteroids. This will determine the efficacy of the therapeutic intervention. If the BMD falls by more than 5% from the baseline antiosteoporotic medication should be added or modified.

The author concluded there is good evidence that bisphosphonates will increase BMD when it is significantly reduced before corticosteroid therapy. He recommended that corticosteroids should be prescribed in the lowest possible dosage and discontinued as soon as possible. Physical activity should be encouraged and immobilization avoided. Factors that increase the risk of falling should be avoided. Calcium should be given in a dosage of at least 1000 mg/day. If hypovitaminosis is likely, such as in house-bound patients, vitamin D (at least 400 iu/day) should be prescribed. The indications for prophylactic bisphosphonates are still not agreed; on the one hand, some physicians will be fairly conservative, only supplying calcium and vitamin D. Alternatively, aggressive early use of bisphosphonates and hormone replacement therapy, irrespective of additional risk factors, has been suggested. Perhaps we should be selective and better define risk factors at the start of corticosteroid treatment and 6 months later.

Effects in children *The literature on the effects of corticosteroid treatment on growth in children has been reviewed (19[R]). There is good evidence that inhaled corticosteroids, especially in dry powder form, can slow growth velocity in some children with asthma. There is a wide range of individual responses and some children have adverse effects with relatively small dosages. It is still not clear whether this is a transient phenomenon, causing a slowing of growth and maturational delay with no adverse effect on adult height, or whether growth can be permanently impaired. Until data are collected in children followed through to adult hood no firm conclusions are possible.*

Collagen type I is the major (90%) structural component of osteoid, the organic matrix of bone. Collagen type III is the predominant collagen of skin and other soft tissues, including bone marrow. Serum concentrations of the terminal procollagen propeptides (amino-terminal propeptide of type I procollagen (PINP), carboxy-terminal propeptide of type I procollagen (PICP), and amino-terminal propeptide of type III procollagen (PIIINP), appear to reflect the rate of collagen synthesis. Carboxy-terminal telopeptide of type I collagen (ICTP) is more specific for collagen degradation. Serum concentrations of these markers can be related to growth velocity in healthy children and those with growth disorders.

Children aged 4.4–11 years from the asthma clinics of four hospitals have been studied (20[C]). The children who used budesonide and beclomethasone dipropionate began treatment at a mean age of 5.8 (4.9–6.3) years, and had taken treatment for a mean of 2.7 years before the study. After 6 months, 52 children were admitted to hospital for a 24-h endocrine study; 13 were not taking corticosteroids, 17 were taking budesonide, 18 beclomethasone dipropionate, and four prednisolone. A fasting blood sample was taken on the morning after admission and PICP, PINP, PIIINP, ICTP, bone-specific alkaline phosphatase (BALP), and osteocalcin were measured. At the end of a year, height velocity over the preceding year was assessed by linear regression of height against age for each child, reducing inaccuracies in measurement by including all intervening observations. All height velocity data were related to reference ranges by conversion to stan-

dard deviation scores. The data were presented as mean standard deviation scores or means, in both cases with 95% confidence intervals.

Markers of collagen synthesis *PINP concentration scores in non-steroid treated patients with asthma (−0.21; CI −0.71, 0.29), were similar to control values, but were lower in children treated with budesonide (−0.64; CI −0.99, 0.29), or beclomethasone dipropionate (−0.9; CI −1.32, 0.48), and this difference was significant. There was no difference between the two groups taking inhaled steroids and the group taking oral steroids (−0.72; CI −1.88, 0.42).*

PICP concentration scores were lower than control values in non-steroid-treated children and tended to rise with steroid use. The differences between the groups were not significant, but PICP was significantly higher in children treated with budesonide (−0.36; CI −0.69, 0.02) or beclomethasone dipropionate (−0.16; CI −0.68, 0.02) compared with non-steroid treated children (−0.67; CI −0.99, 0.36). PIIINP concentration scores in non-steroid treated children were similar to control subjects and significantly lower in children treated with budesonide or beclomethasone dipropionate than in non-steroid treated children.

Markers of collagen degradation *ICTP concentration scores were significantly higher in non-steroid treated children (1.56; CI 0.99, 2.14) than in controls or children treated with inhaled budesonide (0.28; CI −0.38, 0.96) or and beclomethasone dipropionate (−0.52; CI −1.06, 0.03). There were no differences between the inhaled steroids.*

Non-collagenous serum markers of bone metabolism *Mean serum osteocalcin concentrations were lower in patients treated with budesonide (20.9 mg/l; CI 15.0, 26.7), or beclomethasone dipropionate (19.2 mg/l; CI 13.6, 24.7), than in those in the non-steroid group (29.0 mg/l; CI 22.7, 35.4). There were no significant differences between groups in the serum BALP, which was in the reference range in all groups.*

Height velocity *The height velocity score with beclomethasone dipropionate (−1.04; CI −1.4, 0.67) and oral steroids (−1.58; CI −3.19, 0.23) was significantly less than with budesonide (−0.2; CI −0.68, 0.27) or in the non-steroid-treated group (0.03; CI −0.51, 0.58).*

Asthma control, as indicated by the FEV_1 (percent predicted) was similar in all groups 88 (64–112), 89 (63–115), 92 (70–114), and 88 (64–112)% in the non-steroid, budesonide, beclomethasone dipropionate, and oral steroid groups, respectively.

The authors concluded that synthesis of type I and III collagen, as reflected by serum PINP and PIIINP concentrations, is significantly reduced in asthmatic children treated with inhaled corticosteroids. PIIINP showed a positive correlation with height velocity, similar to that seen in other children with disorders of growth. The reduced growth velocity seen in the asthmatic patients was not due to clustering of ages round the peripubertal period, when a physiological decline in growth rate or poor symptom control can occur. Lung function was almost identical in each group, and so impaired growth velocity was attributed to the adverse effects of treatment. Markers of collagen turnover provide a more accurate reflection of growth disturbance than osteocalcin and bone-specific alkaline phosphatase.

Inhaled beclomethasone dipropionate 200 μg bd has been compared with salmeterol 50 μg bd and placebo over 12 months of treatment in 241 children with clinically stable asthma and less than 1 month of prior steroid use (21[C]). Airway responsiveness, assessed by methacholine challenge, was significantly less with beclomethasone dipropionate than with salmeterol or placebo. The effect was lost 2 weeks after the end of treatment. Beclomethasone dipropionate was associated with less variability between morning and evening PEFR, and it also reduced the need for rescue therapy with salbutamol and resulted in fewer withdrawals because of asthma exacerbation. During the 12 months, linear growth was 3.96 cm in the children who used beclomethasone dipropionate, compared with 5.4 cm with salmeterol and 5.04 cm with placebo. The authors concluded that the inhaled steroid was effective in reducing airway hyper-responsiveness and controlling asthma symptoms, but was associated with reduced linear growth. This result is consistent with data reported by others (20[C]).

Conclusions *It appears that low- and medium-dose inhaled corticosteroids are remarkably safe and have little or no effect on bone density and metabolism, particularly compared with oral corticosteroids, which they often replace. It is important that studies are continued for periods of at least 1 year, as biochemical markers of bone metabolism can change over short periods. Assessment of bone mineral density by SXA and DXA is less sensitive than QCT, but because of the radiation dose QCT has been less used, especially in serial studies.*

The finding in two recent studies that inhaled corticosteroids cause diminished growth in children must cause concern. Further studies, carefully designed to avoid the confounding variables of asthma severity and peripubertal age, are needed.

Special senses *Risk of cataract with inhaled corticosteroids* Systemic corticosteroid treatment is a known risk factor for the development of posterior subcapsular cataract. A population-based cross-sectional study of vision and common eye diseases has suggested that inhaled corticosteroids may predispose patients to the development of posterior subcapsular cataract. A total of 3654 people, 49–97 years of age, were recruited to the study (22[C]). Information on potential risk factors for cataracts, including current or prior use of inhaled corticosteroids, was collected by questionnaire. Photographs of each subject's lenses were graded to assess the presence and severity of cortical, nuclear, and posterior subcapsular cataracts. Inhaled corticosteroid use was reported by 370 subjects, of whom 164 reported current use and 206 previous use. After adjustment for age and sex, subjects who reported using inhaled corticosteroids had a higher prevalence of nuclear cataracts (relative prevalence 1.5; 95% CI 1.2, 1.9) and posterior subcapsular cataracts (relative prevalence 1.9; 95% CI 1.3, 2.8). The prevalence of cortical cataracts was not significantly increased. Higher cumulative lifetime doses of beclomethasone were associated with a higher risk of posterior subcapsular cataract. The highest prevalence (27%) was in patients whose lifetime dose was more than 2000 mg (relative prevalence 5.5).

Alternative explanations for these findings have been suggested. If a significant number of the subjects suffered from atopic dermatitis, the topical application of steroids to the face and eyelids could have contributed to cataract development (23[r]). When a multidose inhaler is used without a spacer some portion of the dose may be deposited directly into the eye. Topical application of ophthalmic corticosteroids is thought to increase the risk of cataract (24[r]).

Immunological and hypersensitivity reactions Several case reports have highlighted the occurrence of allergic reactions to corticosteroids.

A 62-year-old woman was treated for a burn with an ointment containing hydrocortisone, without adverse effects. Two years later she was given an intra-articular injection of methylprednisolone acetate into the knee for the relief of arthritis, and developed erythema around the neck. Two years later she was given intravenous hydrocortisone sodium phosphate, 500 mg for 2 days and developed erythema on the neck, trunk, and thighs. Methylprednisolone sodium succinate was substituted for the hydrocortisone. The erythema developed into a generalized rash, which resolved after withdrawal of methylprednisolone. She had positive patch tests with cortisone acetate, methylprednisolone sodium succinate and methylprednisolone acetate (all strongly positive) and with hydrocortisone acetate, prednisolone acetate, prednisolone sodium succinate, and fludrocortisone acetate. Intradermal tests were positive with hydrocortisone and methylprednisolone. After intravenous hydrocortisone 50 mg and methylprednisolone 62.5 mg she developed symmetrical patches of erythema on the neck, chest, axillae, forearms, fingers, and thighs. In addition, after methylprednisolone she had a flare-up at the site of the previous methylprednisolone patch test. Betamethasone produced negative results.

The authors suggested that corticosteroids might cause *contact dermatitis*, as they are widely used both topically and systemically (25[c]).

Severe *anaphylaxis* after parenteral dexamethasone has been confirmed by subsequent challenge (26[c]).

Five minutes after an intramuscular injection of Dalamon® (ALTER, Madrid, Spain) a 48-year-old woman developed intense generalized pruritus, facial angio-edema, hypotension, and loss of consciousness. She was treated with dexchlorpheniramine, epinephrine, methylprednisolone, hydrocortisone, and colloid plasma expander. She was well enough to be discharged after 24 h. Dalamon has several ingredients. Skin tests (prick and intradermal) with each ingredient up to the therapeutic dose were negative, but positive with sodium phosphate dexamethasone 0.4 mg subcutaneously. She tolerated 6-methylprednisolone 40 mg, but had another anaphylactic reaction to hydrocortisone 20 mg subcutaneously.

The authors noted the severe reaction to hydrocortisone, which she had previously received for her original anaphylactic reaction. They believed that she was either in a refractory period or that this treatment had sensitized her to further injection.

It has been suggested that the succinate group may be of importance in reactions to corticosteroids (27[c]).

A 35-year-old woman with dog dander-induced asthma, treated with inhaled budesonide and salbutamol as needed, developed an acute attack of asthma. She received subcutaneous salbutamol and an intramuscular dose of 6-methylprednisolone 60 mg and 20 min later developed dyspnea, wheezing, cyanosis, and stupor. She required endotracheal intubation and assisted ventilation and was given salbutamol, aminophylline, and antibiotics tds and intravenous methylprednisolone every 6 h. Her bronchospasm worsened and seemed to be temporally related to methylprednisolone administration. The steroid was withdrawn and the other treatment continued. There was steady improvement thereafter. Later skin prick testing to prednisolone sodium hemisuccinate and 6-methylprednisolone sodium hemisuccinate was positive. Thirty minutes after intradermal 6-methylprednisolone sodium hemisuccinate 4 mg she developed a dry cough, dyspnea, and wheezing and a 17% fall in FEV_1. IgE antibodies to 6-methylprednisolone sodium hemisuccinate could not be found.

Miscellaneous Dexamethasone has been identified as a probable cause of drug-induced *hiccups* (28[c]).

A 47-year old man receiving chemotherapy for multiple myeloma was given oral dexamethasone 40 mg qds. Within 12 h he developed intractable hiccups four to eight times per minute. Complete physical examination and laboratory studies, including esophagogastroduodenoscopy, were unremarkable. The hiccups ended when dexamethasone was withdrawn and recurred within 12 h of rechallenge on two separate occasions. However, intravenous dexamethasone had no effect and he received six further courses of chemotherapy without incident.

The reflex arc of hiccups has three parts: an afferent limb, comprising the vagus and phrenic nerves and the sympathetic chain from T6 to T12; the central connection; and the efferent limb, which is primarily the phrenic nerves. Stimulation of any of the reflex arc limbs results in hiccups. As the patient's hiccups were caused by oral but not intravenous dexamethasone, the authors proposed that the local gastrointestinal effect of dexamethasone led to reflex arc stimulation.

The course of chickenpox in 13 asthmatic children receiving inhaled budesonide has been documented (29[C]). The duration of fever and rash was documented in each case. The duration of fever was in the normal range. The course of the illness was uneventful. Healing of the rash was within the normal range of 5–20 days.

β_2-ADRENOCEPTOR AGONISTS

(SED-13, 347, 363; SEDA-19, 179; SEDA-20, 167; SEDA-21, 181)

Bambuterol *(SEDA-18, 1–2)*

Bambuterol is the biscarbamate ester prodrug of the β_2-agonist terbutaline (30[R]). It is available in 10- and 20-mg tablets as the hydrochloride salt. It is stable to presystemic elimination and is concentrated in lung tissue after absorption from the gastrointestinal tract. It is hydrolysed to terbutaline primarily by an enzyme, butyrylcholinesterase, that is found in lung tissue, which can form terbutaline from bambuterol in situ. The effect of bambuterol lasts for 24 h. Peak plasma concentrations of terbutaline occur 3.9–6.8 h after administration of bambuterol. Maximum therapeutic benefit occurs 1 week after starting treatment. Except for *suppression of plasma butyrylcholinesterase* the adverse effects of bambuterol are those of a β_2-agonist and are related to the plasma concentration of terbutaline. Plasma butyrylcholinesterase returns to control values about 2 weeks after stopping treatment. Bambuterol may have a better therapeutic:toxic ratio than terbutaline.

In a comparison of oral bambuterol (20 mg) given in the morning (07:00 h) with the same dose given in the evening (22:00 h) in 29 asthmatic patients, the mean 24-h plasma concentration of terbutaline was similar with both administrations, although the C_{max} for evening administration was significantly higher than after a morning dose (17.2 vs 15.5 nmol/l) (31[C]). The 24-h mean FEV_1 was significantly increased by bambuterol (morning 3.2 l; evening 3.4 l) versus placebo (2.9 l); 24-h mean FVC and PEFR showed similar changes, with a maximum effect at 04:00 h independent of dosing time. However, after the evening dose, FEV_1, FEV_{25-75}, and PEFR at 07:00 h were significantly higher. Adverse effects were more frequent with bambuterol than placebo, although the difference was not statistically significant. Thus, although bambuterol was as effective in the morning or evening, evening dosing is preferable for nocturnal asthma.

Bambuterol and modified-release salbutamol have been compared in 152 asthmatics taking at least 800 μg of inhaled corticosteroids (32[C]). All had significant nocturnal symptoms. Both drugs produced a significant 63% reduction in the severity of nocturnal asthma. This was reflected by significant improvements in lung function tests after 3 weeks. Bambuterol caused significantly less tremor. Patients' treatment preferences were bambuterol 49%, modified-release salbutamol 36%, and no preference 15%. The main reason for these preferences was control of asthma symptoms, although a significant subgroup (27%) chose bambuterol because of fewer adverse effects compared with 11% who chose modified-release salbutamol for this reason; 56% of patients preferred once-daily and 7% preferred twice-daily medication.

Oral terbutaline and bambuterol have been compared in elderly patients (mean age 67, range 60–90 years) with chronic reversible airways obstruction in a randomized, double-blind, crossover study consisting of four consecutive 2-week treatment periods (33[C]). Of 84 patients who entered the study, 66 completed all treatment periods; 94% used inhaled/oral corticosteroids in a constant dosage. The treatments were bambuterol solution 20 mg at night, bambuterol 10 mg at night, terbutaline mixture 3 mg tds, and placebo solution. Patients measured daily PEFR, asthma symptoms, use of inhaled β_2-agonist, and tremor. Basal FEV_1 was 1.49 l with 30% reversibility. All treatments were significantly better than placebo. Bambuterol 20 mg resulted in a higher morning PEFR than terbutaline (306 vs 297 l/min); bambuterol 10 mg gave equivalent results. There were no differences in the use of inhaled β_2-agonists. Subjects reported less shortness of breath during the night with bambuterol 20 mg, and during the day with bambuterol 10 mg. Bambuterol 20 mg and terbutaline produced more tremor than bambuterol 10 mg and placebo. The authors concluded that in elderly patients with chronic reversible airways obstruction once-daily bambuterol (10 or 20 mg) has a better therapeutic effect/adverse effect ratio than terbutaline 3 mg tds.

Fenoterol *(SED-13, 363; SEDA-16, 180, 183)*

All β-adrenoceptor agonists can cause *hypokalemia*, and cardiac dysrhythmias can be precipitated by hypokalemia in susceptible patients.

The hypokalemic effect of high-dose fenoterol in premature labor has been documented (34[C]). Data were obtained on 83 patients (aged 28–34 years) who were given an intravenous infusion of fenoterol 0.5–2.0 μg/min. Plasma concentrations of fenoterol and potassium were measured. Pretreatment plasma potassium concentrations were normal (median 4.10, range 4.10–4.40 mmol/l). During the first 2 h the serum potassium fell significantly to 2.88 mmol/l (range 2.80–3.00 mmol/l), but returned to normal within the first day and then remained in the reference range, despite continuous fenoterol administration. No potassium supplements were given. Clinical abnormalities (including cardiac dysrhythmias) due to hypokalemia were not observed.

Salbutamol (albuterol)

Nebulized salbutamol remains part of the initial management of acute severe asthma. In 92 acutely ill asthmatic patients who presented to the emergency department and who were given three doses of salbutamol (2.5 mg) from a wet nebulizer at 20-min intervals, there was a dose-dependent improvement in peak expiratory flow rate (PEFR), but only 66% of the patients were sufficiently improved to go home; 56% of the responders required 5 mg or less to be discharged and the remainder required 7.5 mg (35[C]). In 34% salbutamol was ineffective, and PEFR did not exceed 40% of predicted normal after three doses. The 'non-responders' had more severe disease, as judged by frequency of hospital visits and recurrent hospitalization. It is important to appreciate that a significant proportion of patients who present with asthma will not respond to nebulized salbutamol and will require hospital admission.

A similar result was obtained when salbutamol was dispensed from a multidose pressurized aerosol (PMDI) and a spacer device. In 116 patients who were treated with 4 puffs (400 μg) at 10-min intervals for up to 3 h (total dose of 1200 μg at 30 min) there was a dose-related increase in PEFR, but only 81 patients (70%) improved enough to be discharged home; 70% of the responders needed a cumulative dose of 2.4 mg of salbutamol within 60 min and the others required 3.6 mg or more (36[C]). The 30% of patients who were admitted had little rise in PEFR, which reached 37 (7% of predicted) compared with the discharge group, 67 (14% of predicted). The non-responders had more severe disease, as judged by the length of attack, previous use of β_2-agonists and more severe reduction in lung function, PEFR = 26 (6.2% of predicted) compared with 33 (7.7% of predicted) in the responders. The most significant difference between the two groups was the PEFR after 30 min of treatment, 50 (12% of predicted) in responders and 31 (6.8% of predicted) in non-responders.

A further study has evaluated salbutamol given from a PMDI with spacer device in 100 asthmatics (37[C]). All took 6 puffs (600 μg) initially. Then group 1 ($n = 34$) took a further 6 puffs at 30, 60, and 90 min, group 2 ($n = 33$) 6 puffs every hour, and group 3 ($n = 33$) a second dose at 120 min only. The FEV_1 improved significantly in all three groups. At 120 min, groups 1 and 2 had a significantly greater rise in FEV_1 than group three. Mean heart rates on entry were 99.6, 99.5, and 96.3 beats/min in groups 1, 2, and 3, respectively. The heart rate change in group 1 (+3.4) was significantly different from that in group 3 (−5.8). Blood pressure and serum potassium did not change. The most common adverse effect complained of was *tremor* (six patients in group 1, five in group 2, and five in group 3). *Headache*, *nervousness*, *weakness*, and *palpitation* were much less frequent and occurred in all three groups. The authors concluded that treatments at 60-min intervals were sufficient in most patients, and that 30-min treatments should be reserved for patients with less than a 15% rise in FEV_1 at 15 min. They emphasized that to achieve such good effects with a PMDI and spacer requires adequate instruction. The continued use of nebulized salbutamol in hospital is less cost effective but does not require staff time in instruction and supervision.

A further study has compared salbutamol given by PMDI or nebulizer in 50 patients, of whom 13 had chronic obstructive pulmonary disease and 37 had asthma (38[C]). The patients were treated with either a placebo PMDI (2 puffs) through a 750-ml cone-shaped spacer (Glaxo) plus nebulized salbutamol 2.5 mg in 2 ml (group 1, $n = 25$) or with salbutamol PMDI (2 puffs, 0.2 mg) through a spacer and 2 ml saline by nebulizer (group 2, $n = 25$). The treatments were repeated on three occasions at 15-min intervals. The rise in FEV_1 was similar in the two groups and peaked after 30 min. The authors emphasized the importance of coaching and supervision to achieve an effective result with a PMDI.

These studies, in a total of 323 patients, have emphasized the safety of substantial doses of inhaled salbutamol in asthmatics who are ill enough to attend an emergency department. However, up to a third of such patients may not achieve an adequate response. Failure to respond should result in immediate admission.

Children who presented to an emergency department with severe asthma ($n = 29$) were given nebulized salbutamol, 2.5 mg if 2 years old or younger and 5 mg if over 2 years (39[C]). Children who did not improve entered phase 1 of the study (0–2 h), in which treatment was by a standard protocol: nebulized salbutamol in the same dose; oxygen 4–6 l/min until the oxygen saturation reached 93% in room air for at least 30 min; an intravenous bolus injection of hydrocortisone 5 mg/kg over 3 min; and then intravenous salbutamol 15 μg/kg or saline by random allocation. In phase 2 (2–24 h), the children were given nebulized salbutamol continuously, and then at 30 min, and 1, 2, 3, and 4 h, according to need. The primary endpoints were recovery time (no longer needing nebulized salbutamol) and persistent moderate to severe asthma 2 h after randomization. Recovery time was significantly faster in the 14 children given intravenous salbutamol: 4 h compared with 11.5 h in the 15 children given intravenous saline. Two of the children given intravenous salbutamol needed oxygen to maintain oxygen saturation at 93% on room air, whereas oxygen was needed by eight (53%) of the children who were given saline. The children who were given intravenous salbutamol were able to be transferred from the emergency department 9.7 h earlier than the control group. There were no clinically important adverse effects, although the children who were given intravenous salbutamol had more tremor at 2 h.

Patients with severe asthma appear to tolerate large doses of nebulized salbutamol. A possible reason for this has been suggested from a study in which three groups of subjects were followed after receiving nebulized salbutamol 40 μg/kg: 10 healthy subjects (FEV_1 110% predicted), 10 mild asthmatics (FEV_1 102% predicted), and 10 severe asthmatics (FEV_1 49.2% predicted) (40[C]). Plasma salbutamol concentrations were measured at 5, 10, 20, and 30 min after inhalation. The highest plasma salbutamol concentration (C_{max}) and the average plasma concentration from 0–30 min (C_{av}) were calculated. Plasma C_{av} was 1.31 ng/ml in the severe asthmatics, 2.5 ng/ml in the mild asthmatics, and 2.4 ng/ml in the controls. C_{max} was also lower in the severe asthmatics: 1.7 compared with 2.9 ng/ml in the controls. Tremor and a rise in heart rate were correspondingly less in the severe asthmatics, as was improvement in lung function: FEV_{25-75} increased by 0.3 l/s compared with a rise of 0.74 l/s in mild asthmatics and 0.69 l/s in controls. Baseline airways caliber significantly alters the early lung absorption of nebulized salbutamol, and in severe asthma there is a reduction in early lung absorption of salbutamol after inhalation which does not occur in mild asthma. This is mirrored by lower plasma concentrations of salbutamol, less bronchodilatation, and less tremor.

The pulmonary responses to intravenous fenoterol have been compared with those seen after a low dose (0.4 mg) and a high dose (1.2 mg) of inhaled fenoterol (41[C]). The doses of inhaled fenoterol caused equivalent reductions in airways resistance, reflecting an effect on central airways. Static recoil pressure was reduced by high-dose but not low-dose inhaled fenoterol. Intravenous fenoterol produced similar changes to those seen with high-dose inhaled fenoterol. The authors concluded that the change in static recoil pressure reflected a relaxant effect on alveolar duct muscle. The rapidity of the response showed that the high-dose inhaled fenoterol was absorbed from the bronchial mucosa and reached the alveolar duct muscle via the circulation. It would therefore also be available to cause systemic adverse effects. This is consistent with the effects of inhaled salbutamol in severe obstruction, described above (40[C]), and would explain why intravenous salbutamol may have an additional effect to inhaled salbutamol in severe asthma (39[C]).

Salbutamol via a PMDI (Ventolin) has been compared with salbutamol powder from a dry powder inhaler (Rotacaps with Rotahaler) in 12 patients with mild to moderate asthma in a three-way crossover comparison of Ventolin (two puffs, 90 μg per puff), salbutamol sulfate powder (Rotacaps; two puffs, 100 μg per puff), and lactose powder (placebo; two puffs, 12.5 mg per puff) (42[C]). The salbutamol formulations produced equivalent bronchodilatation, significantly greater than after placebo. There were no changes in serum potassium, blood glucose, or the electrocardiogram before and 30, 60, 90, and 180 min after each treatment, or in blood pressure and heart rate at 15, 30, 45, 60, 90, 120, 180, 240, and 300 min after each treatment.

Salbutamol delivered from a PMDI has been compared with salbutamol from a Turbuhaler (Glaxo-Wellcome) in two studies (43[C]). In the first study 12 patients were given 50, 100, or 200 μg via Turbuhaler or 200 μg via a PMDI (Ventolin) using a four-way crossover design. After correcting for baseline differences the area under the FEV_1 response curve over 0–6 h did not differ significantly between Turbuhaler 50 or 100 μg and salbutamol 200 μg from the PMDI, but salbutamol 200 μg via Turbuhaler produced a significantly higher response than 200 μg via PMDI. There were no adverse events with any of the doses.

In the second study, 50 patients were included in a placebo-controlled five-way crossover trial (43[C]). The doses of salbutamol were 50 and 200 μg via Turbuhaler, and 100 and 200 μg via PMDI (Ventolin). Salbutamol inhaled from the Turbuhaler was 1.98 times (95% CI 1.2, 3.2) more potent than salbutamol inhaled from a Ventolin inhaler in improving the average FEV_1 over 0–6 h. No treatment significantly affected the heart rate, blood pressure, electrocardiogram, or serum potassium. There were 14 reports of tremor in eight patients, four after placebo, one after Turbuhaler 50 μg, one after Turbuhaler 200 μg, and two after PMDI 200 μg.

Endocrine, metabolic Nebulized salbutamol has been reported to cause *increased activity of the renin–angiotensin system* (44[C]). Eight patients with mild asthma were treated with single and multiple doses of 5 mg nebulized salbutamol or placebo in a randomized, double-blind, crossover study. The treatments were given as a single dose or as two doses 30 min apart. Plasma concentrations of renin and angiotensin II rose more after one or two doses of salbutamol than after placebo. Serum potassium concentrations fell from 4.4 mmol/l by a maximum of 0.85 mmol/l 45 min after a single dose and 1.16 mmol/l at 150 min after two doses. The clinical significance of these changes is unclear.

Salmeterol *(SEDA-19, 180; SEDA-21, 184)*

The adverse effects of salmeterol have been previously reviewed (SEDA-21, 184). When salmeterol was given for 1 year to 15 407 patients there were no unexpected major adverse events (45[C]). There were 1022 (6.6%) deaths; 73 patients died of asthma and 39 used salmeterol during the last month of life. Examination of the deaths showed that the majority were due to natural causes. In four of the 39 subjects who died of asthma and who had taken salmeterol the authors thought it possible that death had been related to the use of salmeterol.

Salmeterol aerosol 42 μg bd has been compared with oral theophylline or placebo twice daily for 12 weeks in a multicenter study in 638 patients with moderate asthma (46[C]). Salmeterol was better tolerated and significantly more effective than modified-release theophylline in maintenance treatment. An adverse event was reported in 19, 9, and 19% of those taking placebo, salmeterol, and theophylline, respectively. There was a significant difference between groups only with respect to *gastrointestinal adverse effects*, which occurred in 10% with theophylline, 2% with salmeterol, and 3% with placebo.

Salmeterol 50 μg bd has been compared with fluticasone 250 μg bd and with a combination of these drugs given for 6 weeks (47[C]). The three treatments were equally effective in improving clinical outcome, circadian variation in PEFR and FEV_1, and bronchial hyperresponsiveness to methacholine.

Inhaled salmeterol 50 μg bd has been compared with individually dose-titrated modified-release oral theophylline (48[C]). Sleep quality and cognitive performance were measured in 15 patients. Overnight falls in PEFR were similar with the two drugs. However, with salmeterol there were more nights without waking, fewer nocturnal arousals, and an improved quality of life. Visual vigilance was improved by salmeterol, but otherwise daytime cognition was unaffected. There was no patient preference for either therapy.

Formoterol (6, 12, and 24 μg) has been compared with salmeterol 50 μg in a double-blind, placebo-controlled, crossover study in 28 asthmatic patients (49[C]). FEV_1 was monitored over 12 h. All doses of formoterol had a more rapid onset of effect than salmeterol, as judged by bronchodilatation 3 min after a dose. However, the durations of effect were similar, judging from bronchodilatation at 12 h. Salmeterol 50 μg and formoterol 9 μg (95% CI 3, 19 μg) were of equal potency. There were no significant changes in heart rate compared with placebo. The most common adverse effect was *headache*, observed in six or seven patients after all treatments, including placebo. β_2-Adrenoceptor-mediated adverse effects (tachycardia, palpitation, and tremor) were not reported after placebo or salmeterol but occurred in mild to moderate degree in one, one, and five patients given 6, 12, and 24 μg of formoterol, respectively.

Salmeterol (50 μg bd) has been evaluated for 6 months in a randomized, double-blind, placebo-controlled, crossover study in 87 patients with mild or moderate asthma who were taking beclomethasone dipropionate or budesonide at least 200 μg bd (50[C]). Salmeterol produced a 17% (95% CI 12, 22%) reduction in the use of inhaled steroid. There was no significant difference in the number of patients whose asthma was exacerbated (placebo 25%, salmeterol 16%). Salmeterol was associated with higher morning and evening PEFR and FEV_1, reductions in symptoms and bronchodilator use, and a reduction in airway responsiveness to methacholine. There was no significant change in serum potassium, or heart rate measured over 24 h. The bronchodilator response to an inhaled short-acting β_2-agonist, salbutamol, was unchanged.

Terbutaline *(SED-13, 364; SEDA-18, 188; SEDA-21, 186)*

Intravenous terbutaline has been reported to reverse the allergen-induced late phase reaction in the lung (51[C]). Seven asthmatic subjects developed a pulmonary late-phase reaction to inhaled ragweed extract, the FEV_1 falling to 57% of baseline. Intravenous terbutaline rapidly improved lung function. In a separate study, terbutaline was infused to determine the maximum possible bronchodilatation in the same patients. FEV_1 rose rapidly to a plateau at 40–45 min. At the end of the infusion the FEV_1 was not significantly different from the predicted normal value. With placebo infusion, FEV_1 after allergen dropped from 3 to below 1.7 l and did not recover over 45 min. In contrast, when terbutaline was given FEV_1 began to recover quickly and was still recovering at 45 min when the FEV_1 was not significantly different from that measured before allergen challenge. The authors concluded that the late phase reduction in lung function was due to bronchial smooth muscle spasm, as it was rapidly reversed by terbutaline.

ANTICHOLINERGIC DRUGS
(SED-13, 426; SEDA-20, 167; SEDA-21, 187)

Ipratropium bromide

Inhaled ipratropium bromide is effective and safe in older asthmatic patients with chronic obstructive pulmonary disease who respond inadequately to inhaled β_2-agonists (SEDA-20, 167).

Patients with chronic obstructive pulmonary disease have increased energy expenditure, are often malnourished, and have increased resting energy expenditure. An increase in the work of breathing is thought to be the main cause of this hypermetabolism. Bronchodilators may reduce the work of breathing by relieving airways obstruction but β_2-agonists have a thermogenic effect. Nebulized ipratropium bromide in effective bronchodilator doses did not have a thermogenic effect in patients with chronic obstructive pulmonary disease, while salbutamol produced a sustained increase in resting energy expenditure (52[C]). The clinical importance of the absence of a thermogenic effect with nebulized ipratropium bromide in patients with chronic obstructive pulmonary disease remains to be determined.

Two recent studies have shown that inhaled ipratropium bromide did not add any significant benefit to the effects of salbutamol in acute attacks of asthma (53[C]), (54[C]). In one study (53[C]) patient selection was not described. In the other study patients who were more likely to benefit from inhaled ipratropium (those over 55 years of age, those who had a history consistent with chronic obstructive pulmonary disease, and those who had smoked heavily) were excluded (54[C]). In these younger patients without chronic ob structive pulmonary disease there was a trend towards fewer hospitalizations and greater bronchodilatation when ipratropium was combined with salbutamol, but the difference was not statistically significant.

Another study has shown that nebulized ipratropium significantly augmented the bronchodilatation produced by nebulized salbutamol in asthmatics aged 18–55 years without chronic obstructive pulmonary disease (55[C]).

The patients who obtained the least benefit from the addition of ipratropium were those who had more severe asthma and had taken more β_2-agonist before arrival in the emergency department. In children (mean age 7.3 years) the combination of ipratropium with salbutamol was more effective in treating acute attacks of asthma than either alone (56[C]).

CROMONES *(SED-13, 421; SEDA-19, 183; SEDA-20, 168; SEDA-21, 187)*

Sodium cromoglycate

Sodium cromoglycate is more effective in children than in adults in the prophylactic treatment of asthma (SEDA-19, 183). It is relatively safe, but transient *throat irritation*, *cough*, and mild *bronchospasm* due to local irritation can occur. Reports of more serious adverse effects with sodium cromoglycate are rare and include *urticaria*, *angio-edema*, *anaphylaxis*, and *type III hypersensitivity reactions* (57[cr]).

Urinary system Sodium cromoglycate was associated with *dysuria* and *vesicoureteric reflux* in a 5-year-old asthmatic child (57[cr]). Although the condition improved on withdrawal, the dysuria may have been caused by urinary tract infection unrelated to sodium cromoglycate, and the child was taking a number of other medications, including salbutamol, beclomethasone dipropionate, theophylline, and clemastine for steroid-dependent asthma, chronic otitis media, and chronic sinusitis. The authors of this case report acknowledged that the evidence was merely circumstantial.

Immunological and hypersensitivity reactions Sodium cromoglycate eye drops immediately produced intense *itching*, *burning*, *redness*, and severe *swelling of the conjunctivae* in a 63-year-old man with chronic non-allergic rhinoconjunctivitis (58[c]). There were circulating IgE-specific antibodies to sodium cromoglycate, and skin prick and conjunctival provocation tests were positive. Thus, the acute ocular hypersensitivity reaction to sodium cromoglycate appeared to be produced by an IgE-mediated pathway.

Nedocromil *(SED-13, 422; SEDA-19, 183; SEDA-20, 168; SEDA-21, 187)*

The effect of nedocromil sodium on asthmatic symptoms and bronchial hyper-reactivity has been examined in 20 children with stable non-atopic asthma in a randomized, double-blind, placebo-controlled clinical trial (59[C]). The children using nedocromil sodium took 4 mg (2 puffs) qds from an MDI for 42 days. Nedocromil sodium increased the number of asthma-free days and reduced the severity of asthmatic symptoms and non-specific bronchial hyper-reactivity in non-allergic asthmatic children challenged with nebulized distilled water. These findings suggest that nedocromil sodium can be useful for non-allergic as well as allergic childhood asthma.

ANTIHISTAMINES USED IN ASTHMA

Ketotifen *(SEDA-9, 155; SEDA-10, 137; SEDA-11, 149)*

In a double-blind parallel-group study, 25 patients with atopic asthma took ketotifen (1 mg bd) or a matching placebo for 8 weeks (60[C]). Ketotifen improved airway function and reduced bronchial hyper-reactivity. It also produced significant reductions in activated eosinophils, T cells (CD3+, CD4+, and CD25+ activated cells) in the bronchial mucosa, suggesting that it can reduce allergic inflammation in asthmatic airways. However, in asthmatic children ketotifen 2 mg/day did not have a greater steroid-sparing effect than placebo, even though ketotifen-treated patients were better symptomatically (61[C]). In the 32 children who took ketotifen, headache, increased appetite, and sedation were reported by nine, 10, and four patients, respectively, compared with 13, five, and two, respectively, in the 34 children who took placebo. Hematological and biochemical tests were not significantly affected.

EXPECTORANTS

Potassium iodide *(SED-10, 295; SEDA-7, 191; SEDA-9, 156)*

Delayed hypersensitivity has been attributed to potassium iodide (62[c]).

A 66-year-old man with a history of chronic obstructive pulmonary disease, hypertension, and penicillin allergy developed dyspnea, angio-edema, itching, and erythema of the face and neck a few hours after a second dose of a cough syrup (Elixifilin) containing potassium iodide (130 mg/15 ml), theophylline (80 mg/15 ml), saccharose (2.25 g/15 ml), and ethanol (10%). His symptoms disappeared 24 h after treatment with parenteral corticosteroids. Oral challenge to Elixifilin was then conducted in a single-blind, placebo-controlled trial. About 5 h after Elixifilin challenge, he developed edema of the face and neck, itching of the pharynx and eyes, and a sensation of heat. From the history, alcohol and saccharose were both excluded as causative agents. Challenge with theophylline did not produce an adverse reaction.

The authors concluded that potassium iodide had caused the delayed adverse response. This is consistent with delayed hypersensitivity skin reactions previously observed with iodine.

MUCOLYTIC DRUGS

***N*-Acetylcysteine** *(SEDA-16, 168; SEDA-17, 207; SEDA-20, 170)*

The mucolytic *N*-acetylcysteine is also an antioxidant, and it may protect the lung from free radicals generated by inflammatory cells activated by influenza virus infection (63[C]). The effect of oral *N*-acetylcysteine (600 mg bd for 6 months) on influenza symptoms has been examined in a randomized, double-blind trial of 262 patients, of whom 78% were aged 65 years or older. Patients with chronic respiratory diseases were excluded, to avoid bias. *N*-acetylcysteine significantly reduced the frequency of influenza-like episodes, severity of influenza, and length of time confined to bed. It was generally well tolerated, but some patients complained of *dysuria*, *epigastric pain*, *nausea and vomiting*, *constipation*, or *diarrhea and flushing*. Adverse effects were reported by 9% of patients compared with 5% in the placebo group. Blood pressure, heart-rate, and routine hematological and biochemical measurements were not significantly altered.

Current data do not appear to support the use of *N*-acetylcysteine in children with pulmonary disorders, such as asthmatic bronchitis, bronchitis, excessive mucus production, and dry cough (64[r]). In patients with adult respiratory distress syndrome, intravenous *N*-acetylcysteine did not significantly improve systemic oxygenation nor reduce the need for ventilatory support (65[C]).

Immunological and hypersensitivity reactions The management of anaphylactic reactions to intravenous *N*-acetylcysteine has been reviewed and guidelines developed for their treatment (66[R]). *Anaphylactoid reactions* to intravenous *N*-acetylcysteine appeared to be dose related. Flushing requires no treatment, urticaria should be treated with diphenhydramine, and *N*-acetylcysteine infusion can be continued in both cases. Angio-edema and respiratory symptoms both require diphenhydramine, symptomatic therapy, and the withdrawal of *N*-acetylcysteine. However, when necessary, *N*-acetylcysteine infusion can be started 1 h after the administration of diphenhydramine as symptoms subside.

MISCELLANEOUS DRUGS

Camphor *(SED-13, 433; SEDA-11, 150)*

Camphor is highly toxic, the reported lethal dose being 50–500 mg/kg (67[c]).

A 16-year-old girl took 30 g of camphor dissolved with 250 ml of wine to induce an abortion and started vomiting 45 min later, which may have saved her life (67[c]).

After an attempt at suicide with the camphorated phenol preparation Campho-Phenique (68 mg/kg of camphor and 28.9

mg/kg of phenol) generalized tonic–clonic seizures resulted within minutes (68[c]). The patient fully recovered within 12 h of intubation and supportive medical care.

Eucalyptus *(SED-13, 433; SEDA-16, 171)*

Eucalyptus oil can cause death in doses of 5–560 ml in adults and 15 ml in children (69[c]).

A 73-year-old woman deliberately took about 200–250 ml of eucalyptus oil. She was found unconscious in her home after she had vomited and had been incontinent of urine and feces. On admission to hospital unconscious, she was intubated, ventilated, and given charcoal and polyethylene glycol. The main complication was pneumonitis and aspiration pneumonia. Respiratory support was required for 7 weeks. Three months later she died of pneumonia.

IMMUNOTHERAPY *(SED-13, 424; SEDA-19, 184; SEDA-21, 189)*

Chemical interactions between formaldehyde and the components of standardized allergen extract result in changes in the net charge of the proteins and their tertiary structure. This reduces allergenicity/IgE-binding activity, but immunogenicity is retained. Thus, substantially more 'allergoid' than allergen can be injected into patients before anaphylactic symptoms are induced. As higher doses are tolerated, higher specific IgG concentrations result. Adsorption of allergoids on to aluminium hydroxide suspension gives the benefits of a depot formulation.

Subjects with hypersensitivity to *Parietaria* pollen with symptoms of rhinitis with or without asthma for at least three consecutive years ($n = 40$) were treated in a placebo-controlled trial extending over 2 years (70[C]). All had a positive skin prick response to *Parietaria* pollen extract, a positive nasal provocation response with *Parietaria* pollen extract, and a raised specific IgE concentration. An alum-adsorbed *Parietaria* pollen allergoid (Allergovit, Bracco and Allergopharma, Reinbek) was provided in a treatment set of two vials: vial A contained 1000 TU/ml and vial B 10 000 TU/ml. Maintenance therapy was given using the higher concentration. Immunotherapy caused a reduction in symptoms after natural exposure to the allergen and a reduction in the use of medications. The active treatment group received 547 injections over 2 years. Local immediate skin responses greater than 5 cm in diameter were observed after 13 of 880 injections of the active formulation and occurred in eight patients. This reaction was associated with higher doses of the allergoid, but all subjects were subsequently able to tolerate these doses. There were no immediate systemic reactions. After 27 injections of the active formulation, local late reactions larger than 5 cm in diameter were recorded. Moderate systemic responses were seen after 10 injections in eight of the patients, and the symptoms were controlled by beclomethasone dipropionate (2 puffs of 500 μg) or fenoterol (2 puffs of 400 μg).

Asthmatic patients sensitive to *Dermatophagoides pteronyssinus* ($n = 43$) were given specific immunotherapy over a period of 18 months (71[C]). The patients were divided into two groups: a high-dose immunotherapy (HDI) group (maximum tolerated dose, MTD (4 μg Der p I) and the conventional immunotherapy group (MTD less than 4 μg Der p I). The dose was gradually increased from 0.004 to 16 μg after 20 weeks. The MTD was defined as the highest dose that did not cause a systemic reaction, or the one before that which caused three consecutive large local reactions. In all, 1100 doses were used, 64% in the build-up and 36% in the maintenance periods. There were 54 adverse reactions, 40 of which were systemic, in 30 patients; this represents a frequency of systemic reactions of 4.1%. In only three of the 37 patients who reached the maintenance period was the MTD determined by the appearance of repeated local reactions; therefore, most of the systemic reactions were not preceded by significant local reactions. The most frequent local reactions appeared late ($n = 9$). Systemic reactions appeared only after doses from vials containing 0.4–3.2 μg and 4–16 μg of Der p 1. In the build-up period the frequency of systemic reactions after administering doses from the 4–16 μg vial was 26%, significantly higher than the 4.8% seen with the 0.4–3.2 μg vial. No serious systemic reactions occurred.

There were 13 delayed systemic reactions, including four cases of urticaria and nine of bronchospasm.

A double-blind placebo-controlled trial of multiple allergen immunotherapy has been conducted in 121 allergic children with moderate to severe perennial asthma requiring daily medication (72[C]). Seven treatment allergens for each child were selected on the basis of skin prick tests and measurement of specific IgE concentrations; a preference was given to perennial allergens, such as dust mite and moulds, over seasonal pollens. Treatment mixtures were prepared by combining 1.6 ml of the highest concentration available for each treatment allergen with albumin–saline diluent to a total volume of 9.6 ml per treatment vial. Immunotherapy was started with 0.1 ml of a 1:1000 dilution of this concentrate, and the dose was increased weekly by 0.1 ml until the target maintenance dose of 0.7 ml of concentrate was reached. If a dose produced systemic reactions on two occasions the next lower dose was used for maintenance. Maintenance treatment was given every 2 weeks for 24 months and every 3 weeks thereafter. The principal outcome measure was the amount of asthma medication required to control symptoms and maintain the PEFR within acceptable limits. Both groups were able to reduce their use of medications during the trial; there was a reduction in airway sensitivity to methacholine and a significant increase in the concentration of allergen-specific IgG antibody. Systemic reactions to allergen injection occurred in 21 of 61 children in the immunotherapy group and in four of the 60 in the placebo group. There were 114 systemic reactions in all, 52 of which were treated with adrenergic drugs. All responded to treatment without clinical sequelae. The rate of systemic reaction in the immunotherapy group was 2.6 per 100 injections. However, there was no significant improvement in the control of asthma after immunotherapy: partial or complete remission of asthma occurred in 31% of the immunotherapy group and 28% of the placebo group.

Immunological and hypersensitivity reactions A case of *serum sickness* has been described as a result of immunotherapy for wasp venom hypersensitivity (73[c]).

A man with severe anaphylaxis after a wasp sting had a positive skin test to *Vespula* wasp venom and a raised serum concentration of wasp venom IgE. Immunotherapy was begun. He was given 14 subcutaneous injections of purified venom (ALBAY 550, Vespula Sp, Dome Hollister Stier, Spokane, WA, USA) in increasing doses of 0.001–8 μg on day 1, six injections (4–40 μg) on day 2, three injections (40–50 μg) on day 3, and one injection (100 μg) on day 4. He then had full dose injections on days 9, 16, and 31, then at monthly intervals. After the injection on day 9 he developed erythema at the injection site; this resolved with antihistamines. After injections at 5 and 6 months he had isolated joint pain in both wrists. At 7 months (cumulative dose 1260 μg) he developed motor loss in the left upper limb, weakness of both lower limbs, high grade fever (40°C) of 48 h duration, a transient generalized rash, an indurated erythematous skin lesion over the left forearm, and arthritis of both wrists. There was diffuse flaccid motor loss in all four limbs. The deep tendon reflexes were absent and there was sensory loss to temperature and pain in the left half of the body. The serum concentration of IgE antibody specific to *Vespula* wasp venom, the circulating immune complex concentration, and serum aminotransferase activities were raised. There was evidence of moderate inflammation (raised C-reactive protein and serum fibrinogen). Clinical and electromyographic findings were consistent with a demyelinating polyneuropathy. A provisional diagnosis of serum sickness was made and he was treated with prednisone. There was no improvement after 2 days, but seven plasma exchanges produced dramatic improvement. After 10 days the only residual abnormality was a mild motor deficit and loss of deep tendon reflexes in the left upper limb. Prednisone was tapered off and the immunotherapy protocol was ceased. Six weeks later he suffered a relapse, with fever, erythema over the chest, and arthralgia in both wrists. There was recurrence of the motor deficit, with absent deep tendon jerks in the left upper and lower limbs. The clinical manifestations resolved after three plasma exchanges. Prednisone was again given for 10 days and then tapered off over 1 week. Five weeks later a third episode of serum sickness occurred, with arthralgia of both wrists, fever, and an erythematous rash over the anterior chest. His symptoms resolved after two plasma exchanges 7 days apart. One year later he remained well, with some slight sensory loss in the territory of the median nerve.

REFERENCES

1. Tinkelman DG, Bleecker ER, Ramsdell J, Ekholm BP, Klinger NM, Colice GL, Slade HB. Proventil HFA and Ventolin have similar safety profiles during regular use. Chest 1998;113:290–6.
2. Bleecker ER, Tinkelman DG, Ramsdell J, Ekholm BP, Klinger NM, Colice GL, Slade HB. Proventil HFA provides bronchodilation comparable to ventolin over 12 weeks of regular use in asthmatics. Chest 1998;113:283–9.
3. Dockhorn RJ, Wagner DE, Burgess GL, Hafner KB, Letourneau K, Colice GL, Klinger NM. Proventil HFA provides protection from exercise-induced bronchoconstriction comparable to Proventil and Ventolin. Ann Allergy Asthma Immunol 1997;79:85–8.
4. Poukkula A, Alanko K, Kilpio K, Knuuttila A, Koskinen S, Laitinen J, et al. Comparison of a multidose powder inhaler containing beclomethasone diproprionate (BDP) with a BDP metered dose inhaler with spacer in the treatment of asthmatic patients. Clin Drug Invest 1998;16:101–10.
5. Woodcock A. Effects of inhaled corticosteroids on bone density and metabolism. J Allergy Clin Immunol 1998;101:S456–9.
6. Eastell R. Management of corticosteroid-induced osteoporosis. UK Consensus Group Meeting on Osteoporosis. J Int Med 1995;237:439–47.
7. Pouw EM, Prummel MF, Oosting H, Roos CM, Endert E. Beclomethasone inhalation decreases serum osteocalcin concentrations. Br Med J 1991;302:627–8.
8. Morice AH, Morris D, Lawson-Matthew P. A comparison of nebulized budesonide with oral prednisolone in the treatment of exacerbations of obstructive pulmonary disease. Clin Pharmacol Ther 1996;60:675–8.
9. Kerstjens HA, Postma DS, Van Doormaal JJ, Van Zanten AK, Brand PL, Dekhuijzen PN, Koeter GH. Effects of short-term and long-term treatment with inhaled corticosteroids on bone metabolism in patients with airways obstruction. Dutch CNSLD Study Group. Thorax 1994; 49:652–6.
10. Bootsma GP, Dekhuijzen PN, Festen J, Mulder PG, Swinkels LM, Van Herwaarden CL. Fluticasone propionate does not influence bone metabolism in contrast to beclomethasone dipropionate. Am J Respir Crit Care Med 1996; 153:924–30.
11. Herrala J, Puolijoki H, Impivaara O, Liippo K, Tala E, Nieminen MM. Bone mineral density in asthmatic women on high-dose inhaled beclomethasone dipropionate. Bone 1994;15:621–3.
12. Boulet LP, Giguere MC, Milot J, Brown J. Effects of long-term use of high-dose inhaled steroids on bone density and calcium metabolism. J Allergy Clin Immunol 1994;94:796–803.
13. Hopp RJ, Degan JA, Biven RE, Kinberg K, Gallagher GC. Longitudinal assessment of bone mineral density in children with chronic asthma. Ann Allergy Asthma Immunol 1995;75:143–8.
14. Egan J, Kalra S, Adams J, Eastell R, Maden C, Woodcock A. A randomised double blind study comparing the effects of beclomethasone dipropionate 2000 μg/day versus fluticasone propionate 1000 μg/day on bone density over 2 years. Thorax 1995;50 (Suppl 2):A78.
15. Hughes J, Conry B, Male S, Eastell RA. A phase 3 open parallel group study to compare the efficacy of inhaled fluticasone propionate 500 μg bd and budesonide 800 μg bd on bone density measurements over 1 year in stable chronic asthmatics. Thorax 1996;51 (Suppl 3):A172.
16. Pauwels RA, Yernault JC, Demedts MG, Geusens P. Safety and efficacy of fluticasone and beclomethasone in moderate to severe asthma. Belgian Multicenter Study Group. Am J Respir Crit Care Med 1998;157:827–32.
17. Boutsen Y, Jamart J, Esselinckx W, Stoffel M, Devogelaer JP. Primary prevention of glucocorticoid-induced osteoporosis with intermittent intravenous pamidronate: a randomized trial. Calcif Tissue Int 1997;61:266–71.
18. Bijlsma JW. Prevention of glucocorticoid induced osteoporosis. Ann Rheum Dis 1997; 56:507–9.
19. Shaw NJ, Fraser NC, Weller PH. Asthma treatment and growth. Arch Dis Child 1997; 77:284–6.
20. Crowley S, Trivedi P, Risteli L, Risteli J, Hindmarsh PC, Brook CG. Collagen metabolism and growth in prepubertal children with asthma treated with inhaled corticosteroids. J Pediatr 1998;132:409–13.
21. Simons FE. A comparison of beclomethasone, salmeterol, and placebo in children with asthma. Canadian Beclomethasone Dipropionate-Salmeterol Xinafoate Study Group. New Engl J Med 1997;337:1659–65.
22. Cumming RG, Mitchell P, Leeder SR. Use of inhaled corticosteroids and the risk of cataracts. New Engl J Med 1997;337:8–14.
23. Whitmore SE. Inhaled corticosteroids and the risk of cataracts. New Engl J Med 1997;337:1554.
24. Leiner S. Inhaled corticosteroids and the risk of cataracts. New Engl J Med 1997;337:1554.
25. Murata Y, Kumano K, Ueda T, Araki N, Nakamura T, Tani M. Systemic contact dermatitis caused by systemic corticosteroid use. Arch Dermatol 1997;133:1053–4.
26. Figueredo E, Cuesta-Herranz JI, De Las H, Lluch-Bernal M, Umpierrez A, Sastre J. Anaphylaxis to dexamethasone. Allergy Eur J Allergy Clin Immunol 1997;52:877.
27. Fernandez S, Reano M, Vives R, Borja J, Daroca P, Canto G, Rodriguez J. 6-Methylprednisolone-induced bronchospasm. Allergy Eur J Allergy Clin Immunol 1997;52:780–2.
28. Lossos IS. Comment: drug-induced hiccups. Ann Pharmacother 1997;31:1264–5.

29. Nursoy MA, Bakir M, Barlan IB, Basaran MM. The course of chickenpox in asthmatic children receiving inhaled budesonide. Pediatr Infect Dis J 1997;16:74–7.
30. Sitar DS. Clinical pharmacokinetics of bambuterol. Clin Pharmacokin 1996;31:246–56.
31. D'Alonzo GE, Smolensky MH, Feldman S, Gnosspelius Y, Karlsson K. Bambuterol in the treatment of asthma. A placebo-controlled comparison of once-daily morning vs evening administration. Chest 1995;107:406–12.
32. Gunn SD, Ayres JG, McConchie SM. Comparison of the efficacy, tolerability and patient acceptability of once-daily bambuterol tablets against twice-daily controlled release albuterol in nocturnal asthma. ACROBATICS Research Group. Eur J Clin Pharmacol 1995;48:23–8.
33. McDonald CF, Pierce RJ, Thompson PJ, Allen D, Bowler S, Breslin AB, Bowes G, Saunders N, Murree-Allen K, Frith P, Musk AW. Comparison of oral bambuterol and terbutaline in elderly patients with chronic reversible airflow obstruction. J Asthma 1997;34:53–9.
34. Hildebrandt R, Weitzel HK, Gundert-Remy U. Hypokalaemia in pregnant women treated with the beta$_2$-mimetic drug fenoterol—a concentration and time dependent effect. J Perinat Med 1997;25:173–9.
35. Strauss L, Hejal R, Galan G, Dixon L, McFadden ER Jr. Observations on the effects of aerosolized albuterol in acute asthma. Am J Respir Crit Care Med 1997;155:454–8.
36. Rodrigo C, Rodrigo G. Therapeutic response patterns to high and cumulative doses of albuterol in acute severe asthma. Chest 1998;113:593–8.
37. Karpel JP, Aldrich TK, Prezant DJ, Guguchev K, Gaitan-Salas A, Pathiparti R. Emergency treatment of acute asthma with albuterol metered-dose inhaler plus holding chamber: how often should treatments be administered? Chest 1997;112:348–56.
38. Mandelberg A, Chen E, Noviski N, Priel IE. Nebulized wet aerosol treatment in emergency department—is it essential? Comparison with large spacer device for metered-dose inhaler. Chest 1997;112:1501–5.
39. Browne GJ, Penna AS, Phung X, Soo M. Randomised trial of intravenous albuterol in early management of acute severe asthma in children. Lancet 1997;349:301–5.
40. Lipworth BJ, Clark DJ. Effects of airway calibre on lung delivery of nebulised albuterol. Thorax 1997;52:1036–9.
41. De Troyer A, Yernault JC, Rodenstein D. Influence of beta-2 agonist aerosols on pressure-volume characteristics of the lungs. Am Rev Respir Dis 1978;118:987–95.
42. Kemp JP, Hill MR, Vaughan LM, Meltzer EO, Welch MJ, Ostrom NK. Pilot study of bronchodilator response to inhaled albuterol delivered by metered-dose inhaler and a novel dry powder inhaler. Ann Allergy Asthma Immunol 1997; 79:322–6.
43. Lofdahl CG, Andersson L, Bondesson E, Carlsson LG, Friberg K, Hedner J, Hornblad Y, Jemsby P, Kallen A, Ullman A, Werner S, Svedmyr N. Differences in bronchodilating potency of albuterol in Turbuhaler as compared with a pressurized metered-dose inhaler formulation in patients with reversible airway obstruction. Eur Respir J 1997;10:2474–8.
44. Millar EA, Connell JM, Thomson NC. The effect of nebulized albuterol on the activity of the renin-angiotensin system in asthma. Chest 1997;111:71–4.
45. Mann RD, Kubota K, Pearce G, Wilton L. Salmeterol: a study by prescription-event monitoring in a UK cohort of 15,407 patients. J Clin Epidemiol 1996;49:247–50.
46. Pollard SJ, Spector SL, Yancey SW, Cox FM, Emmett A. Salmeterol versus theophylline in the treatment of asthma. Ann Allergy Asthma Immunol 1997;78:457–64.
47. Weersink EJ, Douma RR, Postma DS, Koeter GH. Fluticasone propionate, salmeterol xinafoate, and their combination in the treatment of nocturnal asthma. Am J Respir Crit Care Med 1997;155:1241–6.
48. Selby C, Engleman HM, Fitzpatrick MF, Sime PM, Mackay TW, Douglas NJ. Inhaled salmeterol or oral theophylline in nocturnal asthma? Am J Respir Crit Care Med 1997;155:104–8.
49. Palmqvist M, Persson G, Lazer L, Rosenborg J, Larsson P, Lotvall J. Inhaled dry-powder formoterol and salmeterol in asthmatic patients: onset of action, duration of effect and potency. Eur Respir J 1997;10:2484–9.
50. Wilding P, Clark M, Coon JT, Lewis S, Rushton L, Bennett J, Oborne J, Cooper S, Tattersfield AE. Effect of long-term treatment with salmeterol on asthma control: a double blind, randomised crossover study. Br Med J 1997; 314:1441–6.
51. Peebles RS Jr, Permutt S, Togias A. Rapid reversibility of the allergen-induced pulmonary late-phase reaction by an intravenous beta$_2$-agonist. J Appl Physiol 1998;84:1500–5.
52. Burdet L, de Muralt B, Schutz Y, Fitting JW. Thermogenic effect of bronchodilators in patients with chronic obstructive pulmonary disease. Thorax 1997;52:130–5.
53. McFadden ER Jr, El Sanadi N, Strauss L, Galan G, Dixon L, McFadden CB, Shoemaker L, Gilbert L, Warren E, Hammonds T. The influence of parasympatholytics on the resolution of acute attacks of asthma. Am J Med 1997;102:7–13.
54. FitzGerald JM, Grunfeld A, Pare PD, Levy RD, Newhouse MT, Hodder R, Chapman KR. The clinical efficacy of combination nebulized anticholinergic and adrenergic bronchodilators vs nebulized adrenergic bronchodilator alone in acute asthma. Canadian Combivent Study Group. Chest 1997;111:311–15.
55. Garrett JE, Town GI, Rodwell P, Kelly AM. Nebulized albuterol with and without ipratropium

bromide in the treatment of acute asthma. J Allergy Clin Immunol 1997;100:165–70.
56. Calvo GM, Calvo AM, Marin HF, Moya GJ. Is it useful to add an anticholinergic treatment to beta$_2$-adrenergic medication in acute asthma attack? J Invest Allergol Clin Immunol 1998;8:30–4.
57. Lester MR, Bratton DL. Adverse reactions to cromolyn sodium: patient report and review of the literature. Clin Pediatr 1997;36:707–10.
58. Valdivieso R, Subiza J, Varela-Losada S, Subiza JL, Narganes MJ, Cabrera M, Serrano L. Severe allergic conjunctivitis and chemosis caused by disodium cromoglycate. J Invest Allergol Clin Immunol 1998;8:58–60.
59. Fiocchi A, Riva E, Santini I, Bernardo L, Sala M, Mirri GP. Effect of nedocromil sodium on bronchial hyperreactivity in children with non-atopic asthma. Ann Allergy Asthma Immunol 1997;79:503–6.
60. Hoshino M, Nakamura Y, Shin Z, Fukushima Y. Effects of ketotifen on symptoms and on bronchial mucosa in patients with atopic asthma. Allergy 1997;52:814–20.
61. Canny GJ, Reisman J, Levison H. Does ketotifen have a steroid-sparing effect in childhood asthma? Eur Respir J 1997;10:65–70.
62. Munoz FJ, Bellido J, Moyano JC, Alvarez MJ, Juan JL. Adverse reaction to potassium iodide from a cough syrup. Allergy 1997;52:111–12.
63. De Flora S, Grassi C, Carati L. Attenuation of influenza-like symptomatology and improvement of cell-mediated immunity with long-term *N*-acetylcysteine treatment. Eur Respir J 1997;10:1535–41.
64. Duijvestijn YC, Gerritsen J, Brand PL. Acetylcysteine in children with lung disorders prescribed by one-third of family physicians: no support in the literature. Ned Tijdschr Geneeskd 1997;141:826–30.
65. Domenighetti G, Suter PM, Schaller MD, Ritz R, Perret C. Treatment with *N*-acetylcysteine during acute respiratory distress syndrome: a randomized, double-blind, placebo-controlled clinical study. J Crit Care 1997;12:177–82.
66. Bailey B, McGuigan MA. Management of anaphylactoid reactions to intravenous *N*-acetylcysteine. Ann Emerg Med 1998;31:710–15.
67. Rabl W, Katzgraber F, Steinlechner M. Camphor ingestion for abortion. Forensic Sci Int 1997;89:137–40.
68. Lahoud CA, March JA, Proctor DD. Campho-Phenique ingestion: an intentional overdose. South Med J 1997;90:647–8.
69. Anpalahan M, Le Couteur DG. Deliberate self-poisoning with eucalyptus oil in an elderly woman. Aust New Zealand J Med 1998;28:58.
70. Tari MG, Mancino M, Ghezzi E, Frank E, Cromwell O. Immunotherapy with an alum-adsorbed *Parietaria*-pollen allergoid: a 2-year, double-blind, placebo-controlled study. Allergy 1997;52:65–74.
71. Olaguibel JM, Tabar AI, Garcia Figueroa BE, Cortes C. Immunotherapy with standardized extract of *Dermatophagoides pteronyssinus* in bronchial asthma: a dose-titration study. Allergy 1997;52:168–78.
72. Adkinson NF Jr, Eggleston PA, Eney D, Goldstein EO, Schuberth KC, Bacon JR, Hamilton RG, Weiss ME, Arshad H, Meinert CL, Tonascia J, Wheeler B. A controlled trial of immunotherapy for asthma in allergic children. New Engl J Med 1997;336:324–31.
73. De Bandt M, Atassi-Dumont M, Kahn MF, Herman D. Serum sickness after wasp venom immunotherapy: clinical and biological study. J Rheumatol 1997;24:1195–7.

J.K. Aronson

17 Positive inotropic drugs and drugs used in dysrhythmias

CARDIAC GLYCOSIDES *(SED-13, 438; SEDA-19, 188; SEDA-20, 173; SEDA-21, 194)*

The effects of digoxin in preventing supraventricular dysrhythmias and in converting atrial fibrillation to sinus rhythm have again been studied (1[C])–(3[C]). In the first study digoxin had no effect on the incidence of postoperative supraventricular dysrhythmias in 35 patients, and one developed a bradydysrhythmia with second-degree heart block attributed to digoxin (since it resolved after withdrawal). In the other two studies, in a total of 258 patients, intravenous digoxin was associated with no higher a rate of conversion to sinus rhythm than placebo. There were adverse effects in very few cases, including *sinus arrest* ($n = 1$), *asymptomatic pauses* ($n = 1$), *asymptomatic bradycardia* ($n = 4$), and *symptomatic self-terminating asystole* for 10 s ($n = 1$). In one patient with previously undiagnosed hypertrophic cardiomyopathy, digoxin caused *left ventricular outflow obstruction*, which resolved with atropine and volume expansion.

Following the DIG study (SEDA-20, 173), there have been several reviews of the usefulness of digoxin in the treatment of heart failure in sinus rhythm (4[R])–(7[R]). A reasonable consensus is that digoxin should be used in patients with heart failure who do not respond completely to diuretics plus either an ACE inhibitor or vasodilators. However, there is a risk of digoxin toxicity, and this is particularly so in patients who are prone to potassium depletion or have renal insufficiency. For the former a potassium-sparing diuretic should be considered if an ACE inhibitor has not provided sufficient potassium retention. In patients whose renal insufficiency is stable digoxin may be used with care, but in those whose renal function is unstable it is better avoided.

Cardiovascular From time to time reports appear confirming the truism that digoxin can cause any type of cardiac dysrhythmia. A recent case of *bidirectional ventricular tachycardia* (8[c]) has illustrated this.

A 71-year-old woman, who had taken digoxin orally for 12 years for atrial fibrillation, was given digoxin intravenously after mitral valve replacement, and developed bidirectional ventricular tachycardia. Her serum digoxin concentration was 4.5 ng/ml and her dysrhythmia responded to treatment with antidigoxin monoclonal antibodies.

Risk factors The use of digoxin in *elderly patients* has been reviewed (9[R]). Elderly patients are at a greater risk of digoxin toxicity, because of lower body-weight, impaired renal function, and a liability to electrolyte imbalance.

Treatment of toxicity The treatment of digoxin toxicity has again been reviewed, parti cularly in relation to elderly patients (10[R]).

Interactions *Amiodarone* The mechanisms whereby amiodarone increases plasma digoxin concentrations are not known, but there is evidence that it reduces the renal and nonrenal clearances of digoxin and its absorption from the gut, without changing its apparent volume of distribution (SEDA-12, 150). However, recent evidence has also suggested that ouabain and amiodarone compete for binding to the Na^+,K^+-ATPase (11). If this happened in man, one would expect a change in apparent volume of distribution, and this seems not to have been reported. However, if the inter-

Side Effects of Drugs, Annual 22
J.K. Aronson, ed.

action occurred only in the heart, say, the change in volume might be too small to be detected. The authors of this report have suggested that an interaction with Na^+, K^+-ATPase in guinea-pig heart may contribute to some of the cardiac actions of amiodarone, such as its prodysrhythmic effects.

Carbimazole In nine of 10 healthy subjects carbimazole reduced the C_{max} of digoxin significantly (from 1.72 to 1.33 ng/ml) without changing the t_{max} or AUC_{0-24} (12[C]). The authors suggested that this was due to a reduction in the rate of absorption, but that is an unlikely explanation, since the t_{max} was unchanged; if the effect on C_{max} was due to a change in the rate of absorption, then the lack of change in t_{max} would have to be explained by a concomitant change in the elimination rate constant, which did not appear to be the case, although serum concentrations were not measured for long enough after the dose to be sure about a change in half-life. A much more likely explanation, if this was a true effect, was that carbimazole increased the volume of distribution of digoxin. In one patient there was a greater than doubling of the C_{max} and a doubling of the AUC_{0-24}. These effects are difficult to explain. If the absorption of digoxin was poor in the absence of carbimazole, an approximate doubling in absorption could be the explanation; however, the absorption of digoxin from the tablets used in this study is usually good (about 67%). A reduction in clearance could have doubled the AUC, but that would have led to a change in half-life, which would have consequently have changed the t_{max}, which did not change in this case. Clearly, these results need to be clarified and confirmed. The authors did not discuss the possibility that carbimazole or a metabolite might have interfered with the fluorescent assay for digoxin that they used.

Eprosartan In 12 healthy men the ATII receptor antagonist eprosartan had no effect on the C_{max} and AUC of digoxin after an oral dose of encapsulated elixir of digoxin (13[C]).

Imidapril In 12 healthy volunteers oral administration of the ACE inhibitor imidapril had no effect on the disposition of digoxin at steady state (14[C]). Digoxin caused a very small reduction in the plasma concentrations of imidapril and a larger reduction in the plasma concentrations of imidaprilat. The authors suggested that this was due to a small reduction in the systemic availability of imidapril (by about 10%). This interaction is probably of little clinical relevance.

Itraconazole Itraconazole increases steady-state serum digoxin concentrations (SEDA-21, 196). One proposed mechanism of this interaction is inhibition of the renal secretion of digoxin by inhibition of P-glycoprotein in the kidney, and this has been bolstered by two further reports suggesting that itraconazole reduces the renal clearance of digoxin, one in a patient taking digoxin for atrial fibrillation (15[c]) and one in 10 healthy volunteers (16[C]). There is also in vitro evidence to support this suggestion (17).

Macrolide antibiotics Macrolide antibiotics reduce the metabolism of digoxin in the gut in some patients before it is absorbed, by inhibiting the growth of *Eubacterium lentum*, an organism that can convert digoxin to less active or inactive metabolites (SEDA-7, 197; SEDA-21, 195). Further anecdotal reports that clarithromycin can do this have recently appeared in six patients (18[c])–(20[c]).

Propafenone Propafenone causes a small increase in plasma digoxin concentrations, but the mechanism is not clear (SEDA-12, 150). Now it has been suggested, from in vitro studies in canine kidney cell monolayers, that propafenone and its two major metabolites, 5-hydroxypropafenone and *N*-depropylpropafenone, inhibit the P-glycoprotein, thus inhibiting the renal clearance of digoxin (21). However, previous studies in man have shown either no effect on renal clearance or a reduction in renal clearance that was attributable to a reduction in glomerular filtration rate, rather than tubular secretion.

Anti-digoxin antibody fragments

The pharmacokinetics of Fab fragments of antidigoxin antibodies have been studied in patients with digoxin or digitoxin intoxication and renal insufficiency (22[c]), (23[C]). The clearance of the Fab fragments was reduced in proportion to the reduction in creatinine clearance. Although some authors have been concerned that prolongation of the presence of digoxin bound to Fab fragments might encourage further exposure to digoxin after dissociation of the complex, the high affinity that Fab fragments have for digoxin and other cardiac glycosides makes this unlikely to be a problem. Indeed, others have suggested that the prolonged presence of excess fragments, unbound to digoxin, would be beneficial in increasing the probability of retrieving digoxin molecules bound to the tissues in toxicity.

OTHER POSITIVE INOTROPIC DRUGS *(SED-13, 447; SEDA-19, 189; SEDA-20, 174; SEDA-21, 196)*

Milrinone

Despite the long-term disadvantages of using milrinone in cardiac failure, with an associated increase in mortality (SEDA-17, 217), reports continue to appear of its beneficial effects after intravenous administration in patients with acute heart failure (SEDA-21, 196); further reports have now appeared. In a prospective, non-randomized study in 71 patients, intravenous milrinone for as long as 8 weeks helped achieve hemodynamic stability, in many cases with successful bridging to heart transplantation (24[C]). Mechanical support from an intra-aortic balloon pump was not often needed in patients treated with milrinone alone, compared with those treated with dobutamine. Adverse effects in those treated with milrinone included a single episode of *ischemic pain* in the setting of hypotension, four cases of *supraventricular dysrhythmias*, and three episodes of sustained *ventricular dysrhythmias*. There was *hypotension* in four patients with renal insufficiency and in one as a result of a drug dosing error. *Thrombocytopenia* (platelet count below 100×10^{12}/l) occurred in three cases, but was attributed to heparin in two.

Milrinone has also been shown to be effective in helping to wean patients from cardiopulmonary bypass (25[C]). In 32 patients with reduced preoperative left-ventricular ejection fractions and/or increased mean pulmonary arterial pressure who were given intravenous milrinone or placebo, bypass support was successfully withdrawn in the 15 patients given milrinone, but in only five of the 15 given placebo (two patients were withdrawn). There were reductions in platelet counts in one patient receiving milrinone and two receiving placebo. One patient receiving milrinone developed a *ventricular tachycardia*, lasting about 1 min, 3 days postoperatively.

DRUGS USED IN DYSRHYTHMIAS

Reviews of the use and adverse effects of antidysrhythmic drugs have appeared in relation to atrial fibrillation (26[R]), (27[R]), paroxysmal supraventricular tachycardia (28[R]), supraventricular tachycardias in children (29[R]), and dysrhythmias after cardiothoracic surgery (30[R]). The adverse effects of Class I antidysrhythmic drugs (31[R]) and of Class III antidysrhythmic drugs (32[R]) have also been reviewed, as has drug-induced *torsade de pointes* (33[R]).

Adenosine *(SED-13, 450; SEDA-19, 190; SEDA-20, 174; SEDA-21, 197)*

The uses and adverse effects of adenosine have been reviewed in its role as an antidysrhythmic drug (34[R]), and in stress echocardiography in the diagnosis of pulmonary artery disease (35[R])–(37[R]).

In a comparison of intravenous adenosine and dipyridamole in 24 patients undergoing thallium scanning, the usual adverse effects of adenosine were observed in 81% (38[C]). The most common adverse effects were *flushing* and *chest pain*. There were severe adverse effects in 4.2%, and in 5% medical intervention (unspecified) was required. However, the adverse effects were transient in all but one case, in which the effects persisted for more than 10 min.

Cardiovascular Transient *atrial fibrillation* has occasionally been reported with adenosine (SEDA-16, 176; SEDA-20, 174). In 200 patients with paroxysmal supraventricular tachycardia, in 198 of whom the dysrhythmia terminated with adenosine, atrial fibrillation or fibrillation and flutter occurred in 24 (12%). An atrial premature complex occurred in all 24, but also in 102 of the 106 patients who did not have atrial dysrhythmias (39[C]). Atrial fibrillation lasted more than 10 min in one-third of the patients. The authors proposed that the mechanism was shortening of the atrial refractory period by adenosine. Most of the patients had a re-entrant tachycardia, either atrioventricular or atrioventricular nodal, and the authors suggested that if the mechanism of a paroxysmal supraventricular tachycardia is unknown and the Wolff–Parkinson–White syndrome is possible, adenosine should be given only if emergency resuscitation is available, because of the potential for a rapid pre-excited ventricular response during atrial fibrillation.

Adenosine has been used in 57 patients to induce transient ventricular asystole during coronary artery bypass grafting (40[C]). During the asystolic pause there was increasing *ventricular dilatation*, due to continuing atrial contractions. During recovery *reflex tachycardia* occurred in about 20% and was controlled with esmolol if necessary. One patient developed a transient episode of *atrial fibrillation*, but there were no other dysrhythmias, apart from occasional *ventricular escape beats*.

Adenosine is a coronary vasodilator, and during exercise ventriculography can cause *myocardial ischemia* through a steal syndrome (SEDA-19, 190). Adenosine, dobutamine, and exercise have been compared as methods for detecting myocardial ischemia during radionuclide ventriculography in 41 patients (41[C]). Myocardial ischemia was judged by the development of new abnormalities of movement of the left ventricular wall. Adenosine-induced ischemia was predicted by the number of stenotic vessels and the peak filling rate; only one of the 14 patients with single-vessel disease developed myocardial ischemic in response to adenosine, suggesting poor sensitivity of adenosine for diagnostic purposes. The corollary of this is that a positive test suggests multivessel disease. This finding has been substantiated by a study in 13 patients, of whom only two had new abnormalities of wall movement during the infusion of adenosine (42[C]). Furthermore, there was little metabolic evidence of ischemia in these patients, only two of whom had evidence of lactate production. The authors suggested that the main mechanism of adenosine-induced defects in thallium scans is heterogeneity of regional blood flow between regions of the myocardium supplied by normal and stenotic arteries.

Two adult patients with structurally normal hearts and normal QT intervals developed *non-sustained polymorphous ventricular tachycardia* after the administration of adenosine for supraventricular tachycardia (43[c]). Adenosine has previously been assumed to cause this rhythm disturbance only in patients with congenital or acquired long QT intervals and was therefore used as a marker of this syndrome.

Risk factors The authors of a recent review of the pediatric use of adenosine as an antidysrhythmic agent have recommended it as the drug of choice in the treatment of paroxysmal tachycardia in *children* (44[R]). Systemic adverse effects, particularly flushing and chest pain, are frequent, but do not require intervention. Severe bronchospasm has occasionally been reported, and adenosine should therefore not be used in patients with reversible airways obstruction. Life-threatening adverse effects are rare, and include prolonged sinus arrest, complete atrioventricular block, atrial fibrillation, ventricular tachycardia, and apnea.

Amiodarone *(SED-13, 452; SEDA-19, 192; SEDA-20, 175; SEDA-21, 198)*

The adverse effects of amiodarone after intravenous administration have been reviewed (45[R]), (46[R]).

The adverse effects of amiodarone in doses of 152–330 mg/day have been analysed in a meta-analysis of four double-blind placebo-controlled trials involving 1465 patients (47[C]). The odds ratios for the different adverse effects (95% CI) were *thyroid* 4.2 (2.0, 8.7), *nervous system* 2.0 (1.3, 3.7), *skin* 2.5 (1.1, 6.2), *eyes* 3.4 (1.2, 9.6), and *bradycardia* 2.2 (1.1, 4.3). There was no increase over placebo in the risk of liver or gastrointestinal effects, and there was only a trend towards pulmonary toxicity, with an odds ratio of 2.0 (0.9, 5.3). Drug withdrawal was necessary in 23% of those taking amiodarone, compared with 15% of those taking placebo, odds ratio 1.5 (1.2, 1.9). There were no cases of dysrhythmias in this analysis.

Cardiovascular Short-term administration of low-dose amiodarone before open-heart surgery and until discharge from hospital in 124 patients reduced the rate of postoperative atrial fibrillation from 53 to 25% (48[C]). In this very brief study (duration of administration 13 days on average) there were no differences in adverse effects between amiodarone and placebo.

In contrast, in 44 patients who were given amiodarone in a mean dose of 205 mg/day preoperatively for up to an average of 231 (range 7–1440) days in a maintenance dosage of 100–420 mg/day (total dose 3–430 g), cardiovascular adverse effects were more common than in 44 controls (49[C]). Adverse effects in the immediate postoperative period were more common in those treated with amiodarone (19 vs 5); these included *atrial fibrillation*, *a need for temporary pacing or an intra-aortic balloon pump*, *myocardial infarction*, and *pulmonary edema*. The patients in the first of these two studies were more highly selected than in the second, and this may have contributed to the differences in results.

Although amiodarone can cause cardiac dysrhythmias, it does so less often than other antidysrhythmic drugs (SEDA-19, 192). Nevertheless, from time to time cases of *polymorphous ventricular tachycardia* are reported (50[c]).

A 77-year old man was given amiodarone 200 mg tds for paroxysmal atrial fibrillation, and 11 days later had an attack of syncope. An electrocardiogram showed self-limiting episodes of a wide complex tachycardia. His QT_c interval had lengthened from 400 to 600 ms. His plasma amiodarone concentration was 0.6 μg/ml, but the plasma concentration of desethylamiodarone was not reported. He was subsequently shown to be having attacks of polymorphous ventricular tachycardia. The dysrhythmia resolved after withdrawal of amiodarone and the administration of magnesium sulfate. There were no electrolyte abnormalities. He was taking no other drugs normally associated with this dysrhythmia.

Respiratory A case of *acute pulmonary toxicity* has recently been reported after the use of intravenous amiodarone in a child with impaired liver function (51[c]).

A 7-month-old boy was given intravenous amiodarone 10 mg/kg as an oral dose followed by a maintenance infusion of 10 mg/kg per day. After 5 days his treatment was changed to oral amiodarone 10 mg/kg per day. By 8 days there was evidence of diffuse nodular and interstitial infiltrates in the chest X-ray, and bronchoalveolar lavage showed foamy macrophages containing lipid. Amiodarone was withdrawn at 11 days, after which improvement occurred rapidly.

This case may have been due to accumulation of amiodarone and its metabolite desethylamiodarone because of hepatic impairment, but unfortunately plasma concentrations were not measured.

Lung damage due to amiodarone usually takes the form of an *interstitial alveolitis* (SEDA-15, 168), as has been illustrated by further case reports (52[c]), (53[c]). In the second of these cases the presentation was rapid and included hemoptysis. However, as another case report has illustrated (54[c]), other types of damage are possible.

A 65-year-old woman was given amiodarone 200 mg bd for paroxysmal atrial fibrillation. Two weeks later she developed acute sinusitis, and over the next few days became breathless and developed a dry cough. A chest X-ray showed bilateral, irregular, nodular opacities, with confluent lesions in the right upper lobe. There was right apical pleural thickening. Consolidation progressed in the right upper lobe and developed in the left lower lobe, while the nodular opacities became generally more prominent. Small bilateral pleural effusions developed, and a CT scan with contrast showed a high degree of attenuation in the nodules, ground-glass opacities in both upper lobes and the right middle lobe, and borderline enlargement of mediastinal lymph nodes. After 9 days amiodarone was withdrawn and prednisone (30 mg/day) was given. A biopsy showed diffuse infiltration of vacuolated histiocytes and lymphocytes in the peribronchiolar interstitium and alveolar walls, consistent with amiodarone-induced pneumonitis. However, there was also necrotizing bronchiolitis and fibrinoid necrosis, consistent with Wegener's granulomatosis.

In this case it appears that Wegener's granulomatosis and amiodarone-induced lung damage co-existed. There was no discussion of the question of whether the primary disease might have exacerbated the lung response to amiodarone.

Nervous system Amiodarone only occasionally causes nervous system effects (SEDA-16, 178), including Parkinsonian-like abnormalities. This has been further confirmed by the report of a case of *akinesia* in a 48-year-old man, who had been given a single loading dose of 3 g. Impaired liver function in this case may have contributed, but plasma concentrations of amiodarone and desethylamiodarone were not measured (55[c]).

Endocrine, metabolic The effects of amiodarone on thyroid function and methods of treating abnormal thyroid function in patients taking amiodarone have been reviewed (56[R]).

Amiodarone-induced *hyperthyroidism* can be very difficult to treat (SEDA-21, 199), and this has been illustrated by two further cases in elderly patients in whom thyroidectomy was required when the thyroid gland became enlarged and nodular, despite treatment with methimazole or propylthiouracil (57[c]). The authors discussed the problems of anesthesia in such cases.

Most cases of thyroid dysfunction in patients taking amiodarone occur during long-term treatment. However, acute abnormalities in thyroid function have now also been reported (58[C]). In 24 patients who were given an intravenous loading infusion of 20 ml/kg on day 1 and 10 mg/kg on day 2, 600 mg/day orally for 7–10 days, and then 200–400 mg/day orally in long-term treatment, the following changes occurred:

(1) a rise in TSH concentration from the first day of treatment, reaching 2.7 times higher than at baseline at 10 days;
(2) a progressive rise in the concentration of reverse T_3 in parallel with TSH, at 10 days reaching about twice as high as at baseline;
(3) a reduction in total T_3 starting on the second day;
(4) progressive increases in total and unbound concentrations of T_4 starting on the fourth day of treatment;
(5) no change in unbound T_3.

It is not clear why amiodarone first caused a rise in serum TSH; however, the authors hypothesized that it might have been due to early inhibition of 5′-deiodinase in pituitary cells, or possibly a direct effect on the secretion of TSH and competition of amiodarone and desethylamiodarone with T_3 for specific nuclear T_3 receptors. The later changes in serum total and unbound T_4 could have been due to direct stimulation of T_4 secretion by the increase in TSH. The changes in T_3 were probably due to inhibition of peripheral conversion of T_4 to T_3, and that might also have contributed to the changes in T_4.

Lithium has been proposed as an alternative to surgical treatment of resistance of hyperthyroidism to conventional drug treatment (59[C]). Of 21 patients with amiodarone-induced hyperthyroidism, five were treated by withdrawal of amiodarone, seven received propylthiouracil 300–600 mg/day, and nine received propylthiouracil 300 mg/day plus lithium 900–1350 mg/day. The time to recovery in the first two groups was about 11 weeks compared with 4 weeks in those given lithium. This was despite the fact that those treated with lithium had more severe symptoms and signs of hyperthyroidism and had been taking amiodarone for significantly longer. The authors concluded that lithium was useful and safe for the treatment of thyrotoxicosis in patients taking amiodarone, but that they would currently reserve it for severe cases only. Lithium inhibits the release of T_4 from the thyroid gland and probably reduces its deiodination.

Liver *Acute severe hepatitis* has occasionally been reported after intravenous amiodarone (SEDA-14, 149; SEDA-15, 170; SEDA-16, 178). Since this has not been reported with oral administration, it may be that the effect is due to the diluent in which amiodarone is prepared, namely polysorbate (Tween) 80. This suggestion has been borne out by the observation that acute hepatitis in a 50-year-old man occurred after the intravenous administration of amiodarone 1.2 g but not during subsequent long-term oral administration (60[c]).

There are many different mechanisms of *microvesicular hepatic steatosis* secondary to drugs, hormones, and cytokines, and these have been reviewed (61[R]). Amiodarone causes this by inhibiting both mitochondrial β-oxidation and the respiratory chain. In lysosomal phospholipidosis the uncharged cationic amphiphilic form of the drug crosses the lysosomal membrane, is trapped in the protonated form, and inhibits the action of intralysosomal phospholipases. A similar effect in mitochondria causes inhibition of electron transfer through the respiratory chain and inhibition of mitochondrial β oxidative enzymes. This in turn can lead to changes similar to those of alcoholic liver disease (SEDA-14, 149).

The effects of amiodarone deposition over many years of treatment on the appearance of the liver on CT scan has been demonstrated in a 66-year-old man in whom there was an abnormally high density of liver tissue (62[c]). Histology showed portal and lobular hepatitis and portal fibrosis and no evidence of increased iron storage.

Pancreas *Pancreatitis* has rarely been reported in patients taking amiodarone (SEDA-21, 199), but a further case has been reported in a 46-year-old woman who had taken amiodarone in a maintenance dose of about 200 mg/day (63[C]).

Skin and appendages Another case of *blue-grey pigmentation* of the skin of the face has been reported in a 61-year-old man who had taken amiodarone in a dose of 200 mg/day for about a year (64[c]).

Interactions In a 52-year-old man taking amiodarone 200 mg bd, plasma concentrations of amiodarone and desethylamiodarone were higher during concurrent therapy with *sertraline* and carbamazepine (65[c]). Since sertraline inhibits CYP3A4 and carbamazepine induces it, the authors attributed this effect to inhibition of the metabolism of amiodarone by sertraline. This was supported by the observation that the change in plasma amiodarone concentration was much greater than the change in the plasma concentration of desethylamiodarone.

Disopyramide *(SED-13, 457; SEDA-19, 194; SEDA-20, 177; SEDA-21, 199)*

Cardiovascular Disopyramide has a marked negative inotropic effect and can therefore cause *hypotension* (SEDA-10, 149). This effect can be potentiated by other drugs with negative inotropic effects, as has been demonstrated in the case of a 54-year-old man, who was treated with disopyramide and metoprolol and developed a severe bradycardia, hypotension, and worsening heart failure associated with hypertrophic obstructive cardiomyopathy (66[c]).

Interactions *Clarithromycin* reduces the clearance of disopyramide (SEDA-21, 200), and this has again been reported in a 74-year-old woman who developed marked prolongation of the QT_c interval in conjunction with a low serum potassium concentration (67[c]). The plasma concentration of disopyramide was at the upper end of the target range and its half-life was markedly prolonged (40 h).

Flecainide *(SED-13, 459; SEDA-19, 195; SEDA-20, 178; SEDA-21, 200)*

Central nervous system adverse effects of flecainide are common (SEDA-15, 176). *Paranoid psychosis*, which has not previously been reported, has now been described (68[c]).

A 62-year-old man was given flecainide 100 mg bd for the treatment of malignant neuropathic pain. After 5 days he became increasingly confused and paranoid. His symptoms disappeared over the 2 weeks after flecainide had been withdrawn. The serum flecainide concentration on admission was greatly raised at 1730 μg/l (target 200–700).

The long duration of recovery in this case suggests that the half-life of flecainide may have been prolonged. However, it was not measured. Other possible causes of psychosis were not ruled out.

Lidocaine (lignocaine) *(SED-13, 460; SEDA-18, 205; SEDA-21, 201)*

Cardiovascular In 100 patients the cardiovascular effects of tracheal extubation were attenuated by the administration of verapamil and lidocaine, both alone and in combination (69[C]). The effects of the combination were greater than the effects of either drug alone. The dose of lidocaine was small (1 mg/kg) and there were no adverse effects attributable to it, although it significantly suppressed coughing and strain.

Nervous system Lidocaine has been used to treat status epilepticus in sporadic studies, mostly in children, and this has been reviewed (70[R]). Despite the use of very high dosages in some of these studies, in a total of 155 patients, adverse effects were rare, and in only one case was toxicity suspected, namely possible *seizure induction or prolongation*.

Risk factors Lidocaine is metabolized to two toxic metabolites, the first step resulting in the formation of monoethylglycinexylidide. The rate of formation of this metabolite from lidocaine is sometimes used as a measurement of liver function, and in 60 children the incidence of adverse effects, largely unspecified, was less in those with *cirrhosis and impaired liver function* than in those who had cirrhosis but normal liver function (71[C]). Since the rate of formation of monoethylglycinexylidide falls with increasing age (72[C]), one would also expect that there would be fewer adverse effects, dose for dose, in elderly patients.

Mexiletine *(SED-13, 462; SEDA-19, 195; SEDA-21, 201)*

In 31 patients randomized to receive either placebo or mexiletine in the treatment of diabetic peripheral neuropathy, adverse effects were more common in those taking mexiletine. The difference was not significant, however, probably because of the small number of subjects studied. However, the expected adverse effects were reported, namely *nausea*, *headache*, *diarrhea*, and *vomiting*. There were also individual cases of *itching*, *pain*, and *palpitation* (73[C]).

Procainamide *(SED-13, 463; SEDA-19, 196; SEDA-20, 178; SEDA-21, 202)*

The short half-life of procainamide means that four times daily dosing is required. To obviate this various modified-release formulations have been developed over the years. A recent twice-daily formulation has been evaluated in 99 patients with ventricular extra beats (74[C]). Adverse effects occurred in 36 patients and were not dose-related; however, the adverse effects that were thought to be associated with procainamide occurred in only 14 patients. There was one death and seven withdrawals due to adverse events associated with the drug. *Chest pain* was more common with procainamide than placebo. Two patients withdrew because of an increased titer of antinuclear antibody, one in association with symptoms of *lupus-like syndrome*. There were no episodes of symptomatic dysrhythmias, and in two cases asymptomatic dysrhythmias were not severe enough to require withdrawal. There were no unexpected abnormalities of laboratory measurements. Blood dyscrasias have previously been reported with procainamide and have been suggested to be more common with modified-release formulations (SEDA-12, 154), although this was not subsequently confirmed (SEDA-21, 202); there were no adverse hematological effects in this study.

Nervous system The handful of reports that procainamide can cause *exacerbation of myasthenia gravis* have been reviewed (75[cR]). The effect seems to be associated with altered postsynaptic binding of acetylcholine to its receptor.

Immunological and hypersensitivity reactions *Antiphospholipid antibodies* have previously been reported in patients with lupus-like syndrome due to procainamide (SEDA-16, 183). In a comparison of 66 patients taking procainamide with 30 similar patients not taking procainamide, 21% of those taking procainamide had moderate to high titers of antiphospholipid antibodies, compared with none of the controls (76[C]). The antiphospholipid antibodies were associated with antinuclear antibodies and antihistone antibodies, but not with clinical manifestations of the lupus-like syndrome.

Propafenone *(SED-13, 465; SEDA-19, 196; SEDA-20, 178; SEDA-21, 202)*

The adverse effects of propafenone in the conversion of recent atrial fibrillation to sinus rhythm or in the treatment of paroxysmal atrial fibrillation have recently been reported in several studies. In a comparison of propafenone with sotalol in the treatment of symptomatic paroxysmal atrial fibrillation in 75 patients, 26% of those treated with propafenone had drug-related adverse effects, including *gastrointestinal discomfort* (10%), *dizziness, blurred vision, and neuralgia* (8%), *a metallic taste* (5%), and *general weakness* (3%); there were no cardiovascular adverse effects (77[C]).

In 240 patients with recent onset atrial fibrillation propafenone was more effective than placebo in converting atrial fibrillation to sinus rhythm (78[C]). Nine of the 119 patients who received propafenone had adverse effects, including *prolongation of the QRS complex* ($n = 3$), *hypotension* ($n = 2$), slight *hypotension and bradycardia* at the moment of conversion ($n = 3$), and episodes of *junctional rhythm* after conversion ($n = 1$). There were no ventricular dysrhythmias. In a similar study in 55 patients, randomized to a single oral dose of propafenone or placebo, transient *hypotension* in three cases was the only adverse effect of propafenone (79[C]). Finally, in a comparison of two different oral loading doses of propafenone (450 or 600 mg) in 105 patients with atrial fibrillation, there were no major adverse effects (80[C]). These three studies suggest that single dose oral propafenone in the conversion of atrial fibrillation to sinus rhythm is very safe.

Nervous system There has been a report of *worsening myasthenia gravis* in a 68-year-man a few hours after he had started to take oral propafenone (75[cR]).

Risk factors Since propafenone is mostly metabolized, one would not expect that its disposition would be altered in *renal insufficiency*. In a study of 28 patients given propafenone for atrial fibrillation associated with chronic renal insufficiency an intravenous bonus dose of 1 mg/kg caused no serious adverse effects or dysrhythmias (81[C]). There was no prolongation of the QT interval, and renal function was not affected by propafenone.

Quinidine *(SED-13, 466; SEDA-19, 196; SEDA-20, 179; SEDA-21, 203)*

Quinidine inhibits the metabolism of *nifedipine* and increases its pharmacological effects (82[C]), (83[C]). In an in vitro study of the interaction of quinidine with nifedipine in binding to a human form of CYP3A4 expressed in insect cells, quinidine was a non-competitive inhibitor of the binding of nifedipine (84).

REFERENCES

1. Amar D, Roistacher N, Burt ME, Rusch VW, Bains MS, Leung DHY, Downey RJ, Ginsberg RJ, Todd TRJ, Curtis JJ. Effects of diltiazem versus digoxin on dysrhythmias and cardiac function after pneumonectomy. Ann Thorac Surg 1997;63:1374–82.
2. Jordaens L, Trouerbach J, Calle P, Tavernier R, Derycke E, Vertongen P, Bergez B, Vandekerckhove Y. Conversion of atrial fibrillation to sinus rhythm and rate control by digoxin in comparison to placebo. Eur Heart J 1997;18:643–8.
3. Hornestam B, Held P, Boman K, Lundstrom T, Peterson M, Karlsson BW, Carlsson T, Falk L, Edvardsson N. Intravenous digoxin in acute atrial fibrillation. Results of a randomized, placebo-controlled multicentre trial in 239 patients. The Digitalis in Acute Atrial Fibrillation (DAAF) Trial Group. Eur Heart J 1997;18:649–54.
4. Reddy S, Benatar D, Gheorghiade M. Update on digoxin and other oral positive inotropic agents for chronic heart failure. Curr Opin Cardiol 1997;12:233–41.
5. Williamson KM, Patterson JH. Is there an expanded role for digoxin in patients with heart failure and sinus rhythm? A protagonist viewpoint. Ann Pharmacother 1997;31:888–92.

6. Campbell RWF. Whither digitalis? Lancet 1997;349:1854–5.
7. Gheorghiade M. Digoxin therapy in chronic heart failure. Cardiovasc Drugs Ther 1997;11 (Suppl 1):279–83.
8. Valent S, Kelly P. Images in clinical medicine. New Engl J Med 1997;336:550.
9. Gosselink ATM, Van Veldhuisen DJ, Crijns HJG. When, and when not, to use digoxin in the elderly. Drugs Aging 1997;10:411–20.
10. Borron SW, Bismuth C, Muszynski J. Advances in the management of digoxin toxicity in the older patient. Drugs Aging 1997;10:18–33.
11. Almotrefi AA, Basco MC, Moorji A, Dzimiri N. Effects of amiodarone on ouabain binding to microsomal Na^+,K^+-ATPase in guinea-pig heart preparations. Gen Pharmacol 1997;29:639–43.
12. Rao BR, Petereit G, Ebert U, Kirch W. Influence of carbimazole on serum levels and haemodynamic effects of digoxin. Clin Drug Invest 1997;13:350–4.
13. Martin DE, Tompson D, Boike SC, Tenero D, Ilson B, Citerone D, Jorkasky DK. Lack of effect of eprosartan on the single dose pharmacokinetics of orally administered digoxin in healthy male volunteers. Br J Clin Pharmacol 1997; 43:661–4.
14. Harder S, Thurmann PA. Pharmacokinetic and pharmacodynamic interaction trial after repeated oral doses of imidapril and digoxin in healthy volunteers. Br J Clin Pharmacol 1997;43:475–80.
15. Alderman CP, Allcroft PD. Digoxin-itraconazole interaction: possible mechanisms. Ann Pharmacother 1997;31:438–40.
16. Jalava K-M, Partanen J, Neuvonen PJ. Itraconazole decreases renal clearance of digoxin. Ther Drug Monit 1997;19:609–13.
17. Ito S, Koren G. Comment: possible mechanism of digoxin-itraconazole interaction. Ann Pharmacother 1997;31:1091–2.
18. Nawarskas JJ, McCarthy DM, Spinler SA. Digoxin toxicity secondary to clarithromycin therapy. Ann Pharmacother 1997;31:864–6.
19. Laberge P, Martineau P. Clarithromycin-induced digoxin intoxication. Ann Pharmacother 1997;31:999–1002.
20. Brown BA, Wallace RJ Jr, Griffith DE, Warden R. Clarithromycin-associated digoxin toxicity in the elderly. Clin Infect Dis 1997;24:92–3.
21. Woodland C, Verjee Z, Giesbrecht F, Koren G, Ito S. The digoxin-propafenone interaction: characterization of a mechanism using renal tubular cell monolayers. J Pharmacol Exp Ther 1997;283:39–45.
22. Caspi O, Zylber-Katz E, Gotsman O, Wolf DG, Caraco Y. Digoxin intoxication in a patient with end-stage renal disease: efficacy of digoxin-specific Fab antibody fragments and peritoneal dialysis. Ther Drug Monit 1997;19:510–15.
23. Renard C, Grene-Lerouge N, Beau N, Baud F, Scherrmann JM. Pharmacokinetics of digoxin-specific Fab: effects of decreased renal function and age. Br J Clin Pharmacol 1997;44:135–8.
24. Mehra MR, Ventura HO, Kapoor C, Stapleton DD, Zimmerman D, Smart FW. Safety and clinical utility of long-term intravenous milrinone in advanced heart failure. Am J Cardiol 1997; 80:61–4.
25. Doolan LA, Jones EF, Kalman J, Buxton BF, Tonkin AM. A placebo-controlled trial verifying the efficacy of milrinone in weaning high-risk patients from cardiopulmonary bypass. J Cardiothorac Vasc Anesth 1997;11:37–41.
26. Maisel WH, Kuntz KM, Reimold SC, Lee TH, Antman EM, Friedman PL, Stevenson WG. Risk of initiating antiarrhythmic drug therapy for atrial fibrillation in patients admitted to a university hospital. Ann Intern Med 1997; 127:281–4.
27. Ganz LI, Antman EM. Antiarrhythmic drug therapy in the management of atrial fibrillation. J Cardiovasc Electrophysiol 1997;8:1175–89.
28. Basta M, Klein GJ, Yee R, Krahn A, Lee J. Current role of pharmacologic therapy for patients with paroxysmal supraventricular tachycardia. Cardiol Clin 1997;15:587–97.
29. Luedtke SA, Kuhn RJ, McCaffrey FM. Pharmacologic management of supraventricular tachycardias in children: Part 1: Wolff–Parkinson–White and atrioventricular nodal reentry. Ann Pharmacother 1997;31:1227–43.
30. Ommen S, Odell JA, Stanton MS. Atrial arrhythmias after cardiothoracic surgery. New Engl J Med 1997;336:1429–34.
31. Caron J, Libersa C. Adverse effects of class I antiarrhythmic drugs. Drug Saf 1997;17:8–36.
32. MacNeil DJ. The side effect profile of class III antiarrhythmic drugs: Focus on d,l-sotalol. Am J Cardiol 1997;80:90G-98G.
33. Jaillon P, Dupuis B, Dahan R, Bottineau G, Caron J, Cazor JL, Chauvenet M, Clement J-P, Escande D, Faisandier Y, Funck-Brentano C, Kolsky H, Koen R, Lacroix D, Leenhardt A, Lehner J-P, Prost JF, Swynghedauw B, Vassort G, Weissenburger J, Wohlhuter C. Drug-induced torsade de pointes: pre-clinical and clinical studies for the prediction of a potential proarrhythmic adverse drug reaction. Thérapie 1997;52:271–80.
34. Wilbur SL, Marchlinski FE. Adenosine as an antiarrhythmic agent. Am J Cardiol 1997;79:30–7.
35. Marwick TH. Adenosine echocardiography in the diagnosis of coronary artery disease. Eur Heart J 1997;18 (Suppl D):D31–6.
36. Iskandrian AE, Heo J. Myocardial perfusion imaging during adenosine-induced coronary hyperemia. Am J Cardiol 1997;79:20–4.
37. Chaudhry FA. Adenosine stress echocardiography. Am J Cardiol 1997;79:25–9.
38. Hilleman DE, Lucas BD Jr, Mohiuddin SM, Holmberg MJ. Cost-minimization analysis of intravenous adenosine and dipyridamole in thallous chloride TI 201 SPECT myocardial perfusion imaging. Ann Pharmacother 1997;31:974–9.
39. Strickberger SA, Man KC, Daoud EG, Goyal R, Brinkman K, Knight BP, Weiss R, Bahu M, Morady F. Adenosine-induced atrial arrhythmia:

a prospective analysis. Ann Intern Med 1997; 127:417–22.

40. Robinson MC, Thielmeier KA, Hill BB. Transient ventricular asystole using adenosine during minimally invasive and open sternotomy coronary artery bypass grafting. Ann Thorac Surg 1997;63 (Suppl):S30–4.
41. Nagaoka H, Isobe N, Kubota S, Iizuka T, Imai S, Suzuki T, Nagai R. Comparison of adenosine, dobutamine, and exercise radionuclide ventriculography in the detection of coronary artery disease. Cardiology 1997;88:180–8.
42. Fenster MS, Feldman MD, Camarano G, Johnson WH, Ellis M, Linden J, Beller GA. Correlation of adenosine thallium 201 perfusion patterns with markers for inducible ischemia. Am Heart J 1997;133:406–12.
43. Smith JR, Goldberger JJ, Kadish AH. Adenosine induced polymorphic ventricular tachycardia in adults without structural heart disease. Pace 1997;20:743–5.
44. Paul T, Pfammatter JP. Adenosine: an effective and safe antiarrhythmic drug in pediatrics. Pediatr Cardiol 1997;18:118–26.
45. Desai AD, Chun S, Sung RJ. The role of intravenous amiodarone in the management of cardiac arrhythmias. Ann Intern Med 1997; 127:294–303.
46. Kowey PR, Marinchak RA, Rials SJ, Filart RA. Intravenous amiodarone. J Am Coll Cardiol 1997;29:1190–8.
47. Vorperian VR, Havighurst TC, Miller S, January CT, Sopher SM, Camm AJ. Adverse effects of low dose amiodarone: a meta-analysis. J Am Coll Cardiol 1997;30:791–801.
48. Daoud EG, Strickberger SA, Man KC, Goyal R, Deeb GM, Bolling SF, Pagani FD, Bitar C, Meissner MD, Morady F. Preoperative amiodarone as prophylaxis against atrial fibrillation after heart surgery. New Engl J Med 1997;337:1785–91.
49. Dimopoulou I, Marathias K, Daganou M, Prapas S, Stavridis G, Khoury M, Geroulanos S, Cokkinos DV. Low-dose amiodarone-related complications after cardiac operations. J Thorac Cardiovasc Surg 1997;114:31–7.
50. Winters SL, Sachs RG, Curwin JH. Nonsustained polymorphous ventricular tachycardia during amiodarone therapy for atrial fibrillation complicating cardiomyopathy: management with intravenous magnesium sulfate. Chest 1997; 111:1454–7.
51. Daniels CJ, Schutte DA, Hammond S, Franklin WH. Acute pulmonary toxicity in an infant from intravenous amiodarone. Am J Cardiol 1997;80:1113–16.
52. Olshansky B. Amiodarone-induced pulmonary toxicity. New Engl J Med 1997;337:1814.
53. Goldstein I, Topilsky M, Seger D, Isakor A, Heller I. Very early onset of acute amiodarone pulmonary toxicity presenting with hemoptysis. Chest 1997;111:1446–7.
54. Scully RE, Mark EJ, McNeely WF, Ebeling SH, Phillips LD. A 65-year-old woman with a dry cough and pulmonary nodules. New Engl J Med 1997;337:1449–59.
55. Malaterre HR, Renou C, Kallee K, Gauthier A. Akinesia and amiodarone therapy. Int J Cardiol 1997;59:107–8.
56. Harjai KJ, Licata AA. Effects of amiodarone on thyroid function. Ann Intern Med 1997; 126:63–73.
57. Klein SM, Greengrass RA, Knudsen N, Leight G, Warner DS. Regional anesthesia for thyroidectomy in two patients with amiodarone-induced hyperthyroidism. Anesth Analg 1997; 85:222–4.
58. Iervasi G, Clerico A, Bonini R, Manfredi C, Berti S, Ravani M, Palmieri C, Carpi A, Biagini A, Chopra IJ. Acute effects of amiodarone administration on thyroid function in patients with cardiac arrhythmia. J Clin Endocrinol Metab 1997;82:275–80.
59. Dickstein G, Shechner C, Adawi F, Kaplan J, Baron E, Ish-Shalom S. Lithium treatment in amiodarone-induced thyrotoxicosis. Am J Med 1997;102:454–8.
60. James PR, Hardman SMC. Acute hepatitis complicating parenteral amiodarone does not preclude subsequent oral therapy. Heart 1997; 77:583–4.
61. Fromenty B, Pessayre D. Impaired mitochondrial function in microvesicular steatosis. Effects of drugs, ethanol, hormones and cytokines. J Hepatol 1997;26 (Suppl):43–53.
62. Beuers U, Heuck A. Images in hepatology. J Hepatol 1997;26:439.
63. Bosch X, Bernadich O. Acute pancreatitis during treatment with amiodarone. Lancet 1997; 350:1300.
64. Sivaram CA, Beckman KJ. Amiodarone-induced skin discoloration. New Engl J Med 1997;337:1813.
65. DeVane CL, Gill HS, Markowitz JS, Carson WH. Awareness of potential drug interactions may aid avoidance. Ther Drug Monit 1997; 19:366–7.
66. Pernat A, Pohar B, Horvat M. Heart conduction disturbances and cardiovascular collapse after disopyramide and low-dose metoprolol in a patient with hypertrophic obstructive cardiomyopathy. J Electrocardiol 1997;30:341–4.
67. Paar D, Terjung B, Sauerbruch T. Life-threatening interaction between clarithromycin and disopyramide. Lancet 1997;349:326–7.
68. Bennett MI. Paranoid psychosis due to flecainide toxicity in malignant neuropathic pain. Pain 1997;70:93–4.
69. Mikawa K, Nishina K, Takao Y, Shiga M, Maekawa N, Obara H. Attenuation of cardiovascular responses to tracheal extubation: comparison of verapamil, lidocaine, and verapamil-lidocaine combination. Anesth Analg 1997;85:1005–10.
70. Walker LA, Slovis CM. Lidocaine in the treatment of status epilepticus. Acad Emerg Med 1997;4:918–22.
71. Reichel C, Nacke A, Sudhop T, Wienkoop G,

Luers C, Hahn C, Pohl C, Spengler U, Sauerbruch T. The low-dose monoethylglycinexylidide test: assessment of liver function with fewer side effects. Hepatology 1997;25:1323–7.
72. Orlando R, Palatini P. The effect of age on plasma MEGX concentrations. Br J Clin Pharmacol 1997;44:206–8.
73. Wright JM, Oki JC, Graves L III. Mexiletine in the symptomatic treatment of diabetic peripheral neuropathy. Ann Pharmacother 1997; 31:29–34.
74. Kerin NZ, Meengs WL, Timmis GC, Salerno D, Haber HE, Singer RM, Switzer D, Zoble R, Carlson M, Weidler D, Raghavan P, Schwartz K, Somberg JC, Kereiakes D, Ellenbogen KA. Activity of Procanbid, procainamide twice-daily formulation, to suppress ventricular premature depolarizations. Cardiovasc Drugs Ther 1997; 11:169–75.
75. Wittbrodt ET. Drugs and myasthenia gravis: an update. Arch Intern Med 1997;157:399–408.
76. Merrill JT, Shen C, Gugnani M, Lahita RG, Mongey A-B. High prevalence of antiphospholipid antibodies in patients taking procainamide. J Rheumatol 1997;24:1083–8.
77. Lee S-H, Chen S-A, Tai C-T, Chiang C-E, Wen Z-C, Chen Y-J, Yu W- C, Huang J-L, Fong A-N, Cheng J-J, Chang M-S. Comparisons of oral propafenone and sotalol as an initial treatment in patients with symptomatic paroxysmal atrial fibrillation. Am J Cardiol 1997;79:905–8.
78. Boriani G, Biffi M, Capucci A, Botto GL, Broffoni T, Rubino I, Della Casa S, Sanguinetti M, Magnani B. Oral propafenone to convert recent-onset atrial fibrillation in patients with and without underlying heart disease: a randomized, controlled trial. Ann Intern Med 1997;126:621–5.
79. Azpitarte J, Alvarez M, Baun O, Garcia R, Moreno E, Martin F, Tercedor L, Fernandez R. Value of single oral loading dose of propafenone in converting recent-onset atrial fibrillation. Results of a randomized, double-blind, controlled study. Eur Heart J 1997;18:1649–54.
80. Botto GL, Capucci A, Bonini W, Boriani G, Broffoni T, Barone P, Espureo M, Lombardi R, Molteni S, Ferrari G. Conversion of recent onset atrial fibrillation to sinus rhythm using a single oral loading dose of propafenone: comparison of two regimens. Int J Cardiol 1997;58:55–61.
81. Napoli C, Sorice P, Di Benedetto A, Di Ieso N, Liguori A. Propafenone in the conversion of atrial fibrillation in patients suffering from chronic renal failure. Am J Ther 1997;4:130–3.
82. Schellens JH, Ghabrial H, Van Der Wart HH, Bakker EN, Wilkinson GR, Breimer DD. Differential effects of quinidine on the disposition of nifedipine, sparteine, and mephenytoin in humans. Clin Pharmacol Ther 1991;50:520–8.
83. Bowles SK, Reeves RA, Cardozo L, Edwards DJ. Evaluation of the pharmacokinetic interaction between quinidine and nifedipine. J Clin Pharmacol 1993;33:727–31.
84. Koley AP, Robinson RC, Markowitz A, Friedman FK. Drug-drug interactions: effect of quinidine on nifedipine binding to human cytochrome P450 3A4. Biochem Pharmacol 1997; 53:455–60.

A.P. Maggioni, M.G. Franzosi and R. Latini

18 β-Adrenoceptor antagonists and antianginal drugs

β-ADRENOCEPTOR ANTAGONISTS *(SED-13, 488; SEDA-19, 201; SEDA-20, 183; SEDA-21, 207)*

ORGANS AND SYSTEMS

Cardiovascular Episodes of *torsade de pointes* have previously been described in patients with renal insufficiency treated with sotalol for supraventricular or ventricular tachycardias (SED-13, 493). Progressive renal insufficiency associated with torsade de pointes has been described in a 47-year-old patient treated chronically with sotalol for paroxysmal atrial flutter (1[c]). The need to adjust the dosage of sotalol according to creatinine concentrations in patients with renal insufficiency should be stressed, as should the fact that sotalol is contraindicated in someone with pre-existing prolongation of the QTc interval. The patient was successfully treated with hemodialysis. In another patient with renal insufficiency torsade de pointes due to sotalol for polymorphic ventricular tachycardia was successfully treated with intermittent peritoneal dialysis (2[c]).

Skin and appendages Adverse cutaneous reactions have previously been described in patients taking atenolol (SEDA 20, 183). *Cutaneous lupus erythematosus* has been described in a patient who had taken atenolol for more than 3 years for hypertension (3[c]).

An eruption on the hands, arms, face, neck, trunk, and legs occurred in a 62-year-old white man with a history of myocardial infarction, hypertension, and diabetes. The eruption was more evident in light-exposed areas. A biopsy specimen showed the characteristic histopathological features of lupus erythematosus. Atenolol was withdrawn and the patient was treated with hydroxychloroquine sulfate, and topical triamcinolone cream. The eruption cleared in 6 months, and the ANA and antihistone titers became undetectable. When the skin lesions had completely disappeared, the patient was rechallenged with atenolol for 3 days. The eruption immediately reappeared.

A case of *Stevens-Johnson syndrome* has been described during carvedilol therapy for heart failure (4[c]).

A 71-year-old man with ischemic cardiomyopathy, NYHA class III, taking ACE inhibitors, diuretics, and digitalis, was given oral carvedilol. After 4 weeks of treatment at a dosage of 6.25 mg bd, rash, pruritus, chills, and dysphagia developed. The rash included purpuric macules, blisters, and target lesions involving the entire skin surface. The tongue and pharynx were swollen. Carvedilol was withdrawn, while all other drugs for heart failure were continued, and the patient was treated with intravenous methylprednisolone and diphenhydramine. There was significant improvement within 2 days and complete resolution within 2 weeks.

Carvedilol therapy is infrequently associated with Stevens–Johnson syndrome. It should be withdrawn at the first evidence of any bullous eruption or the appearance of oral ulceration and the patients should be followed closely.

Side Effects of Drugs, Annual 22
J.K. Aronson, ed.

CALCIUM ANTAGONISTS

(SED-13, 488; SEDA-19, 203; SEDA-20, 185; SEDA-21, 208)

ORGANS AND SYSTEMS

R Long-term safety of calcium antagonists

Controversy about possible adverse effects of calcium antagonists began in 1995, with reports of increases in cardiovascular mortality, myocardial infarction, neoplastic diseases, and gastrointestinal hemorrhage from retrospective case–control and prospective cohort studies, casting doubts on the use of calcium antagonists in the first-line treatment of hypertension (SED-13, 510; SEDA-20, 185).

The findings that have aroused concern about calcium antagonists have also encouraged the institution of a number of important clinical trials in hypertension, some of which have been published in late 1996 and during 1997. Nifedipine has been tested in two trials, the TIBET (5[C]) and the STONE (6[C]) studies, nitrendipine in the Syst-Eur (7[C]) and in HANE (8[C]) studies, and amlodipine in the FACET study (9[C]). The TIBET (Total Ischaemic Burden European Trial) was a double-blind randomized study aimed at assessing the effects of atenolol, modified-release nifedipine, and their combination in 608 patients with mild chronic stable angina. The two drugs, both alone and in combination, caused significant reductions in the number of ischemic episodes during daily activities compared with placebo. During an average follow-up of 2 years, there was a non-significant trend to a lower rate of hard endpoints (cardiac death, non-fatal myocardial infarction, and unstable angina) in the group taking combination therapy. Withdrawal from trial medication was significantly higher in the nifedipine group (40%); the atenolol and combination therapy groups had similar withdrawal rates (27%).

The STONE (Shanghai Trial Of Nifedipine in the Elderly) study assessed the effectiveness of treatment with a Chinese modified-release formulation of nifedipine in 1632 elderly hypertensive patients alternatively allocated to either nifedipine or placebo after a 4-week placebo run-in period over a mean follow-up period of 30 months. There was a significant reduction in the occurrence of severe clinical events in patients treated with nifedipine (77 events with placebo versus 32 with nifedipine). However, the study had several limitations: it was not randomized and reallocation to nifedipine after placebo run-in for patients with severe hypertension was allowed.

In the Systolic Hypertension in Europe (Syst-Eur) randomized trial, nitrendipine was compared with placebo in 4695 elderly patients, followed by the possible addition of enalapril, hydrochlorothiazide, or both. Over a mean follow-up period of 2 years the total stroke rate was reduced by 44%, and fatal and non-fatal cardiac end-points were reduced by 31% compared with placebo. There was no significant difference in cardiovascular mortality (−27%) and total mortality (−14%) or in the rates of cancer and gastrointestinal bleeding.

In the HANE (hydrochlorothiazide, atenolol, nitrendipine, enalapril) study 868 hypertensive patients were randomized to hydrochlorothiazide, atenolol, nitrendipine, or enalapril in a double-blind comparison over 48 weeks. The response rate for atenolol was significantly higher than hydrochlorothiazide and nitrendipine, but not enalapril. The treatment-related dropout rate was significantly higher with nitrendipine (12.8%) compared with enalapril (5.4%), atenolol (5.1%), and hydrochlorothiazide (4.2%).

The FACET (Fosinopril versus Amlodipine Cardiovascular Events Randomised Trial) study compared the effects of fosinopril and amlodipine on serum lipids and diabetes control in 380 diabetic patients with hypertension who were randomly assigned to fosinopril or amlodipine and followed for up to 3.5 years. Both treatments were effective in lowering blood pressure and had similar effects on biochemical measures, but the patients randomized to fosinopril had a significantly lower risk of the combined outcome of major vascular events (acute myocardial infarction, stroke, or hospitalized angina), compared with the patients randomized to amlodipine (14/189 vs 27/191).

Besides these randomized clinical trials, two observational studies deserve to be mentioned. In a case–control study, 189 hypertensive pa-

tients who had had a first cardiovascular event, including all cardiovascular deaths and hospitalizations, were compared with 189 matched controls with regard to any prescribed drug regimen. Compared with those taking β-blocker monotherapy, patients taking long-acting calcium antagonists had no increased risk of a cardiovascular event, whereas patients taking short-acting calcium antagonists were at significantly greater risk (10[C]).

In a cohort of hypertensive patients, all cases of cancer were identified and the risk of cancer among users of calcium antagonists and ACE inhibitors was estimated in a nested case–control study, with users of β-blockers as a reference group (11[C]). The study, based on 446 cases of cancer, showed relative risk estimates for all cancers combined of 1.27 (95% CI 0.98, 1.63) and 0.79 (0.58, 1.06) for users of calcium antagonists and ACE inhibitors, respectively, relative to users of β-blockers. The authors thought that the trend towards a positive association between calcium antagonists and a risk of cancer was unlikely to be causal, since there was no increase in risk with increasing duration of use.

The randomized clinical trials and the retrospective studies mentioned above have provided more insight into the long-term safety and efficacy of calcium antagonists in hypertension. However, the results are still controversial, and there is a need for research to confirm that calcium antagonists reduce morbidity and mortality, as has been shown for diuretics and β-blockers.

The role of calcium antagonists will be further defined by the many large trials that are being planned or are currently under way around the world. On the basis of the current evidence, calcium antagonists should not be recommended as treatments of first choice in comparison with drugs with better proven efficacy.

INDIVIDUAL CALCIUM ANTAGONISTS

Amlodipine

Endocrine, metabolic Amlodipine has been reported to have caused an exacerbation of *acute intermittent porphyria* (12[c]).

A 51-year-old man, with a history of intermittent porphyria, was discharged from the hospital after elective percutaneous transluminal coronary angioplasty taking several drugs, including amlodipine. He presented to the emergency room later on the day of discharge with abdominal pain that had become more severe since discharge. His symptoms resolved 3 days after withdrawal of amlodipine, which was thought to have been responsible for the acute exacerbation. During follow-up visits he was rechallenged with amlodipine unknowingly by different physicians and the same symptoms occurred each time.

The temporal relation between the use of amlodipine and development of the attacks, as well as the resolution of symptoms after withdrawal, supported the association in this case.

Generalized *pruritus* secondary to amlodipine has been reported in two patients, a 59-year-old hypertensive woman and a 69-year-old man, without objective evidence of skin disease (14[c]). In both cases pruritus resolved in 24 h after withdrawal.

Sexual function The effects of five antihypertensive agents on sexual function have been compared with placebo in a post-hoc analysis of a long-term, double-blind, randomized trial, THOMS (15[Cr]). The incidence over 24 and 48 months of *erectile dysfunction* with amlodipine was not different from that with placebo. The other drugs tested (acebutolol, doxazosin, chlorthalidone, and enalapril) also showed incidences not different from placebo, although with chlorthalidone there was a trend to a higher incidence.

Diltiazem

Skin and appendages Skin reactions with diltiazem are not uncommon, and another case of *acute generalized exanthematous pustu-*

lar dermatitis (SED-13, 513; SEDA-18, 215) has been reported, with confirmation of the diagnosis by patch tests 2 months after the resolution of the disease (16[c]).

A 71-year-old woman took oral diltiazem hydrochloride 100 mg for hypertension. After 3 weeks she developed fever and a pruritic erythematous dermatitis involving the abdomen. The eruption gradually worsened and spread to the arms and legs in a few days. A skin biopsy showed a spongiform subcorneal pustule and a superficial perivascular inflammatory cell infiltrate, with evidence of vasculitis. Diltiazem was withdrawn and she was given methylprednisolone and antihistamines, which produced complete resolution within a few days. A marked leukocytosis persisted for more than 4 weeks, then gradually returned to normal.

Interactions In a study in 45 adult patients, 15 of whom were treated with intravenous diltiazem 0.1 mg/kg, 15 with diltiazem 0.2 mg/kg, and 15 with normal saline, the administration of diltiazem before tracheal intubation significantly reduced the time to onset of *vecuronium*-induced neuromuscular blockade, and attenuated changes in blood pressure caused by tracheal intubation (17[c]). However, heart rate did not differ between patients treated and not treated with diltiazem.

Felodipine

Interactions *Grapefruit juice* increases the oral systemic availability of a variety of commonly used medications, including felodipine (SEDA-21, 210). The mechanism of this interaction has been evaluated in a study of the effect of repeated grapefruit juice ingestion on the expression of CYP3A4, a cytochrome P450 present in liver and intestine, assumed to be inhibited by grapefruit juice. Small bowel and colon biopsies were obtained endoscopically in 10 healthy men before and after they had taken grapefruit juice for six days to determine oral felodipine kinetics and measure liver CYP3A4 activity. The authors concluded that grapefruit juice selectively down-regulated CYP3A4 in the small intestine (18[C]). In 12 healthy men the effect of grapefruit juice on the metabolism of felodipine after intravenous and oral administration was investigated with a randomized cross-over design. Grapefruit juice did not significantly alter the pharmacokinetics of intravenous felodipine; however, it caused a marked increase in the AUC and C_{max} of oral felodipine. While the hemodynamic effects of intravenous felodipine were not altered by grapefruit juice, the hemodynamic effects of oral felodipine, as measured by diastolic blood pressure and heart rate, were more pronounced, suggesting that the main acute effect of grapefruit juice on the plasma concentrations of felodipine is mediated by inhibition of gut wall metabolism (19[C]).

An interaction with *cyclosporin*, already reported with several calcium antagonists, including diltiazem, nicardipine, and nifedipine (SED-13, 515, 516), has been reported with felodipine (20[c]). In a double-blind, placebo-controlled, crossover study in 12 healthy men, there were significant increases in AUC and C_{max} of felodipine (58 and 15%, respectively) in subjects who took felodipine together with cyclosporin compared with those who took felodipine alone. The authors suggested that this was due to competitive inhibition of hepatic and/or intestinal metabolism of felodipine by cyclosporin.

Isradipine

An analysis of the database of a multicenter study of isradipine in non-diabetic hypertensive patients (21[cr]) has shown that the excess of serious cardiovascular events in patients taking isradipine (22[Cr]) was largely associated with *impaired glucose metabolism*, as assessed by higher glycosylated hemoglobin concentrations. The hazard ratio for cardiovascular events was 1.11 (95% CI 0.43, 2.90) in patients with glycosylated hemoglobin concentrations below the median, and increased to 2.81 (1.09, 7.26) in those with glycosylated hemoglobin concentrations higher than the median.

Lacidipine

Lacidipine, a long-acting dihydropyridine calcium antagonist, or placebo was added to baseline monotherapy with chlorthalidone in a double-blind cross-over study in 17 patients for 4 weeks (23[Cr]). Besides its hypotensive effect, lacidipine significantly *increased heart rate* on 24 h ambulatory recording. The observed increase in heart rate with lacidipine was unexpected with a long-acting dihydropyridine, although it is a common finding with short-acting compounds.

Mibefradil

Mibefradil is a calcium antagonist with a novel chemical structure and an ability to block T-type calcium channels as well as L-type channels (at higher concentrations). Because of its unique mechanism of action, it has no negative inotropic effects on the heart at therapeutic concentrations and does not cause a reflex increase in heart rate, in contrast to short-acting dihydropyridines (24[R]).

However, recently, because of the high risks of drug–drug interactions, mibefradil has been withdrawn from the market (25[r]), (26[r]). In addition, the large Mortality Assessment in Congestive Heart Failure (MACH) trial (27[C]) has been stopped because of this.

In a double-blind study 205 patients with chronic stable angina pectoris on stable β-blocker therapy were randomized to receive placebo or mibefradil 25 or 50 mg/day (28[Cr]). Mibefradil was well tolerated; two patients withdrew from the trial because of adverse events, *postural hypotension* and *symptomatic bradycardia*. Treatment-related adverse reactions, not reported with placebo, were mild *dizziness* and *light-headedness*. The electrocardiogram showed a dose-related *fall in heart rate* and a slight *increase in the PR interval.*

The safety and tolerability of mibefradil alone or in combination with β-blockers or glyceryl trinitrate (29[R]) has been tested in patients with stable angina pectoris or hypertension. Overall 3430 patients received mibefradil in daily doses of 6.25–200 mg; the most common doses were 50 and 100 mg/day. Compared with placebo, the 100-mg dose caused a slight excess of *dizziness*, *leg edema*, *fatigue*, and *light-headedness*. However, the incidence of these reactions was similar to or lower than that observed with the other calcium antagonists, when tested in comparative trials (30[R]). There were dose-related falls in heart rate and increases in PR interval, leading to an excess of episodes of *sinus bradycardia* (below 45 bpm) and first-degree AV block. Second-degree AV block was infrequent, and complete AV block was observed only in one patient taking the high dose of 150 mg/day. QT interval on average was slightly shortened.

Nicardipine

Use in pregnancy Nicardipine has been compared with salbutamol in an open randomized trial in 90 women with premature labor (31[Cr]). Adverse events were comparable with the two drugs and were mainly *headaches* with nicardipine; neonatal status was comparable, suggesting overall that nicardipine is as safe as salbutamol, with a comparable tocolytic effect.

Nifedipine

Skin and appendages Another case of *telangiectasia* in association with nifedipine (SED-13, 513) has been reported (13[c]).

An 85-year-old woman, who had been given nifedipine 18 months before for hypertension, gradually developed facial non-pruritic telangiectasia over 6 months. There was considerable improvement 4 weeks after nifedipine had been replaced by enalapril, with almost complete resolution 6 months after withdrawal.

Special senses The results of the use of calcium antagonists in the treatment of glaucoma are controversial. In a 6-month study of oral nifedipine (30 mg/day) in a study in 21 patients with normal-tension glaucoma, intraocular pressure and mean visual field sensitivity were unchanged (32[C]). Two patients experienced substantial *reductions in visual fields or contrast sensitivity*; one patient also had *a rise in intraocular pressure*.

Interactions To examine the possible interaction between nifedipine and *tacrolimus*, an immunosuppressive agent approved for use in liver transplant recipients in 1994, the medical records of two groups of hypertensive liver transplant recipients treated or not treated with nifedipine were retrospectively compared (33[C]). In those taking nifedipine the daily dosage of tacrolimus in the nifedipine group was 26, 29, and 38% less at 3, 6, and 12 months, respectively. Blood concentrations of tacrolimus should therefore be monitored during concomitant administration of nifedipine.

NSAIDs blunt the antihypertensive effects of diuretics, β-blockers, and ACE inhibitors. One of the most frequently hypothesized mechanisms for this drug interaction is reduced production of vasodilatory prostaglandins. However, although indomethacin attenuated the hypotensive effect of enalapril, it did not alter that of nifedipine GITS (34[R]). The clinical relevance of this interaction remains to be determined, since it does not occur in all patients, and it has been observed most frequently with indomethacin.

Verapamil

Respiratory Adverse respiratory effects are uncommon with calcium antagonists (SED-13, 511), and a case of *acute bronchospasm* associated with verapamil is unusual (35[c]).

An acute attack of asthma occurred in a 66-year-old white woman with asymptomatic bronchial asthma and hypertension, after she had switched from immediate-release verapamil hydrochloride 40 mg tds to modified-release verapamil 240 mg/day for better hypertension control. She developed dyspnea, cough, and wheezing after taking the first tablet. Despite the administration of anti-asthmatic medications, her symptoms did not improve during the following 6 months. She stopped taking all the drugs and her symptoms disappeared. On four subsequent separate occasions she was rechallenged with modified-release verapamil and similar symptoms developed after each challenge and resolved after withdrawal.

Interactions Previous observations on the use of verapamil to optimize *cyclosporin* immunosuppression in kidney transplant recipients and its nephroprotective effects (SEDA-21, 212) have been confirmed in a trial in 32 heart and lung transplant recipients, randomized to receive a 6-week course of verapamil or a control treatment (atenolol in hypertensive patients and placebo in normotensive patients) 1–2 months after transplantation (36[C]). Verapamil produced an absolute improvement in glomerular filtration rate clearance-time index by 10–15% compared with the control group. Similarly, there was a trend to an improved renal plasma flow clearance-time index with verapamil. Verapamil was also associated with a reduction in cyclosporin dosage requirements, without any significant change in blood concentrations.

NITRATE DERIVATIVES *(SED-13, 488; SEDA-19, 201; SEDA-20, 184; SEDA-21, 208)*

Glyceryl trinitrate (nitroglycerin)

Cardiovascular Glyceryl trinitrate has been used to reduce the hepatic vein pressure gradient in patients with hepatic cirrhosis and portal hypertension, with the aim of lowering the risk of esophageal variceal bleeding. However, marked *hypotension*, *tolerance*, and *reduced oxygen transport* have limited its use (37[Cr]), (38[Cr]). A transdermal patch releasing 5 mg of glyceryl trinitrate over 24 h has been tested in an open, non-placebo-controlled study in 19 patients with cirrhosis and portal hypertension, alone and in combination with spironolactone given for 4 weeks (39[Cr]). Glyceryl trinitrate alone significantly reduced hepatic vein pressure gradient without tolerance over 4 weeks; there were no episodes of hypotension, and headaches subsided within the first 24 h. The combination with spironolactone did not increase therapeutic effectiveness, but two patients withdrew prematurely, one with a severe headache, and the other with increased ascites.

In a double-blind cross-over study in 20 patients with congestive heart failure, in NYHA class III, both nicorandil and glyceryl trinitrate given by intravenous infusion over 24 h significantly reduced pulmonary capillary wedge pressure (40[Cr]). However, there was tolerance to the vasodilatory effects at 24 h with glyceryl trinitrate. All the patients completed the study without major adverse events. The authors concluded that nicorandil might be a useful alternative to glyceryl trinitrate in patients with congestive heart failure, with less potential for tolerance.

The incidence of cardiovascular events has been documented in a double-blind study in 200 patients with unstable angina treated with transdermal glyceryl trinitrate, *N*-acetylcysteine, both, or placebo for 4 months (41[Cr]). Other standard medical therapy (aspirin, β-blockers, and calcium antagonists) was continued. Only the combination significantly reduced the persistence of angina requiring revascularization, compared with placebo. However, there were significantly more withdrawals for adverse events (17 of the 18 cases were for headache) in those taking combined treatment. The authors concluded that although the combination of transdermal glyceryl trinitrate 10 mg/day and oral *N*-acetylcysteine 600 mg tds had greater efficacy, its use is limited by a high incidence (33%) of adverse events requiring drug withdrawal.

Use in pregnancy Recently, glyceryl trinitrate has been used as an antenatal tocolytic, with positive results (42[Cr]) that should be verified in a placebo-controlled trial. There were no adverse effects on the new-born, but *headaches* were often reported by the mothers. Occasionally, *dizziness* and *palpitation* were reported and were dealt with by reducing the dose by patch from 50 to 25 mg (43[c]).

REFERENCES

1. van Uum SHM, van den Merkhof LFM, Lucassen AMJ, Wuis EW, Diemont W. Successful haemodialysis in sotalol-induced torsade de pointes in a patient with progressive renal failure. Nephrol Dial Transplant 1997;12:331–3.
2. Tang S, Lo CY, Lo WK, Tai YT, Chan TM. Sotalol-induced torsade de pointes in a CAPD patient—successful treatment with intermittent peritoneal dialysis. Peritoneal Dial Int 1997; 17:207–8.
3. McGuiness M, Frye RA, Deng JS. Atenolol-induced lupus erythematous. J Am Acad Dermatol 1997;37:298–9.
4. Kowalski BJ, Cody RJ. Stevens–Johnson syndrome associated with carvedilol therapy. Am J Cardiol 1997;80:669–70.
5. Dargie HJ, Ford I, Fox KM. Total Ischaemic Burden European Trial (TIBET). Effects of iscaemia and treatment with atenolol, nifedipine SR and their combination on outcome in patients with chronic stable angina. The TIBET Study Group. Eur Heart J 1996;17:104–12.
6. Gong L, Zhang W, Zhu Y, Zhu J, Kong D, Page V, Ghadirian P, LeLorier J, Hamet P. Shanghai trial of nifedipine in the elderly (STONE). J Hypertension 1996;14:1237–45.
7. Staessen JA, Fagard R, Thijs L, Celis H, Arabidze GG, Birkenhäger WH, Bulpitt CJ, De Leeuw, PW, Dollery CT, Fletcher AE, Forette F, Leonetti G, Nachev C, O'Brien ET, Rosenfeld J, Rodicio JL, Tuomilehto J, Zanchetti A, for the Systolic Hypertension in Europe (Syst-Eur) Trial Investigators. Randomised double-blind comparison of placebo and active treatment for older patients with isolated systolic hypertension. Lancet 1997;350:757–65.
8. Philipp T, Anlauf M, Distler A, Holzgreve H, Michaelis J, Wellek S, on behalf of the HANE trial research group. Randomised, double blind, multicentre comparison of hydrochlorothiazide, atenolol, nitrendipine, and enalapril in antihypertensive treatment: results of the HANE study. Br Med J 1977;315:154–9.
9. Tatti P, Pahor M, Byington RP, DiMauro P, Guarisco R, Strollo F. Results of the Fosinopril Amlodipine Cardiovascular Events Trial (FACET) in hypertensive patients with non-insulin-dependent diabetes mellitus (NIDDM). Circulation 1997;96 (Suppl I):I-764.
10. Alderman MH, Cohen H, Roqué R, Madhavan S. Effect of long-acting and short-acting calcium antagonists on cardiovascular outcomes in hypertensive patients. Lancet 1997;349:594–8.
11. Jick H, Jick S, Derby LE, Vasilakis C, Wald Myers M, Meier CR. Calcium-channel blockers and risk of cancer. Lancet 1997;349:525–8.
12. Kepple A, Cernek PK. Amlodipine-induced acute intermittent porphyria exacerbation. Ann Pharmacother 1997;31:253.
13. Basarab T, Yu R, Russel Jones R. Calcium antagonist-induced photo-exposed telangiectasia. Br J Dermatol 1997;136:974–5.
14. Orme S, Da Costa D, Messenger A. Generalised pruritus associated with amlodipine. Br Med J 1997;315:463.
15. Grimm RH Jr, Grandits GA, Prineas RJ, McDonald RH, Lewis CE, Flack JM, Yunis C, Svendsen K, Liebson PR, Elmer PJ, Stamler J. Long-term effects on sexual function of five antihypertensive drugs and nutritional hygienic treatment in hypertensive men and women. Treatment of mild hypertension study (TOMHS). Hypertension 1997;29:8–14.
16. Vincente-Calleja JM, Aguirre A, Landa N, Crespo V, González-Pérez R, Díaz-Pérez R. Acute generalized exanthematous pustulosis due to diltiazem: confirmation by patch testing. Br J Dermatol 1997; 137:837–9.
17. Saitoh Y, Makita K, Tanaka H. Diltiazem and vecuronium: neuromuscular and cardiovascular effects. Can J Anaesth 1997;44:99–102.

18. Lown KS, Bailey DG, Fontana RJ, Janardan SK, Adair CH, Fortlage LA, Brown MB, Guo W, Watkins PB. Grapefruit juice increases felodipine oral availability in humans by decreasing intestinal CYP3A protein expression. J Clin Invest 1997; 99:2545–53.
19. Lundahl J, Regardh CG, Edgar B, Johnsson G. Effects of grapefruit juice ingestion-pharmacokinetics and haemodynamics of intravenously and orally administered felodipine in healthy men. Eur J Clin Pharmacol 1997;52:139–45.
20. Madsen JK, Jensen JD, Jensen LW, Pedersen EB. Pharmacokinetic interaction between cyclosporine and the dihydropyridine calcium antagonist felodipine. Eur J Clin Pharmacol 1996;50:203–8.
21. Borhani NO, Mercuri M, Borhani PA, et al. Final outcome results of the Multicenter Isradipine Diuretic Atherosclerosis Study (MIDAS). A randomized controlled study. J Am Med Assoc 1996;276:785–91.
22. Byington RP, Craven TE, Furberg CD, Pahor M. Isradipine, raised glycosylated haemoglobin, and risk of cardiovascular events. Lancet 1997; 350:1075–6.
23. Stergiou GS, Malakos JS, Achimastos AD, Mountokalakis TD. Additive hypotensive effect of a dihydropyridine calcium antagonist to that produced by a thiazide diuretic: a double-blind placebo-controlled crossover trial with ambulatory blood pressure monitoring. J Cardiovasc Pharmacol 1997;29:412–6.
24. Lüscher TF, Clozel J-P, Noll G. Pharmacology of the calcium antagonist mibefradil. J Hypertens Suppl 1997;15:S11–18.
25. Anonymous. Roche cites drug interactions in mibefradil withdrawal. Am J Health Syst Pharm 1998;55:1445.
26. Po AL, Zhang WY. What lessons can be learnt from withdrawal of mibefradil from the market? Lancet 1998;351:1829–30.
27. Mahon N, McKenna WJ. Calcium channel blockers in cardiac failure. Prog Cardiovasc Dis. 1998;41:191–206.
28. Alpert JS, Kobrin I, DeQuattro V, Friedman R, Shepherd A, Fenster PE, Thadani U. Additional antianginal and anti-ischemic efficacy of mibefradil in patients pretreated with a beta blocker for chronic stable angina pectoris. Am J Cardiol 1997;79:1025–30.
29. Kobrin I, Charlon V, Lindberg E, Pordy R. Safety of mibefradil, a new once-a-day, selective T-type calcium channel antagonist. Am J Cardiol 1997;80:40C–46C.
30. Davies GJ, Tzivoni D, Kobrin I. Mibefradil in the treatment of chronic stable angina pectoris: comparative studies with other calcium antagonists. Am J Cardiol 1997;80:34C–39C.
31. Jannet D, Abankwa A, Guyard B, Carbonne B, Marpeau L, Milliez J. Nicardipine versus salbutamol in the treatment of premature labor. A prospective randomized study. Eur J Obstet Gynecol Reprod Biol 1997;73:11–16.
32. Harris A, Evans DW, Cantor LB, Martin B. Hemodynamic and visual function effects of oral nifedipine in patients with normal-tension glaucoma. Am J Ophthalmol 1997;124:296–302.
33. Seifeldin RA, Marcos-Alvarez A, Gordon FD, Lewis WD, Jenkins RL. Nifedipine interaction with tacrolimus in liver transplant recipients. Ann Pharmacother 1997;31:571–5.
34. Polónia J. Interaction of antihypertensive drugs with anti-inflammatory drugs. Cardiology 1997;88:47–51.
35. Ben-Noun L. Acute asthma associated with sustained-release verapamil. Ann Pharmacother 1997;31:593–5.
36. Chan C, Maurer J, Cardella C, Cattran D, Pei Y. A randomized controlled trial of verapamil on cyclosporine nephrotoxicity in heart and lung transplant recipients. Transplantation 1997;63: 1435–40.
37. Garcia-Tsao G, Groszmann FJ. Portal hemodynamics during nitroglycerin administration in cirrhotic patients. Hepatology 1987;7:805–9.
38. Moreau R, Roulot D, Braillon A, Guadin C, Hadengu A, Bacq Y, Lebrec D. Low dose of nitroglycerin failed to improve splanchnic hemodynamics in patients with cirrhosis: evidence for an impaired cardiopulmonary baroreflex function. Hepatology 1989;10:93–7.
39. Sugano S, Suzuki T, Nishio M, Makino H, Okajima T. Chronic splanchnic hemodynamic effects of low-dose transdermal nitroglycerin versus low-dose transdermal nitroglycerin plus spironolactone in patients with cirrhosis. Dig Dis Sci 1997;42:529–35.
40. Larsen AI, Goransson L, Aarsland T, Tamby JF, Dickstein K. Comparison of the degree of hemodynamic tolerance during intravenous infusion of nitroglycerin versus nicorandil in patients with congestive heart failure. Am Heart J 1997;134:435–41.
41. Ardissino D, Merlini AP, Savonitto S, Demicheli G, Zanini P, Bertocchi F, Falcone C, Ghio S, Marinoni G, Montemartini C, Mussini A. Effect of transdermal nitroglycerin or N-acetylcysteine, or both, in the long-term treatment of unstable angina pectoris. J Am Coll Cardiol 1997;29:941–7.
42. Rowlands S, Trudinger B, Visva-Lingam S. Treatment of preterm cervical dilatation with glyceryl trinitrate, a nitric oxide donor. Aust NZ J Obstet Gynaecol 1996;36:377–81.
43. Fliegner JR, Gronow M. Treatment of preterm cervical dilatation with glyceryl trinitrate, a nitric oxide donor. Aust NZ J Obstet Gynaecol 1997;37:487.

R. Verhaeghe

19 Drugs acting on the cerebral and peripheral circulations

DRUGS USED IN THE TREATMENT OF ARTERIAL DISORDERS OF THE BRAIN AND LIMBS

Cilostazol

Cilostazol is a phosphodiesterase inhibitor that suppresses platelet aggregation and also acts as a direct arterial vasodilator. Small studies from Japan have suggested that it may be useful for treating chronic arterial disease and the symptoms of intermittent claudication. A recent study in 81 patients with claudication has substantiated this claim: the claudication distance improved by 35% for initial and 41% for absolute claudication distance. There were gastrointestinal complaints in 44% of the patients who took cilostazol and in 15% of those who took placebo. The most commonly reported adverse effects included *diarrhea*, *loose stools*, *flatulence*, and *nausea*; they were usually mild and transient but persisted in some patients. *Headache* occurred in 20% of those who took cilostazol and 15% of those who took placebo (1[C]).

Cinnarizine and flunarizine

(SED-13, 417, 537; SEDA-20, 191)

Parkinsonism, *tardive dyskinesia*, and *depression* have been described in a number of mostly elderly patients taking cinnarizine or flunarizine. In a study of 13 such patients followed for up to 7 years none had full recovery from the extrapyramidal effects, suggesting that long-term prognosis of parkinsonism in such cases is less benign than has been thought. Several patterns of evolution were described: six patients had improvement of their main symptoms, four had persistence or stabilization of their cardinal signs, two had a partially reversible pattern (one cardinal sign remained), and one developed a progressive pattern of parkinsonism. The unsolved question is to what extent flunarizine simply unmasks a pre-existing subclinical 'primary' degenerative process in a number of these patients (2[C]). In another study 66 of 74 patients with cinnarizine-induced parkinsonism recovered completely after drug withdrawal. Four of them later developed Parkinson's disease (3[C]).

So-called *apraxia of eyelid opening* has chiefly been described in the context of extrapyramidal disorders. In one of 10 patients, chronic treatment with flunarizine was a suspected contributing factor; withdrawal led to sustained remission of the eyelid disturbance (4[c]).

Iloprost

Up to now, the prostacyclin analogue iloprost had to be administered intravenously. Its adverse effects are dose-related and predictable from its pharmacological actions: *flushing*, *headache*, *nausea*, *intestinal cramps*, and *diarrhea*. A new oral formulation is currently being investigated in patients with Raynaud's phenomenon secondary to systemic sclerosis and in patients with severe ischemia due to Buerger's disease or atherosclerosis. The first reports have not been particularly encouraging in terms of efficacy. However, tolerance is acceptable: 6% of the patients discontinued iloprost compared with 2% who discontinued placebo (5[c]), (6[c]).

Side Effects of Drugs, Annual 22
J.K. Aronson, ed.

Pentoxifylline *(SED-13, 541; SEDA-21, 215)*

Pentoxifylline suppresses overproduction of tumor necrosis factor-α and improves capillary blood flow, both of which are thought to contribute to the complications of falciparum malaria. Intravenous pentoxifylline was tested for 5 days against placebo in 51 patients but had no effect on the clinical course of the disease. Eleven of 27 patients receiving pentoxifylline (20 mg/kg per day) requested early termination of the infusion because of adverse effects: *nausea*, *vomiting*, and *abdominal discomfort* (7[c]).

DRUGS USED IN THE TREATMENT OF MIGRAINE

Sumatriptan *(SEDA-19, 207; SEDA-20, 192)*

To date, sumatriptan has been available for subcutaneous and oral administration. Subcutaneous doses act rapidly and produce significant relief of migrainous pain within 10–15 min; oral doses need 1–1.5 h to achieve the same effect. Administration by alternative routes is currently being tested. Suppositories and intranasal spray given to healthy volunteers cause only mild to moderate adverse effects (*weakness*, *drowsiness*, *headache*, and *dizziness*), similar to those characteristic of sumatriptan in general (8[c]), (9[c]).

Akathisia occurred in five fairly young patients after subcutaneous or oral administration of sumatriptan (10[C]). The symptoms started early (5–10 min after subcutaneous injection in four and 60 min after oral administration in the last—this patient also had dystonia) and were short-lived. The patients refused further exposure to the drug, but one took sumatriptan again a few weeks later and experienced an identical episode. Increased serotonergic activity leading to inhibition of nigrostriatal dopaminergic neurons and to extrapyramidal symptoms is the postulated mechanism. A similar mechanism is thought to provoke the same symptoms with serotonin reuptake inhibitors.

OTHER PERIPHERAL VASODILATORS

Sildenafil

Sildenafil is a potent inhibitor of cyclic guanosine monophosphate (cGMP) breakdown in the corpus cavernosum, by inhibition of phosphodiesterase type 5. The increased concentration of cGMP leads to relaxation of the smooth muscle cells and vasodilatation in the corpus cavernosum, which is essential for normal penile erection. Thus, sildenafil increases the penile response to sexual stimulation.

Oral sildenafil is highly effective in men with erectile dysfunction (11[Cr]), (12[Cr]) having an NNT of about 2. The main reported adverse effects are *flushing*, *headache*, *dyspepsia*, *visual disturbances*, and *rhinitis*. They are mild, and only 1–2% of the patients discontinue sildenafil because of adverse effects. They show that vasodilatation due to sildenafil is not confined to the corpus cavernosum.

Cardiovascular Since the release of the drug, reports have appeared in the lay press of cases of *sudden death* shortly after administration. One man without a history of previous chest pain or risk factors for cardiovascular disease developed a well-documented myocardial infarction 30 min after he took sildenafil 50 mg and before any attempt at sexual intercourse (13[C]). Two others with severely depressed left ventricular function developed ventricular tachycardia (14[c]). In placebo-controlled trials thus far, there have been no differences in the incidences of myocardial infarction, angina, or coronary artery disorders between sildenafil and placebo (15[R]). Exclusion criteria in clinical trials may have prevented the inclusion of patients at increased risk of adverse events. On the other hand, sexual activity itself increases cardiac workload and the risk of myocardial infarction. Patients with cardiovascular disease should therefore be cautious about using sildenafil.

Interactions The concomitant use of nitrates and sildenafil may precipitate a hypotensive reaction and this combination should therefore be avoided.

REFERENCES

1. Dawson DL, Cutler BS, Meissner MH, Strandness E. Cilostazol has beneficial effects in treatment of intermittent claudication. Results from a multicenter, randomized, prospective, double-blind trial. Circulation 1998;98:678–86.
2. Negrotti A, Calzetti S. A long term follow-up study of cinnarizine- and flunarizine-induced parkinsonism. Mov Disord 1997;12:107–10.
3. Marti-Masso JF, Poza JJ. Cinnarizine-induced parkinsonism: ten years later. Mov Disord 1998; 13:453–6.
4. Defazio G, Livrea P, Lamberti P, De Salvia R, Laddomada G, Giorelli M, Ferrari E. Isolated so-called apraxia of eyelid opening: report of 10 cases and a review of the literature. Eur Neurol 1998;39:204–10.
5. Verstraete M. Oral iloprost in the treatment of thrombangiitis obliterans (Buerger's disease): a double-blind, randomised, placebo-controlled trial. Eur J Vasc Endovasc Surg 1998;15:300–7.
6. Wigley FM, Korn JH, Csuka ME, Medsger TA Jr, Rothfield NF, Ellman M, Martin R, Collier DH, Weinstein A, Furst DE, Jimenez SA, Mayes MD, Merkel PA, Gruber B, Kaufman L, Varga J, Bell P, Kern J, Marrott P, White B, Simms RW, Phillips AC, Seibold JR. Oral iloprost in patients with Raynaud's phenomenon secondary to systemic sclerosis: a multicneter, placebo-controlled, double-blind study. Arthritis Rheum 1998;41:670–7.
7. Hemmer CJ, Hort G, Chiwakata CB, Seitz R, Egbring R, Gaus W, Hogel J, Hassemer M, Nawroth PP, Kern P, Dietrich M. Supportive pentoxifylline in falciparum malaria: no effect on tumor necrosis factor alpha levels or clinical outcome: a prospective, randomized, placebo-controlled study. Am J Trop Med Hyg 1997; 56:397–403.
8. Kunka RL, Hussey EK, Shaw S, Warner P, Aubert B, Richard I, Fowler PA, Pakes GE. Safety, tolerability, and pharmacokinetics of sumatriptan suppositories following single and multiple doses in healthy volunteers. Cephalalgia 1997;17:532–40.
9. Moore KHP, Hussey EK, Shaw S, Fuseau E, Duquesnoy C, Pakes GE. Safety, tolerability, and pharmacokinetics of sumatriptan following ascending single internasal doses and multiple intranasal doses. Cephalalgia 1997;17:541–50.
10. Lopez-Alemany M, Ferrer-Tuset C, Bernacer-Alpera B. Akathisia and acute dystonia induced by sumatriptan. J Neurol 1997;244:131–3.
11. Boolell M, Gepi-Attee S, Gingell JC, Allen MJ. Sildenafil, a novel effective oral therapy for male erectile dysfunction. Br J Urol 1996;78:257–61.
12. Goldstein I, Lue TF, Padma-Nathan H, Rosen RC, Steers WD, Wicker PA, for the Sildafenil Study Group. Oral sildenafil in the treatment of erectile dysfunction. New Engl J Med 1998; 338:1397–404.
13. Feenstra J, van Drie-Pierik RJHM, Laclé CF, Stricker BH CH. Acute myocardial infarction associated with sildenafil. Lancet 1998;352:957–8.
14. Shah PK. Sildenafil in the treatment of erectile dysfunction. New Engl J Med 1998;339:699.
15. Morales A, Gingell C, Collins M, Wicker PA, Osterloh IH. Clinical safety of oral sildenafil citrate (Viagra) in the treatment of erectile dysfunction. Int J Impotence Res 1998;10:69–74.

Faiez Zannad

20 Antihypertensive drugs

Fixed-dose combinations as first-choice therapy for hypertension

Innovation in the area of antihypertensive therapy is based on the discovery of blood pressure-lowering agents that act on new pharmacological targets. This does not necessarily produce more efficacious agents. The response rate to any agent is still around 50% in unselected hypertensive patients. However, tremendous advances have been made when it comes to tolerance profiles. For example, in this chapter the section on the adverse effects of the angiotensin AT1 receptor antagonists, the most recently available agents, is very thin.

An alternative strategy of innovation is based on fixed-dose combination therapy. The rationale for combining two different antihypertensive agents is supported by enhanced antihypertensive efficacy and favorable effects on target organs and/or attenuation of adverse or unwanted effects. Recent evidence has shown that optimal blood pressure control would mandate the use of more than one single antihypertensive agent. Indeed antihypertensive drugs evoke counter-regulatory mechanisms that limit the efficacy of initial pharmacological intervention. For instance, diuretics can activate the renin–angiotensin–aldosterone system, arterial vasodilators can produce reactive stimulation of the sympathetic nervous system and the renin–angiotensin system, and blockade of the sympathetic nervous system can increase plasma volume.

Efficacy *The combination of two antihypertensive agents with complementary modes of action can enhance the efficacy of both agents prescribed separately. The possibility that the dose of the first drug is near or at the top of the dose–response curve, so that less additional effect can be expected from larger doses, favors adding a second drug. On the other hand, if the dose is below of the top of the curve, adverse effects may occur as the dose is increased. Thus, low-dose combinations of two drugs with different modes of action can provide even greater additive effects than would be expected from each drug given separately. In order to be approved for initial therapy, a fixed-dose combination must be shown to be effective and each component of the combination must be shown to contribute to its effect.*

Safety *When thinking about adverse drug reactions, it is useful to distinguish those that are dose related and those that are (within the therapeutic dosing range) dose independent. Fixed-dose combination products expose patients to dose-independent hazards of both drugs. When a combination is used in place of monotherapy, the independent risks of using the second drug must be offset by some commensurate benefit. For approval as first-line therapy, a fixed combination should contain drugs with only dose-dependent adverse effects. This is the case with a combination of a β-blocker and a thiazide diuretic. A physician might reasonably choose to prescribe such a combination before having attempted monotherapy with high doses of one (or each) of the components. In a given patient, the dose-independent risks of the combination of a low dose of a β-blocker and a low dose of a thiazide diuretic might be preferable to the dose-dependent risks associated with monotherapy with a higher dose of either agent.*

Because many of the adverse effects of ACE inhibitors are essentially dose independent within their therapeutic dosing ranges (exceptions being their effects on the kidney and on potassium balance), the risk of low-dose ACE inhibitor monotherapy are no different from the risks of higher dose monotherapy. In other words, the risks of combinations containing an ACE inhibitor are at any dose greater than the risks of ACE inhibitor monotherapy at any

Side Effects of Drugs, Annual 22
J.K. Aronson, ed.

dose. Patients may properly be exposed to the higher risks of such combination therapy, but only when lesser risk monotherapy has been shown to be inadequate. Alternatively, additive efficacy, together with increased benefit related to complementary actions of an ACE inhibitor and a calcium antagonist may produce extra benefit, which may offset the inconvenience of dose-independent adverse reactions when the drugs are used together.

Finally, when monotherapy is ineffective, combinations marketed in single formulations mitigate the problems of adherence to multiple medications. In particular, combinations of long-acting medications that need be taken only once daily will improve compliance compared with formulations that need to be taken more often. Interestingly, analysis of randomized trials of fixed combinations compared with their individual components has consistently shown that the duration of action of the combination exceeds that of each component.

Taking together all the considerations discussed above, the importance of combination therapy for hypertension is now endorsed by several regulatory agencies and by the recent guidelines of the Joint National Committee on Detection, Evaluation, and Treatment of High Blood Pressure (JNC VI) (1[R]), which highly recommends the use of combination therapy as first-line therapy for hypertension.

Sexual function With the advent of sildenafil and other forms of treatment of *erectile dysfunction*, it is likely that more patients will be willing to discuss with their doctors the issue of sexual dysfunction. Patients, as well as physicians, often attribute sexual problems to antihypertensive drugs and modify or discontinue treatment regimens to address this concern. In the Treatment of Mild Hypertension Study (TOMHS) 902 hypertensive patients aged 45–69 years were treated with placebo or an antihypertensive drug for 4 years. The rates of erectile dysfunction at 1 and 2 years, respectively, were: placebo 8.1/16.7%; acebutolol 9.2/11.8%; amlodipine 8.3/15.0%; chlorthalidone 17.1/18.3%, and doxazosin 9.7/14.1%. The rate of reported sexual problems in hypertensive women was low and did not appear to differ by type of drug. The double-blind randomized design and long follow-up of this study adds credibility to these results. The authors cautioned against routine attribution of erectile problems to antihypertensive drugs, at least as far as the drugs investigated in this study are concerned (2[C]).

ANGIOTENSIN-CONVERTING ENZYME INHIBITORS *(SED-13, 546; SEDA-19, 210; SEDA-20, 195; SEDA-21, 219)*

Angio-edema due to ACE inhibitors R

Angio-edema is thought to be a class effect of ACE inhibitors. It usually occurs within hours to days after the start of therapy, although delayed onset has occasionally been described (3[cR]).

Incidence *Black Americans are at increased risk, with an overall rate of 1.6 per 1000 person-years of ACE inhibitor use, and an adjusted relative risk of angio-edema among black American users of ACE inhibitors compared with white users of 4.5 (95% CI 2.9–6.8) (4[CR]). This increase in risk was unrelated to the dosage of ACE inhibitor or the concurrent use of cardiovascular drugs. Moreover, angio-edema appeared to be more severe in black American users. Recent initiation of ACE inhibitor therapy and the use of enalapril or lisinopril were also associated with a higher rate of angio-edema.*

Mechanism *The exact mechanism of angio-edema associated with ACE inhibitors has not been determined. Although the reaction may be immune mediated, IgE antibodies or other specific antibodies have not been detected. Some authors have speculated that it may be related to a deficiency of carboxypeptidase N and complement components, because of its parallel role with that of ACE in the enzymatic inactivation of bradykinin.*

A 66-year-old man with non-insulin-dependent diabetes mellitus, coronary heart disease, hypertension, and atrial fibrillation was admitted because of angio-edema 6 h after enalapril infusion test renography for suspected renovascular hypertension. He had had a similar less severe reaction after starting to take lisinopril a few weeks before. He had a life-long history of episodic swelling of the extremities, face, and lips. In addition, there was a family history of episodic cutaneous angio-edema affecting his father, son, and grandson. A diagnosis of hereditary angio-edema was suspected on the basis of nearly absent hemolytic activity, measured by the CH50 assay, and reduced serum concentrations of C4 and functional C1 esterase inhibitor activity.

The striking correlation in this case between ACE inhibitor administration and the attacks of angio-edema and hypotension suggested that they were probably drug-induced. This is probably the first report of a patient with hereditary angio-edema and recurrent episodes of anaphylactoid reactions precipitated by the administration of an ACE inhibitor (5[c]).

In a case–control study nested within an 8-week open-label study of the use of quinapril for hypertension in 12 275 patients there were 22 cases of angio-edema. They were matched with 48 controls taking quinapril. Patients with angio-edema had significantly lower mean activities of serum carboxypeptidase N and C1 esterase inhibitor compared with controls, but all mean values were within the laboratory's reference range (6[C]). Although this may support the involvement of low activities of carboxypeptidase in the pathogenesis of ACE inhibitor-induced angio-edema, prior testing of patients for low enzyme activities is not likely to be helpful in screening for angio-edema risk in patients in whom ACE inhibitor therapy is being considered. In this study it was also reported that a history of prior episodes of angio-edema was associated with a 6-fold increase in the subsequent risk of angio-edema after ACE inhibitor therapy. Another anecdotal report has pointed out to the risk of recurrence of angio-edema, as it described a case of coincident occurrence of angio-edema on several occasions in one patient after the consecutive administration of captopril, fosinopril, and quinapril (5[c]).

The involvement of high concentrations of bradykinin in the pathogenesis of angio-edema related to the use of ACE inhibitors is still hypothetical, since no definitive increase in bradykinin plasma concentrations during attacks of angio-edema has been shown. However, kinin concentrations are difficult to measure. In a well-documented study, a newly developed reliable assay for specific measurement of plasma bradykinin, excluding other immunoreactive kinins, detected a very high concentration of bradykinin (47 pmol/l) during an acute attack of angio-edema in a patient taking captopril (7[C]). The concentrations fell to 3.2 pmol/l in remission after drug withdrawal. The concentration of bradykinin during chronic ACE inhibition with no angio-edema was not reported. One major contribution of this paper was to demonstrate that plasma bradykinin concentrations were substantially increased in 22 patients with hereditary angio-edema and 22 others with acquired angio-edema, both conditions being associated with inadequate inhibition of the first component of human complement. The infusion of C1 esterase inhibitor immediately lowered bradykinin concentrations in patients with hereditary or acquired C1 esterase inhibitor deficiency. Infusion of C1 esterase inhibitor in ACE inhibitor-induced angio-edema was not investigated.

Individual drugs *Angio-edema has been attributed in case reports to several different ACE inhibitors, including benazepril, captopril, enalapril, lisinopril, quinapril, and ramipril (SEDA-21, 220). Now a further case of angio-edema has been attributed to lisinopril (8[cr]).*

A 41-year-old woman had intermittent recurrent attacks of severe lower quadrant abdominal pain, nausea, vomiting, and watery diarrhea within 48 h of starting lisinopril 5 mg/day for essential hypertension. There were no other signs or symptoms. She did not improve with empirical antiemetics and antispasmodics and had to be admitted 3 weeks later dehydrated. An abdominal CT scan showed bowel edema, ascites, and a prominent adrenal gland. All her symptoms and signs resolved within 2 days of lisinopril withdrawal and the CT scan normalized within 1 week, except for the adrenal gland which took 2 months.

The authors suspected lisinopril-induced abdominal angio-edema and reviewed three previously reported similar cases with enalapril and captopril.

INDIVIDUAL ACE INHIBITORS

Captopril *(SEDA-21, 221)*

Liver *Cholestatic jaundice* has been attributed to captopril in a woman with systemic sclerosis (9[c]).

A 70-year-old woman, who had had systemic sclerosis without renal involvement or hypertension for 2 years, presented with scleroderma renal crisis and secondary acute renal insufficiency and hypertension. Antihypertensive therapy was begun with captopril 25 mg bd and nifedipine. Her blood pressure was controlled and her symptoms improved slightly. Nifedipine was withdrawn 9 days later. After 21 days, she began to show signs of jaundice accompanied by a progressive rise in bilirubin and transaminases. There was no abnormality of gallbladder or biliary tract. Viral serology was negative. Within 72 h of withdrawal of captopril, the jaundice had disappeared and the biochemical parameters indicated a slight degree of *cholestasis*. However, her renal function did not improve and hemodialysis was required. She deteriorated progressively and died 38 days after admission.

The authors referred to numerous other previously reported cases of captopril related hepatotoxicity. They did not discuss the peculiarity of the present case with systemic scleroderma.

Interactions Captopril has been reported to react with *iron* and other transition metals. This interaction has been investigated in vivo in seven healthy adults in a well-designed protocol (10[C]). Each took captopril 25 mg with either ferrous sulfate (300 mg) or placebo. Coadministration of ferrous sulfate and captopril resulted in a 37% reduction in the AUC of unconjugated captopril, with no significant changes in C_{max} or t_{max}. The plasma AUC of total captopril was not altered. The authors suggested that the interaction may be specific to captopril, among ACE inhibitors, because it contains a sulfhydryl group. Therefore, if iron salts were to be taken by a patient requiring an ACE inhibitor one might consider using agents other than captopril.

Enalapril *(SED-12, 479; SEDA-19, 213; SEDA-21, 221)*

Cardiovascular Of all the trials that have investigated the effects of ACE inhibitors on mortality in acute myocardial infarction, only the CONSENSUS II trial did not show a positive effect. In this trial enalaprilat was infused within the 24 h after the onset of symptoms, followed by oral enalapril. The reasons for the negative result of CONSENSUS II remain unresolved, but *hypotension* linked to a poorer prognosis has been reported. In a small substudy of this large trial, a total of 60 patients were investigated for residual *ischemia* before discharge, with exercise testing and Holter electrocardiographic monitoring (11[C]). Episodes of hypotension and pre-discharge ischemia were more common with enalapril than placebo. The authors suggested that enalapril induced a *proischemic* effect in hypotension-prone patients, mediated through exacerbation of the hemodynamic response, inasmuch as the initial blood pressure fall after myocardial infarction is related to residual ischemia and recurrent acute ischemic syndromes. This conclusion is very speculative. The data were derived from a small substudy with multiple subanalyses and cannot support a cause–effect relation between the acute hemodynamic effect and the pre-discharge ischemic conditions. ACE inhibitors should still be used in acute myocardial infarction with the cautious dose titration advocated in the other trials with other ACE inhibitors.

Pancreas Three patients (two men and one women) aged 63–66 developed acute *pancreatitis* while they were taking enalapril 2 mg/day (12[c]). Their serum amylase activities were 900–1100 U/l. Enalapril had been started 3 months to 1 year before the event. In two patients enalapril was the only drug taken immediately before the symptoms began, and other causes were carefully excluded. In the third patient, the relation between enalapril and acute pancreatitis was shown by positive rechallenge. In all three patients the signs and symptoms of pancreatitis resolved after enalapril withdrawal.

Risk factors The long-term safety of enalapril in patients with *severe renal insufficiency* and hypertension has been evaluated in a pooled analysis of three similar randomized placebo-controlled clinical trials totalling 317 patients with serum creatinine concentrations of 10–80 (mean 27) μmol/l (13[R]). Only patients without diabetes were included. Follow up was for 2–3 years. One protocol used a fixed dose (5 mg/day) and the other two allowed titration up to 40 mg/day. Spontaneously reported adverse drug reactions were well documented. Laboratory data were collected at regular intervals. *Cough* occurred in 17.6% of the patients taking enalapril and in 6.1% taking placebo. *Hypotension* (5.9 vs 1.2%) and *paresthesia* (7.8 vs 2.4%) were more frequent with enalapril. *Angio-edema* (1.3 vs 0.6%) and *first-dose hypotension* (1.3 vs 0%) tended to occur more often with enalapril. *Hyperkalemia*, defined as any increase from baseline and left to the judgement of the investigators, was excessive in the enalapril treated patients (28 vs 8.8%). Finally the *hematocrit* fell more often in the enalapril group (7.1 vs 2.0%).

Fosinopril *(SEDA-17, 252; SEDA-18, 224)*

The clinical pharmacology, clinical use, and safety profile of fosinopril have been extensively reviewed (14[R]).

Skin and appendages Two cases of *scleroderma* have been reported, but the relation to fosinopril was very uncertain (15[c]).

In an 83-year-old woman with hypertension, signs of scleroderma appeared acutely 6 months after she started to take fosinopril 20 mg/day. Her signs and symptoms did not improve after withdrawal and despite corticosteroid treatment.

A 59-year-old woman with hypertension developed a dry cough and *eosinophilic fasciitis* with extensive weight loss a few months after she started to take fosinopril 20 mg/day. The authors did not mention improvement after fosinopril withdrawal, despite treatment with prednisolone and cyclosporin.

Lisinopril *(SED-12, 479; SEDA-17, 252; SEDA-18, 225)*

A subgroup analysis of the GISSI-3 trial has been published recently. It showed that early treatment with lisinopril in diabetic patients with acute myocardial infarction is associated with a reduced 6-week mortality (−27%) (16[C]). The result was consistent and homogeneous in type I and type II diabetic patients. The safety profile of lisinopril was not different between the diabetic and non-diabetic patients. This supports the widespread use of ACE inhibitors in diabetic patients with acute myocardial infarction.

Immunological and hypersensitivity reactions *Lupus-like syndrome* has been attributed to lisinopril (17[cr]).

A 73-year-old man with mitral insufficiency and hypertensive heart disease complicated by atrial fibrillation and left ventricular systolic dysfunction developed a lupus-like syndrome during the first month of treatment with lisinopril 5 mg/day. He presented with an erythematous rash, ulcers in the mouth, dysuria, and arthralgia affecting the hands and feet. His ANA titer was positive but other autoantibodies could not be detected. Lisinopril was withdrawn and enalapril substituted. The lupus-like syndrome subsided within a few weeks and the ANA titer fell significantly.

The author emphasized that this is the first such case reported with lisinopril. He stressed the absence of cross-reactivity between lisinopril and enalapril, briefly reviewed previous similar reports with captopril, and pointed out to the more frequent but not clinically significant isolated rise of ANA titers with captopril and enalapril.

A case of *angio-edema* attributed to lisinopril has been mentioned above in the special review.

Perindopril *(SED-13, 549; SEDA-17, 253; SEDA-21, 221)*

Cardiovascular A report of *first-dose hypotension* with perindopril was very controversial and generated a number of letters to the editor (18[c]), (19[r]).

A 61-year-old man had signs of mild heart failure and an acute inferior myocardial infarction was diagnosed. After a single dose of perindopril 2 mg given in mid afternoon of the fifth day he remained normotensive. The next morning he had visual disturbances and a short episode of *hypotension* (90/60 mmHg) which resolved before he complained of any other symptoms. The cerebral CT scan showed a localized ischemic infarction. He was discharged on the ninth day with his visual defect.

The author did not discuss the unusually late occurrence of this first-dose effect. Moreover he recognized, replying to letters to the editor, that one could not rule out an atherosclerotic stoke complicating an acute myocardial infarction.

Pancreas *Pancreatitis* has been attributed to perindopril (20[c]).

A 70-year-old man with non-insulin-dependent diabetes and hypertension presented with typical acute *pancreatitis* 21 days after starting to take perindopril 4 mg/day. The serum amylase activities were up to 3746 IU/l and transaminases, γ-glutamyltransferase, and bilirubin were increased. Imaging showed no dilatation of the biliary or pancreatic ducts and he had had a cholecystectomy at the age of 30. All his signs and symptoms normalized over the 5 days after perindopril withdrawal. He was later involuntarily rechallenged by his general physician and reproduced the same event 20 days after rechallenge. He recovered after drug withdrawal and was still symptom free 2 years later.

The positive rechallenge is a strong argument in favor of a causative role of perindopril in this case.

Ramipril *(SED-13, 549; SEDA-15, 294; SEDA-18, 225)*

The Ramipril Efficacy In Nephropathy (REIN) study included 352 patients with non-diabetic chronic nephropathy with proteinuria of 3 g/day or more. Ramipril safely reduced proteinuria and the rate of fall in the glomerular filtration rate to an extent that seemed to exceed the reduction expected for the degree of blood pressure lowering. The adverse reactions in this study were not different between ramipril and placebo (21[C]).

Skin and appendages A *lichenoid eruption* has been attributed to ramipril (22[c]).

A 55-year-old man with hypertension was given ramipril (dose not reported) and 4 weeks later developed a symmetrical widespread lichenoid eruption affecting the trunk and limbs. He was referred to the hospital with vesicles and bullae and the diagnosed was lichen planus pemphigoides, with consistent clinical, histological, and immunofluorescent findings. Linear basement membrane zone staining with IgG and C3 was only seen at the root of split-skin preparations and there were circulating autoantibodies to the basement membrane zone in a titre of 1/100. Controlled immunoblotting of epidermal extracts detected bullous pemphigoid antigens of 230 and 180 kDa. Ramipril was withdrawn but the signs did not resolve until he was given a 6-week tapering course of prednisolone. There was no recurrence during 1 year of follow-up.

Captopril has been previously reported to cause such a skin reaction, attributed to the sulfhydryl group. This case may have been coincidental and the causal role of ramipril must be questioned.

ANGIOTENSIN II RECEPTOR ANTAGONISTS *(SED-13, 549; SEDA-19, 214; SEDA-20, 196; SEDA-21, 222)*

Losartan *(SEDA-20, 196; SEDA-21, 222)*

There have been several reviews of the clinical efficacy and safety of losartan in essential hypertension. Over a very large database its safety profile seems very good. *Dizziness* is the only consistent adverse effect and that is very much related to its blood pressure lowering effect (23[C]), (24[R]). From a Swedish database of 15 000 patients during a period of surveillance from November 1995 to June 1996, the following types of adverse effects were reported: skin (15), gastrointestinal (13), respiratory (11), neurological (eight), musculoskeletal (five), and miscellaneous reactions (17), a total of 69 reports in 59 patients.

Liver Losartan has been reported to be *hepatotoxic* (25[c]).

A 46-year-old man was admitted because of a 2-week history of malaise, anorexia, nausea, vomiting, low grade fever, and *jaundice*. Examination showed only moderate *hepatomegaly*. Laboratory data showed large rises in AlT, AsT, γ-glutamyltransferase, bilirubin, and alkaline phosphatase. One month before admission he had been given losartan 50 mg/day instead of enalapril, because of a persistent cough. Liver and biliary duct imaging was normal and serology was negative. One month after losartan withdrawal, the AlT and AsT fell substantially and all hepatic tests were normal 4 months after admission. With the patient's consent, losartan was reintroduced. Three weeks later he once more developed signs and symptoms of hepatotoxicity, which disappeared after withdrawal.

This is the first well-documented report of

hepatotoxicity with losartan. The temporal relation, recurrence on re-exposure, and improvement on withdrawal strongly suggest that losartan was responsible.

Pancreas *Pancreatitis* has been attributed to losartan (26[c]).

A 39-year-old man was admitted with a 3-day history of nausea, vomiting, and constant epigastric pain. He had previously taken enalapril for hypertension, but because of a persistent cough, losartan 50 mg/day was substituted 1 week before admission. The diagnosis of acute pancreatitis was based on large rises in the serum activities of amylase and lipase. Serology was negative and a CT scan showed no biliary or pancreatic abnormalities. Five days after admission and losartan withdrawal the laboratory data normalized and the patient was asymptomatic. Three days later, he was re-challenged to losartan 25 mg and again developed acute pancreatitis, which resolved 3 days after withdrawal. The patient continued to take atenolol, and pancreatitis had not recurred 11 months later.

This is the first well-documented reported of pancreatitis with losartan. The temporal relation, recurrence on re-exposure, and improvement on withdrawal strongly suggest that losartan was responsible.

Skin and appendages Two cases of atypical *cutaneous lymphoid hyperplasia* have been reported (27[c]). Both occurred after 2 weeks of treatment with losartan 50 mg/day.

A 77-year-old man developed a T-cell pseudolymphoma, presenting with papular lesions of the thighs, abdomen, and groin. A 74-year-old man presented with erythematous plaques on the back, abdomen and groin. Immunohistochemical studies of the skin showed a T-cell lymphoma. Both patients recovered progressively over a few months after losartan withdrawal.

Immunological and hypersensitivity reactions In an international safety update report based on 200 000 treated patients there were 13 cases of *angio-edema* (28[R]). Two had also taken an ACE inhibitor and three others had previously developed angio-edema when taking ACE inhibitors.

Interactions A study in 10 healthy volunteers has suggested that *rifampicin* has a clinically significant interaction with losartan (29[C]). The AUCs of both losartan and its active metabolite were markedly reduced (about 30 and 40%, respectively) when rifampicin 300 mg bd was given for 1 week. It is uncertain whether this affects the clinical efficacy of losartan.

An interaction of losartan with *lithium* has been reported (30[c]).

A 77-year-old woman was admitted with a 10-day history of ataxia, dysarthria, and confusion. She had been taking lithium carbonate 625 mg/day for several years for bipolar depression. She had always had stable plasma lithium concentrations and had near-normal renal function. Five weeks before admission she had been given losartan 50 mg/day in addition to nifedipine, which she had taken for years. On admission lithium intoxication was diagnosed, as the plasma lithium concentration had risen from 0.63 to 2.0 mmol/l. After losartan withdrawal and progressive reinstitution of the usual dosage of lithium, she recovered and her lithium concentration returned to the usual steady state concentrations.

The authors did not investigate the possible mechanisms of this likely drug interaction.

The pharmacokinetic interaction of *fluconazole* 200 mg/day with losartan 100 mg/day has been investigated in 32 healthy subjects (31[C]). Fluconazole significantly increased (+66%) the steady-state concentration of losartan and inhibited the formation of its active metabolite EXP-3174 (−34%).

DRUGS THAT ACT ON THE SYMPATHETIC NERVOUS SYSTEM *(SED-13, 550; SEDA-19, 214; SEDA-21, 223)*

IMIDAZOLINE RECEPTOR AGONISTS

Moxonidine *(SEDA-21, 223)*

Liver The first case of moxonidine-associated *hepatitis* has been reported (32[c]).

An 83-year-old man developed cholestatic hepatitis after 9 months of continuous therapy with moxonidine. He presented with itching, nausea, jaundice and a maculopapular rash. There was no dilatation of the biliary ducts and no gallstones. Viral serology was negative. Transaminases were higher than 1000 U/l. Bilirubin was increased but γ-glutamyltransferase only slightly so. There was a coagulation disorder and hypoalbuminemia. No autoantibodies were detected and liver biopsy showed features compatible with drug-induced inflammatory intrahepatic cholestasis. The patient recovered fully clinically and his biochemical data normalized 8 weeks after moxonidine withdrawal.

The authors pointed out that this was the first report of suspected moxonidine-induced hepatitis. In a postmarketing surveillance program none of more than 20 000 patients developed cholestatic hepatitis.

Interactions The interaction between moxonidine and *lorazepam* on cognitive function has been investigated in 48 healthy subjects (33[C]). When co-administered with lorazepam, moxonidine 0.4 mg increased the impairment of attentional tasks (choice, simple reaction time and digit vigilance performance, memory tasks, immediate word recall, delayed word recall accuracy, and visual tracking) induced by lorazepam. These effects should be considered when moxonidine is co-administered with lorazepam 1 mg, although they were smaller than would have been produced by a single dose of lorazepam 2 mg alone.

POSTSYNAPTIC α_1-ADRENOCEPTOR ANTAGONISTS *(SED-13, 552; SEDA-19, 215; SEDA-21, 223)*

Doxazosin

Psychiatric Doxazosin has been reported to have caused an *acute psychosis* (34[c]).

A 71-year-old woman with type II diabetes and hypertension was treated with doxazosin 8 mg/day for 9 months. She was also taking nizatidine 150 mg bd and nitrazepam 5 mg at night as long-term prescriptions. One to 2 weeks after the dose of doxazosin was increased to 16 mg/day, she was admitted to a psychogeriatric department with an acute psychosis. She had begun to hear voices and to have auditory hallucinations. Doxazosin was progressively withdrawn over the next 14 days, and by the time the dosage had been reduced to 8 mg/day the psychosis was much less severe; it disappeared completely after withdrawal.

DIRECT VASODILATORS

(SED-13, 553; SEDA-19, 215; SEDA-21, 223)

Minoxidil *(SED-13, 554; SEDA-16, 212; SEDA-17, 254)*

Skin and appendages Topical administration of minoxidil is used in the treatment of women with androgenic alopecia. Severe *hypertrichosis* of the face and the limbs occurred in three women after 2–3 months of treatment with 5% topical minoxidil (35[c]). The hypertrichosis disappeared from the face and arms within 1–3 months and from the legs after 4–5 months of drug withdrawal.

REFERENCES

1. The Sixth Report of the Joint National Committee on Prevention, Detection, Evaluation, and Treatment of High Blood Pressure. Arch Intern Med 1997;157:2413–46.
2. Grimm RH Jr, Grandits GA, Prineas RJ, McDonald RH, Lewis CE, Flack JM, Yunis C, Svendsen K, Liebson PR, Elmer PJ. Long-term effects on sexual function of five antihypertensive drugs and nutritional hygienic treatment in hypertensive men and women: treatment of mild hypertension study (TOMHS). Hypertension 1997;29-I:8–14.
3. O'Mara NB, O'Mara EM. Delayed onset of angioedema with angiotensin-converting enzyme inhibitors: case report and review of the literature. Pharmacotherapy 1996;16:675–9.
4. Brown NJ, Ray WA, Snowden M, Griffin MR. Black Americans have an increased rate of angiotensin converting enzyme inhibitor-associated angioedema. Clin Pharmacol Ther 1996;60:8–13.
5. Ebo DG, Stevens WJ, Bosmans JL. An adverse reaction to angiotensin-converting enzyme inhibitors in a patient with neglected C1 esterase inhibitor deficiency. J Allergy Clin Immunol 1997;99:425–6.
6. Van DeCarr S, Sigler C, Annis K, Cooper K, Haber H. Examination of baseline levels of carboxypeptidase N and complement components as potential predictors of angioedema associated with the use of an angiotensin-converting enzyme inhibitor. Arch Dermatol 1997;133:972–5.
7. Nussberger J, Cugno M, Amstutz C, Cicardi M, Pellacani A, Agostoni A. Plasma bradykinin in angio-oedema. Lancet 1998;351:1693–7.

8. Abdelmalek MF, Douglas DD. Lisinopril-induced isolated visceral angioedema. Review of ACE-inhibitor-induced small bowel angioedema. Dig Dis Sci 1997;42:847–50.
9. Deira JL, Corbacho L, Bondia A, Lerma JL, Gascon A, Martin B, Garcia P, Tabernero JM. Captopril hepatotoxicity in a case of renal crisis due to systemic sclerosis. Nephrol Dial Transplant 1997;2:1717–18.
10. Schaefer JP, Tam Y, Hasinoff BB, Tawfik S, Peng Y, Reimche L, Campbell NRC. Ferrous sulphate interacts with captopril. Br J Clin Pharmacol 1998;46:377–81.
11. Sogaard P, Thygesen K. Potential proischemic effect of early enalapril in hypotension-prone patients with acute myocardial infarction. Cardiology 1997;88:285–91.
12. Maringhini A, Termini A, Patti R, Ciambra M, Biffarella P, Pagliaro L. Enalapril-associated acute pancreatitis: recurrence after rechallenge. Am J Gastroenterol 1997;9:166–7.
13. Keane WF, Polis A, Wolf D, Faison E, Shahinfar S. The long-term tolerability of enalapril in hypertensive patients with renal impairment. Nephrol Dial Transplant 1997;12 (Suppl 2):75–81.
14. Shionoiri H, Naruse M, Minamisawa K, Ueda S, Himeno H, Hiroto S, Takasaki I. Fosinopril: clinical pharmacokinetics and clinical potential. Clin Pharmacokinet 1997;32:460–80.
15. Biasi D, Caramaschi P, Carletto A, Bambara LM. Scleroderma and eosinophilic fasciitis in patients taking fosinopril. J Rheumatol 1997;24:1242.
16. Zuanetti G, Latini R, Maggioni AP, Franzosi M, Santoro L, Tognoni G. Effect of the ACE inhibitor lisinopril on mortality in diabetic patients with acute myocardial infarction: data from the GISSI-3 study. Circulation 1997;96:4239–45.
17. Leak D. Absence of cross-reaction between lisinopril and enalapril in drug-induced lupus. Ann Pharmacother 1997;31:1406–7.
18. Bagger JP. Adverse event with first-dose perindopril in congestive heart failure. Lancet 1997;349:1671–2.
19. MacFadyen RJ, Lees KR, Reid JL, Cleland JGF, Tan LB, Wright DJ, Bagger JP. Adverse event with first-dose perindopril in congestive heart failure. Lancet 1997;350:520–2.
20. Gallego-Rojo FJ, Gonzalez-Calvin JL, Guilarte J, Casado-Caballero FJ, Bellot V. Perindopril-induced acute pancreatitis. Dig Dis Sci 1997;42:1789–91.
21. Ruggenenti P, Perna A, Mosconi L, Matalone M, Garini G, Salvadori M, Zoccali C, Scolari F, Maggiore Q, Tognoni G, Remuzzi G. Randomised placebo-controlled trial of effect of ramipril on decline in glomerular filtration rate and risk of terminal renal failure in proteinuric, non-diabetic nephropathy. Lancet 1997;349:1857–63.
22. Ogg GS, Bhogal BS, Hashimoto T, Coleman R, Barker JNWN. Ramipril-associated lichen planus pemphigoides. Br J Dermatol 1997;136:412–14.
23. Dahlof B, Lindholm LH, Carney S, Pertti J, Ostergren J. Main results of the losartan versus amlodipine (LOA) study on drug tolerability and psychological general well-being. J Hypertens 1997;15:1327–35.
24. McIntyre M, Caffe SE, Michalak RA, Reid JL. Losartan, an orally active angiotensin (AT-1) receptor antagonist: a review of its efficacy and safety in essential hypertension. Pharmacol Ther 1997;74:181–94.
25. Bosch X, Goldberg AL, Smith IS, Stephenson WP. Losartan-induced hepatotoxicity. J Am Med Assoc 1997;278:1572.
26. Bosch X. Losartan-induced acute pancreatitis. Ann Intern Med 1997;127:1043–4.
27. Viraben R, Lamant L, Brousset P. Losartan-associated atypical cutaneous lymphoid hyperplasia. Lancet 1997;350:1366.
28. Hansson L. Medical and cost-economy aspects of modern antihypertensive therapy-with special reference to 2 years of clinical experience with Losartan. Blood Press Supp 1997;6:52–5.
29. Strayhorn VA, Baciewicz AM, Self TH. Update on rifampin drug interactions, III. Arch Int Med 1997;157:2453–8.
30. Blanche P, Raynaud E, Kerob D, Galezowski N. Lithium intoxication in an elderly patient after combined treatment with losartan. Eur J Clin Pharmacol 1997;52:501.
31. Kazierad DJ, Martin DE, Blum RA, Tenero DM, Ilson B, Boike SC, Etheredge R, Jorkasky DK. Effect of fluconazole on the pharmacokinetics of eprosartan and losartan in healthy male volunteers. Clin Pharmacol Ther 1997;62:417–25.
32. Tamm M, Sieber C, Schnyder F, Haefeli WE. Moxonidine-induced cholestatic hepatitis. Lancet 1997;350:1822.
33. Wesnes K, Simpson PM, Jansson B, Grahnen A, Weimann H-J, Kuppers H. Moxonidine and cognitive function: interactions with moclobemide and lorazepam. Eur J Clin Pharmacol 1997;52:351–8.
34. Evans M, Perera PW, Donoghue J. Drug induced psychosis with doxazosin. Br Med J 1997;314:1869.
35. Peluso AM, Misciali C, Vincenzi C, Tosti A. Diffuse hypertrichosis during treatment with 5% topical minoxidil. Br J Dermatol 1997;136:118–20.

Gordon T. McInnes

21 Diuretics

GENERAL

Diuretics were for many years the most widely used of all antihypertensive drugs. Then in the 1980s their popularity waned, because of exaggerated fears of adverse events (1[R]), (2[r]). Now, however, new evidence for the unique benefits of diuretics is stimulating their return to favor. This is reflected in the recommendations of the Sixth Joint National Committee on Prevention, Detection, Evaluation, and Treatment of High Blood Pressure (JNCVI) that diuretics remain a first-choice medication for the management of hypertension (3[r]). The results of numerous randomized, diuretic-based, long-term, controlled clinical trials have shown a reduction in both cerebrovascular and cardiovascular morbidity. In addition, diuretics have been shown to improve quality-of-life measurements at least as much as ACE inhibitors, calcium antagonists, β-blockers, and α-blockers (4[C]).

Risk versus benefit Reasons for the declining use of diuretics in the management of hypertension include the heavy promotion of other medications and the perception that diuretics cause adverse metabolic effects that reduce or eliminate cardiac protection (1[R]). In fact, changes in glucose and cholesterol metabolism are minor, especially with the lower dosages now being used, cardiovascular morbidity and mortality have been reduced in hypertensive patients, even in those with hyperlipidemia or diabetes, and concerns about hypokalemia-induced dysrhythmias have been overstated (SED-13, 559; SEDA-20, 200; SEDA-21, 226).

Most hypertensive patients, including those with hyperlipidemia or glucose intolerance, can be treated effectively with a diuretic as initial therapy or as part of a combination regimen. The use of diuretics would reduce the number of resistant hypertensive patients; these drugs should be used more not less often (1[R]).

In contrast to diuretics, there are few data to confirm specific long-term cardioprotective effects of other antihypertensive agents. The antihypertensive efficacy and effects on cardiovascular morbidity and mortality of diuretics and β-blockers have been compared in a meta-analysis of published data in elderly patients with hypertension (5[C]). Ten randomized trials lasting at least 1 year and involving 16 164 individuals aged at least 60 years were considered. Monotherapy controlled blood pressure in two-thirds of subjects assigned to diuretics and in only one-third of those given β-blockers. Diuretics were superior to β-blockers with regard to all end points (stroke, coronary heart disease events, cardiovascular mortality, and all cause mortality), although not all differences were statistically significant. One prospective, controlled, 2–3-year study suggested that vascular events are more common in hypertensive patients treated with a dihydropyridine calcium antagonist compared with a diuretic (6[C]).

Evidence of the beneficial effects of diuretics in hypertension continues to accumulate. In a substudy from the Systolic Hypertension in the Elderly Program (SHEP) (SED-13, 559; SEDA-20, 200), elderly patients with isolated systolic hypertension had a reduced risk of heart failure when receiving chlorthalidone-based therapy (7[C]). The effect was more marked in patients with prior myocardial infarction. Such patients, older subjects, men and those with higher systolic blood pressure were more likely to develop heart failure; in each category, treatment reduced heart failure. No significant additional protective effect against the development of heart failure was afforded by the addition of atenolol or reserpine to chlorthalidone therapy alone.

Side Effects of Drugs, Annual 22
J.K. Aronson, ed.

Benefits with diuretics are also seen when considering surrogate end points. Diuretics prevent left ventricular hypertrophy, or reduce left ventricular mass if hypertrophy was present before therapy ([8C]). Despite equivalent reduction of diastolic blood pressure, treatment with hydrochlorothiazide 25–50 mg/day for 6 months (n = 43) was associated with a substantial reduction in left ventricular mass, greater than that seen with isradipine 2.5–10 mg bd (n = 89) ([9C]). The superior efficacy of hydrochlorothiazide in reducing left ventricular mass was associated with a greater reduction in systolic blood pressure. Hydrochlorothiazide 12.5–50 mg daily was superior to atenolol 25–100 mg/day, clonidine 0.1–0.5 mg bd, diltiazem 60–180 mg tds, and prazosin 2–10 mg bd in reducing left atrial size in 653 patients treated for up to 2 years ([10C]). There was a similar advantage of hydrochlorothiazide on left ventricular mass in both those with normal left ventricular size and those with left ventricular hypertrophy ([11C]). Therapy with enalapril/hydrochlorothiazide 20/6 mg/day (n = 84) and atenolol 50 mg/day (n = 90) reduced blood pressure similarly in patients with essential hypertension after 12 weeks ([12C]). However, only enalapril and hydrochlorothiazide suppressed urine albumin excretion within the normoalbuminuric range.

Endocrine, metabolic *Glucose metabolism* (SED-13, 565; SEDA-20, 200; SEDA-21, 227) Alteration in hepatic glucose production with high dosages of thiazides may contribute to changes in glucose tolerance in patients with essential hypertension and an increased risk of diabetes mellitus (SEDA-18, 233). In a double-blind crossover study in 15 white hypertensive patients without diabetes mellitus and aged less than 65 years, treatment with captopril (up to 100 mg/day for 12 weeks) plus bendroflumethiazide 5 mg/day raised postabsorptive endogenous glucose production compared with captopril (up to 100 mg/day) alone ([13C]). These findings suggest that combination ACE inhibitor and diuretic therapy is associated with hepatic insulin resistance. Therefore, combined formulations with ACE inhibitors cannot be assumed to ameliorate the adverse effects of high-dose thiazide diuretics on insulin action.

A retrospective analysis of all 4736 patients in SHEP (SED-13, 559; SEDA-20, 200) showed that treatment with low-dose chlorthalidone 12.5–25 mg/day for 3 years, complemented with atenolol or reserpine as necessary, resulted in a non-significant excess of diabetes (8.6 vs 7.5%) compared with placebo ([14C]). Diuretic-based therapy was associated with only minor and mainly non-significant changes in fasting blood sugar (as well as cholesterol, triglycerides, and uric acid). Patients with impaired glucose tolerance (but not overt diabetes mellitus) did not have greater deterioration in carbohydrate metabolism or other risk factors. This suggests that patients with diabetes mellitus are unlikely to have major adverse effects from low-dose chlorthalidone. Low-dose diuretic-based treatment of isolated systolic hypertension has relatively mild effects on cardiovascular risk factors and poses little risk of precipitating excess diabetes mellitus in older patients, at least in the short term. Such treatment can be used safely in most elderly patients with impaired glucose tolerance and diabetes mellitus.

Mineral and fluid balance *Potassium balance* (SED-13, 562; SEDA-20, 202; SEDA-21, 227) Earlier studies suggesting no increased mortality in men with low serum potassium concentrations (SED-13, 563) were not large enough to detect a specific association between serum potassium and the risk of stroke. This has been examined in 43 738 American men aged 40–75 years without diagnosed cardiovascular disease or diabetes mellitus who completed a semiquantitative food frequency questionnaire in 1986 ([15C]). The multivariate relative risk (RR) of stroke of any type in the top quintile of potassium intake compared with the bottom quintile was 0.62 (95% CI 0.43, 0.88). The inverse association was stronger in hypertensives than in normotensives. Use of potassium supplements was also inversely related to stroke among men taking diuretics (RR 0.36; 95% CI 0.18, 0.72). Although earlier findings (SED-13, 563) highlighted the low efficacy and potential risk of potassium supplements, use in diuretics-treated hypertensives may improve outcome.

Thiazide-based treatment in SHEP was associated with a significant mean reduction in serum potassium of 0.3 mmol/l, although severe hypokalemia was rare ([14C]). There were notable reductions in the chronic complications of hypertension, including stroke, in SHEP (SEDA-13, 559). Since potassium supplements were used if the serum potassium concentration fell below 3.5 mmol/l, treatment of hypokalemia may be important in ensuring the cardiovascular benefits of thiazides in the management of hypertension.

Calcium balance (SED-13, 564) The association of renal calcification with furosemide treatment in newborns has often been reported. Four adults in whom nephrocalcinosis appeared to be related to long-term treatment with furosemide have now been observed (16[C]). Ultrasonography showed increased echogenicity of the renal pyramids, correlating perfectly with the findings on CT scan. As in neonates, long-term treatment with furosemide may cause mild medullary nephrocalcinosis, characterized by peripheral deposition of calcium salts in the pyramids, but without apparent modification of renal function.

Withdrawal effects Long-term use of loop diuretics in very old people is common, but may not be easily justified. An assay of dispensing data has been used to identify patients aged at least 75 years using loop diuretics (17[C]). A questionnaire survey of general practitioners (with a 50% response rate) showed that continuation of diuretics was considered unnecessary in 66 of 338 patients (20%). During follow-up, however, the prescription rate in those patients was no different from that in 272 patients for whom continuation of diuretics was considered necessary. Continuation rates were 71 and 75%, respectively, at 12 weeks, and 39 and 47% at 36 weeks. The marked overall reduction in prescribing over the 9 months of follow-up suggests that the assumption that these patients were 'long-term' users may be invalid. Nevertheless, this study suggests that there are substantial opportunities for withdrawal of loop diuretics. There are various reasons why prescription rates were not influenced, but a prominent justification for continuing diuretics is salt and water retention on withdrawal (SEDA-21, 227).

If diuretics are withdrawn suddenly in patients with a normal sodium intake, there will be *rebound retention of sodium and water*, because compensatory mechanisms that maintain sodium balance in the face of diuretics continue to act for several days after the diuresis has worn off (SED-13, 575). There are two methods of mitigating rebound retention of sodium and water: gradual reduction of the dosage or institution of a low sodium diet so that only a small amount of sodium can be retained when the diuretic is withdrawn (18[r]). Rebound retention of sodium and water, with consequent edema, may convince the doctor that continued diuretic therapy is necessary, and the patient is then committed to life-time exposure. Even in patients with heart failure, reduced intake of salt may remove the need for diuretics or allow the use of lower dosages.

Interactions *Non-steroidal anti-inflammatory drugs* (NSAIDs) may reduce the efficacy of diuretics (SED-13, 569, 573; SEDA-17, 268; SEDA-21, 229). The risk of congestive heart failure associated with the use of diuretics and NSAIDs has been investigated in 10 519 patients aged over 55 years (19[C]). There was an increased risk of hospitalization for congestive heart failure during periods of concomitant use (RR 2.2; 95% CI 1.7, 2.9) compared with diuretics alone. After adjustment for age, sex, history of hospitalization, and drug use, the RR was 1.8 (95% CI 1.4, 2.4). Hospitalization for heart failure was usually within 30 days of exposure to an NSAID and the highest frequency was within the first few days. The risk was highest in patients taking thiazides in combination with potassium-sparing diuretics, but there was no increased risk in patients taking loop diuretics. There was no apparent relation with impaired renal function (SED-13, 577), but accurate assessment of the influence of renal capacity on the interaction was precluded, because too few patients had renal impairment. The lack of difference in the risk of hospitalization for different NSAIDs indicated a class effect. Thus, use of NSAIDs in elderly patients taking diuretics leads to a 2-fold increased risk of hospitalization for congestive heart failure. The risk is particularly marked when a potassium-sparing diuretic is co-administered (SED-13, 577).

CARBONIC ANHYDRASE INHIBITORS

Acetazolamide *(SED-13, 571; SEDA-19, 222; SEDA-20, 204; SEDA-21, 228)*

Nervous system *Worsening of neurological deficits* in acute brain ischemia after intravenous acetazolamide has been reported in two men (20[C]).

A 66-year-old man with occlusion of the insular portion of the middle cerebral artery became unconscious with worsened right hemiparesis and aphasia shortly after being given acetazolamide 1000 mg.

A 65-year-old man with vertigo associated with nausea, right hemiparesis, and cerebellar signs due to severe stenosis of the mild portion of the basilar artery became unconscious with tetraplegia shortly after the administration of acetazolamide.

The suggested mechanism is an intracerebral blood flow steal syndrome. However, neurological deterioration in patients with ischemic stroke is not uncommon, and attribution to acetazolamide must be considered uncertain.

Risk factors Acetazolamide inhibits cerebrospinal fluid production, and its effects are augmented by furosemide, suggesting a role for this combination in infants with ventricular dilatation resulting from severe periventricular hemorrhage. The International Posthaemorrhagic Ventricular Drug Trial Group has reported the results of a randomized controlled trial of standard therapy alone or with the addition of acetazolamide plus furosemide in the first 151 of 177 randomized patients (21[C]). The addition of acetazolamide plus furosemide was not only ineffective but also worsened the already poor outcome in these infants. At 1 year, death and the need for shunt placement were substantially commoner in the diuretic-treated group. There were adverse events (e.g. acidosis, nausea, anorexia, and diarrhea) in 37% of those given acetazolamide plus furosemide; in addition, 27% developed *nephrocalcinosis* (SED-13, 571; SEDA-21, 228). *Alteration in cerebral blood flow* due to acetazolamide may have caused additional brain injury.

In a commentary on this trial (22[R]) it was pointed out that the use of acetazolamide alone or with furosemide in the treatment of post-hemorrhagic hydrocephalus is another example of the use of untried therapy in neonatal care. The safety and efficacy of acetazolamide in children has never been established.

Overdosage In patients with impaired renal function, care should be taken to avoid accumulation of acetazolamide.

A 66-year-old woman with chronic renal failure developed acute deterioration of renal function after treatment for 11 days with acetazolamide 500 mg/day for glaucoma (23[C]). She had severe thrombocytopenia and anemia; her stools were strongly positive for occult blood. The serum acetazolamide concentration was raised (77 mg/l, 344 μmol/l). There was extensive hemorrhagic gastritis on gastroscopy. Despite intensive therapy, she died of disseminated intravascular coagulation and septic shock due to severe bone marrow depression 6 days after admission.

It was concluded that overdosage with acetazolamide had destroyed the gastric mucosal barrier by interfering with prostaglandin and bicarbonate release, and had caused thrombocytopenia by bone marrow suppression, eventually leading to hemorrhagic gastritis. Although acetazolamide binds strongly to plasma protein and clearance by hemodialysis is generally poor, this approach and hemoperfusion (without heparin) appeared to be effective in this patient.

LOOP DIURETICS

Bumetanide *(SED-13, 574)*

Musculoskeletal Various musculoskeletal symptoms have been reported with bumetanide, including *pain*, *cramping*, and *weakness*. The symptoms are usually mild and self-limiting, with an incidence of less than 2%, but disabling reactions have occurred after oral administration and intravenous injection of 2–8 mg, and severity correlates with dose. The onset is usually 2–4 h after dosing; the slower onset in this report may have been because of a more gradual increase in plasma concentrations during infusion. Previous reports have suggested that hypoalbuminemia (and consequently higher unbound concentrations) in patients with renal insufficiency may predispose to this reaction.

Eight of 34 patients with heart failure treated with continuous infusions of bumetanide experienced 11 episodes of severe, widespread, disabling musculoskeletal symptoms (24[CR]). Reactions were most severe at infusion rates of about 2 mg/h and were not associated with any specific laboratory abnormality. The onset was gradual over 12–24 h and symptoms resolved 24–48 h after discontinuation. In two patients, the adverse reactions were precipitated by rechallenge. The same patients were given equivalent or larger continuous infusions of furosemide without musculoskeletal symptoms. The symptoms occurred in patients without significant renal impairment or hypoalbuminemia.

Furosemide *(SED-13, 571; SEDA-20, 204; SEDA-21, 229)*

Cardiovascular The efficacy and safety of intravenous furosemide and nitrates has been examined in a randomized trial of patients with severe pulmonary edema (25[C]). After treatment with oxygen, morphine, and furosemide 40 mg, 54 patients were randomized to furosemide 80 mg every 15 min and low-dose isosorbide dinitrate by continuous infusion, and 56 to high-dose isosorbide dinitrate by repeated injection every 5 min. Those given high-dose isosorbide required less mechanical ventilation (13 vs 40%) and had fewer heart attacks (17 vs 30%). Those given high-dose isosorbide dinitrate received an average furosemide dose of 56 mg compared with 200 mg in the other group. The authors concluded that high-dose isosorbide dinitrate, given as repeated intravenous boluses after low-dose intravenous furosemide, is safe and effective in controlling severe pulmonary edema and more effective than high-dose furosemide with low-dose isosorbide nitrate in terms of the need for mechanical ventilation and frequency of myocardial infarction. Whether a further reduction of furosemide dose in the treatment of severe pulmonary edema is possible remains to be determined.

In a commentary on this paper (26[R]) it was suggested that neuroendocrine activation and resultant increased peripheral resistance (afterload) after furosemide reduce cardiac output and stroke volume and increase cardiac work, with the possibility of *worsening myocardial and tissue ischemia*. Since many patients with heart failure have underlying myocardial ischemia or infarction, initial symptomatic benefit from furosemide may be followed by detrimental effects on myocardial perfusion, with extension or completion of myocardial necrosis.

Twenty patients with refractory congestive heart failure despite treatment with a maximum dose of an ACE inhibitor were randomized to treatment with low-dose dopamine and low-dose (80 mg/day) oral furosemide, low-dose dopamine plus medium dose (5 mg/kg per day) furosemide by continuous intravenous infusion, or high dose (10 mg/kg per day) furosemide by infusion (27[C]). There were similar improvements in the signs and symptoms of heart failure, urine output, and weight loss. However, mean arterial pressure and renal function fell (by 14–15 and 41–42%, respectively) with medium- and high-dose furosemide, while blood pressure increased and renal function improved (4 and 14%, respectively) with low-dose furosemide. Changes in mean arterial pressure correlated closely with changes in creatinine clearance. Medium- and high-dose furosemide was associated with more *hypokalemia*. Two patients who received high-dose furosemide developed *oliguric renal insufficiency* and one who received medium-dose furosemide died with *ventricular fibrillation* associated with hypokalemia. The study was discontinued prematurely because of these adverse events. Patients with heart failure tend to have low serum potassium concentrations, even untreated, and dysrhythmias cannot be explained by diuretic-induced hypokalemia in controlled studies (SED-13, 562).

Maintenance of cardiac output in patients with congestive heart failure is highly dependent on preload. Continuous intravenous infusion of medium or high doses of furosemide, by causing dose-dependent venodilatation and diuresis, reduces preload. The consequent reduction in mean arterial pressure and effective blood volume may reduce renal perfusion. Because ACE inhibition impairs renal protection against reduced perfusion, the combination of an ACE inhibitor and high-dose furosemide causes a reduction in glomerular filtration rate linearly related to the change in blood pressure.

Endocrine, metabolic *Lipid metabolism* A randomized, double-blind, placebo-controlled, crossover study in 10 patients has been performed to determine whether there are daily acute rises in lipid and lipoprotein concentrations associated with changes in intravascular volume during long-term furosemide treatment (28[C]). In the 8 h after furosemide administration there were significant increases in serum cholesterol (10%), HDL cholesterol (9.0%), and apolipoprotein b (9.8%). Increases of similar magnitude in triglycerides and apolipoprotein A-I were not significant. The total cholesterol/HDL cholesterol ratio was unchanged. Changes in lipid and lipoprotein concentrations were greater than changes in intravascular volume, albumin, and total protein, suggesting that counter-regulatory hormones (adrenaline and hydrocortisone), stimulated by intravascular volume, may have contributed.

The transience of the increases in lipid concentrations after furosemide during prolonged treatment reflects its brief duration of action. Provided adequate salt and water intake restores intravascular volume, lipid changes are short lived. Such considerations might influence the interpretation of lipid concentrations and cardiac risk with other diuretics. To avoid misinterpretation, blood samples for lipid estimation should be taken in the euvolumic state before diuretic administration.

Miscellaneous An association between furosemide treatment and *fever* (SEDA-20, 204) has been observed in several babies (29[C]). All were in the first year of life and in poor clinical condition because of congestive heart failure barely controlled with digoxin and high dosages of furosemide 2–4 mg/kg per day. They had a fever that lasted several weeks and did not respond to antibiotics. There was a good correlation between body weight and fever, which appeared when the babies had lost 5–7% of their assumed normal body weight. Fever was also associated with raised blood urea nitrogen and hemoconcentration. The authors postulated that fever was due to dehydration, resulting from the intensive diuretic effect of furosemide, similar to the fever observed in neonates in the first days of life when breast milk supply is insufficient. This mechanism is supported by the observations that a lower dose of furosemide did not cause fever and that the same dose of furosemide did not cause fever in the same patients later in life.

A child who had fever, presumably caused by furosemide given postoperatively, did not have fever when ethacrynic acid was used after a second operation, despite a similar diuresis and fluid loss (30[C]).

These anecdotal observations suggest that furosemide can be associated with fever in occasional patients, but the mechanism remains uncertain.

Interactions Co-administration of *meloxicam* for 7 days resulted in increased plasma concentrations and cumulative urinary excretion of furosemide in 19 patients with congestive heart failure (31[C]). However, cumulative urine volume and sodium and potassium excretion were unchanged compared with furosemide alone. Thus, there is no clinically significant interaction between meloxicam and furosemide after repeated administration in patients with heart failure. Meloxicam is an NSAID that is relatively selective for cyclooxygenase-2 (COX-2), sparing the physiologically important COX-1 isoform that mediates vasodilator prostaglandins, which maintain renal function. This might explain the lack of interaction with furosemide in contrast to other NSAIDs (SED-13, 573).

A case report has suggested an interaction between furosemide and *warfarin* (32[CR]).

A 45-year-old man was admitted for acute withdrawal from ethanol and cocaine. Several years earlier he had undergone aortic valve replacement for bacterial endocarditis secondary to intravenous drug abuse. Maintenance therapy was with warfarin 40 mg/week, furosemide 20 mg/day, potassium chloride, and methocarbamol, although he took only the warfarin regularly. His International Normalised Ratio (INR) was 1.93 and his liver enzymes were slightly raised. His prescribed medication was continued and he was given lorazepam, folate, and thiamine. Eight days after admission, the INR was 1.44 and the warfarin dosage was increased. Four days later the INR was 2.08. Thereafter, furosemide was withdrawn and the INR gradually increased over 28 days. There was a significant negative correlation between INR and hematocrit, without evidence of bleeding.

A review of the literature showed that prothrombin time is reduced by about 25% by both chlorthalidone and spironolactone, without changes in plasma warfarin. Reduction in prothrombin time is associated with increased hematocrit. These findings are consistent with a reduced anticoagulant effect of warfarin secondary to diuretic-induced volume depletion, mediating increases in clotting factors. Any effect is therefore likely to be short-lived.

Torasemide (torsemide) *(SED-13, 574; SEDA-21, 229)*

Skin and appendages Cutaneous reactions to torasemide have been described anecdotally and include non-specific *erythematous lesions* and *pruritus*. A *photosensitive lichenoid reaction* to torasemide has been described in an 82-year-old man (33[c]). The overwhelming presence of T-lymphocytes within the lesional skin biopsy specimen and the photodistributed nature of the eruption supported a localized photoallergic cell-mediated hypersensitivity reaction. The temporal association of the skin lesion with treatment, the presence of eosinophils within the biopsy specimen, and resolution after withdrawal of torasemide collectively favored a drug-induced effect.

The presumed epitope targeted in this allergic reaction is unclear, but may represent structural components of the parent drug molecule or its metabolites (or both), or could be the result of an interaction of these molecules with unknown tissue haptens. Torasemide has structural similarities with furosemide, especially the presence of a sulfur-containing moiety in its 16-carbon structure. There is potential for cross-sensitization between torasemide and other sulfonamide-type medications, in particular furosemide, and this may become apparent as the use of torasemide increases. Torasemide should be used cautiously in patients with known hypersensitivity to sulfonamides.

POTASSIUM-SPARING DIURETICS

Spironolactone *(SED-13, 575; SEDA-20, 205; SEDA-21, 230)*

Hematological Spironolactone-induced *agranulocytosis* has been reported in a few isolated cases (SED-13, 575). A further case has been described after the use of spironolactone 20 mg/day for 1 month for cryptogenic cirrhosis (34[CR]). Bone marrow biopsy showed granulocyte hyperplasia with a myeloid/erythroid ratio of 0.02 (normal 3.5). These findings, together with the gradual onset, suggested that agranulocytosis had been caused by a toxic effect of spironolactone on the bone marrow, of which there have been two previous reports. Close monitoring during spironolactone therapy is advised in patients with risk factors for agranulocytosis, such as those of increased age, hepatic or renal impairment, and treatment with high doses for prolonged periods.

Skin and appendages An 82-year-old woman, taking multiple drugs including spironolactone, developed bullous erythematous lesions suggestive of *pemphigoid* on the left thigh (35[c]). The diagnosis was confirmed by histology and direct cutaneous fluorescence. The lesions resolved on withdrawal of spironolactone and did not recur during 18 months of follow-up. A causal effect of spironolactone is plausible but requires confirmation.

Interactions An interaction of spironolactone with *trimethoprim* has been described (36[c]).

A 66-year-old man taking trimethoprim 320 mg/day for recent osteomyelitis and spironolactone 100 mg/day for hypertension developed muscle weakness. His serum potassium concentration was 8.4 mmol/l (4.6 mmol/l before trimethoprim) and there was minor renal impairment. The electrocardiogram showed a regular bradycardia with peaked T waves and prolongation of the QRS complex. His hyperkalemia was treated conventionally and the trimethoprim and spironolactone were discontinued. His blood chemistry normalized over the next 2 days and recovery was uneventful.

Trimethoprim has potassium-sparing properties very similar to those of amiloride (37[R]). It often causes hyperkalemia in high-risk patients and should be added to the list of drugs to be avoided in patients taking potassium-sparing diuretics, especially if there is renal impairment or co-administration of an NSAID.

Triamterene *(SED-13, 577; SEDA-21, 230)*

Interaction An interaction of triamterene with *methotrexate* has been described (38[c]).

A 57-year-old woman presented with pallor, tachycardia, dehydration, profound pancytopenia, and renal impairment. Her serum folate concentration was reduced. Two months earlier, methotrexate 5 mg/week for rheumatoid arthritis had been added to long-term therapy with diclofenac 150 mg/day, atenolol 50 mg/day, and triamterene/hydrochlorothiazide 50/25 mg/day. Her routine medications were withdrawn and she was given oral folinic acid 15 mg qds. Within 1 week, her full blood count and renal function had returned to normal.

Both methotrexate and triamterene inhibit dihydrofolate reductase (SED-13, 577). Thus, there are sound theoretical reasons for marrow toxicity as a result of an interaction between these drugs. Dehydration due to diuretic treatment may have contributed to renal impairment and reduced clearance of methotrexate, further increasing the risk of bone marrow suppression.

REFERENCES

1. Moser M. Why are physicians not prescribing diuretics more frequently in the management of hypertension? J Am Med Assoc 1998;279:1813–6.
2. Freis ED. Current status of diuretics, beta-blockers, alpha-blockers, and alpha-beta-blockers in the treatment of hypertension. Med Clin N Am 1997;81:1305–17.
3. The sixth report of the Joint National Committee on Prevention, Detection, Evaluation and Treatment of High Blood Pressure. Arch Intern Med 1997;157:2413–61 (erratum in 1998;158: 573).
4. Grimm RH Jr, Grandits GA, Cutler JA, Stewart AL, McDonald RH, Svendsen K, Prineas RJ, Leibson PR. Relationship of quality-of-life measures to long-term lifestyle and drug treatment in the treatment of mild hypertension study. Arch Intern Med 1997;157:638–48.
5. Messerli FH, Grossman E, Goldbourt U. Are beta-blockers efficacious as first-line therapy for hypertension in the elderly? A systematic review. J Am Med Assoc 1998;279:1903–7.
6. Borhani NO, Mercuri M, Borhani PA, Buckalew VM, Canossa-Terris M, Carr AA, Kappagoda T, Rocco MV, Schnaper HW, Sowers JR, Bond MG. Final outcome results of the Multicenter Isradipine Diuretic Atherosclerosis Study (MIDAS). J Am Med Assoc 1996;276:785–91.
7. Kostis JB, Davis BR, Cutler J, Grimm RH Jr, Berge KG, Cohen JD, Lacey CR, Perry HM Jr, Blaufox MD, Wassertheil-Smoller S, Black HR, Schron E, Berkson DM, Curb JD, Smith WM, McDonald R, Applegate WB. Prevention of heart failure by antihypertensive drug treatment in older patients with isolated systolic hypertension. J Am Med Assoc 1997;278:212–6.
8. Moser M, Hebert PR. Prevention of disease progression, left ventricular hypertrophy and congestive heart failure in the hypertension treatment trials. J Am Coll Cardiol 1996;27:1214–18.
9. Papademetriou V, Gottdiener JS, Naragan P, Cushman WG, Zachariah PK, Gottdiener PS, Chase GA. Hydrochlorothiazide is superior to isradipine for reduction of left ventricular mass: results of a multicenter trial. J Am Coll Cardiol 1997;30:1802–8.
10. Gottdiener JS, Reda DJ, Williams DW, Materson BJ, Cushman W, Anderson RJ. Effect of single-drug therapy on reduction of left atrial size in mild to moderate hypertension: comparison of six antihypertensive agents. Circulation 1998; 98:140–8.
11. Gottdiener J, Reda D, Massie BM, Materson BJ, Williams DW, Anderson RJ. Effect of single-drug therapy on reduction of left ventricular mass on mild to moderate hypertension: comparison of six antihypertensive agents. Circulation 1997; 95:2007–14.
12. Nielsen S, Dollerup J, Nielsen B, Mogensen CE. Combination of enalapril and low-dose thiazide reduces normoalbuminuria in essential hypertension. J Hypertens 1998;16:1539–44.
13. Hunter SJ, Harper R, Ennis CN, Crothers E, Sheridon B, Johnston GD, Atkinson AB, Bell PM. Effects of combination therapy with an angiotensin converting eznyme inhibitor and thiazide diuretic on insulin action in essential hypertension. J Hypertens 1998;16:103–9.

14. Savage PJ, Pressel SL, Curb JD, Schron EB, Applegate WB, Black HR, Cohen J, Davis BR, Frost P, Smith W, Gonzalez N, Guthrie GP, Oberman A, Rutan G, Probstfield JL, Stamler J. Influence of long-term, low-dose, diuretic-based, antihypertensive therapy on glucose, lipid, uric acid, and potassium levels in older men and women with isolated systolic hypertension: the Systolic Hypertension in the Elderly Program. Arch Intern Med 1998;158:741–51.
15. Ascherio A, Rimm EB, Hernán MA, Giovannucci EL, Kawachi I, Stampfer MJ, Willett WC. Intake of potassium, magnesium, calcium, and fiber and risk of stroke among US men. Circulation 1998;98:1198–204.
16. Solivetti FM, Paganelli C, Zoffoli M, Bacaro D, Quintigliano D, Nasrollah N. Nephrocalcinosis induced by long-term therapy with furosemide. J Clin Ultrasound 1997;25:519–20.
17. Van Kraaij DJW, Jansen RWMM, Gribnau FWJ, Hoefnagels WHL. Loop diuretics in patients aged 75 years or older: general practitioners' assessment of indications and possibilities for withdrawal. Eur J Clin Pharmacol 1998; 54:323–7.
18. Missouris CG, MacGregor GA. Rebound sodium and water retention occurs when diuretic treatment is stopped. Br Med J 1998;316:628.
19. Heerdink ER, Leufkens HG, Herings RMC, Ottervanger JP Stricker BHC, Bakker A. NSAIDs associated with increased risk of congestive heart failure in elderly patients taking diuretics. Arch Intern Med 1998;158:1108–12.
20. Kurokawa Y, Ishiguro M, Takahaski H. Two cases of acute brain ischemia in which neurological deficits were aggrevated by the administration of acetazolamide. Jpn J Clin Radiol 1997; 42:1151–4.
21. International randomised controlled trial of acetazolamide and furosemide in posthaemorrhagic ventricular dilatation in infancy. International PHVD Drug Trial Group. Lancet 1998;352:433–40.
22. Hack M, Cohen AR. Acetazolamide plus furosemide for periventricular dilatation: lessons for drug therapy in children. Lancet 1998;352:418–19.
23. Takeda K, Nakamoto M, Yasunaga C, Nishihara G, Matsuo K, Urabe M, Kitamura M, Nozoi T. Acute hemorrhagic gastritis associated with acetazolamide intoxication in a patient with chronic renal failure. Clin Nephrol 1997;48:266–8.
24. Howard PA, Dunn MI. Severe musculoskeletal symptoms during continuous infusion of bumetanide. Chest 1997;111:359–64.
25. Cotter G, Metzkor E, Kaluski E, Faigenberg Z, Miller R, Simovitz A, Shaham O, Marghity D, Koren M, Blatt A, Moshkovitz Y, Zaidenstein R, Golik A. Randomised trial of high-dose isosorbide dinitrate plus low-dose furosemide versus high-dose furosemide plus low-dose isosorbide dinitrate in severe pulmonary oedema. Lancet 1998;351:389–93.
26. Gammage M. Treatment of acute pulmonary oedema: diuresis or vasodilatation? Lancet 1998;351:382–3.
27. Cotter G, Weissgarten J, Metzkor E, Moshkovitz Y, Litinski I, Tavori U, Perry C, Zaidenstein R, Golik A. Increased toxicity of high-dose furosemide versus low-dose dopamine in the treatment of refractory congestive heart failure. Clin Pharmacol Ther 1997;62:187–93.
28. Campbell N, Brant R, Stalts H, Stone J, Mahallati H. Fluctuations in blood lipid levels during furosemide therapy. A randomized, double-blind, placebo-controlled crossover study. Arch Intern Med 1998;158:1461–3.
29. Garty BZ. Furosemide-associated fever: drug fever or dehydration fever? J Pediatr 1997; 130:499–500.
30. Clegg HW, Riopel DA. Furosemide-associated fever: drug fever or dehydration fever? (Reply). J Pediatr 1997;130:500.
31. Müller FO, Middle MV, Schall R, Terblanché J, Hundt HKL, Groenwoud G, An evaluation of the interaction of meloxicam with frusemide in patients with compensated chronic cardiac failure. Br J Clin Pharmacol 1997;44:393–8.
32. Laizure SC, Madlock L, Cyr M, Self T. Decreased hypoprothrombinemic effect of warfarin associated with furosemide. Ther Drug Monit 1997;19:361–3.
33. Byrd DR, Ahmed I. Photosensitive lichenoid reaction to torsemide—a loop diuretic. Mayo Clin Proc 1997;72:930–1.
34. Whitling AM, Pérgola PE, Sany JL, Talbert RL. Spironolactone-induced agranulocytosis. Ann Pharmacother 1997;31:582–5.
35. Grange E, Scrivener Y, Koessler A, Straub P, Guillaume J-C. Bullous pemphigoid induced by spironolactone. Ann Dermatol Venereol 1997; 124:700–2.
36. Marinella MA. Severe hyperkalemia associated with trimethoprim-sulfamethoxazole and spironolactone. Infect Dis Clin Pract 1997;6:256–60.
37. Perazella MA. Trimethoprim is a potassium-sparing diuretic like amiloride and causes hyperkalemia in high-risk patients. Am J Ther 1997;4:343–8.
38. Richmond R, McRoric ER, Ogden DA, Lambert CM. Methotrexate and triamterene—a potentially fatal combination? Ann Rheum Dis 1997;56:209–10.

Gijsbert B. van der Voet and Frederik A. de Wolff

22 Metals

Aluminium *(SED-13, 583; SEDA-19, 223; SEDA-20, 207; SEDA-21, 232)*

Aluminium compounds continue to be used in antacid therapy and as adjuvants in vaccines. Discussion of the role of aluminium in Alzheimer's disease has for the time being lapsed. Hypersensitivity is being noticed more often than before.

Nervous system Aluminium concentrations in the tissues of six French patients have been reported after the use of aluminium-containing bone cement in otosurgery and neurosurgery (1[c]). In five patients, the mean plasma aluminium concentrations were 1.2, 9.2, 1.0, 2.8, and 2.0 μg/l. In case 1 aluminium concentrations were 176 μg/l in the postauricular cerebrospinal fluid, 34 μg/l in the pontine-cerebellar angle, and 4 and 6 μg/l in the lumbar shunt. As a precautionary measure, in the first three cases the biomaterials were removed soon after the intervention, and no increase in plasma or cerebrospinal fluid aluminium was observed. Measurement of aluminium in these fluids may therefore be considered to be complementary and at times helpful in making decisions. However, care is needed at all stages, from sampling through to analysis, because aluminium is ubiquitous and high results may be due to environmental contamination. The authors called for in-depth pre-marketing trials of these materials in animals.

Skin and appendages Topical zirconium can cause hypersensitivity granulomas in sensitized persons. This has led to the removal of zirconium salts from antiperspirants. However, complexes of zirconium and aluminium are non-sensitizing and are commonly used as active ingredients in topical antiperspirants; nevertheless, a granulomatous reaction has now been reported (2[c]).

A 41-year-old white woman had a 2-year history of asymptomatic discrete and confluent papules in her axillae, some arranged linearly along the axillary creases. She had no history of sensitivity to zirconium, aluminium, or antiperspirants. A biopsy showed well-organized epithelioid granulomas with scattered multinucleated giant cells throughout the dermis. Some granulomas were surrounded by a slight lymphoid infiltrate. Stains for fungi, bacteria, and mycobacteria were negative. There was no gross evidence of foreign material within the granulomas. Polaroscopic examination was negative. Scanning electron microscopy localized foreign material within the organized granulomas, and energy-dispersive X-ray analysis showed significant peaks of zirconium and aluminium. She stopped using topical antiperspirants containing aluminium or zirconium, and topical fluocinonide cream 0.05% led to complete resolution within 3 months.

Immunological and hypersensitivity reactions A 23-year-old man developed dermatitis of the face after using a cream for acne and hyperpigmentation (3[c]). He was patch tested with various allergens, and tested positive to aluminium sulfate and aluminium chloride. Contact sensitization to uninjected aluminium is rare. The typical route of sensitization is the injection of aluminium-adsorbed vaccines, and such patients may present with a granulomatous nodule at the site. The use of antiperspirants and topical medicaments can also lead to allergic contact dermatitis. The diagnosis is usually made accidentally.

Contact sensitivity to nickel and aluminium has been reported to respond to antihistamine therapy (4[c]).

A 19-year-old woman with a history of stress-provoked asthma, allergy to dogs, and periodic hand eczema developed a severe skin reaction when in direct contact with certain metals. She could neither hold coins in the palm of her hand nor touch metal door handles or banisters without a reaction. As a consequence she always wore clothing with long sleeves, which she could pull down over her hands as a form of glove. When in contact with metals erythema and bullae developed. By the following day, these had changed into erosions and ulcerations. Patch tests were performed with nickel sulfate in various concentrations to her forearm and back. Pure aluminium powder in vaseline was applied directly to the skin. Consequently infil-

Side Effects of Drugs, Annual 22
J.K. Aronson, ed.

tration and erythema developed with both nickel and aluminium. She became totally symptom-free when she took cetirizine 10–20 mg/day for 5 days, and continuous usage thereafter kept her symptom-free for 6 years. Test exposures with nickel sulfate and aluminium were repeatedly positive 4 days after withdrawal of cetirizine.

Arsenic *(SED-13, 585)*

Arsenic salts are occasionally still used in skin disease and in dental practice (5[c]), (6[c]). Arsenic compounds are commonly used in semiconductor materials.

Liver Hepatic portal fibrosis and subsequent angiosarcoma has been attributed to long-term arsenic therapy (5[c]).

A 60-year-old man had a history of psoriasis of the palms and soles, which was treated with arsenical salt derivatives from 1972 to 1982. He drank alcohol 100–120 g/day. He had no history of occupational or environmental exposure to vinyl chloride nor had received thorium dioxide or androgenic or anabolic steroids. In 1984 he had an upper gastrointestinal hemorrhage. Only hyperkeratosis and palmar erythema were observed. His liver enzymes were raised. Endoscopy showed an antral ulcer with signs of recent bleeding and grade IV esophageal varices with no evidence of bleeding. Liver biopsy showed preservation of the parenchymal architecture, fibrous expansion of the portal spaces, and minimum lymphocytic infiltrate. The diagnosis was portal fibrosis compatible with idiopathic portal hypertension. When he died of multiorgan failure in 1997, autopsy showed a moderately differentiated multifocal hepatic angiosarcoma with bone, gastric, and splenic metastases.

The authors postulated that the chronic use of arsenical salts had caused the liver damage.

Musculoskeletal Arsenic in dental practice is used for the devitalization of inflamed pulp and sensitive dentine. Two cases of arsenical necrosis of the jawbones have been reported (6[c]).

A 24-year-old man developed bony sequestration associated with his left maxillary second premolar after root treatment by a private practitioner 1 month before. It was later confirmed that an arsenical preparation had been used. A buccal swelling had appeared and gradually extended to involve the whole cheek and the lower eyelid, whilst pus and brown fluid were discharged from the nose. The crown of the left upper second premolar was badly broken down and contained a temporary filling. There was severe destruction of both the buccal and palatal gums, the alveolar bone being exposed and dark in color. The condition was diagnosed as chemical necrosis of the maxilla.

A 41-year-old man complained of trismus, paresthesia of the lip, and right jaw intermittent pain after the extraction of the three lower right molars. The condition had apparently developed after his dentist had inserted a 'pulp killer', which led to necrosis of the gums.

Both patients were treated by removal of the dead bone and teeth involved, various antibiotics, and irrigation of the affected area over an extended period, with excellent results. The authors suggested that conservative treatment of chemical necrosis of the jaws is preferable to more radical treatment.

There is no justification whatsoever for the use of arsenic in modern dental practice.

Bismuth *(SED-13, 585; SEDA-19, 223; SEDA-20, 208; SEDA-21, 233)*

Bismuth salts continue to be used in the eradication of *Helicobacter pylori* (see also Chapter 36). Ranitidine bismuth citrate has been reviewed as a new bismuth compound (7[R]). No new data on the neurotoxic and nephrotoxic effects of bismuth compounds have appeared.

Cardiorespiratory Deposition of bismuth in the heart and lungs has been reported after intravenous injection (8[c]).

A 39-year-old man developed headache, myalgia, weight loss of 4.5 kg, intermittent abdominal pain, back pain, and cough. He had been well until he had had an intravenous injection of a health tonic into his left forearm while in Honduras 2 years before, after which he had been ill for several days with a flu-like illness. He denied any other medical problems, including venereal disease. The chest radiograph showed multiple 2-mm metallic punctate densities scattered throughout the lung fields and lining the contour of the right atrium and ventricle. A CT scan of the chest showed discrete 1-mm dense punctate opacities scattered in both lungs with a subpleural distribution. Alveolar macrophages obtained by bronchoalveolar lavage were evaluated for particles by morphology and energy-dispersive X-ray spectroscopy. Most of the particles gave a single peak for bismuth. Apparently he had been given intravenous bismuth. No follow up was reported.

Skin and appendages Deposition of bismuth

in the skin has been reported after oral administration (9[c]).

A 41-year-old man had a 2-year history of crops of small, black, carbon-like particles (size 0.2–0.5 mm) on the skin. His palms and soles were not involved. These particles appeared at intervals of 15–30 days and persisted for 2 or 3 days if not removed by soap and water. They were located in follicular orifices and caused no symptoms. He denied using any medications except for two bismuth subsalicylate tablets after heavy meals once or twice a month for the last 4 years. Eight black particles, removed from the skin and analysed using an atomic spectrometer, contained bismuth. Biopsy showed a follicular orifice containing black particles and spores of *Plasmodium ovale*. After he stopped taking bismuth subsalicylate, the black granules progressively diminished in number and disappeared a few months later.

Copper *(SED-13, 587; SEDA-19, 224; SEDA-20, 208; SEDA-21, 234)*

Copper is still used in intrauterine contraceptive devices (IUCDs). The role of copper in Wilson's disease and Menkes' disease, both of which involve inherited disturbances in metabolism, continues to be explored.

Hematological A 25-year-old woman who had delivered a healthy child after a normal pregnancy 4 months before, was given tetracycline for a cold (10[c]). A few days later she developed acute severe hemolysis and had signs of hepatic failure, characterized by considerably reduced synthetic capacity of the liver but low serum aminotransferase activity, and a proximal renal tubular disorder. Increased urinary excretion of copper, very high concentrations of copper in the liver and Kayser–Fleischer rings demonstrated Wilson's disease presenting with severe hemolysis. The serum ceruloplasmin concentration was in the lower part of the reference range, and was not helpful in making the diagnosis.

Interactions Anti-platelet aggregation of copper-aspirinate, a copper complex of aspirin, has been studied in vitro and in vivo in rabbits (11). Copper-aspirinate was much more effective than aspirin as an inhibitor of platelet aggregation induced by arachidonic acid, ADP and platelet activating factor. The mechanism of this effect is related to inhibition of platelet cyclo-oxygenase, the release of active substances from platelets, and an increase in PGI_2 concentration in plasma.

Interference with diagnostic routines A CuT380A IUCD (ParaGard), a copper-containing IUCD, and a Signa 1.5T HR system have been subjected to in vitro MRI to evaluate whether exposure to the dynamic magnetic forces generated by MRI resulted in movement, torque, or heat; it did not (12). There appears to be no reason for excluding women with IUCDs of the types examined from MRI examination.

Gallium *(SED-13, 588; SEDA-19, 224; SEDA-20, 209; SEDA-21, 235)*

Gallium (^{67}Ga) is used as a diagnostic tool and gallium nitrate as an antineoplastic agent.

Special senses Gallium has been reported to cause eye damage (13[c]).

After having been given about 2.5 g of intravenous gallium nitrate over 7 days, a 77-year-old man developed bilateral visual loss and optic neuritis with central scotomas on visual field testing and diminished P2-wave amplitude on visual evoked potential examination. The condition worsened after oral corticosteroid therapy. Partial recovery of optic nerve function in both eyes was present after 12 months of oral ferrous sulfate administration.

The authors concluded that partially reversible optic neuritis can be caused by gallium nitrate in the absence of other chemotherapeutic agents. Eye examinations are indicated in patients who receive gallium nitrate.

Interference with diagnostic routines Gallium-67 and abdominal CT scans of a 72-year-old woman who had a malignant lymphoma before, during, and after the administration of gallium nitrate/hydroxyurea combination chemotherapy have been reported (14[c]). During treatment the tumor failed to take up ^{67}Ga despite continuing CT evidence of disease, and the reappearance of ^{67}Ga scan abnormalities after the end of therapy suggested that caution should be taken when interpreting results of ^{67}Ga scintigraphy in patients being given gallium nitrate/hydroxyurea therapy.

Germanium *(SED-13, 588; SEDA-18, 455; SEDA-21, 235)*

Germanium is widely distributed in nature. It is used as a semiconductor and there have been a few attempts to use it in medicine (including cancer chemotherapy).

Overdosage In the past few years 20 cases of germanium overdose have been described, with renal failure and injury to other organs. A 52-year-old man given germanium to prevent recurrence of a brain tumor developed multiple organ dysfunction and died of intractable hyperdynamic shock (15[c]).

Gold *(SED-13, 588; SEDA-19, 224; SEDA-20, 209; SEDA-21, 236)*

There has been a continuous flow of reviews on the use of gold compounds in rheumatoid arthritis, but no new adverse effects have been reported. A critical review of vasomotor reactions to gold compounds has recently appeared (16[R]).

Hematological Thrombocytopenia is an infrequent adverse effect of treatment with auranofin, occurring in 0.7% of patients. Three patients developed serious thrombocytopenia after being given auranofin for 3 months (17[c]). There were no other adverse effects. Auranofin was withdrawn and two of the patients were treated with oral corticosteroids. Platelet counts became normal within 8 weeks. The pathogenesis of the thrombocytopenia is unknown. It is, however, a potentially serious adverse effect and can develop suddenly.

Skin and appendages Chrysiasis of the skin around the eyes has recently been reported in a patient taking gold (18[cr]).

A 70-year-old white woman presented to the clinic complaining of a dark pigmentation around her eyes that became more prominent with exposure to sunlight. She had begun to notice the pigmentation about 3 years before, but had become more concerned when her friends began questioning her about it. She had had long-standing rheumatoid arthritis treated with intramuscular gold sodium thiomalate (Myochrysine®), 50 mg on alternate weeks for 7 years (a total cumulative dose of over 9 g). She had a subtle bluish-gray pigmentation periorbitally and bilaterally on the face. The skin in naturally occurring creases and folds within areas of frank pigmentation was spared. The dorsa of both hands, the intramuscular injection site, and the V area of the neck were not discernibly pigmented. Biopsy showed several small irregular dark granules scattered throughout the dermis, identified as gold by cross-polarized light and electron microscopy with X-ray microanalysis.

The skin toxicity of gold has been reviewed (19[r]). In some countries gold has moved into second place as an allergen, following nickel. Recognition of this is mainly due to improvement of diagnostic methods and to the inclusion of gold in patch testing.

A 34-year-old woman had worn gold and platinum earrings since having her ears pierced when she was 13 years of age (20[c]). She developed painful nodules of both earlobes with mild dermatitis around the places where her ears had been pierced. She did not have gold dental fillings, and had not had therapeutic or occupational exposure to gold salts. Histologically the nodules showed prominent dermal edema with a diffuse dermal lymphocytic infiltrate composed predominantly of plasma cells, small lymphocytes, and histiocytes; there were occasional foreign body type giant cells with a suggestion of lymphoid follicle formation. She had a positive patch test to gold sodium thiosulfate.

A 27-year-old woman who wore gold earrings developed persistent nodules where her ears had been pierced and patch testing showed a positive allergic response to gold sodium thiosulfate (21[c]). Histology of the nodules showed a prominent sarcoid-type granulomatous reaction.

Contact allergy to gold in connection with treatment with gold salts has been sought in 57 patients with rheumatoid arthritis previously treated with gold, with or without cutaneous adverse effects, and in 20 patients intended for such treatment (22[C]). All were exposed to patch and intradermal tests with gold sodium thiosulfate, gold sodium thiomalate, and auranofin. There was contact allergy to gold in eight subjects (10.4%), one of the patients who had already been treated and seven of those intended to be treated. Contact allergy to gold is very frequent among patients with rheumatoid arthritis before gold therapy. In order to avoid early hypersensitivity reactions skin tests should be carried out before gold therapy is begun.

Pemphigus has again been attributed to gold (23[c]).

A 64-year-old woman was treated with gold sodium thiomalate for 18 months for long-standing rheumatoid arthritis with 100 mg/week initially and progressive increases in dosage up to 22.0 g/week. She developed flaccid blisters on the trunk and limbs and numerous erosions and vesicles in the oral cavity. The diagnosis was pemphigus caused by gold. She responded well to methylprednisolone and local antiseptic lotions, and flumethasone pivalate.

Special senses A 71-year-old white woman who had suffered from rheumatoid arthritis for about 15 years and had tried various treatments without benefit (24[c]) was given intramuscular sodium aurothiomalate 50 mg/week. After the third injection she developed widespread exfoliating erythroderma. She was treated with topical betamethasone 0.1% ointment and white soft paraffin and gradually improved. About 10 days later she complained of deafness in both ears accompanied by bilateral discharge and a sensation of irritation, due to otitis externa and bilateral tympanic membrane perforations. The authors implied that the skin of the external auditory canal and the tympanic membrane may have been involved in a generalized reaction to gold.

Iron *(SED-13, 595; SEDA-19, 225; SEDA-20, 211; SEDA-21, 237)*

Reviews continue to be published on iron deficiency anemia and iron overload (especially hemochromatosis), reviewing the search for the genetic basis of this disease and the newer diagnostic and therapeutic measures (25[R])–(27[R]). The toxic effects of native and modified hemoglobins have also been reviewed recently, including the role of iron (28[R]).

Second-generation effects Fetal hypoxic–ischemic encephalopathy can be diagnosed at birth by cerebral ultrasound scanning. The morphological appearance of the lesions depends on the time elapsed between the insult and examination of the brain.

A neonate (29[c]) developed multicystic encephalomalacia and corpus callosum atrophy attributable to an episode of maternal anaphylactic shock at 27 weeks of gestation after intravenous injection of iron. The diagnosis was made by cerebral ultrasound scanning at birth and confirmed by MRI.

This case shows that severe acute maternal hypotension during pregnancy can cause fetal cerebral damage similar to hypoxic–ischemic injuries that occur in the perinatal period.

Overdosage Iron ingestion continues to be one of the major causes of deaths from poisoning in children. In 1995 more than 22 000 children unintentionally took formulations containing iron. Despite child-resistant packaging and education of both the public and medical personnel, the number of deaths has not fallen significantly.

A 13-month-old child ingested prenatal vitamins and despite aggressive efforts died 13 h after the initial presentation (30[c]). His 3-year-old sibling had been evaluated at a local hospital 12 h before for iron ingestion.

Although there have been previous reports of death from iron ingestion, this case report is important because of the sibling's presentation beforehand, illustrating the need for physicians to inquire about other children in the home, possibly preventing further tragic outcomes.

Manganese *(SED-13, 1001; SEDA-19, 225; SEDA-20, 212; SEDA-21, 238)*

The use of mangafodipir trisodium (manganese dipyridoxal diphosphate or MnDPDP), which has been introduced as a hepatobiliary MRI contrast agent (Teslascan®) has been reviewed (31[R]). Its potential for assisting in the characterization of focal liver lesions, the diagnosis of local and global obstructive cholestasis, and the evaluation of hepatic function in diffuse liver diseases has been explored in multiple preclinical experiments in appropriate animals. MnDPDP caused persistent liver enhancement in cholestatic rats, Mn^{2+} was released in vivo after MnDPDP injection, and administration of free Mn^{2+} and bilirubin resulted in intrahepatic cholestasis. This gave concern that in the jaundice that is commonly associated with hepatic and pancreatic tumors, MnDPDP might cause secondary intrahepatic cholestasis on top of the primary cholestatic disease, owing to an interaction between the dissociated Mn^{2+} and increased endogenous bilirubin. It was concluded that MnDPDP is a promising MRI contrast agent for the detection and characterization of focal and diffuse liver disease and that after injection of a single dose of MnDPDP adverse effects will be very unlikely to occur.

Mercury *(SED-13, 598; SEDA-19, 225; SEDA-20, 213; SEDA-21, 239)*

Discussion of the release of mercury from dental amalgams continues, without any clear direction or conclusion. The number of reports of hypersensitivity to mercurials seems to increase, as does the number of reports of intentional and accidental poisoning with metallic mercury, for example from broken thermometers.

Recently the absorbed dose of mercury from amalgams has been reviewed in relation to the potential for adverse effects (32[R]).

Nervous system Despite their potentially disastrous adverse effects, topical mercury salts can still be found as ingredients in some over-the-counter formulations or local remedies. Peripheral polyneuropathy as a result of chronic ammoniated mercury poisoning has been studied and followed over 2 years (33[c]).

A 36-year old man developed a peripheral polyneuropathy after chronic perianal use of an ammoniated mercury ointment. He had very high blood and urine mercury concentrations. Sural nerve biopsy showed mixed axonal degeneration and demyelination. His symptoms gradually improved over 2 years, but neurophysiological examination showed incomplete recovery.

The availability of safer drugs should result in a complete ban of these dangerous compounds.

Immunological and hypersensitivity reactions Data on the immunological effects of mercury in animals and cell cultures have been reviewed (34[R]).

Three cases of mercury hypersensitivity have been reported (35[c]).

A 30-year-old and a 53-year-old woman developed localized allergic contact dermatitis caused by a mercurochrome-containing medical plaster (Mercuroplaster) and a 31-year-old woman developed a systemic eczematous contact dermatitis after breaking a mercury thermometer.

Accidental poisoning There have been several reports of accidental mercury poisoning from broken thermometers.

An 11-month-old Pakistani girl was admitted to the hospital because of drowsiness, malaise, and anorexia (36[c]). She had been well until 6 weeks before admission, when she lost her appetite, stopped crawling or standing up, dribbled from her mouth, sweated profusely, and scratched her skin continually. She had opisthotonus with a generalized pruritic rash and swollen red cold hands and feet with desquamation. She had a persistent tachycardia and hypertension, but a normal body temperature. Her 6-year-old sister came to hospital with similar although less pronounced symptoms, and an environmental cause was suspected. When asked, the mother reported that 2 weeks before the younger child's symptoms had started, mercury from a broken thermometer had dropped onto the carpet in the children's room and had not been retrievable. The urine mercury concentration in the infant was 12.6 μg/l, slightly above the reference value of 10 μg/l. Exposure was confirmed by the mercury content of the hair (1.2 μg/g, reference range below 0.25 μg/g). After 12 days in hospital the urine mercury fell to 4.1 μg/l. Despite the seemingly low concentrations it was decided to treat her with 2,3-dimercaptosuccinic acid 10 mg/kg tds. After 3 months of treatment the symptoms had disappeared totally and the urinary mercury had fallen below 1 μg/l.

A 15-year-old boy fell on a broken mercury thermometer and during the next 5 days a subcutaneous abscess formed on his left forearm (37[c]). He had no signs or symptoms of mercury toxicity. His wound was debrided in the operating room and healed completely after several months without any therapeutic intervention.

Deliberate self-poisoning Although the spontaneous exfoliation of teeth and breakdown of oral tissues from severe mercury intoxication have been noted for over a century, there have been no studies of the mechanisms of these effects. Severe mercury poisoning is rare in modern times, but does occur.

An exfoliated tooth and periodontal and gingival tissues were obtained from a 15-month-old child who had been severely intoxicated with elemental mercury over a period of months and hospitalized for severe neurological and renal effects (38[c]). The tissues were examined both by routine hematoxylin and eosin staining and by autometallography specific for mercury. For comparison, control tissue from an age-matched subject was examined by autometallography. Under light microscopy the gingival tissue showed evidence of moderate to severe acute and chronic inflammation. The tooth pulp tissue showed evidence of moderate vascular dilatation and congestion and was infiltrated by many neutrophils. Autometallography showed intense accumulation of mercury in the soft tissues of the mercury-exposed subject, but not in the tissues of the control subject. The deposits were found primarily in fibroblasts, which are essential in the maintenance of the integrity of the oral tissues.

This, the primary mechanism of the spontaneous sloughing of tissue and loss of teeth may be the cytotoxic effects of the accumulation of mercury in fibroblasts.

Mercury deposition in the tissues can occur after overdosage and can persist for long periods, as the following cases show.

A 35-year-old laboratory technician gave himself elemental mercury intravenously and developed gingivitis, muscular weakness, hyperpyrexia (40°C), abdominal pain, diarrhea, anorexia, and a 6-week weight loss of 5 kg (39[c]). His blood pressure was 110/70 mmHg, heart rate 124/min, and respiratory rate 21/min. Hematology, blood chemistry, urinalysis, electrocardiogram, and neurological parameters were normal. He had bilateral cervical adenopathy and an abscess in the back of the right hand. The abscess was incised and liquid mercury was drained from the wound. X-rays showed globules of metallic density in the lungs and abdomen and at the site of the abscess. A 24-h urine sample contained mercury 500 μg/l. He responded to 2,3-dimercaptopropane-1-sulfonate (Dimaval®) with only the persistent signs of tremor and lower extremity weakness.

A 39-year-old man injected 40 ml of elemental mercury in attempted suicide; 3 years later X-rays showed mercury deposits in the lungs and around the injection site (40[c]). The mercury concentration in his blood was very high (96.3 μg/l; reference range up to 2 μg/l), as was his renal mercury elimination. Despite deposits of mercury in the pulmonary circulation, his pulmonary function was normal, with no reduction in diffusion capacity. There were signs of polyneuropathy. He was given sodium 2,3-dimercaptopropane-1-sulfonate a mercury chelator.

A 16-year-old schoolboy injected himself subcutaneously in both forearms with about 6 ml of metallic mercury and took about 5 ml orally (41[c]). He was admitted to hospital 2 weeks after this incident without any symptoms. Physical examination and all laboratory tests, including chest X-ray, showed no abnormalities, except for granulomata at the injection sites. X-rays showed numerous dispersed globules of mercury in the subcutaneous tissues of both forearms and in the digestive tract, mainly in the appendix. During the next 6 months he showed no toxic effects of mercury, in having high blood and urinary mercury concentrations (132 and 500 μg/l, respectively).

A 27-year-old woman with schizophrenia had intense headaches, loss of vision, and photophobia induced by intraocular injections of mercury (42[cr]). The diagnosis was established once foreign bodies had been seen on skull X-rays. Mercury intoxication, in combination with irreversible damage to the eyes, necessitated bilateral enucleation and the use of sodium-2,3 dimercapto-1-propane sulfonate.

Automutilation is a very rare and dramatic complication of schizophrenia. The psychiatric management was discussed in this report together with a review of the toxicological treatment of mercury intoxication.

Nickel *(SED-13, 599; SEDA-20, 214; SEDA-21, 240)*

Immunological and hypersensitivity reactions Nickel hypersensitivity is an increasing problem in adolescents, especially girls, with a prevalence of up to 30%. The presence of nickel in orthodontic appliances and the possibility of nickel hypersensitivity has been discussed in case reports. A review of the literature on nickel hypersensitivity in relation to orthodontic appliances has shown that the risk is very low in patients who are not nickel hypersensitive at the start of the treatment (43[R]). The slow long-term release of nickel from orthodontic appliances can induce tolerance to nickel in individuals who are not hypersensitive at the start of treatment.

Platinum *(SED-13, 600)*

Nephrotoxicity of platinum compounds remains an issue in anticancer treatment. With regard to occupational exposure to platinum compounds allergic and genotoxic effects apparently are becoming more frequent.

Urinary system The nephrotoxicity of three platinum co-ordination complexes (CPL, KP734, KP735) and three ruthenium co-ordination complexes (KP418, KP692, KP1019) has been tested in rats in comparison with cisplatin (44). There were no renal functional changes (excretion of water, protein, *para*-aminohippurate, and osmolytes) after the administration of 10% of the LD_{50} of the compounds given twice a week for up to 5 weeks. After a relatively high single dose of the substances (50% of the LD_{50}), signs of nephrotoxicity on the day of maximal renal damage decreased in the following order: cisplatin, KP418, CPL, KP734, KP735, KP692, and KP1019. Compared with cisplatin, proteinuria was significantly lower after the administration of any of the compounds, especially KP692 and KP1019. Neither renal lipid peroxidation nor glutathione status was affected. In summary, KP735 in the group of platinum complexes and KP1019 in the ruthenium group had the lowest potential for causing nephrotoxicity.

Genetic effects Platinum and palladium belong to the group of platinum elements and so share many chemical properties. Platinum co-ordination complexes are carcinogenic and genotoxic in mammalian and bacterial cells. However, little is known about palladium genotoxicity. The genotoxic potential of selected platinum and palladium metal salts have been compared in mammalian and bacterial cells using the cytokinesis-block micronucleus test with human lymphocytes and the bacterial SOS chromotest (45). Carboplatin, cisplatin(II), transplantin(II), $PtCl_4$(IV), and K_2PtCl_4(II) caused significantly increased genotoxicity in the micronucleus test and the SOS chromotest. The platinum compounds $PtCl_2$(II) and K_2PtCl_6(IV), and the divalent palladium salts $PdCl_2$(II), K_2PdCl_4(II), $Pd(NH_3)_2J_2$(II), $Pd(NH_3)4Cl_2$(II), and trans-palladium(II) were not genotoxic in the micronucleus test or the SOS chromotest. Thus, there is little evidence of palladium genotoxicity in mammalian and bacterial cells, in contrast to platinum.

Selenium *(SED-13, 600; SEDA-19, 226; SEDA-20, 215; SEDA-21, 240)*

The role of selenium in health and disease, including both deficiency and toxicity, has recently been reviewed (46[R]).

Endocrine, metabolic Selenium is an antioxidant, and is currently being evaluated in patients with inflammatory diseases. However, little is known about the risks of using it in this way. Selenium is a part of a type-I deiodinase which catalyses the conversion of hepatic thyroxine (T_4) to triiodothyronine (T_3). In one case the administration of large doses of selenium led to marked hypothyroidism (47[c]).

A 66-year-old man with chronic glomerulonephritis and no history of thyroid disease was admitted for treatment of severe pneumonia after the removal of a tongue cancer. Thyroid function tests showed serum concentrations of TSH (2.0 mIU/l), free T_3 (1.7 ng/l, 2.6 pmol/l), and free T_4 (0.5 mg/l, 645 nmol/l), consistent with euthyroid sick syndrome. Thyroid autoantibodies were negative. Apart from antibiotics he received intravenous supplementation with selenite (2500 μg in total over 7 days). Six days later his mental status progressively worsened with marked lethargy and poor attention span. Thyroid function tests now showed a rise in free T_3 (2.9 ng/l), a fall in free T_4 (0.4 mg/l), and a raised basal TSH (12.1 mIU/l), suggesting hypothyroidism. In addition, there was marked iodine deficiency, reflected by low 24-h urinary iodine excretion. Selenium-induced hypothyroidism precipitated by marked iodine deficiency was suspected. Following supplementation with iodide (200 μg/day) his mental state and thyroid function normalized within 3 weeks.

Overdosage Reports of acute human selenium toxicity are rare. Two new cases have been reported (48[c]).

One patient ingested a mouthful of selenic acid (30 g/l); he only suffered mild gastrointestinal disturbances. The first plasma selenium concentration, 3 h after ingestion, was the highest (931 μg/l), and the plasma concentrations subsequently fell with a half-life of 17.5 h.

The second patient took 1.7 g of sodium selenite. He had severe gastroenteritis, transient electrocardiographic changes, and a slightly raised serum bilirubin. The first serum concentration, 3 h after ingestion, was 2.7 μg/l.

The authors discussed the prognostic significance of the blood selenium concentration.

Silver *(SED-13, 600; SEDA-19, 226; SEDA-20, 215; SEDA-21, 241)*

Silver is generally considered to present a relatively low toxic threat to humans, because unintentional exposure to large doses is rare. However, as the intentional use of silver pharmaceutical formulations and devices increases, subtle toxic effects of silver are predictable and expected (49[R]). Particular emphasis is given to: (1) the use of silver in topical antimicrobial formulations, as toxicity relates to absorption through dermal wounds into the systemic circulation and possible effects on delayed wound healing; (2) possible local silver toxicity via iontophoretic devices; (3) current theories relating to the toxicological mechanism of action of silver.

Hematological Agranulocytosis has been reported with silver sulfadiazine (50[c]).

A 1-month-old baby was hospitalized in a pediatric intensive care unit after repair of a tracheo-esophageal fistula. She developed gastroesophageal reflux and tracheomalacia in the postoperative period and at 2 months perineal erythema. She was given topical silver sulfadiazine and ketoconazole daily. Five days later agranulocytosis occurred. Silver sulfadiazine was immediately withdrawn. The granulocyte count returned to normal over a few days.

No other cause was found to explain the agranulocytosis. The small surface area of administration, the chronology of the events, and the rapid correction of the disorders after silver sulfadiazine withdrawal all argued for an immunological reaction to this drug. However, it is also possible that it was caused by the sulfonamide.

Risk factors Silver sulfadiazine cream is a potent agent for the treatment of burns, but silver toxicity can occur through topical absorption (51[c]).

A patient with end-stage renal disease had a marked increase in serum silver concentration during treatment for 2 weeks with silver sulfadiazine cream (200 g/day). The serum concentration of silver reached a maximum of 291 ng/ml in association with a rapid deterioration of mental status. Silver sulfadiazine was withdrawn, and hemodialysis, hemofiltration, or plasma exchange were repeatedly performed. Four months later he died. At autopsy, there were very high concentrations of silver in the brain (617 and 824 ng/g wet tissue weight in the cerebrum and cerebellum, respectively). Both plasma exchange and hemofiltration were effective in reducing serum silver, and their effects were additive. By contrast, hemodialysis was ineffective.

This case illustrates that patients with burns and renal insufficiency are at risk of toxic accumulation of silver in serum and tissues. Removal of serum silver can best be effected by plasma exchange, particularly when combined with hemofiltration. In contrast, hemodialysis is not effective.

Titanium *(SEDA-19, 226; SEDA-20, 215; SEDA-21, 241)*

The performance of any implant material in the human body is controlled by two sets of characteristics, biofunctionality and biocompatibility, as has recently been reviewed (52[R]). The role of reactive oxygen derivatives (hydroxyperoxide, hydroxyl radicals, and singlet oxygen molecules) in precipitating inorganic and organic complexes on to the surface of titanium implant alloys has recently been reviewed (53[R]).

Musculoskeletal Endosteal implants fail for a variety of reasons. These include failure to integrate with bone, long-term loss of integration, or invasion of a vital structure. The removal of an implant because of patient discomfort secondary to invasion of the mandibular canal has been reported (54[c]). The histological findings offered a unique opportunity to examine an integrated human dental implant section.

The histological features around three nonsubmerged titanium plasma-sprayed implants, retrieved at autopsy after a 10-month loading period, have been reported (55[c]). At the time of implant insertion, the clinician had noted wide vestibular dehiscence of the central implant, and decided to use a bioabsorbable membrane for guided bone regeneration in this area. After specimen processing, it was possible at low magnification to see that in most of the vestibular slides the central implant was almost completely surrounded by connective tissue, while in most of the lingual slides the quantity of bone around the implant tended to increase. The other two implants had a bone–implant contact percentage of about 60%. In only a few areas was mineralized bone in direct contact with the metal surface, while around the major portion of the implant perimeter there was a layer of unmineralized, red-stained, osteoid material. There was no inflammatory infiltrate in the epithelium or supracrestal connective tissues. The fibers of this tissue had a different orientation: in the most coronal portion of the implants (smooth surface) they tended to run parallel to the implant's surface, while in the most apical region (plasma-sprayed surface) they tended to be arranged in a perpendicular fashion. These results were strikingly similar to those previously reported in dogs and monkeys.

Extensive wear can be caused by titanium alloy implants (56[c]).

A 47-year-old woman with multiple epiphyseal dysplasia had a shoulder hemiarthroplasty for degenerative changes. A hemiprosthesis with a modular nitride-coated titanium head (3M™) fixed on a Morse taper was used to replace the humeral head. The postoperative period was uneventful. However, she had progressive pain during the fourth month after surgery, and the mobility of the shoulder remained restricted. At revision 2 years later the anteroinferior glenoid rim was eroded and the synovium and the glenoid fossa were stained dark owing to accumulation of titanium debris. After the titanium alloy prosthetic head had been removed, a polyethylene glenoid component was implanted and a chromium alloy humeral head was used to replace the titanium component. She made an uneventful recovery.

Apparently, extensive wear can occur on the surface of the titanium alloy head of a shoulder prosthesis after only 2 years of service. Such wear demands withdrawal of titanium alloy articulating surfaces, even in non-weight-bearing joints.

Zinc *(SED-13, 601; SEDA-20, 215; SEDA-21, 242)*

Immunological and hypersensitivity reactions A novel topical formulation of zinc pyrithione has been used to treat psoriasis and appears to be safe and effective (57[c]).

A case of allergic contact dermatitis to a shampoo containing zinc pyrithione associated with an eruption of pustular psoriasis has been reported (58[c]).

A woman who had had stable psoriasis for 5 years, and never any other skin disease, developed severe generalized pustular psoriasis with many lesions where a zinc pyrithione shampoo had been applied a week before. Cyclosporin 200–300 mg/day cleared the eruption within 4 weeks, except for psoriasis of the scalp. Extensive patch testing showed sensitivity to zinc pyrithione.

This case illustrates that generalized pustular psoriasis can be provoked by a substance present in shampoo. Short-term treatment with cyclosporin is valuable in exacerbations of psoriasis caused by allergic contact dermatitis.

REFERENCES

1. Guillard O, Pineau A, Fauconneau B, Chobaut JC, Desaulty A, Angot A, Le Borgne E, Furon O. Biological levels of aluminium after use of aluminium-containing bone cement in post-otoneurosurgery. J Trace Elem Med Biol 1997; 11:53–6.
2. Montemarano AD, Sau P, Johnson FB, James WD. Cutaneous granulomas caused by an aluminum-zirconium complex: an ingredient of antiperspirants. J Am Acad Dermatol 1997;37:496–8.
3. Bajaj AK, Gupta SC, Pandey RK, Misra K, Rastogi S, Chatterji AK. Aluminium contact sensitivity. Contact Dermatitis 1997;37:307–8.
4. Helgesen AL, Austad J. Contact urticaria from aluminium and nickel in the same patient. Contact Dermatitis 1997;37:303–4.
5. Duenas C, Perez-Alvarez JC, Busteros JI, Saez-Royuela F, Martin-Lorente JL, Yuguero L, Lopez-Morante A. Idiopathic portal hypertension and angiosarcoma associated with arsenical salts therapy. J Clin Gastroenterol 1998;26:303–5.
6. Bataineh AB D, Al-Omari MAO, Owais AI. Arsenical necrosis of the jaws. Int Endodont J 1997;30:283–7.
7. Vondracek TG. Ranitidine bismuth citrate in the treatment of *Helicobacter pylori* infection and duodenal ulcer. Ann Pharmacother 1998;32: 672–9.
8. Addrizzo-Harris DJ, Chung A, Rom WN. Radio-opaque punctate opacities on the chest radiograph following intravenous injection of a bismuth compound. Thorax 1997;52:303–4.
9. Ruiz-Maldonado R, Contreras-Ruiz J, Sierra-Santoyo A, Lopez-Corella E, Guevara-Flores A.

Black granules on the skin after bismuth subsalicylate ingestion. J Am Acad Dermatol 1997; 37:489–90.
10. Rath HC, Enger IM, Ruschoff J, Scholmerich J, Holstege A. Acute hemolytic crisis as the initial manifestation of Wilson disease. Z Gastroenterol 1997;35:199–203.
11. Weiping L, Yang YK, Xiong HZ, Cheng XZ, Chen ZH, Shen ZQ, Li L. Coordination of copper with aspirin enhances its anti-platelet aggregation activity. Inflammopharmacology 1997;5:133–8.
12. Pasquale SA, Russer TJ, Foldesy R, Mezrich RS. Lack of interaction between magnetic resonance imaging and the copper-T380A IUD. Contraception 1997;55:169–73.
13. Csaky KG, Caruso RC. Gallium nitrate optic neuropathy. Am J Ophthalmol 1997;124:567–8.
14. Akansel G, Liu Y, Chitambar CR, Kitapci MT, Akansel S, Krasnow AZ, Isitman AT, Collier BD. Effect of gallium nitrate therapy on Ga-67 scintigraphic detection of lymphoma: case report. Clin Nucl Med 1997;22:21–4.
15. Shamir M, Sprung CL. Fatal multiple organ system dysfunction associated with germanium metal used in complementary therapy. Harefuah 1997;133:446–7, 502.
16. Ho M, Pullar T. Vasomotor reactions with gold. Br J Rheumatol 1997;36:154–6.
17. Bakke E, Myklebust G, Gran JT. Thrombocytopenia in association with oral gold treatment (auranofin). Tidsskr Nor Laegeforen 1997;117: 4081–2.
18. Miller ML, Harford RR, Yeager JK, Johnson F. A case of chrysiasis. Cutis 1997;59:256–68.
19. Hostynek JJ. Gold: an allergen of growing significance. Food Chem Toxicol 1997;35:839–44.
20. Fleming C, Burden D, Fallowfield M, Lever R. Lymphomatoid contact reaction to gold earrings. Contact Dermatitis 1997;37:298–9.
21. Armstrong DK, Walsh MY, Dawson JF. Granulomatous contact dermatitis due to gold earrings. Br J Dermatol 1997;136:776–8.
22. Möller H, Svensson A, Björkner B, Bruze M, Lindroth Y, Manthorpe R, Theander J. Contact allergy to gold and gold therapy in patients with rheumatoid arthritis. Acta Dermatol Venereol 1997;77:370–3.
23. Papacharalambous VG, Pramatarov KD, Tsankov NK. Development of pemphigus in a patient with rheumatoid arthritis during a course of gold therapy. Eur J Dermatol 1997;7:65–6.
24. Raza SA, Phillipps JJ. Bilateral tympanic membrane perforation—a result of gold toxicity? Br J Dermatol 1997;136:479–80.
25. Hollan S. Iron overload in light of the identification of a haemochromatosis gene. Haematol Budap 1997;28:109–16.
26. George DK, Powell LW. The screening, diagnosis and optimal management of haemochromatosis. Aliment Pharmacol Ther 1997;11:631–9.
27. Camaschella C, Piperno A. Hereditary hemochromatosis: recent advances in molecular genetics and clinical management. Haematologica 1997;82:77–84.
28. Everse J, Hsia N. The toxicities of native and modified hemoglobins. Free Radic Biol Med 1997;22:1075–99.
29. Luciano R, Zuppa AA, Maragliano G, Gallini F, Tortorolo G. Fetal encephalopathy after maternal anaphylaxis. Case report. Biol Neonate 1997;71:190–3.
30. Morse SB, Hardwick WE Jr, King WD. Fatal iron intoxication in an infant. South Med J 1997;90:1043–7.
31. Ni Y, Marchal G. Clinical implications of studies with MnDPDP in animal models of hepatic abnormalities. Acta Radiol 1997;38:724–31.
32. Mackert JR Jr, Berglund A. Mercury exposure from dental amalgam fillings: absorbed dose and the potential for adverse health effects. Crit Rev Oral Biol Med 1997;8:410–36.
33. Deleu D, Hanssens Y, Al-Salmy HS, Hastie I. Peripheral polyneuropathy due to chronic use of topical ammoniated mercury. J Toxicol Clin Toxicol 1998;36:233–7.
34. Moszczynski P. Mercury compounds and the immune system: a review. Int J Occup Med Environ Health 1997;10:247–58.
35. Matsumoto J, Natsuaki M. Three cases of mercury allergy. Skin Res 1997;39:48–52.
36. Velzeboer SCJM, Frenkel J, De Wolff FA. A hypertensive toddler. Lancet 1997;349:1810.
37. Smith SR, Jaffe DM, Skinner MA. Case report of metallic mercury injury. Pediatr Emerg Care 1997;13:114–16.
38. Martin MD, Williams BJ, Charleston JD, Oda D. Spontaneous exfoliation of teeth following severe elemental mercury poisoning: case report and histological investigation for mechanism. Oral Surg Oral Med Oral Pathol Oral Radiol Endodont 1997;84:495–501. Comment in: Oral Surg Oral Med Oral Pathol Oral Radiol Endodont 1998; 85:349.
39. Torres-Alanis O, Garza-Ocanas L, Pineyro-Lopez A. Intravenous self-administration of metallic mercury: report of a case with a 5-year follow-up. J Toxicol Clin Toxicol 1997;35:83–7.
40. Hohage H, Otte B, Westermann G, Witta J, Welling U, Zidek W, Heidenreich S. Elemental mercurial poisoning. South Med J 1997;90:1033–6.
41. Chodorowski Z, Sein-Anand J, Nowicki A, Galant K. Subcutaneous self-injection and oral self-administration of metallic mercury-case report. Przegl Lek 1997;54:759–62.
42. Auer C, Ducrey N, Uffer S, Othenin-Girard P, Herbort CP. Self-mutilating intraocular injection of metallic mercury. Arch Ophthalmol 1997;115:556–7.
43. Lindsten R, Kurol J. Orthodontic appliances in relation to nickel hypersensitivity. A review. J Orofac Orthop 1997;58:100–8.
44. Kersten L, Braunlich H, Keppler BK, Gliesing C, Wendelin M, Westphal J. Comparative nephrotoxicity of some antitumour-active platinum and ruthenium complexes in rats. J Appl Toxicol 1998;18:93–101.
45. Gebel T, Lantzsch H, Plessow K, Dunkelberg

H. Genotoxicity of platinum and palladium compounds in human and bacterial cells. Mutat Res 1997;389:183–90.
46. Foster LH, Sumar S. Selenium in health and disease: a review. Crit Rev Food Sci Nutr 1997;37:211–28.
47. Hofbauer LC, Spitzweg C, Magerstad RA, Heufelder AE. Selenium-induced thyroid dysfunction. Postgrad Med J 1997;73:103–4.
48. Gasmi A, Garnier R, Galliot-Guilley M, Gaudillat C, Quartenoud B, Buisine A, Djebbar D. Acute selenium poisoning. Vet Hum Toxicol 1997;39:304–8.
49. Hollinger MA. Toxicological aspects of topical silver pharmaceuticals. Crit Rev Toxicol 1996; 26:255–60.
50. Viala J, Simon L, Le Pommelet C, Philippon L, Devictor D, Huault G. Agranulocytosis application of silver sulfadiazine in a 2-month old infant. Arch Pediatr 1997;4:1103–6.
51. Iwasaki S, Yoshimura A, Ideura T, Koshikawa S, Sudo M. Elimination study of silver in a hemodialyzed burn patient treated with silver sulfadiazine cream. Am J Kidney Dis 1997; 30:287–90.
52. Gotman I. Characteristics of metals used in implants. J Endourol 1997;11:383–9.
53. Eliades T. Passive film growth on titanium alloys: physicochemical and biologic considerations. Int J Oral Maxillofac Implants 1997;12:621–7.
54. Cranin AN, Baraoidan M, DeGrado J. A human clinical and histologic report of an osseointegrated titanium alloy root form implant. J Oral Implantol 1997;23:21–4.
55. Piattelli A, Scarano A, Piattelli M, Bertolai R, Panzoni E. Histologic aspects of the bone and soft tissues surrounding three titanium non-submerged plasma-sprayed implants retrieved at autopsy: a case report. J Periodontol 1997;68:694–700.
56. Simon JP, de Smet L, Fabry G. Wear of a titanium-alloy shoulder prosthetic head. Acta Orthop Belg 1997;63:126–7.
57. Crutchfield CE 3rd, Lewis EJ, Zelickson BD. The highly effective use of topical zinc pyrithione in the treatment of psoriasis: a case report. Dermatol Online J 1997;3:3.
58. Nielsen NH, Menne T. Allergic contact dermatitis caused by zinc pyrithione associated with pustular psoriasis. Am J Contact Dermatitis 1997;8:170–1.

R.H.B. Meyboom

23 Metal antagonists

Deferiprone *(SED-13, 624; SEDA-20, 221; SEDA-21, 249)*

In a long-term follow-up study of 56 transfusion-dependent patients using deferiprone (75 mg/kg), most of whom had thalassemia major, 29 patients continued the drug until the time of analysis, and 12 continued for over 36 months (1[CR]). Since in only 25% of the patients tested were liver iron concentrations low enough for organ damage to be likely, the authors concluded that only a minority of patients taking deferiprone were adequately chelated in the long term.

Hematological The risk of *agranulocytosis* is a major limiting factor to the use of deferiprone, with an estimated frequency of 1.6% (SED-13, 624; (2[CR])). In five of the 13 patients so far reported deferiprone was restarted, and granulocytopenia recurred (2[CR]). After rechallenge granulocytopenia developed in 2–4 weeks, a much shorter interval compared with the original episode. Once the granulocyte counts started to fall, agranulocytosis developed in 5–7 days. The available evidence ethically precludes the rechallenge of future patients. Oxidation of deferiprone with hypochlorous acid, the major oxidant of neutrophil leukocytes, results in the formation of a chemically reactive species, consistent with the quinone metabolite of deferiprone. The authors concluded that deferiprone agranulocytosis may result from a T cell-mediated immunological reaction, induced by a reactive metabolite of deferiprone.

Agranulocytosis and systemic vasculitis have been described in association with deferiprone (3[cR]).

A 24-year-old woman with thalassemia developed malaise, arthritis, and purpuric lesions after using deferiprone 50 mg/kg per day for 6 months. Her symptoms subsided within a few days of withdrawal. After 1 month, deferiprone was restarted in al lower dose of 40 mg/kg. Four months later a sore throat and fever prompted a leukocyte count and agranulocytosis was found. Circulating immune complexes were present and the T cell subset analysis, which had been normal 1 year before, showed a reduced T suppressor cell count with a ratio T helper/T suppressor of 3.7. Circulating immune complexes were present; antinuclear antibodies, anti-DNA antibodies, and extractable nuclear antigens, which had previously been absent, were detected. After withdrawal of deferiprone the neutrophils recovered, but 2 weeks later there was a new episode of severe arthritis and palpable purpura of the legs; the palms and soles were diffusely erythematous and there was desquamation over the distal phalanges. Later, transverse fissures of the nails appeared, secondary to vascular changes in the nail beds.

In addition to agranulocytosis, a diagnosis of deferiprone-induced systemic vasculitis was made.

Skin and appendages In 61 patients who had a bone marrow transplant because of thalassemia and received deferoxamine to accelerate the clearance of iron deposits, local skin reactions were the only adverse effect reported (4[cr]).

Special senses Eight patients with deferoxamine-related *hearing loss* were switched to deferiprone (dose not specified). In five there was a deterioration of hearing impairment (5[c]).

Deferoxamine (desferrioxamine) *(SED-13, 619; SEDA-19, 232; SEDA-20, 221; SEDA-21, 248)*

The effect of subcutaneous deferoxamine on the prognosis of thalassemia has been evaluated (6[CR]). In the 1960s the median survival in thalassemia major was 17 years. Since the introduction of iron chelation by subcuta-

Side Effects of Drugs, Annual 22
J.K. Aronson, ed.

neous deferoxamine, the median survival time has reached 29 years. By 29 years of age nearly 73% of patients are free of diabetes mellitus and hypothyroidism and 51% are without cardiac decompensation.

Nervous system and special senses Reversible *sensorimotor neurotoxicity* has been described in two thalassemic patients during the intravenous administration of high dosages of deferoxamine (120 mg/kg per day) for iron overload (7[cR]).

A 20-year-old woman developed paresthesia of the left hand and arm after 6 months, followed by bilateral marked upper extremity weakness. Deep tendon reflexes were absent and there was reduced vibration and position sense. There were also disturbances of vision and hearing. Audiometry showed bilateral sensorineural hearing loss. Visual acuity was 20/20 (right eye) and 10/400 (left eye), with a central scotoma. Visual evoked potentials showed marked prolongation of conduction times and complete extinction of the left eye. There was swelling of the left optic disc, a left visual superior quadrant defect, and bilateral hearing deficit. The symptoms improved after withdrawal of deferoxamine.

A 34-year-old woman, developed paresthesia and weakness of the hands and feet after 5 months. There was proximal weakness of both arms, areflexia, hyperesthesia to pin-prick and temperature, and reductions in position and vibratory sense. EMG of the upper extremities was consistent with neuropathy. There were no abnormalities of hearing or vision. She recovered fully after withdrawal of deferoxamine. Later, deferoxamine had to be discontinued for a second time because of recurrence of paresthesia.

The *ototoxicity* of deferoxamine has been studied in 70 adult transfusion-dependent patients (5[CR]). There was hearing loss attributable to deferoxamine in 22 patients. Of the 70 patients, 59 had thalassemia; 21 of them had deferoxamine-attributable hearing loss. Characteristically, these patients had high-frequency sensorineural hearing loss—seven had a notch at 6 kHz and one at 3 kHz; less frequently they had tinnitus. The authors concluded that regular audiometric follow-up with special attention to the frequencies of 3 and 6 kHz may help to detect and prevent permanent hearing loss.

Opportunistic infections *Mucormycosis* has been described in a patient taking deferoxamine (8[c]).

A 33-year-old man, who 1 year before had had a bone marrow transplant for relapsed acute leukemia, presented with a dry cough and hemoptysis. Chronic graft-versus-host disease was treated with azathioprine 75 mg/day. Because of transfusion iron overload he also received deferoxamine, 2000 mg/day for 5 days a week (route not stated, probably subcutaneous). Bronchial washings showed hyphae and a diagnosis of mucormycosis was made; *Candida* and *Aspergillus* species also were found. Owing to the localized nature of the infection, the left lower lobe of the lung was surgically resected for diagnosis and therapy, and he was given amphotericin; deferoxamine was withdrawn. Long-term follow-up showed no recurrence of the fungal infection.

In addition to deferoxamine, leukemia and azathioprine immune suppression may have facilitated mucormycosis in this case. Mucormycosis has a high fatality rate (SED-13, 623). The importance of this case report is that it illustrates that mucormycosis can have a favorable prognosis if diagnosed early and treated aggressively.

Edetic acid (ethylene diamine tetra-acetic acid; EDTA) and its derivatives *(SED-13, 626; SEDA-20, 222; SEDA-21, 250)*

Intramuscular dimercaptopropanol (BAL) plus intravenous calcium disodium EDTA has been compared with oral *meso*-2,3-dimercaptosuccinic acid (DMSA) plus intravenous EDTA in 45 children with lead poisoning (9[c]). Vomiting and increased alanine aminotransferase activity during therapy occurred more often with BAL + EDTA compared with DMSA + EDTA. All eight children with abnormal AlT values had received BAL. Nine of 23 who received BAL vomited, compared with four of 22 children treated with DMSA.

Solvents have been used to treat stones in the common bile duct, by giving them via a nasobiliary catheter in 41 patients after papillotomy and via a T-tube in three patients (10[c]). Two alternative solvents (26 mmol/l edetic acid, 40 mmol/l sodium deoxycholate, and 30% dimethylsulfoxide in an alkaline aqueous solution; and a 70/30 mixture of dimethylsulfoxide and methyl *tert*-butyl ether) were infused continuously for 2 h. Adverse effects were frequent but not serious and included *abdominal pain* (68%), *nausea* (72%), *vomit-*

ing (52%), *diarrhea* (50%), and *sleepiness* (50%).

Immunological and hypersensitivity reactions The results of a patch test study have underlined the sensitizing properties of derivatives of edetic acid, such as ethylenediamine, diethylenetriamine, and triethylenetetramine, components of plastics and glues (11[cr]).

Penicillamine *(SED-13, 605; SEDA-19, 229; SEDA-20, 219; SEDA-21, 251)*

Serious intercurrent diseases in patients with rheumatoid arthritis can be mistaken for complications of treatment with penicillamine or other drugs (SEDA-21, 252). In this respect it is of interest to note a case of pure red cell anemia in a patient with long-standing rheumatoid arthritis, probably not related to the use of drugs (12[cr]).

Nervous system Penicillamine can cause a remarkable variety of peripheral and central nervous system disorders (SED-13, 607).

The unusual adverse effect of *internuclear ophthalmoplegia* has been described as the first sign of *cerebral necrotizing vasculitis* (13[cR]), emphasizing the treacherous nature of adverse reactions to penicillamine and the importance of early diagnosis.

A 33-year-old woman who had used penicillamine (dose not specified) for 7 years for Wilson's disease, presented with nausea, headaches, intermittent diplopia, and tinnitus. Neurological examination and brain MRI were normal. Trientine was substituted and her symptoms resolved. Normal electromyography and acetylcholine receptor antibody titers excluded penicillamine-induced myasthenia. Shortly after reinstitution of penicillamine she noticed oscillations of the environment. She had a right internuclear ophthalmoplegia, upbeat nystagmus, limitation of upward gaze, and dissociation of accommodation and pupillary constriction. Soon afterwards, she developed right hemiparesis and a fever. The cerebrospinal fluid contained 62 red blood cells and 15 leukocytes per mm^3, mostly polymorphonuclear cells, glucose 2.9 mmol/l, and protein 8.1 g/l. Magnetic resonance angiography of the intracranial circulation showed multiple areas of narrowing of the left middle cerebral artery. Over the next week she developed severe bilateral sciatic and ulnar neuropathies. A sural nerve biopsy showed multifocal interstitial perivascular and intramural inflammatory infiltrates, with areas containing necrotizing inflammatory and thrombosing vasculitis, involving medium and small arteries, consistent with a periarteritis nodosa-like vasculitis.

The authors concluded that this patient had a penicillamine-induced necrotizing vasculitis and that the syndrome of internuclear ophthalmoplegia had resulted from involvement of the cerebral medial longitudinal fascicle. In the single previous case report of a similar (less serious) condition, pseudo-internuclear ophthalmoplegia was caused by penicillamine-induced myasthenia (SED-13, 607).

Drug-induced *myasthenia gravis* has been reviewed (14[R]). In contrast with other drug causes, it is characteristic of penicillamine that about 90% of patients have *antiacetylcholine receptor antibodies*. Two more cases of penicillamine-induced myasthenia gravis have been described (15[cr]), (16[cr]).

A 53-year-old Chinese woman noticed gradual weakness in both upper limbs, blurring of vision, and diplopia, in the course of 6 months of treatment with penicillamine (600 mg/day) for biliary cirrhosis. An edrophonium test was positive and antiacetylcholine receptor antibodies were detected. Complete resolution occurred when the drug was withdrawn.

Myasthenia gravis developed in a 54-year-old woman taking penicillamine (200 mg/day) for eosinophilic fasciitis. After 11 months she developed bilateral ptosis (but not diplopia), dysarthria with nasal speech, dysphagia, and mild facial paresis. Myasthenia was confirmed by electromyography; her anti-acetylcholine receptor antibody titer was very high. There was marked improvement after withdrawal of penicillamine and treatment with prednisolone and pyridostigmine.

Deterioration of the neurological symptoms of Wilson's disease is a well-known phenomenon early in treatment with penicillamine (SED-13, 607). Precipitation of neurological abnormalities by penicillamine has now been described in a boy with Wilson's disease, without previous neurological involvement (17[cR]).

A 9-year-old boy developed a tremor of the upper limbs, seriously impairing fine motor activity, after taking penicillamine (20/mg/kg per day) for 10 weeks. The tremor was rhythmic, with variable oscillation, increased with movement, became accentuated as the limb approached its target, and disappeared during sleep. It became progressively more severe over 2 weeks. The serum transaminase activities increased to twice pretreatment values. Replacement of penicillamine by oral zinc sulfate (300 mg/day) was followed by prompt disappearance of the tremor.

Hematological Data on drug-related *thrombocytopenia* in 309 spontaneous case reports, collected by the Danish Committee on Adverse Drug Reactions from 1968 to the end of 1991 (cytotoxic drugs excluded), have been reviewed ([18cr]). Important general findings were that there was no difference in recovery between patients treated with and without corticosteroids, and that the mortality rate due to hemorrhage was 3.6%. In this series penicillamine was the fifth most commonly suspected drug (18 cases, 6%).

A placebo-controlled second-line drug discontinuation and resumption study has been reported in 51 patients with rheumatoid arthritis, 25 of whom were treated with antimalarial drugs, 10 with parenteral gold, four with penicillamine, eight with sulfasalazine, two with azathioprine, and two with methotrexate ([19CR]). In the treatment group 78% of patients had a sustained remission, compared with 62% in the placebo group. Of those who required resumption of the (same) second-line drug only two had significant adverse effects, including transient thrombocytopenia and anemia in association with penicillamine in one, but discontinuation was not required.

Gastrointestinal Although it is benign, *stomatitis* is a troublesome adverse effect of disease-modifying anti-rheumatic drugs (DMARDs). In 2% of patients stomatitis led to discontinuation of these drugs; for penicillamine the figure was 3.1% ([20R]). The authors concluded that stomatitis during treatment with a DMARD may be a consequence of multiple factors, including hematinic deficiency, viral or *Candida* infection, recurrent aphthous ulceration, or Sjögren's syndrome. Resolution of stomatitis can be achieved by considering, investigating, and treating these factors, so that the use of penicillamine (or another suspected drug) can be maintained. Reducing the dosage or temporary withdrawal of the drug can also help settle the stomatitis, and reinstitution is usually successful. However, stomatitis during the use of penicillamine can also be a sign of drug-induced pemphigus, cicatricial pemphigoid, or a lichenoid eruption (SED-13, 609).

Urinary system Penicillamine is a relatively frequent cause of *membranous glomerulonephropathy* (SED-13, 609). Proteinuria, and less often the nephrotic syndrome, is the characteristic clinical manifestation; full recovery is the rule. A series of case reports has shown that rarely more serious and progressive renal injury may occur (SED-13, 610). We have previously discussed the difficulties in distinguishing rheumatoid nephropathy from adverse reactions to penicillamine (SEDA-21, 252). Further observations in two patients have been described, providing details of serious renal injury, probably occurring as *late complications of pre-existent penicillamine nephropathy*.

A 65-year-old woman with autoimmune thyroiditis, scleroderma, and a radical mastectomy for mucinous breast carcinoma took d-penicillamine (750 mg/day), L-thyroxine (0.1 mg/day), and nifedipine (10 mg/day) for scleroderma-related Raynaud's phenomenon, and a multivitamin formulation ([21CR]). For several years repeated urinalyses showed mild proteinuria, always under 1 g/day, without hypertension or renal failure (creatinine clearance 80 ml/min). She had previously had a leukocytoclastic vasculitis, attributed to the use of naproxen. After 4 years she developed persistent anorexia, weight loss, fatigue, and fever. Her serum creatinine was 999 μmol/l and urine microscopy showed many red cells and occasional granular and hyaline casts. She also had new circulating antihistone antibodies and perinuclear antineutrophil cytoplasmic antibodies, identified to be antimyeloperoxidase antibodies. A renal biopsy showed extensive glomerular crescent formation and collapse of the glomerular tufts. There were granular C3 and IgG deposits in most glomeruli. Electron microscopy showed numerous electron-dense deposits in the glomerular basement membrane and a few in the mesangium, but none in the subendothelium, and there was effacement of the podocyte foot processes. A diagnosis was made of acute evolving crescentic glomerulonephritis, in addition to underlying stage II–III membranous glomerulonephritis. Penicillamine was withdrawn and she was given immunosuppressives and hemodialysis, resulting in partial recovery of renal function.

A 65-year-old man developed the nephrotic syndrome after taking penicillamine 600 mg/day for 10 years for rheumatoid arthritis ([22CR]). Penicillamine was withdrawn and within 18 months his proteinuria disappeared. Some time later (interval not specified) he became dyspneic, with a serum creatinine of 146 μmol/l, associated with proteinuria (1.8 g/24 h), hematuria, and hemoglobinemia (127 mg/l). Two days later he developed gross hematuria, followed by total anuria, and hemodialysis was started. A renal biopsy showed severe glomerular necrosis with a ruptured Bowman's capsule, surrounded by a strong inflammatory reaction. Immunofluorescence of the residual fragments of the basement membrane showed IgG linear fixation, and circulating antiglomerular basement membrane antibodies were detected, directed against the NC1 domain of the α-3 chain forming collagen IV, as is usual in membranous nephropathy, but also against the NC1 domain of the α-1 and α-4 chains forming collagen IV. This unusual target for antiglomerular basement antibodies would be explained by previous modification of the basement membrane.

The authors of the second report suggested that pre-existing membranous nephropathy had modified the antigenicity of the glomerular basement membrane and induced susceptibility to the development of secondary anti-basement membrane antibodies. It is noteworthy that the patient's HLA haplotype included the DR15 antigen (susceptibility for Goodpasture's syndrome) and B8/DR3 antigen (susceptibility for drug-induced glomerulonephritis). In spite of treatment with high-dose corticosteroids no recovery was observed in a 1-year follow-up period.

About 20 cases of penicillamine-induced *crescentic glomerulonephritis* have been described, often combined with alveolar hemorrhage (i.e. *Goodpasture's syndrome*) (SED-13, 610; (21[R])). Renal involvement was severe and many patients required dialysis. Patients who received immunosuppressive therapy had a comparatively good outcome.

Skin and appendages *Transient acantholytic dermatosis* (*Grover's disease*) has been reported as a suspected adverse reaction to penicillamine (23[cR]). Transient acantholytic dermatosis is a papulovesicular eruption in elderly people, characterized histologically by focal acantholytic dyskeratosis. Its cause is unknown, but it has been reported in association with several other dermatoses and internal malignancies.

A 62-year-old white woman who had taken penicillamine 250 mg/day for progressive systemic sclerosis for 5 years developed an itching eruption, with several indistinct 2–3-mm skin-coloured to pinkish papules and papulovesicles scattered on the extensor surfaces of the extremities and on the trunk. Histological examination showed a well-circumscribed area of suprabasal acantholysis and dyskeratotic cells. Direct and indirect immunofluorescence tests were negative, making an autoimmune reaction unlikely.

Although transient acantholytic dermatosis has not previously been described in association with penicillamine, it does cause acantholysis in vitro (SED-13, 612). The case observation remained inconclusive, however, since penicillamine was not discontinued and new lesions continued to appear, while the old lesions regressed gradually without treatment.

Type II bullous *systemic lupus erythematosus* has been attributed to penicillamine (24[cr]).

A 34-year-old woman, had a generalized vesicobullous eruption, erosive lesions on the malar and periorbital regions, severe orogenital ulcerations, and vasculitic lesions on the digits. ANF was positive at a dilution of 1:320 and there were antiplatelet and antineutrophil antibodies, but anti-double-stranded DNA was negative. There was a pancytopenia. A biopsy showed subepidermal bullae with a predominantly neutrophilic infiltrate in the upper dermis. Direct immunofluorescence showed granular deposition of IgG, IgM, and C3 in the basement membrane. Immunoblotting on urea extracts of normal skin recognized proteins of 220 and 285 kDa.

This case report was unusual, in that the reaction developed within only 6 days of the introduction of penicillamine. Unfortunately the dosage was not mentioned, and further explanation is needed regarding the (perhaps erroneously) cited leukocyte count of $900 \times 10^9/l$ and a single reference to the use of dapsone.

Pemphigus is a bullous autoimmune disorder of the skin, characteristically associated with antidesmoglein antibodies (25[r]). Desmogleins are members of the cadherin family of calcium-dependent cell adhesion molecules. Cadherins are subdivided into the classical and desmosomal cadherins. Desmogleins and desmocollins belong to the latter group and are linked to the intracellular network of keratin intermediate filaments through desmoplakin and plakoglobin. Pemphigus is either idiopathic or drug-induced. Penicillamine is by far the most frequent cause of the drug-related variant. The clinical behavior of the reaction allows divisions into two main groups. Pemphigus that continues after drug withdrawal is referred to as triggered pemphigus, whereas a reaction that clears soon after withdrawal is called induced pemphigus. Antibodies in patients with (idiopathic) pemphigus vulgaris recognize desmoglein-3 (130 kDa) and those with pemphigus foliaceus recognize desmoglein-1 (160 kDa). Details on antidesmoglein autoantibodies have been provided in relation to a recent case report (25[cR]).

A 33-year-old woman took penicillamine, first 250 mg/day and later 500 mg/day, for mixed connective tissue disease. The other drugs used were prednisone and nifedipine. About 2 months later she developed an erosive eruption on her face, arms, trunk, abdomen, arms, and legs. There were multiple crusted plaques with an erythematous halo measuring 0.5–1.5 cm, together with erosions and erythematous macules. Nikolsky's sign was positive. Biopsy specimens showed acantholysis in the spinous and granular cell layers and a scanty inflammatory infiltrate. Direct immunofluorescence showed IgG and C3 in the intercellular epidermal spaces, and indirect immunofluorescence was positive for IgG4 pemphigus foliaceus antibodies in a titer of 1:640, with intercellular epidermal and nuclear epidermal patterns. There was a negative immunoblot of the 160-kDa band (desmoglein-1), which occurs in about two-thirds of patients with idiopathic pemphigus foliaceus, but her serum immunoprecipitated the 62- and 45-kDa fragments of desmoglein. These bands represent proteolytic fragments of the extracellular domain of desmoglein 1, the major pemphigus foliaceus antigen. Penicillamine was withdrawn and the dosage of prednisone increased. After 1 month the lesions started to disappear and over the next 2 years there was no recurrence.

The antibody reactivity in the sera of 10 patients with drug-related pemphigus has been compared with that in patients with idiopathic pemphigus (26[CR]). The autoantibody response was similar in the two groups. In pemphigus vulgaris antibodies react with desmoglein 3 and in pemphigus foliaceus with desmoglein 1. These findings suggest a similar basic molecular mechanism of spontaneous and drug-induced disease. The authors distinguished three groups of pemphigus-inducing drugs: thiol drugs (e.g. penicillamine), 'masked thiol drugs' (sulfur-containing drugs undergoing metabolic changes to form thiol groups, e.g. piroxicam, β-lactam compounds), and drugs with an active amide group (e.g. dipyrone, enalapril). Thiol-related pemphigus usually presents as the foliaceus variant, with comparatively few immunofluorescence findings and a good prognosis, whereas drugs with an active amide group can provoke pemphigus vulgaris with a less favorable prognosis on drug withdrawal. However, in a recent case of penicillamine-induced pemphigus foliaceus, new lesions continued to develop for several months despite drug withdrawal and treatment with prednisone (27[cr]). Histological examination showed an intragranular layer and cell-poor split with scattered acantholytic cells. There were polymorphonuclear leukocytes and eosinophils in the upper dermis. Direct immunofluorescence showed intercellular staining in the epidermis for IgG and C3 and nucleolar staining with IgG.

A thorough histopathological study of a patient with the characteristic *tardive degenerative dermatosis*, known to occur with high doses of penicillamine, has been reported ((28[cR]), SED-13, 611).

A 20-year-old man took penicillamine for Wilson's disease for 12 years in a usual dosage of about 1 g/day, with a day off every 3 days. He developed a circular or serpiginous arrangement of nuchal papules, characteristic of elastosis perforans serpiginosa. In addition, there were yellowish scar-like changes inside the circular arrangement of the papules. On the skin of the axillae and groin there was thickening, wrinkling, and pigmentation of the skin. Elastic fibers were increased and enlarged in the dermis and had characteristic thorn-like projections. Next to the transepidermal channels giant cells formed granulomatous reactions engulfing the degenerative elastic fibers. In the dermis of the scar-like tissue, on the other hand, there was almost no evidence of elastic fibers but there were massive aggregations of collagen fibers. Electron microscopy showed oval or club-shaped elastic fibers with thorn-like extrusions. These degenerative 'lumpy-bumpy' elastic fibers had a 'core' and a 'coat', and the zebra skin pattern of normal elastic fibers was abolished. Giant cells surrounded such degenerative elastic fibres. The patient stopped taking penicillamine, but suffered a serious relapse of Wilson's disease. Penicillamine was therefore restarted in a lower dosage and no new lesions have formed.

A case report from Spain has renewed interest in the penicillamine-associated *yellow nail syndrome* ((29[cR]), SEDA-9, 223; SED-13, 612).

A 28-year-old woman took penicillamine 375 mg/day for rheumatoid arthritis. After about 2 years she noticed yellowish discoloration, thickening, opacification, transverse stripes, and hyperconvexity of the nails of the hands and toes. There were no associated respiratory or other symptoms. She recovered fully after stopping penicillamine.

Musculoskeletal Penicillamine can cause *arthralgia* or *arthritis*, with or without a lupus-like syndrome. It has been emphasized that Wilson's disease may itself be associated with a polyarthritis resembling rheumatoid arthritis, but without immunological features, in the context of a patient in whom arthritis recovered when Wilson's disease was effectively treated with penicillamine (30[cr]). The authors pointed out that arthropathy in Wilson's disease is rare and that when it develops during the use of penicillamine it may be easily mistaken for an adverse reaction to the drug.

REFERENCES

1. Hoffbrand AV, Al-Refaie F, Siritanaratkul N, Davies B, Wonke B. Long term follow-up of 56 patients commencing deferiprone therapy. Bone Marrow Transplant 1997;19 (Suppl 2):20–1.
2. Loebstein R, Diav-Citrin O, Atanackovic G, Olivieri NF, Koren G. Deferiprone-induced agranulocytosis. A critical review of five rechallenged cases. Clin Drug Invest 1997;13:345–9.
3. Castriota-Scanderbeg A, Sacco M. Agranulocytosis, arthritis and systemic vasculitis in a patient receiving the oral iron chelator L1 (deferiprone). Br J Haematol 1997;96:254–5.
4. Giardini C, Galimberti M, Lucarelli G, Polchi P, Angelucci E, Baronciani D, Gaziev D, Erer B, Ripalti M, Rapa S, Muretto P. Desferrioxamine therapy of secondary hemochromatosis after BMT for thalassemia. Bone Marrow Transplant 1997;19 (Suppl 2):119–22.
5. Chiodo AA. Alberti PW, Sher GD, Francombe WH, Tyler B. Desferrioxamine ototoxicity in an adult transfusion-dependent population. J Otolaryngol 1997;26:116–22.
6. Giardina PJ, Ehlers KH, Grady RW, Lesser ML, New MI, Hilgartner MW. Progress in the management of thalassemia: over a decade and a half of experience with subcutaneous desferrioxamine. Bone Marrow Transplant 1997;19 (Suppl 2):9–10.
7. Levine JE, Cohen A, MacQueen M, Martin M, Giardina PJ. Sensorimotor neurotoxicity associated with high-dose deferoxamine treatment. J Pediatr Hematol Oncol 1997;19:139–41.
8. Venkattaramanabalaji GV, Foster D, Greene JN, Muro-Cacho CA, Sandin RL, Saez R, Robinson LA. Mucormycosis associated with deferoxamine therapy after allogeneic bone marrow transplantation. Cancer Control 1997;4:168–71.
9. Besunder JB, Super DM, Anderson RL. Comparison of dimercaptosuccinic acid and calcium disodium ethylenediaminetetraacetic acid versus dimercaptopropanol and ethylenediaminetetraacetic acid in children with lead poisoning. J Pediatr 1997;130:966–71.
10. Takacs T, Lonovics J, Caroli-Bosc F-X, Montet A-M, Montet S-C. Litholyse de contact des calculs de la voie biliaire principale. Etude chez 44 malades. Gastroenterol Clin Biol 1997;21:655–9.
11. Holness DL, Nethercott JR. Results of patch testing with a specialized collection of plastic and glue allergens. Am J Contact Dermatitis 1997; 8:121–4.
12. Tsai C-Y, Yu C-L, Tsai Y-Y, Kung Y-Y, Wu T-H, Tsai S-T. Pure red cell aplasia in a man with RA. Scand J Rheumatol. 1997;26:329–31.
13. Pless M, Sandson T. Chronic internuclear ophthalmoplegia: a manifestation of d-penicillamine cerebral vasculitis. J Neuro Ophthalmol 1997;17:44–6.
14. Wittbrodt ET. Drugs and myasthenia gravis: an update. Arch Intern Med 1997;157:399–408.
15. Chuah SY, Wong NW, Goh KL. Lethargy in a patient with cirrhosis. Postgrad Med J 1997; 73:177–9.
16. Kato Y, Naito Y, Narita Y, Kuzuhara S. d-Penicillamine-induced myasthenia gravis in a case of eosinophilic fasciitis. J Neurol Sci 1997;146:85–6.
17. Porzio S, Iorio R, Vajro P, Pensati P, Vegnente A. Penicillamine-related neurologic syndrome in a child affected by Wilson disease with hepatic presentation. Arch Neurol 1997;54:1166–8.
18. Pedersen-Bjergaard U, Andersen M, Hansen PB. Drug-induced thrombocytopenia: clinical data on 309 cases and the effect of corticosteroid therapy. Eur J Clin Pharmacol 1997;52:183–9.
19. Ten Wolde S, Hermans J, Breedveld FC, Dijkmans BAC. Effect of resumption of second line drugs in patients with rheumatoid arthritis that flared up after treatment discontinuation. Ann Rheum Dis 1997;56:235–9.
20. Carpenter EH, Plant MJ, Hassell AB, Shadforth MF, Fisher J, Clarke S, Hothersall TE, Dawes PT. Management of oral complications of disease-modifying drugs in rheumatoid arthritis. Br J Rheumatol 1997;36:473–8.
21. Karpinski J, Jothy S, Radoux V, Levy M, Baran D. d-Penicillamine-induced crescentic glomerulonephritis and antimyeloperoxidase antibodies in a patient with scleroderma. Case report and review of the literature. Am J Nephrol 1997;17:528–32.
22. Bindi P, Gilson B, Aymard B, Noel LH, Wieslander J. Antiglomerular basement membrane

glomerulonephritis following d-penicillamine-associated nephrotic syndrome. Nephrol Dial Transplant 1997;12:325–7.
23. Zvulunov A, Grunwald MH, Avinoach I, Halevy S. Transient acantholytic dermatosis (Grover's disease) in a patient with progressive systemic sclerosis treated with d-penicillamine. Int J Dermatol 1997;36:476–7.
24. Condon C, Phelan M, Lyons JF. Penicillamine-induced type II bullous systemic lupus erythematosus. Br J Dermatol 1997;136:474–5.
25. Penas PE, Buezo GF, Carvajal I, Dauden E, Lopez A, Diaz LA. d-Penicillamine-induced pemphigus foliaceus with autoantibodies to desmoglein-1 in a patient with mixed connective tissue disease. J Am Acad Dermatol 1997;37:121–3.
26. Brenner S, Bialy-Golan A, Anhalt GJ. Recognition of pemphigus antigens in drug-induced pemphigus vulgaris and pemphigus foliaceus. J Am Acad Dermatol 1997;36:919–23.
27. McGovern TW, Bennion SD. Diffuse blisters and erosions in a patient with limited scleroderma. Penicillamine-induced pemphigus foliaceus (PIPF). Arch Dermatol 1997;133:499 + 504.
28. Iozumi K, Nakagawa H, Tamaki K. Penicillamine-induced degenerative dermatoses: report of a case and brief review of such dermatoses. J Dermatol 1997;24:458–65.
29. Garcia-Nieto AV, Fernandez Roldan JC, Martinez-Sanchez F, Gonzalez Gomez J, Moreno Gimenez JC. Yellow nail syndrome by d-penicillamine. Actas Dermo-Sifiliogr 1997;88:191–5.
30. Narvaez J, Alegre-Sancho JJ, Juanola X, Roig-Escofet D. Arthropathy of Wilson's disease presenting as noninflammatory polyarthritis. J Rheumatol 1997;24:2494.

Pam Magee

24 Antiseptic drugs and disinfectants

BISBIGUANIDES

Chlorhexidine *(SED-13, 651; SEDA-19, 235; SEDA-20, 225; SEDA-21, 254)*

Anaphylactic shock caused by chlorhexidine-containing lubricants has been described after cystoscopy or urinary catheterization (SEDA-18, 225; SEDA-19, 235; SEDA-20, 225). Anaphylaxis has also been reported after chlorhexidine has been applied to open wounds (SED-13, 651).

Two patients developed *skin eruptions and severe hypertension* immediately after their leg wounds had been cleaned using a 4% chlorhexidine solution. Both showed a positive skin scratch test for chlorhexidine. Neither had a positive lymphocyte transformation test, and one had a previous history of exposure to chlorhexidine (1[c]).

Several antiseptics have recently been used to coat central venous catheters. *Anaphylactic shock* due to a chlorhexidine-coated central venous catheter was confirmed on rechallenge (2[c]).

A 47-year-old woman with a history of uterine myoma was scheduled for hysterectomy. She was a well-controlled diabetic with no history of allergic reactions. She received 5 mg oral diazepam as premedication. Before induction of anesthesia, an epidermal catheter was placed in the second lumbar interspace, and 2 ml of 1% mepivacaine was given as a test dose. Her preinduction blood pressure was 126/82 mmHg, with a heart rate of 82 beats/min in sinus rhythm. Anesthesia was induced with propofol (1.5 mg/kg) and tracheal intubation was facilitated with vecuronium (0.1 mg/kg). Anesthesia was maintained with sevoflurane in nitrous oxide and oxygen. After induction of anesthesia a central venous catheter coated with chlorhexidine and silver sulfadiazine was introduced via the right subclavian vein. During placement of the catheter her arterial blood pressure fell to 70/40 mmHg and she had a tachycardia of 120 beats/min. Her hypotension was refractory to vasoactive agents, fluid replacement, and corticosteroids. There was no evidence of bronchoconstriction, but a generalized irregular raised erythema was noted. Her blood pressure rose after 30 min with dopamine and the erythema gradually subsided after 2 h. The central venous catheter remained in situ for a further 2 days and no further anaphylaxis occurred. Prick tests for propofol, mepivacaine, vecuronium, atropine, Ringer's acetate, povidone iodine, chlorhexidine, silver sulfadiazine, and latex were all negative 1 week after the reaction. A repeat prick test 6 weeks later was significantly positive for chlorhexidine. However, this was not reported and at a subsequent operation the same agents were used for induction and the same chlorhexidine silver sulfadiazine-coated catheter type was inserted. Severe hypotension and tachycardia occurred as soon as the central venous catheter was inserted. The catheter was removed immediately. Her blood pressure recovered within 15 min with epinephrine and norepinephrine. Once she was hemodynamically stable a non-coated central venous catheter was inserted without incident. Biochemistry immediately after the hypotensive episode showed raised histamine 540 nmol/l (0.1–0.5) reduced C3, C4, and lymphocyte count. Her serum IgE concentration was low at 15 u/ml before induction.

It was considered that this patient may have had a low IgE trait, in which individuals are prone to hypersensitivity reactions. A possible explanation of why allergy did not continue after the first event, while the catheter was in place, could be the exhaustion of circulating antibody or immunoglobulin.

This is the first report of anaphylactic shock induced by a chlorhexidine-coated central venous catheter. Although this may be a rare reaction it is a significant adverse event and demonstrates the importance of using a prick test at an optimal time.

Side Effects of Drugs, Annual 22
J.K. Aronson, ed.

IODOPHORS *(SED-13, 655; SEDA-17 294; SEDA-18, 256; SEDA-20, 226)*

Povidone iodine

The use of intraperitoneal povidone iodine as an agent for peritoneal lavage in colorectal surgery is controversial. It has a wide range of antimicrobial activity and is rapidly lethal to dissociated colorectal cancer cells. However, severe *anaphylaxis* associated with the lavage or installation of povidone iodine into wounds or body cavities had been reported (SED-13, 655; SEDA-17, 294; SEDA-18, 256). It is usually used in colorectal surgery as a 1% solution. Sclerosing encapsulated peritonitis has been reported in two cases after the intraperitoneal use of a 5 and 10% povidone iodine solution (3[c]). In both patients significant morbidity resulted from the postoperative development of sclerosing encapsulated peritonitis. In one patient an ileo-anal pouch could not be fashioned after an initial colectomy, and in the second a small bowel obstruction required a laparotomy and a period of intravenous nutrition. The use of povidone iodine in uncomplicated colorectal surgery cannot be recommended and solutions greater than 1% should not be used.

Povidone iodine has also been used to reduce the incidence of exit-site infections in 130 patients undergoing continuous ambulatory peritoneal dialysis (CAPD) (4[C]). A randomized trial was performed to assess any additional benefits conferred by the use of povidone iodine dry powder spray at dressing changes over an existing strict protocol of exit care. Exit infections occurred in 14 (18%) of 77 patients who used the spray and in 15 (21%) of 72 patients who did not. The risk of peritonitis was also similar in each group. The proportion of infections caused by *Staphylococcus aureus* was reduced in the spray group, but infections caused by *Pseudomonas aeruginosa* were increased. Rash occurred in 6% of those using the spray. The rash lasted for a median of 19 (range 8–79) days before resolution. The use of a povidone iodine spray does not therefore seem justified.

Endocrine, metabolic Cardiopulmonary bypass has profound effects on thyroid function. These effects can be exacerbated in infants, because they are able to absorb large amounts of iodine transcutaneously. *Hypothyroidism* has been reported in neonates exposed to povidone iodine in several ways (SEDA-17, 294; SEDA-18, 256; SEDA-20, 226). In a prospective, randomized, controlled trial of 37 infants undergoing repair of congenital cardiac abnormalities, the use of povidone iodine as a preoperative antiseptic was assessed to determine if it contributed to suppression of thyroid function (5[C]). During cardiopulmonary bypass two groups of children received either povidone iodine or chlorhexidine as a topical preoperative antiseptic. A third group required thoracotomy but not cardiopulmonary bypass and received povidone iodine as a preoperative antiseptic. Thyrotropin (TSH), total tri-iodothyronine (T_3), and thyroxine (T_4) were measured on four occasions: (a) before preparation for surgery; (b) immediately after surgery; (c) at 2 days after surgery; (d) at 5–8 days after surgery. There was a significant fall in TSH concentrations immediately after surgery in the two bypass groups. This change was significantly greater than in the change in TSH concentration in the thoracotomy group. Total T_3 and T_4 concentrations fell by postoperative day 2 in both bypass groups, and the changes were significant when compared with the thoracotomy group. Total T_3 and T_4 concentrations rose significantly in all groups after postoperative day 2, with no significant differences. This suggests that cardiopulmonary bypass has a more significant effect on thyroid metabolism than does preoperative antiseptic.

ORGANIC MERCURY COMPOUNDS *(SED-13, 598; SEDA-21, 255)*

Merbromin

Merbromin (Mercurochrome) is a weak topical mercurial antiseptic previously believed to be poorly absorbed from the gastrointestinal tract. However, a single case report of *mercury intoxication* after self-poisoning has been reported (SEDA-18, 256). Two more reports of mercury poisoning, one after mistaken ingestion of 100 ml of 2% merbromin solution (6[c]) and one after self-poisoning with 20 ml of 2% merbromin (7[c]) suggest that merbromin can be significantly absorbed from the gastrointestinal tract, resulting in toxic blood mercury concentrations.

PHENOLIC COMPOUNDS

(SED-13, 600; SEDA-18, 257; SEDA-21, 255)

Phenol

Phenolic disinfectants (Meytol, Dettol) are widely used for domestic purposes, often in concentrations higher than those recommended. If the cleaning equipment is stored without prior rinsing, phenol can concentrate, as it evaporates more slowly than water. *Phenol burns* have been reported after a moist mop that had previously been used with a phenol disinfectant for cleaning was handled (7[c]).

A 65-year-old man sustained painless full-thickness burns to his right hand after using a phenolic household disinfectant for carpet-cleaning 6 days before. The solution was made up of about 150 ml of phenolic disinfectant (Meytol) and 3 l of water. The composition of the disinfectant, according to the label on the bottle, was soap 0.5%, halogenated phenol 0.5%, and pine oils 0.5%. The patient used a mop for cleaning and used his bare hands to squeeze it. At the end of cleaning the mop was left to dry. During the next 2 days he did not notice anything wrong with his hands, and on the morning of the third day he picked up the moist mop with his right hand. On day 4 the skin of his right hand became pale and blistered and he developed full thickness chemical burns and digital tip gangrene. The affected areas were completely painless and anesthetic. The wounds were thoroughly irrigated with 0.9% saline and treated conservatively using a Flammazine hand bag and early physiotherapy. The dead tissue eventually sloughed off and was replaced with granulation tissue, which epithelialized uneventfully.

Precautions are advisable for the use of phenol disinfectants: gloves should be worn when performing domestic cleaning and all cleaning equipment should be washed with plenty of fresh water after use.

QUATERNARY AMMONIUM COMPOUNDS

Cetrimonium bromide, cetrimonium chloride, and steartrimonium chloride are quaternary ammonium salts used in concentrations of up to 10% in cosmetic products as biocides. In a safety assessment of these agents by the US Cosmetic Ingredient Review Expert Panel it was concluded on the basis of animal and clinical data that cetrimonium chloride, cetrimonium bromide and steartrimonium chloride are safe for use in rinse-off products and are safe in concentrations of up to 0.25% in leave-on products (8[R]).

REFERENCES

1. Fujita S, Sumita S, Kawana S, Iwasaki H, Namiki A. Two cases of anaphylactic shock induced by chlorhexidine. Jpn J Anesthesiol 1997;46: 1118–21.
2. Oda T, Hamasaki J, Kanda N, Mikami K. Anaphylactic shock induced by an antiseptic-coated central venous catheter. Anaesthesiology 1997; 87:1242–4.
3. Keating JP, Nuell M, Hill GL. Sclerosing encapsulating peritonitis after intraperitoneal use of povidone iodine. Aust New Zealand J Surg 1997;67:742–4.
4. Wilson APR, Lewis C, O'Sullivan, Shetty N, Neild GH, Mansell M. The use of povidone iodine in exit site care for patients undergoing continuous ambulatory peritoneal dialysis (CAPD). J Hosp Infect 1997;35:287–93.
5. Brogan TV, Bratton SL, Lynn AM. Thyroid function in infants following cardiac surgery: comparative effects of iodinated and noniodinated topical antiseptics. Crit Care Med 1997;25:1583–7.
6. Hirsch M, Jochle W, Spahr A. Quecksilbervergiftung durch Merbromin. Munch Med Wochenschr 1997;139:39–40.
7. DeBono R, Laitung G. Phenolic household disinfectants–further precautions required. Burns 1997;23:182–5.
8. Anderson FA. Final report on the safety assessment of cetrimonium chloride, cetrimonium bromide and steartrimonium chloride. Int J Toxicol 1997;16:195–220.

T. Midtvedt

25 Penicillins, cephalosporins, other β-lactam antibiotics, and tetracyclines

℞ *Increasing bacterial resistance*

The topic of the increasing rate of antibiotic resistance in an increasing number of bacterial species world-wide has been addressed several times in these volumes (SEDA-12, 206; SEDA-16, 273; SEDA-19, 237; SEDA-20, 228) and, as underlined in SEDA-21 (p. 257), it is certainly not the time to stop worrying.

But it is time to admit that we—and I include all the groups involved in health care, from local practitioners to multinational pharmaceutical companies—are the ones to blame. In other words, it is our use—to a certain extent misuse as well as overuse—of these drugs that had stimulated the microbial world to defend itself by increasing its defence against our weapons. It is amazing how much we have succeeded in altering and destroying. On a personal note, I can relate the fact that my father was the first patient in Norway to receive in all more than 1 000 000 International Units of penicillin when he was treated in 1945 for a very serious streptococcal septicemia. Nowadays, the equivalent of 1 000 000 IU of penicillin might be an ordinary evening dose for a streptococcal sore throat.

It should be admitted that very often too potent antibiotics have been used to treat mild to moderate infections in too 'healthy' patients. Of course, 'mene, mene, tekel, upharsin' (Daniel 5:25) has been written over and over again on the wall, but we have not paid enough attention to the moving finger.

Accepting the sad fact that we have been weighed in the scales and found wanting, it is certainly time to ask: were do we go from here?

Side Effects of Drugs, Annual 22
J.K. Aronson, ed.

It is encouraging to appreciate that World Health Organization has realized the problem (1^R), and with a new General Secretary (a medical doctor trained in microbiology) in charge, there is every reason to believe, to expect, and to demand that WHO will increase its efforts to create a better antibiotic policy world wide. It is also encouraging to recognize that the European Union has realized the problem. In September 1998, Copenhagen hosted a European Union Conference: The Microbial Threat. Close to 400 delegates from all over Europe convened and succeeded in producing a pamphlet entitled Conclusions of responding to the European Union Conference on 'The Microbial Threat' (2^R). It is good news indeed when they state that The European Community and member states must recognise that antimicrobial resistance is a major European and global problem and when they recommend that the EU should collect data on the supply and consumption of antibiotics as well as to set up a 'European surveillance system of antimicrobial resistance' and to make research on antimicrobial resistance a high priority.

Thus, and at last, nearly everybody realizes that the microbial threat does exist. The key question is: are we doing enough? To be rude, on this point the Copenhagen Recommendation can be characterized as a mountain that has given birth to a mouse; i.e. virtually nothing of protective value has happened. While we are collecting and recording data, the microbial world will continue to develop resistance. The time has come to be far more active. That means that the time has come for every doctor to ask himself: am I using antibiotics optimally? and: am I receiving adequate information from the pharmaceutical companies and leading experts?

Looking back to over the twentieth century, there is one group of leaders that should be left behind, and that is the members of the international jet-set of experts travelling from one manufacturer-sponsored congress or symposium to another. Sad to relate, the outcome of such meetings can, as a rule, be given in advance. After a certain number of 'positive' lectures about the new drug, the chairman ends the section by stating that the new drug is very promising, and is certainly a drug for future trials and use. The memory among the members in the jet-set is remarkably short, i.e. it is likely that they have told precisely the same story about another drug some few months earlier. These false prophets were there when the third generation of cephalosporins started to flood the market, they were on top of the waves when new macrolides and fluoroquinolones were introduced, and their names are on a close to endless number of publications dealing with new antibiotics. Again allowing myself to be personal, having been in the business of writing about adverse effects of antibiotics for more than 15 years, I am sorry to say that I hardly, if ever, have seen any of the members of the jet-set writing anything of solid value regarding possible adverse effects when new drugs have been introduced.

Let us try entering the new millennium with the simple goal of obtaining a reduction instead of an increase in antimicrobial resistance. Then our antibiotics will be of value to future generations.

PENICILLINS *(SED-13, 693; SEDA-19, 239; SEDA-20, 229; SEDA-21, 259)*

Liver Drug-induced *hepatic injury* can present as hepatocellular, cholestatic, or a mixed pattern of acute or chronic onset (3[R]). Concerning penicillins, there is old and ample evidence linking semisynthetic penicillins like oxacillin (4[C]), flucloxacillin (5[C]) and amoxicillin–clavulanic acid (SEDA-15, 255) to drug-induced liver injury. The first report of liver toxicity after penicillin came as early as 1946 (6[c]). However, in the following years there were very few cases of liver injury after administration of penicillin G (7[R]), (8[R]). In relation to their large consumption, penicillins G and V have been considered to be nearly free of liver toxicity. However, recent data from a new case, very carefully investigated, has underlined the importance of not forgetting the penicillins as hepatotoxic drugs (9[c]).

A 54-year-old man with low back pain and fever, preceded by 3 months of general malaise, had a pyogenic vertebral spondylitis (L5/S1) due to *Streptococcus agalactiae*, and was given penicillin G, 5 000 000 IU qds. After a month there was a marked increase in transaminases associated with a high peripheral eosinophil count and increased concentrations of eosinophilic cationic protein, indicating eosinophilic activation and the presence of an allergic reaction. Skin tests and assays for specific antibodies to penicillin G were negative, but lymphocyte transformation tests showed T-cell sensitization to penicillin G, although not to amoxicillin and ceftriaxone. Penicillin G was replaced by ceftriaxone, and 4 days later his liver enzymes and eosinophil count began to fall. One year later he was in perfect health with normal liver function tests.

The authors classified their report as a probable case of drug-induced liver injury. The rapid response to withdrawal of penicillin obviated the need for liver biopsy. The time course and enzyme pattern fulfilled the criteria of drug-induced hepatocellular liver damage, as defined by an International Consensus Meeting (10[R]).

Urinary system The naturally occurring β-lactams have high target specificity for groups of bacterial proteins that are not present in mammalian cells. This is thought to be the major reason for their low toxicity. Over the years new and more effective β-lactams have been developed, but unfortunately sometimes with an increase in adverse effects.

There has, for example, been increased nephrotoxicity, expressed as *acute proximal tubular necrosis* after β-lactam therapy. For more than 25 years, this has been the main interest of Tune and his group at Stanford University and their experiences have recently been summarized (11[R]).

The major mechanisms of β-lactam toxicity include: (1) transport into the tubular cell, mainly by the antiluminar organic anion secretory carrier; (2) acetylation of target proteins, causing respiratory intracellular toxicity by inactivation of mitochondrial anionic substrate carriers; (3) lipid peroxidation.

Cephaloridine is the most nephrotoxic β-lactam, and it has therefore been extensively studied. Briefly summarized: its transport into the tubular cell is followed by minimal cell to luminal fluid movement, resulting in 'extreme intracellular sequestration' (11[R]), it attacks the mitochondrial carriers of pyruvate and the short-chain fatty anions, and it causes significant oxidative damage. Other nephrotoxic β-lactams, such as cephaloglycin and imipenem, undergo less intracellular trapping than cephaloridine, but have sufficient tubular cell uptake and toxicity to mitochondrial substrate carriers to be nephrotoxic.

Carbapenems have become a major focus for pharmaceutical development. Unfortunately, some nephrotoxicity has been seen with nearly all carbapenems so far tested (12[R])–(14[R]). However, new carbapenems continue to be developed. At the 1998 ICAAC meeting, more than 10 novel carbapenems, at varying stages of development, were presented.

A logical method of minimizing renal toxicity would be to develop penems that undergo little or no tubular uptake (15[R]). Another way would be to introduce organic anion transport inhibitors. Cilastatin, developed to prevent the hydrolysis of imipenem by a renal peptidase, also reduces its tubular secretion and nephrotoxicity (16[R]). Betamipron, developed specifically to inhibit the secretory transport of the penems, seems to be nephroprotective when used together with panipenem and cephaloridine, through reduction of their tubular cell uptake (16[R])

Historically, the development of β-lactams lacking features that promote renal toxicity has occurred mostly by chance. A recent approach has been to have a carbon-for-sulfur substitution in cephalosporins. The first of these carbacephems to be studied in greater detail underwent greater tubular cell uptake and was more toxic than its cephalosporin analog (17[R]). At present, it is not known whether this pattern holds true for the other carbacephems.

Giving an organic anion transport inhibitor, such as betamipron, will also reduce nephrotoxicity. However, it may also reduce the movement of β-lactams out of the central nervous system, thereby potentially increasing the risk of neurotoxicity (18[R]). As usual, it is difficult to sail between Scylla and Charybdis.

CEPHALOSPORINS *(SED-13, 711; SEDA-19, 242; SEDA-20, 229; SEDA-21, 260)*

Cefepime

Hematological *Neutropenia* occurs rarely during cephalosporin therapy, but it should not be forgotten that each derivative has its own incidence rate. Recently, two cases of possible cefepime-induced neutropenia have been reported (19[C]).

A 42-year-old man with osteomyelitis was given a 42-day course of intravenous cefepime, 2 g every 12 h. On day 28, his white cell count had fallen to 1.7×10^9/l and with only 6% banded neutrophils. Cefepime was withdrawn and the white cell count rose to 5.7×10^9/l after a week, and with 47% segmented neutrophils.

A 48-year-old woman received cefepime 2 g bd for a wound infection. After 30 days she developed fever neutropenia (white cell count 1.5×10^9/l, with 10% segmented neutrophils). Cefepime was withdrawn and her blood count rose to normal within a week.

Since cefepime is a relatively new cephalosporin, the author stated that health care professionals should diligently report cefepime-related adverse reactions. It is worth noting that cefepime is being increasingly used in patients with neutropenia, and it might be wise not to change too quickly to cefepime therapy in such patients.

CARBACEPHEMS

Carbacephems are closely related to cephalosporins (sulphur is substituted by carbon in the 6-ring). Loracarbef is a carbacephem that can be taken orally. It has been recommended for treatment of a variety of community-acquired infections. However, as usual, it takes some time before the specific profile of adverse effects has been satisfactorily evaluated.

Liver In a recent report from Sweden, loracarbef was associated with *acute liver damage* (20[c]).

A 75-year-old man developed itching, jaundice, pale stools, and right upper quadrant pain after recently having finished 4 weeks of treatment with loracarbef 400 mg bd for pneumonia. Before the start of treatment his liver enzymes had been within the reference range. Biochemical investigations showed: total bilirubin 330 μmol/l, AsT 1.3 μkat/l, AIT 1.2 μkat/l, alkaline phosphatase 13 μkat/l, all significantly raised. Virological tests and tests for autoantibodies were all negative, as was retrograde endoscopic cholangiography. Liver biopsy showed swollen hepatocytes and rather severe cholestasis in the cytoplasm and in the canaliculi. After withdrawal of loracarbef the liver functions tests improved and became normal after about 10 weeks.

The authors stated that the acute liver injury in this patient suggests a cholestatic reaction to loracarbef according to international criteria (10[R]). They also mentioned that the Swedish Adverse Drug Reactions Adversary Committee has received two other reports of liver injury probably caused by loracarbef. One patient had a hepatocellular type of reaction after 10 days of loracarbef and positive rechallenge. The other had a mixed hepatocellular/cholestatic type of reaction after 7 days of loracarbef with slow recovery after withdrawal. The authors calculated the incidence of loracarbef-induced acute liver injury to be in the order of 1:70 000 prescriptions, which is far above the incidences after the use of other oral β-lactams.

TETRACYCLINES *(SED-13, 725; SEDA-20, 231; SEDA-21, 261)*

℞ *Comparative toxicity of tetracycline, doxycycline, and minocycline*

Over the years, adverse effects related to minocycline have been reported far more often in SEDA than adverse effects related to other tetracycline derivatives. This is of course related to the high number of published reports, but may not reflect a real difference in safety. Questions about this have recently been discussed in a comprehensive review article (21[R]).

The authors stated that minocycline has been reported to cause several adverse events, including a hypersensitivity syndrome reaction, a serum sickness-like reaction, and a drug-induced lupus-like syndrome, in addition to various types of single organ dysfunction. The hypersensitivity syndrome reaction was defined by fever, skin eruption, and internal organ involvement within 8 weeks after the start of therapy; the serum sickness-like reaction was defined by fever, skin eruption (most commonly urticarial or erythema multiforme), and arthralgia, with or without lymphadenopathy, within 6 weeks of treatment; drug-induced lupus-like syndrome was defined by the presence of antinuclear antibodies, at least one clinical feature of systemic lupus erythematosus (SLE) that resolves with drug discontinuation, and the absence of idiopathic SLE; single organ dysfunction was defined as the presence of severe disease in one major organ, e.g. pancreatitis, hepatitis.

They intended to evaluate whether similar events were associated with other tetracycline antibiotics, such as tetracycline and doxycycline. Their search was based on several sources, including reports in MEDLINE for the period 1966–1996 and information held by the Adverse Drug Reaction Monitoring Division of the Health Protection Branch in Ottawa, Canada, for the same period of time. They also went through all tetracycline-related records of all patients referred to the Glaxo-Wellcome Drug Safety Clinic, Toronto, Canada, for the period January 1985 to October 1996. A total number of 77 published papers were commented on in their review.

Their search produced the numbers of reports related to minocycline, tetracycline and doxycycline shown in Table 1.

In the articles reviewed, the kidney was never involved in a case of single organ dysfunction when minocycline was used, although alterations in renal function have been observed when several organs were involved. None of the tetracyclines is free of adverse renal effects; however, the risk is probably least with doxycycline.

Obviously minocycline is involved in far more reports of adverse effects than the two other tetracyclines. However, the authors went further and discussed whether this may relate to the unique structure and metabolism of min-

Table 1. *Numbers of reports of adverse effects of minocycline, tetracycline, and doxycycline (21[R])*

	Minocycline	Tetracycline	Doxycycline
Hypersensitivity syndrome reaction	19	2	1
Serum sickness-like reaction	11	3	2
Drug-induced lupus-like syndrome	32	0	0
Single organ dysfunction	40	37	6
Totals	102	42	9

ocycline. All tetracyclines have the same basic four-ring carbocyclic structure, but they differ in substituents. Minocycline is the only one with a substituent dimethylamino group in the 7 position. The authors suggested that an iminoquinonone derivative may be generated that is a potential reactive electrophilic intermediate; since neither tetracycline nor doxycycline contains this amino acid side chain, they have not the potential to form this reactive metabolite.

The authors applied this theory to several types of minocycline-induced adverse effects. Black pigmentation in the thyroid gland is relatively commonly seen in patients taking long-term minocycline, and is not seen with other tetracyclines. They suggested that this is because the strongly electron-donating dimethylamino group in minocycline increases its reactivity to oxidation. This is supported by previous findings (22[R]) that treatment of minocycline-induced black pigmentation with thyroid peroxidase resulted in the formation of a black product, whereas other members of the tetracycline family were not oxidized to dark products by the same system.

The authors mentioned another difference between various tetracyclines in the formation of metabolites, that a minocycline–gluthathione conjugate is formed when minocycline is incubated in vitro with hypochlorous acid, as is found in neutrophils. When tetracycline or doxycycline were incubated in the same system no gluthathione conjugates were detected. This in vitro system serves as a surrogate for oxidative reactions in the liver.

The potential reactive metabolites generated by minocycline may bind to tissue molecules, thereby causing cell damage directly, or they may act as haptens, eliciting an immune response secondarily (23[R]). A similar 'hapten' theory is used to explain hypersensitivity reactions seen with sulfonamides, aromatic anticonvulsants, and some other drugs, including cefaclor (24[R]).

Reviewing the literature, the authors found no cases of lupus-like syndrome related to members of the tetracycline family other than minocycline. Of the many theories for the mechanisms behind the lupus-like syndrome, they focused on the possibility that a reactive metabolite binds to the class II major histocompatibility antigen and induces an autoimmune reaction analogous to a graft-versus-host reaction (25[R]). A reactive metabolite may bind directly to histones and act as a hapten, producing an antigenic complex capable of stimulating autoantibody formation (26[R]). Factors that have been implicated in causing the lupus-like syndrome include long-term use of the drug, dose dependency, and the presence of a functional group that is easily oxidized to a reactive metabolite, such as we hypothesized occurs with minocycline (21[R]).

In fact, the way minocycline is given may influence its adverse effects profile. Of all the members of the tetracycline family, minocycline is more commonly used in long-term treatment, especially for acne vulgaris, whereas doxycycline and tetracycline are more likely to be described for acute infections, for which the duration of treatment is relatively short. Going through more than 18 million prescriptions for tetracyclines in Canada, the authors found repeat prescriptions in close to two-thirds of the patients taking minocycline compared with about 32 and 9% in patients taking tetracycline or doxycycline, respectively.

Apparently minocycline differs in several ways from the other members of the family, and it might be reasonable to assume that patients with serious adverse reactions to minocycline can subsequently be safely treated with other tetracycline derivatives. Although the authors underlined the fact that there is minimal evidence to support this claim, there have been some supporting anecdotes. For example, a patient who developed a minocycline-induced pneumonitis on two occasions tolerated doxycycline without relapse (27[c]). Another patient who developed minocycline-induced lupus-like syndrome, later tolerated doxyxyline (28[c]). The authors ended their review by stating that because of the severity of these reactions, patients who experience a serious adverse event while receiving one of these tetracycline antibiotics should be advised to avoid all tetracyclines until more information regarding potential cross-reactivity is known (21[R]).

Tetracycline

Interactions Tetracycline, metronidazole, and bismuth subsalicylate are widely used in combination for treatment of *Helicobacter pylori* infection. It has been generally assumed that bivalent and trivalent cations, including *bismuth*, impair the absorption of tetracycline owing to the formation of poorly soluble chelates. This was the background for a recent investigation to determine whether the observed decrease in tetracycline bioavailability is due to the active drug bismuth subsalicylate via complexation, or to magnesium aluminium silicate (Veegum) an inactive excipient present only in the liquid formulation of bismuth subsalicylate, which might absorb the tetracycline, rendering it unavailable for systemic absorption (29[C]). In 11 healthy volunteers, who took part in a randomized, three-period, three-treatment, complete crossover study with a 7-day wash-out period between treatments, the mechanism for the interaction was not complexation between tetracycline and bismuth subsalicylate, but rather adsorption of tetracycline to magnesium aluminium silicate.

Minocycline

Nervous system *Intracranial hypertension* or pseudotumor cerebri is a well-known adverse effect of tetracyclines, especially in children. Minocycline is lipophilic and passes the blood–brain barrier more readily than other tetracyclines, attaining higher concentrations in the cerebrospinal fluid, and this may contribute to its mechanism of action. Among the reported cases related to minocycline, raised intracranial pressure has been more often seen in women; neurological and ophthalmological symptoms develop 1 month after therapy begins, and signs mitigate after withdrawal (30[R]), (31[c]). Two new cases fit well into that description.

A 19-year-old healthy woman took minocycline 100 mg/day for acne vulgaris and 2 weeks later developed severe headache, nausea, and visual disturbance (32[c]). She had severe bilateral papilledema with visual field damage. Minocycline was withdrawn and the papilledema disappeared. However, the visual fields and visual acuity were permanently damaged.

A 15-year-old girl taking minocycline 100 mg bd for acne vulgaris developed headaches (33[c]). She had bilateral papilledema with multiple cottonwool spots and enlarged blind spots. Minocycline was withdrawn, and within a month there was only a trace of papilledema, which subsequently resolved.

Skin and appendages Nine cases of *scleral pigmentation* probably induced by minocycline have been reviewed (34[R]). The characteristic scleral pattern is a blue-gray band of 3–5 mm starting at the limbus, usually enhanced in the palpebral aperture, possible due to the photosensitizing properties of minocycline. These changes may or may not be associated with minocycline-induced pigmentary changes in other tissues, and they can appear after relatively small total doses of minocycline (as low as 18 g). The scleral pigmentation may resolve within years, or may be permanent.

Cutaneous pigmentation due to minocycline may be present in up to 14% of patients treated for facial dermatoses. In most cases the pigment fades over time, but in some patients it may persist for years.

A 62-year-old woman had taken a cumulative dose of 440 g of minocycline when she started to develop perioral and malar blue-black pigmentation (35[c]). Minocycline was withdrawn and she was treated with a hydroquinone cream for 6 months without any effect. The pigmented areas were then exposed to laser therapy at 532 nm wavelength with an excellent response.

General exanthematous pustulosis has been attributed to minocycline (36[c]).

A 52-year-old woman with well-controlled generalized pustular psoriasis and Sjögren's syndrome, developed several folliculitis-like papules limited to the perioral area and was given minocycline (100 mg/day). Three hours after the first dose, she developed erythroderma with numerous superficial pustules over her body and a fever of 39°C. She said that she had had similar pustulation 5 years before, and old records showed that that outbreak had started on the seventh day of minocycline therapy. She also has abnormal serum AsT, AlT, LDH, γ-GTP, alkaline phosphatase, and total bilirubin, and raised sedimentation rate and C-reactive protein. Serum concentrations of IL-6, IL-8, and endothelial-leukocyte adhesion molecule 1 (ELAM-1) were raised, whereas IL-2 and TNF-α were both within the reference ranges. Minocycline was withdrawn; the pustules resolved within 10 days and the raised liver enzymes and serum cytokine concentrations fell gradually.

The authors argued that the spontaneous rapid clinical resolution, with transiently raised serum enzymes, suggested that the symptoms were of an acute generalized exanthematous pustulosis in a patient with generalized pustular psoriasis and not an exacerbation of her psoriasis. This has been supported by another report (37[R]).

Immunological and hypersensitivity reactions Drug-induced *lupus-like syndrome* was mentioned above and was also commented upon in SEDA-21 (p. 262). However, new reports continue to appear, of which the following are a few.

A 14-year-old girl, who had taken minocycline 100–200 mg/day for 5 months for acne vulgaris, developed symptoms of myalgia, arthralgia, polyarthritis, and flushed face (38[c]). A test for antinuclear antibodies was positive. Minocycline was withdrawn and her conditions dramatically improved within 7 days.

A 22-year-old woman, who had taken minocycline for 2 years for acne vulgaris, developed generalized arthralgia and joint swelling (39[c]). Minocycline was withdrawn and all clinical and laboratory abnormalities returned rapidly to normal. Three weeks later she took one minocycline tablet and had an abrupt severe exacerbation, which resolved within 2 days.

A report (28[c]) referred to in SEDA-21 (p. 262), prompted several letters in which new cases of lupus-like syndrome were described (40[c]). In their reply, the original authors stated that practitioners should cease medication as soon as the patient develops malaise, arthralgias, joint stiffness, rash, livedo, fever, or other symptoms. Faced with a difficult decision, a physician should ask, What would be my advice? Would I prescribe a powerful drug such as minocycline to a member of my own family? for example, to one of my teenaged children?

Very simple but suitable advice might be: if you can use another tetracycline derivative, use it.

REFERENCES

1. Anonymous. WHO report. Geneva: World Health Organization, 1998.
2. Midtvedt T. The microbial threat—the Copenhagen recommendation. Microb Ecol Health Dis 1998;10:65–7.
3. Koch HK, Gropp A, Oehlert W. Drug-induced liver injury in liver biopsies of the years 1981 and 1983, their prevalence and type of presentation. Pathol Res Pract 1985;179:469–77.
4. Bruckstein AH, Attia AA. Oxacillin hepatitis. Two patients with liver biopsy and review of the literature. Am J Med 1978;64:519–22.
5. Victorino RMM, Maria VA, Correia AP, De Moura MC. Floxacillin- included cholestatic hepatitis with evidence of lymphocyte sensitization. Arch Intern Med 1987;147:987–9.
6. Felder SL, Felder L, Unusual reaction to penicillin. J Am Med Assoc 1950;143:361–2.
7. Valdivia-Barriga V, Feldman A, Orellana J, Generalized hypersensitivity with hepatitis and jaundice after the use of penicillin and streptomycin. Gastroenterology 1963;45:114–17.
8. Girard JP, Haenni B, Bergoz R, Kapanci Y, Cruchaud A. Lupoid hepatitis following administration of penicillin. Helv Med Acta 1967;34:23–35.
9. Bauer TM, Bircher AJ. Drug-induced hepatocellular liver injury due to benzylpenicillin with evidence of lymphocyte sensitization. J Hepatol 1997;26:429–32.
10. Report of an International Consensus Meeting. Criteria of drug-induced liver disorders. J Hepatol 1990;11:272–6.
11. Bruce MT. Nephrotoxicity of beta-lactam antibiotics: mechanisms and strategies for prevention. Pediatr Nephrol 1997;11:768–72.

12. Birnbaum J, Kahan FM, Kropp H, MacDonald JS. Carbapenems. A new class of beta-lactam antibiotics. Discovery and improvment of imipenem/cilastatin. Am J Med 1985;78 (Suppl 6A):3–21.
13. Topham JC Murgatroyd LB, Jones DV, Goonetilleke UR, Wright J. Safety evaluation of meropenem in animals: studies on the kidney. J Antimicrob Chemother 1989;24 (Suppl A):287–306.
14. Brughera M, Scampinini G, Ferrari ML, Nava A, Mazué G. Toxicologic profile of FCE 22101 and its orally available ester FCE 22891. J Antimicrob Chemother 1989;23 (Suppl C):129–35.
15. Tune BM, Hsu C-Y. Prevention of nephrotoxicity of betalactam antibiotics. In: De Broe ME, Verpooten GA, editors. Prevention in Nephrology. Dordrecht: KlHwer, 1991:39–49.
16. Hirouchi Y, Naganuma H, Kawahara Y, Okada R, Kamiya A, Inui K, Hori R. Preventive effect of betamipron on nephrotoxicity and uptake of carbapenems in rabbit renal cortex. Jpn J Pharmacol 1994;66:1–6.
17. Tune BM, Hsu C-Y, Fravert D. Cephalosporin and carbacephem nephrotoxicity: roles of tubular cell uptake and acylating potential. Biochem Pharmacol 1996;51:557–61.
18. Blaszczak L, Brown R, Cook G, Hornback W, Hoying R, Indelicato J, Jordan C, Katner A, Kinnick M, McDonald JI, Morin JM, Munroe JE, Pasini CE. Comparative reactivity of 1-carba-1-dethiacephalosporins with cephalosporins. J Med Chem 1990;33:1656–62.
19. Dahlgren AF. Two cases of possible cefepime-induced neutropenia. Am J Health Syst Pharm 1997;54:2621–2.
20. Bjornsson E, Olsson R. Acute liver injury due to loracarbef. J Hepatol 1997;26:739–40.
21. Sharpiro LE, Knowles SR, Shear NH. Comparative safety of tetracycline, minocycline, and doxycycline. Arch Dermatol 1997;133:1224–30.
22. Taurog A, Dorris M, Doerge D. Minocycline and the thyroid: antihyroid effects of the drug, and the role of thyroid peroxidase in minocycline-induced black pigmentation of the gland. Thyroid 1996;6:211–19.
23. Shear N, Spielberg S. Anticonvulsant hypersensitivity syndrome: in vitro assessment of risk. J Clin Invest 1988;82:1826–32.
24. Kearns G, Wheeler J, Childress S, Letzig L. Serum sickness-like reactions to cefaclor: role of hepatic metabolism and individual susceptibility. J Pediatr 1994;125:805–11.
25. Uetrecht J. The role of leukocyte-generated metabolites in the pathogenesis of idiosyncratic drug reactions. Crit Rev Toxicol 1992;20:299–366.
26. Hess E. Drug-related lupus. New Engl J Med 1988;318:1460–2.
27. Sitbon O, Bidel N, Dussopt C, Azarian R, Braud ML, Lebargy F, Fourme T, De Blay F, Piard F, Camus P. Minocycline pneumonitis and eosinophilila: a report on eight patients. Arch Intern Med 1994;154:1633–40.
28. Masson C, Chevailler A, Pascaretti C, Legrand E, Bregeon C, Audran M. Minocycline related lupus. J Rheumatol 1996;23:2160–1.
29. Healy DP, Dansereau RJ, Dunn AB, Clendening CE, Mounts A, Deepe JRGS. Reduced tetracycline bioavailability caused by magnesium aluminium silicate in liquid formulations of bismuth subsalicylate. Ann Pharmacother 1997;31:1460–4.
30. Lubetzki C, Sanson M, Cohen D, Schaison-Cusin M, Lhermitte F, Lyon-Caen O. Benign intracranial hypertension and minocycline. Rev Neurol Paris 1988;144:218–20.
31. Le-Bris P, Glacet-Breard A, Coscas G, Meyrignac C. Papilledema caused by minocycline: apropos of a case. J Fr Ophthalmol 1988;11:681–4.
32. Shiri J, Amichai B. Intracranial hypertension and minocycline. Ann Intern Med 1997;127:168.
33. Lewis PA, Kearney PJ. Pseudotumor cerebri induced by minocycline treatment for acne vulgaris. Acta Dermatol Venereol 1997;77:83.
34. Fraunfelder F T, Randall J A. Minocycline-induced scleral pigmentation. Ophthalmology 1997;104:936–8.
35. Wilde JL, English JC III, Finley EM. Minocycline-induced hyperpigmentation: treatment with the neodymium YAG laser. 1997;133:1344–6.
36. Yamamoto T, Minatohara K. Minocycline-induced acute generalized exanthematous pustulosis in a patient with generalized pustular psoriasis showing elevated level of sELAM-1. Acta Dermatol Venereol 1977;77:168–9.
37. Spencer JM, Silvers DN, Grossman ME. Pustular eruption after drug exposure: is it pustular psoriasis or a pustular drug eruption? Br J Dermatol 1994;130:514–19.
38. Farver D K. Minocycline-induced lupus. Ann Pharmacother 1997;31:1160–3.
39. Crosson J, Stillman MT. Minocycline-related lupus erythematosus with associated liver disease. J Am Acad Dermatol 1997;36 (Suppl II):867–8.
40. Emery P, Gough A, Griffiths B, Pointud P, Masson C, Laine P. Minocycline related lupus. J Rheumatol 1997;24:1850–2.

J.K. Aronson

26 Miscellaneous antibacterial drugs

GENERAL

The uses and clinical pharmacology of miscellaneous antibiotics have been reviewed in various circumstances: (1) dermatology (1[R]), (2[R]); (2) pregnancy (3[R]), (4[R]); (3) neonates (4[R]); (4) critical care (5[R]); (5) in patients with an acute abdomen (6[R]); (6) in patients with infections due to methicillin-resistant staphylococci (7[R]).

The adverse effects and interactions of antibiotics in Japanese children have been reviewed (8[R]). Macrolide and azalide antibiotics commonly caused gastrointestinal symptoms, such as *diarrhea* and *loose stools* (1–6%), and hypersensitivity reactions, such as *rash* and *fever* (0.2–1.6%). *Eosinophilia*, *thrombocythemia*, and *raised serum transaminase activities* were common abnormal laboratory findings.

Neuropsychiatric Neuropsychiatric reactions to antibiotics have been reviewed (9[R]). Psychiatric adverse effects of antibiotics include *anxiety* and *panic*, *major depression*, *psychosis*, and *delirium* in patients with and without a premorbid psychiatric history. Risk factors include prior psychopathology, co-existing medical conditions, slow acetylator status, advanced age, concomitant medications, and increased permeability of the blood–brain barrier, as well as high antibiotic dosage and intrathecal or intravenous administration. Psychiatric toxicity can result from various mechanisms of action, including antagonism of the actions of GABA or pyridoxine, adverse interactions with alcohol, or inhibition of protein synthesis. Adverse pharmacokinetic and pharmacodynamic interactions can occur between antibiotics and other drugs, including lithium, benzodiazepines, carbamazepine, valproate, neuroleptic drugs, antidepressants, methadone, and disulfiram. However, accurate epidemiological data on their incidence are not available.

Liver Evidence on antibiotic-associated *acute liver damage* has been reviewed (10[R]). Antituberculous, antimycotic, antiviral, antiprotozoal, and antiseptic compounds were excluded. Only case reports, series, and epidemiological data were used; results from clinical trials were reviewed only when no other information was available. Antibiotic-associated acute liver injury is rare (incidence not over one case per 10 000 users for most drugs). The hepatotoxic effects of all erythromycin salts was confirmed, and recent evidence has suggested that roxithromycin should be added to the list of antibiotics that can cause liver damage. Among fluoroquinolones, only ciprofloxacin has been associated with serious hepatitis. Co-trimoxazole-induced hepatitis is often reported, but trimethoprim alone can also cause acute liver damage. Finally, *acute bile duct injury* and *ductopenia* have been described with several antibiotics.

Immunological and hypersensitivity reactions Compared with penicillins, macrolides, cefalosporins, tetracyclines and other antibiotics rarely cause immunological reactions, which have been reviewed (11[R]). Most reactions are pathophysiologically not IgE-mediated immediate-type reactions, and the sensitivity of skin tests is low.

Side Effects of Drugs, Annual 22
J.K. Aronson, ed.

AMINOGLYCOSIDE ANTIBIOTICS *(SED-13, 744; SEDA-19, 245; SEDA-20, 234; SEDA-21, 265)*

Once daily dosage regimens Reviews of once daily dosing of aminoglycoside antibiotics (SEDA-21, 265) continue to appear, both in general (12[R]) and in relation to their use in critical care (13[R]) and in immunocompromised patients (14[R]). Although there is relatively little information about immunocompromised patients, the available evidence suggests that once-daily regimens are as effective and safe as standard regimens (14[R]). In a review of eight separate meta-analyses it has been suggested that for many infections the case has been proven for once-daily aminoglycosides (i.e. equal efficacy and equal or perhaps reduced toxicity) and that further meta-analyses are not necessary, although further large-scale randomized trials would be useful in children, pregnant women, and patients with endocarditis (15[R]).

Urinary system Aminoglycoside *nephrotoxicity* has again been reviewed (16[R]), (17[R]), (18[r]). Nephrotoxicity complicates 10–20% of therapeutic courses. Important risk factors include age and previous renal insufficiency, which can lead to overdosing (because of a reduced glomerular filtration rate), dehydration, hypovolemia, potassium and magnesium depletion, liver disease, sepsis itself, and the concomitant administration of other drugs (including cefalosporins, cyclosporin, cisplatin, non-steroidal anti-inflammatory drugs, ACE inhibitors, loop diuretics, methoxyflurane, and any basic amino acid, such as lysine) (SEDA-21, 266). Polycationic aminoglycosides bind to anionic, brush-border, phospholipid membranes and are transported intracellularly. They disrupt normal phospholipid trafficking within the cell, consistent with aminoglycoside injury, although similar changes occur with other drugs that do not cause renal insufficiency.

Trough aminoglycoside concentrations are thought to be related to nephrotoxicity, although this is a subject of controversy. In 1238 febrile patients with neutropenia treated with netilmicin plus a cefalosporin, nephrotoxicity occurred in similar proportions of patients with high, normal, or low peak or trough concentrations of netilmicin. However, in patients who received netilmicin with concomitant amphotericin and vancomycin, both themselves nephrotoxic, nephrotoxicity was associated with high peak and trough netilmicin concentrations; however, the numbers of cases were too few for definitive conclusions to be reached (19[c]).

In 200 patients with established *acute renal insufficiency* (4.9/1000 admissions), renal ischemia (50%) and nephrotoxic drugs (21%) were the main causes; of the drug-induced cases, 86% were due to aminoglycosides, the rest being due to iodinated radiocontrast media and cisplatin (20[C]). Histological investigation in 43 cases showed acute tubular necrosis (53%), tubular hydropic degeneration (16%), glomerulopathies (16%), and other lesions (15%). Dialysis was required in 101 patients. The mortality rate was 47% and the most important causes of death were sepsis (38%), respiratory insufficiency (19%), and multiple organ failure (11%). Mortality was higher in oliguric patients (63%) than non-oliguric (35%), and in ischemic renal failure (57%) than in nephrotoxic renal failure (15%).

In a prospective study of 835 cases of *chronic renal insufficiency* the most common causes were glomerulonephritis (29%), diabetic nephropathy (23%), and interstitial nephritis (17%), followed by obstructive nephropathy (6.4%), benign nephrosclerosis (4.1%), and polycystic kidney disease (2%) (21[C]). However, in patients over 40, diabetic nephropathy was the most common cause (37%). In 121 patients, acute deterioration of their underlying renal dysfunction was most commonly due to accelerated hypertension (26%), infection (22%), volume depletion (20%), and drugs (15%); the most common drugs responsible were NSAIDs, ACE inhibitors, and aminoglycosides.

Fanconi syndrome due to aminoglycosides is rare. Three further cases related to the administration of high doses (3.6 × 15 g), with normal renal function, have been reported (22[c])r. The pattern of aminoaciduria showed large increases in neutral amino acids, followed by dibasic and near-normal acidic amino acids. There was reduced tubular reabsorption of phosphate and a very high clearance rate of potassium in association with hypokalemia. The urinary excretion of β_2-microglobulin was greatly increased.

Special senses Genetic susceptibility to aminoglycoside-induced *ototoxicity* (SEDA-21, 267) has been further studied in relation to a mitochondrial mutation at nucleotide 1555.

In five Japanese families with aminoglycoside-induced hearing loss there was a mitochondrial mutation at nucleotide 1555 in 28 of 32 subjects; 100 American control subjects did not have any evidence of this mutation, suggesting that the 1555 A→G (A1555G) mitochondrial mutation may be more frequent among Asian populations (23[c]). Many subjects with this mitochondrial mutation have a mild, high-frequency, progressive hearing loss, even without the administration of aminoglycosides, suggesting that the A1555G mutation may play a more general role in hearing loss.

In China the widespread use of aminoglycoside antibiotics accounts for about 25% of profound deafness in some areas. In three Mongolian pedigrees from Ulan Bator, all of which included several individuals with streptomycin-induced deafness in a pattern consistent with matrilineal transmission, amplified mtDNA, obtained from transformed lymphoblastoid cell lines, showed the A→G point mutation in the 12S rRNA gene in two families (24[c]). There was no other example of this substitution among 400 control samples from Mongolians with normal hearing. The authors concluded that genetic counselling and screening of high risk families before the use of these drugs could have a dramatic effect on the incidence of deafness.

The nucleotide 1555 A→G mutation was identified in seven of 41 unrelated ethnically diverse American individuals (Caucasians, Hispanics, and Asians) with hearing loss after aminoglycoside exposure (25[C]). None of the other known mutations was found. Four of the seven patients had a family history of aminoglycoside-induced ototoxicity. Particularly unexpected was the late onset of hearing loss in three of these patients, years after aminoglycoside exposure; in one of these patients there was a second sequence change in the 12S ribosomal RNA gene, which could have been responsible for the milder phenotype.

Although ototoxicity usually occurs with systemic administration of aminoglycosides, it has also been reported after the topical application of aminoglycosides to the ears (26[c]).

The ototoxic effect of aminoglycosides has been harnessed in the treatment of intractable Menière's disease (27[C]). In 21 patients treated with intratympanic gentamicin, 17 patients had complete elimination of vertigo at 2-year follow-up, three reported a 60–99% reduction in frequency, and 19 described themselves as having no impairment secondary to dizziness. However, average hearing thresholds and word-recognition scores worsened after gentamicin.

Interactions Aminoglycoside-induced nephrotoxicity may be enhanced or mitigated by other antibiotics. Combinations (gentamicin plus placebo, ticarcillin/clavulanate, piperacillin, or ceftazidime) were given for 7 days to groups of eight young, healthy, men, in whom 24-h urine collections were analyzed for the renal tubular enzymes alanine aminopeptidase and *N*-acetyl-β-D-glucosaminidase (NAG) (28[C]). Enzymuria was reduced by *ticarcillin/clavulanate* and increased by *ceftazidime*; piperacillin had no effect. The authors concluded that ticarcillin/clavulanate may be renal protective and that ceftazidime may enhance aminoglycoside-induced renal injury.

FOSFOMYCIN *(SED-13, 760; SEDA-18, 269)*

Fosfomycin tromethamine is a phosphonic acid bactericidal agent with in vitro activity against most urinary tract pathogens, particularly *Escherichia coli* and *Citrobacter*, *Enterobacter*, *Klebsiella*, *Serratia*, and *Enterococcus* spp. (29[R]), (30[R]), (31[r]). It is used in a single dose to treat urinary tract infections. There is little cross-resistance between fosfomycin and other antibacterial agents, possibly because its chemical structure and site of action are different. As the oral tromethamine salt it is 34–41% systemically available. It has a half-life of 5.7 h and is primarily excreted unchanged in the urine. It is well tolerated, with few adverse events. In one analysis, 52 of 848 subjects (6.1%) had adverse effects, 75% of which were gastrointestinal: *diarrhea* (4%), *vomiting* (1%), and *nausea* (0.4%); these are usually transient, mild, and self-limiting. In US studies the only adverse effects that were reported in over 1% of patients were *diarrhea* (9%), *vaginitis* (5.5%), *nausea* (94.1%), *headache* (3.9%), *dizziness* (1.3%), *weakness* (1.1%), and *dyspepsia* (1.1%), and these were generally similar to those in patients who did not receive fosfomycin.

GLYCOPEPTIDES *(SED-13, 757; SEDA-19, 251; SEDA-20, 245; SEDA-21, 276)*

Comparisons of teicoplanin with vancomycin have been reviewed (32[R]). In 18 studies involving 1420 patients, teicoplanin caused adverse effects in 73/715 (10%), compared with 129/705 (18%) with vancomycin. In particular, *nephrotoxicity* seems to be more common with vancomycin and has been estimated at 1.5–15%. The lower of these two estimates may be more correct, since the high incidence in some studies has been attributed to impurities in earlier formulations. In 15 comparative studies involving 1861 patients there was nephrotoxicity with teicoplanin in 43/946 (4.5%) compared with 83/915 (9.1%) with vancomycin. *Red man syndrome* is common with vancomycin, particularly when it is infused at a high rate, but it has also been reported with teicoplanin.

Teicoplanin

The uses of antibiotics in patients with infections due to methicillin-resistant staphylococci have been reviewed, with special emphasis on teicoplanin (7[R]). In four randomized controlled trials in which 1140 patients were given teicoplanin, 5.1% experienced adverse events; in 1% of cases the event was attributable to the drug. The adverse effects that were highlighted were *abnormal liver enzymes* and *thrombophlebitis* (occasional effects) and *rashes* and *neutropenia* (rare effects).

The adverse effects of teicoplanin have been summarized from the results of several trials (33[R]). In 3377 patients there were adverse effects in 10% of patients: *hypersensitivity* (2.6%), *hepatic dysfunction* (1.7%), *local intolerance* (1.6%), *fever* (0.8%), *altered renal function* (0.6%), and *ototoxicity* (0.3%). In 1219 patients in the US the occurrence of adverse effects was different: *hypersensitivity* (14%), *nausea* (5%), *diarrhea* (3%), *thrombocytopenia* (2.4%), *disturbances of balance or hearing* (1.4%), and *nephrotoxicity* (0.9%). Teicoplanin was associated with significantly fewer adverse effects and less nephrotoxicity than vancomycin.

Patients with acute exacerbations of chronic osteomyelitis ($n = 44$) or endocarditis ($n = 10$) were given intravenous teicoplanin; the mean loading dose was 15 mg/kg/day for 3–10 days followed by 15 mg/kg three times a week, individualized to achieve serum trough concentrations of about 10 mg/l for osteomyelitis and 20 mg/l for endocarditis (34[C]). Treatment duration was 28–150 days for patients with osteomyelitis and 28–88 days for those with endocarditis. There were averse events in nine patients: *rash* ($n = 3$), *thrombocytopenia* (n = 3), and drug *fever*, *pseudomembranous colitis*, *nausea*, *leukopenia*, and *transient hearing impairment* ($n = 1$ each).

Teicoplanin + ciprofloxacin has been compared with ceftriaxone in the treatment of community-acquired pneumonia severe enough to require hospital admission. In a multicenter, open, randomized, parallel-group comparison in 240 patients (158 over 65 years, 82 with other underlying diseases, and 71 who had previously been treated with other antibiotics without cure or improvement) (35[C]), there was cure or improvement in 85% of the patients given teicoplanin compared with 73% who were given ceftriaxone; there were failures in 5.8 and 24%, respectively. Adverse events were mild. There were *raised serum transaminases* in three patients given teicoplanin and four given ceftriaxone and *rashes* in three and two, respectively. One other patient given teicoplanin had *stomatitis* and one had *thrombocythemia*.

Hematological *Leukopenia* rarely occurs with teicoplanin (0.3%). The mechanism is unknown. Two patients who were treated with teicoplanin for bone and/or joint infections had severe febrile leukopenia after 14 and 21 days of therapy (36[c]). Vancomycin was given to one of these patients with no adverse effect.

Skin and appendages In a multicenter randomized comparison of teicoplanin + tobramycin with cefalothin + tobramycin in 68 patients, the incidence of clinical failure was 4.6 times higher in those given cefalothin + tobramycin than in those given teicoplanin + tobramycin (7/28 vs 2/37) (37[C]). There was no significant difference in bacterial eradication between the two groups. Local and systemic tolerability were good for both regimens. One patient who received teicoplanin had *transitory erythema and prurigo*.

Special senses Seven patients with enterococcal endocarditis were treated with teicoplanin (7–10 mg/kg per day for 28–105 days) alone (one case) or in combination with aminoglycosides (six cases); all were cured (38[C]). One patient developed *gustatory anesthesia* during the last week of therapy.

Interactions Resistance to *warfarin* has been reported in a 60-year-old woman who was given teicoplanin for methicillin-resistant *Staphylococcus aureus* septicemia (39[c]). The authors hypothesized that teicoplanin had increased the rate of clearance of warfarin.

Vancomycin

In 26 cancer patients with chemotherapy-related neutropenic fever treated intravenously with vancomycin 30 mg/m^2 per day, imipenem 1500 mg/day, and pefloxacin 800 mg/day, no adverse effects were reported (40[C]).

Hematological Hematological adverse effects due to vancomycin are rare. Vancomycin-induced *neutropenia* has previously been believed to be due to a hypersensitivity reaction, since antibodies against circulating neutrophils have been detected in some patients. However, concentration-dependent suppression of hemopoietic bone marrow progenitor cells has been demonstrated in a patient with vancomycin-induced neutropenia after autologous stem cell transplantation for multiple myeloma (41[c]). Further reports of vancomycin-associated neutropenia have appeared (42[c]), (43[c]).

Thrombocytopenia has also been associated with vancomycin (44[c]), (45[c]). In one case drug-dependent platelet antibodies were detected (45[c]).

Urinary system *Nephrotoxicity* of vancomycin and its potential interaction with cilastatin have been studied in rabbits (46). Vancomycin alone (300 mg/kg intravenously) caused increases in serum creatinine and blood urea nitrogen and morphological changes in the kidneys. There was no nephrotoxicity when vancomycin was given with cilastatin. The total clearance of vancomycin was dose-dependently accelerated by cilastatin. These results suggest that cilastatin may reduce or eliminate the nephrotoxic effects of vancomycin.

Skin and appendages In a retrospective study of adverse skin reactions associated with intravenous vancomycin over a 14-month period, two different brands of vancomycin were compared in 224 adults, 12 (5.4%) of whom had infusion-related reactions (47[C]). Ten (5.7%) of 174 patients who received vancomycin for more than 1 day had delayed skin reactions. Risk factors for the reactions were age below 40 years (for both infusion-related and delayed reactions) and duration of therapy over 7 days (for delayed reactions). There was a significant increase in adverse skin reactions associated with the use of one batch of vancomycin, although analytical testing of this batch failed to identify any difference from other batches associated with routine rates of adverse reactions.

In 15 patients with urological disorders in whom MRSA infections were treated with vancomycin and imipenem/cilastatin there was moderate *erythema* in one patient, but this disappeared several days after the completion of treatment (48[C]).

Immunological and hypersensitivity reactions A 34-year-old man had an allergic reaction after inhaling decontaminating drugs for bone marrow transplantation; challenge tests showed that vancomycin repeatedly caused *dyspnea*, *fever*, *hypoxia*, *eosinophilia*, and a *raised CRP* (49[c]).

A 51-year-old man received vancomycin 1.75 g/day intravenously for 4 weeks and developed a syndrome characterized by *high fever*, *erythema multiforme*, *eosinophilia*, and presumed *interstitial nephritis*; this delayed hypersensitivity reaction resolved with withdrawal of the drug and treatment with methylprednisolone (50[c]).

Miscellaneous Following an increase in the incidence of *chemical peritonitis* when a new vancomycin formulation was used a prospective study was carried out in 26 consecutive patients undergoing CAPD (51[C]). Vancoled (Lederle) was used on 30 occasions: 12 were for exit-site infections and chemical peritonitis occurred on four of those occasions; 18 were for peritonitis and chemical peritonitis occurred on three of those occasions. Thus, the overall incidence of chemical peritonitis was 23%. The inflammatory response was associated with a predominance of neutrophils in the peritoneal fluid, without eosinophils. The authors had previously noted a less than 1% incidence of chemical peritonitis when using Vancocin (Eli Lilly). The authors suggested that the peritonitis had been due to the direct effects of impurities in the formulation.

Interactions Vancomycin and *amikacin* are both nephrotoxic. In 2-month-old rats given intraperitoneal injections of amikacin (80 mg/kg) alone or with vancomycin (100 mg/kg) there were similar morphological and biochemical features (52). The authors concluded that vancomycin did not influence the nephrotoxic effect of amikacin and that the drugs could be used in combination.

Interference with diagnostic routines *Topical eosin*, which has been used in the treatment of patients with burns, has been found to interfere with a fluorometric polarization immunoassay for serum vancomycin (53). The cause of the interference was not elucidated, but was thought to have resulted from a direct interaction between the two compounds. The authors recommended ultrafiltration of the sample to remove eosin before assay.

LINCOMYCINS

Clindamycin *(SED-13, 756; SEDA-19, 245; SEDA-20, 238; SEDA-21, 268)*

Drug rashes are more frequent in patients with HIV infection than in the general population and have been reviewed (54[R]). In seven studies involving 322 patients taking clindamycin + primaquine, 163 (51%) had a rash; in contrast, in one study involving 52 patients taking prophylactic clindamycin, only 11 (21%) had a rash. In seven studies involving 225 patients with cerebral toxoplasmosis taking clindamycin + pyrimethamine, 51 (23%) had a rash. The rashes usually consisted of a spontaneously resolving benign *maculopapular rash*.

MACROLIDES *(SED-13, 734; SEDA-19, 246; SEDA-20, 239; SEDA-21, 269)*

The uses and adverse effects of macrolides have again been reviewed (55[R])–(60[R]). A relatively new macrolide, dirithromycin, has been the subject of a short review (61[r]).

Immunological and hypersensitivity reactions A case of *Churg-Strauss syndrome* has been attributed to azithromycin in a 49-year-old man (62[c]).

Interactions The drug interactions of dirithromycin have been compared with those of other macrolides (63[R]). Erythromycin and clarithromycin are metabolized by cytochrome P450 and can inhibit the metabolism of other drugs. Azithromycin and dirithromycin do not inhibit cytochrome P450. In studies with *cyclosporin*, *theophylline*, *terfenadine*, *warfarin*, and *ethinylestradiol*, dirithromycin, like azithromycin, was much less likely to cause the interactions that clarithromycin and erythromycin do.

Digoxin The interaction of macrolides with *digoxin* (see Chapter 17) has been reviewed (64[r]).

Pimozide The FDA has reported two sudden deaths when clarithromycin was added to *pimozide* therapy; the mechanism was thought to be inhibition of pimozide metabolism by clarithromycin, resulting in prolongation of the QT interval (65[r]).

Tacrolimus Interactions of macrolides with tacrolimus have been reviewed (66[r]). Clarithromycin, erythromycin, josamycin, and triacetyloleandomycin all inhibit the metabolism of tacrolimus, causing increased plasma concentrations and immunosuppression.

Miscellaneous *Toxic shock syndrome* in a 43-year-old man who was HIV positive has been attributed to ciprofloxacin (69[cr]).

Interactions Interactions with quinolones have been reviewed (70[R]). Interactions of importance include: chelation interactions with various cations (*calcium*, *aluminium*, *magnesium*, *iron*, *zinc*) and cation-containing formulations (*sucralfate*, *didanosine*, and *mineral--containing multivitamins*); malabsorption problems during co-administration with *dairy products* and *enteral feeding solutions*; and inhibition of the hepatic metabolism of *methylxanthines* and perhaps other drugs that depend on hepatic metabolism for elimination.

POLYPEPTIDES

Bacitracin *(SED-13, 760; SEDA-18, 171)*

Bacitracin is used topically, but contact allergy is rare (SEDA-18, 171). Recently a case of *anaphylaxis* with topical use has been reported (67[c]).

A 21-year-old man had a bleeding tattoo, to which a mixture of bacitracin and polymixin was applied. He developed abdominal cramps, paresthesia in the tongue, tongue swelling, intense pruritus in the face and head, flushing, and urticaria. Two weeks later skin tests showed hypersensitivity to bacitracin but not polymixin.

QUINOLONES *(SEDA-19, 248; SEDA-21, 272)*

Liver Quinolones can occasionally cause liver damage (SEDA-19, 249). *Hepatitis* has now been reported in a man who took ofloxacin followed by ciprofloxacin (68[c]).

A 21-year-old man with Wegener's granulomatosis, who had taken cyclophosphamide, prednisolone, ranitidine, and domperidone for 18 months, was given ofloxacin for 5 days and two doses of ciprofloxacin. He became jaundiced, with hepatomegaly but no splenomegaly or ascites. Ultrasonography was normal and serology for viral hepatitis was negative. His hepatitis resolved slowly after withdrawal of the quinolones.

SULFONAMIDES, TRIMETHOPRIM, AND CO-TRIMOXAZOLE *(SED-13, 826; SEDA-19, 268; SEDA-20, 264; SEDA-21, 274)*

Recent reviews have included the following: (1) the clinical pharmacokinetics of sulfonamides (71[R]); (2) current indications for co-trimoxazole (72[R]); (3) treatment of *Pneumocystis carinii* pneumonia in adults with AIDS (73[R]).

In 20 healthy volunteers who took a 10-day course of trimethoprim, adverse effects occurred in 75% of those who took 20 mg/kg per day, compared with 11% of those who took 10 mg/kg per day (74[C]).

Psychiatric Three cases of *psychotic reactions* have been reported in patients with AIDS taking co-trimoxazole for secondary prophylaxis of *Pneumocystis carinii* pneumonia (75[c]).

Mineral and fluid balance Trimethoprim in therapeutic doses can cause *hyperkalemia* (SEDA-21, 274), since it has potassium-sparing actions like those of amiloride, blocking luminal sodium channels in the distal convoluted tubule (76[R]).

In a comparison of co-trimoxazole ($n = 64$), trimethoprim + dapsone ($n = 58$), and clindamycin + primaquine ($n = 57$), there was a significantly higher incidence of hyperkalemia of grades I (5.6–6.0 mmol/l) and II (6.1–6.5 mmol/l) in the patients who took trimethoprim (77[c]). There was only one case of more severe hyperkalemia (6.6–7.0 mmol/l) in a patient who took trimethoprim + dapsone. The mean plasma potassium concentration was higher in those who took co-trimoxazole than in those who took trimethoprim + dapsone, suggesting that the sulfonamide may in some way potentiate the hyperkalemic action of trimethoprim.

Not surprisingly, other potassium-sparing drugs can enhance the hyperkalemic effect of trimethoprim, as has been demonstrated with spironolactone (78[c]) and the ACE inhibitor ramipril (79[c]), (80[c]).

Hematological It has been suggested that *pure red cell aplasia* in two patients with AIDS may have been due to co-trimoxazole (81[c]).

In 20 healthy volunteers there was a significant *fall in serum folate concentration* during a 10-day course of trimethoprim (20 mg/kg per day) (74[C]). However, blood counts were not reported.

Urinary system In 20 healthy volunteers a 10-day course of trimethoprim (10 or 20 mg/kg per day) significantly *increased serum creatinine concentrations and reduced creatinine clearance* by 16–20 ml/min (74[C]). The effect was the same at both dosages. This effect was attributed to the well-known effect of trimethoprim in inhibiting tubular creatinine secretion and not to any nephrotoxic effect.

Skin and appendages In 20 healthy volunteers who took a 10-day course of trimethoprim, *skin rashes* occurred in 60% of those who took 20 mg/kg per day, compared with 10% of those who took 10 mg/kg per day (74[C]).

Adverse skin reactions that occurred in the divisions of general internal medicine of three different hospitals between 1974 and 1993 have been reported (82[C]). The skin reactions were classified into four groups: maculopapular rashes, urticaria, vasculitis, and nonhomogeneous but clinically well-defined rashes. There were 1317 definite or probable drug-induced skin reactions in 48 005 consecutively hospitalized patients: 1201 cases of maculopapular rashes (91%), 78 cases of urticaria (5.9%), 18 cases of cutaneous vasculitis (1.4%), and 20 cases of other rashes (1.5%; five of erythema multiforme minor, six of fixed eruption, one of photosensitivity, and eight of acneiform eruptions). The main drugs involved did not differ for the first three types of reactions: first penicillins, then sulfonamides (most often combined with trimethoprim), and third NSAIDs. There were no severe events, such as erythema multiforme/-Stevens-Johnson syndrome or toxic epidermal necrolysis. In 5789 patients taking sulfonamides, there were 137 cases of maculopapular rashes, and five each of urticaria and vasculitis.

In addition to the six cases of fixed drug eruption in this study, other cases have been reported (83[C]), (84[c]), (85[c]). In 34 patients with a history of fixed drug eruption caused by co-trimoxazole ($n = 29$) or any other sulfonamide ($n = 5$), trimethoprim was confirmed by rechallenge as the cause in six, all of whom tolerated sulfonamides (83[C]). In three of these patients there was a positive patch test to trimethoprim and in one the diagnosis was confirmed by histological study of the lesion induced by the patch test. In five patients challenge with pyrimethamine was negative, suggesting that there is no cross-reactivity between diaminopyrimidines. Thus, not all cases of fixed drug eruption in patients taking co-trimoxazole are due to the sulfonamide component, but to trimethoprim.

Skin hyperpigmentation was the first sign of folate deficiency in an 18-year-old woman who took pyrimethamine and co-trimoxazole for 2 weeks (86[c]).

Drug rashes are more frequent in patients with HIV infection than in the general population and have been reviewed (54[R]). The incidence was higher in patients with *Pneumocystis carinii* pneumonia than in patients taking prophylactic treatment: in 15 studies involving 697 patients with *Pneumocystis carinii* pneumonia taking co-trimoxazole, 247 (35%) had a rash, and in three studies involving 75 patients taking trimethoprim + dapsone, 32 (43%) had a rash; in contrast, in 10 studies involving 1204 patients taking prophylactic co-trimoxazole, 201 (17%) had a rash. In seven studies involving 351 patients with cerebral toxoplasmosis taking sulfadiazine + pyrimethamine, 103 (29%) had a rash. The rashes usually consist of a spontaneously resolving benign maculopapular rash. Treatment can be continued in over 50% of cases. Signs that require discontinuation are either mucocutaneous signs (mucosal lesions, spots, Nikolski's sign) or related to hematological, hepatic, or renal lesions. Lyell's syndrome and Stevens-Johnson syndrome are 1000 times more frequent than in the general population, but have an identical prognosis. The main drugs that have been incriminated are sulfadiazine, trimethoprim + dapsone, co-trimoxazole, and aminopenicillins. Corticosteroid therapy may play a preventive role, but there have been no prospective studies. Some authors recommend desensitization, but there have been serious adverse events during challenge.

Toxic epidermal necrolysis occurred in a 34-year-old man with AIDS who was taking co-trimoxazole (87[c]).

Special senses *Uveitis* with aseptic meningitis has been reported in an 18-year-old woman who took trimethoprim for 7 days for a urinary tract infection, having previously taken a 7-day course without complications (88[c]). On a subsequent occasion she developed a uveitis with aseptic meningitis 4 h after a single dose of trimethoprim.

A 45-year-old woman who had recurrent urinary tract infections treated with co-trimoxazole, trimethoprim alone, and ciprofloxacin developed bilateral anterior uveitis after taking co-trimoxazole and trimethoprim and retinal haemorrhages after taking trimethoprim (89[c]).

Immunological and hypersensitivity reactions Hypersensitivity reactions to co-trimoxazole are common in patients with AIDS. Sulfonamides are partly detoxified by the action of glutathione-*S*-transferases, of which there are two major genotypes, M1 and T1. These genotypes are absent in 55 and 15% of Caucasians, respectively. In 80 Caucasian patients and 205 healthy controls the distribution of the M1 and T1 genotypes was similar. However, in the patients with AIDS the M1 genotype was absent in significantly more patients who were sulfonamide intolerant (72%) than in those who were tolerant (48%); there was no such association with the T1 genotype (90[C]). The authors suggested that deficiency of glutathione and absence of M1 glutathione-*S*-transferase activity might favor the accumulation of nitrososulfonamide derivatives, the covalent binding of which to cellular macromolecules could mediate hypersensitivity reactions.

Desensitization with a combination product of sulfamethoxazole and trimethoprim has been performed over 2 days in 48 patients infected with HIV with a history of allergic reactions (e.g., rash) to co-trimoxazole (91[C]). Of the 48 patients, 37 (77%) tolerated co-trimoxazole desensitization without adverse effects and continued to take co-trimoxazole daily. Desensitization failed in 11 patients, one of whom developed acute hypotension and a non-fatal myocardial infarction. The factors that were predictive of failure were a high CD4+ cell percentage (11 vs 8%) and a high CD4+/CD8+ ratio (0.27 vs 0.12). The authors concluded that desensitization with co-trimoxazole was effective and was more often successful in patients with lower CD4+ cell percentages and CD4+/CD8+ ratios. However, they suggested that co-trimoxazole should be reintroduced carefully.

Interactions *Pindolol* In eight young men (22–33 years) and seven elderly men (62–79 years) who took pindolol 10 mg bd, trimethoprim 200 mg od reduced the renal clearance of *R*(+)-pindolol in the young subjects by 37% and in the elderly subjects by 26%; trimethoprim reduced the renal clearance of *S*(−)-pindolol in a similar fashion (92[C]). Stereoselective renal excretion of pindolol was unaffected by trimethoprim, and the *R*(+)/*S*(−)-pindolol renal clearance ratio was unchanged from control in all of the subjects. The mechanism of the effect of trimethoprim on pindolol renal clearance was inhibition of organic base secretion.

Tolbutamide Sulfonamides inhibit tolbutamide hydroxylation by inhibition of CYP2C9. In goat hepatic microsomes the K_i for the sulfonamides was 205–4546 μmol/l, sulfadoxine having the lowest K_i, followed by sulfadimethoxine, sulfamoxole, sulfadimidine, and sulfaphenazole; however, in hepatocytes sulfaphenazole was the most potent inhibitor (93).

REFERENCES

1. Chapel KL, Rasmussen JE. Pediatric dermatology: advances in therapy. J Am Acad Dermatol 1997;36:513–26.
2. Epstein ME, Amodio-Groton M, Sadick NS. Antimicrobial agents for the dermatologist. II. Macrolides, fluoroquinolones, rifamycins, tetracyclines, trimethoprim-sulfamethoxazole, and clindamycin. J Am Acad Dermatol 1997;37:365–81.
3. Dashe JS, Gilstrap III LC. Antibiotic use in pregnancy. Obstet Gynecol Clin North Am 1997;24:617–29.
4. Edwards MS. Antibacterial therapy in pregnancy and neonates. Clin Perinatol 1997;24:251–66.
5. Foxworth J. Recognizing and preventing antibiotic-associated complications in the critical care setting. Crit Care Nurs Q 1997;20:1–11.
6. Farber MS, Abrams JH. Antibiotics for the acute abdomen. Surg Clin North Am 1997; 77:1395–417.
7. Mini E, Nobili S, Periti P. Methicillin-resistant staphylococci in clean surgery. Is there a role for prophylaxis? Drugs 1997;54 (Suppl 6):39–52.
8. Iwata S, Akita H. Adverse effects of antibiotics. Acta Paediatr Jpn Overs Ed 1997;39:143–54.
9. Sternbach H, State R. Antibiotics: neuropsychiatric effects and psychotropic interactions. Harv Rev Psychiatry 1997;5:214–26.
10. Vial T, Biour M, Descotes J, Trepo C. Antibiotic-associated hepatitis: update from 1990. Ann Pharmacother 1997;31:204–20.
11. Eichler G, Merk HF. Unerwünschte Arzneimittelreaktionen durch Antibiotika. Allergologie 1997;20:368–74.
12. Craig WA, Andes D. Aminoglycosides are useful for severe respiratory tract infections. Semin Respir Infect 1997;12:271–7.
13. Berg JM, Nahum A, Tschida SJ. Novel approaches to drug delivery in critical care. Semin Respir Crit Care Med 1997;18:65–78.
14. Hatala R, Dinh TT, Cook DJ. Single daily dosing of aminoglycosides in immunocompromised adults: a systematic review. Clin Infect Dis 1997;24:810–16.
15. Gilbert DN. Editorial response: meta-analyses are no longer required for determining the efficacy of single daily dosing of aminoglycosides. Clin Infect Dis 1997;24:816–19.
16. Swan SK. Aminoglycoside nephrotoxicity. Semin Nephrol 1997;17:27–33.
17. Choudhury D, Ahmed Z. Drug-induced nephrotoxicity. Med Clin North Am 1997;81:705–17.
18. Bennett WM. Drug nephrotoxicity: an overview. Renal Fail 1997;19:221–4.
19. Kemery V Jr, Halko J, Kralovicova K, Grausova S, Stopkova K, Netriova J. Netilmicin serum levels in 138 cancer patients. Do they predict nephrotoxicity or therapeutic failure? Int J Antimicrob Agents 1997;8:215–16.
20. Barretti P, Soares VA. Acute renal failure: clinical outcome and causes of death. Renal Fail 1997;19:253–7.
21. Mittal S, Kher V, Gulati S, Agarwal LK, Arora P. Chronic renal failure in India. Renal Fail 1997;19:763–70.
22. Gainza FJ, Minguela JI, Lampreabe I. Aminoglycoside-associated Fanconi's syndrome: an underrecognized entity. Nephron 1997;77:205–11.
23. Usami S-I, Abe S, Kasai M, Shinkawa H, Moeller B, Kenyon JB, Kimberling WJ. Genetic and clinical features of sensorineural hearing loss associated with the 1555 mitochondrial mutation. Laryngoscope 1997;107:483–90.
24. Pandya A, Xia X, Radnaabazar J, Batsuuri J, Dangaansuren B, Fischel-Ghodsian N, Nance WE. Mutation in the mitochondrial 12S rRNA gene in two families from Mongolia with matrilineal aminoglycoside ototoxicity. J Med Genet 1997;34:169–72.
25. Fischel-Ghodsian N, Prezant TR, Chaltraw WE, Wendt KA, Nelson RA, Arnos KS, Falk RE. Mitochondrial gene mutation is a significant predisposing factor in aminoglycoside ototoxicity. Am J Otolaryngol Head Neck Med Surg 1997;18:173–8.
26. Hui Y, Park A, Crysdale WS, Forte V. Ototoxicity from ototopical aminoglycosides. J Otolaryngol 1997;26:53–6.
27. Corsten M, Marsan J, Schramm D, Robichaud J. Treatment of intractable Menière's disease with intratympanic gentamicin: review of the University of Ottawa experience. J Otolaryngol 1997;26:361–4.
28. Nix DE, Thomas JK, Symonds WT, Spivey JM, Wilton JH, Gagliardi NC, Schentag JJ. Assessment of the enzymuria resulting from gentamicin alone and combinations of gentamicin with various beta-lactam antibiotics. Ann Pharmacother 1997;31:696–703.
29. Patel SS, Balfour JA, Bryson HM. Fosfomycin tromethamine. A review of its antibacterial activity, pharmacokinetic properties and therapeutic efficacy as a single-dose oral treatment for acute uncomplicated lower urinary tract infections. Drugs 1997;53:637–56.
30. Gelfand M, Johnson R. Single-dose fosfomycin tromethamine: evaluation in the treatment of uncomplicated lower urinary tract infection. Adv Ther 1997;14:49–63.

31. Anonymous. Fosfomycin for urinary tract infections. Med Lett Drugs Ther 1997;39:66–8.
32. Zeckel ML. A closer look at vancomycin, teicoplanin, and antimicrobial resistance. J Chemother 1997;9:311–35.
33. Grüneberg RN. Anti-Gram-positive agents. What we have and what we would like. Drugs 1997;54 (Suppl 6):29–38.
34. Graninger W, Presterl E, Wenisch C, Schwameis E, Breyer S, Vukovich T. Management of serious staphylococcal infections in the outpatient setting. Drugs 1997;54 (Suppl 6):21–8.
35. Rizzato G, Allegra L, on behalf of the Multicentre Italian Study Group coordinated by Centro Thorax. Efficacy and tolerability of a teicoplanin- ciprofloxacin combination in severe community-acquired pneumonia. Comparison with ceftriaxone in a Multicentre Italian Study. Clin Drug Invest 1997;14:337–45.
36. Bréchignac X, Boibieux A, Bernard P, Peyramond D. Toxicité hématologique sévère de la teicoplanine: deux observations. Méd Mal Infect 1997;27:1034–6.
37. Lupo A, Rugiu C, Bernich P, Laudon A, Marcantoni C, Mosconi G, Cantaluppi MC, Maschio G. A prospective, randomized trial of two antibiotic regimens in the treatment of peritonitis in CAPD patients: teicoplanin plus tobramycin versus cephalothin plus tobramycin. J Antimicrob Chemother 1997;40:729–32.
38. Venditti M, Tarasi A, Capone A, Galié M, Menichetti F, Martino P, Serra P. Teicoplanin in the treatment of enterococcal endocarditis: clinical and microbiological study. J Antimicrob Chemother 1997;40:449–52.
39. Acosta FG, Liberato NL, Chiofalo F. Warfarin resistance induced by teicoplanin. Haematologica 1997;82:637–8.
40. Casali A, Santini S, Della Giulia M, Di Lauro L, Vici P, Gionfra T, Sega FM. Triple combination antimicrobial regimen in the treatment of infections of neutropenic cancer patients. J Exp Clin Cancer Res 1997;16:321–4.
41. Meehan KR, Verma UN, Esteva-Lorenzo F, Mazumder A. Suppression of progenitor cell growth by vancomycin following autologous stem cell transplantation. Bone Marrow Transplant 1997;19:1029–32.
42. Shuster J. Reversible neutropenia associated with iv vancomycin. Hosp Pharm 1997;32:824–6.
43. Mandl DL, Garrison MW, Palpant SD. Agranulocytosis induced by vancomycin or ticarcillin/-clavulanate. Ann Pharmacother 1997;31:1321–4.
44. Howard CE, Adams LA, Admire JL, Chu MA, Alred GL. Vancomycin-induced thrombocytopenia: a challenge and rechallenge. Ann Pharmacother 1997;31:315–18.
45. Mizon P, Kiefel V, Mannessier L, Mueller-Eckhardt C, Goudemand J. Thrombocytopenia induced by vancomycin-dependent platelet antibody. Vox Sang 1997;73:49–51.
46. Toyoguchi T, Takahashi S, Hosoya J, Nakagawa Y, Watanabe H. Nephrotoxicity of vancomycin and drug interaction study with cilastatin in rabbits. Antimicrob Agents Chemother 1997;41:1985–90.
47. Korman TM, Turnidge JD, Grayson ML. Risk factors for adverse cutaneous reactions associated with intravenous vancomycin. J Antimicrob Chemother 1997;39:371–81.
48. Imai T, Tanaka K, Chokyu H, Miyazaki S, Matsui T, Arakawa S, Kamidono S, Saito H, Harada K, Tachibana Y, Kataoka N, Takenaka A, Kobayashi M, Omae H, Shinozaki M, Mizuno Y, Tatsumi N, Ogawa T, Yamanaka K, Kondo K, Nakagawa H, Shirakawa T, Goto K. Fundamental and clinical studies on the effect of combination therapy with imipenem/cilastatin and vancomycin in patients with MRSA infections in the urological field. Ishinihon J Urol 1997;59:192–8.
49. Kahata K, Hashino S, Imamura M, Mori A, Kobayashi S, Asaka M. Inhaled vancomycin-induced allergic reaction in decontamination of respiratory tracts for allogeneic bone marrow transplantation. Bone Marrow Transplant 1997; 20:1001–3.
50. Marik PE, Ferris N. Delayed hypersensitivity reaction to vancomycin. Pharmacotherapy 1997;17:1341–4.
51. Wong P-N, Mak S-K, Lee K-F, Fung LH, Wong AKM. A prospective study of Vancomycin-(Vancoled-) induced chemical peritonitis in CAPD patients. Peritoneal Dial Int 1997;17:202–4.
52. Ergür AT, Onarlioglu B, Günay Y, Çetinkaya O, Bulut HE. Does vancomycine increase aminoglycoside nephrotoxicity? Acta Paediatr Jpn Overs Ed 1997;39:422–7.
53. Leal T, Dupret P, Hassoun A, Wallemacq PE. Topical application of eosin to burns produces interference in measurement of serum vancomycin by fluorescence polarization immunoassay. Clin Chem 1997;43:1238–40.
54. Bocquet H, Chosidow O. Les toxidermies cours du SIDA. Rev Fr Allergol Immunol Clin 1997;37:678–84.
55. Vergis EN, Yu VL. Macrolides are ideal for empiric therapy of community-acquired pneumonia in the immunocompetent host. Semin Respir Infect 1997;12:322–8.
56. Tarlow MJ, Block SL, Harris J, Kolokathis A. Future indications for macrolides. Pediatr Infect Dis J 1997;16:457–62.
57. Tarlow MJ. Macrolides in the management of streptococcal pharyngitis/tonsillitis. Pediatr Infect Dis J 1997;16:444–8.
58. Klein JO. History of macrolide use in pediatrics. Pediatr Infect Dis J 1997;16:427–41.
59. Amsden GW, Peloquin CA, Berning SE. The role of advanced generation macrolides in the prophylaxis and treatment of *Mycobacterium avium* complex (MAC) infections. Drugs 1997;54:69–80.
60. Charles L, Segreti J. Choosing the right macrolide antibiotic. A guide to selection. Drugs 1997;53:349–57.

61. Anonymous. Dirithromycin. Prescrire Int 1997;6:69–71.
62. Hübner C, Dietz A, Stremmel W, Stiehl A, Andrassy K. Macrolide-induced Churg-Strauss syndrome in a patient with atopy. Lancet 1997;350:563.
63. Watkins VS, Polk RE, Stotka JL. Drug interactions of macrolides: emphasis on dirithromycin. Ann Pharmacother 1997;31:349–56.
64. Bizjak ED, Mauro VF. Digoxin-macrolide drug interaction. Ann Pharmacother 1997; 31:1077–9.
65. Anonymous. Pimozide and macrolide antibiotics contraindicated. P T 1997;22:17.
66. Pauwels O. Tacrolimus (FK506) et interactions médicamenteuses. J Pharm Clin 1997;16:75–81.
67. Dyck ED, Vadas P. Anaphylaxis to topical bacitracin. Allergy Eur J Allergy Clin Immunol 1997;52:870–1.
68. Jones SE, Smith RH. Quinolones may induce hepatitis. Br Med J 1997;314:869.
69. Zompi S, Bocquet H, Houhou S. Syndrome de choc toxique d'origine médicamenteuse chez un patient séropositif pour le VIH. Med Ther 1997;3:419–23.
70. Guay DRP. Implications of quinolone pharmacokinetic drug interactions. Hosp Pharm 1997;32:677–60.
71. Vree TB, Van Der Ven AJAM. Clinical pharmacokinetics of sulphonamides. Chemother J 1997;6:21–7.
72. Tauchnitz Ch. Stellung der Trimethoprim-Sulfonamid Kombination heute. Chemother J 1997;6:17–20.
73. Deresinski SC. Treatment of *Pneumocystis carinii* pneumonia in adults with AIDS. Semin Respir Infect 1997;12:79–97.
74. Naderer O, Nafziger AN, Bertino JS Jr. Effects of moderate-dose versus high-dose trimethoprim on serum creatinine and creatinine clearance and adverse reactions. Antimicrob Agents Chemother 1997;41:11.
75. Geit M, Simma R, Wimberger F. Psychotische Reaktionen nach hochdosierter Gabe von Sulfametrol-Trimethoprim. Chemother J 1997;6:169.
76. Perazella MA. Trimethoprim is a potassium-sparing diuretic like amiloride and causes hyperkalemia in high-risk patients. Am J Ther 1997;4:343–8.
77. Safrin S, Finkelstein D. Comparison of oral agents for treatment of *Pneumocystis carinii* pneumonia. Ann Intern Med 1997;126:407–8.
78. Marinella MA. Severe hyperkalemia associated with trimethoprim-sulfamethoxazole and spironolactone. Infect Dis Clin Pract 1997;6:256–60.
79. Bugge JF. Severe hyperkalaemia induced by trimethoprim in combination with an angiotensin-converting enzyme inhibitor in a patient with transplanted lungs. J Intern Med 1996;240:249–52.
80. Jolobe OMP. Severe hyperkalaemia induced by trimethoprim in combination with an angiotensin-converting enzyme inhibitor in a patient with transplanted lungs. J Intern Med 1997;242:88–9.
81. Stricker RB, Goldberg B. AIDS and pure red cell aplasia. Am J Hematol 1997;54:264.
82. Hunziker Th, Kunzi U-P, Braunschweig S, Zehnder D, Hoigné R. Comprehensive hospital drug monitoring (CHDM): adverse skin reactions, a 20-year survey. Allergy Eur J Allergy Clin Immunol 1997;52:388–93.
83. De Barrio M, Herrero T, Tornero P, Armentia L, Rubio M. Exantema fijo por trimetoprim: incidencia, diagn-stico y reactividad cruzada. Rev Esp Allergol Inmunol Clin 1997;12:106–10.
84. Willms-Jones JCh, Jenke S, Feuker W, Schultz-Ehrenburg U. Multilokuläres fixes Arzneimittelexanthem. H G Z Hautkr 1997;72:852–3.
85. Özkaya-Bayazit E, Baykal C. Trimethoprim-induced linear fixed drug eruption. Br J Dermatol 1997;137:1028–9.
86. Jucgla A, Sais G, Berlanga J, Servitje O. Hyperpigmentation of the flexures and pancytopenia during treatment with folate antagonists. Acta Derm-Venereol 1997;77:165–6.
87. Quintas S, Do Carmo G, Gama R, Norberto A, Xavier R, Coutinho VS. Sindrome de Lyell num doente com SIDA. Acta Med Port 1997; 10:509–16.
88. Gilroy N, Gottlieb T, Spring P, Peiris O. Trimethoprim-induced aseptic meningitis and uveitis. Lancet 1997;350:112.
89. Kristinsson JK, Hannesson OB, Sveinsson O, Thorleifsson H. Bilateral anterior uveitis and retinal haemorrhages after administration of trimethoprim. Acta Ophthalmol Scand 1997;75:314–15.
90. Deloménie C, Mathelier-Fusade P, Longuemaux S, Rozenbaum W, Leynadier F, Krishnamoorthy R, Dupret J-M. Glutathione S-transferase (*GSTM 1*) null genotype and sulphonamide intolerance in acquired immunodeficiency syndrome. Pharmacogenetics 1997;7:519–20.
91. Caumes E, Guermonprez G, Lecomte C, Katlama C, Bricaire F. Efficacy and safety of desensitization with sulfamethoxazole and trimethoprim in 48 previously hypersensitive patients infected with human immunodeficiency virus. Arch Dermatol 1997;133:465–9.
92. Ujhelyi MR, Bottorff MB, Schur M, Roll K, Zhang H, Stewart J, Markel ML. Aging effects on the organic base transporter and stereoselective renal clearance. Clin Pharmacol Ther 1997;62:117–28.
93. Zweers-Zeilmaker WM, Horbach GJ, Witkamp RF. Differential inhibitory effects of phenytoin, diclofenac, phenylbutazone and a series of sulfonamides on hepatic cytochrome P4502C activity in vitro, and correlation with some molecular descriptors in the dwarf goat (*Caprus hircus aegagrus*). Xenobiotica 1997;27:769–80.

Robert G. Irwin, Andreas H. Groll and Thomas J. Walsh

27 Antifungal drugs

AMPHOTERICIN B *(SED-13, 774; SEDA-19, 257; SEDA-20, 250; SEDA-21, 282)*

Amphotericin remains the most important drug for the treatment of life-threatening invasive fungals in immunocompromised patients. While the results of phase I/II studies with the novel lipid formulation are now being published, at the same time more detailed information on the safety and tolerability of amphotericin B deoxycholate also has become available, allowing better assessment of its toxicity profile.

Amphotericin B deoxycholate (D-AmB)

In a multicenter, randomized, double-blind trial designed and co-ordinated by the NIAID Mycoses Study Group, the effectiveness of 14 days of higher-dose D-AmB (0.7 mg/kg per day) with or without flucytosine (100 mg/kg per day) as induction therapy was investigated in 381 adults with AIDS-associated cryptococcal meningitis (1[C]). Compared with regimens used in previous studies, higher-dose D-AmB plus flucytosine was associated with an increased rate of cerebrospinal fluid sterilization (60%) and reduced mortality (5.5%) at 2 weeks. A total of 11 patients (2.9%; 5 vs 6 for both groups) had toxic effects requiring the withdrawal of study drug (*raised serum creatinine*, three; *nausea*, two; *hypokalemia*, two; *rash*, *headache*, *hemolytic anemia*, and *gastrointestinal hemorrhage*, one each). Among the patients with normal serum creatinine concentrations at baseline, 1% in each group had values that were more than three times the upper limit of the reference range during the 2 weeks of treatment. Overall, the combination of D-AmB plus flucytosine was well tolerated.

In a comparison of D-AmB (1 mg/kg per day over 2 h on days 1–41 and 61–80) with sodium antimony gluconate in the treatment of Indian post-kala-azar dermal leishmaniasis, 11 patients were given D-AmB and all developed *fever and chills* during infusion (2[c]). However, these events were considered mild and were observed only during the first 20 days of treatment. Three patients had *increases in serum creatinine* not exceeding 167 μmol/l (2.0 mg/dl). D-AmB achieved a 100% cure rate with no relapse after 12 months of follow-up, compared with 63% in patients treated with sodium antimony gluconate.

Cardiovascular *Raynaud's syndrome* in the legs during inhalation of an aerosolized D-AmB solution in water (5 mg/ml; target dose 10 mg) has been reported in two children with cancer. The symptoms were reversible and did not recur when the patients were rechallenged with intravenous L-AmB (3[C]). The authors proposed that constriction of peripheral blood vessels mediated by thromboxane A2 was the underlying mechanism.

Acute *hypertension* can occur in association with D-AmB therapy (SEDA-21, 282). Exacerbation of underlying hypertension during D-AmB infusion (0.7 mg/kg over 2 h) has recently been reported in an adult with AIDS-associated cryptococcal meningitis that was eventually fatal (4[r]). Increases in blood pressure occurred with each of 26 daily infusions of D-AmB. Extension of the infusion time to 6 h did not prevent the hypertensive response. This report underscores the need for close monitoring of the blood pressure in patients receiving D-AmB, at least during the first infusion.

Mineral and fluid balance A 17-year-old boy with chronic granulomatous disease devel-

Side Effects of Drugs, Annual 22
J.K. Aronson, ed.

oped magnesium loss with tetany, despite apparent correction of hypomagnesemia, after being given D-AmB (5[c]). The authors pointed to the predominantly intracellular distribution of magnesium and the need for sufficient amounts of supplementary $MgSO_4$ for correcting long-standing hypomagnesemia.

Urinary system In a randomized, prospective multicenter comparison in Canada of fluconazole with amphotericin B deoxycholate (D-AmB) in the treatment of candidemia, 106 non-neutropenic adults were randomized to receive fluconazole 400 mg/day for 4 weeks or D-AmB 0.6 mg/kg per day to complete a cumulative dose of 8 mg/kg (20 mg/kg in the case of evidence of a metastatic site) (6[C]). Enrolment was stratified by disease severity. For the intention-to-treat group ($n = 103$), the mean daily dose of fluconazole was 466 mg and that of D-AmB 0.53 mg/kg, and the median durations of treatment were 21 (range 1–89) and 15 (range 1–53) days, respectively. The intention-to-treat analysis showed no differences in clinical response rates (50 vs 58%) or mortality (26 vs 21%) at day 14. *Nephrotoxicity*, however, defined as an increase in the serum creatinine concentration to ≥1.5 times baseline, occurred significantly more often with D-AmB (43 vs 19%). There were no differences with respect to other adverse drug effects.

In vitro studies have shown that D-AmB, which distributes into high-density lipoproteins (HDL) and low-density lipoproteins (LDL) in plasma after intravenous administration, is less toxic to the kidney when it is associated with HDL cholesterol than with LDL cholesterol (7). The results of a small pilot investigation in critically ill patients have suggested that patients with raised concentrations of LDL cholesterol may indeed be more susceptible to the nephrotoxic effects of D-AmB, when an undefined threshold in the cumulative dose is reached (8[c]).

Intravenous D-AmB causes vasoconstriction, ischemia, and oliguria in animals (9). Since adenosine is excreted in the urine by the ischemic kidney, urinary adenosine excretion has been measured in 20 adults who were receiving D-AmB (15–75 mg intravenously), before and for 2 h during the infusion on 1 day during the first 4 days of treatment (10[C]). Infusion of D-AmB was associated with a significant reduction in mean urinary output, both in patients who were loaded with isotonic saline (500 ml before D-AmB) and in those who were not. The mean urinary adenosine excretion was unchanged in the saline-loaded group and, surprisingly, was reduced in the comparator group. Development of renal insufficiency later during treatment did not correlate with changes in urinary output or adenosine excretion during the first days of therapy.

Risk factors *Children* The toxic effects of D-AmB in infants of very low birth weight (<1500 g) have been evaluated retrospectively (11[C]). Of the patients with systemic candidiasis 18 received D-AmB once daily over 4–6 h. The initial dose was 0.25 mg/kg and the dose was increased in daily increments of 0.25 mg/kg to a maximum of 1 mg/kg; the mean cumulative dose was 20 mg/kg. Two infants with pre-existing raised BUN concentrations had *a fall in urinary output* (less than 1 ml/kg per h), which improved after interruption of therapy for 24 h. *Hypokalemia* was observed on a single occasion in each of two infants and resolved without treatment. Six infants had thrombocytopenia before therapy, which resolved within the first week of treatment. There was no evidence of hepatic toxicity. None of the infants had fever (over 37.5°C).

The infusion-related adverse effects of D-AmB (0.5 mg/kg) administered over 1 or 4 h have been studied in 24 immunocompromised children (12[C]). All were premedicated with diphenhydramine and paracetamol. Although *chills* appeared to be more severe in the rapid infusion group on day 1, the mean chill score in both groups after day 1 was similar. One patient in the standard 4-h infusion arm developed *bradycardia*, and there were also more patients with *diastolic hypotension* in this group. There were no differences in renal and hepatic function. The authors suggested that a larger trial might be warranted to investigate the short infusion regimen, which may be beneficial for multimorbid patients and outpatient treatment options.

Aerosolized amphotericin Two studies have provided data on the adverse effects of aerosolized D-AmB in the prevention of invasive mycoses of the lung.

In 126 patients who had receiving a lung, heart-lung, or heart transplant aerosolized D-AmB B 20 mg tds caused *nausea*, the only adverse effect, in 10 (7.9%), leading to withdrawal of treatment in two patients ([13c]).

Of 42 neutropenic patients with hematological malignancies, only 48% managed to complete the scheduled regimen of D-AmB (2 ml of a 5 mg/ml solution given over 20 min) and 52% had adverse effects, which consisted of *cough*, *dyspnea*, *pulmonary obstruction*, *nausea*, and *vomiting*; five patients stopped treatment because of adverse effects ([14C]).

The efficacy of aerosolized D-AmB has not yet been investigated in a randomized, prospective, comparison. In the first of the studies discussed here there was a significant reduction in invasive fungal infections compared with a historical control group. However, historically controlled comparisons in aspergillosis may be difficult to interpret if populations are not carefully balanced for risk factors and environmental exposure. To illustrate this point, the second uncontrolled trial of aerosolized D-AmB showed poor tolerability and a high rate of proven or possible invasive fungal infections (28%).

Amphotericin B Colloidal Dispersion (ABCD)

A combined safety analysis from five open-label Phase I/II studies of 572 adults and children, mostly pretreated immunocompromised patients, reported infusion-related adverse effects with at least one infusion in 62% of patients; other, non-acute adverse effects recorded in under 10% of patients were *abdominal pain* (11%), *thrombocytopenia* (11%), *hypertension* (11%), *headache* (11%), and *raised creatinine concentrations* (10%) ([15C]). Mean serum creatinine concentrations at the end of therapy were not different from those at baseline. Adverse effects attributable to ABCD and requiring withdrawal occurred in 70 patients (12%). The most frequent of these were *infusion-related adverse events* (5.4%), followed by *raised serum creatinine concentrations* (3.3%) and *abnormal liver function tests* (1.4%). The mean daily dose in the analysed trials was 3.9 (range 0.1–9.1) mg/kg and the median total number of treatment days was 16 (range 1–409); the median cumulative dose of ABCD was 58 (range 0.1–1378) mg/kg. The maximum tolerated dose was 7.5 mg/kg.

Urinary system A pooled retrospective subgroup analysis was performed on 82 mostly adult patients with proven or probable aspergillosis who were treated with ABCD in a daily dose of 0.5–8 mg/kg (median duration of treatment, 24 days; median cumulative dose, 5.9 g; range 0.4–34) ([16C]). There was *nephrotoxicity*, defined as a doubling of the serum creatinine concentration from baseline, an increase of at least 1 mg/dl, or a 50% fall in calculated creatinine clearance, in six of 73 ABCD recipients (8.2%); the median serum creatinine concentration at the end of therapy was unchanged compared with baseline. Overall responses (49%) and survival rates (50%) were better than those observed in 261 patients treated with D-AmB at six cancer or transplant centers between 1990 and 1994.

Amphotericin B Lipid Complex (ABLC)

The efficacy and safety of 68 courses of ABLC (5 mg/kg) have been evaluated in 64 adults with hematological malignancies and presumed or proven fungal infections; half of the patients were recipients of an allogeneic ($n = 23$) or autologous ($n = 9$) bone marrow transplant ([17C]). Seven patients, who were not premedicated, developed *febrile reactions* to ABLC, and the drug was stopped in five of those. Another patient developed tachycardia and tachypnea and was withdrawn from study after 8 days. There was a doubling in serum creatinine in seven of 53 evaluable courses (13%), necessitating withdrawal of the drug in three patients (6%). The overall response rate in 53 evaluable courses was 71%.

In an analysis of 95 bone marrow transplant recipients with presumed or confirmed invasive fungal infections who received ABLC in an emergency use program at a daily target dose of 5 mg/kg (mean cumulative dose 6314 mg; range 80–40 700; mean duration of treatment 25 days; range 1–198), 53% of 59 clinically evaluable patients responded (18[C]). There was a doubling in serum creatinine at some time during therapy in 12 of 90 evaluable patients; however, only two patients discontinued therapy because of kidney-related adverse events. Patients who entered the study with raised serum creatinine concentrations had a statistically significant fall in the mean serum creatinine at 3 and 6 weeks from baseline. Altogether, 10 patients discontinued therapy because of an adverse event (*anemia*, two; *renal insufficiency*, *raised serum creatinine*, *altered mental state*, *bilirubinemia*, *sepsis*, *chills*, *anaphylactic reaction*, *respiratory failure*, one case each).

The efficacy and safety of ABLC have also been analysed in 13 liver transplant patients who received the drug in dosages of 1.25–5 mg/kg per day (mean duration of treatment 6.5 weeks; range 1–16; mean total dose 11.3 g, range 1.76–26.0) (19[C]). The baseline serum creatinine in 12 patients was over 220 μmol/l (2.5 mg/dl), and all of these patients were on hemodialysis when ABLC was begun. Of the seven survivors, six discontinued dialysis within 1 week of completion of therapy, and all had improved renal function during treatment. The remaining patient had a third liver transplant and a kidney transplant; his serum creatinine improved during treatment with ABLC. Of the six non-survivors, two had significant improvements in renal function while receiving ABLC. There were infusion-related *fever and chills* in two patients each (15%). The overall response rate to ABLC therapy was 65%.

The minimal effective dose of ABLC against visceral leishmaniasis unresponsive to antimony has been evaluated in an randomized open-label study in 60 patients who were given ABLC once daily by 2 h infusion on 5 consecutive days (20[c]). The patients were randomly assigned to receive 1, 2, or 3 mg/kg to a total dose of 5, 10, and 15 mg/kg. While almost all of these unpremedicated patients had *fever and chills* during the first infusion, these reactions diminished with subsequent infusions, and 42% had no infusion-related reactions with the fifth dose. Laboratory investigation of renal function on day 19 showed no abnormalities. Responses to treatment ranged from 84 to 100% and were dose dependent.

Risk factors *Children* The safety and tolerance of ABLC have been studied in children with cancers (21[C]). Six children with hepatosplenic candidiasis received ABLC 2.5 mg/kg for 6 weeks to a total dose of 105 mg/kg. Compared with baseline, the mean serum creatinine was stable at the end of therapy and at follow-up at 1 month. *Hypokalemia* and *hypomagnesemia* occurred in one and two patients, respectively. There were no abnormalities of hepatic transaminases, bilirubin, alkaline phosphatase, or hematological measurements attributable to ABLC. Five of the six patients had infusion-related toxicity (*fevers*, *chills*, *rigors*, *nausea*, *headache*) with the first 2.5 mg/kg dose before administration of premedication. These reactions were mild to moderate and were well controlled thereafter by conventional premedications, including paracetamol, diphenhydramine, meperidine, and lorazepam. All five evaluable patients had a partial or complete response to treatment.

Liposomal Amphotericin B (AmBisome)

A combined analysis of two parallel, prospective, open-label, randomized, multicenter comparisons of liposomal amphotericin (L-AmB) and D-AmB as empirical antifungal therapy in 338 persistently febrile neutropenic adults and children has been published (22[C]). They received either D-AmB (1 mg/kg per day, which is higher than the recommended dose of 0.5–0.6 mg/kg per day for this indication) or L-AmB (1 or 3 mg/kg per day). While the results of these studies provided evidence for at least equivalent efficacy, there were significantly fewer drug-related adverse effects with L-AmB. There were severe drug-related adverse effects in 11 of the 102 patients who received D-AmB: *nephrotoxicity* ($n = 7$), *rigors*, *fevers*, and *skin rash* ($n = 2$), and *hypokalemia* and *dyspnea* ($n = 1$ each); in contrast, only three of 236 patients who received L-AmB developed severe drug-related adverse reactions: *encephalopathy*, *con-*

vulsions, and *hypokalemia* ($n = 1$ each). Dosage reduction or withdrawal was required on 35 occasions with D-AmB and on 15 occasions with L-AmB. There was significantly less hypokalemia in patients treated with L-AmB, despite freely prescribed potassium supplements or potassium-sparing diuretics. Nephrotoxicity, defined as a 100% or more increase in serum creatinine from baseline, occurred significantly more often with D-AmB (24%) compared with L-AmB (11%), independent of other concomitant nephrotoxic drugs, such as platinum derivatives, aminoglycosides, vancomycin, and cyclosporin. Moreover, the time to develop nephrotoxicity was significantly longer with L-AmB than with D-AmB.

In a small, open-label, randomized comparison of L-AmB with D-AmB for induction therapy of AIDS-associated cryptococcal meningitis, patients received either L-AmB 4 mg/kg per day ($n = 15$) or D-AmB 0.7 mg/kg per day ($n = 13$) for 3 weeks, followed by fluconazole 400 mg/day for 7 more weeks (23[c]). The time to and the rate of clinical response were identical in the 28 evaluable patients (L-AmB 15, D-AmB 13), but there was more rapid clearance of cerebrospinal fluid by L-AmB. Amphotericin was prematurely discontinued because of toxicity in one patient receiving L-AmB (mild somnolence) and in two patients receiving D-AmB (increase in serum creatinine and abnormal liver function tests). There were acute reactions during the first infusion of L-AmB in two patients (*tachycardia*, *hypotension*, *facial flushing*, *tickling cough* in one patient; *tachycardia*, *shortness of breath*, and *fever* in the other). These reactions did not recur when the infusion was continued at a lower rate. Serum creatinine concentrations rose significantly more during treatment with D-AmB. D-AmB and L-AmB caused hypokalemia in three and four patients, respectively.

Safety data are also available from 74 patients with bone marrow transplants who received L-AmB in an initial median dose of 2.8 (range 0.6–5.1) mg/kg for 13 (range 1–55) days for a variety of reasons (24[c]). There were adverse effects in three patients, requiring withdrawal in one patient who presented with *fever and severe chills*. The other two patients had *headache*, *abdominal pain*, and *fever*. The serum creatinine rose to more than 200% of baseline values in eight patients. Most of the patients had increases in serum bilirubin and hepatic transaminases, but the frequency of high-grade graft-versus-host disease and/or veno-occlusive disease was high, precluding any definitive conclusions about hepatotoxicity.

Risk factors *Children* The safety of L-AmB has been investigated in 15 children with bone marrow transplants and primary immunodeficiencies (25[C]). The mean daily dose was 5 (range 2–6) mg/kg and the mean duration of treatment 43 (range 6–195) days. Except for a low-grade *fever* in one patient, a significant *increase in serum creatinine* in one, and mild *hypokalemia* in four, L-AmB was well tolerated.

L-AmB (1–3 mg/kg, cumulative dose up to 30 mg/kg) was well tolerated when it was used as first-choice treatment of *L. infantum* visceral leishmaniasis in 106 immunocompetent children (3 months to 14 years of age) in an endemic area in Italy (26[c]). No clinical or biochemical adverse effects were noted.

Two premature infants (birth weights 2600 and 590 g) with underlying renal impairment and candidemia (associated with meningitis in the second case) were successfully treated with L-AmB (3 and 5 mg/kg per day for 26 and 27 days, respectively) (27[c]). Except for a slight transient rise in serum transaminases in one case and hyperbilirubinemia in the other, L-AmB was well tolerated, without evidence of infusion-associated reactions or renal toxicity.

Amphotericin B deoxycholate formulated in parenteral lipid emulsions

In an open study, the immediate tolerability and *nephrotoxicity* of D-AmB prepared in Intralipid 20% (1 mg/ml) (Il-D-AmB) has been evaluated in 45 courses of empirical treatment for suspected fungal infections in 38 patients with hematological malignancies (28[C]). Il-D-AmB was given over 4 h and patients were prospectively monitored before, during, and after the infusion. The mean duration of therapy was 11 (range 2–29) days and the total dosage of the formulation was 365 (range 90–3500) mg. There were *fevers* and/or *rigors* during 30 of 45 treatment courses (66%) and premedications for their control or prevention were required in 26 of the 45 courses (58%). There were pre- and post-infusion variations in blood pressure and pulse rate exceeding 10% in 40 and 45% of infusions, respectively. Serum creatinine increased by over 44 (range 55–99) μmol/l in eight treatment courses (18%). Most patients were receiving other concomitant nephrotoxic drugs, such as aminoglycosides, vancomycin, and cyclosporin. Thus, this carefully conducted study failed to show that administration of D-AmB in Intralipid 20% improved its immediate tolerability. On the other hand, there was little effect on renal function at the relatively low doses of 0.5–0.6 mg/kg per day.

The pharmacokinetics of amphotericin have been studied after the administration of D-AmB and IL-D-AmB in 13 patients (29[c]). IL-D-AmB resulted in significantly lower peak plasma concentrations and AUC of amphotericin. The authors proposed that these pharmacokinetic differences could at least in part explain the reduced toxicity of IL-D-AmB in some series.

Risk factors *Children* The renal tolerance of IL-D-AmB (as a solution of 0.5–1 mg/ml in Intralipid 20% administered over 4–6 h) has been evaluated in a population of low-birth-weight (infants under 1250 g) (30[C]). Over 2 years, 52 patients received IL-D-AmB in 58 courses lasting 310 days; 23 episodes were randomly accessed and reviewed. All patients received a daily dose of 1 mg/kg by day 2 of therapy and the mean total dose was 20 (range 10–26) mg/kg. Only one patient had a rise in serum creatinine of more than 26 μmol/l; overall, serum creatinine fell significantly after day 10 of IL-D-AmB therapy. Serial urine output, serum potassium, and potassium supplementation data showed no significant differences from baseline. There were no infusion-related reactions. Crude mortality was comparatively low (8.6%), but under half of the patients had a documented invasive infection.

Stability The compatibility and chemical stability of D-AmB in two concentrations (0.05 and 0.5 mg/ml) prepared in a 20% fat emulsion or in 5% dextrose have been investigated (31[r]). The solutions were either protected from light or exposed to fluorescent room light; all were stored at room temperature. At 0, 4, 8, and 24 h after preparation, the containers were inverted several times and the contents were inspected for color, clarity, and precipitation; an aliquot was removed at each time for assay of the amphotericin concentration. D-AmB and IL-D-AmB 0.05 and 0.5 mg/ml were chemically stable for up to 23–25 h at room temperature, with or without protection from light; there was no precipitation. Although IL-D-AmB separated over time (by 8 h), slight agitation of the container reversed this.

D-AmB prepared in Intralipid 10%, Intralipid 20%, or Lipofundin 20% to a final concentration of 0.2 mg/ml by vigorous agitation for 18 h results in stable emulsions with association of D-AmB with the lipid phase for at least 1 month at 4°C (32[r]). In addition, the MICs of all mixtures against various *Candida* species were similar to those of D-AmB and did not change after storage for at least 2 weeks at 4°C. Furthermore, human red blood cell hemolysis was much lower than with D-AmB.

It has been pointed out that the infusion rate may affect the tolerability of Il-D-AmB (33[c]). *Pulmonary toxicity*, which was noted in association with IL-D-AmB in a number of patients in a previous study, might have been related to the rapid infusion of a large amount of lipid or to aggregation created by combining D-AmB with the lipid.

ALLYLAMINES *(SED-13, 793; SEDA-19, 240; SEDA-21, 288)*

Terbinafine

The synthetic allylamine terbinafine is a potent fungicide in the systemic treatment of dermatomycoses caused by filamentous fungi. It acts by inhibiting the biosynthesis of ergosterol at the activity of squalene epoxidase; ergosterol depletion and accumulation of toxic squalenes in the fungal cell membrane lead to growth inhibition and cell death (34[R]). Terbinafine is usually well tolerated in dosages of 250–500 mg/day, and has a relatively low incidence of adverse effects. The primary adverse effects associated with terbinafine include *gastrointestinal upsets* and *skin reactions* in 2–7% of patients. Terbinafine can cause *hepatitis*; potentially severe hepatotoxicity can occur in 1:120 000 patients, and asymptomatic rises in liver enzyme activities are likely to occur in 1:200. Less common significant adverse effects have included *reversible loss of taste*, *severe skin eruptions*, *Stevens–Johnson syndrome*, and *blood dyscrasias* (35[r]). There is no evidence that these idiosyncratic effects are increasing in incidence with increasing use of terbinafine (36[C]).

The safety of terbinafine has been monitored in four open, uncontrolled, post-marketing surveillance studies in four European countries, the results of which have been analysed collectively (37[C]). The studies included 25 884 patients (mean age 48, range 1–98 years) treated with terbinafine for dermatophyte infections of the skin and its appendages at dermatology, general, and family practices. Follow-up data were available on 25 091 patients. The recommended daily dose of 250 mg was prescribed for 99% of the cohort. The median duration of treatment was 12 weeks (range 1 day to almost 3 years); 40% of the patients took treatment for more than 12 weeks. About 40% of the subjects had one or more concomitant illnesses and were treated for these conditions with one or more co-medications. The main end-point of the analysis was the incidence of adverse events, as reported by physicians, with their opinion regarding the relation to terbinafine therapy.

During the course of the study, 2717 patients (11%) reported adverse events; there was no evidence of drug–drug interactions. The most frequently reported adverse events were related to the gastrointestinal tract (4.9%), the skin (2.3%), the whole body (1.5%), the central or peripheral nervous system (1.2%), the respiratory system (1.0%), and the musculoskeletal system (0.8%). Of all events, 56% were considered by the investigators to be possibly or probably related to terbinafine. A total of 1370 patients (5.3%) discontinued terbinafine therapy early because of adverse events.

Hepatobiliary events were reported in 55 (0.2%) of all patients; 45 of these had *asymptomatic rises in hepatic enzymes*. Of the other 10 patients, five reported non-specific symptoms, such as *diarrhea*; the other five had *cholestasis*, potentially related to terbinafine in two cases. Altogether 186 patients (0.7%) had either *distortion or loss of taste*; the available information suggested that these disturbances were reversible on withdrawal. Five patients reported parosmia, in three cases associated with taste loss.

Terbinafine was considered a possible or probable cause of 11 (0.04%) serious adverse events; these included *thrombocytopenia* (n = 3); *severe skin reactions* (n = 2); *large bowel obstruction and duodenal ulceration*, *cholestatic hepatitis*, *bronchospasm*, *neutropenia*, *thrombocytopenia with pancreatitis*, *severe urticaria/angio-edema* and *unilateral leg edema* (n = 1 each). The overall mortality during the study was 0.09%, and none of the 24 deaths was considered to have been related to terbinafine.

The safety and efficacy of oral terbinafine 250 mg/day for 12 or 24 weeks has been evaluated in 358 patients with toenail onychomycosis in a North American multicenter, double-blind, placebo-controlled study (38[c]). Terbinafine was well tolerated; there were nine (2.5%) serious, possibly or probably drug-related adverse effect, all involving the gastrointestinal tract or the skin and necessitating withdrawal of the drug in five instances (1.4%). There were no changes in hematological and biochemical measurements.

In a double-blind comparison of therapy for 6 or 12 weeks with terbinafine 250 mg/day for onychomycosis in 148 German patients, there was a similar tolerability profile of both regimens, with symptoms related to the gastrointestinal tract and skin leading the list of possibly drug-related events (39[c]).

In a double-blind, placebo-controlled, multicenter study in Denmark and Iceland, 148 patients with toenail onychomycosis were randomized to treatment with either terbinafine 250 mg/day or placebo for 3 months and were followed for 12 months (40[c]). There were adverse effects in 14% of those who took terbinafine compared with 5.4% with placebo;

adverse effects possibly associated with terbinafine included one case each of *urticaria*, *erythema multiforme*, and *progressive psoriasis*. All adverse effects were considered moderate to mild and all disappeared rapidly after withdrawal.

The safety and efficacy of terbinafine 250 mg/day for 12, 18, and 24 weeks for onychomycosis of the toenail have been evaluated in an open label multicenter study in 1508 patients (41[c]). Possibly or definitely related adverse events occurred in 117 patients (7.8%). Most events involved the skin, the gastrointestinal system, or the respiratory system. There was at least one serious adverse event in 57 patients (3.8%); in no case did the investigator believe that the event had a definite relation to treatment with terbinafine and in one case it was considered uncertain. Nevertheless, 88 (5.8%) of patients withdrew because of adverse events, irrespective of whether or not they were related to terbinafine. Elderly patients (over 60 years of age) and patients with diabetes mellitus had a similar frequency and distribution of adverse effects to the entire study population.

In 21 HIV-infected patients treated with terbinafine 250 mg/day for 16 weeks for toenail onychomycosis, possibly related adverse effects were limited to one instance of moderate *gastric pain* (42[C]). There were no laboratory changes attributable to terbinafine, and there were no clinically significant drug interactions.

Liver and biliary Hepatobiliary reactions (see also above), including *cholestasis*, are uncommon adverse events associated with the use of terbinafine and appear to be idiosyncratic.

An otherwise healthy 40-year-old patient developed severe cholestatic jaundice 6 weeks after starting to take terbinafine 250 mg/day for onychomycosis (43[c]). Liver biopsy showed centrilobular and canalicular bile stasis and mild lymphocytic infiltration of some portal tracts. Withdrawal resulted in full clinical and biochemical recovery within 10 weeks.

Prolonged cholestasis with reduction of interlobular bile ducts occurred in a 75-year-old woman shortly after discontinuation of a 3-week course of terbinafine 250 mg/day for cutaneous candidiasis (44[c]). She had also taken long-standing nicergoline (a vasodilator) and fenofibrate. Although her serum bilirubin returned to normal 10 weeks after withdrawal of terbinafine, anicteric cholestasis persisted. A percutaneous liver biopsy 6 months later showed a reduction in interlobular biliary ducts and mild bile duct proliferation, periportal fibrosis, and mononuclear infiltration. There was mild canalicular cholestasis and minimal intralobular hepatocyte necrosis. Serum γGT activity remained moderately raised 17 months after withdrawal of terbinafine.

Skin and appendages *Acute generalized exanthematous pustulosis* has clinical and histological features that resemble pustular psoriasis. Drugs and viruses have been implicated in its pathogenesis. Histologically documented acute generalized exanthematous pustulosis has been attributed to terbinafine (45[c]). Generalized pustulosis and fever occurred 2 weeks after the start of terbinafine 250 mg/day. After withdrawal of terbinafine and the addition of oral methylprednisolone (1 mg/kg) all the symptoms resolved within 3 weeks.

Psoriasis has been described in four patients who took oral terbinafine (46[c]). Two had preexisting plaque-type psoriasis that flared up at 12 and 17 days after starting terbinafine. Another developed pustular-type psoriasis de novo after 27 days of terbinafine therapy. The fourth had psoriasis with stable plaque disease and had a pustular flare after taking terbinafine for 21 days. In all cases the psoriasis cleared or abated after withdrawal of terbinafine and the institution of antipsoriatic therapy.

Special senses *Anterior uveitis* has been reported in a patient with late-stage AIDS after 12 days of treatment with oral terbinafine for refractory oral candidiasis (47[c]). The presenting symptoms consisted of extreme redness of both eyes and blurred vision. After withdrawal of terbinafine, the patient's ocular symptoms reduced slightly, but rapidly worsened when the drug was restarted after 4 days. Treatment with terbinafine was eventually withdrawn, and all the signs resolved with ocular steroid drops within 2 weeks.

Immunological and hypersensitivity reactions An otherwise healthy, 35-year-old patient had *a hypersensitivity reaction* with fever, rash, lymphadenopathy, and mildly raised γ-glutamyltransferase activity 10 days after starting to take oral terbinafine 250 mg/day (48[c]). The patient's symptoms resolved with corticosteroid treatment over 2 weeks. The mechanism of this reaction is unclear. The authors pointed out that after withdrawal terbinafine can persist in skin and plasma for several weeks in concentrations that may play a role in sustaining such adverse reactions.

Risk factors *Children* In most countries, terbinafine has not been licensed for use in children. However, several studies have included over 200 patients, and these have been summarized (49[r]). Three additional small series have been published on the use of systemic terbinafine in the treatment of *tinea corporis* or *tinea capitis* in children (50[c]), (51[C]), (52[c]). Daily doses were 62.5 mg for children weighing under 18.5 kg, 125 mg for 18.5–25 kg, and 250 mg for children over 25 kg. The first study (50[c]) included 15 children (14 months to 11 years) who took treatment for 2–10 weeks. The only reported possible adverse event was acute *urticaria* in one child and that disappeared despite continued administration of terbinafine. The second study (51[c]) included 18 patients who took a 2-week course of terbinafine. Three patients had possibly drug-related adverse events: *malaise*, *epigastric pain*, *diarrhea*, and a slight *rise in hepatic transaminase activities*, which were reversible and did not recur after re-exposure; *a papular facial rash* thought to be a dermatophytid reaction; and *axillary folliculitis* (one patient each). The third study (52[c]), performed in an orphanage in Bangkok, included 82 patients treated for 1–3 weeks for *tinea capitis*. In this study, there were no laboratory or clinical adverse effects.

Interactions The metabolism of terbinafine is not mediated by cytochrome P450, and so the potential for drug interactions is low. The possible consequences of concurrent administration of various therapeutic agents with oral antifungal agents, including terbinafine, have been reviewed (53[r]).

Terbinafine can increase *caffeine* concentrations when caffeine is given intravenously.

Cimetidine can increase terbinafine plasma concentrations.

Concurrent *rifampicin* can reduce terbinafine plasma concentrations.

Terbinafine can reduce the trough *cyclosporin* concentration in transplant patients (53[r]), (54[c]).

Placebo-controlled crossover studies have shown no evidence of significant pharmacokinetic interactions of terbinafine with digoxin (55[C]) or warfarin (56[C]).

AZOLE DERIVATIVES *(SED-13, 782; SEDA-19, 259; SEDA-20, 252; SEDA-21, 282)*

Fluconazole

The clinical pharmacokinetics and drug interactions of fluconazole have been reviewed (57[R]).

A prospective, multicenter, randomized comparison of the safety and efficacy of fluconazole 800 mg intravenously followed by 400 mg/day for 4 weeks versus amphotericin B deoxycholate (D-AmB) 0.6 mg/kg per day (cumulative dose 8 mg/kg) for candidemia in non-neutropenic patients ($n = 106$) showed significantly fewer adverse events in the fluconazole group (6[C]). Patients with *Candida glabrata* or *Candida krusei* were withdrawn from the study and treated with D-AmB. *Renal impairment*, defined as an increase in the serum creatinine concentration to more than 1.5 times the baseline concentration, occurred significantly more often with D-Amb (in 23 patients) than with fluconazole (10 patients). There was *hypokalemia* in 17 of the fluconazole-treated patients and 17 of those treated with D-AmB.

The efficacy and safety of fluconazole have been assessed in the treatment of 587 adult patients with fungal infections in a large, multicenter, prospective, single-arm study (58[CR]). A loading dose of fluconazole (200 or 400 mg) was given orally or intravenously, followed by 100 or 200 mg/day. Candidiasis was cured or improved in 96% of 73 patients with AIDS and in 79% of 218 patients without AIDS. *Cryptococcus* responded clinically in 69% of 29 patients with AIDS and in all seven patients without AIDS. Adverse events were reported in 11% of 580 patients, and 54 (9.3%) were judged to be treatment-related.

The adverse events were for the most part mild or moderate. There was *cholestatic jaundice* in 13 patients, *hepatocellular damage* in nine, *nausea* in 11, *rash* in five, and *maculopapular rash* in four. There were abnormal laboratory tests as follows: alkaline phosphatase (5.1%); AlT (4.8%); AsT (4.7%); total bilirubin (2.9%); platelet count (2.5%). There were 13 withdrawals from the study because of adverse drug reactions.

The treatment of cryptococcal meningitis associated with AIDS has been evaluated in a double-blind, multicenter trial (59[C]). Treatment began with D-AmB (0.7 mg/kg per day) with or without flucytosine (100 mg/kg per day) for 2 weeks followed by 8 weeks of treatment with itraconazole (400 mg/kg per day, $n = 155$) or fluconazole (400 mg/kg per day, $n = 151$). At 2 weeks of treatment, significantly more patients treated with flucytosine had sterile cerebrospinal fluid cultures (60%) than those treated with D-AmB alone (51%). Clinical responses to fluconazole and itraconazole were similar (68 and 70%, respectively); however, at 10 weeks, negative cultures were more common with fluconazole than itraconazole (72 and 60%, respectively). Six patients in each group withdrew because of toxicity. Six patients had *nausea and vomiting*, and two of those had a *raised serum creatinine*. Two patients had *rashes*, including one taking fluconazole who had *Stevens–Johnson syndrome* and survived. One patient each had *headache*, *neutropenia*, *hyperkalemia*, and *hepatic failure*. The last two patients, both taking itraconazole, died. There were hematological adverse effects in 20% of patients, 7% had hepatotoxicity, and 4% had nephrotoxicity.

The adverse effects of chronic, high-dose fluconazole have been reported in an analysis of a multicenter, dose-escalating study of the treatment of invasive mycoses in 93 patients treated for at least 6 months with at least 300 mg/day (60[CR]). Therapy was discontinued owing to adverse events possibly related to fluconazole in two cases, one with *premature ejaculation*, and one with *arthralgia*. Adverse effects possibly attributable to the drug occurred in 27% of patients, but no adverse effect occurred in over 3%. Asymptomatic laboratory abnormalities were common (in 42%). The most common laboratory abnormalities were *eosinophilia* (12%), *increased AsT* (10%), and *increased blood urea nitrogen or creatinine* (8%).

The safety and efficacy of fluconazole and griseofulvin have been compared in a prospective, multicenter, double-blind randomized trial in the treatment of *tinea corporis* and *tinea cruris* (1[C]). Fluconazole-treated patients ($n = 114$) took 150 mg once a week orally for 6 weeks; the griseofulvin-treated patients ($n = 116$) took 500 mg/day for 4–6 weeks. Treatment-related adverse events occurred more often with griseofulvin. Nine fluconazole-treated patients had 10 adverse events: *gastrointestinal complaints* (five), *CNS symptoms* (two), *increased sweating* (two), and *a transient rash* (one). There were 19 adverse events in 15 griseofulvin-treated patients: *CNS symptoms* (nine), *gastrointestinal complaints* (seven), and *urticaria*, *photosensitivity*, and *transient taste loss* (one each). Three patients discontinued griseofulvin owing to adverse events, two with *headache* and one with *urticaria*.

Interactions Fluconazole inhibits CYP3A4 and CYP2C9, which are found in the liver and intestine. The interaction of fluconazole with the angiotensin II receptor antagonists *eprosartan* and *losartan* has been assessed in 16 healthy men (61[c]). Eprosartan is rapidly absorbed orally and is not metabolized by cytochrome P450. Losartan is well absorbed orally and undergoes extensive first-pass metabolism by cytochrome P450. Fluconazole did not alter the eprosartan AUC and C_{max}. However, it increased the AUC and C_{max} of losartan by 66 and 30%, respectively.

Midazolam is a benzodiazepine that is metabolized by CYP3A4. The effect of the route of administration of fluconazole on the interaction of fluconazole with oral midazolam has been assessed in nine healthy adults in a randomized, double-blind, crossover study (62[c]). Both oral and intravenous fluconazole increased the AUC (2–2.5 times), the elimination half-life (2.5 times), and the C_{max} (2.5 times). The AUC and C_{max} of midazolam were significantly higher after oral than intravenous fluconazole.

The effect of fluconazole on the steady-state pharmacokinetics of *delavirdine* has been assessed in eight HIV-positive patients and five controls (63[c]). Delavirdine is metabolized by cytochrome P450, and it was given in a dosage of 300 mg every 8 h for 30 days. Fluconazole 400 mg/day dose was given on days 16–30. Fluconazole did not alter the pharmacokinetics of delavirdine.

Ritonavir is an HIV protease inhibitor that is metabolized by CYP3A4. In a multiple dosing, crossover study in eight healthy volunteers, fluconazole increased (64[c]) the C_{max} and AUC of ritonavir by under 15%. Although the increase was statistically significant it is probably clinically unimportant.

The effect of fluconazole on the metabolism of *rifabutin* and its metabolite LM565 has been assessed in human liver microsomes and recombinant human CYP3A4 (65[cr]). Rifabutin was metabolized by the liver microsomes, but not by CYP3A4. However, LM565 was metabolized by CYP3A4. This suggests that the change in rifabutin exposure with fluconazole is not due to inhibition of CYP3A4, but that the increased exposure to LM565 is.

Itraconazole

The efficacy and safety of intermittent therapy with itraconazole has been evaluated in a multicenter, randomized placebo-controlled, double-blind study in fingernail onychomycosis in 73 patients (66[C]). Itraconazole was given in a dosage of 200 mg bd during the first week of each month for 2 months. Adverse events were reported in 10 itraconazole-treated patients and in nine placebo-treated patients. There was *headache* in 8% with both itraconazole and placebo. *Gastrointestinal symptoms* occurred next most often: four events with itraconazole and three with placebo. There were no clinically significant laboratory abnormalities.

Intermittent and continuous itraconazole have been compared in a multicenter, double-blind, parallel-group study in the treatment of toe-nail onychomycosis (67[C]). It was given as either 200 mg/day for 3 months ($n = 65$) or 400 mg/day for 1 week per month for 3 months ($n = 64$). There were no statistically significant differences in efficacy, mycological cure, or overall response. Adverse events were most often *gastrointestinal*: 17% with continuous treatment and 14% with intermittent treatment. Two patients taking continuous treatment withdrew owing to adverse events possibly due to itraconazole, one with moderately severe *dermatitis*, and one with *increased AlT activity* (more than three times the reference value). One patient taking intermittent treatment withdrew with *impotence* that was possibly drug related.

Itraconazole 400 mg/day for 1 week has been compared with itraconazole 100–200 mg/day for 2–4 weeks in *tinea pedis* infection in a multicenter, prospective study ($n = 484$) (68[C]). The overall incidence of adverse events was 5%. They included *nausea* (1.2%), *abdominal pain* (1%), *dyspepsia* (0.7%), *headache* (0.7%), *vomiting* (0.4%), *pruritus* (0.3%), *gastritis* (0.2%), *fatigue* (0.2%), and *rash* (0.1%). No adverse events were reported in the 400 mg/day group. No patient withdrew because of adverse events.

Itraconazole oral solution 100–200 mg/day has been compared with fluconazole tablets 100–200 mg/day in esophageal candidiasis in immunocompromised patients in a multicenter, randomized, double-blind study (69[C]). There were adverse events in 48% (30/62) of itraconazole-treated patients and 51% (32/63) of fluconazole-treated patients. Gastrointestinal events were the most common in both groups. Fluconazole-treated patients reported a higher incidence of *vomiting* (14 vs 6.5%) and *abdominal pain* (9.5 vs 3.2%). Itraconazole-treated patients had a higher incidence of *fever* (15 vs 6.3%). Adverse events that required removal from the study occurred in only three patients: one itraconazole-treated patient with moderate *nausea*, *vomiting*, and *dehydration*, one fluconazole-treated patient with *mild soft stools and moderate generalized malaise*, and one fluconazole-treated patient with *mild weakness*, *dizziness*, and *shakiness*.

Compassionate-use itraconazole in 125 patients for invasive aspergillosis produced a complete response in 27%, improvement in 36%, no change in 16%, and deterioration in 21% (70[C]). Adverse events due to itraconazole did not provide new information on toxicity and were not detailed.

The pharmacokinetics and safety of intravenous itraconazole for 1 week followed by oral itraconazole for 2 weeks have been evaluated in prophylaxis in 16 adults in an intensive care unit (71[C]). They received itraconazole 200 mg intravenously four times for 2 days, and then once daily for 5 days. Oral itraconazole solution 200 or 400 mg/day was then given for 2 weeks. The mean target plasma concentration was 500 ng/ml. From 96 to 168 h of intravenous therapy the mean plasma concentration was 605–658 ng/ml. After 2 weeks of oral administration at 200 mg/day the mean concentration was 245 ng/ml and at 400 mg/day it was 805 ng/ml. Gastrointestinal adverse events, mainly *diarrhea*, were dose-related. Therapy was discontinued in one of seven patients taking 400 mg/day of itraconazole solution. The severe adverse events were one case of *respiratory depression* and one of *albuminuria* during intravenous infusion, and three severe gastrointestinal events in the 400 mg/day oral therapy group (one *diarrhea*, one *abdominal pain*, and one *nausea*, *vomiting*, and *diarrhea*). Other adverse events were noted in 11 of 16 patients, but most were considered to be related to the disease and not the drug. There were no abnormalities in creatinine clearance. No consistent laboratory abnormalities were found.

Itraconazole maintenance therapy for the treatment of histoplasmosis in 46 patients with AIDS has been evaluated in a prospective, multicenter, open-label study (72[C]). Patients with mild to moderate disseminated histoplasmosis were treated with itraconazole 200 mg/day ($n = 42$) or 400 mg/day ($n = 4$) after completing 12 weeks of itraconazole induction therapy. Therapy was discontinued in three patients because of *hepatotoxicity*. One had resolution of hepatitis after withdrawal, the second had a liver biopsy that suggested viral hepatitis, the third was terminally ill and did not have follow-up testing after withdrawal. One patient developed *nephrotic syndrome* that did not resolve on withdrawal, and one developed a *maculopapular rash*. Adverse effects that did not necessitate drug withdrawal included *anemia* (17 patients), *neutropenia* (16), *raised AsT* (11), and *fever* (10).

Skin and appendages *Acute generalized exanthematous pustulosis* has been attributed to itraconazole (73[cr]).

A 27-year-old Korean woman with a history of psoriasis developed fever, neutrophilia, and a rash after taking itraconazole for 1 week. Skin biopsy was performed and was consistent with acute generalized exanthematous pustulosis. One month after withdrawal of itraconazole and clearance of the symptoms, a scratch/patch test with itraconazole failed to elicit a reaction. An oral dose of itraconazole resulted in pustules within 2 h of administration. She had no further pustules during 2 years of follow-up.

There has been only one previous report of acute generalized exanthematous pustulosis associated with itraconazole, in a patient who did not have psoriasis and was not challenged with itraconazole after the event.

Desensitization to an itraconazole-induced skin reaction has been reported (74[c]).

A 30-year old woman with hay fever, asthma, and atopic dermatitis had culture-proven *Aspergillus* and *Curvularia* sinusitis. She was given itraconazole 100 mg bd. After 1 week of therapy she developed a confluent erythematous rash over her face, neck, and shoulders. The rash faded within a few days of withdrawal, but returned on rechallenge. Skin testing was negative. Because of little clinical improvement, oral desensitization was performed uneventfully. She tolerated 6 weeks of itraconazole and made an excellent recovery.

Interactions Itraconazole is a potent inhibitor of CYP3A4. *Felodipine* undergoes first-pass metabolism by CYP3A4. In 10 healthy volunteers itraconazole greatly increased felodipine plasma concentrations and effects (75[C]). Itraconazole increased the C_{max} of felodipine nearly 8-fold, the AUC 6-fold, and the elimination half-life 2-fold. Systolic blood pressure and heart rate were affected more during co-administration of itraconazole.

Itraconazole moderately increased the AUC and C_{max} of *oxybutynin* in healthy volunteers (76[c]). There was no statistically significant change in the concentration of the active metabolite of oxybutynin, *N*-desethyl-oxybutynin. There were no significant adverse events.

The non-benzodiazepine anxiolytic *buspirone* increased the AUC of itraconazole 19-fold and its C_{max} 13-fold (77[c]). There were no significant adverse events.

The P glycoprotein multidrug transporter, also known as the multidrug resistance (MDR) protein, is a unidirectional pump found in renal and biliary epithelia, where it extrudes drugs such as cyclosporin, vinca alkaloids, verapamil, and digoxin into the urine. Itraconazole inhibits P glycoprotein, and this interaction is the proposed mechanism for the interaction of itraconazole with *digoxin* (78[c]), as it is for other drugs that inhibit the P glycoprotein (SED-13, 444).

Ketoconazole

Ketoconazole inhibits cytochrome P450 enzyme-dependent 14-demethylation of lanosterol to cholesterol and thus suppresses gonadal and adrenal androgen synthesis. Ketoconazole 200 mg tds produces rapid and reversible medical castration, which has specific usefulness in patients with prostate cancer. An evaluation of 50 consecutive patients with progression of advanced prostate cancer despite flutamide withdrawal showed that ketoconazole retained significant activity (79[C]). After treatment, 63% of patients had a greater than 50% fall in prostate-specific antigen, and 48% had a greater than 80% fall. Adverse effects included *nausea* (10%), *fatigue* (6.3%), *edema* (6.3%), *hepatotoxicity* (4.2%), *rash* (4.2%), and *anorexia* (2%). There was one case of *congestive heart failure*, but a causal relation to ketoconazole could not be established.

In a single-arm trial in 20 consecutive patients with progressive advanced prostate cancer despite antiandrogen therapy simultaneous antiandrogen withdrawal and treatment with ketoconazole have been evaluated (80[C]). Prostate-specific antigen fell by over 50% in 55% of patients. Adverse effects included *nausea and vomiting* (15%), *fatigue* (10%), reversible *hepatotoxicity* (10%), and *rash* (20%).

Endocrine, metabolic Ketoconazole-induced *adrenal crisis* has been reported (81[cR]).

A 77-year-old man with nerve root compression due to spinal metastases from prostate cancer took ketoconazole 200 mg qds after refusing orchidectomy. He experienced significant pain relief over several days, but 9 days later developed generalized weakness, abdominal pain, nausea and vomiting, severely diminished mentation, hypotension, and a fever of 38.1°C. He was given a bolus of 400 ml intravenous crystalloid and corticosteroids for the possibility of cerebral hemorrhage with increased intracranial pressure. After 1 h he became alert and recovered verbal responsiveness and his vital signs returned to normal. Although an initial serum cortisol concentration was not obtained, the presumptive diagnosis of adrenal insufficiency was made based on the clinical presentation, neurological changes, electrolyte abnormalities, the absence of bacterial sepsis, and the prompt response to corticosteroid administration.

No previous case of overt adrenal insufficiency in a patient with prostate cancer taking ketoconazole has been reported. However, the so-called asthenia syndrome, consisting of weakness, fatigue, apathy, and anorexia, is seen in many of these patients and may represent a subtle manifestation of adrenal compromise. The asthenia syndrome reverses readily with the addition of prednisone or withdrawal of ketoconazole.

Liver and biliary The incidence, severity, and course of ketoconazole-associated hepatic toxicity in patients with onychomycosis have been evaluated (82[CR]). Patients were randomized to ketoconazole (n = 137) or griseofulvin (n = 74) in a ratio of 2:1. No biochemical or overt hepatitis developed in patients treated with griseofulvin. Of the patients who took ketoconazole, 24 developed *asymptomatic transaminase rises* without a change in bilirubin, and four developed *jaundice* or clinical symptoms of *hepatitis* after 2–10 weeks of therapy. Of the 24 patients with asymptomatic enzyme rises, 17 had adequate follow up; they continued therapy with ketoconazole, and their liver enzymes tended to return to normal. The four patients with jaundice or symptoms discontinued ketoconazole and their liver function tests returned to normal. No patient had fulminant hepatitis. The authors recommended that ketoconazole may be continued with caution in patients with asymptomatic and anicteric hepatic injury, and that it should be withdrawn in patients with overt hepatitis. However, the author of an editorial expressed two concerns about this approach: that retrospective reviews of ketoconazole-associated liver injury had case fatality rates of 1/33 and 1/16, and that three patients have been reported who developed fulminant hepatic failure after a delay in the withdrawal of ketoconazole in the face of liver enzyme abnormalities (83[r]).

REFERENCES

1. Van Der Horst C, Saag MS, Cloud GA, Hamill RS, Graybill JR, Sobel JD, Johnson PC, Tuazon CU, Kerkering T, Moskovitz BL, Powderly WG, Dismukes WE. Treatment of cryptococcal meningitis associated with the acquired immunodeficiency syndrome. New Engl J Med 1997; 337:15–21.
2. Thakur CP, Narain S, Umar N, Hassan SM, Jha DK, Kumar A. Amphotericin B is superior to sodium antimony gluconate in the treatment of Indian post-kala-azar dermal leishmaniasis. Ann Trop Med Parasitol 1997;91:611–16.
3. Zernikow B, Fleischhack G, Hasan C, Bode U. Cyanotic Raynaud's phenomenon with conventional but not with liposomal amphotericin B: three case reports. Mycoses 1997;40:359–61.
4. Ferreira E, Perreault MM. Hypertension exacerbated by amphotericin B administration. Ann Pharmacother 1997;31:1407–8.
5. Narita M, Itakura O, Ishiguro N, Togashi T. Hypomagnesemia-associated tetany due to intravenous administration of amphotericin B. Eur J Pediatr 1997;156:421–2.
6. Phillips P, Shafran S, Garber G, Rotstein C, Smaill F, Fong I, Salit I, Miller M, Williams K, Conly JM, Singer J, Ioannou S. Multicenter randomized trial of fluconazole versus amphotericin B for treatment of candidemia in non-neutropenic patients. Eur J Clin Microbiol Infect Dis 1997; 16:337–45.
7. Wasan KM, Rosenblum MG, Cheung L, Lopez-Berestein G. Influence of lipoproteins on renal cytotoxicity and antifungal activity of amphotericin B. Antimicrob Agents Chemother 1994;38:223–7.
8. Wasan KM, Conklin JS. Enhanced amphotericin B nephrotoxicity in intensive care patients with elevated levels of low-density lipoprotein cholesterol. Clin Infect Dis 1997;24:78–80.
9. Reiner NE, Thompson WL. Dopamine and saralasin antagonism of renal vasoconstriction and oliguria caused by amphotericin B in dogs. J Infect Dis 1979;140:564–75.
10. Carlson MA, Ferraz AAB, Condon RE. Urinary adenosine excretion in patients receiving amphotericin B. Surgery 1997;121:190–3.
11. Kingo ARM, Smyth JA, Waisman D. Lack of evidence of amphotericin B toxicity in very low birthweight infants treated for systemic candidiasis. Pediatr Infect Dis J 1997;16:1002–3.
12. Dele Davies H, King SM, Doyle J, Matlow A, Koren G, Hamilton R, Portwine C. Controlled pilot study of rapid amphotericin B infusions. Arch Dis Child 1997;76:165–6.
13. Reichenspurner H, Gamberg P, Nitschke M, Valantine H, Hunt S, Oyer PE, Reitz BA. Significant reduction in the number of fungal infections after lung-, heart-lung-, and heart-transplantation using aerosolized amphotericin B prophylaxis. Transplant Proc 1997;29:627–8.
14. Erjavec Z, Woolthius GMH, DeVries-Hospers HG, Sluiter WJ, Daenen SMGJ, De Pauw B, Halie MR. Tolerance and efficacy of amphotericin B inhalations for prevention of invasive pulmonary aspergillosis in hematological patients. Eur J Clin Microbiol Infect Dis 1997;16:364–8.
15. Herbrecht R. Safety of amphotericin B colloidal dispersion. Eur J Clin Microbiol Infect Dis 1997;16:74–80.
16. White MH, Anaissie EJ, Kusne S, Wingard JR, Hiemenz JW, Cantor A, Gurwith M, Du Mond C, Mamelok RD, Bowden RA. Amphotericin B colloidal dispersion vs. amphotericin B as therapy for invasive aspergillosis. Clin Infect Dis 1997;24:635–42.
17. Mehta J, Kelsey S, Chu P, Powles R, Hazel D, Riley U, Evans C, Newland A, Treleaven J, Singhal S. Amphotericin B lipid complex (ABLC) for the treatment of confirmed or presumed fungal infections in immunocompromised patients with hematological malignancies. Bone Marrow Transplant 1997;20:39–43.
18. Wingard JR. Efficacy of amphotericin B lipid complex injection (ABLC) in bone marrow transplant patients with life-threatening systemic mycoses. Bone Marrow Transplant 1997;19:343–7.
19. Merhav H, Mieles L. Amphotericin B lipid complex in the treatment of invasive fungal infections in liver transplant patients. Transplant Proc 1997;29:2670–4.
20. Sundar S, Agrawal NK, Sinha PR, Horwith GS, Murray HW. Short course, low-dose amphotericin B lipid complex therapy for visceral leishmaniasis unresponsive to antimony. Ann Intern Med 1997;127:133–7.
21. Walsh TJ, Whitcomb P, Piscitelli S, Figg WD, Hill S, Chanock SJ, Jarosinski P, Gupta R, Pizzo PA. Safety, tolerance, and pharmacokinetics of amphotericin B lipid complex in children with hepatosplenic candidiasis. Antimicrob Agents Chemother 1997;41:1944–8.
22. Prentice HG, Hann IM, Herbrecht R, Aoun M, Kvaloy S, Catovsky D, Pinkerton CR, Schey SA, Jacobs F, Oakhill A, Stevens RF, Darbyshire PJ, Gibson BES. A randomized comparison of liposomal versus conventional amphotericin B for the treatment of pyrexia of unknown origin in neutropenic patients. Br J Haematol 1997;98:711–18.
23. Leenders ACAP, Reiss P, Portegies P, Clezy K, Hop WCJ, Hoy J, Borleffs JCC, Allworth T, Kauffmann RH, Jones P, Kroon FP, Verbrugh HA, De Marie S. Liposomal amphotericin B (AmBisome) compared with amphotericin and both followed by oral fluconazole in the treatment of AIDS-associated cryptococcal meningitis. AIDS 1997;11:1463–71.
24. Kruger W, Stockschlaeder M, Sobottka I, Betker R, deWit M, Kroeger N, Grimm J, Arland M, Fiedler W, Erttmann R, Zander AR. Antimycotic therapy with liposomal amphotericin B for patients undergoing bone marrow or peripheral

blood stem cell transplantation. Leuk Lymphoma 1997;24:491–9.
25. Pasic S, Flannagan L, Cant AJ. Liposomal amphotericin B (AmBisome) is safe in bone marrow transplantation for primary immunodeficiency. Bone Marrow Transplant 1997;19:1229–32.
26. Di Martino L, Davidson RN, Giacchino R, Scotti S, Raimondi F, Castagnola E, Tasso L, Cascio A, Gradoni L, Gramiccia M, Pettoello-Mantovani M, Bryceson ADM. Treatment of visceral leishmaniasis in children with liposomal amphotericin B. J Pediatr 1997;131:271–7.
27. Al Arishi H, Frayha HH, Kalloghlian A, Al Alaiyan S. Liposomal amphotericin B in neonates with invasive candidiasis. Am J Perinatol 1997; 14:573–6.
28. Laverdiere M, Habel F, Weiss K, Delorme J, Dubois G, Gagnon N, Belanger R. Poor immediate tolerability of amphotericin B lipid emulsion in patients with hematological malignancies. J Antimicrob Chemother 1997;40:910–12.
29. Heinemann V, Kaehny B, Jehn U, Muehlbayer D, Debus A, Wachholz K, Bosse D, Kolb H-J, Wilmanns W. Serum pharmacology of amphotericin B applied in lipid emulsions. Antimicrob Agents Chemother 1997;41:728–32.
30. Friedlich PS, Steinberg I, Fujitani A, DeLemos RA. Renal tolerance with the use of intralipid-amphotericin B in low-birth-weight neonates. Am J Perinatol 1997;14:377–83.
31. Owens D, Fleming RA, Restino MS, Cruz JM, Hurd DD. Stability of amphotericin B 0.05 and 0.5 mg/ml in 20% fat emulsion. Am J Health-Syst Pharm 1997;54:683–6.
32. Shadkhan Y, Segal E, Bor A, Gov Y, Rubin M, Lichtenberg D. The use of commercially available lipid emulsions for the preparation of amphotericin B-lipid admixtures. J Antimicrob Chemother 1997;39:655–8.
33. Herbrecht R, Letscher V. Safety and efficacy of intralipid emulsions of amphotericin B. J Antimicrob Chemother 1997;40:137–9.
34. Groll AH, Piscitelli SC, Walsh TJ. Clinical pharmacology of systemic antifungal agents: a comprehensive review of agents in clinical use, current investigational compounds, and putative targets for antifungal drug development. Adv Pharmacol 1998;44:343–500.
35. Abdel-Rahman S, Nahata MC. Oral terbinafine: a new antifungal agent. Ann Pharmacother 1997;31:445–56.
36. O'Sullivan DP, Needham CA, Bangs A, Atkin K, Kendall FD. Postmarketing surveillance of oral terbinafine in the UK: report of a large cohort study. Br J Clin Pharmacol 1996;42:559–65.
37. Hall M, Monka C, Krupp P, O'Sullivan D. Safety of oral terbinafine. Results of a postmarketing surveillance study in 25884 patients. Arch Dermatol 1997;133:1213–19.
38. Drake LA, Shear NH, Arlette JP, Cloutier R, Danby FW, Elewski BE, et al. (29 authors). Oral terbinafine in the treatment of toenail onychomycosis: North American multicenter trial. J Am Acad Dermatol 1997;37:740–5.
39. Tausch I, Brautigam M, Weidinger G, Jones TC. Evaluation of 6 weeks treatment of terbinafine in tinea unguium in a double-blind trial comparing 6 and 12 weeks therapy. The Lagos V Study Group. Br J Dermatol 1997;136:737–42.
40. Sveijgaard EL, Brandrup F, Kragballe K, Larsen PO, Veien NK, Holst M, et al. (21 authors). Oral terbinafine in toenail dermatophytosis. A double-blind, placebo-controlled multicenter study with 12 months' follow-up. Acta Dermatol Venereol 1997;77:66–9.
41. Pollak R, Billstein SA. Safety of oral terbinafine for toenail onychomycosis. J Am Podiatr Med Assoc 1997;87:565–70.
42. Herranz P, Garcia J, deLucas R, Gonzalez J, Pena JM, Diaz R, Casado M. Toenail onychomycosis in patients with acquired immune deficiency syndrome: treatment with terbinafine. Br J Dermatol 1997;137:577–80.
43. Dwyer CM, White MI, Sinclair MS. Cholestatic jaundice due to terbinafine. Br J Dermatol 1997;136:976–7.
44. Mallat A, Zafrani ES, Metreau JM, Dhumeaux D. Terbinafine-induced prolonged cholestasis with reduction of interlobular bile ducts. Dig Dis Sci 1997;42:1486–8.
45. Kempinaire A, DeRaeve L, Merckx L, DeConinck A, Bauwens M, Roseeuw D. Tebinafine-induced acute generalized exanthematous pustulosis confirmed by a positive patch-test result. J Am Acad Dermatol 1997;37:653–5.
46. Gupta AK, Sibbald RG, Knowles SR, Lynde CW, Shear NH. Terbinafine therapy may be associated with the development of psoriais de novo or its exacerbation: four case reports and a review of drug-induced psoriasis. J Am Acad Dermatol 1997;36 (Suppl II):858–62.
47. Price T, Stallman J, Dretler RH. Anterior uveitis in a patient with AIDS who was treated with terbinafine for oral candidiasis: a potential drug-induced reaction. Clin Infect Dis 1997; 25:752–3.
48. Gupta AK, Kopstein JB, Shear NH. Hypersensitivity reaction to terbinafine. J Am Acad Dermatol 1997;36:1018–19.
49. Jones TC. Overview of the use of terbinafine (Lamisil) in children. Br J Dermatol 1995;132: 683–9.
50. Bruckbauer HR, Hofmann H, Systemic antifungal treatment of children with terbinafine. Dermatology 1997;195:134–6.
51. Krafchik B, Pelletier J. The use of oral terbinafine (Lamisil®) in children. Dermatology 1997;194 (Suppl 1):43–4.
52. Kullavanijaya P, Reangchainam S, Ungpakorn R, Randomized single-blind study of efficacy and tolerability of terbinafine in the treatment of tinea capitis. J Am Acad Dermatol 1997;37:272–3.
53. Katz HI. Possible drug interactions in oral

treatment of onychomycosis. J Am Podiatr Med Assoc 1997;12:571–4.

54. Lo ACY, Lui S-L, Lo W-K, Chan DTM, Cheng IKP. The interaction of terbinafine and cyclosporine A in renal transplant patients. Br J Clin Pharmacol 1997;43:340–1.
55. Tarral A, Franchetau P, Guerret M. Effects of terbinafine on the pharmacokinetics of digoxin in healthy volunteers. Pharmacotherapy 1997; 17:791–5.
56. Guerret M, Franchetau P, Hubert M. Evaluation of effects of terbinafine on single oral dose pharmacokinetics and anticoagulant actions of warfarin in healthy volunteers. Pharmacotherapy 1997;17:767–73.
57. Debruyne D. Clinical pharmacokinetics of fluconazole in superficial and systemic mycoses. Clin Pharmacokinet 1997;33:52–77.
58. Troke PF. Large-scale multicentre study of fluconazole in the treatment of hospitalised patients with fungal infections. Multicentre European Study Group. Eur J Clin Microbiol Infect Dis 1997;16:287–95.
59. Faergemann J, Mörk NJ, Haglund A, Ödegård T, Back O, Ekholm E, et al. (32 authors). A multicentre (double-blind) comparative study to assess the safety and efficacy of fluconazole and griseofulvin in the treatment of *tinea corporis* and *tinea cruris*. Br J Dermatol 1997;136:575–7.
60. Stevens DA, Diaz M, Nergoni R, Montero-Gei F, Castro LGM, et al. (19 authors). Safety evaluation of chronic fluconazole therapy. Chemotherapy 1997;43:371–7.
61. Kazierad DJ, Martin DE, Blum RA, Tenero DM, Ilson B, Boike SC, Etheredge R, Jorkasky DK. Effect of fluconazole on the pharmacokinetics of eprosartan and losartan in healthy male volunteers. Clin Pharmacol Ther 1997;62:417–25.
62. Ahonen J, Olkkola KT, Neuvonen PJ. Effect of route of administration of fluconazole on the interaction between fluconazole and midazolam. J Clin Pharmacol 1997;51:415–19.
63. Borin MT, Cox SR, Herman BD, Carel BJ, Anderson RD, Freimuth WW. Effect of fluconazole on the steady-state pharmacokinetics of delvirdine in human immunodeficiency virus-positive patients. Antimicrob Agents Chemother 1997;41:1892–7.
64. Cato A III, Cao G, Hsu A, Cavanaugh J, Leonard J, Granneman R. Evaluation of the effect of fluconazole on the pharmacokinetics of ritonavir. Drug Metab Dispos 1997;25:1104–6.
65. Trapnell CB, Jamis-Dow C, Klecker RW, Collins JM. Metabolism of rifabutin and its 25-desacetyl metabolite, LM565, by human liver microsomes and recombinant human cytochrome P-450 3A4:relevance to clinical interaction with fluconazole. Antimicrob Agents Chemother 1997; 41:924–6.
66. Odom RB, Aly R, Scher RK, Daniel CR III, Elewski BE, Zaias N, DeVillez R, Jacko M, Oleka N, Moskovitz BL. A multicenter, placebo-controlled, double-blind study of intermittent therapy with itraconazole for the treatment of onychomycosis of the fingernail. J Am Acad Dermatol 1997;36:231–5.
67. Havu V, Brandt H, Heikkilä H, Hollmen A, Oksman R, Rantanen T, Saari S, Stubb S, Turjanmaa K, Piepponen T. A double-blind, randomized study comparing itraconazole pulse therapy with continuous dosing for the treatment of toenail onychomycosis. Br J Dermatol 1997;136:230–4.
68. Gupta AK, De-Doncker P, Heremans A, Stoffels P, Pierard GE, Decroix J, Heenen M, Degreef H. Itraconazole for the treatment of *tinea pedis*: a dosage of 400 mg/day given for 1 week is similar in efficacy to 100 or 200 mg/day given for 2 to 4 weeks. J Am Acad Dermatol 1997;36:789–92.
69. Wilcox CM, Darouiche RO, Laine L, Moskovitz BL, Mallegol I, Wu J. A randomized, double-blind comparison of itraconazole oral solution and fluconazole tablets in the treatment of esophageal candidiasis. J Infect Dis 1997;176:227–32.
70. Stevens DA, Lee JY. Analysis of compassionate use itraconazole therapy for invasive aspergillosis by the NIAID mycoses study group criteria. Arch Intern Med 1997;157:1857–62.
71. Vandewoude K, Vogelaers D, Decruyenaere J, Jaqmin P, De-Beule K, Van-Peer A, Woestenborghs R, Groen K, Colardyn F. Concentrations in plasma and safety of 7 days of intravenous itraconazole followed by 2 weeks of oral itraconazole solution in patients in intensive care units. Antimicrob Agents Chemother 1997;41:2714–18.
72. Hecht FM, Wheat J, Korzun AH, Hafner R, Skahan KJ, Larsen R, Limjoco MT, Simpson M, Schneider D, Keefer MC, Clark R, Kwan-Kew-Lai, Jacobson JM, Squires K, Bartlett JA, Powderly W. Itraconazole maintenance treatment for histoplasmosis in AIDS: a prospective, multicenter trial. J AIDS Hum Retrovirol 1997;16:100–7.
73. Young-Min-Park, Jin-Wou-Kim, Chung-Won-Kim. Acute generalized exanthematous pustulosis induced by itraconazole. J Am Acad Dermatol 1997;36:794–6.
74. Douglas R, Spelman D, Czarny D, O'Hehir R. Desensitization to itraconazole. J Allergy Clin Immunol 1997;99:269.
75. Jalava K-M, Olkkola KT, Neuvonen PJ. Itraconazole greatly increases plasma concentrations and effects of felodipine. Clin Pharmacol Ther 1997;61:410–15.
76. Lukkari E, Juhakoski A, Aranko K, Neuvonen PJ. Itraconazole moderately increases serum concentrations of oxybutynin but does not affect those of the active metabolite. Eur J Clin Pharmacol 1997;52:403–6.
77. Kivistö KT, Lamberg TS, Kantola T, Neuvonen PJ. Plasma buspirone concentrations are greatly increased by erythromycin and itraconazole. Clin Pharmacol Ther 1997;62:348–54.
78. Ito S, Koren G, Alderman CP, Allcroft P. Possible mechanism of digoxin-itraconazole interaction. Ann Pharmacother 1997;31:1091–2.
79. Small EJ, Baron AD, Fippin L, Apodaca D. Ketoconazole retains activity in advanced prostate

cancer patients with progression despite flutamide withdrawal. J Urol 1997;15:1204–7.

80. Small EJ, Baron A, Bok R. Simultaneous antiandrogen withdrawal and treatment with ketoconazole and hydrocortisone in patients with advanced prostate carcinoma. Cancer 1997;8: 1755–9.

81. Sarver RG, Dalkin BL, Ahmann FR. Ketoconazole-induced adrenal crisis in a patient with metastatic prostatic adenocarcinoma: case report and review of the literature. Urology 1997; 49:781–5.

82. Chien R-N, Yang L-J, Lin P-Y, Liaw Y-F. Hepatic injury during ketoconazole therapy in patients with onychomycosis: a controlled cohort study. Hepatology 1997;25:103–7.

83. Bernuau J, Durand F, Pessayre D, Chien R-N, Liaw Y-F. Ketoconazole-induced hepatotoxicity. Hepatology 1997;26:802.

Isabela Ribeiro, Charles Woodrow and Sanjeev Krishna

28 Antiprotozoal drugs

ANTIMALARIAL DRUGS

(SED-13, 799; SEDA-19, 262; SEDA-20, 257; SEDA-21, 293)

The current recommendations on the prevention and treatment of malaria have been reviewed (SEDA-20, 257; (1[R]), (2[R])).

Drug combinations As with other antimicrobial agents, the combination of two or more antimalarial drugs in treatment regimens for primary infections is being developed as a strategy to limit the emergence of drug resistance. Two related advantages accrue with combination regimens: the use of existing antimalarials to which resistance is developing may be prolonged, and resistance to new classes of antimalarials may be delayed. The potential disadvantage of combination regimens results from toxicity, which may arise through drug interactions as well as adverse effects of individual drug. The artemisinin derivatives seem to be relatively free from major toxicity, and for these and other reasons are now being studied in combination with a number of other, longer-acting antimalarials in many parts of the world. Chlorproguanil–dapsone and atovaquone–proguanil are also combinations under intensive investigation.

Artemisinin and derivatives

(SED-13, 818; SEDA-19, 262; SEDA-20, 259; SEDA-21, 293)

For reviews of the safety of artemisinin derivatives, see SEDA-21 (p. 293) and (3[R]).

The artemisinin family of antimalarial drugs comprises a number of derivatives that are effective in the treatment of both uncomplicated and severe *P. falciparum* malaria. Five compounds are available in an array of formulations: artesunate (intravenous, rectal, and oral), artemisinin (intramuscular, rectal, and oral), dihydroartemisinin (oral), artemether (intramuscular, rectal, and oral), and arteether (intramuscular).

Until recently there was a paucity of pharmacokinetic studies on these derivatives, hampered by the non-availability of adequate analytical methods. However, in the last 2 years several studies have been published (4[C])–(11[C]). Comparative studies on the antimalarial activity of these compounds have shown that short treatment courses are associated with significant incidence of recrudescence; regimens lasting 5–7 days minimize this risk. Shorter courses may achieve higher efficacy when combined with a longer-acting antimalarial, such as mefloquine (12[C])–(24[C]). The combination of mefloquine (25 mg/kg) and 3 days artesunate (12 mg/kg) remains an effective treatment in areas of multi-drug resistance (18[C]), (24[C]), but concerns about the tolerability of mefloquine have led to a search for alternative partners for artemisinin derivatives, such as benflumetol (see below).

Recent reviews of clinical trials have confirmed the benign safety profile of artemisinin derivatives (3[R]), (5[R]). Most adverse events were mild and transient, none resulted in discontinuation of treatment, and no adverse drug interactions were observed. Indeed, the incidence of *vomiting* induced by mefloquine appears to be lower when it is given after artesunate (3[R]). Although most artemisinin derivatives produce a highly characteristic neurological lesion in several animal species, so far there is no convincing evidence of neurotoxicity in man.

The drug known as CGP 56697 includes a variety of oral formulations of artemether and benflumetol in a fixed ratio of 1:6. Benflumetol (lumefantrine) is a Chinese fluorene derivative conforming to the arylamino alcohol group of antimalarials (which includes quin-

Side Effects of Drugs, Annual 22
J.K. Aronson, ed.

ine, mefloquine, and halofantrine) and has an elimination half-life of 4–5 days. CGP 56697 was efficacious and well tolerated in adults with uncomplicated malaria in China (25[C]). A phase II study in children and adults in Thailand (26[C]) showed that CGP 56697 was less efficacious but better tolerated than the standard artesunate–mefloquine regimen. There were no serious adverse effects, although 4% of patients in the CGP 56697 arm experienced *pruritus* and/or a *rash*. In Gambian children CGP 56697 was efficacious and did not cause neurodevelopmental delay (27[C]), (28[C]). In Tanzania this drug combination was much more effective than chloroquine alone, although this study was carried out in an area of high chloroquine resistance (29[C]). Artemether–benflumetol is a promising option for the treatment of uncomplicated malaria in areas of multi-drug resistance.

Atovaquone *(SED-13, 828; SEDA-19, 266; SEDA-20, 259; SEDA-21, 294)*

Atovaquone is considered under the section on the treatment and prophylaxis of *Pneumocystis carinii* pneumonia. The combination of atovaquone with proguanil is safe and effective in malaria and has recently been shown to be prophylactic in African children (30[C]).

CHLOROQUINE AND CONGENERS *(SED-13, 801; SEDA-19, 262; SEDA-20, 260; SEDA-21, 294)*

Chloroquine and hydroxychloroquine

The efficacy of chloroquine in *P. falciparum* infection is now limited by parasite resistance in most parts of the world, and several African countries no longer use chloroquine as routine first-line treatment. However, it is still used to treat *P. malariae*, *P. ovale*, and *P. vivax* infections and as prophylaxis (in combination with proguanil) in pregnant women or when mefloquine is inappropriate.

Skin and appendages '*Pruritus*' or severe *skin discomfort*, predominantly in the palmar and plantar areas occurs in 20% of Africans. Prednisolone (10 mg, single dose) can mitigate this adverse effect (31[C]). Other cutaneous reactions include *eruptions*, *mucocutaneous hyperpigmentation*, and *exacerbation of psoriasis*. *Acute generalized exanthematous pustulosis* has been reported to be associated with chloroquine (100 mg/day) plus proguanil (32[c]).

Immunological and hypersensitivity reactions *Immunosuppression* has been documented in soldiers taking chloroquine as long-term prophylaxis (33[C]), although the likelihood of opportunistic infections is low. An area of immediate practical concern to physicians managing travellers is the potential for antimalarials to interfere with vaccination, as previously exemplified by depressed immune responses to live rabies vaccination. Chloroquine and chlorproguanil, respectively, interfere with immunization with the live cholera vaccine CVD103-HgR (34[C]) and the live typhoid vaccine Ty21a. The mechanism of this interference may involve inhibition of antigen presentation and does not represent direct antibacterial activity of antimalarials. Chloroquine had no significant effect on tetanus–diphtheria vaccination (35[C]).

Amodiaquine *(SED-13, 807; SEDA-20, 260)*

Amodiaquine, a 4-aminoquinoline, has been used to treat and prevent malaria in the past. In the mid-1980s reports of fatal adverse reactions appeared, including *agranulocytosis*, *hepatotoxicity*, and *aplastic anemia*, and its licence for prophylaxis and first-line treatment was withdrawn. However, a review of amodiaquine treatment for uncomplicated malaria (36[R]) showed that tolerability was no worse than chloroquine or pyrimethamine–sulfadoxine and that life-threatening adverse reactions were reported only when the drug was used as prophylaxis. This conclusion was based on retrospective data only. Although there is partial cross-resistance between chloroquine and amodiaquine, amodiaquine remains a valuable drug that may have potential as first-line treatment of malaria.

Halofantrine *(SED-13, 820; SEDA-19, 263; SEDA-20, 260; SEDA-21, 295)*

Halofantrine is a phenanthrene methanol belonging to the arylaminoalcohol family. It is used as an alternative treatment for uncomplicated *P. falciparum* malaria in areas with a high prevalence of multiple drug resistance. No cross-resistance with chloroquine and atovaquone has been documented (37[C]), but there may be cross-susceptibility with quinine, mefloquine, and artemether (38[C]). Over the past year, there has been a sharp fall in susceptibility in isolates from Gabon (39[C]) and Burkina Faso (40[C]). In view of its potential for *cardiotoxicity*, cautious use of halofantrine has been advocated, particularly as a stand-by treatment for febrile illness among travellers (41[r]) or as a second-line treatment of *P. falciparum* malaria (42[c]), (43[c]). A combination regimen of halofantrine with primaquine was superior to chloroquine for the treatment of uncomplicated *P. falciparum* and *P. vivax* infections in Indonesia, with 100% cure rates at 28-day follow-up (44[C]). The regimen was well tolerated with no serious adverse effects.

Cardiovascular Halofantrine prolongs cardiac repolarization and prolongs the QT interval. It causes dose-related life-threatening *cardiac dysrhythmias*, such as torsade de pointes (SEDA-20, 263; SEDA-21, 295; (41[r])). A recent review of the literature and databases of the FDA has shown clear sex differences in the incidence of this phenomenon, women being at a higher risk for the development of halofantrine-related ventricular dysrhythmias (45[r]). The case of a young woman with no predisposing prolongation of the QT_c interval has recently been reported (46[c]).

Hematological *Hemolysis* imitating blackwater fever can follow treatment with halofantrine, as illustrated in two patients with a history of previous uncomplicated quinine treatment (47[c]).

Hypersensitivity and immunological reactions The first case of *anaphylactic shock* with halofantrine has been reported (48[c]).

Mefloquine *(SED-13, 808; SEDA-19, 265; SEDA-20, 261; SEDA-21, 296)*

Mefloquine remains useful in the treatment of uncomplicated malaria in areas of chloroquine resistance. The recommendations for mefloquine as prophylaxis in travellers are under constant review. An examination of the value of mefloquine prophylaxis has prompted debate about the tolerability of the drug (49[C]).

Cardiovascular Mefloquine pre-treatment *exacerbated the QT_c prolongation* caused by halofantrine (50[C]), but mefloquine itself does not prolong the QT_c interval (51[C]), (52[C]). Two recent reports have described *abnormalities of atrial and nodal conduction* associated with mefloquine (53[c]), (54[c]).

A 32-year-old man with no previous cardiac history took weekly mefloquine at the recommended dose during a trip to Thailand. Two days after each of the fourth, fifth, sixth, and seventh doses he had palpitation, dizziness, and vertigo. These symptoms disappeared within 2 days on all occasions. An electrocardiogram 3 days after the seventh dose showed aberrantly conducted beats, each followed by an aberrantly conducted echo-beat. There was no prolongation of the QT_c interval. Cardiac enzymes, echocardiography, and stress ECG showed no evidence of coronary insufficiency. The coupled aberrantly conducted beats occurred less often after withdrawal of mefloquine. Cardiograms later showed a relatively short PR interval, possibly related to a hitherto symptom-free Lown–Ganong–Levine syndrome.

A 63-year-old man, with a short history of bouts of palpitation 35 years before, presented with palpitation and chest discomfort 2 days after taking a first dose (250 mg) of mefloquine for a planned journey to Thailand. His electrocardiogram showed a regular narrow-complex tachycardia of 260/min. Administration of adenosine revealed atrial activity, confirming a diagnosis of atrial flutter with 1:1 A:V conduction. Administration of digoxin and sotalol changed A:V conduction to 2:1 before sinus rhythm was restored. Electrolytes, thyroid hormone concentrations, and echocardiogram were all normal.

Nervous system Disabling neuropsychiatric reactions after treatment and as prophylaxis have been reported in a child for the first time (55[c]). A comparison of artesunate–mefloquine with artemether–benflumetol (26[C]) has given an estimate of the true incidence of mefloquine-attributable neurological adverse effects (overall 10%), such as *dizziness*, *sleep disorders*, *abnormal gait*, *paresthesia*, *tremor*, *nystagmus*, and *ataxia*. The association of the postmalaria neurological syndrome with mefloquine treatment suggests that mefloquine should not be used in the treatment of severe malaria.

Skin and appendages Mefloquine has previously been associated with *erythema multiforme and Stevens–Johnson syndrome*. The first case of *toxic epidermal necrolysis* associated with mefloquine prophylaxis has now been reported (56[c]).

A 6-year-old healthy Nigerian girl, resident in the UK, began to take 125 mg mefloquine weekly a week before travelling to Nigeria. Five weeks later she developed blistering of the oral mucosa with periorbital and facial swelling. The blistering worsened and progressed to exfoliation of 95% of the body surface over 48 h. There was ulceration of the mucosal surfaces and her hair and nails were shed. She developed several complications of severe skin loss and was managed in a pediatric intensive care unit. Measures included careful attention to fluid balance, broad-spectrum antibiotics, and total parenteral nutrition. Although her pyrexia resolved and re-epithelialization began, cardiac asystole occurred and resuscitation attempts were unsuccessful. Necropsy was refused.

Use in pregnancy Mefloquine is teratogenic in animals given 5–20 times the recommended human dose. However, analysis of 1627 spontaneous reports of mefloquine exposure (data collected by the manufacturer) immediately before or during pregnancy has failed to demonstrate any particular type or increased prevalence of malformations (57[C]). In the US mefloquine is considered by the FDA as class III, i.e. it may be appropriate prophylaxis in pregnant women who travel to malarial areas, since the benefit of prophylaxis outweighs the risk of teratogenicity.

Interactions The combination of mefloquine with *quinine* may be encountered in self-medication polypharmacy or when failed mefloquine treatment requires a course of quinine (or vice versa). Understandably, there has been concern that the two drugs may have a clinically significant pharmacodynamic interaction, but there was no evidence for this in one small study (58[c]).

Primaquine and congeners (8-aminoquinolines) *(SED-13, 810; SEDA-19, 264; SEDA-21, 296)*

Primaquine is an 8-aminoquinoline antimalarial used to eradicate the hepatic stages of *P. vivax* and *P. ovale* and as prophylaxis against *P. falciparum*. It is less immunosuppressive than chloroquine (33[c]). Primaquine prophylaxis enhanced anti-tetanus antibody titres after diphtheria–tetanus immunization (35[C]).

Etaquine (WR 238605) *(SED-13, 811)*

Etaquine, an analog of primaquine with a half-life of 14 days, had greater efficacy and less toxicity than primaquine in preclinical studies. Initial studies in healthy volunteers showed only mild, transient *gastrointestinal adverse effects* at doses of 300–600 mg (59[C]). The relative hemolytic potential of WR 238605 compared with primaquine is unknown, since individuals with G6PD deficiency were excluded. In a subsequent efficacy study a single dose of 300 mg had good efficacy, protecting three of four subjects challenged with malaria (60[C]). In the subject who developed malaria, patency was delayed for 3 weeks compared with controls, and symptoms were less severe. These safety, efficacy, and pharmacokinetic properties make etaquine a strong candidate for further testing as a prophylactic, radical curative, and terminal eradication drug.

Proguanil and congeners *(SED-13, 811)*

Hematological The potential of proguanil to cause serious *bone marrow toxicity* when it accumulates in patients with chronic renal failure has again been demonstrated (61[c]).

Immunological and hypersensitivity reactions Chlorproguanil *interferes with immunization* with the live typhoid vaccine Ty21a, as noted above.

Chlorproguanil–dapsone

The antifolate combination chlorproguanil–dapsone is cleared more rapidly from the body than the pyrimethamine–sulfadoxine combination and may therefore exert less long-term selection pressure on parasites. Furthermore, the mutation that is thought to confer resistance to chlorcycloguanil (the active metabolite of chlorproguanil) is relatively rare in Africa, and chlorproguanil–dapsone is more potent in vitro than pyrimethamine–sulfadoxine. A pharmacokinetic study (62[C]) and a trial (63[C]) in Kenya have shown that a 3-day course of daily chlorproguanil–dapsone is safe and effective in children with uncomplicated malaria. A comparable regimen had a high failure rate in Thailand, where multidrug resistance is more prevalent. Chlorproguanil–dapsone is a relatively cheap drug combination that may find use as an effective alternative to pyrimethamine–sulfadoxine in areas such as East Africa, where resistance to antifolates is present but not so entrenched as in South-East Asia.

Pyronaridine *(SEDA-21, 297)*

Pyronaridine is an acridine antimalarial with a relatively slow action that has been used to treat uncomplicated *P. falciparum* and *P. vivax* malaria in China for the past 20 years. Pyronaridine was efficacious and safe for the treatment of uncomplicated chloroquine-resistant falciparum malaria in children in Cameroon; adverse effects associated with it were minor, transient, and mainly limited to the gastrointestinal tract (64[C]). Pyronaridine was also effective against *P. ovale* and *P. malariae* infections in this population (65[C]). However, on the China–Laos PDR border the average defervescence time of falciparum malaria treated by pyronaridine has increased from 33 to 56 h, with recrudescence rates rising from 15 to 38% in 1995 (66[C]).

Quinine and congeners *(SED-13, 814; SEDA-19, 265; SEDA-20, 261; SEDA-21, 297)*

Overdosage Quinine is widely prescribed as symptomatic treatment for leg cramps, and cases of self-poisoning appear to be common (67[c]). Acute intoxication is associated with *blindness*, *cardiotoxicity*, and *acute renal failure*; *death* has been reported with a dose of as little as 8 g. Management consists of measures to reduce quinine absorption. Hyperbaric oxygen has been proposed as specific therapy for blindness.

Malaria vaccines *(SED-13, 822; SEDA-21, 298)*

For reviews of the current strategies for vaccine development, see (68[R])–(70[R]).

Candidate malaria vaccines have failed to elicit consistently protective immune responses against challenge with P. falciparum *(71[C])–(76[C]). To circumvent difficulties due to parasite polymorphism and genetic restriction of T-cell responses, new strategies are being devised, such as the use of DNA vaccines. Phase I studies of a DNA vaccine containing sequence from 10 peptides demonstrated good cytotoxic T-lymphocyte responses (77[C]); the toxicity profile will be reported in the near future. Optimization of multigene* P. falciparum *DNA vaccines will require extensive clinical trials during coming years (78[C]).*

Another vaccine candidate is the multiple antigen peptide (MAP) system consisting of multiple copies of a B-cell epitope from the central repeat region of the P. falciparum *circumsporozoite protein (PfCSP), in combination with a universal T-cell epitope, the P2P30 portion of tetanus toxin. Rodent studies showed high immunogenicity of this vaccine formulated with a different adjuvant, specifically in liposomes, lipid A, and aluminium hydroxide (79[C]).*

Recombinant constructs representing both major allelic forms of the P. falciparum *merozoite surface antigen (MSA-2) have been formulated with a range of adjuvants, with good results (80[C]). The merozoite surface protein-1 (MSP-1) has also emerged as a potential target.*

Two new types of vaccines are under preliminary clinical evaluation. One is directed against sexual-stage surface antigens of P. falciparum *(Pfs25 and Pfs28) and can block the transmission of the disease (81[C])–(83[C]). The other is an antisporozoite vaccine with a new immunogen (RTS, S) in which the circumsporozoite protein is fused to the hepatitis B surface antigen and can protect against infection (84[C]), (85[C]).*

Another strategy in vaccine development is the use of enhancers, such as recombinant vaccinia viruses (86[C]) and GM-CSF (87[C]). NYVAC-Pf7, a highly attenuated vaccinia virus with fragments of seven P. falciparum *genes inserted into its genome, was recently tested in a phase I/IIa trial in healthy volunteers, who received three immunizations of two different dosages of NYVAC-Pf7 (88[C]). The vaccine was safe and well tolerated but variably immunogenic. While antibody responses were generally poor, cellular immune responses were detected in over 90% of the volunteers.*

DRUGS USED FOR *PNEUMOCYSTIS CARINII* PNEUMONIA

The drugs used for the treatment and prophylaxis of *Pneumocystis carinii* pneumonia have been reviewed (SEDA-20, 266; (89[R])–(92[R])).

Atovaquone *(SED-13, 828; SEDA-19, 266; SEDA-20, 264; SEDA-21, 298)*

Atovaquone is a hydroxynaphthaquinone compound active in the prevention and treatment of *Pneumocystis carinii* pneumonia, *P. falciparum* malaria, and *Toxoplasma gondii* infections.

The oral suspension of micronized atovaquone is under investigation in infants and children. A recent Phase I study conducted by the Pediatric AIDS Clinical Trials Group has shown that this formulation is safe and well tolerated in children. A single daily dose of 30 mg/kg may be adequate for therapy of *P. carinii* pneumonia, but infants aged 3–24 months may require a dosage of 45 mg/kg per day (93[C]).

Co-trimoxazole (trimethoprim–sulfamethoxazole) *(SED-13, 826; SEDA-19, 268; SEDA-20, 264; SEDA-21, 299)*

Co-trimoxazole remains the mainstay for the prophylaxis and treatment of a variety of opportunistic infections in HIV-infected patients (89[R])–(91[R]). Nevertheless, it is underused because of the high incidence of adverse events. A recent meta-analysis has been published on the relative efficacy and toxicity of *P. carinii* prophylactic regimens (94[R]). Regardless of dose, co-trimoxazole was almost universally effective for patients who tolerated it. Substituting one double-strength tablet (1600/320 mg) three times a week instead of the standard tablet daily led to a reduction of 43% (95% CI 30–54%) in the number of patients who had to discontinue the drug because of adverse effects.

Nervous system Co-trimoxazole-induced *aseptic meningitis* has been described before (SEDA-19, 269; SEDA-21, 299). A similar adverse effect reported in a patient treated solely with trimethoprim was also associated with *uveitis* (95[c]). Although the trimethoprim component has been implicated as a cause of aseptic meningitis in the past (96[c]), (97[c]), uveitis has so far been attributed to sulfonamides (98[c]).

An 18-year-old woman presented with a recent history of recurrent urinary tract infections. During her second episode of urinary tract infection treated with trimethoprim, she developed headache, red and sore eyes, and neck ache within hours of the first dose. She was given amoxicillin–clavulanate instead and completed a 7-day course. Her eye pain persisted for 2 weeks. Two months later, she developed headache, fever, painful red eyes, and photophobia after having been given trimethoprim for urinary tract symptoms. She had neck stiffness and a positive Kernig's sign. A slit lamp examination showed white cells in the anterior chamber and a proteinaceous 'flare', consistent with a diagnosis of bilateral anterior uveitis.

Other neurological adverse effects include *headaches, ataxia, peripheral neuritis, sei-*

zures, *hallucinations*, and *tremor*. The first case of isolated tremor ascribed to co-trimoxazole has been reported in a patient with AIDS (99[c]).

A 46-year-old man with a 6-year history of AIDS was evaluated for 'shakes'. He had taken co-trimoxazole for PCP for 13 days and had experienced increasing tremulousness over the preceding 10 days. His other medications included paroxetine, didanosine, prednisone, leucovorin, clotrimazole, and diazepam, none of which had been started recently. He had no known AIDS-related neurological complication, except for mild sensory neuropathy, thought to be associated with didanosine. Neurological examination showed a bilateral, high frequency, low amplitude postural tremor, greater in the arms than the legs. It was less prominent on finger–nose and heel–shin testing and absent at rest. He had a similar tremor of the head. His handwriting was markedly impaired. His gait was hesitant but not wide-based. He was slightly unsteady but did not tend to fall to one side or the other. The remainder of the physical examination was unremarkable. A cranial CT scan and lumbar puncture were within normal limits. A tentative diagnosis of co-trimoxazole-induced tremor was made, and the drug was withheld. His symptoms resolved within 3 days.

Endocrine, metabolic Because they are structurally similar to sulfonylureas, sulfonamides may cause *hypoglycemia* in susceptible individuals by increasing pancreatic secretion of insulin. Hypoglycemia resulting from a combination of sulfonylureas and sulfonamides is well recognised. Nine cases of hypoglycemia have been reported with the isolated use of co-trimoxazole alone. Over the past year, two further cases have been described, one in a patient with acute renal failure and another in a malnourished patient with severe infection (100[c]), (101[c]).

Urinary system The trimethoprim component of co-trimoxazole can cause mild reversible *increases in serum creatinine*, reportedly by inhibiting its renal tubular secretion (102[c]).

Mineral and fluid balance Trimethoprim has also been implicated in an amiloride-like action on the distal tubule, leading to *hyperkalemia* with both high and low doses (103[c]), (104[C]), (105[c]). Severe symptomatic hyperkalemia has recently been reported in a patient with hyporeninemic hypoaldosteronism taking a standard dose of co-trimoxazole (106[c]). This case highlighted the importance of careful follow-up of patients with disturbances of potassium homeostasis, and especially of renal potassium handling, who are treated with co-trimoxazole. A new mechanism of hyperkalemia has also been described in a patient taking a standard dose of co-trimoxazole for prolonged treatment of a urinary tract infection: voltage-dependent renal tubular acidosis with consequent hyperkalemia and hyperchloremic metabolic acidosis (107[c]).

Liver and biliary The first case of *vanishing bile duct syndrome* has been reported with co-trimoxazole (108[c]). This rare syndrome is characterized by progressive cholestasis, caused by the irreversible loss of bile ducts, which can lead to progressive liver failure.

A 57-year-old Samoan-American man with no significant past medical history developed jaundice within 5 days of taking a therapeutic course of co-trimoxazole (800/160 mg) for prostatitis. Before therapy, liver enzymes and hematological tests had been within normal limits. Five days after the start of co-trimoxazole the AsT was 205 U/l (reference range 10–45 U/l), the AlT was 465 U/l (10–45 U/l), the alkaline phosphatase 295 U/l (30–130 U/l), and the total bilirubin 34 μmol/l (under 20 μmol/l). Prothrombin, partial thromboplastin, serum iron concentration, and iron-binding capacity were normal. Drug-induced cholestasis was suspected and co-trimoxazole was withdrawn. A liver biopsy 12 weeks later showed severe intrahepatic cholestasis and bile ducts in fewer than 25% of the portal tracts. Antinuclear and antimitochondrial antibodies, hepatitis A, B, and C virus serology, HIV testing, abdominal CT scan, and endoscopic retrograde cholangiopancreatography were normal. Anti-smooth muscle antibodies were positive (1:640). Prednisone 40 mg/day produced no significant response. After orthotopic liver transplantation, histology showed extensive fibrosis and almost complete loss of bile ducts from the portal tracts.

Drug-induced ductopenia can progress long after the offending drug is withdrawn. Although the titers of anti-smooth muscle antibodies were raised in this case, the diagnosis of autoimmune hepatitis was felt to be unlikely, given the histological features and the absence of response to steroids.

Skin and appendages Two reports of *fixed drug eruption* have appeared, one described as linear (extending from the lateral aspect of the fourth and fifth finger, along the wrist and lateral aspect of the extensor surface of the arm) and the other post-coitally on the coronal sulcus of the penis (109[c]), (110[c]).

Immunological and hypersensitivity reactions Some cutaneous reactions to co-trimoxazole may be immunologically mediated and may be due to common antigenic determinants between drug and viruses or the build-up of toxic hydroxyalamine metabolites of sulfamethoxazole that can function as haptens. There is increasing confidence in the efficacy of desensitization protocols for non-life-threatening adverse reactions to co-trimoxazole, with success rates of 45–97% (111[R])–(113[R]), (114[C]), (115[C]). Some questions, however, still remain. It is unclear whether reinstitution of full-dose therapy (rechallenge) or a dose escalation regimen ('desensitization') is better. However, desensitization, although useful, is not entirely safe.

There have been reports of *anaphylactoid reactions* (113[R]), consisting of erythematous rash, conjunctivitis, acute fever, intense pruritus, and hypotension on re-exposure, occasionally associated with pulmonary infiltrates, dyspnea, hypoxemia, and renal failure.

A co-trimoxazole *desensitization syndrome* with delayed hematological toxicity has also been described (116[R]).

Interactions A case of hyperpigmentation of flexures and pancytopenia has been reported with the combined used of co-trimoxazole and *pyrimethamine* (117[c]). This reaction was thought to be a manifestation of folate deficiency caused by the use of the two folate antagonists.

Dapsone *(SED-13, 826)*

The use of dapsone for the treatment and prevention of *P. carinii* infection has recently been reviewed (118[R]).

Dapsone, with or without trimethoprim or pyrimethamine, has strong activity against *P. carinii*, as demonstrated by in vitro methods, animal studies, and clinical trials. Dapsone blocks folic acid synthesis in *P. carinii* by inhibition of dihydropteroate synthetase activity. It also has activity against other human pathogens, e.g. *Mycobacterium leprae*, and has been used in the treatment of chronic autoimmune thrombocytopenic purpura. Dapsone is well absorbed (70%–80%) from the gastrointestinal tract, reaches a peak serum concentration in 2–6 h, and is adequately distributed to the fluid of the alveolar spaces. The combination with trimethoprim is recommended for therapeutic use for *P. carinii* pneumonia in patients who cannot tolerate co-trimoxazole. Dapsone is also active against *P. falciparum* and is used in combination with proguanil (see above) and pyrimethamine.

Evidence from more than 40 studies of dapsone as prophylaxis for *P. carinii* pneumonia in AIDS patients has shown that dapsone, either alone or in combination with pyrimethamine, is as effective as aerosolized pentamidine or atovaquone but slightly less effective than co-trimoxazole (118[R]). A recent meta-analysis (94[R]) has shown that among 100 patients given dapsone 100 mg/day instead of twice a week for 1 year for primary prophylaxis of *P. carinii*, seven fewer patients would develop it, but 17 more would have significant toxic reactions. Thus, low doses of dapsone reduce toxic effects, but at the expense of some loss of efficacy. Adverse effects include *rash*, *anemia*, *methemoglobinemia*, *agranulocytosis*, *hepatic dysfunction*, and dose-dependent *hemolysis*, particularly in patients with glucose-6-phosphate dehydrogenase deficiency. There has been a recent report of *urinary tract carcinoma* among 12 leprosy patients treated with dapsone for long periods (2–25 years); however, all these patients had also taken phenacetin-containing analgesics (119[C]).

DRUGS USED FOR TOXOPLASMOSIS

Sulfadiazine

Sulfadiazine–pyrimethamine is the drug combination of choice in the treatment of toxoplasmosis.

Urinary system Sulfonamide-induced *crys-*

talluria with renal failure is well documented and there have been several case reports of this complication among patients with AIDS treated for cerebral toxoplasmosis. A third case of sulfadiazine-induced obstructive renal failure secondary to crystalluria, requiring surgical intervention has now been described (120[C]).

Salivary glands The first case of *sialadenitis* induced by sulfadiazine has been described (121[c]).

A 50-year-old man, a long-time smoker with a history of chronic bronchitis and allergy to β-lactam antibiotics, was given Bronco-aseptilex® (sulfadiazine 350 mg/5 ml, cyclamate, and guaiacol) for an exacerbation of chronic bronchitis. Two hours after the first dose (5 ml of syrup), he noted a swelling in his throat and the floor of his mouth, and plugging of his ears. He was treated with antihistamines and prednisone and Bronco-aseptilex® was discontinued. He recovered completely after 3 days. Prick testing with an undiluted solution of Bronco-aseptilex® and diluted sulfadiazine was negative. There was bilateral swelling of the parotid and submandibular glands after single-blind oral challenges with Bronco-aseptilex® and sulfadiazine.

DRUGS FOR VISCERAL LEISHMANIASIS

Pentavalent antimonials have been the mainstay in the treatment of visceral leishmaniasis (kala-azar). These drugs commonly cause *myalgia* and *arthralgia*, and case reports have emphasized the potential of sodium antimony gluconate to cause *cardiotoxicity* (122[c]), (123[c]).

Cardiovascular Lot-to-lot variations occur in the manufacture of antimony formulations, and these may influence clinical efficacy and toxicity. All eight cases of visceral leishmaniasis treated with sodium antimony gluconate 20 mg/kg per day from one relatively high osmolarity lot developed cardiotoxicity 3–28 days after starting therapy. This consisted of *congestive cardiac failure*, *prolongation of the QT_c interval*, and *ventricular extra beats followed by ventricular tachycardia*, *torsade de pointes*, and *ventricular fibrillation*; three patients died. No patient had taken a total dose of more than 600 mg/kg. The authors proposed that the osmolarity of formulations should be measured to help identify inappropriately manufactured drug (124[C]).

Visceral leishmaniasis is becoming increasingly resistant to sodium antimony gluconate in Bihar State, India, so that new drugs (or preferably combinations of drugs to prevent the emergence of resistance) are urgently needed (125[r]). Amphotericin B is efficacious, but has a poor safety profile in this population (in addition to which the lipid complex form is prohibitively expensive) and furthermore increases the cardiotoxicity associated with sodium antimony gluconate. In a study of patients treated with amphotericin B after failure to respond to sodium antimony gluconate, amphotericin B precipitated ventricular dysrhythmias and cardiac arrest on the first day of infusion in three of seven patients who still had electrocardiographic evidence of antimonial-related cardiotoxicity (126[C]). Patients given a 10-day rest period after treatment with sodium antimony gluconate before starting amphotericin B, allowing the cardiogram to stabilize, did not develop any cardiac problem. In patients with visceral leishmaniasis who fail to respond to sodium antimony gluconate but have electrocardiographic evidence of cardiotoxicity, amphotericin B should be delayed for at least 10 days to allow resolution of antimonial-related cardiotoxicity. It must be noted that this interaction could reasonably have been predicted in advance, given the potential of amphotericin B to cause hypokalemia, itself a cause of a long QT interval. Intravenous aminosidine (a 21-day course of 16 or 20 mg/kg) is highly efficacious in this area (127[C]), but its adverse effects profile is not fully documented, particularly in terms of neuro-ototoxicity. Furthermore, intravenous aminosidine is not currently being marketed.

OTHER COMPOUNDS

Furazolidone *(SED-13, 837)*

Psychiatric A prolonged course of furazolidone given to a patient with AIDS for the treatment of giardiasis resistant to metronidazole was associated with an episode of *hypomania* (128[c]). The mechanism may have involved cumulative monoamine oxidase inhibition.

Metronidazole *(SED-13, 831; SEDA-19, 270; SEDA-21, 301)*

Neuropsychiatric Metronidazole can cause a number of neuropsychiatric adverse effects, such as *encephalopathy*, *cerebellar dysfunction*, *seizures*, *states of confusion*, *excitation*, and *depression*. An episode of major psychosis has been attributed to a 5-day course of intravenous metronidazole (129[c]).

Use in pregnancy Metronidazole readily crosses the placenta, and its use in pregnancy is controversial. It is classified according to the FDA risk categories for drug use during pregnancy as a B risk drug: i.e. either animal reproduction studies have not shown risk to the fetus but there are no controlled studies in pregnant women, or animal studies have shown an adverse effect on the fetus that was not confirmed in controlled studies in women in the first trimester of pregnancy. The manufacturer and the Centers for Disease Control have stated that metronidazole should not be used during the first trimester. However, since there are no options for the treatment of trichomoniasis, metronidazole is often used to treat this infection during pregnancy (130[r]). A recent meta-analysis did not show any relation between metronidazole exposure during the first trimester of pregnancy and birth defects (131[R]).

REFERENCES

1. Bradley DJ, Warhurst DC. Guidelines for the prevention of malaria in travellers from the United Kingdom. Commun Dis Rep CDR Rev 1997;7:R137–52
2. White NJ. The treatment of malaria. New Engl J Med 1997;335:800–6.
3. Ribeiro I, Olliaro P. Safety of artemisinin and its derivatives. A systematic review of published and unpublished clinical trials. Paper presented at 'The rational use of qinghaosu and its derivatives', a conference convened by the International Laveran Association, Annecy, France, 19–22 April 1998.
4. Hassan-Alin M, Ashton M, Kihamia CM, Mtey GJ, Bjorkman A. Multiple dose pharmacokinetics of oral artemisinin and comparison of its efficacy with that of oral artesunate in falciparum malaria patients. Trans R Soc Trop Med Hyg 1996;90:61–5.
5. Alin MH, Ashton M, Kihamia CM, Mtey GJB, Bjorkman A. Clinical efficacy and pharmacokinetics of artemisinin monotherapy and in combination with mefloquine in patients with falciparum malaria. Br J Clin Pharmacol 1996; 41:587–92.
6. Batty KT, Thu LTA, Davis TME, Ilett KF, Mai TX, Hung NC, Tien NP, Powell SM, Thien HV, Binh TQ, Kim NV. A pharmacokinetic and pharmacodynamic study of intravenous vs. oral artesunate in uncomplicated malaria. Br J Clin Pharmacol 1998;45:123–9.
7. Benakis A, Paris M, Loutan L, Plessas CT, Plessas ST. Pharmacokinetics of artemisinin and artesunate after oral administration in healthy volunteers. Am J Trop Med Hyg 1997;56:17–23.
8. Benakis A, Paris M, Loutan L, Plessas CT, Plessas ST. Pharmacokinetic study of a new pharmaceutical form of artesunate (Plasmotrim 200 Rectocaps) administered in healthy volunteers by rectal route. Jpn J Trop Med Hyg 1996;24 (Suppl 1):39–45.
9. Bethell DB, Teja-Isavadharm P, Phuong CXT, Thuy PTT, Mai TTT, Thuy TTN, Ha NTT, Phuong PT, Kyle D, Day NPJ, White NJ. Pharmacokinetics of oral artesunate in children with moderately severe *Plasmodium falciparum* malaria. Trans R Soc Trop Med Hyg 1997;91:195–8.
10. De Vries PJ, Tran Khac Dien, Nguyen Xuan Khanh, Le Nguyen Binh, Pham Thi Yen, Dao Din Duc, Van Boxtel CJ, Kager PA. The pharmacokinetics of a single dose of artemisinin in patients with uncomplicated falciparum malaria. Am J Trop Med Hyg 1997;56:503–7.
11. Benakis A, Paris M, Anh TK, Binh TQ, Plessas CT, Plessas ST. Pharmacokinetic study of dihidroartemisinin in malaria patients in Vietnam. Jpn J Trop Med Hyg 1996;24 (Suppl 1):71–6.
12. Looareesuwan S, Viravan C, Vanijanonta S, Wilairatana P, Suntharasamai P, Charoenlarp P, Arnold K, Kyle D, Canfield C, Webster K. Randomised trial of artesunate and mefloquine alone and in sequence for acute uncomplicated falciparum malaria. Lancet 1992;339:821–4.
13. Looareesuwan S, Viravan C, Vanijanonta S, Wilairatana P, Pitisuttithum P, Andrial M. Comparative clinical trial of artesunate followed by mefloquine in the treatment of acute uncomplicated falciparum malaria: two- and three-day regimens. Am J Trop Med Hyg 1996;54:210–13.
14. Looareesuwan S, Vanijanonta S, Viravan C, Wilairatana P, Charoenlarp P, Andrial M. Ran-

domised trial of mefloquine alone and artesunate followed by mefloquine for the treatment of acute uncomplicated falciparum malaria. Ann Trop Med Parasitol 1994;88:131–6.
15. Luxemburger C, ter Kuile FO, Nosten F, Dolan G, Bradol JH, Phaipun L, Chongsuphajaisiddhi T, White NJ. Single day mefloquine-artesunate combination in the treatment of multidrug resistant falciparum malaria. Trans R Soc Trop Med Hyg 1994;88:213–17.
16. Nosten F Artemisinin: large community studies Trans R Soc Trop Med Hyg 1994;88 (Suppl 1):S45–6.
17. Looareesuwan S, Wilairatana P, Vanijanonta S, Viravan C, Andrial M. Efficacy and tolerability of a sequential, artesunate suppository followed by mefloquine, treatment of severe falciparum malaria. Ann Trop Med Parasitol 1995;89:469–75.
18. Sabchareon A, Attanath P, Chanthavanich P, Phanuaksook, Prarinyanupharb V, Poonpanich Y, Mookamanee P, Teja-Isavadharm P, Heppner DG, Brewer TG, Chongsuphajaisiddhi T. Comparative clinical trial of artesunate suppositories and oral artesunate in combination with mefloquine in the treatment of children with acute falciparum malaria. Am J Trop Med Hyg 1998;58:11–16.
19. Looareesuwan S, Wilairatana P, Molunto W, Chalermrut K, Olliaro P, Andrial M. A comparative clinical trial of sequential treatments of severe malaria with artesunate suppository followed by mefloquine in Thailand. Am J Trop Med Hyg 1997;57:348–53.
20. Bhatt KM, Bhatt SM, Omonge E, Oteko L, Andrial M. Efficacy and tolerability of a sequential artesunate suppository-mefloquine treatment of severe falciparum malaria. Jpn J Trop Med Hyg 1996;24 (Suppl 1):59–63.
21. Gómez-Landires EA. Efficacy of artesunate suppository followed by oral mefloquine in the treatment of severe falciparum malaria in endemic areas where resistance to chloroquine exists in Ecuador. Jpn J Trop Med Hyg 1996;24 (Suppl 1):17–24.
22. Thwe Y, Than M, Phay S, Oo AZ, Soe AY. Artesunate suppository-mefloquine tablets (Plasmotrim, Rectocaps, Mefloquine, Lactab) in the treatment of severe falciparum malaria. Jpn J Trop Med Hyg 1996;24 (Suppl 1):25–32.
23. Kyaw W, Than M, Thwe Y, Gyi KK, Soe AY, Sabai, Ye H, Tint K, Aye KM. Efficacy of artemether and artesunate suppositories (Rectocaps) in the treatment of uncomplicated falciparum malaria. Jpn J Trop Med Hyg 1996;24 (Suppl 1):55–8.
24. Price RN, Nosten F, Luxemburger C, van Vugt M, Phaipun L, Chongsuphajaisiddhi T, White NJ. Artesunate/mefloquine treatment of multi-drug resistant falciparum malaria. Trans R Soc Trop Med Hyg 1997;91:574–7.
25. Jiao X, Liu GY, Shan CO, Zhao X, Li XW, Gathmann I, Royce C. Phase II trial in China of a new, rapidly-acting and effective oral antimalarial, CGP 56697, for the treatment of *Plasmodium falciparum* malaria. Southeast Asian J Trop Med Public Health 1997;28:476–81.
26. Van Vugt M, Brockman A, Gemperli B, Luxemburger C, Gathmann I, Royce C, Slight T, Looareesuwan S, White NJ, Nosten F. Randomized comparison of artemetherbenflumetol and artesunatemefloquine in treatment of multidrug-resistant falciparum malaria. Antimicrob Agents Chemother 1998;42:135–9.
27. Von Seidlein L, Jaffar S, Pinder M, Haywood M, Snounou G, Gemperli B, Gathmann I, Royce C, Greenwood B. Treatment of African children with uncomplicated falciparum malaria with a new antimalarial drug, CGP 56697. J Infect Dis 1997;176:1113–16.
28. Von Seidlein L, Bojang K, Jones P, Jaffar S, Pinder M, Obaro S, Doherty T, Haywood M, Snounou G, Gemperli B, Gathmann I, Royce C, McAdam K, Greenwood B. A randomized controlled trial of artemether/benflumetol, a new antimalarial and pyrimethamine/sulfadoxine in the treatment of uncomplicated falciparum malaria in African children. Am J Trop Med Hyg 1998;58:638–44.
29. Hatz C, Abdulla S, Mull R, Schellenberg D, Gathmann I, Kibatala P, Beck H-P, Tanner M, Royce C. Efficacy and safety of CGP 56697 (artemether and benflumetol) compared with chloroquine to treat acute falciparum malaria in Tanzanian children aged 1–5 years. Trop Med Int Health 1998;3:498–504.
30. Lell B, Luckner D, Ndjave M, Scott T, Kremsner PG. Randomised placebo-controlled study of atovaquone plus proguanil for malaria prophylaxis in children. Lancet 1998;351:709–13.
31. Adebayo RA, Sofowora GG, Onayemi O, Udoh SJ, Ajayi AA. Chloroquine-induced pruritus in malaria fever: contribution of malaria parasitaemia and the effects of prednisolone, niacin, and their combination, compared with antihistamine. Br J Clin Pharmacol 1997;44:157–61.
32. Janier M, Froidevaux D, Lons-Danic D, Daniel F. Acute generalized exanthematous pustulosis due to the combination of chloroquine and proguanil. Dermatology 1998;196:271.
33. Fryauff DJ, Church LW, Richards AL, Widjaja H, Mouzin E, Ratiwayanto S, Hadiputranto H, Sutamihardja MA, Richie TL, Subianto B, Tjitra E, Hoffman SL. Lymphocyte response to tetanus toxoid among Indonesian men immunized with tetanus-diphtheria during extended chloroquine or primaquine prophylaxis. J Infect Dis 1997;176:1644–8.
34. Kollaritsch H, Que JU, Kunz C, Wiedermann G, Herzog C, Cryz SJ Jr. Safety and immunogenicity of live oral cholera and typhoid vaccines administered alone or in combination with antimalarial drugs, oral polio vaccine, or yellow fever vaccine. J Infect Dis 1997;175:871–5.
35. Fryauff DJ, Cryz SJ, Widjaja H, Mouzin E, Church LW, Sutamihardja MA, Richards AL, Subianto B, Hoffman SL. Humoral immune response to tetanus-diphtheria vaccine given during

extended use of chloroquine or primaquine malaria chemoprophylaxis. J Infect Dis 1998; 177:1762–5.
36. Olliaro P, Nevill C, LeBras J, Ringwald P, Mussano P, Garner P, Brasseur P. Systematic review of amodiaquine treatment in uncomplicated malaria. Lancet 1996;348:1196–201.
37. Gay F, Bustos D, Traore B, Jardinel C, Southammavong M, Ciceron L, Danis MM. In vitro response of *Plasmodium falciparum* to atovaquone and correlation with other antimalarials: comparison between African and Asian strains. Am J Trop Med Hyg 1997;56:315–7.
38. Pradines B, Rogier C, Fusai T, Tall A, Trape JF, Doury JC. In vitro activity of artemether against African isolates (Senegal) of *Plasmodium falciparum* in comparison with standard antimalarial drugs. Am J Trop Med Hyg 1998;58:354–7.
39. Philipps J, Radloff PD, Wernsdorfer W, Kremsner PG. Follow-up of the susceptibility of *Plasmodium falciparum* to antimalarials in Gabon. Am J Trop Med Hyg 1998;58:612–18.
40. Ouedraogo JB, Dutheil Y, Tinto H, Traore B, Zampa H, Tall F, Coulibaly SO, Guiguemde T. In vitro sensitivity of *Plasmodium falciparum* to halofantrine compared with chloroquine, quinine and mefloquine in the region of Bobo-Dioulasso, Burkina Faso (West Africa). Trop Med Int Health 1998;3:381–4.
41. Touze JE, Fourcade L, Peyron F, Heno P, Deharo JC. Is halofantrine still advisable in malaria attacks? Ann Trop Med Parasitol 1997; 91:867–73.
42. Touze JE, Perret JL, Nicolas X, Fourcade L, Bernard J, Keundjian A, Soares JM, Doury JC. Efficacy of low-dose halofantrine for second treatment of uncomplicated falciparum malaria. Lancet 1997;349:255–6.
43. Tish KN, Pillans PI. Recrudescence of *Plasmodium falciparum* malaria contracted in Lombok, Indonesia after quinine/doxycycline and mefloquine: case report. New Zealand Med J 1997;110:255–6.
44. Fryauff DJ, Baird JK, Basri H, Wiady I, Purnomo, Bangs MJ, Subianto B, Harjosuwarno S, Tjitra E, Richie TL, Hoffman SL. Halofantrine and primaquine for radical cure of malaria in Irian Jaya, Indonesia. Ann Trop Med Parasitol 1997; 91:7–16.
45. Ebert SN, Liu X-K, Woosley RL. Female gender as a risk factor for drug-induced cardiac arrhythmias: evaluation of clinical and experimental evidence. J Womens Health 1998;7:547–57.
46. Gundersen SG, Rostrup M, von der Lippe E, Platou ES, Myrvang B, Edwards G. Halofantrine-associated ventricular fibrillation in a young woman with no predisposing QT_c prolongation. Scand J Infect Dis 1997;29:207–8.
47. Van den Ende J, Coppens G, Verstraeten T, Van Haegenborgh T, Depraetere K, Van Gompel A, Van den Enden E, Clerinx J, Colebunders R, Peetermans WE, Schroyens W. Recurrence of blackwater fever: triggering of relapses by different antimalarials. Trop Med Int Health 1998; 3:632–9.
48. Fourcade L, Gachot B, De Pina JJ, Heno P, Laurent G, Touze JE. Anaphylactic shock associated with halofantrine treatment for malaria. Presse Med 1997;26:559.
49. Croft A, Garner P. Mefloquine to prevent malaria: a systematic review of trials. Br Med J 1997;315:1412–16.
50. Nosten F, Ter Kuile FO, Luxemburger C, Woodrow C, Kyle DE, Chongsuphajaisiddhi T, White NJ. Cardiac effects of antimalarial treatment with halofantrine. Lancet 1993;341:1054–6.
51. Davis TM, Dembo LG, Kaye-Eddie SA, Hewitt BJ, Hislop RG, Batty KT. Neurological, cardiovascular and metabolic effects of mefloquine in healthy volunteers: a double-blind, placebo-controlled trial. Br J Clin Pharmacol 1996; 42:415–21.
52. Evans SJ, Waller PC. Neurological, cardiovascular and metabolic effects of mefloquine in healthy volunteers: a double-blind, placebo-controlled trial. Br J Clin Pharmacol 1997;43:665.
53. Richter J, Burbach G, Hellgren U, Dengler A, Bienzle U. Aberrant atrioventricular conduction triggered by antimalarial prophylaxis with mefloquine. Lancet 1997;349:101–2.
54. Fonteyne W, Bauwens A, Jordaens L. Atrial flutter with 1:1 conduction after administration of the antimalarial drug mefloquine. Clin Cardiol 1996;19:967–8.
55. Clattenburg RN, Donnelly CL. Case study: neuropsychiatric symptoms associated with the antimalarial agent mefloquine. J Am Acad Child Adolesc Psychiatry 1997;36:1606–8.
56. McBride SR, Lawrence CM, Pape SA, Reid CA. Fatal toxic epidermal necrolysis associated with mefloquine antimalarial prophylactics. Lancet 1997;349:9045.
57. Vanhauwere B, Maradit H, Kerr L. Post-marketing surveillance of prophylactic mefloquine (Lariam) use in pregnancy. Am J Trop Med Hyg 1998;58:17–21.
58. Supanaranond W, Suputtamongkol Y, Davis TME, Pukrittayakamee S, Teja-Isavadharm P, Webster HK, White NJ. Lack of a significant adverse cardiovascular effect of combined quinine and mefloquine therapy for uncomplicated malaria. Trans R Soc Trop Med Hyg 1997;91:694–6.
59. Brueckner RP, Lasseter KC, Lin ET, Schuster BG. First-time-in-humans safety and pharmacokinetics of WR 238605, a new antimalarial. Am J Trop Med Hyg 1998;58:645–9.
60. Brueckner RP, Coster T, Wesche DL, Shmuklarsky M, Schuster BG. Prophylaxis of *Plasmodium falciparum* infection in a human challenge model with WR 238605, a new 8-aminoquinoline antimalarial. Antimicrob Agents Chemother 1998; 42:1293–4.
61. Sirsat RA, Dasgupta A. Haematological complications of proguanil in a patient with chronic renal failure. Nephron 1997;75:108.
62. Winstanley P, Watkins W, Muhia D, Szwandt S, Amukoye E, Marsh K. Chlorproguanil/dapsone for uncomplicated *Plasmodium falciparum*

malaria in young children: pharmacokinetics and therapeutic range. Trans R Soc Trop Med Hyg 1997;91:322–7.

63. Amukoye E, Winstanley PA, Watkins WM, Snow RW, Hatcher J, Mosobo M, Ngumbao E, Lowe B, Ton M, Minyiri G, Marsh K. Chlorproguanil-dapsone: effective treatment for uncomplicated falciparum malaria. Antimicrob Agents Chemother 1997;41:2261–4.

64. Ringwald P, Bickii J, Basco LK. Efficacy of oral pyronaridine for the treatment of acute uncomplicated falciparum malaria in African children. Clin Infect Dis 1998;26:946–53.

65. Ringwald P, Bickii J, Same Ekobo A, Basco LK. Pyronaridine for treatment of *Plasmodium ovale* and *Plasmodium malariae* infections. Antimicrob Agents Chemother 1997;41:2317–19.

66. Yang HL, Liu DQ, Yang YM, Huang KG, Dong Y, Yang PF, Liao MZ, Zhang CY. In vitro sensitivity of *Plasmodium falciparum* to eight antimalarials in China-Myanmar and China-Lao PDR border areas. Southeast Asian J Trop Med Public Health 1997;28:460–4.

67. Mackie MA, Davidson J, Clarke J. Quinine-acute self-poisoning and ocular toxicity. Scott Med J 1997;42:8–9.

68. Hoffman SL, Doolan DL, Sedegah M, Wang R, Scheller LF, Kumar A, Weiss WR, Le TP, Klinman DM, Hobart P, Norman JA, Hedstrom RC. Toward clinical trials of DNA vaccines against malaria. Immunol Cell Biol 1997;75:376–81.

69. Doolan DL, Hedstrom RC, Wang R, Sedegah M, Scheller LF, Hobart P, Norman JA, Hoffman SL. DNA vaccines for malaria: the past, the present, and the future. Indian J Med Res 1997;106:109–19.

70. Kwiatkowski D, Marsh K. Development of a malaria vaccine. Lancet 1997;350:1696–707.

71. Bojang KA, Obaro SK, Leach A, D'Alessandro U, Bennett S, Metzger W, Ripley-Ballou W, Targett GAT, Greenwood BM. Follow-up of Gambian children recruited to a pilot safety and immunogenicity study of the malaria vaccine SPf66. Parasite Immunol 1997;19:579–81.

72. Migasena S, Heppner DG, Kyle DE, Chongsuphajaisiddhi T, Gordon DM, Suntharasamai P, Permpanich B, Brockman A, Pitiuttutham P, Wongsrichanalai C, Srisuriya P, Phonrat B, Pavanand K Viravan C, Ballou WR. SPf66 malaria vaccine is safe and immunogenic in malaria naive adults in Thailand. Acta Trop 1997;67:215–27.

73. Nosten F, Luxemburger C, Kyle DE, Gordon DM, Ballou WR, Sadoff JC, Brockman A, Permpanich B, Chongsuphajaisiddhi T, Heppner DG. Phase I trial of the SPf66 malaria vaccine in a malaria-experienced population in Southeast Asia. Am J Trop Med Hyg 1997;56:526–32.

74. Urdaneta M, Prata A, Struchiner CJ, Tosta CE, Tauil P, Boulos M. Evaluation of SPf66 malaria vaccine efficacy in Brazil. Am J Trop Med Hyg 1998;58:378–85.

75. Bojang KA, Obaro SK, D'Alessandro U, Bennett S, Langerock P, Targett GA, Greenwood BM. An efficacy trial of the malaria vaccine SPf66 in Gambian infants: second year of follow-up. Vaccine 1998;16:62–7.

76. Alonso PL, Lopez MC, Bordmann G, Smith TA, Aponte JJ, Weiss NA, Urassa H, Armstrong Schellenberg JR, Kitua AY, Masanja H, Thomas MC, Oettli A, Hurt N, Hayes R, Kilama WL, Tanner M. Immune responses to *Plasmodium falciparum* antigens during a malaria vaccine trial in Tanzanian children. Parasite Immunol 1998; 20:63–71.

77. Wang R, Doolan DL, Le TP, Hedstrom RC, Coonan KM, Charoenvit Y, Jones TR, Hobart P, Margalith M, Ng J, Weiss WR, Sedegah M, de Taisne C, Norman JA, Hoffman SL. Induction of antigen-specific cytotoxic T lymphocytes in humans by a malaria DNA vaccine. Science 1998;282:476–80.

78. Hoffman SL, Doolan DL, Sedegah M, Aguiar JC, Wang R, Malik A, Gramzinski RA, Weiss WR, Hobart P, Norman JA, Margalith M, Hedstrom RC. Strategy for development of a pre-erythrocytic *Plasmodium falciparum* DNA vaccine for human use. Vaccine 1997;15:842–5.

79. Le TP, Church LW, Corradin G, Hunter RL, Charoenvit Y, Wang R, de la Vega P, Sacci J, Ballou WR, Kolodny N, Kitov S, Glenn GM, Richards RL, Alving CR, Hoffman SL. Immunogenicity of *Plasmodium falciparum* circumsporozoite protein multiple antigen peptide vaccine formulated with different adjuvants. Vaccine 1998; 16:305–12.

80. Pye D, Vandenberg KL, Dyer SL, Irving DO, Goss NH, Woodrow GC, Saul A, Alving CR, Richards RL, Ballou WR, Wu MJ, Skoff K, Anders RF. Selection of an adjuvant for vaccination with the malaria antigen, MSA-2. Vaccine 1997;15:1017–23.

81. Duffy PE, Kaslow DC. A novel malaria protein, Pfs28, and Pfs25 are genetically linked and synergistic as falciparum malaria transmission-blocking vaccines. Infect Immun 1997;65:1109–13.

82. Gozar MMG, Price VL, Kaslow DC. *Saccharomyces cerevisiae*-secreted fusion proteins Pfs25 and Pfs28 elicit potent *Plasmodium falciparum* transmission-blocking antibodies in mice. Infect Immun 1998;66:59–64.

83. Ambroise Thomas P. Vaccination against malaria. Disappointments and hopes. Bull Acad Natl Med 1997;181:1637–48.

84. Stoute JA, Slaoui M, Heppner DG, Momin P, Kester KE, Desmons P, Wellde BT, Garcon N, Krzych U, Marchand M, Ballou WR, Cohen JD. A preliminary evaluation of a recombinant circumsporozoite protein vaccine against *Plasmodium falciparum* malaria. New Engl J Med 1997;336:86–91.

85. Wang R, Doolan DL, Charoenvit Y, Hedstrom RC, Gardner MJ, Hobart P, Tine J, Sedegah M, Fallarme V, Sacci JB Jr, Kaur M, Klinman DM, Hoffman SL, Weiss WR. Simultaneous induction of multiple antigen-specific cytotoxic T lymphocytes in nonhuman primates by immuniza-

tion with a mixture of four *Plasmodium falciparum* DNA plasmids. Infect Immun 1998;66:4193–202.
86. Sedegah M, Jones TR, Kaur M, Hedstrom R, Hobart P, Tine JA, Hoffman SL. Boosting with recombinant vaccinia increases immunogenicity and protective efficacy of malaria DNA vaccine. Proc Natl Acad Sci USA 1998;95:7648–53.
87. Weiss WR, Ishii KJ, Hedstrom RC, Sedegah M, Ichino M, Barnhart K, Klinman DM, Hoffman SL. A plasmid encoding murine granulocyte-macrophage colony-stimulating factor increases protection conferred by a malaria DNA vaccine. J Immunol 1998;161:2325–32.
88. Ockenhouse CF, Sun PF, Lanar DE, Wellde BT, Hall BT, Kester K, et al. (27 authors). Phase I/IIa safety, immunogenicity, and efficacy trial of NYVAC-Pf7, a poxvectored, multiantigen, multistage vaccine candidate for *Plasmodium falciparum* malaria. J Infect Dis 1998;177:1664–73.
89. Miller RF, Le Noury J, Corbett EL, Felton JM, De Cock KM. *Pneumocystis carinii* infection: current treatment and prevention. J Antimicrob Chemother 1996;37 Suppl B:33–53.
90. Warren E, George S, You J, Kazanjian P. Advances in the treatment and prophylaxis of *Pneumocystis carinii* pneumonia. Pharmacotherapy 1997;17:900–16.
91. Santamauro JT, Stover DE. *Pneumocystis carinii* pneumonia. Med Clin North Am 1997; 81:299–318.
92. Fishman JA. Treatment of infection due to *Pneumocystis carinii*. Antimicrob Agents Chemother 1998;42:1309–14.
93. Hughes W, Dorenbaum A, Yogev R, Beauchamp B, Xu J, McNamara J, Moye J, Purdue L, van Dyke R, Rogers M, Sadler B. Phase I safety and pharmacokinetics study of micronized atovaquone in human immunodeficiency virus-infected infants and children. Pediatric AIDS Clinical Trials Group. Antimicrob Agents Chemother 1998; 42:1315–18.
94. Ioannidis JP, Cappelleri JC, Skolnik PR, Lau J, Sacks HS. A meta-analysis of the relative efficacy and toxicity of *Pneumocystis carinii* prophylactic regimens. Arch Intern Med 1996;156:177–88.
95. Gilroy N, Gottlieb T, Spring P, Peiris O. Trimethoprim-induced aseptic meningitis and uveitis. Lancet 1997;350:112.
96. Carlson J, Wilholm B-E. Trimethoprim associated aseptic meningitis. Scand J Infect Dis 1987;19:687–91.
97. Derbes SJ. Trimethoprim-induced aseptic meningitis. J Am Med Assoc 1984;252;2865–6.
98. Northrop CV, Moore Shepherd S, Abbuhl S. Sulphonamide-induced iritis. Am J Emerg Med 1996;14:577–9.
99. Van Gerpen JA. Tremor caused by trimethoprim-sulfamethoxazole in a patient with AIDS. Neurology 1997;48:537–8.
100. Lee AJ, Maddix DS. Trimethoprim/sulfamethoxazole-induced hypoglycemia in a patient with acute renal failure. Ann Pharmacother 1997; 31:727–2.
101. Hekimsoy Z, Biberoglu S, Comlekci A, Tarhan O, Mermut C, Biberoglu K. Trimethoprim/sulfamethoxazole-induced hypoglycemia in a malnourished patient with severe infection. Eur J Endocrinol 1997;136:304–6.
102. Naderer O, Nafziger AN, Bertino JS. Effects of moderate-dose versus high-dose trimethoprim on serum creatinine and creatinine clearance and adverse reactions. Antimicrob Agents Chemother 1997;41:2466–70.
103. Safrin S, Finkelstein DM, Feinberg J, Frame P, Simpson G, Wu A, Cheung T, Soeiro R, Hojczyk P, Black JR. Comparison of three regimens for treatment of mild to moderate *Pneumocystis carinii* in patients with AIDS. A double-blind, randomised trial of oral trimethoprim-sulfamethoxazole, dapsone-trimethoprim, and clindamycin-primaquine. Ann Intern Med 1996; 124:792–802.
104. Alappan R, Perazella MA, Buller GK. Hyperkalemia in hospitalised patients treated with trimethoprim-sulfamethoxazole. Ann Intern Med 1996;124:316–20.
105. Safrin S, Finkelstein D. Comparison of oral agents for treatment of *Pneumocystis carinii* pneumonia. Ann Intern Med 1997;126:407–8.
106. Elisaf M, Terrovitou C, Tomos P, Siamopoulos KC. Severe hyperkalaemia after co-trimoxazole administration in a patient with hyporeninaemic hypoaldosteronism. Nephrol Dial Transplant 1997;12:1254–5.
107. Lin S-H, Kuo AA, Yu F-C, Lin Y-F. Reversible voltage-dependent distal renal tubular acidosis in a patient receving standard doses of trimethoprim-sulphamethoxazole. Nephrol Dial Transplant 1997;12:1031–3.
108. Yao F, Behling CA, Saab S, Li S, Hart M, Lyche KD. Trimethoprim-sulfamethoxazole-induced vanishing bile duct syndrome. Am J Gastroenterol 1997;92:167–9.
109. Gruber F, Stasic A, Lenkovic M, Brajac I. Postcoital fixed drug eruption in a man sensitive to trimethoprim-sulfamethoxazole. Clin Exp Dermatol 1997;22:144–5.
110. Ozkaya-Bayazit E, Baykal C. Trimethoprim-induced linear fixed drug eruption. Br J Dermatol 1997;137;1028–9.
111. Everson-Mays RE, Weidle PJ. Restarting trimethoprim-sulfamethoxazole after a hypersensitivity reaction in patients with the human deficiency virus. Am J Health-Syst Pharm 1997; 54:1545–50.
112. Stein GE. Trimethoprim/sulfamethoxazole-induced hypersensitivity syndrome. Ann Pharmacother 1997;31:1259.
113. Carr A. Role of desensitisation for drug hypersensitivity in patients with HIV infection. Drug Saf 1997;17:119–26.
114. Rieder MJ, King SM, Read S. Adverse reactions to trimethoprim-sulfamethoxazole among children with human immunodeficiency virus infection. Pediatr Infect Dis J 1997;16:1028–31.
115. Caumes E, Guermonprez G, Lecomte C, Katlama C, Bricaire F. Efficacy and safety of de-

sensitization with sulfamethoxazole and trimethoprim in 48 previously hypersensitive patients infected with human immunodeficiency virus. Arch Dermatol 1997;133:465–9.
116. Stricker RB, Gullet JH, Williams LE, Goldberg B. Co-trimoxazole desensitization syndrome: delayed hematologic toxicity complicating prophylactic therapy in AIDS patients. AIDS 1996;10:927–9.
117. Jucgla A, Sais G, Berlanga J, Servitje O. Hyperpigmentation of the flexures and pancytopenia during treatment with folate antagonists. Acta Dermatol Venereol 1997;77:165–6.
118. Hughes WT. Use of dapsone in the prevention and treatment of *Pneumocystis carinii* pneumonia: a review. Clin Infect Dis 1998;1:191–204.
119. Hironaka K, Mizushima M, Tsuzi C, Makino H. Urinary tract carcinoma in leprosy patients treated with dapsone for a long period. Nephron 1997;76:358–9.
120. Mir N, O'Farrell N, Creagh TA, Knowles C. Obstructive renal failure requiring surgical intervention in an AIDS patient being treated with sulfadiazine. Int J STD AIDS 1997;8:61–2.
121. Anibarro B, Fontela JL. Sulfadiazine-induced sialadenitis. Ann Pharmacother 1996; 30:59–60.
122. Ortega-Carnicer J, Alcazar R, De la Torre M, Benezet J. Pentavalent antimonial-induced torsade de pointes. J Electrocardiol 1997;30:143–5.
123. Nazmul-Ahasan HAM, Jalil-Chowdhury MA, Azhar MA, Rafiqueuddin AKM, Fakrul-Islam M. Conduction defect following pentavalent antimony therapy in visceral leishmaniasis. Trop Doct 1997;27:59–61.
124. Sundar S, Sinha PR, Agrawal NK, Srivastava R, Rainey PM, Berman JD, Murray HW, Singh VP. A cluster of cases of severe cardiotoxicity among kala-azar patients treated with a high-osmolarity lot of sodium antimony gluconate. Am J Trop Med Hyg 1998;59:139–43.
125. Lockwood DNJ. Some good news for treatment of visceral leishmaniasis in Bihar. Br Med J 1998;316:1205.
126. Thakur CP. Sodium antimony gluconate, amphotericin, and myocardial damage. Lancet 1998;351:1928–9.
127. Jha TK, Olliaro P, Thakur CP, Kanyok TP, Singhania BL, Singh IJ, Akhoury S, Jha S. Randomised controlled trial of aminosidine (paromomycin) v sodium stibogluconate for treating visceral leishmaniasis in North Bihar, India. Br Med J 1998;316:1200–5.
128. Elliott AM, Klaus BD, North DS, Martin HP. Furazolidone-induced mood disorder during the treatment of refractory giardiasis in a patient with AIDS. Clin Infect Dis 1998;26:1015.
129. Schreiber W, Spernal J. Metronidazole-induced psychotic disorder. Am J Psychiatry 1997; 154:1170–1.
130. Sobel JD. Vaginitis. New Engl J Med 1997;337:1896–1903.
131. Caro-Paton T, Carvajal A, De Diego IM, Martin-Arias LH, Alvarez-Requejo A, Rodriguez-Pinilla E. Is metronidazole teratogenic? A meta-analysis. Br J Clin Pharmacol 1997;44:179–82.

P. Reiss and M.D. de Jong

29 Antiviral drugs

COMPOUNDS ACTIVE AGAINST RNA VIRUSES

R *Lipodystrophy and insulin resistance with HIV-protease inhibitors*

Clinical description *A newly reported adverse event of the use of all currently available members of the class of HIV-protease inhibitors is a syndrome of peripheral lipodystrophy, central adiposity, breast hypertrophy in women, hyperlipidemia, and insulin resistance. Peripheral lipodystrophy in patients is characterised by fat wasting of the face, limbs, buttocks and upper trunk, while central adiposity may manifest itself as increase in belly size and an increase in the dorsocervical fat pad, creating the appearance of a 'buffalo hump' (1*[C]*). The increase in belly size is often associated with symptoms of abdominal fullness, distension, and bloating. This is probably due to a change in body fat distribution, with selective accumulation of fat intra-abdominally (2*[C]*).*

Incidence and biochemical findings *The largest series of patients with the syndrome reported so far was the result of a cross-sectional study performed in the out-patient clinic of a university teaching hospital. HIV-infected patients taking at least one protease inhibitor (*n = *116) were compared with protease inhibitor-naive patients (*n = *32) and healthy men (*n = *47). Lipodystrophy was assessed by physical examination and questionnaire, and body composition by dual-energy X-ray absorptiometry (DEXA-scan). HIV protease inhibitor-naive patients had similar body composition to healthy men. HIV protease inhibitor therapy was associated with substantially lower total body fat (13.2 vs 18.7 kg) and significantly higher total cholesterol and triglyceride concentrations. There was lipodystrophy in 74 (64%) protease inhibitor recipients after a mean of 13.9 months, compared with one patient among those not taking a protease inhibitor. Fat loss occurred in all regions except the abdomen after a median 10 months. Patients with lipodystrophy had a relative weight loss of 0.5 kg/month, had significantly higher triglyceride, cholesterol, insulin, and C-peptide concentrations, and were more insulin resistant than the protease inhibitor recipients without lipodystrophy. Patients taking ritonavir and saquinavir in combination had significantly lower body fat, higher lipid concentrations, and a shorter time to lipodystrophy than patients taking indinavir. Three patients developed new or worsening diabetes mellitus (3*[C]*).*

Mechanism *It has been postulated that this syndrome is mediated by the interaction of HIV protease inhibitors with two proteins involved in normal body metabolism, cytoplasmic retinoic acid-binding protein type 1 (CRABP-1) and low density lipoprotein receptor-related protein (LRP), as a result of molecular homology between these two particular proteins and the HIV-protease enzyme (4*[C]*).*

Nelfinavir

Nelfinavir is the most recent HIV protease inhibitor. The main adverse event that has been consistently reported is *diarrhea* and *loose stools* in 20–30% of patients (5[R]). The frequency with which diarrhea is truly dose-limiting is not yet clear, but clinical experience suggests that in many cases treatment can be continued in conjunction with non-specific anti-diarrheal medication.

Side Effects of Drugs, Annual 22
J.K. Aronson, ed.

Nevirapine *(SEDA-19, 277; SEDA-21, 308)*

Skin and appendages As reported previously, the principal dose-limiting adverse effect of the non-nucleoside reverse transcriptase inhibitor nevirapine is *skin rash*. In a study of the safety and antiretroviral efficacy of nevirapine, 20 previously untreated HIV-infected patients were treated with nevirapine in a dosage of 400 mg/day, after a 2-week lead-in period at a dosage of 200 mg/day to reduce the risk of skin rash (6[CR]). However, the most frequent adverse effects were skin rash and fever, frequently coincident, occurring within the first 4 weeks of treatment in 20 and 25% of patients, respectively. One patient developed a mild skin rash during the low-dose lead-in period, but it progressed to a Stevens-Johnson syndrome when the dose was increased to 400 mg/day. Nevirapine was withdrawn and corticosteroids given; recovery was complete within 25 days. Severe skin rashes associated with fever and edema were observed in two other patients, both of whom recovered on withdrawal.

Ritonavir *(SEDA-20, 272; SEDA-21, 309)*

Ritonavir is an HIV-protease inhibitor. Its most common dose-limiting adverse effects are *nausea*, *vomiting*, and *diarrhea*, which have been reported to occur in over 20% of patients in trials and even more in clinical practice. These adverse effects are especially seen during the early stages of therapy, and to some extent may be prevented by using a step-up approach, increasing to the full treatment dose in gradual fashion over 6 days. Other adverse effects, which occur in 5–10% of patients but are seldom treatment-limiting, are *circumoral paresthesia*, *taste disturbance*, and *generalized weakness*.

Laboratory abnormalities with the use of HIV protease inhibitors that are increasingly being reported at conferences, and that seem to be most pronounced with ritonavir, are *asymptomatic increases in cholesterol*, *triglycerides, and hepatic transaminases*. Whether persistent hypercholesterolemia and/or hypertriglyceridemia will translate into an increased incidence of atherosclerotic cardiovascular disease or pancreatitis remains to be determined.

Interactions An important consideration in the use of all HIV-protease inhibitors, but of ritonavir in particular, is their potential for drug interactions through their effects on the hepatic cytochrome P450 oxidase system. The use of HIV protease inhibitors (saquinavir, indinavir, and ritonavir), including the issue of drug–drug interactions, has recently been reviewed (7[R]). Ritonavir is a potent inhibitor of CYP3A4, by which it is also primarily metabolized. Thus, ritonavir will slow the metabolism of drugs through this system, which may lead to important increases in the serum concentrations of other drugs and result in significant adverse effects. Inducers of CYP3A4 will increase the metabolism of ritonavir, which may result in reduced ritonavir exposure, thereby increasing the chance of viral ritonavir resistance. A list of drugs that are contraindicated or should be used with caution or in a reduced dosage are listed in Table 1 (8[R]).

Table 1. *Drugs that are contraindicated in patients taking ritonavir (8[R])*

Alprazolam
Amfebutamone (bupropion)
Amiodarone
Astemizole
Bepridil
Cisapride
Clorazepate
Clozapine
Dextropropoxyphene
Diazepam
Dihydroergotamine
Encainide
Ergotamine
Estazolam
Flecainide
Flurazepam
Midazolam
Pethidine
Pimozide
Piroxicam
Propafenone
Quididine
Rifabutin
Terfenadine
Triazolam
Zolpidem

Stavudine (2′,3′-didehydro-3′-deoxythymidine, D4T) *(SEDA-20, 273)*

The most important adverse effects of stavudine are *peripheral neuropathy* and *increases in hepatic transaminases*, both of which usually resolve upon discontinuation of the drug.

Hematological Modest *macrocytosis* without associated anemia can occur during treatment with stavudine. In a retrospective study of 17 HIV-infected persons, there were progressive increases in mean corpuscular volume in all individuals during treatment with stavudine, reaching a mean increase of 10.5 fl after 12–20 weeks (9[C]).

Immunological and hypersensitivity reactions A case of stavudine-associated drug *fever* has been reported (10[C]).

A 29-year-old HIV-infected woman was given stavudine (40 mg bd) on the first day post-partum. The next day she developed fever without localizing signs or symptoms. Physical, laboratory, and radiographic evaluation did not reveal a source of infection, and a diagnosis of stavudine-induced drug fever was made. Treatment with stavudine was discontinued, and her body temperature became normal within 28 h.

Liver A case of presumed stavudine-induced *hepatic steatosis and lactic acidosis* has been reported(11[CR]).

A 32-year-old HIV-infected woman was admitted to hospital with a 6-week history of progressive nausea, vomiting, anorexia, and general malaise. She had a tachycardia and a mild fever with massive tender hepatomegaly. She had lactic acidosis (blood lactate concentration 6.6 mmol/l; reference range 0.3–1.3 mmol/l). Liver function tests were abnormal, with a slight reduction in serum albumin and a slight increase in alanine aminotransferase. Her renal function was normal. Hematological investigation showed a macrocytosis, a CD4+ lymphocyte count of 35×10^6/l, and lymphopenia. Bacterial, viral, fungal, and mycobacterial cultures were negative. Serological studies did not show evidence of active infection with hepatitis virus, cytomegalovirus, or Epstein–Barr virus. Her history included zidovudine-induced anemia, presumed didanosine-induced hepatic steatosis without hepatomegaly or lactic acidosis, and drug-induced bronchiolitis obliterans. Her medications included stavudine (40 mg bd, begun 6 months before), lamivudine (150 mg bd, begun 1 year before), azithromycin (1.25 g/week), aciclovir (200 mg tds), co-trimoxazole (960 mg twice a week), and temazepam (10 mg od). She had started to take indinavir 3 months before, but had stopped taking it 2 weeks before admission. Lamivudine and stavudine were withdrawn. She was given intravenous hydrocortisone and co-enzyme Q, which has potential benefit in congenital encephalomyopathies (12[C]) and in an animal model of zidovudine-induced mitochondrial dysfunction (13). She rapidly improved, with total resolution of symptoms and improvement of biochemical parameters by 48 h, followed by gradual improvement in hepatic tenderness and a reduction in liver size. After 2 weeks lamivudine and indinavir were reintroduced without problems.

Fulminant hepatic steatosis with lactic acidosis has been reported in HIV-infected patients during treatment with zidovudine, didanosine, or zalcitabine, and is thought to result from interference by these agents of mitochondrial DNA synthesis through inhibition of mitochondrial γ DNA polymerase. Since stavudine had been the most recent addition to her medication, and since both indinavir and lamivudine were reintroduced without problems, the authors concluded that stavudine can also induce hepatic steatosis and lactic acidosis by this mechanism. The fact that this patient had previously had other possible nucleoside analog-induced mitochondrial cytopathies (zidovudine-induced anemia, didanosine-induced hepatic steatosis) suggests a predisposition to this problem.

REFERENCES

1. Lo JC, Mulligan K, Tai VW, Algren H, Schambelan M. 'Buffalo hump' in men with HIV infection. Lancet 1998;351:867–70.
2. Miller K, Jones E, Yanovski JA, Shankar R, Feuerstein I, Falloon J. Visceral abdominal-fat accumulation associated with use of indinavir. Lancet 1998;351:871–5.
3. Carr A, Samaras K, Burton S, Law M, Freund J, Chisholm DJ, Cooper DA. A syndrome of peripheral lipodystrophy, hyperlipidemia and insulin resistance in patients receiving HIV protease inhibitors. AIDS 1998;12:F51–8.
4. Carr A, Smaras K, Chisholm DJ, Cooper DA. Pathogenesis of HIV-1 protease inhibitor-associated peripheral lipodystrophy, hyperlipidemia, and insulin resistance. Lancet 1998;352:1881–3.
5. Perry CM, Benfield P. Nelfinavir. Drugs 1997;54:81–7.

6. de Jong MD, Vella S, Carr A, Boucher CAB, Imrie A, French M, et al. (23 authors). High dose nevirapine in previously untreated HIV-1 infected persons does not result in sustained suppression of viral replication. J Infect Dis 1997;175:966–70.
7. Oliphant CM, Bonnema SM. New advances in the pharmacologic treatment of human immunodeficiency virus (HIV) infection: focus on protease inhibitors. J Pharm Pract 1997;10:20–51.
8. Lea A P, Faulds D. Ritonavir. Drugs 1996; 52:541–6.
9. Ahmad S, Sukthankar A. Stavudine induced macrocytosis. Genitourin Med 1997;73:421–3.
10. Wax JR, Mueller S. Puerperal febrile morbidity associated with the reverse transcriptase inhibitor stavudine. J Matern Fetal Med 1997; 6:118–19.
11. Lenzo NP, Garas BA, French MA. Hepatic steatosis and lactic acidosis associated with stavudine treatment in an HIV patient: a case report. AIDS 1997;11:1294–6.
12. Peterson PL. The treatment of mitochondrial myopathies and encephalomyopathies. Biochim Biophys Acta 1995;1271:275–80.
13. Linnane AW, Degli Aposti M, Generowicz M, Luff AR, Nagley P. The universality of bioenergetic disease and amelioration with redox therapy. Biochim Biophys Acta 1995;1271:191–4.

C.J. Ellis

30 Drugs used in tuberculosis and leprosy

COMBINATION THERAPY FOR TUBERCULOSIS

Liver It is well established that *hepatic necrosis* is the most important adverse effect of first-line antituberculous therapy, at least in patients without HIV infection. Asymptomatic rises in transaminases are common and not by themselves justification for stopping medication, since they settle spontaneously in most patients while treatment continues. Identifying those patients who are at increased risk of significant hepatotoxicity is important, since prompt withdrawal of medication is vital if serious illness and even death is to be prevented, but it is no substitute for warning all patients taking antituberculous drugs that they should report all new illnesses, especially when associated with vomiting.

Work in China (1[C]) has shown that hepatitis B carriers were no more likely to react adversely to antituberculous medication than non-carriers, but has confirmed the general finding that older patients (over 35 years) do suffer hepatotoxicity more often. An earlier study from India had shown that low body mass also predicted hepatotoxicity (2[C]).

Skin and appendages In HIV-positive individuals, adverse reactions to all types of medication are common, and skin reactions are especially frequent and often severe. Thiacetazone is now well recognised as a cause of severe reactions, some of them fatal (see below), but even in combination antituberculous regimens that exclude thiacetazone the incidence of adverse skin reactions is much higher in HIV-positive than HIV-negative patients: 23% against 1% in one study from Cameroon (3[C]).

Side Effects of Drugs, Annual 22
J.K. Aronson, ed.

INDIVIDUAL ANTITUBERCULOUS AND ANTILEPROTIC DRUGS

Dapsone *(SED-13, 894; SEDA-19, 284)*

Nervous system Dapsone *neuropathy* is not common, in spite of the now widespread use of this drug in a variety of unrelated disorders. It was first reported in a patient with pyoderma gangrenosum treated with dapsone 40 mg/day (4[c]). It has not previously been reported in patients with leprosy, but it would be easy to miss, since worsening neuropathy in this context would readily be attributed to the underlying disease, it being well recognised, for example, that antibacterial therapy can cause nerve-damaging hypersensitivity reactions in the host. An Indian patient who took dapsone in a dosage of 300 mg/day, three times the intended dosage, developed tingling in the hands and feet and progressive weakness of the muscles of the hands and feet (5[c]). Nerve conduction studies showed reduced action potentials. A hypersensitivity reaction was initially diagnosed. However, there was no improvement with prednisolone, but complete recovery 10 weeks after withdrawal of dapsone. Dapsone neuropathy has not been reported in patients with leprosy taking the usually recommended dosage of 100 mg/day.

Risk factors In some cases acetylator phenotype is related to variation in clinical response and to susceptibility to adverse reactions. Brazilian workers who tested 30 patients with leprosy for acetylator status found that 13 were slow acetylators and 13 fast acetylators (6[C]). They had been taking dapsone for at least 6 months when tested, and 13 were anemic, with hemoglobin concentrations of 7.2–10.9 g/dl. However, there was no correlation with acetylator status. This confirms the findings of a study of patients taking dapsone for rheumatoid arthritis (7[C]).

Rifamycins *(SED-13, 892; SEDA-21, 313)*

Hematological A 46-year-old woman died of severe *disseminated intravascular coagulation* which followed her third monthly dose of rifampicin, given with daily dapsone for the treatment of leprosy (8[c]).

Urinary system A further case of *acute renal insufficiency* associated with hemolytic anemia has been described in a 70-year-old woman (9[c]). Hemolysis started after the second dose of rifampicin (for *M. tuberculosis* infection), and the patient's blood contained rifampicin-dependent IgG and IgM antibodies, which caused red cell lysis through interaction with the 1 antigen on the red cell surface. This antigen is also expressed on renal tubular epithelium. The authors noted that had been 37 other reports of patients in whom acute renal insufficiency had developed suddenly, most of whom also developed hemolytic anaemia and/or thrombocytopenia. Intermittent or interrupted treatment appears to predispose to this complication, and the patient described had completed a conventional continuous course of treatment for *M. tuberculosis* infection 2 years before its re-introduction.

Immunological and hypersensitivity reactions The drug-induced *lupus-like syndrome* has been linked to isoniazid therapy but not previously to rifampicin or other types of rifamycin. Seven cases of the syndrome have now been reported in patients, six of them women, who were taking rifampicin ($n = 4$) or rifabutin ($n = 3$) in standard dosages for mycobacterial infections (10[C]). None of the patients was HIV-1 positive, none was simultaneously taking isoniazid, and, although they were taking other antimycobacterial drugs, their symptoms disappeared with withdrawal of the rifamycin alone. All of the patients had two or more of fever, malaise, myalgia, and arthralgia and all had positive antinuclear antibodies. All were also taking either ciprofloxacin or clarithromycin, and the authors speculated that these drugs, which are cytochrome P450 enzyme inhibitors, could have increased the serum concentrations of the rifamycins.

Pyrazinamide *(SED-13, 890)*

Cardiovascular Acute symptomatic *hypertension* consistently followed the administration of pyrazinamide to a 65-year-old woman with pulmonary tuberculosis (11[c]). The association was clear: headache with tachycardia and hypertension (supine blood pressure 170/110 mmHg) followed the first dose of a tablet of rifampicin, isoniazid, and pyrazinamide in combination, recurred on re-challenge with the combination and after subsequent challenge with pyrazinamide alone, but did not recur when the other two were given alone.

Risk factors *Children* Although pyrazinamide is a part of conventional combination therapy for children with tuberculosis, as in adults (12[R]), there is little published information on its safety. Now the question of safety in children has been prospectively studied in 114 Spanish children treated with conventional short-course chemotherapy (13[C]). Liver transaminases and uric acid were measured before and 1, 3, and 5 months after the start of therapy. In those with raised transaminases before the start of therapy there was no increase during therapy, and concentrations normalized in all patients after its conclusion. In 11 children there was a modest rise during therapy, in six cases after 1 month, in three cases after 3 months, and in two cases after 5 months. The maximum AlT value was 193 IU/l. These results are not unexpected and support accepted practice.

Thiacetazone *(SED-13, 892; SEDA-19, 282)*

In SEDA-19 (p. 282) arguments were advanced for the abandonment of thiacetazone as an antituberculous drug, despite its undoubted cheapness, on the grounds of the very high incidence of severe skin reactions, some rapidly fatal, in patients infected with HIV-1. However, some practitioners continue to use it in poorer countries, where few alternatives are affordable or regularly available. In an attempt to predict which patients can be treated with comparative safety, doctors in Kampala, Uganda, examined a variety of risk factors and found that only anergy to tuberculin and lymphocytopenia were associated with increased risk of adverse reactions in 90 patients who took thiacetazone (14^{C}). These parameters also correlated with advanced immune deficiency, i.e. advanced HIV disease.

REFERENCES

1. Hwang SJ, Wu JC, Lee CN, Yen FS, Lu CL, Lim TP, Lee SD. A prospective clinical study of isoniazid-rifampicin-pyrazinamide-induced liver injury in an area endemic for hepatitis B. J Gastroenterol Hepatol 1997;12:87–91.
2. Singh J, Arora A, Garg PK, Thakur VS, Pande JN, Tandon RK. Antituberculous treatment-induced hepatoxicity: role of predictive factors. Postgrad Med J 1995;71:359–69.
3. Kuaban C, Bercion R, Koulla-Shiro S. HIV seroprevalence rate and incidence of adverse skin reactions in adults with pulmonary tuberculosis receiving thiacetazone-free treatment. East African Med J 1997;74:474–7.
4. Saqueton AC, Lorincz AL, Vick NA, Hamer RD. Dapsone and peripheral neuropathy. Arch Dermatol 1969;100:214–17.
5. Pavithram K, Satish TC. Dapsone-induced motor polyneuropathy in a patient with leprosy. Int J Lepr 199;65:262–3.
6. Queiroz RHC, Souza AM, Melchior E, Vouveria EG. Carvallo D. Influence of acetylator phenotype on the hematological and biochemical effects associated with dapsone in leprosy patients. Lepr Rev 1997;68:212–17.
7. Kelly C, Griffiths ID. Dapsone in rheumatoid arthritis. Ann Rheum Dis 1981;40:630.
8. Souza CS, Alberto FL, Foss NT. Disseminated intravascular coagulopathy as an adverse reaction to intermittent rifampicin. Int J Lepr 1997;65:366–71.
9. De Vriese AD, Robbrecht DL, Vanholder RC, Vogelaers DP, Lameire NH. Rifampicin-associated acute renal failure. Am J Kidney Dis 1998;31:108–15.
10. Berning SE, Iseman MD. Rifamycin-induced lupus syndrome. Lancet 1997;349:1521–2.
11. Goldberg J, Moreno F, Barbara J. Acute hypertension as an adverse effect of pyrazinamide. J Am Med Assoc 1977;277:1356.
12. British Medical Association and Royal Pharmaceutical Society of Great Britain. Antituberculous drugs. Br Natl Formulary 1998;35:160–265.
13. Sanchez S-A, Vidal ML, Joya-Verde G, Del Castillo F, de Jose MI, Garcia-Hortelano J. Tolerance of pyrazinamide in short course chemotherapy for pulmonary tuberculosis in children. Paediatr Infect Dis J 1997;16:760–3.
14. Okwera A, Johnson JL, Vjecha MJ, Wolski K, Whalen CC, Hom D, Huebner R, Mugerwa RD, Ellner JJ. Risk factors for adverse drug reactions during thiacetazone treatment of pulmonary tuberculosis in human immunodeficiency virus infected adults. Int J Tuberc Lung Dis 1997;15:441–5.

A.G.C. Bauer

31 Antihelminthic drugs

Albendazole *(SED-13, 912; SEDA-19, 286; SEDA-20, 280; SEDA-21, 315)*

Albendazole is a benzimidazole used in the treatment of strongyloidiasis, larva migrans cutanea, neurocysticercosis, and in high doses in echinococcosis. In the past year several papers have appeared on its use in both neurocysticercosis (1[C])–(5[C]) and human echinococcosis (6[R]), (7[R]), (8[C]).

Albendazole and human echinococcosis A recent extensive review of all aspects of human echinococcosis included medical treatment (6[R]). It was concluded that albendazole 10 mg/kg per day for 4 weeks, with a 2-week rest period, for six cycles is the most effective treatment of human echinococcosis, with up to 70–80% of patients experiencing a partial response, with a significant reduction in cyst size but with complete cure of the disease in only one-third. Calcified and complex cysts respond poorly to treatment. Adverse effects, *neutropenia* (on average less than 1%), alopecia (on average less than 1%), and *disturbances of liver function* (1–5%), are rare and usually transient.

In another report of 12 years of experience of albendazole in human echinococcosis, the results of treatment of 3560 patients in several clinical trials have been reviewed (7[R]). Comparable conclusions were drawn, with a partial response in 70–80% and cure rates around 30%. Efficacy appears to increase with the length of treatment, but continuous versus cyclical treatment is still controversial. The adverse effects noted were also comparable. There was a *mild self-limiting increase in liver enzymes* in 10–20% of the patients, necessitating withdrawal, but only in 12 of 316 patients (3.8%) in the European studies reviewed. All cases of liver function abnormality were reversible and may have been caused by a local effect on the liver parenchyma by an inflammatory reaction to the decaying hepatic cyst (8[C]), since there is a much lower frequency of liver function disturbances in patients treated with prolonged courses of albendazole for neurocysticercosis (9[C]). The second most important adverse effect was *bone marrow suppression*, usually transient, mainly affecting white cell production, which occurred in 1% of cases. Clinical serious agranulocytosis is even more rare, but fatalities have occurred. The third most frequent adverse effect was alopecia, usually in the form of thinning hair and rarely total; in all cases complete regrowth of hair occurred after withdrawal.

These low frequencies of adverse effects contrast with a recent study from Italy (10[C]), of 12 patients treated for human echinococcosis of the liver with albendazole given either in doses of 400 mg bd for 6 months or in 6-week cycles of 400 mg bd with 2 weeks between cycles. Three patients had abnormalities of liver function. In one of these the reaction progressed to *hepatitis*, necessitating withdrawal. *Alopecia* developed in two of 12 patients.

Skin and appendages Adverse effects of albendazole on the skin mainly consist of minor rashes. However, a more serious case of *Stevens–Johnson syndrome* has recently been described (11[C]).

A 57-year-old man was admitted with widespread target eruptions, painful oral and ocular erosions, a high fever, and arthralgia, consistent with Stevens–Johnson syndrome, 2 weeks after starting to take albendazole 400 mg/day for toxocariasis. His ESR and CRP were raised and his serum transaminases slightly increased. The symptoms and laboratory abnormalities subsided within 20 days after withdrawal. He had not taken any other drugs at the time.

Albendazole and neurocysticercosis In a pro-

Side Effects of Drugs, Annual 22
J.K. Aronson, ed.

spective double-blind trial (1[C]) 55 patients were randomized to receive oral albendazole 400 mg bd for 7 days followed by placebo for 7 days or oral albendazole 400 mg bd for 14 days. Both groups received dexamethasone 1.5 mg tds for 5 days, tapered over 3 days. Any antiepileptic treatment was continued. All the patients were admitted to the hospital and electroencephalography and CT scanning was performed at 15, 90, and 360 days. There was no difference in efficacy between the two regimens, with an overall reaction rate of 78%, although only 35–40% of the patients were free of lesions at 3 months. Outcome was correlated with the number of cysts and was especially poor in patients with more than 20 cysts. In patients with fewer than 20 cysts, three-quarters of the cysts disappeared, but in the four patients with more than 20 cysts, all the cysts cleared in only one case. The presenting symptoms at the start of treatment were headache (90%) and seizures (82%). Other symptoms were memory loss (30%) and symptoms of intracranial hypertension, such as headache and vomiting (12%). Minor adverse effects after treatment with albendazole occurred in 19 of 50 patients (38%) and consisted of *nausea* in 13 patients, *abdominal pain* in three, and *diarrhea* in three. Four patients developed a *transient skin rash*. One had persistent *hiccup* and one had *mild loss of hair* for 1 month after treatment. Neurological adverse effects after treatment occurred frequently. Most patients complained of *headache* (46/50 patients, 92%), starting in the first 2 days in 17 patients and between 3 and 5 days in 11 cases. *Seizures* occurred in 12 patients with a history of epileptic seizures, but in none of the other patients. One patient had worsening of pre-existent *extrapyramidal symptoms* and developed generalized rigidity. The symptoms diminished after day 12 and improved slowly over the following months. A control CT scan at 90 days showed moderate *hydrocephalus*, which had not been present before treatment. Another patient had *acute intracranial hypertension* 3 days after treatment, which subsided after the reintroduction of corticosteroids and treatment with mannitol; a CT scan on day 15 showed a significant inflammatory reaction. No patients died during treatment, but two died in the first year of follow-up; both deaths were attributed to a *bacterial ventriculitis* after the placement of ventriculo-peritoneal catheters.

A somewhat higher efficacy of albendazole in the treatment of neurocysticercosis has been found in a study from Ecuador in 17 patients treated with albendazole 15 mg/kg per day for 8 days, combined with intravenous dexamethasone (2[C]). All were heavily infected, and several patients had very large cysts (over 5 cm) and had chronic neurological symptoms (seizures in 14 patients, hemiparesis in 10, headache and vomiting in five, dementia in three, papilledema in two, and optic atrophy in one). Brain CT scans 3 months after treatment showed complete resolution of 22 out of 30 cysts (90% efficacy), while 14 patients (82%) had total resolution of all cysts. Albendazole was not associated with severe adverse effects. Ten patients had *headaches* during treatment. Two patients with giant cysts had a transient *rise in intracranial pressure*, which had to be treated with mannitol. Three patients had transient *worsening of their hemiparesis* and one had *generalized seizures*.

In another study 10 patients with neurocysticercosis of the fourth ventricle were treated with albendazole 15 mg/kg per day for 2 weeks (3[C]). Six of these patients presented with acute hydrocephalus requiring immediate ventriculoperitoneal shunting. Nine patients improved after a first round of treatment, with disappearance of the cysts in three patients and a reduction in size in five patients, with further disappearance of cysts in four of these five patients after a second course of treatment. The remaining patient had a further reduction in cyst size. Six patients, all with ventricular drains, had no further adverse effects during treatment, while four patients had headaches, which were satisfactorily treated with paracetamol and corticosteroids. One patient had breakthrough *epileptic seizures* which were controlled with corticosteroids and an increase in the dosage of antiepileptic drugs.

These results all suggest that the adverse effects experienced after treatment with albendazole for neurocysticercosis are caused by a transient rise in intracranial pressure due to an inflammatory reaction to the degenerating cyst. The additional administration of corticosteroids prevented or reduced adverse effects considerably in all cases. The authors suggested that treatment with corticosteroids should be started before treatment with albendazole and be continued for at least 1 week afterwards (4[C]). The recommended dosages are 1 mg/kg per day of prednisone orally for patients with small subarachnoid cysts located within the cortical sulci and intravenous dexamethasone (up to 12 mg/day) for patients with large cysts located in the Sylvian fissure or in the basal cisterns. In this context a study of the pharmacokinetic interaction of dexamethasone with albendazole sulfoxide in 24 patients with active neurocysticercosis showed that dexamethasone may increase plasma concentrations of albendazole sulfoxide due to inhibition of albendazole elimination (5[C]). It is unclear whether this finding has implications for albendazole dosages.

Amocarzine

Although ivermectin is very effective in the treatment of onchocerciasis, an effective and safe macrofilaricidal drug is still lacking. In earlier studies of rodent and bovine filarial infections amocarzine showed promise as a macrofilaricidal drug and was afterwards extensively tried in humans. Promising results were obtained in the early 1990s in Ecuador, with reported death rates of both male and female worms of around 80% after treatment with 3 mg/kg bd for 3 days and with acceptable adverse effects, including *dizziness*, *itching*, and *rash*. There were reversible neurological symptoms, such as *impaired co-ordination* and a *positive Romberg's sign*, in 4–12% of patients (12[C]). Amocarzine was later tried in Africa in higher doses, with much less positive results. Nevertheless, a new study of the efficacy of amocarzine in combination with ivermectin in the treatment of onchocerciasis has been conducted in Ghana in 100 men from a highly endemic area for onchocerciasis who were randomized to receive a single dose of ivermectin 150 μg/kg on day 1 followed by amocarzine 3 mg/kg bd at meals for 3 days on days 8, 9, and 10, or to ivermectin, or amocarzine alone (13[C]). Unlike ivermectin, amocarzine did not affect the female worms or the intrauterine embryos and was a less potent microfilaricidal drug. The combination of ivermectin and amocarzine was not more effective than ivermectin alone. Adverse effects were more severe with amocarzine alone compared with ivermectin alone or to amocarzine preceded by ivermectin. Mazotti-type reactions, such as *itching*, *rash*, *peripheral sensory phenomena*, and *swellings*, were all more severe or frequent after amocarzine than after ivermectin. Pretreatment with ivermectin markedly reduced these adverse reactions but did not affect other symptoms, such as *dizziness* and *gaze-evoked nystagmus*, suggesting that these adverse effects were probably directly drug-related and not a reaction to dying worms. The authors concluded that amocarzine cannot be recommended for West African patients with onchocerciasis.

Diethylcarbamazine *(SED-13, 905; SEDA-19, 286; SEDA-21, 315)*

Although diethylcarbamazine is increasingly being replaced by ivermectin in the treatment of most forms of human filariasis, it is still widely used in developing countries, especially in the treatment of loiasis and lymphatic filariasis, but to a lesser extent also in onchocerciasis. In a large study of risk factors for the development of optic nerve disease in an area endemic for onchocerciasis in Kaduna state in Nigeria, eye examinations were performed on 6831 individuals aged 5 years or more (14[C]). *Optic nerve disease* was found in 9% of the population. There was a statistically significant relation between optic nerve disease and the previous use of diethylcarbamazine, with a possible causal relation in 30% of all cases of optic nerve disease. However, this finding does not necessarily indicate a toxic effect of diethylcarbamazine on the optic nerve, but more probably indicates more severe disease and/or incomplete treatment.

Ivermectin *(SED-13, 906; SEDA-19, 287; SEDA-20, 280; SEDA-21, 315)*

Ivermectin is a very effective microfilaricidal drug in the treatment of strongyloidiasis and all types of filariasis (except *Dipalonema perstans* infections); it is also used in the treatment of scabies. Although severe adverse effects can occur, especially in the more heavily infected patients (owing to allergic reactions to the dying worms), it is considered to be safe, with generally only minor adverse effects.

Ivermectin and lymphatic filariasis In a meta-analysis of the results of 15 published trials, the efficacy and adverse effects of a single dose of ivermectin were studied in a total of 748 microfilaremic patients with filariasis bancrofti (15[CR]). All doses of ivermectin almost completely eradicated microfilaremia within 1 week (about 90% of the patients becoming microfilaria negative), but higher doses (200–400 μg/kg) were more effective in maintaining low microfilaria levels. After treatment, 316 of 395 patients (80%) had at least one adverse effect: a *flu-like illness* (66%), *headache* (72%), *weakness* (49%), *myalgia* (48%), *chills* (51%), and *lethargy* (74%). Other less frequently reported adverse effects were *sweating*, *arthralgia*, *dizziness*, *anorexia*, *vomiting*, *abdominal pain*, *sore throat*, and *dyspnea*. Most of the adverse effects occurred within 24 h after the start of treatment and subsided within 3 days. These adverse effects were generally mild and usually did not need medication. A more severe adverse effect was *postural hypertension*, which occurred in 7.5% of patients but required only symptomatic treatment. Local reactions were reported in only 11 patients in only three studies and consisted of *epididymitis*, *lymphadenitis/lymphangitis*, and *scrotal swelling*. The authors concluded that ivermectin is a safe and effective drug in the treatment of lymphatic filariasis and is also effective in doses of 200–400 μg/kg in maintaining low microfilaria levels, possibly because it has also some effect on the adult worm, comparable to the effect it has on the adult onchocerca worm. A yearly single dose of 400 μg/kg can be a safe and effective strategy for the control of filariasis bancrofti.

Ivermectin and loiasis In loiasis more severe adverse effects, especially encephalopathy, can occur after treatment with ivermectin, mainly in the more heavily infected individuals, as a result of an intense immune reaction to antigens of the dying microfilaria. In view of this serious complication mass treatment with ivermectin in loiasis-endemic areas is not advised. This point has been further emphasized by a report of severe adverse effects after mass treatment with ivermectin for onchocerciasis in an area in which *Loa loa* is also endemic (16[C]). Although the incidence of severe effects was small in absolute terms and occurred in only 22 patients out of a total of 17 877 individuals treated, this still made mass treatment with ivermectin for onchocerciasis problematic. Age and pretreatment levels of *Loa loa* and *Dipalonema perstans* microfilaria were significantly higher in the individuals with the more severe reactions after treatment. Two patients, both with very high *Loa loa* microfilaria counts developed serious neurological reactions, consisting of *disorders of consciousness* progressing to *coma*, which persisted for 2–3 days with motor and sensory deficits. Both patients made a full recovery after 1 month. It has been recommended (17[R]) that the Mectizan Expert Committee specific criteria for ivermectin programs in loiasis (18[R]) should be carefully followed.

Meanwhile, two reports have shown that a single dose of ivermectin is effective in lowering *Loa loa* microfilaremia 12 months after treatment. In a study from Cameroun a single dose of ivermectin 150 μg/kg caused a mean lowering of microfilaria levels of 74% at 1 year (19[C]), while in a study from Gabon (20[C]) a single dose of ivermectin 200 μg/kg given to 71 patients resulted in a substantial fall in *Loa loa* microfilaremia. Of these patients 43 (63%) had no circulating microfilaria at 1 year and the geographical mean peripheral microfilaria count had fallen by 89%. Half of these patients (36/74) had adverse effects: *pruritus* (36), *skin rash* (six), *arthralgias* (four), and *calabar-like swellings* (seven). These adverse effects were treated successfully with antihistamines. There were no cases of encephalopathy.

Ivermectin and *Mansonella streptocerca* infections *Mansonella streptocerca* is a more obscure filaria. It primarily infects primates, who are the main reservoir. The disease is transferred by midges and mainly involves the skin, comparable to onchocerciasis. The diagnosis is made by a skin snip. In a mass treatment study from Western Uganda 700 patients with and without positive skin snips for *M. streptocerca* were treated with a single oral dose of ivermectin 150 μg/kg (21[C]). Six and 12 days after treatment no microfilaria were found in the skin of 53 of 96 microfilaria carriers, while the mean density of microfilaria in the remaining carriers fell to 33–40% of the levels before treatment. Adverse effects included *itch*, which occurred in almost all treated individuals, and skin problems, most often an *acute papular dermatitis* on the trunk or arms and more rarely on the lower part of the body. On the second day after treatment six of 40 microfilaria carriers (15%) and six of 55 microfilaria-negative patients developed acute dermatitis, which increased to 45% of 86 microfilaria carriers on the sixth day. Of the microfilaria carriers 72% had no skin lesions before the start of treatment. In most cases the dermatitis abated within a few days. Therapy with antihistamine tablets and corticosteroid cream sufficed, even in the more severe cases. A few patients developed larger papules after treatment with ivermectin, probably as an allergic reaction to the adult female worms. Comparable skin reactions have been described after treatment with diethylcarbamazine for this condition, suggesting that these adverse effects are caused by allergic reactions to antigens of the dying worms.

Ivermectin and scabies In a puzzling report from Canada an excess of deaths has been described in a ward of 47 mostly demented patients, mean age 73 years, treated with a single oral dose of ivermectin (150–200 μg/kg) for scabies; within 6 months 15 of the 47 had died (22[C]). All who died developed a *sudden change in behavior, with lethargy, anorexia, and listlessness before death*. In this same ward only 28 deaths had been recorded in the 3 years before. In all other wards of the same facility (163 beds), in which no-one was treated with ivermectin, there were 10 deaths in the same period and 144 in the 3 years previous. It is at present unclear whether this excess of deaths after ivermectin was a real effect, and if so if it was attributable to the drug itself, or to concomitant disease or treatment. In reaction to this report two other groups reported no excess of deaths after treatment with ivermectin in elderly patients (23[c]), (24[c]).

Levamisole *(SED-13, 1135; SEDA-19, 354; SEDA-20, 348; SEDA-21, 317)*

Levamisole was originally developed as an antihelminthic drug, but is now mainly used as an immunomodulating drug in the adjuvant chemotherapy of Dukes B and C colonic cancer in combination with 5-fluorouracil, in the treatment of rheumatic diseases, and in the treatment of nephrosis in children. Lately the combination of 5-fluorouracil and levamisole for the adjuvant chemotherapy of Dukes B and C colonic cancer has lost favor compared with adjuvant chemotherapy with calcium folinate (leucovorin) and 5-fluorouracil, which is at least as effective with a shorter duration. Nevertheless during the past year several reviews of the use of adjuvant chemotherapy for Dukes B and C colonic cancer with the combination of 5-fluorouracil and levamisole have appeared (25[R])–(28[R]). One can conclude from these studies that the combination of 5-fluorouracil and levamisole is usually well tolerated, although about 5% of patients do not complete the full course, owing to adverse effects.

Adverse effects described after monotherapy with levamisole include *abnormalities in taste*, *arthralgia*, and *myalgia*. The most frequent adverse effects reported after combination treatment are those that can be expected after cytostatic treatment and consist of gastroenterological and hematological effects.

Nervous system Neurological adverse effects include *anxiety*, *sleep disturbances*, and *depression* (25[R]), (28[R]), but also the rare but more serious syndrome of *multifocal leukoencephalopathy*, which occurs in about 0.04% of patients and leads to severe, often permanent, neurological damage (25[R]).

Hematological Hematological adverse effects mainly consist of *neutropenia/agranulocytosis* (25[R]), (28[R]), which is usually transient after withdrawal.

Liver Mild reversible liver function disturbances have been reported in about 40% of cases and are often associated with *fatty infiltration of the liver* (26[R]), (28[R]). These liver function abnormalities are usually attributed to combination treatment with 5-fluorouracil and not to levamisole alone. However, there has been a recent report of liver toxicity after treatment with levamisole in a child with nephrosis (29[c]), suggesting that disturbances of liver function can also be seen after treatment with levamisole alone.

A 14-year-old boy with frequently relapsing minimal change nephrotic syndrome taking maintenance prednisone was given levamisole 50 mg tds on alternate days. Four weeks later he developed pruritus. He had an increased AlT but his bilirubin, γ-glutamyltransferase, and alkaline phosphatase remained normal. After 4 weeks the AlT had increased further, but the other liver function tests remained normal and the pruritus had disappeared. Levamisole was nevertheless withdrawn and the AlT returned to normal.

Gastrointestinal *Nausea* occurs in about 57% of patients, *diarrhea* in 47%, *vomiting* in 17%, and *constipation and upper abdominal complaints* in 10%.

Skin and appendages Levamisole has previously been associated with necrotizing vasculitis (30[c]). Now *ischemic necrosis* has also been reported (31[c]).

A 10-year-old boy, taking levamisole 2 mg/kg per day for nephrotic syndrome, suddenly developed bullous hemorrhagic lesions on both earlobes due to ischemic necrosis caused by the occlusion of large vessels in the deep plexus by thrombotic material and cellular debris, and occlusion of the small vessels of the superficial dermis with fibrin deposits around these vessels. The lesions healed completely, without sequelae, within 25 days of withdrawal of levamisole.

Metrifonate *(SED-13, 836, 914)*

Metrifonate is effective in the treatment of schistosomiasis hematobium infections, for which it is almost as effective as praziquantel, with only minor adverse effects. It is therefore used if praziquantel is not available or is contraindicated. Because of its prolonged inhibition of brain cholinesterase and increased steady-state concentrations of acetylcholine in the cortex and the hippocampus, all of which may be disturbed in Alzheimer's disease, it is now also increasingly used in the treatment of this condition (32[r]). The use of metrifonate has been reviewed (33[R]). Statistically significant improvements in cognitive performance were obtained by the administration of a single daily dose of metrifonate (loading dose 2 mg/kg per day, maintenance dosage 0.65 mg/kg per day), while lower dosages and placebo were not effective. Reported adverse effects were mainly mild-to-moderate dose-dependent cholinergic effects, such as *nausea*, *vomiting*, *abdominal discomfort*, *diarrhea*, *weakness*, and *muscle cramps*. In elderly volunteers there was no correlation between acetylcholinesterase and butyrylcholinesterase activities and adverse events. In 55 children given three doses of metrifonate 7.5–10 mg/kg at 2-week intervals there was no significant change in neuromuscular transmission. No significant hematological disturbances or abnormalities of liver function have been reported after metrifonate, although significant falls in serum albumin concentrations have been described. However, very high doses of metrifonate, or additional exposure to insecticides with anticholinesterase activity, can cause more severe neurotoxicity. Metrifonate is currently being used in Phase III trials in the treatment of Alzheimer's disease.

Praziquantel *(SED-13, 909; SEDA-20, 282; SEDA-21, 318)*

In 130 children in Northern Senegal treatment with praziquantel 40 mg/kg for schistosomiasis mansoni resulted in disappointing cure rates, and the patients were randomized to receive either a single dose of praziquantel 40 mg/kg or two oral doses of 30 mg/kg at 6-h intervals (34[C]). There was no significant difference in the rather disappointing efficacy of both treatments, with negative stools in 34 and 44% 6 weeks after treatment, although mean egg counts were reduced by 90% in both groups. Adverse effects after treatment were more frequent in the single-dose group. Adverse effects for which there was a significant difference were: *diarrhoea* (22 vs 2%), *general malaise* (48 vs 12%), *myalgia* 10 vs 0%), and *fever* (34 vs 2%). Other adverse effects that did not differ between the groups were: *abdominal pain* (76 vs 51%), *nausea* (22 vs 12%), *vomiting* for under 2 h (28 vs 12%), vomiting for more than 2 h (36 vs 15%), bloody *diarrhea* (9 vs 14%), *drowsiness* (49 vs 24%), *headache* (40 vs 39%), and *skin rash* (13 vs 8%). In addition there were a few cases of *edema*, *urticaria*, *heartburn*, or *dizziness*. There were no serious adverse effects. It seems advisable to give praziquantel in two doses of 30 mg/kg instead of a single dose of 40 mg/kg, since efficacy is comparable and adverse effects less frequent.

Suramin *(SED-13, 915; SEDA-19, 289; SEDA-20, 283; SEDA-21, 318)*

Suramin is rarely used as a macrofilaricidal drug in the treatment of onchocerciasis because of serious toxicity. Its wide range of adverse effects include hematological, neurological, ophthalmological, endocrine, and skin abnormalities. Lately however it has been used in the treatment of hormone-refractory prostate cancer, in which it has shown some anti-tumor effect, although again accompanied by extensive and sometimes severe adverse effects. Renewed interest in suramin has led to a recent review (35[R]) focusing on its biological and therapeutic properties as well as its clinical toxicity. The authors concluded that both the clinical and toxic effects of suramin are probably caused by interaction of the sulfonated groups of the drug with various biological molecules.

In a Phase II trial suramin was added to leuprolide and flutamide in previously untreated metastatic prostate cancer in 50 patients (36[C]). Suramin was given by infusion in doses designed to maintain plasma concentrations at 175–300 μg/ml. There was severe *thrombocytopenia* in five patients (10%) and *neutropenia* in four (8%), normalizing after withdrawal of suramin and the administration of granulocyte stimulating factor (G-CSF). Three patients developed grade 3 neurotoxicity; two had *proximal muscle weakness* and the third developed *phrenic nerve paralysis*. Other severe adverse effects included *pain*, *raised transaminases*, *infection*, *acute renal failure*, *disseminated intravascular coagulopathy*, *weight loss*, and *vortex keratopathy* in individual patients. In all, 14 of 50 patients (38%) had grade 3–4 toxicity. There were no deaths and all the adverse effects were reversible.

Nervous system The administration of suramin to patients with hormone-refractory prostate cancer has been previously associated with several neurological abnormalities, including distal axonal polyneuropathy, motor neuropathy, paresthesia, and a Guillain-Barré-like syndrome. The neurological adverse effects of suramin have recently been studied in 41 patients with treatment-refractory cancer, 84% of whom had hormone-refractory prostate cancer (37[CR]). The patients were given suramin by intermittent infusions designed to provide constant peak plasma concentrations. Two different types of neurological symptoms occurred. Six patients (15%) developed a *demyelinating neuropathy* like Guillain-Barré syndrome, and one asymptomatic patient showed electrophysiological evidence suggestive of a demyelinating neuropathy. Four patients developed electrophysiological signs of *axonal polyneuropathy*, while a fifth, who had had mild axonal neuropathy before the start of treatment, deteriorated after the administration of suramin. In the patients who developed a Guillain-Barré-like syndrome, the symptoms and signs of motor weakness developed subacutely and were maximally severe after 2–6 weeks. Most of the patients recovered spontaneously after withdrawal, although at a variable rate, except two patients with severe symptoms. One patient had plasmapheresis five times and had to be ventilated for 6 months, after which there were still persistent, but less severe, symptoms; a second patient refused further treatment and died. In one patient a sural biopsy showed the mixed axonal and demyelinating neuropathy described previously after the administration of suramin. The total cumulative dose of suramin was 7.13 g/m^2 (n = 7) in patients who developed demyelinating neuropathy, 5.79 g/m^2 (n = 5) in patients who developed clinical or subclinical axonal neuropathy, and 5.78 g/m^2 (n = 29) in patients without neurotoxicity. Although these results were not statistically significant, they were consistent with earlier findings that associated the development of a Guillain-Barré-like syndrome with higher dosages.

Interactions In 26 patients treated with suramin for hormone-refractory prostate cancer *furosemide* reduced the total body clearance of suramin by 36% (38^C). In view of the increased risk of severe adverse effects after treatment with higher plasma concentrations of suramin, it would be prudent to adapt dosage schemes in patients treated with both suramin and furosemide.

Tiabendazole (thiabendazole)

(SED-13, 911)

Tiabendazole is a benzimidazole that is effective and often used in the treatment of strongyloidiasis. Severe *cholestasis* has previously been reported, sometimes ending in death or liver transplantation. Recently another case of severe liver dysfunction after treatment with tiabendazole for strongyloidiasis has been described (39^c).

A 26-year-old Cambodian man became icteric a month after taking tiabendazole 25 mg/kg per day for 3 days for strongyloidiasis, with a second course 20 days later. He had pruritus and symptoms of sicca syndrome, and raised bilirubin, transaminases, and alkaline phosphatase. Markers for hepatitis A, B, and C were all negative, as were antinuclear, smooth muscle and antimitochondrial antibodies. A liver biopsy showed centrilobular cholestasis with necrosis and discrete cholangitis, and no bile ducts. After liver transplantation, the voluminous liver (2600 g) showed extensive portal and periportal fibrosis, extensive intracanalicular and intrahepatocytic cholestasis, and absent intralobular bile ducts in almost all portal fields.

In view of this and earlier reports it is advisable not to prescribe tiabendazole for strongyloidiasis.

REFERENCES

1. Garcia HH, Gilman RH, Horton J, Martinez M, Herrera G, Altamirano J, Cuba JM, Rios-Saaverdra N, Verastegui M, Boero J, Gonzalez AE. Albendazole therapy for neurocysticercosis: a prospective double-blind trial comparing 7 vs 14 days of treatment. Neurology 1997;48:1421–7.
2. Del Brutto OH. Albenazole therapy for subarachnoid cysticerci: clinical and neuroimaging analysis of 17 patients. J Neurol Neurosurg Psychiatry 1997;62:659–61.
3. Proano JV, Madrazo I, Garcia L, Garcia-Torres E, Correa D. Albendazole and praziquantel treatment in neurocysticercosis of the fourth ventricle. J Neurosurg 1997;87:29–33.
4. Del Brutto OH. Clues to prevent cerebrovascular hazards of cysticidal drug therapy. Stroke 1997;28:1088.
5. Takayanagui OM, Lanchote VL, Marques MPC, Bonato PS. Therapy for neurocysticercosis: pharmacokinetic interaction of albendazole sulfoxide with dexamethasone. Ther Drug Monit 1997;19:51–5.
6. Bhatia G. Echinicoccus. Semin Respir Infect 1997;12:171–86.
7. Horton RJ. Albendazole in the treatment of human cystic echinococcosis: 12 years of experience. Acta Trop 1997;64:79–93.
8. Teggi A, Lastilla MG, Grossi G, Franchi C, de Rosa F. Increase of serum-glutamic-oxaloacetic and glutamic-pyruvic transaminases in patients with hydatid cysts treated with mebendazole and albendazole. Mediterr J Infect Parasit Dis 1995;10:85–90.
9. Chagnon A, Galzin M, De Jaureguiberry JP, Boyer B, Paris JF, Marlier S, Carli P. Prolonged treatment of recurrent neurocysticercosis by sequential courses of albendazole and praziquantel. Med Trop 1994;54:275–6.
10. Luchi S, Vincenti A, Mesima F, Parenti M, Scasso A, Campetelli A. Albendazole treatment of human hydatid disease. Scand J Infect Dis 1997;29:165–7.
11. Dewerdt S, Machet L, Jan-Lamy V, Lorette G, Thérizol-Feily M. Stevens–Johnson syndrome after albendazole. Acta Dermatol Venereol 1997; 77:411.
12. Guderian RH, Anselmi M, Proano R, Naranjo A, Poltera AA, Moran M, Lecaillon JB, Zak F, Carcante S. Onchocercicidal effects of three drug regimens of amocarzine in 148 patients of two races and both sexes from Esmeraldas, Equador. Trop Med Parasitol 1991;42:263–85.
13. Awadzi K, Opoku NO, Attah SK, Addy ET, Duke BOL, Nyama PK, Kshissagar NA. The safety and efficacy of amocarzine in African onchocerciasis and the influence of ivermectin on the clinical and parasitological response to treatment. Am Trop Med Parasitol 1997;91:282–96.
14. Cousens SN, Yahaya H, Murdoch I, Samaila E, Evans J, Babalola OE, Zakari M, Abiose A, Jones BR. Risk factors for optic nerve disease in communities mesoendemic for savannah onchocerciasis, Kaduna state, Nigeria. Trop Med Int Health 1997;2:89–98.
15. Cao W-C, Van Der Ploeg CPB, Plaisier AP,

Van Der Sluijs J, Habbema JDF. Ivermectin for the chemotherapy of bancroftian filariasis: a meta-analysis of the effect of single treatment. Trop Med Int Health 1997;2:393–403.
16. Gardon J, Gardon-Wendel N, Demanga-Ngangue, Kamguo J, Chippaux J-P, Boussinesq M. Serious reactions after mass treatment of onchocerciasis with ivermectin in area endemic for *Loa loa* infections. Lancet 1997;350:18–22.
17. Burnham GM. Ivermectin where *Loa loa* is endemic. Lancet 1997;350:2–3.
18. The Mectizan Expert Committee. Central nervous complications of Loiasis and adverse CNS events following treatment. Atlanta: Mectizan Donation Program 1996.
19. Gardon J, Kamngo J, Folefack G, Gardon-Wendel N, Bouchite B, Boussinesq M. Marked decrease in *Loa loa* microfilaraemia six and twelve months after a single dose of ivermectin. Trans R Soc Trop Med Hyg 1997;91:593–4.
20. Duong TH, Kombila M, Ferrer A, Bureau P, Gaxotte P, Richard-Lenoble D. Reduced *Loa loa* microfilaria count ten to twelve months after a single dose of ivermectin. Trans R Soc Trop Med Hyg 1997;91:592–3.
21. Fischer P, Bamuhiiga, Buttner DW. Treatment of human *Mansonella streptocerca* infection with ivermectin. Trop Med Int Health 1997; 2:191–9.
22. Barkwell R, Shields S. Deaths associated with ivermectin treatment of scabies. Lancet 1997; 349:1144–5.
23. Diazgranados JA, Costa JL. Deaths after ivermectin treatment. Lancet 1997;349:1698.
24. Reintjes R, Hoek C. Deaths associated with ivermectin for scabies. Lancet 1997;350:215.
25. Vaughn DJ, Haller DG. The role of adjuvant chemotherapy in the treatment of colorectal cancer. Hematol Oncol Clin North Am 1997; 11:699–719.
26. Vaughn DJ, Haller DG. Adjuvant therapy for colorectal cancer: past accomplishments, future directions. Cancer Invest 1997;15:435–47.
27. MacDonald JS. Adjuvant therapy for colon cancer. Ca Cancer J Clin 1997;47:243–56.
28. Kluting A. Levamisole in the adjuvant treatment of colon cancer. Pharm Ztg 1997;142:30–4, 36.
29. Bulugahapitiya DTD. Liver toxicity in a nephrotic patient treated with levamisole. Arch Dis Child 1997;76:289.
30. Scheinberg MA, Gomez Bezerra JB, Almeida FA, Silveira LA. Cutaneous necrotising vasculitis induced by levamisole. Br Med J 1978;1:408.
31. Menni S, Pistritto G, Gianotti R, Ghio L, Edefonti A. Ear lobe bilateral necrosis by levamisole-induced occlusive vasculitis in a pediatric patient. Pediatr Dermatol 1997;14:477–9.
32. Giacobini E. Metrifonate: a viewpoint. Drugs Aging 1997;11:497.
33. Lamb HM, Faulds D. Metrifonate. Drugs Aging 1997;11:490–6.
34. Guisse F, Polman K, Stelma FF, Mbaye A, Talla I, Niang M, Deelder AM, Ndir O, Gryseels B. Therapeutic evaluation of two different dose regimens of praziquantel in a recent *Schistosoma mansoni* focus in Northern Senegal. Am J Trop Med Hyg 1997;56:511–14.
35. Baghdiguian S, Fantini J. Suramin: a molecule with a broad spectrum of biological and therapeutic properties. Cancer J 1997;22:31–7.
36. Dawson NA, Figg WD, Cooper MR, Sartor O, Bergan RC, Senderowicz AM, Steinberg SM, Tompkins A, Weinberger B, Sausville EA, Reed E, Myers CE. Phase II trial of suramin, leuprolide and flutamide in previously untreated metastatic prostate cancer. J Clin Oncol 1997;15:1470–7.
37. Soliven B, Dhand UK, Kobayashi K, Arora R, Martin B, Petersen MV, Janisch L, Vogelzang NJ, Vokes EE, Ratain MJ. Evaluation of neuropathy in patients on suramin treatment. Muscle Nerve 1997;22:31–4.
38. Piscitelli SC, Forrest A, Lush RM, Ryan N, Whitfield LR, Figg WD. Pharmacometric analysis of the effect of furosemide on suramin pharmacokinetics. Pharmacotherapy 1997;17:431–7.
39. Skandrani K, Richardet J-P, Duvoux C, Cherqui D, Zafrani ES, Dhumeaux D. Transplantation hépatique pour ductopénie sévère associée la prise de thiabendazole. Gastroenterol Clin Biol 1997;21:623–5.

S. Dittmann

32 Vaccines

GENERAL

Surveillance of adverse events after immunization

The Programme on International Drug Monitoring of the World Health Organization currently numbers 50 members. In all member countries, national Drug Reaction Monitoring Centers collect reports from health professionals and pass them on for entry into the international database housed at the WHO Collaborating Center for International Drug Monitoring in Uppsala, Sweden. Currently, there are some 1 600 000 reports on file, and each year almost 200 000 new reports are added. The database generates signals of potentially severe drug toxicity and provides confirmation of signals generated in specific countries. The center also acts as the guardian of the standardized terminology of adverse drug reactions in computerized systems. Although vaccines are considered to be safe, the work of the center underlines the importance of collecting information on the safety of vaccines to provide sound reference data in the event of a problem. Since vaccines are administered to healthy people, mostly children, the impact of a perceived problem can be enormous. Because of these considerations, many countries have already established specific programmes for the monitoring of adverse events after immunization (1[R]).

Drug-related mortality reported between 1984 and 1994 has been analysed in Canada (2[C]). For non-suicide drug-related deaths, the most commonly reported suspect drugs were classified as nervous system agents (557 reports out of a total of 1086 reports); in comparison, 13 deaths occurred in which vaccines were reported as the suspect drug (diphtheria–tetanus–pertussis vaccine; oral poliovirus vaccine, measles–mumps–rubella vaccine, influenza vaccine, Hemophilus influenzae type b vaccine).

The 1996 Update on vaccine side effects, adverse reactions, contraindications, and precautions elaborated and published by the US Advisory Committee on Immunization Practices includes summarized conclusions of evidence for the possible association between specific adverse effects and childhood vaccines (Tables 1 and 2). The conclusions are based on the reports of the Institute of Medicine (cited at length in SED-12 (p. 817) and SEDA-18 (p. 325)) (3[R]), (4[R]).

Reported adverse events after immunization in New Zealand from 1990 to 1995 have been presented (5[C]). Reactions at the injection site following adult tetanus–diphtheria vaccine was the most commonly reported adverse effect of the vaccine and the vaccine was the most common cause of this effect (68 reports per 100 000 immunizations). The rates for the other childhood vaccines were as follows.

1. *'Abnormal crying' after diphtheria–tetanus–pertussis/Hemophilus influenzae type b vaccine: 29 reports per 100 000 immunizations compared with three per 100 000 after diphtheria–tetanus–pertussis vaccine.*
2. *Reactions at the injection site after diphtheria – tetanus – pertussis/Hemophilus influenzae type b vaccine: 25 reports per 100 000 immunizations compared with 17 per 100 000 after diphtheria–tetanus–pertussis vaccine.*
3. *Fever after Hemophilus influenzae type b vaccine: 16 reports per 100 000 immunizations compared with two per 100 000 after hepatitis B vaccine and one per 100 000 after influenza vaccine.*
4. *The most common reports after measles–mumps–rubella vaccine were rash (17 per 100 000), fever (12 per 100 000), and*

Side Effects of Drugs, Annual 22
J.K. Aronson, ed.

Table 1. *Evidence for possible associations between adverse events and childhood vaccines* (3^R)

Evidence	DT/Td/tetanus toxoid	Measles vaccine	Mumps vaccine	OPV/IPV	Hepatitis B vaccine	Hemophilus influenzae type b (Hib) vaccine
None available to establish a casual relation	None	None	Neuropathy Residual seizure disorder	Transverse myelitis (IPV) Thrombocytopenia (IPV) Anaphylaxis (IPV)	None	None
Inadequate to accept or reject a causal relation	Residual seizure disorder other than infantile spasms Demyelinating diseases of the central nervous system Mononeuropathy Arthritis Erythema multiforme	Encephalopathy Subacute sclerosing panencephalitis Residual seizure disorder Sensorineural deafness (MMR) Optic neuritis Transverse myelitis Guillain–Barré syndrome Thrombocytopenia Insulin-dependent diabetes mellitus	Encephalopathy Aseptic meningitis Sensorineural deafness (MMR) Insulin-dependent diabetes mellitus Sterility Thrombocytopenia Anaphylaxis	Transverse myelitis (OPV) Guillain–Barré syndrome (IPV) Death from SIDS	Guillain–Barré syndrome Demyelinating diseases of the central nervous system Arthritis Death from SIDS	Guillain–Barré syndrome Transverse myelitis Thrombocytopenia Anaphylaxis Death from SIDS
Favored rejection of a causal relation	Encephalopathy Infantile spasms (DT only) Death from SIDS (DT only)	None	None	None	None	Early-onset Hib disease (conjugate vaccines)
Favored acceptance of a causal relation	Guillain–Barré syndrome Brachial neuritis	Anaphylaxis	None	Guillain–Barré syndrome (OPV)	None	Early-onset Hib disease in children ages 18 months whose first Hib vaccination was with unconjugated PRP vaccine
Established a causal relation	Anaphylaxis	Thrombocytopenia (MMR) Anaphylaxis (MMR) Death from measles infection	None	Poliomyelitis in recipient or contact (OPV) Death from polio infection	Anaphylaxis	None

See the original paper for extensive notes to this table. OPV, oral poliovirus vaccine; IPV, inactivated poliovirus vaccine; DT, diphtheria and tetanus toxoids for pediatric use; Td, diphtheria and tetanus toxoids for adult use; SIDS, sudden infant death syndrome.

Table 2. *Evidence for possible associations between adverse effects and DTP and MMR vaccines (3[R])*

Evidence	Adverse event	
	DTP vaccine	RA 27/3 MMR
None available to establish a causal relation	Autism	None
Inadequate to accept or reject a causal relation	Aseptic meningitis Chronic neurological damage Erythema multiforme or other rash Guillain-Barré syndrome Hemolytic anemia Type 1 diabetes Learning disabilities and attention-deficit disorder Peripheral mononeuropathy Thrombocytopenia	Radiculoneuritis and other neuropathies Thrombocytopenic purpura
Favored rejection of a causal relation	Infantile spasms Hypsarrhythmia Reye's syndrome Sudden infant death syndrome	None
Favored acceptance of a causal relation	Acute encephalopathy Shock and unusual shock-like state	Chronic arthritis
Established a causal relation	Anaphylaxis Protracted inconsolable crying	Acute arthritis

DTP, diphtheria, tetanus toxoids, and pertussis vaccine; MMR, measles, mumps, and rubella vaccine.

inflammation at the injection site (five per 100 000).

(5) There were very few reports of adverse effects after poliovirus vaccine; rash, fever, and headache were all reported at less than one per 100 000 immunizations.

The authors concluded that the picture confirmed the overall safety of vaccines and the value of an adverse events monitoring system.

Recognizing the need to improve the capability to study vaccine safety, the US Centers for Disease Control and Prevention (CDC) participated during the late 1980s in two pilot studies using large linked databases of computerized immunization and medical records (SEDA-20, 286). This participation prompted the CDC to initiate planning for the Vaccine Safety Datalink in 1989. The design of the project and preliminary results and limitations have now been described (6[C]).

Nervous system MRI scanning has been found to be useful in the diagnosis of meningoencephalitis following mumps immunization (Urabe AM vaccine strain) (7[C]). The authors therefore recommended the incorporation of MRI scanning of brain and spinal cord into the investigation of adverse events of vaccines suspected to include involvement of the central nervous system.

Respiratory It has been suggested that there is accumulating evidence that immunization causes *asthma* (8[C]), but it has been pointed out (9[R]) that the cohort study cited in this study had many important limitations. In a British cohort study (10[C]), (11[c]) there was no association between immunization and wheeze.

Endocrine, metabolic To address concerns raised in the media regarding the relation between type 1 *diabetes mellitus* and immunization, the Institute for Vaccine Safety at the Johns Hopkins School of Public Health held a workshop on 20 March 1998 in Baltimore, Maryland (12[R]). All available data on the pathogenesis of diabetes, autoimmunity, epidemiology, biostatistics, and adverse events following immunization were analysed. The workshop found no evidence that changing the routine childhood immunization would increase or decrease the risk of developing type 1 diabetes. A similar meeting was held on 14–15 May 1998 in Bethesda, Maryland. The consensus was that existing studies in humans do not show an increase in type 1 diabetes attributable either to any vaccine or to the timing of the vaccine (13[R]).

In a study of about 116 000 Finnish children immunization started at birth was associated with a reduced risk of insulin-dependent diabetes (14[C]). The children were randomized to receive either four doses of the vaccine, starting at 3 months of age, or one dose at 24 months of age. However, when the data were discussed at the Baltimore meeting mentioned above, the panel concluded that the analytical methods had been incorrect.

Hematological Clinical data on 309 cases of *thrombocytopenia* reported between 1968 and 1991 to the Danish Committee on Adverse Drug Reactions have been presented (15[R]). Measles–mumps–rubella vaccine (nine cases) and diphtheria–tetanus–polio vaccine (two cases) have been reported as causative.

Urinary system Macroscopic *hematuria* has been reported after immunization with tetanus toxoid and oral poliovirus vaccine in a 15-year-old boy (16[c]). The episode occurred 48 h after administration of the vaccine and resolved spontaneously without recurrence. The UK Medicines Control Agency had received five previous unpublished cases of hematuria associated with tetanus immunization.

Special senses Drug-induced *uveitis* has been reviewed (17[R]). The authors stated that evidence is scarce on uveitis associated with vaccines such as BCG vaccine, hepatitis B vaccine and with intravenous immunoglobulin.

Immunological and hypersensitivity reactions Allergic reactions to vaccines have been reviewed, including pathogenesis, clinical features, diagnosis, prevention, and treatment (18[R]).

BACTERIAL VACCINES

Bacille Calmette-Guérin (BCG) vaccine *(SED-13, 920; SEDA-20, 287; SEDA-21, 326)*

Disseminated infections Two cases of *disseminated BCG infection* have been reported in children suspected to be immune-deficient (19[c]). The children recovered after surgical and antituberculous treatment. In another fatal case of disseminated BCG infection in a child with secondary immune deficiency a previously healed BCG scar ulcerated (20[c]). Cases of lupus vulgaris 6 months after immunization in a 24-year-old woman (21[c]) and osteomyelitis 2 months after vaccination in a 1-year-old Japanese girl (22[C]) have been described. Redness and other local signs at the site of BCG vaccination is a common feature of Kawasaki disease, and *necrotic ulcerations* at the BCG vaccination site have been described in one such case (23[C]).

In relation to cases of disseminated BCG infection in India and Croatia (24[C]), (25[C]), it has been recommended that a family history of primary immunodeficiency should be sought before the administration of BCG vaccine, since that would be a contraindication.

Intravesical BCG Intravesical BCG has become the most widely used immunostimulant in the non-specific immunotherapy of bladder cancer, particularly superficial transitional cell carcinoma. However, the treatment is not free from adverse effects (SED-13, 925). Updates on the indications, limits, and contraindications, as well as the efficacy, strains, route of administration, dosage, schedule, toxicity, and ways of improving BCG therapy have recently been published (26[R]), (27[R]).

The extent and duration of the systemic influence of intravesical BCG therapy on the peripheral blood lymphocyte subset and monocyte counts of 30 patients has been examined (28[C]). A systemic response began 3 months after the start of treatment and was most marked at 12 months, featuring *a significant reduction in the number of T helper cells and an increase in T suppressor subsets.*

The effects of *isoniazid* on the incidence and severity of adverse effects of intravesical

BCG therapy have been analysed in patients who received BCG with ($n = 289$) and without ($n = 190$) isoniazid (29[C]). The authors concluded that prophylactic oral administration of isoniazid (300 mg/day at every BCG instillation) caused no reduction in any adverse effect of BCG. In contrast, transient liver function disturbances occurred slightly more often when isoniazid was used.

The polymerase chain reaction has been used to monitor BCG in the blood after intravesical BCG instillation (22 patients) as well as after antituberculous therapy (30[C]). The early and fast diagnosis of BCG in the blood was considered to be potentially valuable in initiating specific early treatment of BCG complications.

Reports of complications after intravesical BCG therapy continue to appear: (1) *disseminated pulmonary granulomas* which recovered after antituberculous treatment in a 62-year-old man (31[c]); (2) *Reiter's syndrome* in a 35-year-old woman (the second case reported in the international literature (32[c])); (3) *miliary tuberculosis* after the seventh treatment in a 64-year-old man (33[c]); (4) a *granulomatous renal mass* at the left upper pole occurring after the sixth treatment in a 54-year-old man (34[c]); (5) *reactive arthritis* before the fourth treatment in a 70-year-old woman (35[c]).

In eight patients with *arthritis* after BCG immunotherapy, BCG-induced arthritis was considered to be an immunopathological model of migration of T cells into inflammatory sites (36[C]).

Granulomatous prostatitis was identified in seven of nine patients (37[C]). The authors considered the complication to be a common occurrence of BCG immunotherapy.

***Mycobacterium vaccae* vaccine** Several lines of evidence have suggested that natural or vaccine-induced immunity may be effective in the prevention of infections due to *Mycobacterium avium complex* (MAC). Protection against disseminated MAC infection would require immunization before the development of immunosuppression. *Mycobacterium vaccae* vaccine is a heat-killed vaccine prepared from a rapidly growing environmental mycobacterium that expresses antigens common to many mycobacteria. When this experimental vaccine was administered in a three-dose intradermal schedule to 10 healthy adult volunteers at 0, 2, and 10 months, the immunization was well tolerated and induced measurable immunological responses to mycobacterial antigens (38[c]).

Diphtheria vaccine (including diphtheria–tetanus vaccine) *(SED-13, 926; SEDA-20, 288; SEDA-21, 328)*

In the study of adverse events after immunizations in New Zealand in 1990–1995 mentioned above (5[C]), reactions at the injection site after adult tetanus–diphtheria vaccine (68 reports per 100 000 immunizations) were reported five times more often than with tetanus vaccine

In a 2-year-old boy who developed *urticaria* after his third diphtheria–tetanus–polio immunization the histamine release results suggested that he had had a specific reaction to the purified diphtheria toxoid in the vaccine (39[C]). The authors excluded a reaction to tetanus toxoid or the polio component of the combination vaccine.

Hemophilus influenzae type b (Hib) vaccine *(SED-13, 927; SEDA-19, 293; SEDA-20, 288; SEDA-21, 329)*

In a study of tolerability and immunogenicity of *Hemophilus influenzae* type b vaccines, 30 volunteers aged 69–84 years were immunized with either Pedvax-Hib (a conjugate of Hib polysaccharide and an outer membrane protein complex of *Neisseria meningitidis*-PRP-OMP) or Hib TITER (a conjugate of Hib oligosaccharide and a non-toxic mutant diphtheria toxin, CRM_{197}-HbOC) (40[C]). The volunteers received a pediatric dose. Before immunization, 40% of the volunteers had serum anti-PRP antibody concentrations below 1.0 μg/ml. Four weeks after immunization, all the volunteers had concentrations over 1.0 μg/ml, which is generally considered to be protective. Adverse effects of immunization were mild, except in one volunteer given

HbOC, who developed extensive *erythema and swelling at the injection site*.

The immunogenicity and safety of a diphtheria–tetanus–pertussis–Hib combination vaccine (tetanus-conjugated Hib vaccine) have been compared with those of the same combination obtained by the reconstitution of lyophilized Hib vaccine with liquid DTP vaccine in 262 healthy infants randomized to receive injections at 2, 4, and 6 months of age, a subgroup of 134 of whom received a booster dose at 12 months (41[C]). Systemic and local reactions were generally mild and did not differ significantly between the two groups. With regard to Hib antibodies, the combination vaccine was at least as immunogenic as the lyophilized formulation.

Meningococcal vaccine *(SED-13, 938; SEDA-20, 288; SEDA-21, 329)*

What is probably the first case of *acute disseminated encephalomyelitis* after immunization with meningococcal A + C vaccine has been reported (42[c]). Encephalomyelitis developed 4 weeks after immunization in a 23-year-old woman; she recovered with steroid treatment.

Pertussis vaccine (including diphtheria–tetanus–pertussis vaccine [DTP]) *(SED-13, 940; SEDA-19, 297; SEDA-20, 289; SEDA-21, 329)*

Acellular pertussis vaccine The safety and immunogenicity of a new DTP vaccine (DTaP) including a recombinant acellular pertussis component in 2000 infants have been evaluated in a comparison with 498 controls who received whole cell pertussis–diphtheria–tetanus vaccine (DTwP) at 2, 4, and 6 months of age (43[C]). In addition, the safety and immunogenicity of the same new DTaP vaccine were evaluated as a booster dose in a subset of the same population treated at 15–18 months of age and compared with a licensed DTaP vaccine. The new vaccine was associated with fewer local and systemic reactions after primary immunization compared with DTwP, and the local and systemic reactions after booster immunization were similar after either acellular vaccine (Table 3). When comparing the immunogenicity of the new vaccine with DTaP vaccine, the vaccines were equivalent for the antidiphtheria response, the DTwP vaccine produced a higher antitetanus response, and the new vaccine was significantly more immunogenic for the pertussis antigens tested. After the booster dose, the new vaccine had equal or improved immunogenicity for the antigens tested compared with the other DTaP vaccine, except for a higher antifilamentous hemagglutinin response with the other DTaP vaccine.

In a study of the humoral and cellular immunogenicity and safety of full-strength and half-strength acellular pertussis components of TdaP vaccines 80 medical personnel were divided into three groups who received either a full strength TdaP vaccine (pertussis toxin 1 μg/0.5 ml; filamentous hemagglutinin 4 μg/0.5 ml), or a half-strength TdaP vaccine, or a Td vaccine without acellular pertussis component (44[C]). Local and systemic reactions were minimal and there were no differences among the three groups. The recipients of both full-strength and half-strength TdaP vaccines had a strong antibody response; there were higher anti-pertussis toxin and anti-filamentous hemagglutinin antibody titers in volunteers who received the full-strength TdaP vaccine. There was no significant pertussis toxin-specific proliferative response after immunization, but there was a filamentous hemagglutinin-specific proliferative response.

The safety and immunogenicity of 12 acellular pertussis vaccines and one whole-cell pertussis vaccine given as a fourth dose have been compared in 1293 children aged 15–20 months (45[C]). The trial was a follow-up of an earlier multicenter trial (SEDA-18, 332), in which the same vaccines were given as a primary series at 2, 4, and 6 months of age. As a fourth dose, the children received the same vaccine as in the primary series. There were variations in the occurrence of reactions among DTaP vaccines. In general, DTaP vaccines were associated with fewer adverse events than a US-licensed DTwP vaccine. Redness and swelling at the injection site oc-

Table 3. *Local and systemic reactions to two types of DTP vaccine within 48 h of the third of three injections (43[C])*

Reaction	C-aPDT		wDPT	
	%	n	%	n
Any redness	9.8	1637	28.7	418
Redness ⩾1 inch	0.4	1637	5.0	418
Any swelling	6.4	1638	18.4	419
Swelling ⩾1 inch	0.7	1637	6.9	418
Any tenderness	4.6	1628	21.0	414
Tenderness interferes with leg movement	3.9	1627	13.0	414
Fever >38°C	6.7	1644	25.3	419
Irritability	39.7	1644	57.5	419
Restless sleep	15.9	1643	20.3	419
Hives	0.2	1645	0.2	419
Gray/ashen tone	0.0	1645	0.0	419
Lethargic/limp	0.0	1645	0.0	419
Convulsions	0.0	1645	0.0	419

C-aPDT, recombinant acellular pertussis–diphtheria–tetanus; wDPT, whole cell diphtheria–pertussis–tetanus.

curred more often in DTaP-primed than in DTwP-primed children. For DTaP vaccines, *fever*, *irritability*, and *pain*, *redness*, *and swelling at the injection site* occurred more often after the fourth dose than after the third dose of the same vaccine in the primary series. Most DTaP vaccines stimulated comparable or higher serum antibody responses than DTwP for those antigens contained in the vaccine (Table 4).

A randomized controlled comparison of two-, three, and five-component acellular pertussis vaccines and a whole-cell pertussis vaccine has been carried out in 82 892 infants who were immunized either at age 3, 5, and 12 months, or at 2, 4, and 6 months (46[C]). They were randomly assigned to a two-component DTaP vaccine (pertussis toxin, filamentous hemagglutinin; 20 697 infants), a three-component DTaP vaccine (recombinant pertussis toxin, filamentous hemagglutinin, pertactin; 20 728 infants), a five-component DTaP vaccine (pertussis toxin, filamentous hemagglutinin, pertactin, fimbriae antigens; 20 747 infants), or a UK-made DTwP vaccine (20 720 infants). The serological responses to the acellular vaccines were similar to those previously reported. The whole-cell vaccine was highly immunogenic for fimbriae, pertactin, and filamentous hemagglutinin, but had a low antipertussis toxin response. The relative risks of pertussis with or without cough are shown in Table 5. High fever and seizures occurred more often after whole-cell vaccine than after any of the acellular vaccines. *Hypotonic–hyporesponsive episodes* also occurred significantly more often in the whole-cell group (34 events) and were more frequent in the acellular groups (22 events in the two-component group, 16 in the three-component group, and 29 in the five-component group) than previously reported.

Implementation of acellular pertussis vaccines

Table 4. *Percent of infants who at 15–20 months had reactions after the fourth administration of pertussis vaccine (45[C])*

Vaccine	Fever		Irritability		Redness		Swelling		Pain	
	⩾100.1°F	>102°F	Any	Severe	Any	>20 mm	Any	>20 mm	Any	Severe
DTaP/DTaP (*n* = 1079)	22.6	1.9	37.8	1.1	29.5	5.5	23.2	6.7	30.3	0.7
WCL/WCL (*n* = 16)	31.3	0.0	68.8	0.0	56.3	18.8	43.8	18.8	87.5	18.8
WCL/DTaP (*n* = 187)	21.4	2.1	32.6	1.6	15.5	1.6	15.0	2.1	26.2	1.1

DTaP, diphtheroid, tetanus, and acellular pertussis vaccine; WCL, DTwP (whole cell pertussis) vaccine manufactured by Lederle Laboratories.

Table 5. *Relative risks of pertussis with different types of vaccine (46[C])*

Variable	Three-component acellular vaccine	Five-component acellular vaccine	Whole-cell vaccine
Relative risk of pertussis with cough (95% CI)			
3 doses	1.38 (0.71–2.69)	0.85 (0.41–1.79)	1.00
≥1 dose	1.65 (1.12–2.45)	1.25 (0.82–1.89)	1.00
Relative risk of pertussis with or without cough (95% CI)			
3 doses	2.55 (1.50–4.33)	1.40 (0.78–2.52)	1.00
≥1 dose	1.84(1.36–2.51)	1.25 (0.90–1.75)	1.00

in various countries Since 1997, the American Academy of Pediatrics has recommended licensed DTaP as the preferred vaccine for all five doses in the immunization schedule (47[C]). As of 1 July 1997, Ontario, Prince Edward Island, and Alberta were the first provinces in Canada to switch from using the combination vaccine containing whole-cell pertussis vaccine, diphtheria and tetanus toxoids, inactivated poliovirus vaccine, and *Hemophilus influenzae* type b conjugate vaccine to using a similar five-component product containing the same antigens but including a five-component acellular pertussis component (48[C]). In 1996 a comparison of a DTaP vaccine (containing pertussis toxin, filamentous hemagglutinin, and pertactin as pertussis antigens) licensed in Austria with DTwP vaccines used for long in the country showed a lower rate of adverse effects caused by the acellular vaccine in infants (49[C]). In 1997, the Swedish Medical Products Agency analysed adverse reaction reports for the first year of use (1966) of a DTaP vaccine (containing pertussis toxin, filamentous hemagglutinin, and pertactin as pertussis antigens). Of the 89 reports received, 52 were of a general nature, including 25 cases of fever and 18 injection site reactions. Other reactions included prolonged crying episodes, restlessness, cramps, and two cases of muscle hypotonia. In addition, there were 18 cases of hypotonic–hyporesponsive episodes, which usually occurred on the first day after immunization. The children suddenly became pale, unresponsive, and impossible to communicate with, often for hours. The mechanism behind this reaction is unknown. The reaction seemed to be harmless, although it was an unpleasant experience for the families concerned. The Agency stated that it did not expect this vaccine to cause hypotonic–hyporesponsive episodes (1[R]).

It has been pointed out that the optimal composition of acellular vaccines has not yet been determined: the number of antigens varies from one to five (pertussis toxin, filamentous hemagglutinins, pertactin, fimbria antigens) and antigen amounts are also different (50[C]). Therefore, studies that follow licensing will be of the utmost importance in studying the induction of herd immunity and possible rare adverse events. The current status of acellular pertussis vaccines in practice has been reviewed (51[R]).

Whole-cell pertussis vaccine The immunogenicity and reactogenicity of a reformulated Australian DTwP vaccine have been compared with those of the currently marketed DTwP vaccine in 634 infants who received a primary series of the new DTwP vaccine and 208 who received the currently marketed DTwP vaccine (52[C]). The reformulation became necessary because the currently available vaccine was not suitable for combination with other components, such as conjugated Hib vaccine and hepatitis B vaccine. The new vaccine had both a slightly improved adverse effects profile, and a somewhat better pertussis antibody response.

Two cases of *brachial neuritis* have been reported after DTwP immunization in infants (53[c]).

A 6-month-old girl received her second DTwP immunization in her right thigh. A week later she stopped moving her left arm; the arm was abducted at the shoulder and extended at the elbow, spontaneous movement was minimal, and the biceps and triceps reflexes were absent. Recovery was complete within 1 month.

A 4-month-old child stopped moving both arms 3 weeks after a second DTwP immunization. Recovery was complete within 4 months.

In both cases other causes of brachial neuritis, such as trauma, were excluded. Taking into account the well-known brachial neuritis that can occur after tetanus immunization, the authors suspected that tetanus component had caused the complication. Because the affected limb is often not the one injected, it is believed that the neuritis is immune-mediated.

A case of *Nicolau syndrome* (livedo-like skin necrosis) has been reported (54[C]). In the 1920s, the syndrome was a well-known adverse effect of bismuth salts used to treat syphilis. There have been no previous reports associated with immunization.

Acellular pertussis vaccine versus whole-cell pertussis vaccine An informal consultation of invited epidemiologists, infectious disease clinicians, immunologists, representatives of regulatory agencies for biological products, and other scientists and public health officials was held in Geneva on 18–19 May 1998 on the control of pertussis using whole-cell and acellular pertussis vaccines. The consultation was called jointly by the Children's Vaccine Initiative and the World Health Organization Global Programme on Vaccines. They reviewed: (1) current data available on the global epidemiology and surveillance of pertussis and the relevance of apparent increases in reported disease; (2) current data available on possible correlates of immunity to clinical efficacy and evidence of antigenic variation as it effects efficacy; (3) the roles and means of the WHO and national control authorities in evaluating pertussis vaccines; (4) current control of pertussis in selected developed and developing countries; (5) economic implications of vaccine choice for local vaccine production in developing countries.

The meeting made the following recommendations:

(1) The WHO is encouraged to develop and promulgate new case definitions for pertussis for surveillance purposes, with consideration of all available information on the sensitivity and specificity of clinical and laboratory case criteria in children.
(2) In developed countries with diagnostic capabilities, special surveillance studies are encouraged to examine the extent and relative importance of *B. pertussis* infection in adolescents and adults in various settings, and the field effectiveness of the various vaccines and schedules in use.
(3) The WHO should consider the development of new models to estimate the current burden of pertussis and disease averted at global, regional, and national levels.
(4) A WHO working group may be helpful in defining the questions to address some aspects of the above three points.
(5) The WHO should support a strong collaborating laboratory or laboratory network for the characterization (antigenic heterogeneity, antibiotic sensitivity) of *B. pertussis* isolates from around the world and for long-term storage of isolates.
(6) The current control regulations and recommendations for pertussis vaccines (whole-cell and acellular) needs thorough review in the light of recently available scientific data, and appropriate revisions should be made.
(7) National immunization programmes should be aware that with the use of all vaccines, but particularly with the use of whole-cell pertussis vaccines, there is an opportunity for adverse events after immunization to be reported. These events may be coincidental, provoked, or vaccination-caused (due to dilution/injection method or common to rare inherent effects of the vaccine). Surveillance of adverse events after immunization can be useful in detecting rare serious adverse events to monitor overall vaccine safety, but are particularly useful in monitoring vaccination programme functioning. Programme personnel first need full preparation for such surveillance. This preparation includes: (a) public education in expected common and uncommon adverse events; (b) investigation of reported illnesses after vaccination and collection of additional information; (c) advice on the clinical management of anaphylaxis and other rare medical events; (d) appropriate public health responses; (e) appropriate responses to

the public, medical personnel, and the media.

(8) Manufacturers are encouraged to continue and further collaborative relationships with local producers for technology transfer, quality control, and issues in the manufacturing process, with full involvement of the relevant national control authority.

(9) Whole-cell vaccines of documented quality have proved to be highly effective tools for preventing pertussis. Acellular pertussis vaccines are valuable alternatives to whole-cell vaccines for primary immunization in infancy. Because of their safety profiles, acellular vaccines may be preferred alternatives in industrialized countries, in which pertussis vaccination with whole-cell vaccines is not widely accepted. In each country, recommendations for the use of pertussis vaccines will be based on local risk–benefit and cost–benefit analyses.

(10) Further use of acellular vaccines in many circumstances can be further considered for booster doses (fourth and fifth doses) in improving pertussis control after evaluation by local authorities of the epidemiological, cost, and programmatic issues. Additional data on the potential benefit of booster doses using acellular pertussis vaccines in adolescence or older ages are needed (55[R]).

Combination vaccines: DTaP or DTwP vaccine combined with other antigens such as hepatitis B or *Hemophilus influenzae* type b [Hib] or inactivated polio virus or simultaneous administration of these vaccines; other combination vaccines *(SEDA-20, 290; SEDA-21, 330)*

Four-, five- and even six-component combination vaccines based on DTaP or DTwP vaccine, and including other antigens such as hepatitis B or Hib or inactivated poliovirus vaccine, will play an important role in future immunization programmes. Other combination vaccines, such as hepatitis A/hepatitis B or Hib/hepatitis B, will also be used. Because combinations based on DTP will be of particular interest, the safety and immunogenicity of combination vaccines will be mainly discussed here. Some of these combination vaccines have already been licensed in some countries, and others are expecting licensure soon or are being evaluated in clinical trials. In general, there are similar results when comparing both seroconversion rates and mean geometric antibody titers as well as reactogenicity after the administration of combination vaccines or separate injections of DTaP/DTwP vaccine and other single-antigen vaccines. However, some studies have shown that the development of combination vaccines requires careful research and evaluation.

Combination vaccines or simultaneous administration of various vaccines: DTP and *Hemophilus influenzae* type B (Hib) vaccines In infants who simultaneously received DTaP vaccine at 3, 4, and 5 months and Hib (HbOC) vaccine at 3 and 5 months into either contralateral arms or collateral thighs, there was no difference in the immunogenicity of any of the four vaccine antigens. However, administration of either of the two vaccines into the arms was associated with significantly more local adverse effects than administration into the thighs (Table 6) (56[C]). Of 98 pre-term infants who were monitored for *apnea* and *bradycardia* in the 24-h periods before and after immunization, only one developed apnea or bradycardia before immunization compared with 17 after immunization. The authors recommended that cardiorespiratory function in pre-term infants born at less than 31 weeks gestation should be monitored for 48 h after immunization so that supplementary oxygen can be provided if needed (57[C]). In an evaluation of a similar study of 97 pre-term infants, the authors made the same recommendation for cardiorespiratory monitoring (58[C]).

DTP and hepatitis B vaccines No serious adverse events were reported in 119 children who received a primary series of DTwP and hepatitis B vaccines during the first year of life and a booster dose of combination DTwP/HB

Table 6. *Local and systemic reactions in the arms and thighs after two different types of H. influenzae vaccine* (56[C])

	Thigh (n = 54) (%)	Arm (n = 54) (%)
HbOC		
Erythema	15	40
Swelling	3.6	9.1
Induration	3.6	22
Pain on pressure	1.8	5.5
DTaP		
Erythema	29	66
Swelling	7.3	30
Induration	26	50
Pain on pressure	1.8	17
General symptoms		
Temperature >38.0°C	9.1	15
Respiratory	13	15
Weariness	16	11
Crying	9.1	9.1
Rash	9.1	9.1

HbOC, Hib oligosaccharide diphtheria toxin conjugate; DTaP, diphtheroid, tetanus, and acellular pertussis vaccine.

vaccine at 18 months (59[C]). The majority of local and systemic reactions were mild. After the booster dose, all the children were seroprotected against diphtheria and tetanus (0.1 IU/ml), and seroresponded to pertussis (15 ELISA units/ml); the hepatitis B seroconversion rate was over 97%.

After a full immunization course in 106 infants, who were randomized to receive three doses of DTwP or combination DTwP/HB vaccines at 3, 5, and 7 months of age, all the children in both groups had seroprotective titers against diphtheria and tetanus (0.1 IU/ml), seroresponded to *B. pertussis* (15 ELISA units/ml), and had seroprotective concentrations of antihepatitis B antibodies (10 mIU/ml) (60[C]). There were no significant differences between the groups in relation to the incidence of local and general symptoms. The authors concluded that the hepatitis B component in the DTwP/HB combination vaccine did not interfere with the immune response to the three other components of the vaccine.

DTP/polio and *Hemophilus influenzae* type B (Hib) vaccines In a randomized comparison, infants aged 2, 4, 6, and 12 months were given one of two combination DTP/IPV (inactivated poliovirus vaccine) vaccines, containing either acellular components (aP group, n = 100) or whole-cell pertussis components (wP group, n = 101) mixed with a tetanus-conjugated Hib vaccine (61[C]). Immunogenicity was comparable for the diphtheria, tetanus, and Hib components, but significantly superior for pertussis toxin, filamentous hemagglutinin, pertactin, and polioviruses 1, 2, 3 in the aP group. The incidence of local adverse reactions was two to three times lower in the aP group after the primary series and booster dose. *Fever* was reported more than twice as often after wP immunization than after aP immunization in the primary series, and almost four times as often after the booster dose. Severe fever (39.5°C) was also more frequent in the wP group, 3.8 times after the primary series and twice after the boosters. Two serious adverse events were thought to have been possibly related to immunization: *convulsions* after the first dose in a child in the wP group and *a pruritic rash* over the face, front of the ears, and hands with a fever of 38.5°C one day after the booster dose in a child in the aP group.

DTP/IPV and rabies vaccines Pre-exposure immunization against rabies could be beneficial to children in countries where the disease is enzootic. In a Vietnamese study 84 infants were randomly assigned to receive three doses of DTP/IPV vaccine at 2, 3, and 4 months of age either alone or with two doses of purified Vero cell rabies vaccine at 2 and 4 months (62[C]). All the infants developed protective antibody titers against diphtheria, tetanus, pertussis, and polio. All who received the rabies vaccine developed protective antibody concentrations against rabies. Local and systemic reactions did not differ between the groups; no serious reactions were reported.

Various combinations and simultaneous administrations Travellers to tropical countries are recommended to be protected against various diseases through immunization and malaria prophylaxis. Thus, the safety and immunogenicity of simultaneous administration of live oral cholera and typhoid vaccines, administered alone or in combination with oral poliovirus vaccine, yellow fever vaccine, and antimalarial drugs has been evaluated (63[C]). The results suggested that *chloroquine* and *proguanil* should not be given simultaneously with cholera vaccine (*Vibrio cholerae* CVD103-HgR strain) or typhoid vaccine (Ty21a strain). The reported adverse events are shown in Table 7.

Pneumococcal vaccine *(SED-13, 942; SEDA-21, 330)*

Among the barriers to wider use of pneumococcal vaccines in elders and other people at risk are persistent concerns regarding vaccine-associated adverse effects. In a cross-sectional survey of 1006 elderly and/or high-risk persons pneumococcal vaccine was not associated with an increase in systemic adverse effects during the week after immunization compared with symptoms reported during a control period (64[C]). However, pneumococcal immunization was associated with local symptoms in 28% of the vaccinees, mostly pain but occasionally redness and/or swelling. These local symptoms were almost always mild to moderate and of short duration (Table 8).

Of 384 patients at risk, 133 reported adverse effects (65[C]). Most were minor and local, but systemic and more severe local reactions (*extensive swelling or very sore arms*) were reported in 10 patients.

Simultaneous immunization with influenza and pneumococcal vaccine In a study of the interaction between 23-valent pneumococcal polysaccharide vaccine and influenza vaccine, 152 adults with chronic respiratory disease were randomized to receive both vaccines either simultaneously or with an interval of 1 month (66[C]). There were no significant differences in serological responses between the groups. The incidence and severity of both local and systemic adverse effects were also similar: there were mild local reactions in 38 and 36%, and systemic reactions in five and three of the vaccinees, respectively.

In an evaluation of simultaneous immunization in 85 elderly subjects, pre-immunization pneumococcal antibodies were associated with more reactions, both local and systemic, after vaccination (67[C]). A *rise in temperature* (9% of vaccinees), and *pain at the injection site* (5% of vaccinees) were significantly associated with raised preimmunization pneumococcal polysaccharide antibody concentrations.

Conjugated pneumococcal polysaccharide vaccines Pneumococcal polysaccharides are not immunogenic in infants, but improved immunogenicity of polysaccharide-protein conjugates has been demonstrated. A vaccine containing serotype 6B pneumococcal polysaccharide conjugated with tetanus toxoid has been administered to healthy infants at 3, 4, and 6 months (21 infants) and at 7 and 9 months (19 infants) (68[C]). A booster injection was given at 18 months. There were no significant adverse reactions. Local reactions were mild and infrequent. A temperature of 38°C occurred after 13 injections; on three occasions it was higher (38.7°C), and in all cases coincided with a respiratory infection. This study showed that the vaccine elicits functional antibodies and induces memory response in infants.

Tetravalent pneumococcal vaccine containing 6B, 14, 19F, and 23F polysaccharides conjugated to either tetanus or diphtheria toxoid has been evaluated in 75 infants who received conjugated tetanus toxoid, conjugated diphtheria toxoid, or placebo at 2, 4, and 6 months of age (69[C]). At 12 months of age all vaccinated children were boosted with a 23-valent non-conjugate polysaccharide pneumococcal vaccine. Both vaccines were well tolerated and did not differ at each injection between the groups. Both vaccines induced serotype-specific anticapsular antibodies and induced immunological memory.

VIRAL VACCINES

Hepatitis A vaccine *(SED-13, 928; SEDA-20, 290; SEDA-21, 330)*

Hepatitis and hepatitis A prevention through immunization has been reviewed (70[R]).

A new liposomal hepatitis A vaccine has been investigated in 117 healthy adults, mainly students, using a single-dose primary

Table 7. *Adverse events after the administration of combinations of two types of Vibrio cholerae vaccine with antimalarial drugs or other vaccines (63[C])*

		% reporting adverse reaction						
n	Concomitant treatment	Diarrhea	Nausea	Vomiting	Abdominal discomfort	Headache	Malaise	Cutaneous
CVD 103-HgR								
45	None	22	20	0	22	51	44	6.7
30	Mefloquine	33	13	0	17	37	37	10
30	Chloroquine	10	13	3.3	28	37	33	3.3
30	Proguanil	30	37	6.7	23	57	50	6.7
30	Yellow fever vaccine	10	10	0	3.3	47	63	20
30	Oral poliovirus vaccine	10	10	0	6.7	30	47	3.3
CVD-HgR/Ty21a2								
45	None	31	16	2.2	13	40	51	11
30	Mefloquine	40	20	3.3	17	50	53	3.3
30	Chloroquine	20	23	0	23	63	30	0
30	Proguanil	30	33	0	10	40	53	10
30	Yellow fever vaccine	30	6.7	0	10	33	43	13
30	Oral poliovirus vaccine	30	3.3	0	13	30	40	6.7

CVD, *Vibrio cholerae* vaccines.

Table 8. *Systemic adverse reactions to pneumococcal vaccine (64[C])*

Symptom	Comparison period (n = 1006) n	Postvaccination period (n = 1006) n
Fever	26	19
Rash	48	7
Myalgias	111	14
Fatigue	183	35
Malaise	84	26
Headache	46	9
Decrease in usual activities	50	12
Coincidental URI symptoms	147	38
Overall health		
Same as usual	906	985
Better than usual	29	11
Worse than usual	71	9

schedule and a booster injection after 1 year (71[C]). The vaccine was well tolerated and highly immunogenic. Seroconversion 14 and 28 days after the first dose was 97 and 99%, respectively, and 100% after the second dose. There were local reactions in 48 vaccinees; they were usually mild and lasted 1–2 days. There were mild-to-moderate systemic reactions, mostly headache, in 38 vaccinees.

Hepatitis B vaccine *(SED-13, 928; SEDA-19, 299; SEDA-21, 331)*

Hepatitis B vaccine and multiple sclerosis

Although the current hepatitis B vaccine is one of the safest ever produced, concerns are still sometimes expressed, particularly since 1996 when a French neurologist publicized that he had seen several cases of multiple sclerosis or demyelinating disease in women who had received hepatitis B vaccine, and this has been picked up by the media and anti-immunization groups.

In 1998 the French Health Authorities invited leading experts in the fields of immunization and possible adverse effects to meet in Paris and discuss scientific studies carried out in France on the possible relation between hepatitis B vaccine and multiple sclerosis. The conclusion of the meeting was that there is no evidence of a causal link between multiple sclerosis and hepatitis B vaccine. Nevertheless, the Minister of Health decided to stop hepatitis B immunization of schoolchildren aged 11–12 years, but to continue immunizing adults at high risk and infants. The rationale for this decision was the limited opportunity for full discussion to reach informed consent during immunization sessions carried out in schools. It was recommended that immunization of school children and adolescents would in future be performed by general practitioners, who have a better opportunity to discuss the benefits and risks of immunization on an individual basis and to obtain informed consent.

The impact of this decision, or any other to curtail an immunization programme, should not be underestimated. It raises concerns not only about the safety of the hepatitis B vaccine, but also about the safety of vaccines in general. In view of this, the WHO took strong action, and its Global Programme on Immunization issued a statement in 1997 (when the French media had picked up the issue) that there was no evidence that hepatitis B vaccine causes multiple sclerosis (72[R]). This was based on the following considerations:

(1) A comparison of the geographical incidence and prevalence of hepatitis B with that of multiple sclerosis, which show large differences: Scandinavia and Northern Europe have the highest rates of multiple sclerosis and the lowest rates of hepatitis B infection, whereas in Africa and in Asia there are very low rates of multiple sclerosis and the highest rates of hepatitis B infection. If the virus does not cause multiple sclerosis, it is unlikely that the vaccine can do so.

(2) The WHO also looked at all the post-marketing surveillance studies from the different vaccine manufacturers in North America. Such post-marketing studies are highly relevant sources of knowledge of adverse effects. None of these studies showed any evidence of an increased risk of multiple sclerosis.

(3) The WHO also analysed the French data. The notification rate of demyelinating diseases in terms of association with the administration of the hepatitis B vaccine was 0.6 cases per 100 000 vaccinees, which is a lower rate than the expected incidence in the same population, which in France is estimated as 1.7 cases per 100 000. In other words, these data give no cause for suspicion of a link between hepatitis B vaccine and multiple sclerosis.

When the French Minister of Health took the decision in 1998 to stop hepatitis B immunization in schools, a scientific conference was organized by the Viral Hepatitis Prevention Board in collaboration with the WHO, at which all the available data were carefully analysed with the help of external experts from many disciplines. Their final conclusion, published in a press release, was that the available scientific data do not demonstrate a causal association between hepatitis B vaccine and central nervous system diseases, including multiple sclerosis (73[R]). It was stated, moreover, that since 1981 more than a billion doses of hepatitis B vaccine have been used world wide, with an outstanding record of safety and efficacy. The WHO also warned of the consequences of stopping immunization on the basis of unfounded worries, as happened with pertussis vaccine in the UK, when due to such unfounded publications pertussis immunization was stopped and major epidemics of natural pertussis immediately followed. The WHO therefore strongly recommended that all countries should use the hepatitis B vaccine in routine immunization in their national immunization programmes.

A recent statement from the National Multiple Sclerosis Society in the US (74[R]) should also be mentioned. Referring to anecdotal reports suggesting that immunization against hepatitis B may increase the risk of multiple sclerosis, the Board stated: (1) such reports have NOT been confirmed by any statistically significant scientific studies to date; (2) because of the potential for public concern about this issue, further studies of the possibility of association of hepatitis B vaccine and demyelinating disease, including multiple sclerosis, are under way in the US and Europe; (3) hepatitis B infection can result in serious, sometimes fatal, disease and immunization is effective in its prevention; (4) in the view of the Board, there is no evidence of a link between hepatitis B immunization and multiple sclerosis; (5) people with multiple sclerosis are encouraged to discuss the small general risks of any immunization with their physicians.

The Board considered that the cause of multiple sclerosis remains unknown, but it is believed to be due to the impact of an environmental or infectious trigger on the immune system of an individual who carries a genetic predisposition. After decades of searching, no environmental or infectious trigger has been identified. There is no indication that infection with hepatitis B leads to multiple sclerosis, and there are no statistically significant data to support a link between hepatitis B and multiple sclerosis.

Summarizing the review, it is important that the message that hepatitis B vaccine is still among the safest and most powerful vaccines in immunization programmes should be spread worldwide.

Skin and appendages *Alopecia* after immunization has been evaluated in 60 reports submitted since 1984 (75[C]). In 16 cases re-immunization had resulted in repeated hair loss. In four cases evidence of a causal relation had been considered, and in 12 cases a causal relation had been considered possible or probable. Of the 60 cases, 46 had received hepatitis B vaccine. The majority of patients recovered.

Anetoderma (a disorder characterized by loss of dermal substance clinically and loss of elastic substance histologically) has been described after hepatitis B immunization in two siblings (76[c]). The lesions were multiple, discrete, soft, elevated, light-colored, 2–5 mm papules, without surrounding erythema on the trunk, arms, and legs, and they began 2 weeks after the first dose of vaccine. The cause of anetoderma is unknown; however, this report further supports the concept that an immunological mechanism may be causative.

Special senses *Optic neuritis* has been attributed to hepatitis B vaccine (77[c]).

A 28-year-old man developed end-stage renal insufficiency. He was treated with maintenance hemodialysis and given recombinant hepatitis B vaccine (following a negative result of testing for hepatitis B antibodies). His health improved. One week after immunization he developed bilateral retrobulbar optic neuritis. After treatment with prednisone 1 mg/kg per day his bilateral visual acuity improved and his visual fields normalized.

Two cases of *hearing loss* have been reported (78[c]), (79[c]).

A 42-year-old man developed no antibodies after a primary series and was therefore given hepatitis B vaccine again 13 years later. After the first dose he experienced disabling tinnitus associated with a sensation of fullness in his right ear. The symptoms disappeared quickly. Four weeks later he received a second injection and the same evening the same symptoms recurred, together with hearing loss in the right ear without vertigo. After steroid treatment for 5 months his hearing loss improved gradually. However, once or twice a month he had sudden abrupt auditory impairment accompanied by intense tinnitus.

An 11-year-old boy complained of tinnitus and sudden left-sided deafness associated with vertigo and nausea 48 h after a second injection of recombinant hepatitis B vaccine. Despite treatment with corticosteroids, carbogen, and vitamin B_{12} his hearing loss improved only slightly. After 2 years, he was still left with marked neurosensory left hypoacusia.

Musculoskeletal *Juvenile chronic polyarthropathy* involving the ankles, joints of the hands and feet, wrists, shoulders, and hips has been attributed to hepatitis B vaccine in a 9-year-old boy 3 weeks after a second dose of recombinant hepatitis B vaccine (80[c]).

Immunological and hypersensitivity reactions *Lymphocytic vasculitis* has been attributed to hepatitis B vaccine (81[c]).

A 26-year-old woman developed diffuse subcutaneous edema 10 days after a second dose of hepatitis B vaccine. She complained of 4 days of rectal bleeding, ill-defined abdominal discomfort, and bilateral leg pains and tightness. Later on she developed swelling of the lower legs and hands. She was eventually found to have a lymphocytic vasculitis in the muscles. She did not mount an immune response to the vaccine, having undetectable hepatitis B surface antigen (HBsAg), anti-HBsAg, and anti-hepatitis B core antigen.

A causal relation between vasculitis and hepatitis B immunization has rarely been reported elsewhere and is doubtful in this case.

An immunological reaction to hepatitis B vaccine has been associated with *acute respiratory distress syndrome* (82[C]).

A 50-year-old man, 24 h after immunization, developed angiectasis and erythema on the center of the face, on the forehead, and on the back of the hands, severe malaise, and a slight persistent fever. Two days later he became dyspneic and a chest radiograph showed atelectasis of the lower and medium right lobes. He died with intractable hypoxemia and shock. Post-mortem examination showed acute inflammatory reactions in the liver and kidney. There was deposition of HBsAg and HBcAg in the lung, liver and kidney.

The authors assumed that the second dose of vaccine had caused excessive production of antibodies, giving rise to immune complex deposition.

Hepatitis A and B vaccines

Reviews of viral hepatitis and vaccines against hepatitis A and hepatitis B, including current knowledge on efficacy and adverse effects, have appeared (83[R]), (84[R]).

Human immunodeficiency virus vaccine (including other immunization in HIV-infected people) *(SED-13, 930; SEDA-19, 299; SEDA-20, 291; SEDA-21, 334)*

Immunization of HIV-infected people Skin papules appeared all over the body of a 10-month-old boy who had been born to a mother with unknown HIV infection and who had been immunized with BCG at birth; *Mycobacterium bovis*, BCG strain, was cultured from a lymph node and blood, and HIV infection had been diagnosed 2 months before BCG infection had been disseminated (85[c]).

Response to immunization in HIV-infected persons In 90 HIV-infected homosexual men and 44 HIV-uninfected men who received two doses of hepatitis A vaccine (720 ELISA units/ml) either 1 month or 6 months apart, the seroconversion rate was significantly greater in uninfected men (100 vs 82%), and the geometric mean anti-HAV titer after two doses was also significantly greater in the same group (1086 vs 101 IU/l) (86[C]). Local symptoms were reported by 10% of the HIV-positive and by 9% of the HIV-negative men; mild systemic symptoms were reported by 33% of the HIV-positive and by 15% of the HIV-negative men.

New vaccines Organisms of the *Mycobacterium avium* complex (MAC) commonly cause disseminated bacterial infection among patients with AIDS. There is evidence that immunoprophylaxis against MAC infection may be possible. A heat-killed *Mycobacterium vaccae* vaccine was given in a three-dose schedule to 12 HIV-infected adults with CD4 cell counts below 300×10^6/l (87[C]). The vaccine was well tolerated and produced detectable immunological responses in three of 11 subjects who completed the trial.

In 24 patients who received three doses of a prototype human HIV type 1 synthetic peptide vaccine, the vaccine was well tolerated without any serious adverse effects and HIV-1-specific responses were detected (88[C]).

Influenza vaccine *(SED-13, 932; SEDA-19, 300; SEDA-21,334)*

Influenza vaccines, particularly their efficacy, safety, and tolerability, have been reviewed (89[R]).

Nervous system The reported neurological complications of natural influenza and influenza immunization have been compared; *Guillain–Barré syndrome* was the only neurological complication after immunization (90[R]).

Guillain–Barré syndrome was also the focus of another recent publication (91[C]). The number of reports of influenza vaccine-associated Guillain–Barré syndrome to the (US) Vaccine Adverse Event Reporting System increased from 37 in 1992–3 to 74 in 1993–4, raising concerns about a possible increase in vaccine-associated risk. Detailed data analyses showed that the relative risk of Guillain–Barré syndrome associated with influenza immunization (swine flu vaccine), adjusted for age, sex, and vaccine season, was 2.0 for the 1992–3 season and 1.5 for the 1993–4 season. For the two seasons combined, the adjusted relative risk of 1.7 suggested a rate of slightly more than one additional case of Guillain–Barré syndrome per million vaccinees. An accompanying editorial also referred to the occurrence of Guillain–Barré syndrome during the 'swine flu' immunization campaign in 1976 (92[R]). The authors considered the results of this study as epidemiological evidence that immunization against strains of influenza other than swine flu may increase the risk of Guillain–Barré syndrome, albeit minimally.

Skin and appendages A 4-year-old child developed *erythromelalgia* (a rare disease characterized by palmar and plantar erythema, burning pain, and a local increase in temperature) 10 days after influenza immunization. After treatment the child quickly recovered (93[c]).

Special senses *Optic neuritis* occurred in a 59-year-old man 2 weeks after influenza immunization (94[c]).

Immunological and hypersensitivity reactions A case of severe microscopic *polyangiitis* involving the skin and joints has been reported in a 34-year-old man (95[c]). A causal relation was supported by markedly raised titers of anti-influenza A antibody in the synovial fluid relative to those in the serum.

An acute symmetrical *polyarthropathy*, *orbital myositis*, and *posterior scleritis* occurred 2 h after influenza immunization in a 78-year-old man (96[c]). The authors believed that this represented a hypersensitivity reaction. No other underlying infective, inflammatory, or systemic causes were discovered.

New vaccines and approaches to increase immunogenicity In 77 elderly volunteers immunized with either liposomal or control subvirion vaccine containing 12 mg/dose of hemagglutinin from influenza A/Taiwan/1/86

(H1N1) virus, both serological responses as well as local and systemic adverse reactions were infrequent and did not differ between vaccine groups (97[C]).

Steroid hormones, such as dehydroepiandrosterone (DHEA) and its sulfated prohormone (DHEAS), are among the soluble mediators that are thought to influence the immune response in humans. In a double-blind, randomized, placebo-controlled trial of DHEAS injection with 1993/94 and 1994/95 influenza vaccine in 78 older individuals, DHEAS was well tolerated in 49 cases (98[C]). In 12 individuals (33%) who received DHEAS there was minimal to moderate arm soreness on day 2, compared with 10 (24%) who reported these symptoms after placebo. A one-time supplemental dose of DHEAS with influenza immunization enhanced the specific antibody response to the 1993/94 H3N2 antigen. However, additional investigations on the role of DHEAS in the ageing human immune response are warranted.

In a similar study of 66 patients with chronic obstructive pulmonary disease and chronic asthma using a bacterial immunostimulant, 32 received influenza vaccine (A/Johannesburg/33/94 [H3N2], A/Singapore 86 [H1N1], B/Beijing/184/93) and 34 received influenza vaccine and a bacterial immunostimulant (one tablet containing ribosomal fractions of *Klebsiella pneumoniae*, *Streptococcus pneumoniae*, *Streptococcus pyogenes*, *Hemophilus influenzae*; equivalent to 0.525 mg of RNA) (99[C]). After immunization, no systemic reactions were reported and only a few volunteers reported pain at the injection site and slight increases in temperature.

Japanese encephalitis vaccine

(SED-13, 934; SEDA-20, 291; SEDA-21, 334)

In a review of the indications, benefits, and risks of Japanese encephalitis immunization, it has been recommended that the vaccine should remain restricted to travellers with an increased risk of acquiring Japanese encephalitis, defined as travellers who spend a month or longer in endemic areas, especially rural areas, during the season of transmission (100[R]).

Biken vaccine (killed mouse brain-derived vaccine) is available internationally, although in insufficient quantities to meet world-wide needs. In 1988 a live attenuated primary hamster kidney-derived Japanese encephalitis vaccine (SA14–14–2) was licensed in China. This vaccine has been evaluated in a randomized trial in 26 239 children, half of whom received the vaccine and half of whom served as controls. The adverse events observed within 30 days are presented in Table 9. Immunogenicity was not evaluated during this trial, because the live attenuated vaccine is known to be effective (101[C]).

Nervous system Neurological complications were seen in Japan in 1965–73 in the order of one per 2.3 million vaccinees, and in Denmark in three per 175 000 immunized individuals (one of them with a predisposition to multiple sclerosis) (102[R]).

A 14-year-old boy developed *acute disseminated myelitis* 2 weeks after receiving Japanese encephalitis vaccine (a highly purified vaccine derived from the Beijing strain) (103[c]). The authors referred to other reports of central nervous complications after administration of the Beijing strain: two cases of acute disseminated encephalomyelitis in children (104[c]) and a further case in Japan (105[c]).

Skin and appendages In Denmark, immunization against Japanese encephalitis with vaccine from Biken (Nakayama-NIH strain) has been used in travellers since 1983. In the period 1983–95, 350 000 doses of vaccine were delivered and 101 adverse reactions have been reported, including 73 allergic mucocutaneous reactions (106[C]). The highest frequency of such reactions were seen in the period 1989–92. Three batches distributed before 1992 caused the majority of reactions. The highest incidence rate of *urticaria/angio-edema* was seen in 1992 (17/10 000 vaccinees) and fell to three per 10 000 in 1995. In 30% of cases the reactions occurred after the first dose, 62% after the second dose, and 6% after revaccination. Of the 68 patients of whom detailed clinical descriptions were available, 35 had urticaria and angio-edema, 21 had urticaria

Table 9. *Number (%) of subjects with complete follow-up who experienced adverse events in the 30 days after immunization with Japanese encephalitis vaccine (101[C])*

Event	Vaccinated (n = 13 266)	Unvaccinated (n = 12 951)	Risk ratio (95% CI)
Encephalitis	0 (0.0)	0 (0.0)	Undefined
Meningitis	0 (0.0)	0 (0.0)	Undefined
Hospital admission	82 (0.6)	114 (0.9)	0.70 (0.43–1.15)
Severe reaction consistent with anaphylaxis	0 (0.0)	0 (0.0)	Undefined
Seizure	14 (0.1)	15 (0.1)	0.91 (0.37–2.22)
Fever lasting —3 days	357 (2.7)	442 (3.4)	0.79 (0.56–1.11)
Diarrhea	12 (0.1)	11 (0.1)	1.06 (0.46–2.49)
Upper respiratory infection	292 (2.2)	353 (2.7)	0.81 (0.55–1.18)
Bronchitis	38 (0.3)	44 (0.3)	0.84 (0.49–1.44)

only, eight had angio-edema only, and four had *erythema multiforme or erythema nodosum*. The median duration from immunization until reaction was 2 days (range 0–12 days). The cause of the reactions was unclear.

When Japanese encephalitis vaccine from the same manufacturer was used in US Marine Corps personnel, of 38 reactors, 26 had *urticaria and/or angio-edema*, and 11 had *pruritus* (107[C]). The reaction rate was 267 per 100 000 vaccinees.

An association between reactions to Japanese encephalitis vaccine and a history of *urticaria or allergic rhinitis* has been identified (108[C]). In Japan, three children experienced immediate-type reactions to Japanese encephalitis vaccine. All had antigelatin IgE in their sera and the authors assumed that the allergic reactions to Japanese encephalitis vaccines might have been caused by the gelatin used as a stabilizer in the vaccine.

Measles–mumps–rubella (MMR) vaccine (including measles–mumps and measles–rubella vaccine) and combination measles–mumps–rubella–varicella vaccine *(SED-13, 937; SEDA-19, 300; SEDA-20, 291; SEDA-21, 335)*

The safety and immunogenicity of a measles–mumps–rubella vaccine (including the Edmonston measles strain, the Jeryl–Lynn mumps strain, the Wistar RA 27/3 rubella stain) mixed with the Oka *Varicella zoster* vaccine strain have been evaluated in 494 healthy children, 1–2.5 years of age (109[C]). The children were randomized to receive either the mixed vaccine plus placebo or MMR vaccine plus varicella vaccine at two separate sites. All vaccines in the study were generally well tolerated (Table 10). The overall rates of seroconversion for measles, mumps, rubella, and varicella were over 95% in both groups. In a second study it was found that the mixed measles–mumps–rubella–varicella vaccine can be safely and effectively given concomitantly with diphtheria–tetanus–pertussis and oral poliovirus vaccine.

A Vaccine Safety Datalink project has been used to compare adverse events after measles–mumps–rubella immunization either at 4–5 or at 10–12 years (110[C]). Information on events that are plausibly associated with MMR immunization (*seizures*, *pyrexia*, *malaise/fatigue*, *musculoskeletal symptoms*, *rash*, *edema*, *induration*, *lymphadenopathy*, *thrombocytopenia*, *aseptic meningitis*, *joint pain*) has been collected from 8514 children who received the vaccine at preschool age and from 18 036 schoolchildren. The results suggested that the risk of events is greater in those aged 10–12 years.

Hematological Several cases of recurrent *thrombocytopenic purpura* have recently been reported after repeated MMR immunization (111[C]), (112[C]). The Advisory Committee on Immunization Practices (ACIP) of the Centers for Disease Control and Prevention (CDC) has therefore recommended avoiding subsequent doses of MMR if the previous episode of thrombocytopenia occurred in close temporal proximity to the previous immunization, i.e. within 6 weeks (113[C]), (114[C]).

Table 10. *Adverse effects of MMRV plus other vaccines vs MMR plus other vaccines, vs VARIVAX (109[C])*

Vaccine(s)	n	Percentage of recipients with			
		Local reactions	Measles/rubella-like rash	Varicella-like rash	Fever ≥102°F
MMRV + placebo	239	13	9.2	7.1	25
MMRV + DTaP + OPV	158	18	17	2.5	23
MMR + VARIVAX	239	13	3.3	7.1	22
MMR + DTaP + OPV	158	18	13	0	24
VARIVAX	145	17	0	2.1	15

DTaP, diphtheroid, tetanus, and acellular pertussis vaccine; MMRV, measles, mumps, rubella, and varicella vaccine; MMR, measles, mumps, and rubella vaccine; OPV, oral poliovirus vaccine; VARIVAX, varicella vaccine.

Mumps vaccine *(SED-13, 938; SEDA-19, 301; SEDA-20, 291; SEDA-21, 336)*

Nervous system The risk of *aseptic meningitis* is increased after the administration of MMR vaccine that contains the Urabe mumps vaccine strain (SED-13, 938). Now the incidence of aseptic meningitis after immunization with MMR containing the Jeryl–Lynn mumps vaccine strain has been assessed in a Vaccine Safety Datalink project (115[C]). The overall rate of confirmed cases in the study population (children aged 1–2 years) was 172 cases per million children, very close to the background rate of 162 naturally occurring cases per million children aged 1–4 years in Olmsted County, MN. The authors concluded that there is no increased risk of aseptic meningitis after vaccination with MMR, including the Jeryl–Lynn mumps vaccine strain.

Nucleotide sequence analyses of various mumps virus strains, including the commercially produced Jeryl–Lynn and Urabe AM9 vaccine strain, have been published (116).

Poliomyelitis vaccine *(SED-13, 943; SEDA-19, 302; SEDA-21, 336)*

℞ *Vaccine-associated poliomyelitis*

Reports of vaccine-associated paralytic poliomyelitis and encephalitis in different circumstances continue to appear.

Vaccine-associated paralytic poliomyelitis occurred in an immunocompetent 27-year-old man who had previously received oral poliovirus vaccine during infancy (117[C]). He acquired the infection from a recently immunized household contact.

Infantile weakness has been reported as a manifestation of vaccine-associated paralytic poliomyelitis (118[C]), and encephalitis has been reported after polio immunization in a 6-month-old boy with underlying hypogammaglobulinemia (119[C]).

Safety of live vaccine strains *The safety of poliovirus vaccine strains has been comprehensively reviewed, with particular reference to the vaccine virus strain type 2, discussing the possibility of developing an attenuated bivalent type 1 and type 3 Sabin strain poliovirus vaccine (120[R]). The type 2 Sabin strain is mainly associated with vaccine-associated paralytic poliomyelitis in contacts and experience gained during the poliomyelitis elimination campaign in the Americas showed that type 2 poliovirus was the first of the three types to disappear.*

Sabin type 1 poliovirus strains isolated from patients with vaccine-associated paralytic poliomyelitis have been characterized (121[C]). Surprisingly, none of the strains analysed were as neurovirulent in transgenic mice as was the wild-type parent of Sabin 1 (Mahoney strain).

Changes in immunization policies *There is no doubt that oral poliovirus vaccine is very effective and safe and the tool to be used in world-wide efforts to eradicate polio. However, it carries a very low risk of vaccine-associated paralytic poliomyelitis. Therefore, in some countries in which wild poliomyelitis has long been eliminated, changes in immunization strategies have been discussed or implemented. The alternatives are the replacement of oral poliovirus vaccine by inactivated poliovirus vaccine or to use a sequential immunization strategy (inactivated poliovirus vaccine to be* *followed by oral poliovirus vaccine). In 1997, the American Academy of Pediatrics issued a recommendation that regimens of sequential inactivated poliovirus vaccine and oral poliovirus vaccine, inactivated poliovirus vaccine only, or oral poliovirus vaccine only are currently acceptable. Nevertheless, assuming continued progress toward global polio eradication and the development of new combination vaccines that contain inactivated poliovirus vaccine, the routine use of an inactivated vaccine-only regimen is considered to be the alternative for the future (122[R]).*

Sequential parenteral–oral vaccine has also been recommended as carrying as a reasonable balance of risks and benefits and as the preferred regimen for routine immunization of healthy children (123[R]).

Miller et al. suggested that the Delphi panel had assumed that no immunodeficient people receiving immunization will avoid vaccine-associated paralytic poliomyelitis by receiving two doses of inactivated poliovirus vaccine before oral poliovirus vaccine (124[C]). Commenting on this statement and referring to a review of 105 cases of vaccine-associated paralytic poliomyelitis, including 11 immunodeficient recipients with vaccine-associated paralytic poliomyelitis, Brown calculated that vaccine-associated paralytic poliomyelitis will be reduced by 27% among immunodeficient recipients if the sequential schedule of two doses of inactivated poliovirus vaccine and two doses of oral poliovirus vaccine is adopted (125[C]). Others have justified the statement made by Miller et al. and have explained why the panel decided not to predict any reduction in the approximately one to two cases per year of vaccine-associated paralytic poliomyelitis that occur in the US among immunologically abnormal recipients of oral poliovirus vaccine by switching to the sequential schedule of two doses of inactivated poliovirus vaccine followed by two doses of oral poliovirus vaccine (126[C]).

From an analysis of various data on vaccine-associated paralytic poliomyelitis in Germany and elsewhere, it has been suggested that a change from a long-standing and well-established oral poliovirus vaccine immunization programme to another strategy could have a negative impact on compliance in the population (127[R]). The authors proposed that pregnant women be immunized during the last trimester of pregnancy in order to transfer antibodies to their neonates. However, it has been argued that immunization of pregnant women with live vaccines is usually contradicted because of possible damage to the baby (128[R]).

Provocation vaccine-associated poliomyelitis *Provocation poliomyelitis is a well-known phenomenon, characterized by paralysis due to natural poliomyelitis in a person who has received an injection before the onset of the disease. In most cases the paralysis occurs in the limb in which the injection has been administered or that limb and others are affected. Seven cases of neurological disease occurring between 1976 and 1985 in Germany have been reported in young children after simultaneous administration of oral poliovirus vaccine and diphtheria–tetanus toxoids or diphtheria–tetanus–pertussis vaccine (129[C]). However, the virological data were incomplete, only one case having been confirmed by the isolation of a vaccine-like polio virus, and in three cases the clinical symptoms did not correspond to poliomyelitis. The author concluded that in some cases the simultaneous administration of injectable vaccines cannot be excluded as a cause for paralysis.*

Rabies vaccine *(SED-13, 946; SEDA-19, 303; SEDA-21, 337)*

A 14-year-old boy had a *seizure* after the administration of human diploid rabies cell vaccine simultaneously with rabies immune globulin (130[c]). The symptoms developed within minutes after injection. Following treatment and about 2 h later, his mental status returned to normal.

Rubella vaccine *(SED-13, 947; SEDA-20, 292; SEDA-21, 337)*

The association between adverse musculoskeletal and neurological events and rubella immunization has been investigated in 546 healthy postpartum rubella-seronegative women (131[C]). They received either mono-

Table 11. *Number (%) of acute and persistent adverse reactions to rubella vaccine (131[C])*

Reaction	Treatment		Odds ratio (95% CI)
	Placebo (n = 275)	Vaccine (n = 268)	
Sore throat	88 (32%)	91 (34%)	1.09 (0.75–1.59)
Cervical lymphadenopathy	27 (10%)	52 (19%)	2.21 (1.31–3.76)
Rash	31 (11%)	66 (25%)	2.57 (1.58–4.21)
Arthralgia	44 (16%)	57 (21%)	Not tested
Arthritis	11 (4%)	24 (9%)	Not tested
Arthralgia or arthritis	55 (20%)	81 (30%)	1.73 (1.17–2.57)
Myalgia	44 (16%)	55 (21%)	1.36 (0.88–2.10)
Paresthesia	19 (7%)	20 (7%)	1.09 (0.57–2.09)
Arthralgia or arthritis	41 (15%)	58 (22%)	1.58 (1.01–2.45)
Myalgia	26 (9%)	40 (15%)	1.68 (0.99–2.84)
Paresthesia	12 (4%)	13 (5%)	1.12 (0.50–2.50)

valent rubella vaccine (n = 270) or saline placebo (n = 276). In all, 543 women completed a 1-month follow-up, and 456 women completed the 12-month assessment. There was a significantly higher incidence of *acute joint manifestations* with rubella vaccine (30%) than with placebo (20%). The frequency of *chronic or recurrent arthralgia or arthritis* was only marginally significant (Table 11).

Tick-borne encephalitis vaccine

(SED-13, 949; SEDA-20, 292)

Referring to the licensure of the first tick-borne encephalitis vaccine (TBE vaccine) in France, an overview on potential neurological effects of the vaccine has been provided (132[R]): some cases of *neuritis*, a case of *encephalomyelitis* leaving the patient with a gait disorder, 11 cases of miscellaneous and generally transient neurological disorders reported from Switzerland between 1987 and 1992, and a case of facial palsy and sensory deficit in a limb occurring after simultaneous immunization against TBE and tetanus.

Varicella vaccine *(SED-13, 950; SEDA-20, 292; SEDA-21, 338)*

The indications, efficacy, and safety of varicella vaccine have been reviewed (133[R]), (134[R]).

Transmission of the varicella vaccine virus from a toddler to his pregnant mother has been reported (135[c]) and discussed (136[R]).

A toddler with a history of an allergic diathesis developed 30 generalized lesions 24 days after varicella immunization. His mother subsequently had about 100 lesions. There was no evidence of fetal transmission.

Nervous system In an experimental model of multiple sclerosis, repeated high doses of antigen (myelin basic protein) have deleted both the clinical and pathological manifestations of the disease. The effects of varicella vaccine on 50 patients with chronic progressive multiple sclerosis have therefore been studied (137[C]). The patients were immunized with varicella vaccine and followed for 1 year. All were seropositive for varicella before immunization and all had rises in varicella antibodies after being given the vaccine. There was improvement in 14 patients, four became worse, and 29 were unchanged. Four patients developed mild chickenpox after immunization. No other untoward adverse effects occurred.

Immunological and hypersensitivity reactions Two weeks after varicella immunization a 26-year-old man developed about 50 macular lesions on the trunk (138[c]). Skin biopsy showed *a hypersensitivity vasculitis*. Therapy with prednisone cleared the lesions within 1 week.

Yellow fever vaccine *(SED-13, 951)*

The possibility of dengue hemorrhagic fever after yellow fever immunization has been discussed (139[R]). Knowledge that the pathogenesis of dengue hemorrhagic fever may stem from previous host sensitization by dengue viral antigens and the close taxonomic relation between yellow fever and dengue viruses has raised concern and reluctance to recommend yellow fever immunization by many Ecuadorian physicians.

HUMAN IMMUNOGLOBULIN

Leukocytoclastic vasculitis has been attributed to human immunoglobulin (140^c).

A 30-year-old woman with chronic inflammatory demyelinating polyneuropathy was treated with intravenous human immunoglobulin 0.4 g/kg per day for 5 days. On the third day she developed a papular facial rash, which extended to her upper back and palms over the next week. Some lesions developed non-blanching purpura and others painful superficial skin necrosis. A skin biopsy specimen showed a leukocytoclastic vasculitis. Following treatment, the rash resolved, leaving a few areas of scarring.

INJECTION TECHNIQUES

When 50 chronic dialysis patients who failed to produce antibodies after the primary hepatitis B vaccine series were revaccinated either by intradermal or intramuscular administration, there was a higher seroprotection rate with intradermal than with intramuscular administration (141^C). There was no difference in reactogenicity.

In a comparison in 97 young healthy adults of the reactogenicity of a recombinant hepatitis B vaccine when injected with the Biotect jet-gun (a pneumatically powered drug delivery system using disposable syringes) or with conventional syringes and needles, the jet-gun produced significantly more local symptoms (142^C).

Use of jet injectors A new type of needleless jet-injector (Mini-Imojet) administers liquid vaccines from a single-use, pre-filled cartridge named Imule, avoiding the risk of cross-contamination. Administration of various vaccines by jet-injector has been compared with standard syringe technique. All the jet-administered vaccines were of equivalent or superior immunogenicity. The most common reactions were mild (minor bleeding, superficial papules, erythema, induration). The technical and safety advantages of the Mini-Imojet reinforces the interest of this new technique for mass immunization (143^C).

REFERENCES

1. Anonymous. Adverse drug reaction monitoring: new issues. WHO Drug Inf 1997;11:1–4.
2. Mittmann N, Liu BA, Iskedjian M, Bradley CA, Pless R, Shear NH, Einarson TR. Drug-related mortality in Canada (1984–1994). Pharmacoepidemiol Drug Saf 1997;6:157–68.
3. ACIP issues update on potential adverse events from vaccines. Am Fam Phys 1997;55:702–4.
4. Recommendations of the Advisory Committee on Immunization Practices (ACIP). Update: vaccine side effects, adverse reactions, contraindications, and precautions. Morb Mortal Wkly Rep 1996;45 (RR-12).
5. Mansoor O, Pillans PI. Vaccine adverse events reported in New Zealand 1990–5. New Zealand Med J 1997;110:270–2.
6. Chen RT, Glasser JW, Rhodes PH, Davis RL, Barlow WE, Thompson RS, Mullooly JP, Black SB, Shinefield HR, Vadheim CM, Marcy SM, Ward JI, Wise RP, Wassilak SG, Hadler SC, Swint E, Hardy JR, Payne T, Benson P, Draket J, Drew L, Mendius B, Ray P, Lewis N, Fireman BH, Jing J, Wulfsohn M, Lugg MM, Osborne P, Rastogi S, Patriarca P, Caserta V. Vaccine safety datalink project: a new tool for improving vaccine safety monitoring in the United States. Pediatrics 1997;99:765–73.
7. Arya SC. Mumps vaccine-associated neurological involvement and magnetic resonance imaging of the vaccinees. Pharmacoepidemiol Drug Saf 1997;6:429.
8. Blomfield R. Childhood vaccination should have been included in asthma study. Br Med J 1998;317:205.
9. Mansoor OD. Selective evidence was used to support link between immunisation and asthma. Br Med J 1999;318:193.
10. McIntyre PB, O'Brien ED, Heath TC. Immunisation and asthma. Commun Dis Intell 1998; 22:38.
11. Butler NR, Golding J, editors. From birth to five: a study of the health and behaviour of Britain's 5-year-olds. Oxford, Pergammon Press, 1986.
12. Halsey N. Personal communication.
13. Rabinovich R. Personal communication.
14. Classen DC. Public should be told that vaccines may have long term adverse events. Br Med J 1999;318:193.

15. Pedersen-Bjergaard U, Andersen M, Hansen PB. Drug-induced thrombocytopenia: clinical data on 309 cases and the effect of corticosteroid therapy. Eur J Clin Pharmacol 1997;52:183–9.
16. Doughty IM, Price DA, Webb NJA. Macroscopic haematuria following immunisation with tetanus toxoid and oral polio vaccine. Eur J Pediatr 1997;156:898.
17. Fraunfelder FW, Rosenbaum JT. Drug-induced uveitis. Incidence, prevention and treatment. Drug Saf 1997;17:197–207.
18. Aberer W, Kranke B. Allergic reactions to vaccines. Allergologie 1997;20:407–11.
19. Karnak I, Senocak ME, Buyukpamukcu N, Gocmen A. Is BCG vaccine innocent? Pediatr Surg Int 1997;12:220–3.
20. Eregie CO. Ulceration of a previously healed BCG scar in suspected disseminated BCG infection. Ann Trop Paediatr 1997;17:135–9.
21. Deprez P. BCG vaccine-induced lupus vulgaris. Nouv Dermatol 1997;16:116.
22. Nishi J-I, Kamenosono A, Sarker KP, Yoshino S, Ikei J, Matsuda Y. Bacille Calmette-Guerin osteomyelitis. Pediatr Infect Dis J 1997;16:332–3.
23. Kuniyuki S, Asada M. An ulcerated lesion at the BCG vaccination site during the course of Kawasaki disease. J Am Acad Dermatol 1997;37 (Suppl II):303–4.
24. Arya SC, Al Harfi H. Post-vaccination disseminated bacille Calmette-Guerin (BCG) infection. Ann Saudi Med 1997;17:262–3.
25. Banac S, Franulovic J. Familial liability to complications after BCG vaccination. Acta Paediatr Int J Paediatr 1997;86:899–902.
26. Martinez-Pineiro JA, Martinez-Pineiro L. BCG update: intravesical therapy. Eur Urol 1997;31 (Suppl 1):31–41.
27. Nseyo UO, Lamm DL. Immunotherapy of bladder cancer. Semin Surg Oncol 1997;13:342–9.
28. Yoshimura K, Yamauchi T. Influence of intravesical bacillus Calmette-Guerin therapy on systemic immunological status. Int J Urol 1997; 4:456–60.
29. Vegt PDJ, Van der Meijden APM, Sylvester R, Brausi M, Holtl W, De Balincourt C, Andriole GL. Does isoniazid reduce side effects of intravesical bacillus Calmette-Guerin therapy in superficial bladder cancer? Interim results of European Organization for Research and Treatment of Cancer Protocol 30911. J Urol 1997;157:1246–9.
30. Tuncer S, Tekin MI, Ozen H, Bilen C, Unal S, Remzi D, Lamm DL. Detection of bacillus Calmette-Guerin in the blood by the polymerase chain reaction method of treated bladder cancer patients. J Urol 1997;158:2109–12.
31. De Diego A, Rogado MC, Prieto M, Nauffal D, Perpina M. Disseminated pulmonary granulomas after intravesical bacillus Calmette-Guerin immunotherapy. Respiration 1997;64:304–6.
32. Saporta L, Gumus E, Karadag H, Kuran B, Miroglu C. Reiter syndrome following intracavitary BCG administration. Scand J Urol Nephrol 1997;31:211–2.
33. Foster DR. Miliary tuberculosis following intravesical BCG treatment. Br J Radiol 1997; 70:429.
34. Siskron IV FT, Venable DD, Gonzalez E, Eastham JA. Granulomatous mass in a nonrefluxing renal unit after bacillus Calmette-Guerin therapy for bladder cancer. J Urol 1997;158:882–3.
35. Smith MD, Chandran G, Parker A, Youssef PP, Ahren M, Coleman M, Macardle P, Roberts-Thomson P. Synovial membrane cytokine profiles in reactive arthritis secondary to intravesical bacillus Calmette-Guerin therapy. J Rheumatol 1997;24:752–8.
36. Farahat MNM. Selective migration of the human helper/inducer T-cell subset (CD4+) in BCG-induced arthritis. Biochem Soc Trans 1997;25:371S.
37. LaFontaine PD, Middleman BR, Graham SD Jr, Sanders WH. Incidence of granulomatous prostatitis and acid-fast bacilli after intravesical BCG therapy. Urology 1997;49:363–6.
38. Von Reyn CF, Arbeit RD, Yeaman G, Waddell RD, Marsh BJ, Morin P, Modlin JF, Remold HG. Immunization of healthy adult subjects in the United States with inactivated *Mycobacterium vaccae* administered in a three-dose series. Clin Infect Dis 1997;24:843–8.
39. Skov PS, Pelck I, Ebbesen F, Poulsen LK. Hypersensitivity to the diphtheria component in the Di-Te-Pol vaccine. A type I allergic reaction demonstrated by basophil histamine release. Pediatr Allergy Immunol 199;8:156–8.
40. Kantor E, Luxenberg JS, Lucas AH, Granoff DM. Phase I study of the immunogenicity and safety of conjugated *Hemophilus influenzae* type b vaccines in the elderly. Vaccine 1997;15:129–32.
41. Amir J, Melamed R, Bader J, Ethevenaux C, Fritzell B, Cartier JR, Arminjon F, Dagan R. Immunogenicity and safety of a liquid combination of DT-PRP-T vs lyophilized PRP-T reconstituted with DTP. Vaccine 1997;15:149–54.
42. Py MO, Andre C. Acute disseminated encephalomyelitis: association with meningococcal A and C vaccine. Case report. Arq Neuro-Psiquiatr 1997;55:632–5.
43. Black SB, Shinefield HR, Bergen R, Hart C, Kremers R, Lavetter A, Lemesurier J, Morozumi PA, Ray P, Lewis EM, Fireman B, Schwalbe J, Hallam P, Shandling M, Dekker C, Granoff DM, Izu A, Podda A. Safety and immunogenicity of Chiron/Biocine recombinant acellular pertussis-diphtheria-tetanus vaccine in infants and toddlers. Pediatr Infect Dis J 1997;16:53–8.
44. Lin T-Y, Chiang B-L. Specific immune response in adult medical personnel immunized with acellular pertussis vaccine with special emphasis on T helper cell response. Vaccine 1997;15:1917–21.
45. Pichichero ME, Deloria MA, Rennels MB, Anderson EL, Edwards KM, Decker MD, Englund JA, Steinhoff MC, Deforest A, Meade BD. A safety and immunogenicity comparison of 12

acellular pertussis vaccines and one whole-cell pertussis vaccine given as a fourth dose in 15- to 20-month-old children. Pediatrics 1997;100:772–88.

46. Olin P, Rasmussen F, Gustafsson L, Hallander HO, Heijbel H, Norrby R, Winberg J, Holmgren J, Melander H, Olin P, Storsaeter J, Hallander H, Reizenstein E, Hellstrom GW, Rasmussen F, Romanus V, Ostlund B, Wigzell H, Nordenfelt E, Gothefors L, Kornfalt R, Einemo I, Netterlid E, Olcen P, Klein D, Barreto L, Stellfeld M, Meschievitz C, Bogaerts H. Randomised controlled trial of two-component, three-component, and five-component acellular pertussis vaccines compared with whole-cell pertussis vaccine. Lancet 1997;350:1569–77.
47. Halsey NA, Chesney PJ, Gerber MA, Gromisch DS, Kohl S, Marcy SM, Marks MI, Murray DL, Overall JC Jr, Pickering LK, Whitley RJ, Yogev R, Peter G, Hall CB, Hadler S, Breiman R, Hardegree MC, Jacobs RF, MacDonald NE, Orenstein WA, Rabinovich NR, Schwartz B. Acellular pertussis vaccine: recommendations for use as the initial series in infants and children. Pediatrics 1997;99:282–8.
48. Halperin SA. Acellular pertussis vaccine has arrived in Canada, finally. Can Fam Phys 1997;43:1581–2.
49. Spork KD. Evaluation of the first pertussis vaccine 'Infanrix-™ DTPa' registered in Austria. Pediatr Padol 1997;32:25–7.
50. Trollfors B, Taranger J. Towards better pertussis vaccines. Ann Med 1997;29:87–9.
51. Lopez AL, Blumberg DA. An overview of the status of acellular pertussis vaccines in practice. Drugs 1997;54:189–96.
52. Nolan T, Hogg G, Darcy M-A, Varigos J, McEwen J. Primary course immunogenicity and reactogenicity of a new diphtheria-tetanus-whole cell pertussis vaccine (DTP(w)). J Paediatr Child Health 1997;33:413–17.
53. Hamati-Haddad A, Fenichel GM. Brachial neuritis following routine childhood immunization for diphtheria, tetanus, and pertussis (DTP): Report of two cases and review of the literature. Pediatrics 1997;99:602–3.
54. Nagore E, Torrelo A, Gonzalez-Mediero I, Zambrano A. Livedoid skin necrosis (Nicolau syndrome) due to triple vaccine (DTP) injection. Br J Dermatol 1997;137:1030–1.
55. Children's Vaccine Initiative (CVI) and Global Programme on Immunization of the World Health Organization (WHO). Informal Consultation on control of pertussis with whole cell and acellular vaccines. Report (in press) on a meeting May 18–19, 1998, Geneva. World Health Organization, Geneva, 1999.
56. Schmitt HJ, Wirsing von Konig CH, Zepp F, Huff J, Jahn K, Schmidtke P, Meyer C, Habermehl P, Uhlenbusch R, Angersbach P. Immunogenicity and reactogenicity of HbOC vaccine administered simultaneously with acellular pertussis vaccine (DTaP) into either arms or thighs of infants. Infection 1997;25:298–302.
57. Botham SJ, Isaacs D, Henderson-Smart DJ. Incidence of apnoea and bradycardia in preterm infants following DTP(w) and Hib immunization: a prospective study. J Paediatr Child Health 1997;33:418–21.
58. Sanchez PJ, Laptook AR, Fisher L, Sumner J, Risser RC, Perlman JM. Apnea after immunization of preterm infants. J Pediatr 1997;130:746–51.
59. Poovorawan Y, Theamboonlers A, Sanpavat S, Chumdermpadetsuk S, Safary A, Vandepapeliere P. Long-term antibody persistence after booster vaccination with combined tetravalent diphtheria, tetanus, whole-cell *Bordetella pertussis* and hepatitis B vaccine in healthy infants. Ann Trop Paediatr 1997;17:301–8.
60. Diez-Delgado J, Dal-Re R, Llorente M, Gonzalez A, Lopez J. Hepatitis B component does not interfere with the immune response to diphtheria, tetanus and whole-cell *Bordetella pertussis* components of a quadrivalent (DTPw-HB) vaccine: A controlled trial in healthy infants. Vaccine 1997;15:1418–22.
61. Dagan R, Igbaria K, Piglansky L, Melamed R, Willems P, Grossi A, Kaufhold A. Safety and immunogenicity of a combined pentavalent diphtheria, tetanus, acellular pertussis, inactivated poliovirus and *Haemophilus influenzae* type b-tetanus conjugate vaccine in infants, compared with a whole cell pertussis pentavalent vaccine. Pediatr Infect Dis J 1997;16:1113–21.
62. Lang J, Hoa DQ, Gioi NV, Tho LT, Vien NC, Kesmedjian V, Plotkin S. A randomised feasibility trial of pre-exposure rabies vaccination with DTP-IPV in infants. Lancet 1997;349:1663–5.
63. Kollaritsch H, Que JU, Kunz C, Wiedermann G, Herzog C, Cryz SJ Jr. Safety and immunogenicity of live oral cholera and typhoid vaccines administered alone or in combination with antimalarial drugs, oral polio vaccine, or yellow fever vaccine. J Infect Dis 1997;175:871–5.
64. Nichol KL, MacDonald R, Hauge M. Side effects associated with pneumococcal vaccination. Am J Infect Control 1997;25:223–8.
65. McDonald P, Friedman EHI, Banks A, Anderson R, Carman V. Pneumococcal vaccine campaign based in general practice. Br Med J 1997;314:1094–8.
66. Fletcher TJ, Tunnicliffe WS, Hammond K, Roberts K, Ayres JG. Simultaneous immunisation with influenza vaccine and pneumococcal polysaccharide vaccine in patients with chronic respiratory disease. Br Med J 1997;314:1663–5.
67. Sankilampi U, Honkanen PO, Pyhala R, Leinonen M. Associations of prevaccination antibody levels with adverse reactions to pneumococcal and influenza vaccines administered simultaneously in the elderly. Vaccine 1997;15:1133–7.
68. Sigurdardottir ST, Vidarsson G, Gudnason T, Kjartansson S, Kristinsson KG, Jonsson S, Valdimarsson H, Schiffman G, Schneerson R, Jonsdottir I. Immune responses of infants vaccinated with serotype 6B pneumococcal polysaccharide conjugated with tetanus toxoid. Pediatr Infect Dis J 1997;16:667–74.

69. Dagan R, Melamed R, Zamir O, Leroy O. Safety and immunogenicity of tetravalent pneumococcal vaccines containing 6B, 14, 19F and 23F polysaccharides conjugated to either tetanus toxoid or diphtheria toxoid in young infants and their boosterability by native polysaccharide antigens. Pediatr Infect Dis J 1997;16:1053–9.
70. Sjogren MH. Hepatitis A virus. Prog Liver Dis 1997;15:171–80.
71. Ambrosch F, Wiedermann G, Jonas S, Althaus B, Finkel B, Gluck R, Herzog C. Immunogenicity and protectivity of a new liposomal hepatitis A vaccine. Vaccine 1997;15:1209–13.
72. Anonymous. Wkly Epidemiol Rec 1997; 72:149–52.
73. World Health Organization. Press Release WHO/67, 2 October 1998.
74. Medical Advisory Board of the National Multiple Sclerosis Society: Statement from 14 August 1998. National Multiple Sclerosis Society: News Desk Research Bulletins, 3 September 1998.
75. Wise RP, Kiminyo KP, Salive ME. Hair loss after routine immunizations. J Am Med Assoc 1997;278:1176–8.
76. Daoud MS, Dicken CH. Anetoderma after hepatitis B immunization in two siblings. J Am Acad Dermatol 1997;36:779–80.
77. Albitar S, Bourgeon B, Genin R, Fen-Chong M, N'Guyen P, Serveaux M-O, Atchia H, Schohn D. Bilateral retrobulbar optic neuritis with hepatitis B vaccination. Nephrol Dial Transplant 1997;12:2169–70.
78. Biacabe B, Erminy M, Bonfils P. A case report of fluctuant sensorineural hearing loss after hepatitis B vaccination. Auris Nasus Larynx 1997;24:357–60.
79. Orlando MP, Masieri S, Pascarella MA, Ciofalo A, Filiaci F. Sudden hearing loss in childhood consequent to hepatitis B vaccination: a case report. Ann NY Acad Sci 1997;830:319–21.
80. Bracci M, Zoppini A. Polyarthritis associated with hepatitis B vaccination. Br J Rheumatol 1997;36:300–1.
81. Drucker Y, Prayson RA, Bagg A, Calabrese LH. Lymphocytic vasculitis presenting as diffuse subcutaneous edema after hepatitis B virus vaccine. J Clin Rheumatol 1997;3:158–61.
82. Ranieri VM, Dell'Erba A, Gentile A, Bruno F, La Gioia V, Spagnolo A, Sacco R, Caruso G, Antonaci S, Schiraldi O, Brienza A. Liver inflammation and acute respiratory distress syndrome in a patient receiving hepatitis B vaccine: a possible relationship? Intensive Care Med 1997;23:119–21.
83. Lemon SM, Thomas DL. Vaccines to prevent viral hepatitis. New Engl J Med 1997;336:196–204.
84. Feely M. Hepatitis and hepatitis immunisation. J R Soc Health 1997;117:41–6.
85. Raton JA, Pocheville I, Vicente JM, Gonzalez R, Bilbao I, Gutierrez C, Diaz-Perez JL. Disseminated bacillus calmette-guerin infection in an HIV-infected child: a case with cutaneous lesions. Pediatr Dermatol 1997;14:365–8.
86. Neilsen GA, Bodsworth NJ, Watts N. Response to hepatitis A vaccination in human immunodeficiency virus-infected and -uninfected homosexual men. J Infect Dis 1997;176:1064–7.
87. Marsh BJ, Von Reyn CF, Arbeit RD, Morin P. Immunization of HIV-infected adults with a three-dose series of inactivated *Mycobacterium vaccae*. Am J Med Sci 1997;313:377–83.
88. Phanuphak P, Teeratakulpixam S, Sarangbin S, Nookhai S, Ubolyam S, Sirivichayakul S, Leesavan A, Forrest BD, Hanson CV, Li M, Wang CY, Koff WC. International clinical trials of HIV vaccines: I. Phase I trial of an HIV-1 synthetic peptide vaccine in Bangkok, Thailand. Asian Pac J Allergy Immunol 1997;15:41–8.
89. Palache AM. Influenza vaccines. A reappraisal of their use. Drugs 1997;54:841–56.
90. Hayase Y, Tobita K. Influenza virus and neurological diseases. Psychiatry Clin Neurosci 1997; 51:181–4.
91. Lasky T, Terraciano GJ, Magder L, Koski CL, Ballesteros M, Nash D, Clark S, Haber P, Stolley PD, Schonberger LB, Chen RT. The Guillain–Barré syndrome and the 1992–1993 and 1993–1994 influenza vaccines. New Engl J Med 1998;339:1797–802.
92. Ropper AH, Victor M. Influenza vaccination and the Guillain–Barré syndrome. New Engl J Med 1998;339:1845–6.
93. Confino I, Passwell JH, Padeh S. Erythromelalgia following influenza vaccine in a child. Clin Exp Rheumatol 1997;15:111–13.
94. Hull TP, Bates JH. Optic neuritis after influenza vaccination. Am J Ophthalmol 1997; 124:703–4.
95. Kelsall JT, Chalmers A, Sherlock CH, Tron VA, Kelsall AC. Microscopic polyangiitis after influenza vaccination. J Rheumatol 1997;24:1198–202.
96. Thuirairajan G, Hope-Ross MW, Situnayake RD, Murray PI. Polyarthropathy, orbital myositis and posterior scleritis: an unusual adverse reaction to influenza vaccine. Br J Rheumatol 1997;36:120–3.
97. Powers DC. Summary of a clinical trial with liposome-adjuvanted influenza A virus vaccine in elderly adults. Mech Ageing Dev 1997;93:179–88.
98. Degelau J, Guay D, Hallgren H. The effect of DHEAS on influenza vaccination in aging adults. J Am Geriatr Soc 1997;45:747–51.
99. Centanni S, Pregliasco F, Bonfatti C, Mensi C, Tarsia P, Guarnieri R, Allegra L. Clinical efficacy of a vaccine-immunostimulant combination in the prevention of influenza in patients with chronic obstructive pulmonary disease and chronic asthma. J Chemother 1997;9:273–8.
100. Jelinek T, Nothdurft HD. Japanese encephalitis vaccine in travellers. Is wider use prudent? Drug Saf 1997;16:153–6.
101. Liu Z-L, Hennessy S, Strom BL, Tsai TF, Wan C-M, Tang S-C, Xiang C-F, Bilker WB, Pan X-P, Yao Y-J, Xu Z-W, Halstead SB. Short-term safety of live attenuated Japanese encephalitis vaccine (SA14–14–2): results of a randomized

trial with 26,239 subjects. Infect Dis 1997; 176:1366–9.
102. Anonymous. Vaccination against Japanese encephalitis for all travellers not currently recommended. Drugs Ther Perspect 1997;10:11–13.
103. Fukuda H, Umehara F, Kawahigashi N, Suehara M, Osame M. Acute disseminated myelitis after Japanese B encephalitis vaccination. J Neurol Sci 1997;148:113–15.
104. Ohtaki E, Murakami Y, Komori H, Yamashita Y, Matsuishi T. Acute disseminated encephalomyelitis after Japanese B encephalitis vaccination. Pediatr Neurol 1992;8:137–9.
105. Ohtaki E, Matsuishi T, Hirano Y, Maekawa K. Acute disseminated encephalomyelitis after treatment with Japanese encephalitis vaccine (Nakayama-Yoken and Beijing strains). J Neurol Neurosurg Psychiatry 1995;59:316–17.
106. Plesner A-M, Ronne T. Allergic mucocutaneous reactions to Japanese encephalitis vaccine. Vaccine 1997;15:1239–43.
107. Berg SW, Mitchell BS, Hanson RK, Olafson RP, Williams RP, Tueller JE, Burton RJ, Novak DM, Tsai TF, Wignall FS. Systemic reactions in US Marine Corps personnel who received Japanese encephalitis vaccine. Clin Infect Dis 1997;24:265–6.
108. Sakaguchi M, Yoshida M, Kuroda W, Harayama O, Matsunaga Y, Inouye S. Systemic immediate-type reactions to gelatin included in Japanese encephalitis vaccines. Vaccine 1997; 15:121–2.
109. White CJ, Stinson D, Staehle B, Cho I, Matthews H, Ngai A, Keller P, Eiden J, Kuter B. Measles, mumps, rubella, and varicella combination vaccine: safety and immunogenicity alone and in combination with other vaccines given to children. Clin Infect Dis 1997;24:925–31.
110. Davis RL, Marcuse E, Black S, Shinefield H, Givens B, Schwalbe J, Ray P, Thompson RS, Chen R, Glaser JW, Rhodes PH, Swint E, Jackson LA, Barlow WE, Immanuel VH, Benson PJ, Mullooly JP, Drew L, Mendius B, Lewis N, Fireman BH, Ward JI, Vadheim CM, Marcy SM, Jing J, Wulfson M, Lugg M, Osborne P, Wise RP. MMR2 immunization at 4 to 5 years and 10 to 12 years of age: a comparison of adverse clinical events after immunization in the vaccine safety datalink project. Pediatrics 1997;100:767–71.
111. Drachtman RA, Murphy S, Ettinger LH. Exacerbation of chronic idiopathic thrombocytopenic purpura following MMR immunization. Arch Pediatr Adolesc Med 1994;148:326–7.
112. Vlacha V, Forman EN, Miron D, Peter G. Recurrent thrombocytopenic purpura after repeated MMR vaccination. Pediatrics 1996; 97:738–9.
113. Rollan AR, Pool V, Chen R, Rhodes P. Indications for measles-mumps-rubella vaccination in a child with prior thrombocytopenia purpura. Pediatr Infect Dis J 1997;16:423–4.
114. Centers for Disease Control and Prevention. Update: vaccine side effects, adverse reactions, contraindications and precautions. Recommendations of the Advisory Committee on Immunization Practices (ACIP). Morb Mort Wkly Rep 1996;45 (RR-12):14.
115. Black S, Shinefield H, Ray P, Lewis E, Chen R, Glasser J, Hadler S, Hardy J, Rhodes P, Swint E, Davis R, Thompson R, Mullooly J, Marcy M, Vadheim C, Ward J, Rastogi S, Wise R. Risk of hospitalization because of aseptic meningitis after measles-mumps-rubella vaccination in one- to two-year-old children: an analysis of the Vaccine Safety Datalink (VSD) project. Pediatr Infect Dis J 1997;16:500–3.
116. Mori C, Tooriyama T, Imagawa T, Yamanishi K, Brown EG, Dimock K, Wright KE. Nucleotide sequence at position 1081 of the hemagglutinin-neuraminidase gene in the mumps virus urabe vaccine strain. J Infect Dis 1997;175:1548.
117. Tate CA, Johnson GD. Case report: acute vaccine-associated paralytic poliomyelitis. Muscle Nerve 1997;20:253–4.
118. David WS, Doyle JJ. Acute infantile weakness: a case of vaccine-associated poliomyelitis. Muscle Nerve 1997;20:747–9.
119. Yeung WL, Ip M, Ng HK, Fok TF. An infant with encephalitis. Lancet 1997;350:1594.
120. Parkman PD. An assessment of the safety and efficacy implications of removing the type 2 strain from the trivalent oral poliovirus vaccine. Vaccine Res 1997;6:49–66.
121. Georgescu M-M, Balanant J, Ozden S, Crainic R. Random selection: a model for poliovirus infection of the central nervous system. J Gen Virol 1997;78:1819–28.
122. Halsey NA, Chesney PJ, Gerber MA, Gromisch DS, Kohl S, Marcy SM, Marks MI, Murray DL, Overall JC Jr, Pickering LK, Whitley RJ, Yogev R, Peter G, Hall CB, Breiman R, Hardegree MC, Jacobs RF, MacDonald NE, Orenstein WA, Rabinovich NR, Schwartz B. Poliomyelitis prevention: recommendations for use of inactivated poliovirus vaccine and live oral poliovirus vaccine. Pediatrics 1997;99:300–5.
123. Conrad DA, Jenson HB. New recommendations for poliovirus vaccination: combination regimen captures best effects of available vaccines. Postgrad Med 1997;102:45–62.
124. Miller MA, Sutter RW, Strebel PM, Hadler SC. Cost effectiveness of incorporating inactivated poliovirus vaccine into the routine childhood immunization schedule. J Am Med Assoc 1996;276:967–71.
125. Brown B. Inactivated poliovirus vaccine and vaccine-associated paralytic poliomyelitis. J Am Med Assoc 1997;277:295.
126. Sutter RW, Strebel PM, Miller MA, Hadler SC. Inactivated poliovirus vaccine and vaccine-associated paralytic poliomyelitis. J Am Med Assoc 1997;277:295.
127. Fescharek R, Budde RK, Arras C. OPV vs IPV—could placental immunity reduce the number of vaccine-associated paralytic poliomyelitis? Vaccine 1997;15:1707–9.
128. Minor PD. OPV vs IPV—could placental immunity reduce the number of vaccine-associated paralytic poliomyelitis? Vaccine 1997;15:1709.

129. Ehrengut W. Role of provocation poliomyelitis in vaccine-associated poliomyelitis. Acta Paediatr Jpn Overs Ed 1997;39:658–62.
130. Mortiere MD, Falcone AL, Plotkin SA, Loupi E, Lang J. An acute neurologic syndrome temporally associated with postexposure treatment of rabies. Pediatrics 1997;100:718–21.
131. Tingle AJ, Mitchell LA, Grace M, Middleton P, Mathias R, MacWilliam L, Chalmers A. Randomised double-blind placebo-controlled study on adverse effects of rubella immunisation in seronegative women. Lancet 1997;349:1277–81.
132. Anonymous. Tick-borne encephalitis vaccine. Prescrire Int 1997;6:135–7.
133. White CJ. Varicella-zoster virus vaccine. Clin Infect Dis 1997;24:753–63.
134. Duff P. Varicella vaccine. Infect Dis Obstet Gynecol 1997;4:63–5.
135. Salzman MB, Sharrar RG, Steinberg S, LaRussa P. Transmission of varicella vaccine virus from a healthy 12-months-old child to his pregnant mother. J Pediatr 1997;131:151–4.
136. Long SS. Toddler-to-mother transmission of varicella-vaccine virus: How bad is that? J Pediatr 1997;131:10–12.
137. Ross RT, Nicolle LE, Cheang M. The varicella zoster virus: a pilot trial of a potential therapeutic agent in multiple sclerosis. J Clin Epidemiol 1997;50:63–8.
138. Gerecitano J, Friedman-Kien A, Chazen GD. Allergic reaction to varicella vaccine. Ann Intern Med 1997;126:833–4.
139. Guzman RJ, Kron MA. Threat of dengue haemorrhagic fever after yellow fever vaccination. Lancet 1997;349:1841.
140. Howse M, Bindoff L, Carmichael A. Facial vasculitic rash associated with intravenous immunoglobulin. Br Med J 1998;317:1291.
141. Fabrizi F, Andrulli S, Bacchini G, Corti M, Locatelli F. Intradermal versus intramuscular hepatitis B re-vaccination in non-responsive chronic dialysis patients: a prospective randomized study with cost-effectiveness evaluation. Nephrol Dial Transplant 1997;12:1204–11.
142. Mathei C, Van Damme P, Meheus A. Hepatitis B vaccine administration: comparison between jet-gun and syringe and needle. Vaccine 1997;15:402–4.
143. Parent Du Chatelet I, Lang J, Schlumberger M, Vidor E, Soula G, Genet A, Standaert SM, Saliou P, Gueye A, Julien H, Lafaix C, Lemardeley P, Monnereau A, Spiegel A, Soke M, Varichon JP. Clinical immunogenicity and tolerance studies of liquid vaccines delivered by jet-injector and a new single-use cartridge (Imule): comparison with standard syringe injection. Vaccine 1997;15:449–58.

H.W. Eijkhout and W.G. van Aken

33 Blood, blood components, plasma, and plasma products

NON-INFECTIOUS ADVERSE EFFECTS OF BLOOD TRANSFUSION

Respiratory *Transfusion-related acute lung injury* (TRALI) is characterized by hypoxia and respiratory failure after infusion. Leukoagglutinating granulocyte or lymphocytotoxic antibodies in the plasma of donors cause neutrophil aggregation and trapping in the lungs, with complement activation. The neutrophil inflammatory response results in pulmonary capillary damage. TRALI has been related to transfusion of whole blood, red cell concentrates, and fresh frozen plasma.

In addition, TRALI has been observed after transfusion of random platelet concentrates (1[c]). Testing for HLA and granulocyte antibodies is recommended in suspected cases.

Immunological and hypersensitivity reactions Patients with severe aplastic anemia who have received blood transfusions before hemopoietic cell transplantation have an increased risk of *graft rejection*. It is therefore recommended that leukocyte-depleted blood components be used in these patients (2[R]). Leukocyte-depleted blood components are also used to prevent febrile non-hemolytic transfusion reactions in patients with hemoglobinopathies who require long-term transfusion support (2[R]).

Platelet transfusion can cause antibodies against alloantigens, resulting in *refractoriness to platelet transfusion* (3[C]). Alloimmunization can be prevented through leukocyte reduction by filtration and ultraviolet B irradiation (to remove or inactivate cells bearing alloantigens).

An association between allogeneic transfusion and postoperative bacterial infection has been suggested (4[C]). In 63 transfused patients wound infection was observed in 39 (11.4%) compared with 24 (3.9%) of 63 patients who had not been transfused. The authors concluded that allogeneic transfusion results in a small increase in the risk of postoperative wound infection. Randomized controlled trials are required to establish this effect.

TRANSMISSION OF INFECTIOUS AGENTS IN BLOOD TRANSFUSIONS

Bacterial infections transmitted by blood transfusion The incidence of bacteria in red cell concentrates and platelet concentrates is about 0.3–0.4% (5[r]). Whether contaminating micro-organisms cause septic complications depends on the number of bacteria and their ability to cause damage via exotoxins or endotoxins released during storage (5[r]).

About half of the serious septic complications after red cell concentrate transfusion are caused by *Yersinia enterocolitica* (5[r]). This complication can be avoided by removing leukocytes from blood components.

Blood components can be contaminated by non-sterile containers, the donor's skin or blood, or during the collection, preparation, or storage of blood components (5[r]).

Transfusion of a red cell concentrate contaminated with *Serratia liquefaciens* caused endotoxic shock and disseminated intravascular coagulation in a 60-year-old woman (6[c]). The source of contamination was not found.

A pooled platelet preparation contaminated with *Clostridium perfringens* caused a fatal septic reaction in a man with acute myeloid leukemia (7[c]). The arm of one of the donors who had contributed towards the platelet pool was contaminated with

Side Effects of Drugs, Annual 22
J.K. Aronson, ed.

this organism, possibly because the arm skin had not been disinfected effectively.

Viral infections transmitted by blood transfusion Blood transfusion can result in the transmission of several blood-borne viruses, such as *human immunodeficiency virus (HIV 1–2)*, *HTLV*, *hepatitis C (HCV)*, and *hepatitis B virus (HBV)* (8[C]). The greatest risk to the safety of blood supply is donation by seronegative donors during the infectious window period between the time of infection and seroconversion. The adjusted incidence rates of HIV, HTLV, HCV, and HBV seroconversion are small among people who donated blood more than once during a study period (combined incidence of 18.61 per 100 000 person-years). The seroconversion rate is the highest for HBV, followed by HCV. These viruses both have a long window period. New screening tests, which shorten the window period, will reduce the risk of transfusion-transmitted viral infections. In addition anti-HBc testing in HBsAg-negative first-time donors can identify a high risk group with a prevalence of 0.02% (9[C]).

Transfused patients with β-thalassemia major *are at high risk of blood-borne viral infections* (10[C]). More than 60% of Italians with thalassemia are infected with hepatitis C. Recently the prevalence of hepatitis G virus in 40 such patients has been assessed; HGV-RNA was detected in nine (22.5%) (10[C]). In addition, all were positive for HCV. Concurrent hepatitis G infection can occur in about 10% of cases with hepatitis C virus (11[r]), (12[C]). In healthy controls and blood donors the prevalence of hepatitis G virus is 1.4% (11[r]). So far, it has been concluded that hepatitis G virus can be transmitted by blood components, but is not a significant cause of post-transfusion hepatitis (11[r]), (13[r]). In addition there is no evidence that hepatitis G virus affects hemopoietic recovery (14[c]). In 50% of infected individuals hepatitis G virus is cleared from the circulation by the development of an immune response (12[C]).

Infection with *cytomegalovirus* (CMV) can cause significant morbidity and mortality in immunocompromised CMV-seronegative patients (2[R]). It has been recommended that CMV-negative or leukocyte-depleted blood components should be used to prevent CMV transmission and to prevent reactivation of latent CMV infection (2[R]).

Human *parvovirus B19* can be transmitted by factor VIII concentrates and other blood products (15[R]). So far, intravenous immunoglobulin and albumin have not been associated with parvovirus B19. Parvovirus B19 is the causative agent of fifth disease, a rash-like disease of childhood. In adults parvovirus B19 can cause arthralgia and chronic arthritis (15[R]), (16[c]). However, it has more serious consequences in pregnant women, in patients with raised red cell counts, and in patients with chronic or acquired immunodeficiency (15[R]). In these patients parvovirus B19 infection can cause acute aplastic or hypoplastic anemia, pancytopenia, chronic neutropenia, thrombocytopenia, or lymphocyte deficiency (15[R]), (16[c]). To prevent transmission of parvovirus B19 it is necessary to develop well-validated screening assays and new techniques to inactivate the virus during the production of blood products (15[R]).

B-cell lymphoma after autologous bone marrow transplantation for T-cell acute lymphoblastic leukemia has been reported (17[c]). *Epstein-Barr virus* proteins and genome have been demonstrated in post-transplantation lymphoma, suggesting a causative role.

Parasitic infections transmitted by blood transfusion *Trypanosoma cruzi*, a protozoan parasite endemic in Mexico, Central America, and South America, is the causative agent in Chagas' disease and can be transmitted by blood products. A study in two Red Cross regions (Los Angeles and Miami) has determined the prevalence of *Trypanosoma cruzi* antibodies in 23 978 at-risk blood donors and 25 587 controls (18[C]). *T cruzi* antibodies were found in 34 donors (33 and one, respectively). Seropositive donors shared one risk factor: they had been born or spent an extensive time in an endemic area. To prevent the transmission of *Trypanosoma cruzi* it is necessary to test all donors, but no tests have been so far licensed in the US.

INTRAVENOUS IMMUNOGLOBULINS

Intravenous immunoglobulins are used for the treatment of primary and secondary immunodeficiencies, autoimmune disorders (such as immune thrombocytopenia, dermatomyositis), neurological diseases (such as Guillain-Barré syndrome, chronic inflammatory demyelinating polyneuropathy), and for the prevention of bacterial infections, notably in immunosuppressed patients (19[c]), (20[c]), (21[R]). Various mechanisms of the immunomodulatory effects of intravenous immunoglobulin have been proposed. Intravenous immunoglobulin contains a variety of anti-idiotypic antibodies that bind to and neutralize pathogenic autoantibodies, thus preventing their interaction with self-antigens (20[r]). Other immunomodulatory effects that have been proposed include inhibition of complement deposition, neutralization of cytokines, and modulation of Fc-receptor-mediated phagocytosis (22[R]).

The different intravenous immunoglobulin formulations are equivalent with regard to therapeutic effectiveness and adverse effects (19[c]), which occur in 1–15% of patients. Most of the adverse effects are mild, such as *fever*, *chills*, *rash*, *headache*, *myalgia*, *hypertension*, and *thoracic pain*, and have been attributed to complement activation by IgG aggregates (19[c]), (23[R]). These adverse effects usually resolve within 1 h of stopping or slowing the infusion and respond to symptomatic treatment (analgesics, antihistamines) (21[R]), (24[c]). Severe complications are rare and often other predisposing risk factors are present (25[R]).

Cardiovascular Intravenous immunoglobulin has been associated with *thrombotic complications*, such as cerebral infarction, pulmonary embolism, and deep venous thrombosis (25[R]). Myocardial ischemia has also been reported, possibly due to increased serum IgG, which causes increased blood viscosity (26[c]). Although the frequency of thromboembolic events after intravenous immunoglobulin is unknown, it appears that patients often have risk factors, such as intracardiac thrombus and long-term immobilization (25[R]), (27[c]).

In a 17-year-old man bilateral central retinal vein occlusion occurred during treatment with high-dosage intravenous immunoglobulin (500 mg/kg per day for 14 days) (28[c]). Immunoglobulin treatment was withheld, and high serum viscosity and serum IgG normalized after 1 month. The authors suggested that to prevent increased serum viscosity and visual disturbances the concentration of immunoglobulin be reduced or the interval of intravenous immunoglobulin administration be increased.

To avoid rapid *fluid overload* in patients with a compromised cardiovascular system or congestive heart failure, a slower infusion rate is recommended (22[R]).

Respiratory A 37-year-old man with cancer-associated thrombotic thrombocytopenic purpura–hemolytic uremic syndrome developed non-cardiogenic *pulmonary edema* during intravenous immunoglobulin treatment (29[c]). As result of hydrostatic pulmonary edema he died of respiratory failure 72 h after the last immunoglobulin infusion. The authors suggested that instead of solubilizing existing circulating immune complexes, the high dosage of immunoglobulins had led to enhanced immune complex formation and/or deposition (29[c]).

Nervous system *Aseptic meningitis* after intravenous immunoglobulin infusion has been reported in several conditions, such as idiopathic thrombocytopenic purpura and chronic inflammatory demyelinating polyneuropathy. This adverse effect occurs within 24 h of infusion and is associated with severe headache, nuchal rigidity, and spinal fluid pleocytosis (30[R]). In several studies the incidence has been 11–17% (24[c]). The symptoms usually start at 6–48 h after infusion and clear within 3–5 days. Similar symptoms will recur after rechallenge with immunoglobulins, irrespective of the infusion rate, extension of treatment over several hours, or the use of different intravenous immunoglobulin formulations (24[c]). Analysis of cerebrospinal fluid shows leukocyte pleocytosis with raised protein and IgG concentrations. In 3% of cases cerebrospinal fluid eosinophilia has been reported (24[c]). The mechanism of aseptic meningitis remains unclear, but a reaction to stabilizers or hypersensitivity mediated by entry of immunoglobulin molecules into the cerebrospinal fluid compartment have been held responsible (SEDA-21, 344).

Patients with a history of migraine have an increased risk of aseptic meningitis (25[R]). Injection of intravenous immunoglobulin can trigger *a migraine attack* in a patient with a history of migraine. This can be prevented by propranolol prophylaxis (22[R]).

Hematological A severe complication of intravenous immunoglobulin treatment is *hemolytic anemia*, due to isoantibodies present in immunoglobulin formulations (25[R]). Hemolytic anemia can probably be prevented by using intravenous immunoglobulins that lack anti-D antibodies as well as anti-A and anti-B antibodies (SEDA-21, 345).

Transient *neutropenia* has been documented (25[R]), (31[C]). The mechanism of neutrophil damage is unclear (25[R]). This is a rare and clinically insignificant complication of intravenous immunoglobulin therapy.

Leukocytopenia induced by intravenous immunoglobulin (32[c]) has been reported and appears to be dose related (32[c]).

Mild transient *increases in liver enzymes* (AsT, AlT) have been reported (25[R]), (33[R]), but it is still debated if this effect is causally linked to intravenous immunoglobulin (25[R]).

Urinary system *Acute renal insufficiency* is an uncommon adverse effect of intravenous immunoglobulin (19[c]). In most cases serum creatinine concentrations increase during intravenous immunoglobulin therapy, accompanied by a gradual reduction in urine output (34[c]). After withdrawal of intravenous immunoglobulin serum creatinine and diuresis return to pretreatment values (19[c]). In less than one-third of cases, hemodialysis is required (23[R]).

In most cases of acute renal insufficiency renal biopsy shows swelling and vacuolization of the epithelial cells of the proximal tubules, with preservation of the brush border. Immune deposits have not been observed (23[R]).

Although the cause of intravenous immunoglobulin-associated acute renal insufficiency is unknown, it has been suggested that it is related to the stabilizing agent used in the intravenous immunoglobulin formulation (21[R]), (23[R]) (SEDA-21, 345). Of the reported cases, 82% occurred after infusion of Sandoglobulin, which contains sucrose as a stabilizer. The renal lesions found in the majority of biopsy specimens are identical to those described with sucrose nephropathy (23[R]). Most patients who developed acute renal failure after intravenous immunoglobulin containing sucrose did not develop renal disturbances when maltose-containing intravenous immunoglobulin was used. Other potential mechanisms of acute renal insufficiency due to intravenous immunoglobulin have been proposed, for example renal artery vasoconstriction resulting in ischemic renal injury and abnormal glomerular hemodynamics due to increased plasma oncotic pressure (23[R]).

There are several proposed risk factors for intravenous immunoglobulin-associated acute renal insufficiency, such as pre-existing renal impairment, older age, hypertension, and underlying paraproteinemia with rheumatoid factor activity (SEDA-21, 345) (23[R]).

Skin and appendages Skin reactions to intravenous immunoglobulin are rare. Recently a cutaneous reaction to immunoglobulin, typical of *pompholyx*, has been reported (35[c]). Other skin reactions include *urticaria*, *palmar pruritus*, *petechiae*, and *leukocytoclastic vasculitis*; these reactions can be the result of an allergic reaction to intravenous immunoglobulin or immunological reactions between infused IgG and skin antigens (35[c]).

Special senses In a 70-year-old woman *Wegener's granuloma* with ocular involvement, retinal vasculitis, and uveitis developed on two separate occasions after intravenous immunoglobulin (36[c]). The authors suggested that these complications were an adverse effect of intravenous immunoglobulin therapy.

Immunological and hypersensitivity reactions Severe *anaphylactic reactions* have been observed in patients with underlying IgA deficiency with anti-IgA antibodies (23[R]). Intravenous immunoglobulin is therefore contraindicated in these patients. However, because of the low prevalence of patients with selective IgA deficiency and anti-IgA antibodies, routine screening for IgA deficiency before intravenous immunoglobulin therapy is generally not recommended (21[R]).

Immune-complex *arthritis* and hypersensitivity myocarditis have been associated with intravenous immunoglobulin therapy (25[R]).

Transmission of viral infections Transmission of *hepatitis C* by intravenous immunoglobulin was reported several years ago (25[R]). Subsequently, several manufacturers have changed the purification protocol and have added a viral inactivation step, e.g. the solvent and detergent step (22[R]), (25[R]). Transmission of HIV and other viral diseases has not been documented. Intravenous immunoglobulin formulations are considered relatively safe (21[R]), (25[R]).

CLOTTING FACTOR CONCENTRATES

Hemophilia A and B, deficiencies of clotting factors VIII and IX, respectively, are characterized by spontaneous bleeding into muscles, mucocutaneous membranes, and joints (SEDA-21, 342). To arrest bleeding and prevent bleeding complications, hemophiliacs are treated with clotting factor concentrates. Important adverse effects of these concentrates include inhibitor formation, immunosuppression, and thrombotic complications.

Hematological Prolonged infusion of high-dosage porcine factor VIII in hemophiliacs with inhibitors is associated with *thrombocytopenia* (37[c]). In most patients platelet counts fall at 18–24 days after the start of continuous infusion. Platelet counts, which may fall to $11–87 \times 10^9/l$, normalize within 2.5–7 days after stopping the infusion (37[c]).

Treatment of bleeding episodes in hemophiliacs with inhibitors using high dosages of activated prothrombin complex concentrates has been associated with *thrombosis*, *myocardial infarction*, and *disseminated intravascular coagulation* (38[C]), (39[r]). The thrombogenicity of prothrombin complex concentrates has been ascribed to the presence of factor IXa and factor Xa (39[r]). However, high concentrations of factor VIIa have been found in prothrombin complex concentrates that were used when thromboembolic events occurred (40[r]). To determine the significance of high factor VIIa concentrations in prothrombin complex concentrates for increased thrombotic risks, in vivo thrombogenicity studies have to be performed (39[r]). To prevent such complications, infusion of a maximum of 200 U/kg per day of activated prothrombin complex has been recommended (40[C]).

Urinary system Recently *nephrotic syndrome* associated with hypocomplementemia has been described in a patient with hemophilia B with inhibitor (41[c]). In addition, anaphylactoid reactions occurred after the infusion of three different factor IX concentrates. Hypocomplementemia, allergic reactions, and administration of foreign proteins (factor IX concentrates) suggested a diagnosis of immune complex-mediated glomerulopathy.

Immunological and hypersensitivity reactions In patients with hemophilia, *inhibitor formation* generally occurs when they are young (37[c]). The incidence of inhibitors in patients with hemophilia A is 5–20% (37[c]), and is high when the disease is severe. It is suspected that there is a genetic predisposition for inhibitor formation and that factor VIII products may vary in their propensity to induce inhibitor formation (37[c]), (42[c]). Factor VIII gene inversion of intron 22 represents a high-risk abnormality for the development of anti-factor VIII antibodies (43[c]). Hemophiliacs with inhibitors can be treated with factor VIII concentrates or with products (e.g. factor VIIa) that activate the clotting cascade without the need to administer factor VIII. In patients with factor VIII inhibitors treated with continuous infusion of porcine factor VIII, alloantibodies to porcine factor VIII can develop (37[c]). In a patient with an antiporcine inhibitor titre of 0.8 BU, anaphylaxis reaction occurred after re-exposure with porcine factor VIII (37[c]). It has recently been observed that heating of lyophilized factor VIII, which is used to eliminate the risk of viral contamination, does not seem to alter the activity or immunoreactivity of the factor VIII molecule (42[C]).

In contrast to hemophilia A, the incidence of inhibitors in hemophilia B is only 1–3% (44[C]). Patients with hemophilia B who have complete gene deletions or major derangements of the factor IX gene may develop anaphylactic reactions after factor IX infusion. The occurrence of anaphylaxis is related to the formation of factor IX antibodies (44[C]). These patients can be safely treated with recombinant factor VIIa.

Transmission of infections Most adult hemophiliacs who were treated with commercial clotting factor concentrates before 1985 are infected with blood-borne viruses, such as *HIV* and *hepatitis C* (45[R]). Since the introduction of virucidal methods for plasma-derived clotting factor concentrates, including vapor heating and mixtures of solvent and detergent, infections with hepatitis viruses and HIV have become rare among patients with hemophilia (46[C]). However, it has recently been shown that hepatitis G virus can be transmitted by blood products without hepatitis C virus transmission (45[R]).

In a study of a recombinant factor VIII *seroconversion for parvovirus B19* occurred in five of 16 susceptible patients (47[C]). Several explanations for this have been given, for example community-acquired infections or oversensitivity of the serological tests used. However, it is also possible that albumin in recombinant factor VIII was responsible for the seroconversions.

So far, transmission of Creutzfeldt-Jakob disease and new-variant Creutzfeldt-Jakob disease by blood or blood products has not been found (48[R]), (49[r]). The CNS tissues of 30 hemophiliacs who died with CNS symptoms have been examined; Creutzfeldt-Jakob disease was not detected in any of these cases (48[R]). The risk of transmission of new-variant Creutzfeldt-Jakob disease in patients treated with blood products (48[R]), (49[r]) has led to the introduction of certain safety measures-the application of donor exclusion criteria and, in some countries, a ban on plasma and routine leukodepletion.

ERYTHROPOIETIN (EPOETIN)

Recombinant human erythropoietin stimulates erythropoiesis. In patients with chronic renal insufficiency, erythropoietin increases the number of red cells, improves well-being, and reverses some uremic symptoms such as malaise and fatigue (50[c]). It is also indicated for autologous blood donation in non-anemic patients, anemia of prematurity, AIDS-associated anemia, myeloma-associated anemia, and anemia in rheumatoid arthritis (51[C]), (52[R]), (53[C]), (54[c]), (55[R]), (56[C]).

Treatment with erythropoietin improves anemia and eliminates or reduces the number of blood transfusions and thereby the risks of iron overload, sensitization, and transmission of viral diseases (58[R]).

Erythropoietin should be given subcutaneously, because this route allows a dosage reduction of about 30% compared with the intravenous route (55[R]), (57[R]). Subcutaneous administration results in lower peak plasma erythropoietin concentrations, but a longer half-life of about 19–22 h compared with 4–5 h after intravenous administration (55[R]).

Hyporesponsiveness to erythropoietin is caused by iron deficiency, blood loss, hyperparathyroidism, aluminium intoxication, inflammation, and malignancy (57[R]).

Adequate iron stores and availability are required for proper erythropoiesis and hemoglobin synthesis (58[C]). Iron supplementation is necessary in many uremic patients treated with erythropoietin (58[C]). Intravenous iron has also been recommended for patients with autologous blood donation receiving erythropoietin (59[R]).

Cardiovascular *Hypertension* develops in about 30–35% of dialysis patients receiving erythropoietin (60[C]). The most important risk factors for the development of hypertension or worsening of hypertension in patients with renal failure are pre-existing hypertension and high doses of erythropoietin (60[C]). To avoid hypertension it has been recommended that the dosage of erythropoietin be modified so that the hematocrit increases gradually (60[C]).

Increased peripheral vascular resistance, which has been observed in patients receiving erythropoietin (57[R]), is the main cause of hypertension. Factors that contribute to increased peripheral vascular resistance are increased blood viscosity and improved hypoxia, which reduces hypoxic vasodilatation (57[R]).

In hemodialysed patients treated with erythropoietin, *fistula thrombosis* has been described (61[C]), (62[C]). It has been proposed that thrombosis of the fistula during erythropoietin treatment can be prevented by antiplatelet therapy (62[C]). Erythropoietin modulates endothelial secretion by reducing prostacyclin and enhancing the production of thromboxane A_2 and endothelin-1 (62[C]). It has been suggested that a significant reduction in free protein S antigen activity (but not protein C activity), antithrombin III activity, fibrinogen activity, and plasminogen activity during the early phase of erythropoietin treatment may predispose to thrombotic events (61[C]), (63[C]).

Hematological Erythropoietin has been associated with the development of *acute leukemia*. It has been suggested that it may stimulate extramedullary hemopoiesis, with secondary transformation to leukemia (64[c]). In both murine and human systems, genetic alterations of the erythropoietin receptor gene, which are not rare, could be involved in the occurrence of the erythroleukemic process (64[c]).

Rapid and transitory *leukopenia*, especially lymphocytopenia has been reported after high doses erythropoietin (65[c]).

In a 63-year-old man with end-stage renal disease, antibodies to erythropoietin developed after treatment with erythropoietin, resulting in *pure red cell aplasia* (66[c]). Parvovirus infection was ruled out. Over the course of several months the antibodies spontaneously disappeared and red cell precursors reappeared.

Skin and appendages Subcutaneous injection of erythropoietin is painful. Administration of erythropoietin at the site of an arteriovenous fistula is more painful than in an arm without a fistula (67[C]).

A new multidose formulation of epoetin-β (water for injection containing benzalkonium chloride 0.002% and benzyl alcohol 0.4%) did not cause more adverse effects after subcutaneous injection than epoetin in the standard monodose solvent (water for injections) (68[C]).

Spinal abscess formation subsequent to *pyoderma gangrenosum* after subcutaneous administration of erythropoietin has been reported (69[c]). Pyoderma gangrenosum has been described after the administration of other hemopoietic colony-stimulating factors (70[c]), although it has also been reported to have responded to treatment with GM-CSF (71[c]).

Special senses Several ophthalmic adverse affects, such as *visual disturbances*, *visual hallucinations*, *conjunctival inflammation*, and *iritis-like reactions*, have been described after treatment with erythropoietin (SEDA-21, 348). In a 63-year-old woman, treated with erythropoietin for aplastic anemia, retinal hemorrhages occurred during erythropoietin therapy and disappeared after withdrawal (72[c]).

Immunological and hypersensitivity reactions So far, only four cases of *antibodies against erythropoietin* have been reported (55[R]).

A common adverse effect of erythropoietin is a *flu-like syndrome*, which has been encountered in 4–21% of patients (51[C]), (61[c]). It has been suggested that increased IL-β and TNF-α production, induced by the administration of erythropoietin may be the cause of fever and flu-like symptoms (61[c]).

REFERENCES

1. Ramanathan RK, Triulzi DJ, Logan TF. Transfusion-related acute lung injury following random donor platelet transfusion: a report of two cases. Vox Sang 1997;73:43–5.
2. Chapman JF, Forman K, Kelsey P, Knowles SM, Murphy MF, Williamson LM, Wood JK;Working Party: Murphy MF, Kinsey S, Murphy W, Pamphilon D, Warwick R, Williamson LM, Wood JK. Guidelines on the clinical use of leucocyte-depleted blood components. Transfus Med 1998;8:59–71.
3. The Trial to Reduce Alloimmunization to Platelets Study Group. Leukocyte reduction and ultraviolet B irradiation of platelets to prevent alloimmunization and refractoriness to platelet transfusions. New Engl J Med 1997;26:1861–9.
4. Vamvakas EC, Carven JH. Transfusion of white-cell-containing allogeneic blood compo-

nents and postoperative wound infection: effect of confounding factors. Transfus Med 1998;8:29–36.

5. Högman CF, Engstrandt L. Serious bacterial complications from blood components-how do they occur? Transfus Med 1998;8:1–3.
6. Boulton FE, Chapman ST, Walsh TH. Fatal reaction to transfusion of red-cell concentrate contaminated with *Serratia liquefaciens*. Transfus Med 1998;8:15–18.
7. McDonald CP, Hartley S, Orchard K, Hughes G, Brett MM, Hewitt PE, Barbara JAJ. Fatal *Clostridium perfringens* sepsis from a pooled platelet transfusion. Transfus Med 1998;8:19–22.
8. Schreiber GB, Busch MP, Kleinman SH, Korelitz JJ for the Retrovirus Epidemiology Donor Study. The risk of transfusion-transmitted viral infections. New Engl J Med 1996;334:1685–90.
9. Molijn MHJ, van der Linden JM, Ko LK, Gorgels J, Hop W, van Rhenen DJ. Risk factors and anti-HBc reactivity among first time blood donors. Vox Sang 1997;72:207–10.
10. Sampietro M, Corbetta N, Cerino M, Fabiani P, Ticozzi A, Orlandi A, Lunghi G, Fargion S, Fiorelli G, Cappellini MD. Prevalence and clinical significance of hepatitis G virus in adult beta-thalassaemia major patients. Br J Haematol 1997; 97:904–7.
11. Nakamura S, Takagi T, Matsuda T. Hepatitis G virus RNA in patients with B-cell non-Hodgkin's lymphoma. Br J Haematol 1997;98:1048–51.
12. Wilde JT, Ahmed MM, Collingham KE, Skidmore SJ, Pillay D, Mutimer D. Hepatitis G virus infection in patients with bleeding disordes. Br J Haematol 1997;99:285–8.
13. Barbara JAJ. Does GB virus C ('hepatitis G virus') threaten the safety of our blood supply? Transfus Med 1997;7:75–6.
14. Moriyama K, Okamura T, Nakano S. Hepatitis GB virus C genome in the serum of aplastic anaemia patients receiving frequent blood transfusions. Br J Haematol 1997;96:864–7.
15. Prowse C, Ludlam CA, Yap PL. Human parvovirus B19 and blood products. Vox Sang 1997;72:1–10.
16. Biesma DH, Nieuwenhuis HK. Life-threatening anaemia caused by B19 parvovirus infection in a non-immunocompromised patient. Neth J Med 1997;50:81–4.
17. Briz M, Forés R, Regidor C, Busto M-J, Cajal SRY, Cabrera R, Díez J-L, Sanjuán I, Fernández M-N. Epstein-Barr virus associated B-cell lymphoma after autologous bone marrow transplantation for T-cell acute lymphoblastic leukemia. Br J Haematol 1997;98:485–7.
18. Leiby DA, Read EJ, Lenes BA, Yund AJ, Stumpf RJ, Kirchhoff LV, Dodd RY. Seroepidemiology of *Trypanosoma cruzi*, etiologic agent of Chagas' disease in US blood donors. J Infect Dis 1997;176:1047–52.
19. Michail S, Nakopoulou L, Stavrianopoulos I, Stamatiadis D, Avdikou K, Vaiopoulos G, Stathakis C. Acute renal failure associated with immunoglobulin administration. Nephrol Dial Transplant 1997;12:1497–9.
20. Gupta S. Intravenous immune globulin in neuromuscular disorders. West J Med 1997;167:349–50.
21. Stangel M, Gold R. Treatment with intravenous immunoglobulins in critical care of neuromuscular disorders. Infus Ther Transfusionsmed 1997;24:171–7.
22. Dalakas MC. Intravenous immune globulin therapy for neurologic diseases. Ann Intern Med 1997;126:721–30.
23. Cayco AV, Perazella MA, Hayslett JP. Renal insufficiency after intravenous immune globulin therapy: a report of two cases and an analysis of the literature. J Am Soc Nephrol 1997;8:1788–94.
24. Picton P, Chisholm M. Aseptic meningitis associated with high dose immunoglobulin: case report. Br Med J 1997;315:1203–4.
25. Stangel M, Hartung HP, Marx P, Gold R. Side effects of high-dose intravenous immunoglobulins. Clin Neuropharmacol 1997;20:385–93.
26. Fishman DN, Smilovitch M. Intravenous immunoglobulin, blood viscosity and myocardial infarction. Can J Cardiol 1997;13:775–7.
27. Rosenbaum JT. Myocardial infarction as a complication of immunoglobulin therapy. Arthritis Rheum 1997;40:1732–3.
28. Oh KT, Boldt HC, Danis RP. Iatrogenic central retinal vein occlusion and hyperviscosity associated with high-dose intravenous immunoglobulin administration. Am J Ophthalmol 1997;124:416–18.
29. Suassuna JHR, da Costa MADL, Faria RA, Melichar AC. Noncardiogenic pulmonary edema triggered by intravenous immunoglobulin in cancer associated thrombotic thrombocytopenic purpura-hemolytic uremic syndrome. Nephron 1997;77:368–70.
30. Stiehm ER. Human intravenous immunoglobulin in primary and secondary antibody deficiencies. Pediatr Infect Dis J 1997;16:696–707.
31. Heyneman CA, Gudger GA, Beckwith JV. Intravenous immune globulin for inducing remissions in systemic lupus erythematosus. Ann Pharmacother 1997;31:242–4.
32. Sica REP, Genovese O. Leukopenia induced by intravenous immune globulin. Eur J Neurol 1997;4:197–8.
33. Vollmer-Conna U, Hickie I, Hadzi-Pavlovic D, Tymms K, Wakefield D, Dwyer J, Lloyd A. Intravenous immunoglobulin is ineffective in the treatment of patients with chronic fatigue syndrome. Am J Med 1997;103:38–43.
34. Blanco R, González-Gay MA, Ibáñez D, Sánchez-Andrade A, Gonzalez-Vela C. Paradoxical and persistent renal impairment in Henoch-Schönlein purpura after high-dose immunoglobulin therapy. Nephron 1997;76:247–8.
35. Catteau B, Delaporte E, Piette F. Meningitis and skin reaction after intravenous immune globulin therapy. Ann Intern Med 1997;127:1130.
36. Blum M, Andrassy K, Adler D, Hartmann M, Völker HE. Early experience with intravenous immunoglobulin treatment in Wegener's granulomatosis with ocular involvement. Graefe's Arch Clin Exp Ophthalmol 1997;235:599–602.

37. Rubinger M, Houston DS, Schwetz N, Woloschuk DMM, Israels SJ, Johnston JB. Continuous infusion of porcine factor VIII in the management of patients with factor VIII inhibitors. Am J Hematol 1997;56:112–18.
38. Hay CRM, Negrier C, Ludlam CA. The treatment of bleeding in acquired haemophilia with recombinant factor VIIa: a multicentre study. Thromb Haemostasis 1997;78:1463–7.
39. Hellstern P, Beeck H, Fellhauer A, Fischer A, Faller-Stöckl B. Factor VII and activated-factor-VII content of prothrombin complex concentrates. Vox Sang 1997;73:155–61.
40. Negrier C, Goudemand J, Sultan Y, Bertrand M, Rothschild C, Lauroua P and the members of the French FEIBA study group. Factor Eight Bypassing Activity. Multicenter retrospective study on the utilization of FEIBA in France in patients with factor VIII and factor IX inhibitors. Thromb Haemostasis 1997;77:1113–19.
41. Constantinescu AR, Weiss LS, Saidi P, Eisele J, Ettinger LJ. Nephrotic syndrome associated with hypocomplementemia in a 4-year-old boy with hemophilia. J Pediatr Hematol Oncol 1997;19:345–7.
42. Gilles JG, di Giambattista M, Laub R, Saint-Remy JMR. Heating lyophilised factor VIII does not alter its recognition by specific antibodies. Vox Sang 1997;73:16–23.
43. Vianello F, Radossi P, Tison T, Dazzi F, Tagariello G, Davoli PG, Girolami A. Prevalence of anti-FVIII antibodies in severe haemophilia A patients with inversion of intron 22. Br J Haematol 1997;97:807–9.
44. Warrier I, Ewenstein BM, Koerper MA, Shapiro A, Key N, DiMichele D, Miller RT, Pasi J, Rivard GE, Sommer SS, Katz J, Bergmann F, Ljung R, Petrini P, Lusher JM. Factor IX inhibitors and anaphylaxis in hemophilia. J Pediatr Hematol Oncol 1997;19:23–7.
45. Tong CYW, Sallam TA, Williams H, Mutton KJ, Gilmore IT, Toh CH. Hepatitis G virus RNA and its relation to hepatitis C infection in adult haemophilic patients. Br J Haematol 1997; 99:295–7.
46. Uhle C, Zimmermann R, Goeser T, Seelig R. Virus inactivation and prevalence of GBV-C in haemophiliacs. Br J Haematol 1997;99:837–8.
47. Aygören-Pürsün E, Scharrer I, The German Kogenate Study Group. A multicenter pharmacosurveillance study for the evaluation of the efficacy and safety of recombinant factor VIII in the treatment of patients with hemophilia A. Thromb Haemost 1997;78:1352–6.
48. Evatt BL. Prions and haemophilia: assessment of risk. Haemophilia 1998;4:628–33.
49. Ludlam CA. New-variant Creutzfeldt-Jakob and treatment of haemophilia. Lancet 1997; 350:1704.
50. Yagil Y for the Multicenter Study Group Israel. Proposed therapeutic algorithm for the treatment of anemia of chronic renal failure in predialysis patients with low dose once weekly sybcutaneous r-HuEPO. Isr J Med Sci 1997;33:36–44.
51. Cazenave JP, Irrmann C, Waller C, Sondag D, Baudoux E, Genetet B, Laxenaire MC, Dupont E, Sundal E, Obrist R, Stocker H. Epoetin alfa facilitates presurgical autologous blood donation in non-anaemic patients scheduled for orthopaedic or cardiovasculair surgery. Eur J Anaesthesiol 1997;14:432–42.
52. Meyer MP. Anaemia of prematurity;epidemiology, management and costs. Pharmacoeconomics 1997;12:438–45.
53. Balfour HH Jr. Recombinant human erythropoietin for treatment of anemia in persons with AIDS not receiving zidovudine. Int J Antimicrob Agents 1997;8:189–92.
54. Mittelman M, Zeidman A, Fradin Z, Magazanik A, Lewinski UH, Cohen A. Recombinant human erythropoietin in the treatment of multiple myeloma-associated anemia. Acta Haematol 1997;98:204–10.
55. Cazzola M, Mercuriali F, Brugnara C. Use of recombinant human erythropoietin outside the setting of uremia. Blood 1997;89:4248–67.
56. Nordström D, Lindroth Y, Marsal L, Hafström I, Henrich C, Rantapää-Dahlqvist S, Engström-Laurent A, Fyhrquist F, Friman C. Availability of iron and degree of inflammation modifies the response to recombinant human erythropoietin when treating anemia of chronic disease in patients with rheumatoid arthritis. Rheumatol Int 1997;17:67–73.
57. Valderrbano F. Recombinant erythropoietin: 10 years of clinical experience. Nephrol Dial Tranplant 1997;12 (Suppl 1):2–9.
58. Tarng D-C, Huang T-P, Chen TW. Mathematical approach for estimating iron needs in hemodialysis patients on erythropoietin therapy. Am J Nephrol 1997;17:158–64.
59. Mercuriali F. Erythropoietin and iron in autologous haemotherapy. Bailliere's Clin Anaesthesiol 1997;11:351–62.
60. Yalçinkaya F, Tümer N, Çakar N, Özkaya N. Low-dose erythropoietin is effective and safe in children on continuous ambulatory peritoneal dialysis. Pediatr Nephrol 1997;11:350–2.
61. Takemasa A, Yorioka N, Yamakido M. Investigation of the influenza-like symptoms associated with recombinant human erythropoietin therapy. J Int Med Res 1997;25:127–34.
62. Viron B, Chamma F, Jaar B, Michel C, Mignon F. Thrombosis of angioaccess in haemodialysed patients treated with human recombinant erythopoietin. Nephrol Dial Transplant 1997; 12:368–70.
63. Jaar B, Denis A, Viron B, Verdy E, Chamma F, Siohan P, Mignon F. Effects of long-term treatment with recombinant human erythropoietin on physiologic inhibitors of coagulation. Am J Nephrol 1997;17:399–405.
64. Mazzarella V, Splendiani G, Tozzo C, Casciani CU. Acute leukemia in a uremic patient undergoing erythropoietin treatment. Nephron 1997;76:361.
65. Buemi M, Allegra A, Corica F, Cavallaro G, Aloisi C, Pettinato G, Frisina N. Rapid and tran-

sient lymphocytopenia after i.v. administration of high doses of human recombinant erythropoietin. Hematopathol Mol Hematol 1998;11:13–17.
66. Prabhakar SS, Muhlfelder T. Antibodies to recombinant human erythropoietin causing pure red cell aplasia. Clin Nephrol 1997;5:331–5.
67. Teruel JL, Sánchez FJL, Ortuño J. Estudio comparativo del dolor entre las inyecciones subcutáneas de la nueva formulación de la eritropoyetina alfa y de la eritropoyetina beta. Nefrologia 1997;17:214–20.
68. Franke W, Scherhag R. Tolerability and efficacy of multidose formulations of epoetin beta. Clin Drug Invest 1997;13:199–206.
69. Park CW, Shin YS, Shin MJ, Koh SH, Chang KU, Ahn YB, Chang YS, Bang BK. Pyoderma gangrenosum and spinal epidural abscess after subcutaneous administration of recombinant human erythropoietin. Nephrol Dial Transplant 1997;12:1506–8.
70. Lewerin C, Mobacken H, Nilsson Ehle H, Swolin B. Bullous pyoderma gangrenosum in a patient with myelodysplastic syndrome during granulocyte colony-stimulating factor therapy. Leuk Lymphoma 1997;26:629–32.
71. Bulvik S, Jacobs P. Pyoderma gangrenosum in myelodysplasia responding to granulocyte macrophage-colony stimulating factor (GM-CSF). Br J Dermatol 1997;136:637–8.
72. Nishimura Y, Okamoto N, Akaki Y, Nishikawa N, Fukuda M. A central retinal vein occlusion presumed to be induced by erythropoietin. Folia Ophthalmol Jpn 1997;48:472–5.

P.I. Folb

34 Intravenous infusions: solutions and emulsions

PLASMA SUBSTITUTES

Hydroxyethyl starch *(SED-13, 992; SEDA-20, 311; SEDA-21, 351)*

The syndrome of acute hypotension, non-cardiogenic pulmonary edema, anemia, and coagulopathy following surgery and administration of dextran 70 is called the '*dextran syndrome*' (1[cr]). Factors other than acute volume overload due to intravascular absorption of dextran are thought to account for it. A combination of diverse pathophysiological factors may be responsible, namely, direct pulmonary toxicity, activation of the coagulation cascade, release of vasoactive mediators, hypotension, pulmonary edema, intravascular intravasation of fluids, dilution of blood, and impaired renal and hepatic clearance.

Hematological High-molecular weight hydroxyethyl starch can cause *coagulation disorders*, although its effects are controversial and conflicting, according to a review of the literature of the last 30 years (2[R]). Reports have ranged from no effects, to laboratory but not clinical abnormalities, to outright clinical effects with coagulation disturbances. The authors suggested that hydroxyethyl starch reduces platelet function by coating the platelet surface or damaging the platelet. It is now generally agreed that hydroxyethyl starch is contraindicated when there is established coagulopathy, and that it should be used with caution in intracranial procedures, major trauma, cases in which blood loss would be poorly tolerated, and patients with history of a bleeding disorder.

Side Effects of Drugs, Annual 22
J.K. Aronson, ed.

In 10 patients with cerebrovascular diseases the administration of 10% hydroxyethyl starch 200/0.62 (500 ml/day for 11 days) impaired coagulation (3[c]). There was a significant 43% increase in activated partial thromboplastin time. Factor VIII:C, von Willebrand ristocetin co-factor, and von Willebrand factor antigen fell below the limit required for hemostasis (30%), and in some patients below 10%. This was thought to be due to accumulation of large molecules that are difficult to break down and which affect rheological function and coagulation unfavorably. The pathogenetic mechanism that affects factor VIII/von Willebrand factor complex has not been elucidated; there may be accelerated elimination after attachment of the complex to starch molecules. The significant falls in factor XI and factor XII show that impairment of the intrinsic system of coagulation is not limited to the factor VIII/von Willebrand factor complex.

Even a small total volume of 6% hydroxyethyl starch (2500 ml in 3 days) (average molecular weight 450 kDa) can cause significant coagulation disturbance (4[c]).

In a controlled study of 189 patients undergoing coronary bypass grafting, hydroxyethyl starch infused intraoperatively caused significant *reductions in hematocrit and platelet count, prolongation of the prothrombin time*, and *increases in blood loss and hemostatic drug requirements* (5[C]). There were trends towards greater transfusion requirements and re-exploration rates for bleeding. Hemorrhagic complications after the infusion of large volumes of hydroxyethyl starch can be avoided if a starch with low in vivo molecular weight is used (6[C]). This is not only because of a smaller effect on the coagulation system and avoidance of an acquired Type 1 von Willebrand syndrome, but also because of a smaller reduction in platelet volume, since platelet volume and function are correlated. In addition, high-molecular weight macromolecules affect plasma viscosity and erythrocytes negatively.

Urinary system Hydroxyethyl starch can cause *increasing serum creatinine concentrations*. Associated symptoms and signs include *pain in the renal region and swelling of the kidney parenchyma*. In 25 patients randomly allocated to no treatment or hydroxyethyl starch 10% (12 ml/kg) the hydroxyethyl starch caused *changes in renal tubular function*, with increased excretion of α1-microglobulin, Tamm-Horsfall protein, and brush border enzyme acetyl-β-glucosaminidase (7[C]). There were no significant differences in glomerular function. These findings suggest that hydroxyethyl starch causes a primary renal tubular lesion.

Of 211 patients with acute ischemic stroke, stages III or IV, treated with daily intravenous infusion of 500–1000 ml of low-molecular weight dextran (dextran 40) over 4 days, 10 (4.7%) developed *acute renal failure* associated with dextran infusion (8[C]). Oliguria developed after 3–6 days. The incidence of dextran-induced acute renal failure was significantly higher in patients with pre-existing reduction of glomerular filtration rate below 30 ml/min per 1.73 m^2. Five of the patients with acute renal failure died within 4–12 days after hemodilution therapy with dextran 40; this high mortality was attributable to non-renal complications.

In another report of two cases of anuric acute renal failure caused by dextran 40, diuresis and renal function were quickly restored to normal after plasmapheresis (9[c]). Renal biopsy showed normal kidneys, except for swelling and vacuolation of renal tubules, suggestive of osmotic nephrosis.

Conclusions have differed as to whether the use of hydroxyethyl starch in brain-dead organ donors causes *reduced kidney graft function* at 1, 3, and 6 months after transplantation (10[c])–(12[c]). In one report (13[c]), reduced kidney graft function, increases in creatinine, or increased hemodialysis requirements have been described in those given hydroxyethyl starch during the first 10 days after transplantation. However, others have not confirmed this (5[c]), (6[c]).

Skin and appendages Severe *pruritus* after infusion of hydroxyethyl starch is common. In three patients with persistent pruritus after hydroxyethyl starch during and after heart surgery there was histopathological evidence of storage vacuoles containing hydroxyethyl starch in the dermis (14[c]). Hydroxyethyl starch solutions are heterogeneous, and contain molecules with a wide range of molecular weights. The smaller molecules (under 50 kDa) are rapidly excreted by the kidneys, whereas larger molecules persist intravascularly until they are slowly hydrolysed or taken up by the mononuclear phagocyte system and other cells in various tissues. The mechanism by which storage of hydroxyethyl starch causes pruritus is not adequately understood. It does not seem to be an allergic hypersensitivity reaction mediated by the immune system, as there is usually little or no inflammatory cell infiltrate, and the incidence of pruritus is dose related. Whether macrophages, endothelial cells, keratinocytes, Langerhans cells, or other cells in which the starch molecules are deposited release mediators that cause itching, or whether there is a more direct effect on sensory nerve fibres is uncertain. In this small series the number of mast cells was increased and mast cells were degranulated on electron microscopy. These features have not been seen in other studies. The resistance of the pruritus to treatment suggests that it is not simply mediated by histamine.

In skin biopsies from 93 patients who had received hydroxyethyl starch, half of whom presented with pruritus, immuno-electron microscopical investigation was conducted using an antibody highly specific for hydroxyethyl starch (15[C]). There were intracytoplasmic storage vacuoles in the skin in all patients who had received hydroxyethyl starch. Dose-dependent uptake of hydroxyethyl starch was first detectable in macrophages and afterwards in endothelial and epithelial cells. There were hydroxyethyl starch-reactive vacuoles in the Schwann cells of unmyelinated and small myelinated nerve fibres, and in endoneural and perineural cells. Neural devacuolization paralleled the clinical improvement in pruritus. The authors of this study suggest that deposits of hydroxyethyl starch in cutaneous nerves, as a consequence of a high cumulative dose, may account for itching after hydroxyethyl starch infusion.

TOTAL PARENTERAL NUTRITION *(SED-13, 994; SEDA-19, 318; SEDA-20, 310; SEDA-21, 353)*

Many of the safety issues in the administration of total parenteral nutrition (TPN) relate to the fact that the process is inherently unphysiological (16[R]). Instead of periodic ingestion of nutrients via the gastrointestinal tract, resulting in gradual entry of nutrients into the blood, nutrients are infused directly at a constant rate. The gastrointestinal tract as a mediator of nutrient absorption, the periodicity of nutrient administration, and the natural biorhythms of hormone secretion are all lost.

Cardiovascular *Peripheral venous thrombosis* is the principal complication of peripheral TPN. It necessitates removal and replacement of the catheter. It rarely occurs as a result of bacterial colonization and is usually due to the mechanical effects of the cannula and the properties of the infusate, in particular, the osmolality and pH of the fluid. With the use of a fine-bore polyurethane catheter and all-in-one feeds the overall incidence of peripheral venous thrombosis was 30%, and it occurred at a mean of 5.2 days (17[c]). Lines were used for an average of 6.5 days, which is in the clinically useful range, since the majority of courses of TPN are given for less than 7–14 days.

Respiratory In a retrospective cohort study of the use of TPN in 51 patients, five of 11 who had received FreAmine as a source of amino acids had a respiratory event (*chest pain*, *dyspnea*, *cardiopulmonary arrest*, or new *interstitial infiltrates* on chest radiograph), in contrast to none of 39 who received Travasol (18[c]). The events apparently resulted from infusion of calcium phosphate precipitate in an opaque admixture. It was most likely that calcium phosphate crystals deposited in the pulmonary microvasculature.

Nervous system Considerable recent interest has been stimulated in the pathogenesis of *critical illness polyneuropathy* during the course of artificial nutrition (19[c]). Critical illness polyneuropathy is common in intensive care units, and it is an important cause of failure to wean. The neurological disability can last 6 months. There is a strong association with sepsis and multiple organ dysfunction syndrome, the nervous system being yet another focus of organ failure. The authors noted that neurological function improved after the withdrawal of nutrition in patients whose condition was worsening. Critical illness polyneuropathy is an axonal polyneuropathy, demonstrable after death by histological evidence of axonal degeneration. A functional disorder is likely to precede structural changes. The autonomic nervous system is commonly involved, and all patients with critical illness polyneuropathy had early cardiovascular instability requiring antihypotensive medication. It seems that artificial feeding after starvation leads to reduced activity of the enzymes for glucose oxidation, with the result that nutrient glucose causes accumulation of phosphorylated glycolytic intermediates; this in turn causes a block in the energy cascade that is an essential element in the development of axonal polyneuropathies.

Although the mechanism responsible for the polyneuropathy is not known, there is evidence that disturbances of microcirculation and increased microvascular permeability can lead to endoneural edema, resulting in primary axonal degeneration of peripheral nerves (20[r]). Hyperalimentation may favor the metabolic disturbances that arise during sepsis, but it is by no means clear that nutrition is the only cause of critical illness polyneuropathy. A sensitive bioassay capable of identifying a low-molecular weight fraction toxic to rat spinal motor neurones has been identified in the sera of patients with critical illness polyneuropathy (21[r]), (22[C]).

A 24-year-old patient developed an acute hemiplegia and seizures after accidental catheterization of the right common carotid artery and TPN infusion (23[c]). MRI of the brain showed lesions in the frontal lobe and putamen consistent with an ischemic stroke. Angiography through the central venous catheter confirmed its intra-arterial location. The patient's weakness improved after hyperbaric oxygen treatment.

Endocrine, metabolic *Non-ketotic hyperglycemia* developed in a dog treated inadvertently within 2 h of receiving 1800 ml hyperosmolar solution for a pancreatic abscess (24[c]). The blood glucose concentration reached 44 mmol/l and the plasma osmolality was more than 334 mOsm/l. Lipemia was severe and persisted for several days. The dog developed nausea, vomiting, severe hyperglycemia, polyuria, glucosuria, and hypokalemia, but recovered without long-term sequelae. Intravenous glucose had been infused at a rate of 107 mg/kg per min, quite sufficient to overload metabolic pathways by an excess of glucose. The glycemia exceeded the renal ability to retain glucose, and there was glycosuria associated with osmotic diuresis.

Micronutrient deficiencies *Thiamine deficiency* Optic neuropathy has been attributed to thiamine deficiency during TPN (25[c]).

A 22-year-old man treated with intravenous hyperalimentation without vitamin supplementation for 4 weeks suddenly developed deterioration in his vision and oscillating vision. His visual acuity was under 0.1 in both eyes. The optic fundi were normal. There was no response to treatment for 2 days with high-dose corticosteroids. Over the next few days he developed the full-blown clinical picture of Wernicke's encephalopathy, confirmed by characteristic findings on brain MRI scan. His serum vitamin B1 concentration was 110 ng/l (reference range 200–500 ng/l). He responded fully to thiamine 300 mg/day plus betamethasone for 4 weeks. There were no residual neurological deficits and no long-term memory disturbance.

In a comprehensive review of reports of 33 patients with TPN-induced fulminant beriberi, and the authors' experience of another 10 cases, a characteristic syndrome has emerged (26[CR]). TPN-induced fulminant beriberi becomes evident 4–40 days after the start of TPN, and is more likely to develop in patients with malignancies, ulcerative colitis, or short bowel syndrome, and in those receiving chemotherapy. Although the patients have various symptoms, few develop the classical signs of beriberi or the characteristic findings seen in alcoholic patients. The severity of metabolic acidosis is high and refractory to bicarbonate, but it responds quickly to intravenous thiamine. Rapid intravenous administration of thiamine is imperative, and the patient should be transferred urgently to an intensive care unit when TPN-induced beriberi develops.

In a Japanese study of six cases of TPN-associated lactic acidosis the patients developed hypotension, Kussmaul respiration, and clouding of consciousness, as well as abdominal pain not directly related to the underlying disease (27[C]). During TPN there was blockade of oxidative decarboxylation of α-keto acids, such as pyruvate and α-ketoglutarate, resulting in pyruvate accumulation and massive lactate production. None of the patients responded to sodium bicarbonate or other conventional emergency treatment for shock and lactic acidosis. Thiamine replenishment intravenously, 100 mg every 12 h, resolved the lactic acidosis and improved the clinical condition of three patients. This report has emphasized the need (i) to supplement TPN with thiamine-containing vitamins in patients whose food intake does not meet nutritional requirements; (ii) to monitor patients routinely, measuring serum thiamine concentration and erythrocyte transketolase activity during TPN; and (iii) to replenish thiamine intravenously using high doses urgently with the first symptoms and signs of lactic acidosis. In this review, patients were characterized by comparatively old age, underlying disease requiring extensive abdominal surgery, minimal preoperative food intake, and postoperative TPN with no food intake and no supplemental multivitamins. Thiamine cannot achieve the desired effect, even with a large dose, if hepatic function is severely disturbed, because thiamine is not phosphorylated and remains physiologically inactive in this situation.

Choline deficiency Liver dysfunction has been attributed to choline deficiency during TPN (28[c])

A 41-year-old woman with advanced cervical cancer developed clinical and biochemical evidence of liver dysfunction 2 months after starting TPN. She had jaundice, nausea, and vomiting. Her serum choline concentration was 5.77 mmol/l. She responded well to oral choline 3 g/day and glutamine 15 g/day. The repeat serum choline concentration 4 months later was 12.8 mmol/l, a 45% improvement. There was histological evidence of hepatic steatosis, and the case shows the possible importance of choline deficiency in its pathogenesis.

Phosphatidylcholine is an essential component of the very low-density lipoprotein (VLDL) complex that facilitates the transport of triacylglycerols out of the liver. Choline is most effectively synthesized from methionine when it enters the liver via the portal vein. This first-pass effect is bypassed with parenteral infusion of methionine. However, in this case the improvement in liver function could not be attributed solely to correction of choline deficiency. Glutamine supplementation, which is necessary for gut integrity, may also have contributed. Intravenous fat emulsions contain choline, but not in sufficient amounts to prevent choline deficiency. The authors concluded that a low plasma choline concentration is a potential causative factor in the development of hepatic steatosis, and that choline deficiency should be considered when the condition develops.

Although choline is not regarded as an essential nutrient for humans, there is evidence that it is 'conditionally essential' in patients receiving TPN. Choline is a methyl group donor, a component of phospholipids, and a precursor of acetylcholine and lecithin. In animals and healthy humans, choline deficiency impairs liver function. In patients receiving long-term TPN low concentrations of plasma choline are common and are associated with hepatic steatosis. Treatment of these patients with oral choline improves plasma choline concentrations and reduces hepatic fat content. Intravenous administration of choline for TPN-associated hepatic steatosis with documented subnormal plasma unbound choline concentrations is effective treatment (29[r]).

Mineral and fluid balance *Manganese*- Neurological and radiological disorders have been reported in patients receiving long-term TPN (30[c]). On the basis of raised serum manganese concentrations these abnormalities have been attributed to manganese intoxication. Alterations in basal ganglia signal intensity detected by MRI have been reported, but the precise nature of the abnormalities is uncertain.

A 63-year-old patient who received TPN developed neurological disorders after several months of treatment, and there was a hypersignal in the basal ganglia and in cerebral white matter on MRI. At post mortem, high concentrations of manganese were found in the radiologically abnormal areas. Serum manganese concentrations were not a reliable indicator of cerebral concentrations.

This is believed to be the first reported case showing a relation between high intracerebral manganese concentrations, radiological abnormalities, and neurological disorders during prolonged TPN.

Phosphate Hyperphosphatemia complicated by calcification of subcutaneous arteries and skin infarcts has been reported in a 31-year-old woman with sepsis who received an unintended excess of phosphate in TPN (31[c]). She did not have chronic renal failure or hyperparathyroidism. She had unintentionally received total elemental phosphorus infused over a 7-week period in a daily amount of 1.8–4.2 g, over three times the normal daily requirement. Serum phosphorus increased to 3 mmol/l (reference range 0.76–1.46 mmol/l). Calcification of subcutaneous arteries was complicated by widespread infarcts of the anatomically related skin and subcutis, apparently the result of hypoperfusion of these vessels during an episode of septic shock. The infarcts were characterized by blotchy skin discoloration.

Hematological Parenteral nutrition with lipid emulsions is associated with *impaired monocyte and neutrophil functions*. However, in a blind, randomised, crossover study of the effects of long-chain triglycerides and a mixture containing 50% medium-chain triglycerides and 50% long-chain triglycerides in 10 malnourished patients with gastric cancer and 10 matched healthy subjects, there were no effects on ex vivo human neutrophil and monocyte chemotaxis, phagocytosis, bacterial killing, and oxidative metabolism measured by a nitroblue tetrazolium reduction test (22[C]). However, the authors maintained that there should be very few inhibitory effects on phagocytic cells if lipid emulsion rates are kept at around 0.08 g/kg per h.

In preterm infants it has been argued, from in vitro evidence (32[c]), that administration of intralipid may interfere with the binding of IL-2 to specific receptors on activated lymphocytes, with suppression of the immune response. Such interference with IL-2 binding to its specific receptor might account for the greater susceptibility to infections in this age group associated with TPN.

Sea-blue histiocytes have been reported in the bone marrow in seven patients with severe thrombocytopenia receiving long-term TPN for management of extensive small bowel resection (33[c]). All received intravenous fat emulsion (Intralipid 20%) for 3–18 months. Bone marrow biopsy showed sea-blue histiocytes dispersed amongst hemopoietic cells or arranged in aggregates adjacent to osseous lamellae and blood vessels or separated from bone trabeculae. The significance of these histological findings in association with TPN and thrombocytopenia is not known.

A 22-year-old woman receiving long-term TPN for short bowel syndrome presented with *pancytopenia* and hepatosplenomegaly (34[c]). Her bone marrow was infiltrated with sea-blue histiocytes, and cytochemistry confirmed that these were lipid-laden macrophages. The total amount of fat in the regimen was subsequently reduced, and there was partial hematological improvement. In sea-blue histiocytosis macrophages containing intracytoplasmic phospholipid, such as ceroid, lipofuscin, and sphingomyelin, are found in the bone marrow and liver, causing pancytopenia and hepatosplenomegaly. It can develop as a result of abnormal metabolism and accumulation of lipid in macrophages, analogous to Gaucher's disease and Niemann-Pick disease.

The *activation of coagulation* that occurs during TPN is thought to be aggravated by coincidental infection. To test this hypothesis, seven healthy subjects were injected intravenously with endotoxin (2 ng/kg) after 1 week of standard TPN compared with standard enteral feeding (35[c]). Parenteral nutrition was associated with a selectively enhanced activation of the coagulation system (manifested by raised plasma concentrations of thrombin–antithrombin III complexes). Activation of the fibrinolytic system was similar in the groups. The conclusion was that in patients receiving TPN, bacterial infection may facilitate the occurrence of venous thrombosis by synergistic stimulation of the coagulation system.

Cholestasis associated with TPN

Incidence *TPN-associated cholestasis has recently been reviewed (36[R]). It is a major cause of morbidity and mortality in neonates. Although the association of cholestasis with TPN has long been known, little is known of its cause or treatment. There is an inverse relation between the incidence of cholestasis and both gestational age and birth weight. For infants with a birth weight of less than 1000 g the incidence of cholestasis increases considerably. About 50% of infants under 1000 g at birth develop TPN-associated cholestasis, whereas the incidence falls to less than 10% in infants who weigh more than 1500 g. The longer TPN is used in neonates the greater is the risk of cholestasis, and the risk approaches 100% in neonates who receive TPN for more than 8 weeks. Sepsis can also aggravate the risk and severity of cholestasis. There is a higher incidence of cholestasis in neonates who received TPN earlier in life. In one study, TPN-induced liver disease developed in 40–60% of infants who required long-term TPN for intestinal failure (37[R]).*

Pathogenesis *The pathogenesis is multifactorial, and related to prematurity, low birth weight, and duration of TPN. Lack of enteral feeding leads to reduced gut hormone secretion, reduced bile flow, and biliary stasis, all of which may be important mechanisms in the development of cholestasis, biliary sludge, and cholelithiasis. There is no evidence that lipid emulsions themselves cause cholestasis, although excess lipid calorie intake can lead to hepatic steatosis.*

The possible causes of TPN-associated cholestasis include:

(1) a direct toxic effect of TPN solutions (an essential factor missing from the TPN solution; for example, taurine, is needed to solubilize bile salts and which may be necessary for adequate excretion of bile);

(2) lack of enteral stimulation leading to failure of normal hormonal stimulation

in the hepatobiliary tree (cholecystokinin, for example, is needed for both intrahepatic bile flow as well as gallbladder contraction);

(3) lack of enteral feeding, leading to mucosal barrier breakdown causing bacterial translocation, which in turn can lead to an increase in endotoxins, tumor necrosis factor, IL-6 or IL-1β in the portal blood stream, all of which can cause hepatic injury.

Phytosterols have been linked with a high incidence of cholestatic liver disease in infants. Affected infants have high plasma concentrations of phytosterols (compounds that resemble cholesterol but with an alkylated side chain). The phytosterols that accumulate in patients receiving TPN are derived from soya oil and/or soya lecithin used to make the intravenous lipid emulsions. There is a close association between phytosterolemia and cholestatic liver disease. In experiments in neonatal piglets phytosterols given without any other components of TPN reduce bile flow. Increasing the content of phytosterols in cell membranes may interfere with the function of important transport proteins involved in the secretion of bile (38[c]), and the authors proposed that the amount of phytosterols infused in standard TPN regimens is such that the infant's capacity to clear phytosterols by biliary secretion, loss from the skin and gut mucosa and metabolism is exceeded. With increasing duration of TPN there is a steady increase in the phytosterol content of plasma lipoproteins and cell membranes. This affects membrane fluidity and the function of hepatic membrane-bound transport, such as canalicular ATP-dependent bile acid transport and sodium–potassium ATPase. The phytosterols can also inhibit cholesterol 7α-hydroxylase and thereby reduce bile acid synthesis. This contributes to a reduced bile acid pool size and bile acid-dependent bile flow. Phytosterols cannot be metabolized to bile acids and are less soluble in bile than cholesterol. Thus, when biliary acid concentrations are low, they can precipitate, contributing to the characteristic sludge or stones seen in children receiving TPN. Phytosterol-induced changes in the erythrocyte membrane (perhaps coupled with altered macrophage function) lead to accelerated breakdown of erythrocytes and an increased load of bilirubin presented to the liver. Precipitation of bilirubin in the bile contributes to biliary sludge and stones. Phytosterol-induced changes in neutrophil function lead to impaired phagocytosis of bacteria and an increased risk of sepsis; the latter is responsible for further damage to hypatocytes (38).

In an experimental study of TPN-associated cholestasis and the role of plant sterols in neonatal piglets, daily injection of phytosterols led to their progressive accumulation in serum, liver, and bile (39). Serum bile acid concentrations were significantly higher in the sterol-treated piglets and maximal bile acid excretion was lower. Phytosterols caused inhibition of secretory function in isolated rat hepatocyte couplets. Plant sterols appear to act at an early stage of canalicular accumulation, i.e. affecting one or a combination of uptake, transcytosis, and canalicular transport of the cholephile.

In vitro, phytosterols inhibit cholesterol 7α-hydroxylase, the rate-limiting step in bile acid synthesis. This could lead to reduced bile acid-dependent bile flow. Phytosterols can be metabolized to polar bile acids, and these are potentially cholestatic. Phytosterols can bind to sterol carrier proteins, impairing movement of cholesterol, bile acid precursors, and other lipids across the cell. Finally, the similarity in structures between cholesterol and the major plant sterols can lead to substitution of cholesterol in the liver cell membranes by phytosterols, thus interfering with membrane function.

In neonates who are at a high risk of developing TPN-associated cholestasis when receiving a prolonged course of TPN, lack of gastrointestinal hormone formation, including cholecystokinin, may be responsible. In a prospective controlled study patients who received cholecystokinin prophylaxis had direct bilirubin concentrations significantly lower than in the untreated group (40[c]).

Presentation *The clinical manifestations of TPN-associated cholestasis include a progressively rising conjugated bilirubin concentration starting after 2 weeks of TPN. Liver biopsy characteristically shows bile duct proliferation, bile plugs, and congestion. The laboratory and histological findings, although characteristic, are non-specific and can occur with other cholestatic processes. No single test is definitive for the diagnosis, which must be based on a* *process of exclusion of other diseases. The clinical consequences include increased rates of sepsis, cirrhosis, and mortality. Liver failure develops with end-stage cholestasis.*

Pancreas The effects of TPN on endocrine and exocrine functions of the pancreas have been investigated in rats (41). Glucose tolerance after intravenous glucose tolerance testing was unchanged in rats who received TPN for 7 or 14 days, compared with controls. Basal plasma insulin concentrations were slightly lower and the insulin secretory response to intravenous glucose was markedly impaired in the TPN-treated animals at both 7 and 14 days, compared with controls. The weight of pancreas, total content and concentration of pancreatic protein, and total amylase content of the pancreas were lower, whereas the total content of both chymotrypsin and trypsin was higher. The conclusion was that after TPN treatment *the insulin secretory response to glucose is impaired, the exocrine pancreas is hypoplastic, and the storage pattern of pancreatic exocrine enzymes is altered.*

℞ *Effects of TPN on bone*

Metabolic bone disease in children as a result of TPN has recently been thoroughly reviewed (16[R]). It mainly results in osteopenia and occasionally fractures. The cause is multifactorial. Calcium and phosphate deficiency play a major role in the preterm infant, but the part played by aluminium toxicity is unknown in this age group. Lack of reference ranges of bone histomorphometry in premature infants and inadequate reference data for biochemical markers of bone turnover contribute to the uncertainty. Other factors that may play a role in the pathogenesis of bone disease associated with total parenteral nutrition include lack of periodic enteral feeding, underlying intestinal disease (including malabsorption and inflammation), neoplasms, and drug-induced alterations in calcium and bone metabolism.

The mandible and forearm bone mineral content and dental and periodontal state in 15 patients, aged 26–65 years, on home parenteral nutrition for short bowel syndrome, have been compared with findings in healthy subjects (42[C]). Bone mineral content was measured by dual-photon absorptiometry. All patients were eating freely to supplement their parenteral nutrition. There was mandibular osteoporosis in 47%; 33% had osteoporosis in the forearm and radiographic changes of osteoporotic fractures in the vertebral column. The dental and periodontal state did not differ from that of the healthy age-matched population.

There is evidence that TPN itself might adversely affect bone, especially bone density. In adults receiving long-term TPN there is no improvement in bone density, despite the anabolic effects of TPN on other tissues, even though TPN solutions may contain little or no aluminium. Infants treated with TPN from birth develop low bone density for their age, suggesting that TPN in some way contributes directly to osteopenia (16[R]). A 17% long-term increase in spinal bone mineral content has been found in patients who have received TPN solutions without additional vitamin D (43[C]). However, this rise was balanced by a 15% fall in hip bone mineral content. No mention was made in the report of bone mineral density in these patients, and the overall changes in their bone density are uncertain.

Depletion of bone mineral occurs in patients who depend on long-term TPN. However, much of the older information is confounded by the presence of unknown aluminium burdens or by overt aluminium toxicity. Many patients dependent on TPN have metabolic bone disease at the start of therapy. Several factors are likely to influence the magnitude of calcium loss in the urine with TPN infusion, including protein, glucose, and sodium loads, phosphate and base intake, and the infused dose of calcium. In a non-human primate study it was not possible to show a negative calcium balance with the use of TPN in the absence of underlying disease (44). At higher rates of intravenous nutrition support (343 kJ/kg per day, 82 kcal/kg per day, or 46 mmol N/kg per day) there was negative calcium balance in a non-human model. The implication of this is that if TPN contributes directly to the osteopenia that occurs during long-term TPN, it may in selected individuals be due to impairment of the normal regulation of parathyroid hormone and impaired renal tubular handling of calcium.

In general, the question of whether parenteral nutrition adversely affects calcium regulation remains unclear. Human studies are confounded by uncontrolled variables such as how much food is eaten, gut absorption, underlying disease, medications that adversely affect bone (including corticosteroids), and aluminium contamination of parenteral nutrients. In a study in non-human primates that controlled for underlying clinical variables and mobility TPN resulted in weight maintenance and positive nitrogen and calcium balance (45[c]). The net calcium balance was lowest at the beginning of TPN and it improved progressively with time. Calciuria in response to TPN was raised initially, but fell within 2 weeks of the start of therapy; it resulted from an initial increase in urine-filtered calcium. Calcium balance in prolonged TPN was preserved by a reduction in the fraction of calcium filtered by the kidney that was excreted in the urine (45[c]). The conclusion from these experimental findings is that current TPN formulations do not have deleterious effects on bone health.

Cytokines, such as interleukin (IL) 1, IL-6, and tumour necrosis factor-α (TNF-α), influence bone resorption and they have been invoked as a cause of type 1 osteoporosis. TPN in experimental rats enhances the catabolic effect of TNF-α (46). The role of TPN-induced cytokine release or activity, especially of IL-1, IL-6, and TNF-α, in causing hypercalciuria and reduced mineralization in patients receiving TPN needs to be clarified.

A premature infant with necrotizing enterocolitis who needed prolonged administration of TPN sustained a rachitic fracture (47[c]). After high calcium-fortified TPN supplementation the fracture healed well, and serum alkaline phosphatase activity fell. This suggested that during prolonged TPN the mixture should contain higher calcium and phosphorus concentrations in prematurity than in childhood. A rise in serum alkaline phosphatase may imply an impending risk of rachitic fracture.

No effective treatment has been established for aluminium-loaded patients other than identifying the primary source of aluminium contamination and reducing or eliminating it with an appropriate substitute constituent. Prospective studies of serum aluminium concentration and urinary aluminium excretion in children receiving long-term TPN would allow better definition of the extent to which aluminium loading remains a problem (16[R]).

Immunological and hypersensitivity reactions There have been rare cases of severe allergic reactions to parenterally administered lipid solutions. These reactions can be mistaken for symptoms of the underlying disease or the adverse effects of cytostatic chemotherapy (48[c]). In three patients re-exposure to long-chain fatty acids and exposure to medium-chain fatty acids solutions with no soybean lecithin added were well tolerated. The data suggested that traces of soybean proteins were the allergenic agents responsible.

Anaphylaxis has been reported in a 4-year-old child when TPN was resumed after a 5-day interruption in therapy after a prior 16-day treatment following surgery for Wilms' tumour. The authors considered the reaction to have been a type 1 IgE-mediated allergic response, although the causative agent was not identified. It was considered unlikely that individual amino acids had stimulated the allergic response, although the possibility that aggregated amino acids had acted as potential sensitizers could not be excluded. A component of the multivitamin mixture was considered the more likely explanation; the vitamin mixture contained vitamin E for intravenous injection, vitamin K_1, the preservatives butylated hydroxyanisole and butylated hydroxytoluene, and polysorbate emulsifiers (49[c]).

Infections associated with TPN ℞

Bacterial invasion *Enteral nutrition prevents the development of gut barrier failure through several mechanisms. In the first place, it provides an important source of energy to integral parts of cellular membranes, epithelial cells, and organelles in the mucosa. It blocks local submucosal macrophage function, including the transport of adherent and/or invading enteric bacteria to extraintestinal sites, or the production of inflammatory mediators (tumor necrosis factor, interleukins). Finally, it furnishes a mucosal surfactant cover to the* *intestinal mucosal surface, which protects against adherence of enteric microflora to the brush border. Failure of gut endothelial barrier function, as evidenced by an increase in endothelial permeability, resulting in tissue edema and epithelial dysfunction, can lead to bacterial invasion. It is also possible that pathophysiological changes caused by liver resection delay the repair of superficial injuries of the intestinal mucosa. Loss of intestinal mucosal integrity is thought to predispose to bacterial translocation across the intestinal epithelium (50[r]).*

Infecting organisms *In rats there was greater bacterial translocation with parenteral feeding than with enteral feeding in controls. The same happened after partial hepatectomy, with a correspondingly increased risk of sepsis, principally due to E. coli, enterococci, and Klebsiella, and to a lesser degree Proteus mirabilis. It is likely that the normal intestinal flora, especially the strictly anaerobic microflora, which do not readily translocate, function to control intestinal colonization and translocation of potential pathogenic species, such as E. coli and other Enterobacteriaceae, Pseudomonas, and enterococcus species. Significant alterations in the strict anaerobic flora of the gut may potentiate the process of translocation (51[c]).*

Contamination *Since the introduction of TPN in hospital care the potential microbiological risks associated with manufacture, preparation, and administration have fallen but not disappeared (52[r]). Fatal infectious complications still occur. The TPN mixture remains a good growth medium for micro-organisms, more conducive to microbial growth than glucose alone or amino acid solutions. Storage of mixtures allows time for microbial multiplication, often to counts of millions per ml. Even organisms such as Staphylococcus epidermidis and Bacillus species, relatively non-pathogenic in normal circumstances, can multiply in the infusion to such large numbers as to have disastrous effects. Many of these commensal organisms tend to be insensitive to antibiotics. In an open-system aseptic process of preparation the estimated risk of contamination, according to the World Health Organization, is one in 3000. In the UK standards of aseptic compounding are under the statutory control of the National Licensing Authority (the Medicines Control Agency), which has set high environmental requirements for TPN compounding. Microbiological and environmental quality control assurance need to be assured.*

Catheter-mediated infections *The average rate of episodes of catheter-related bacteremia in patients receiving TPN is 3–5%. Higher rates have been reported during long-term therapy. Patients with nosocomial infection have an 11-fold higher risk of acquiring an additional nosocomial infection compared with those with no infection. Prompt removal of the catheter and targeted antimicrobial treatment remains the standard approach for febrile episodes in these circumstances. However, many catheter-related infections caused by coagulase-negative staphylococci can be successfully treated with the catheter still in place. Commonly isolated organisms from TPN solutions are coagulase-negative staphylococci, Staphylococcus aureus, Candida species. Serratia species, and Enterobacter species. Infection with Malassezia furfur is a rare but serious complication strongly associated with TPN in young children. Candida infection is a particular problem in patients receiving TPN (53[R]).*

Risk factors *Independent risk factors have been determined for nosocomial coagulase-negative staphylococcal bacteremia in very low birth weight neonates, after adjusting for severity of the underlying disease in 590 consecutively admitted neonates with birth weights less than 1500 g (54[C]). Two procedures were independently associated with a subsequent risk of coagulase-negative staphylococcal bacteremia: intravenous lipids and any surgical or percutaneously placed central venous catheter. Of the cases of bacteremia reviewed 85% were attributable to lipid therapy. By contrast, the relative importance of intravenous catheters as independent risk factors has fallen over the last 10 years.*

Malassezia furfur is an emerging systemic pathogen in neonates receiving intravenous lipid emulsions, judging by more than 50 case reports. However, a recent systematic study of M. furfur in 928 study samples did not show a single positive culture, suggesting that the risk of M. furfur to hospitalized patients may be less than was previously thought. The findings do not support routine inclusion of special cul-

tures for M. furfur in skin site surveillance programs among hospitalized patients receiving TPN (55[C]).

Of 378 children in Taipei, who received TPN for a total of 6562 patient days over a 20-month period, 56 developed clinical sepsis and positive blood cultures (56[C]). Significant features in those with sepsis included longer duration of TPN, age under 3 months, use of central venous catheters, gastrointestinal disease as an indication for TPN, low birth weight, and a short gestational age in prematurity. The authors concluded that considering the high incidence of sepsis during TPN every attempt should be made to minimize the duration of TPN therapy and to encourage early enteral feeding.

Miscellaneous Two adult cases of local extravasation of TPN fluid have been reported (57[c]). Both patients developed an *intense inflammatory reaction* that was successfully controlled with repeated local administration of the hyaluronidase analog chondroitin sulfatase. Although the exact mechanism of tissue damage by extravasated TPN is not understood, it is probably related to osmolarity, pH, and ion concentrations. In children the effects of extravasation can be devastating. Special care should be taken when high-osmolarity (1000–1700 mOsm/l) peripheral TPN is given, as fluids of this osmolarity are likely to cause severe tissue damage if they extravasate. In general, fluid osmolarity should not exceed 600–900 mOsm/l, to minimize the risk of this complication. The position of the catheter needs to be checked regularly.

Use in pregnancy Maternal and embryo/fetal toxicity have been assessed in rats and rabbits given a 20% lipid solution containing medium-chain triglycerides and a long-chain lipid emulsion in a ratio of 3:1, with once daily intravenous administration during organogenesis (58). There were no adverse effects in fetal rats, even in the presence of maternal toxicity. However, there were embryo and fetal toxicity (resorptions) and skeletal abnormalities in rabbits. The authors considered that these adverse fetal effects were probably the result of dietary deprivation, maternal toxicity, or both, rather than direct teratogenic effects.

Interactions *Warfarin* resistance developed in a 39-year-old woman with severe Crohn's disease during high-dose infusion of propofol, which contains 10% emulsified soybean oil (59[c]). Despite an increase in dosage of warfarin to 30 mg/day, anticoagulation was not achieved until propofol was withdrawn. Lipid emulsions may interfere pharmacodynamically with warfarin activity by enhancing the production of clotting factors, facilitating platelet aggregation, or supplying vitamin K. They also enhance warfarin binding to albumin. The authors recommended that until further information about the mechanism of interference is elucidated, heparin should be considered for initial anticoagulation in patients with intestinal absorptive deficiencies who receive high-dose lipid emulsions and require reliable anticoagulation. If warfarin is used, the INR should be monitored daily to ensure adequate anticoagulation.

DIALYSIS FLUIDS

Adverse effects of peritoneal dialysis fluids on the peritoneum

R

Giant and atypical mesothelial cells can develop in response to irritation caused by peritoneal dialysis solutions. Mesothelial hyperplasia without an increase in mesothelial cell size, cytological atypia in mesothelial cells, polynucleate cells with nucleoles, and enlarged mesothelial cells with a flat small nucleus and without evident nucleoles have been described (60[Cr]). In a study of 22 patients who had been on chronic ambulatory peritoneal dialysis for at least 6 months, the mesothelial cells were studied morphologically and characterized histochemically. Giant mesothelial cells with evident nuclei or multiple nuclei were found, probably in association with the stimulating effect of peritoneal dialysis solutions on mesothelial cell turnover. Besides an acceleration of mesothelial replication, the chemical and physical stress of peritoneal dialysis could also cause cytological changes. These giant cells are not found unless there is peritonitis. During peritonitis mesothelial cells detach en masse from the basal lamina. These alterations in mesothelial cells are not associated with an increased risk of malignant transformation.

Continual exposure of the peritoneum over a period of years to conventional peritoneal dialysis fluids contributes to loss of membrane function in two ways: (i) by compromising peritoneal host defense mediated by resident and infiltrating leukocytes and the resident cells of the peritoneal membrane; (ii) by directly contributing to structural changes in the peritoneal membrane (61[R]). Peritoneal dialysis fluids have significant modulatory, and in some cases toxic, effects on peripheral and peritoneal cell functions. The impact of long-term exposure of the peritoneum to peritoneal dialysis fluids, and how its function as a dialysing organ is affected, are less well understood. From a comprehensive review of the literature it has emerged that lactate-buffered peritoneal dialysis fluids inhibit many leukocyte and peritoneal cell functions, even when exposure times are short. This suggests the need for more biocompatible peritoneal dialysis fluids. Neutral pH bicarbonate- or bicarbonate/lactate-buffered fluids are superior in all test systems to lactate-buffered fluids, irrespective of the concentration of glucose in the solution. The cell inhibitory and stimulatory effects of high glucose remain, and this issue will have to be addressed before the perfect biocompatible alternative is produced. It is not clear whether the long-term use of bicarbonate-containing fluids will improve patient outcome by reducing infection rates and better preserving the integrity of the peritoneal membrane.

The adverse effects of peritoneal dialysis fluids on the peritoneum have been succinctly summarized as part of the argument that a new, less toxic, and less acidic fluid is required for peritoneal dialysis (62[r]). A low pH, high osmolality, high lactate concentration, and the presence of several toxic contaminants may all contribute to impaired cellular function in the peritoneal membrane. In conventional peritoneal dialysis the pH is deliberately lowered to 5.0–5.6 in order to prevent caramelization of the glucose (i.e., the production of glucose degradation products) during heat sterilization and storage. Low pH, especially in combination with tissue fluid hyperosmolality and high lactate concentrations, will cause vasodilatation and recruitment of capillaries in microvascular beds. In the peritoneal membrane, acidic solutions cause an increased 'effective' vascular surface area and a more rapid loss of glucose gradient than a neutral solution. Thus, a neutral solution would theoretically behave more favorably with regard to transperitoneal ultrafiltration (glucose-induced osmosis) than a conventional acidic solution. This is because the glucose osmotic gradient will be better preserved over time with neutral solutions. Even neutralized peritoneal dialysis solutions seem to be cytotoxic in vitro. This cytotoxicity is related less to hyperosmolality and the presence of lactate in the fluid than the toxicity that occurs at a low pH. Glucose degradation products formed during heat sterilization and storage include acetaldehyde, methylglyoxal, 2-furaldehyde, formaldehyde, 5-hydroxymethylfurfural, and formic acid. All may, in the long term, affect the peritoneum adversely and lead to a deterioration of peritoneal membrane function. The risk of losing ultrafiltration capacity after 6 years of continuous ambulatory peritoneal dialysis is as high as 31%. Glucose degradation products can also cause abdominal discomfort and pain, and may be responsible for acute losses in ultrafiltration capacity.

In a review of the infectious complications of peritoneal dialysis (63[r]) it was confirmed that peritonitis contributes to death in 5% of peritoneal dialysis patients. The common organisms causing peritonitis are Staphylococcus epidermidis, Staphylococcus aureus, streptococci, Gram-negative bacilli, and fungi. Predisposing factors are exit-site infections leading to tunnel infections, catheter infections, and nasal carriage S. aureus which is associated with exit-site and tunnel infections and peritonitis. Coagulase-negative staphylococci are often resistant to methicillin, and methicillin-resistant S. aureus was the cause of 13% of all episodes of peritonitis, and in one study for 30% of catheter infections (63[r]). Vancomycin is required for treatment (but not prophylaxis) of such cases.

Icodextrin

Icodextrin is a maltodextrin glucose polymer with a mean molecular weight of 20 kDa.

It is broken down to maltose and is increasingly being used as an alternative to glucose as the active osmotic agent for peritoneal dialysis. Icodextrin is similar in structure to dextran. It has improved ultrafiltration properties owing to reduced absorption of icodextrin compared with glucose.

Skin and appendages Severe *cutaneous hypersensitivity* has been reported with icodextrin (45[c]).

A 48-year-old woman with a long history of insulin-dependent diabetes mellitus developed a maculopapular rash 10 days after changing to 7.5% icodextrin in order to improve ultrafiltration. The rash affected most parts of her body and was associated with severe pruritus. By 13 days it had become exfoliative and erythrodermic. There was rapid improvement in the first few days after the icodextrin dialysate was stopped and she reverted to conventional glucose peritoneal dialysate.

Hypersensitivity to icodextrin was the most likely explanation for the severe skin reaction. The epitope(s) for allergic reactions to dextrans have not been identified, although they are undoubtedly immunogenic. It is possible that the same or a similar epitope is responsible for hypersensitivity to icodextrin.

CATHETERS

A preterm infant developed *acute focal lung edema* due to central venous catheter migration into the right pulmonary vein (64[c]). The substances aspirated from the endotracheal tube contained TPN fluid. After the catheter was withdrawn into the right atrium recovery was quick and uncomplicated.

REFERENCES

1. Ellingson TL, Aboulafia DM. Dextran syndrome: acute hypotension, noncardiogenic pulmonary edema, anemia, and coagulopathy following hysteroscoopic surgery using 32% dextran 70. Chest 1997;111:513–18.
2. Warren BB, Durieux ME. Hydroxyethyl starch: safe or not? Anesth Analg 1997;84:206–12.
3. Treib J, Haass A, Pindur G, Grauer MT, Jung F, Wenzel E, Schimrigk K. Increased hemorrhagic risk after repeated infusion of highly substituted medium molecular weight hydroxyethyl starch. Arzneim Forsch Drug Res 1997;47:18–22.
4. Baldassarre S, Vincent J-L. Coagulopathy induced by hydroxyethyl starch. Anesth Analg 1997;84:451–3.
5. Cope JT, Banks D, Mauney MC, Lucktong T, Shockey KS, Kron IL, Tribble CG. Intraoperative hetastarch infusion impairs hemostasis after cardiac operations. Ann Thorac Surg 1997;63:78–83.
6. Treib J, Haass A. Hydroxyethyl starch. J Neurosurg 1997;86:574–5.
7. Dehne MG, Muhling J, Sablotzki A, Papke G, Kuntzsch U, Hempelman G. Effect of hydroxyethyl starch solution on kidney function in surgical intensive care patients. Anasthesiol Intensivmed Notfallmed Schmerzther 1997;32:348–54.
8. Biesenbach G, Kaiser W, Zazgornik J. Incidence of acute oligoanuric renal failure in dextran 40 treated patients with acute ischemic stroke stage III or IV. Renal Fail 1997;19:69–75.
9. Ferraboli R, Malheiro PS, Abdulkader RCRM, Yu L, Sabbaga E, Burdmann EA. Anuric acute renal failure caused by dextran 40 administration. Renal Fail 1997;19:303–6.
10. Holzheimer R. Hydroxyethylstarch and renal function in kidney transplant recipients. Lancet 1997;349:883–4.
11. Coronel B, Mercatello A, Martin X, Lefrancois N. Hydroxyethylstarch and renal function in kidney transplant recipients. Lancet 1997; 349:884.
12. Cittanova ML, Legendre C. Hydroxyethylstarch and renal function in kidney transplant recipients. Lancet 1997;349:884.
13. Cittanova M, Leblanc I, Legendre C, Mouquet C, Riou B, Coriat P. Effect of hydroxyethylstarch in brain-dead kidney donors on renal function in kidney-transplant recipients. Lancet 1996;348:1620–2.
14. Speight EL, MacSween RM, Stevens A. Persistent itching due to etherified starch plasma expander. Br Med J 1997;314:1466–7.
15. Metze D, Reimann S, Szepfalusi Z, Bohle B, Kraft D, Luger TA. Persistent pruritus after hydroxyethyl starch infusion therapy: a result of long-term storage in cutaneous nerves. Br J Dermatol 1997;136:553–9.
16. Klein GL. Metabolic bone disease of total parenteral nutrition. Nutrition 1998;14:149–52.
17. Kane KF, Lowes JR. Peripheral parenteral nutrition and venous thrombophlebitis. Nutrition 1997;13:577–8.
18. Shay DK, Fann LM, Jarvis WR, and the Hospital Infections Program, Centers for Disease Control and Prevention. Respiratory distress and sudden death associated with receipt of a peri-

pheral parenteral nutrition admixture. Infect Control Hosp Epidemiol 1997;18:814–17.
19. Waldhausen E, Mingers B, Lippers P, Keser G. Critical illness polyneuropathy due to parenteral nutrition. Intensive Care Med 1997; 23:922–3.
20. Berek K, Margreiter J, Willeit J, Berek A, Schmutzhard E, Mutz N. Critical illness polyneuropathy—only due to parenteral nutrition? Intensive Care Med 1997;23:923–4.
21. Bolton CF, Young GB. Critical illness polyneuropathy due to parenteral nutrition. Intensive Care Med 1997;23:924–5.
22. Waitzberg DL, Bellinati-Pires R, Salgado MM, Hypolito IP, Colleto GMDD, Yagi O, Yamamuro EM, Gama-Rodrigues J, Pinotti HW. Effect of total parenteral nutrition with different lipid emulsions on human monocyte and neutrophil functions. Nutrition 1997;13:128–32.
23. Bohlega S, McLean DR. Hemiplegia caused by inadvertent intra-carotid infusion of total parenteral nutrition. Clin Neurol Neurosurg 1997;99:217–19.
24. Moens NMM, Remedios AM. Hyperosmolar hyperglycaemic syndrome in a dog resulting from parenteral nutrition overload. J Small Anim Pract 1997;38:417–20.
25. Suzuki S, Kumanomido T, Nagata E, Inoue J, Niikawa O. Optic neuropathy from thiamine deficiency. Intern Med 1997;36:532.
26. Kitamura K, Yamaguchi T, Tanaka H, Hashimoto S, Yang M, Takahashi T. TPN-induced fulminant beriberi: a report on our experience and a review of the literature. Surg Today 1996;26:769–76.
27. Nakasaki H, Ohta M, Soeda J, Makuuchi H, Tsuda M, Tajima T, Mitomi T, Fujii K. Clinical and biochemical aspects of thiamine treatment for metabolic acidosis during total parenteral nutrition. Nutrition 1997;13:110–17.
28. Hager L. Choline deficiency and TPN associated liver dysfunction: a case report. Nutrition 1998;14:60–2.
29. Shronts EP. Essential nature of choline with implications for total parenteral nutrition. J Am Diet Assoc 1997;97:639–46, 649.
30. Alves G, Thiebot J, Tracqui A, Delangre T, Guedon C, Lerebours E. Neurologic disorders due to brain manganese deposition in a jaundiced patient receiving long-term parenteral nutrition. J Parenter Enter Nutr 1997;21:41–5.
31. Janigan DT, Perey B, Marrie TJ, Chiasson PM, Hirsch D. Skin necrosis: an unusual complication of hyperphosphatemia during total parenteral nutrition therapy. J Parenter Enter Nutr 1997;21:50–2.
32. Sirota L, Straussberg R, Notti I, Bessler H. Effect of lipid emulsion on IL-2 production by mononuclear cells of newborn infants and adults. Acta Paediatr Int J Paediatr 1997;86:410–13.
33. Maier-Redelsperger M, Girot R. Sea-blue histiocytes in bone-marrow due to a long-term total parenteral nutrition including fat-emulsions. Br J Haematol 1997;97:685–92.
34. Meiklejohn DJ, Baden H, Greaves M. Sea-blue histiocytosis and pancytopaenia associated with chronic total parenteral nutrition administration. Clin Lab Haematol 1997;19:219–21.
35. Van Der Poll T, Levi M, Braxton CC, Coyle SM, Roth M, Ten Cate JW, Lowry SF. Parenteral nutrition facilitates activation of coagulation but not of fibrinolysis during human endotoxemia. J Infect Dis 1998;177:793–5.
36. Teitelbaum DH. Parenteral nutrition-associated cholestasis. Curr Opin Pediatr 1997;9:270–5.
37. Kelly DA. Liver complications of pediatric parenteral nutrition-epidemiology. Nutrition 1998;14:153–7.
38. Clayton PT, Whitfield P, Iyer K. The role of phytosterols in the pathogenesis of liver complications of pediatric parenteral nutrition. Nutrition 1998;14:158–64.
39. Iyer KR, Spitz L, Clayton P. New insight into mechanisms of parenteral nutrition-associated cholestasis: role of plant sterols. J Pediatr Surg 1998;33:1–6.
40. Teitelbaum DH, Han-Markey T, Drongowski RA, Coran AG, Bayar B, Geiger JD, Uitvlugt N, Schork MA. Use of cholecystokinin to prevent the development of parenteral nutrition-associated cholestasis. J Parenter Enter Nutr 1997;21:100–3.
41. Fan BG, Salehi A, Sternby B, Axelson J, Lundquist I, Andren-Sandberg A, Ekelund M. Total parenteral nutrition influences both endocrine and exocrine function of rat pancreas. Pancreas 1997;15:147–53.
42. Von Wowern SN, Klausen B, Moller EH. Bone loss and oral health status in patients on home parenteral nutrition. Ugeskr Laeger 1997; 159:4982–5.
43. Verhage AH, Cheong WK, Allard JP, Jeejeebhoy KN. Increase in lumbar spine bone mineral content in patients on long-term parenteral nutrition without vitamin D supplementation. J Parenter Enter Nutr 1995;19:431–6.
44. Lipkin EW. A longitudinal study of calcium regulation in a nonhuman primate model of parenteral nutrition. Am J Clin Nutr 1998;67:246–54.
45. Lam-Po-Tang MKL, Bending MR, Kwan JTC. Icodextrin hypersensitivity in a CAPD patient. Peritoneal Dial Int 1997;17:82–4.
46. Jeejeebhoy KN. Metabolic bone disease and total parenteral nutrition: a progress report. Am J Clin Nutr 1998;67:186–7.
47. Tsai JR, Yang PH. Rickets of premature infants induced by calcium deficiency: a case report. Chang Keng I Hsueh 1997;20:142–7.
48. Weidmann B, Lepique C, Heider A, Schmitz A, Niederle N. Hypersensitivity reactions to parenteral lipid solutions. Supportive Care Cancer 1997;5:504–5.
49. Market AD, Lew DB, Schropp KP, Hak EB. Parenteral nutrition-associated anaphylaxis in a 4-year-old child. J Pediatr Gastroenterol Nutr 1998;26:229–31.

50. Andersson R, Wang X. Experimental hepatectomy: the effect on the intestine and influence of various supplements. Nutrition 1997;13: 473–4.
51. Jian-Guang-Qiu JG, Delany HM, Teh EL, Freundlich L, Gliedman ML, Steinberg JJ, Chee-Jen-Chang, Levenson SM. Contrasting effects of identical nutrients given parenterally or enterally after 70% hepatectomy: bacterial translocation. Nutrition 1997;13:431–7.
52. Allwood MC. Microbiological risks in parenteral nutrition compounding. Nutrition 1997; 13:60–1.
53. Widmer AF Management of catheter-related bacteremia and fungemia in patients on total parenteral nutrition. Nutrition 1997;13 Suppl 4:18S-25S.
54. Avila-Figueroa C, Goldmann DA, Richardson DK, Gray JE, Ferrari A, Freeman J. Intravenous lipid emulsions are the major determinant of coagulase-negative staphylococcal bacteremia in very low birth weight newborns. Pediatr Infect Dis J 1998;17:10–17.
55. Jatoi A, Hanjosten K, Ross E, Mason JB. A prospective survey for central line skin-site colonization by the pathogen *Malassezia furfur* among hospitalized adults receiving total parenteral nutrition. J Parenter Enter Nutr 1997;21:230–2.
56. Yeung CY, Lee HC, Huang FY, Wang CS. Sepsis during total parenteral nutrition: exploration of risk factors and determination of the effectiveness of peripherally inserted central venous catheters. Pediatr Infect Dis J 1998;17:135–42.
57. Gil ME, Mateu J. Treatment of extravasation from parenteral nutrition solution. Ann Pharmacother 1998;32:51–5.
58. Henwood S, Wilson D, White R, Trimbo S. Developmental toxicity study in rats and rabbits administered an emulsion containing medium chain triglycerides as an alternative caloric source. Fundam Appl Toxicol 1997;40:185–90.
59. MacLaren R, Wachsman BA, Swift DK, Kuhl DA. Warfarin resistance associated with intravenous lipid administration: discussion of propofol and review of the literature. Pharmacotherapy 1997;17:1331–7.
60. Di Paolo N, Garosi G, Monaci G, Brardi S. Biocompatibility of peritoneal dialysis treatment. Nephrol Dial Transplant 1997;12 Suppl 1:78–83.
61. Jorres A, Williams JD, Topley N. Peritoneal dialysis solution biocompatibility: inhibitory mechanisms and recent studies with bicarbonate-buffered solutions. Peritoneal Dial Int 1997;17 (Suppl 2):S42–6.
62. Rippe B, Simonsen O, Wieslander A, Landgren C. Clinical and physiological effects of a new, less toxic and less acidic fluid for peritoneal dialysis. Peritoneal Dial Int 1997;17:27–34.
63. Piraino B. Infectious complications of peritoneal dialysis. Perit Dial Int 1997;17 (Suppl 3):S15–8.
64. Yeoh HA, Chou YH, Wong HF. Migration of a central venous catheter into pulmonary vein complicated with lung edema in a premature infant. Acta Paediatr Sin 1997;38:303–5.

K. Peerlinck and J. Vermylen

35 Drugs affecting blood coagulation, fibrinolysis, and hemostasis

COUMARIN CONGENERS

(SED-13, 1033; SEDA-19, 321; SEDA-20, 312; SEDA-21, 358)

Warfarin treatment of deep vein thrombosis is a possible cause of *venous limb gangrene* in patients with heparin-induced thrombocytopenia, perhaps because of acquired failure of the protein C anticoagulant pathway to regulate thrombin generation (1[C]).

In three patients mutations in the factor IX propeptide were found to cause severe *bleeding* during coumarin therapy, despite therapeutic ranges of the prothrombin time and International Normalized Ratio (INR). In all three cases coumarin treatment caused an unusually selective reduction in factor IX activity, and analysis of the factor IX gene showed mis-sense mutations in the factor IX propeptide at a position that is essential for the carboxylase recognition site. In coumarin-treated patients with an uncommon bleeding pattern, determination of activated partial thromboplastin time and factor IX, in addition to the prothrombin time and INR, is recommended (2[C]).

HEPARINS *(SED-13, 1028; SEDA-19, 322; SEDA-20, 313; SEDA-21, 358)*

Hematological The incidence and major risk factors of *bleeding complications* in patients admitted to a cardiology service and treated with intravenous heparin have been studied in 416 consecutive patients (3[C]). There were 23 hemorrhagic complications in 21 heparin-treated patients (5.5%); 12 of these were directly related to a vascular access site and 11 were spontaneous. There was no apparent relation between the dose or duration of heparin therapy and hemorrhagic complications. In a multivariate analysis, female sex, recent thrombolytic therapy, and a reduced hemoglobin concentration on admission were significantly predictive of a hemorrhagic event.

Skin and appendages *Skin necrosis* has been attributed to enoxaparin (4[c]).

A 43-year-old woman who had first developed localized skin necrosis and thrombocytopenia (with a positive serotonin release test) secondary to subcutaneous administration of unfractionated heparin, developed skin necrosis at injection sites during subsequent enoxaparin therapy, although her platelet counts remained stable.

The authors advised against the use of low-molecular weight heparins in patients with a previous history of heparin-associated thrombocytopenia or heparin-induced skin necrosis.

Mineral and fluid balance There were significant *increases in serum potassium* in 116 patients treated with a prophylactic dose (3075 U) of nadroparin subcutaneously (5[C]). Hypoaldosteronism and hyperkalemia caused by unfractionated heparin (6[R]) and high doses of low-molecular weight heparins have been documented (7[C]). The authors concluded that even the lowest dose of nadroparin increases serum potassium concentration and recommended measurement of the serum potassium during the administration of low-molecular weight heparin in patients with potassium con-

Side Effects of Drugs, Annual 22
J.K. Aronson, ed.

centrations over 5 mmol/l. In an 86-year-old woman with impaired renal function the serum potassium increased from 4.3 to 6.1 mmol/l during treatment with low-dose (20 mg) enoxaparin (8[c]).

DRUGS THAT ALTER PLATELET FUNCTION

Abciximab *(SED-13, 1039; SEDA-21, 359)*

Four of 744 patients treated with abciximab at a single center developed acute profound *thrombocytopenia* within 11–26 h after treatment (9[C]). Platelet counts responded to platelet transfusion in each patient. Platelet counts remained depressed for at least 3 days but returned to baseline within 2 weeks.

Dipyridamole *(SED-13, 1466)*

Radionuclide scanning is being increasingly used to assess myocardial perfusion, and dipyridamole is the most commonly used stress agent.

Cardiovascular Two cases of *asystole* have been reported in patients being given intravenous dipyridamole (10[r]).

Respiratory There have been several incidents of acute bronchospasm in asthmatic patients given intravenous dipyridamole. Now there has been a report of *respiratory arrest* in a patient with emphysema (11[c]).

A 59-year-old woman with a recent anterior myocardial infarction was referred for a dipyridamole–tetrofosmin myocardial perfusion scan. Previous pulmonary function testing had shown severe emphysema with no reversibility after inhaled bronchodilators. About half way through the administration of intravenous dipyridamole (0.56 mg/kg over 4 min) and before the injection of the radioisotope, her breathing became erratic and her level of consciousness fell. The infusion was terminated, but she deteriorated rapidly and had an acute respiratory arrest. She was resuscitated and recovered spontaneous respiration without requiring endotracheal intubation.

Biliary An 85-year-old patient developed recurrence of dipyridamole-containing *gallstones* 18 months after endoscopic removal of a gallstone and sphincterotomy (12[c]). Physicochemical analysis of the gallstones showed the presence of dipyridamole, representing 15% of the dry weight in the first stone and 35% in the second stone. The authors had previously identified dipyridamole in biliary stones from nine patients.

Ticlopidine *(SED-13, 1039; SEDA-19, 323; SEDA-20, 314; SEDA-21; 359)*

Hematological complications, especially neutropenia, are well known during treatment with ticlopidine. Three Chinese patients with ticlopidine-induced *aplastic anemia* have been reported and 13 other cases reviewed (13[cr]). Older patients seem to be especially at risk of this complication (all but one patient were over 60 years) and mortality was high (six out of 16).

ANTIFIBRINOLYTIC DRUGS

Aprotinin *(SED-13, 1060; SEDA-20, 314; SEDA-21, 359)*

The frequency of *anaphylactic reactions* on re-exposure to high-dose aprotinin has been studied in 240 patients with 248 re-exposures. There were seven adverse reactions to aprotinin. The risk was greater in patients in whom the previous exposure had occurred less than 6 months before (14[C]).

THROMBOLYTIC DRUGS

(SED-13, 1035; SEDA-19, 323; SEDA-20, 314; SEDA-21, 359)

The frequency of *intracranial hemorrhage* among 312 patients undergoing thrombolysis for pulmonary embolism was 1.9% (six of 312) (15[C]). Two of six intracranial hemorrhages were fatal. Diastolic hypertension was a risk factor, as was pre-existing intracranial disease.

In the NINDS tPA Stroke Trial, intravenous rtPA was given to 312 stroke patients within 3 h of onset; it increased the absolute risk of symptomatic intracerebral hemorrhage by 6%, but was associated with a reduction in the absolute risk of 3-month mortality of 4% compared with placebo-treated patients (16[C]). The variables that were independently associated with an increased risk of symptomatic intracerebral hemorrhage were the severity of neurological deficit and brain edema or mass effect on CT scan before treatment.

REFERENCES

1. Warkentin TE, Elavathil LJ, Hayward CPM, Johnson MA, Russett JI, Kelton JG. The pathogenesis of venous limb gangrene associated with heparin-induced thrombocytopenia. Ann Intern Med 1997;127:804–12.
2. Oldenburg J, Quenzel E-M, Harbrecht U, Fregin A, Kress W, MHller CR, Hertfelder H-J, Schwaab R, Brackmann H-H, Hanfland P. Missense mutations at ALA-10 in the factor IX propeptide: an insignificant variant in normal life but a decisive cause of bleeding during oral anticoagulant therapy. Br J Haematol 1997;98:240–4.
3. Juergens CP, Semsarian C, Keech AC, Beller EM, Harris PJ. Hemorrhagic complications of intravenous heparin use. Am J Cardiol 1997; 80:150–4.
4. Tonn ME, Schaiff RA, Kollef MH. Enoxaparin-associated dermal necrosis: a consequence of cross-reactivity with heparin-mediated antibodies. Ann Pharmacother 1997;31:323–6.
5. Canova CR, Fischler MP, Reinhart WH. Effect of low-molecular-weight heparin on serum potassium. Lancet 1997;349:1447–8.
6. Oates JA, Wood AJJ. Heparin. New Engl J Med 1991;324:1565–74.
7. Levesque H, Verdier S, Cailleux N, Elie-Legrand MC, Gancel A, Basuyau JP, Borg JY, Moore N, Courtois H. Low molecular-weight heparins and hypoaldosteronism. Br Med J 1990;300:1437–8.
8. Longhurst JG. Mania. Lancet 1997;350:292.
9. Berkowitz SD, Harrington RA, Rund MM, Tcheng JE. Acute profound thrombocytopenia after c7E3 Fab (abciximab) therapy. Circulation 1997;95:809–13.
10. Frossard M, Weiss K, Gossinger H, Zeiner A, Leitha T. Asystole during dipyridamole infusion in patients without coronary artery disease or beta-blocker therapy. Clin Nucl Med 1997;22:97–100.
11. Hillis GS, Al-Mohammed A, Jennings KP. Respiratory arrest during dipyridamole stress testing. Postgrad Med J 1997;73:301–2.
12. Sautereau D, Moesch C, Letard J-C, Cessot F, Gainant A, Pillegand B. Recurrence of biliary drug lithiasis due to dipyridamole. Endoscopy 1997;29:421–3.
13. Kao T-W, Hung C-C, Chen Y-C, Tien H-F. Ticlopidine-induced aplastic anemia: report of three Chinese patients and review of the literature. Acta Haematol 1997;98:211–13.
14. Dietrich W, Späth P, Ebell A, Richter JA. Prevalence of anaphylactic reactions to aprotinin: analysis of two hundred forty-eight reexposures to aprotinin in heart operations. J Thorac Cardiovasc Surg 1997;113:194–201.
15. Kanter DS, Mikkola M, Patel SR, Parker JA, Goldhaber SZ. Thrombolytic therapy for pulmonary embolism. Frequency of intracranial hemorrhage and associated risk factors. Chest 1997; 111:1241–5.
16. The NINDS t-PA Stroke Study Group. Intracerebral hemorrhage after intravenous t-PA therapy for ischemic stroke. Stroke 1997;28:2109–18.

H.J. de Silva

36 Gastrointestinal drugs

ANTIEMETICS

Cisapride *(SED-13, 1067; SEDA-19, 325; SEDA-20, 316; SEDA-21, 361)*

The use of cisapride in patients in intensive care has been reviewed (1[R]). Adverse effects are rare and are unlikely to be apparent in most patients. Those reported include *abdominal cramps*, *diarrhea*, *headache*, *dystonic reactions*, *convulsions*, and *hypersensitivity*.

Cisapride in dosages of 10 mg qds and 20 mg bd were equally effective and safe in the treatment of reflux esophagitis (2[c]). About 20% of patient arms had adverse effects, in reducing order of frequency: *diarrhea*, *abdominal pain*, and *constipation*. In a randomized, double-blind, placebo-controlled study of 535 patients, cisapride in dosages of 20 mg bd or 20 mg at night had no benefit over placebo in maintaining symptomatic remission in patients with gastro-esophageal reflux disease who were initially made symptom-free with potent antisecretory drugs (3[c]). Cisapride 20 mg bd caused significantly more adverse effects than placebo, including *diarrhea*, *constipation*, *abdominal pain*, and *flatulence*. In another randomized double-blind study in 70 patients, cisapride 10 mg qds was effective in the treatment of non-specific esophageal motility disorders (4[C]). *Loose stools* (6%) and *borborygmi* (4%) were common.

Interactions Faster rates of gastric emptying can cause reduced absorption of drugs from the stomach and increase the rate of absorption from the small intestine; for example, increased absorption of *morphine*, *diazepam*, and *cimetidine* (1[R]). Cisapride also accelerates the absorption of a new broad-spectrum aminofluoroquinolone, *sparfloxacin*, but without a significant effect on the extent of systemic availability (in contrast sucralfate caused a 44% reduction in the availability of sparfloxacin) (5[C]).

Several drugs, such as *ketoconazole*, *itraconazole*, *miconazole*, *erythromycin*, and *clarithromycin*, inhibit the metabolism of cisapride by inhibiting CYP3A4, causing a marked increase in plasma cisapride concentrations, which can lead to abnormal cardiac conduction, especially prolongation of the QT_c interval, which is probably mediated via 5-HT4 receptors in the atria and sinoatrial node (1[R]).

Two cases of cisapride cardiotoxicity in association with *erythromycin* have been reported (6[c]). In both there was prolongation of the QTc interval and one developed runs of torsade de pointes. These changes resolved completely on withdrawal.

Risk factors Cisapride should also be used with caution in patients with severe *cardiac disease* or other risk factors for developing dysrhythmias, particularly *hypokalemia* and *hypomagnesemia* (1[R]). Its safety in *pregnancy* has still not been ascertained. Cisapride should not be given to patients with *intestinal obstruction*, *perforation*, or *hemorrhage*.

Domperidone *(SED-13, 1069)*

The effects of chronic oral domperidone on gastrointestinal symptoms and gastric emptying have been assessed in 11 patients with Parkinson's disease (7[C]) and 17 patients with gastroparesis of various causes (8[C]). Domperidone reduced symptoms and accelerated gastric emptying in both studies. Among the 11 patients with Parkinson's disease who took domperidone for an average of 3 years, one had nipple tenderness. Serum prolactin concentrations were raised in all patients after 2 weeks of treatment. Among the patients with gastroparesis, who took domperidone for 4

Side Effects of Drugs, Annual 22
J.K. Aronson, ed.

years, three developed *gynecomastia*, and the serum prolactin concentrations were again increased in all patients.

Metoclopramide *(SED-13, 1069; SEDA-20, 316)*

In adults metoclopramide has been reported to cause *gynecomastia* and *galactorrhea* due to hyperprolactinemia secondary to its dopamine antagonist action. A male neonate with gynecomastia and galactorrhea after 3 weeks of metoclopramide therapy, and a 18-year-old boy on long-term metoclopramide who developed asymmetrical gynecomastia have been described (9[c]). In both cases withdrawal of the drug led to normalization of serum prolactin concentrations and resolution of gynecomastia. There has also been a report of a 16-year-old girl who developed an acute dystonic reaction followed by respiratory arrest after a single dose of metoclopramide 10 mg intravenously (10[c]).

5-HT$_3$ receptor antagonists *(SED-13, 1070; SEDA-19, 325; SEDA-20, 316)*

A randomized double-blind trial has shown that the addition of metopimazine, a dopamine receptor antagonist, increased the efficacy of a combination of ondansetron and methylprednisolone in controlling vomiting in patients receiving cisplatin-based chemotherapy (11[c]). There were no serious adverse effects. Minor adverse effects attributable to therapy included *abdominal pain*, *constipation*, and *headache*, and the frequency of these adverse effects were similar, whether or not metopimazine was used. Likewise, ondansetron 8 mg tds, when combined with metoclopramide and methylprednisolone, improved control of acute and delayed onset emesis in patients undergoing chemotherapy (12[c]). Adverse effects attributable to antiemetic therapy were *facial rash*, *constipation*, *headache*, and *weakness*, but none was severe.

The 5-HT3 receptor antagonist tropisetron was more effective than metoclopramide in preventing nausea and vomiting in patients receiving abdominal radiotherapy for seminoma (13[c]). Two of 11 patients who were given tropisetron developed *constipation*, and one of them discontinued the drug.

ULCER HEALING DRUGS *(SED-13, 1071; SEDA-19, 326; SEDA-20, 317; SEDA-21, 362)*

The efficacy of on-demand histamine H_2 receptor antagonists for gastro-esophageal reflux disease has been investigated in two trials. In a comparison of single doses of fast-dissolving famotidine wafers and ranitidine tablets for on-demand therapy for gastro-esophageal reflux disease in 930 patients, both drugs were equally effective and only minor adverse effects, unpleasant taste and nausea, were reported, with a similar frequency for both drugs (14[c]). In another study low-dose famotidine used on demand in a dose of 10 mg to be taken within 30 min of an episode of heartburn was compared with chewable alginate tablets (15[c]). Famotidine was more effective in preventing recurrence of symptoms than alginate. The frequency of adverse effects was similar in the two groups (8% with famotidine and 9% with alginate), the most common being *headache*, *abdominal pain*, and *nausea*.

Liver In a matched case–control study of 108 981 people who had received prescriptions for cimetidine, ranitidine, famotidine, or omeprazole, 33 were considered to have had liver injury for which no cause other than these drugs could be implicated (16[C]). The adjusted relative risk (confidence intervals) for *acute liver injury* with cimetidine was 5.5 (1.9–15.9), with omeprazole 2.1 (0.2–19.2), and with ranitidine 1.7 (0.5–5.8). The risk with cimetidine was especially high in the first 2 months of therapy at a dosage of 800 mg/day or more.

HISTAMINE H_2-RECEPTOR ANTAGONISTS *(SED-13, 1071; SEDA-19, 326; SEDA-20, 317; SEDA-21, 362)*

Cimetidine

Liver The rate of *acute liver injury* due to cimetidine 800 mg/day in the UK has been estimated at greater than 10 per 100 000 users (17[R]). The increased risk was seen mainly in the first 2 months of use. The risks of liver injury due to ranitidine and omeprazole were much lower.

Gastrointestinal There has been one case report suggesting a link between the use of ranitidine and *lymphocytic colitis* (18[c]). Now a case of *collagenous colitis* has been described in a patient who had taken cimetidine for 5 days (19[c]). However, response of the diarrhea to withdrawal of cimetidine was not satisfactory, making a causal relation difficult to establish.

Tumor-inducing effects Gynecomastia and a *lobular carcinoma of the breast* has been reported in a man with a chronic gastric ulcer who had been taking cimetidine in a dosage of 400 mg/day for 17 years (20[c]).

Ranitidine

The safety of ranitidine has been reviewed using data from 189 controlled trials, in which more than 26 000 patients took daily ranitidine for 4 weeks or more; 87 of the trials were placebo-controlled (21[R]). The prevalence of adverse effects was similar in patients taking ranitidine (20%) or placebo (27%). The common adverse effects reported were *headache*, *nausea*, *vomiting*, *abdominal pain*, *diarrhea*, and *dizziness*.

Hematological Hematological adverse effects of ranitidine are extremely rare, but include *leukopenia*, *thrombocytopenia*, *aplastic anemia*, *hemolytic anemia*, and *pancytopenia*. Thrombocytopenia has been reported in a patient who had taken ranitidine for 1 day (22[c]). The platelet count improved gradually after withdrawal.

Tolerance Intravenous omeprazole (8 mg/h for 24 h after a bolus of 80 mg) was superior to intravenous ranitidine (0.25 mg/kg per h for 24 h after a bolus of 50 mg) in maintaining a consistently high intragastric pH over 24 h, in 40 patients with bleeding peptic ulcers (23[C]). Ranitidine was less effective during the second half of the 24-h treatment period. This loss of effectiveness was probably due to *tolerance*. Continuous infusions of H_2 receptor antagonists increase the concentration of proton pump protein in experimental animals (24. As the level of gene expression remains unchanged, the mechanism may be by a reduction in the rate of enzyme turnover. In addition, alternative pathways of stimulation of acid secretion may also contribute to development of tolerance in man (25[R]).

PROTON PUMP INHIBITORS *(SED-13, 1075; SEDA-19, 327; SEDA-20, 318; SEDA-21, 363)*

Lansoprazole *(SED-13, 1076; SEDA-19, 327; SEDA-20, 319)*

In a randomized double-blind trial in 105 patients, lansoprazole 30 mg/day was superior to ranitidine 150 mg bd for the treatment of erosive reflux esophagitis (26[C]). The frequencies of adverse effects were similar in the two groups. The most commonly reported adverse effects with lansoprazole were *headache*, *diarrhea* and *weakness*.

In another randomized double-blind trial, lansoprazole for 8 weeks was effective in healing erosive reflux esophagitis resistant to treatment with H_2 receptor antagonists in 84% of 105 patients compared with only 32% of 54 patients who were randomized to continue taking ranitidine (27[C]). The frequencies of adverse effects were similar with lansoprazole and ranitidine. The common adverse effects attributable to lansoprazole were *headache and diarrhea*. Lansoprazole caused a significant *rise in serum gastrin concentrations*, but there was no significant difference in gastrin concentrations between patients taking lansoprazole 30 or 60 mg/day.

Omeprazole *(SED-13, 1075)*

Gastrointestinal Six patients developed histologically confirmed *gastric fundic gland polyps* while taking omeprazole 20 mg/day for 1–5 years for Barrett's esophagus (28[c]). None had *Helicobacter pylori* infection. Serum gastrin concentrations were normal in four and slightly raised in two.

Skin and appendages Several well-documented case reports have suggested an association between omeprazole and *diffuse hair loss*. In a 48-year-old woman diffuse hair loss occurred twice, on both occasions within 3–4 weeks of starting omeprazole and resolving within 2–3 weeks of withdrawal (29[c]).

Liver *Severe hepatitis* occurred on two occasions, when a 30-year-old man with advanced renal insufficiency secondary to diabetic nephropathy was treated for esophagitis with omeprazole (30[c]).

Nervous system *Drowsiness and lethargy* occurred in a 64-year-old man on two occasions when he took omeprazole (31[c]).

Urinary system Two case reports, in a 70-year-old woman and a 71-year-old man, have added further evidence to the association between omeprazole and *interstitial nephritis* (32[c]).

Interactions The interaction of omeprazole with *warfarin* is slight and probably clinically irrelevant. In a controlled retrospective study of 118 patients taking long-term *acenocoumarol* combined with omeprazole and 299 age- and sex-matched controls there was no evidence of an interaction, even though it has been suggested that these drugs are both metabolized by the same cytochrome P450 enzymes (33[C]). Omeprazole and acenocoumarol can therefore be safely administered in combination.

OTHER ULCER HEALING DRUGS

Bismuth compounds *(SED-13, 1077; SEDA-19, 328; SEDA-20, 320; SEDA-21, 364)*

Bismuth, which forms a viscous soluble complex with carbomer, may interfere with bacterial adherence. In 12 patients with chronic resistant mucosal inflammation in ileal reservoirs (pouchitis) after restorative proctocolectomy with ileal pouch anal anastomosis, who were treated with enemas containing elemental bismuth complexed with carbomer every night for 45 nights, remission was achieved in 10 (34[C]). Serum bismuth concentrations were negligible in all patients and no adverse effects were reported.

Sucralfate *(SED-13, 1078; SEDA-19, 328; SEDA-20, 320)*

Bezoars, masses of wholly undigested materials that form within the gut lumen, can form from drugs. They can occur with sucralfate in patients with other risk factors for their development, such as dehydration and impaired gastric motility, as has been reported in an 11-year-old girl with encephalitis (35[c]).

Helicobacter pylori eradication regimens *(SEDA-20, 320; SEDA-21, 362)*

Helicobacter pylori eradication regimens include drugs that suppress gastric acid secretion (proton pump inhibitors or H2 receptor antagonists) and one or two antibiotics (usually from among amoxicillin, metronidazole, tinidazole, clarithromycin, and tetracycline), with or without a bismuth compound. The choice of treatment depends on several factors, including reported efficacy, adverse effects, cost, and convenience of dosing. Bacterial resistance, particularly to metronidazole, is another factor that may affect eradication rates and influence the choice of antibiotics (36[c]).

Seven-day antibiotic regimens are more effective than shorter (2-day) regimens (37[c]), and there is a tendency for thrice-daily antibiotic regimens to be better than twice-daily regimens, without a significant increase in the frequency of adverse effects (36[c]), (38[c]). Adverse effects relate to the individual drugs used. In one study there was a significantly higher frequency of adverse effects with a bismuth-based regimen (32%) compared with omeprazole (4%) (39[c]). Common adverse effects encountered with the bismuth-based regimen included *nausea*, *vomiting*, *diarrhea*, *abdominal discomfort*, *headache*, and *a metallic taste*.

LAXATIVES *(SED-13, 1080; SEDA-21, 361)*

Cascara

A woman who intermittently abused cascara for 2 years developed a well-defined area of *bluish pigmentation in the stomach* with a similar histological appearance to melanosis coli in patients who abuse laxatives; the authors termed this 'melanosis gastri' (40[c]).

Lactulose

In 75 cirrhotic patients with hyperammonemia, lactulose 45 ml/day improved psychometric tests in 36 patients with subclinical hepatic encephalopathy (41[c]). Adverse effects attributable to lactulose occurred in 26% of patients and included *diarrhea*, *soft stools*, *anorexia*, *abdominal pain*, *vomiting*, and in one patient *glycosuria*.

Phenolphthalein

The use of phenolphthalein-containing laxatives has been studied in relation to the occurrence of adenomatous colorectal polyps in data from three case–control studies involving 866 patients with polyps and 1066 controls (42[C]). The data suggested that phenolphthalein does not increase the risk of adenomatous colorectal polyps.

Phosphates

In a survey of Canadian colonoscopists, in which 268 out of 400 who were sent a questionnaire responded, sodium phosphate was found to be used more frequently than polyethylene glycol for colonic cleansing (43[C]). A greater number reported complications with sodium phosphate than with polyethylene glycol. These included symptoms suggestive of *hypovolemia*, *renal failure*, *small unexplained colonic mucosal aphthous ulcers*, and *excessive luminal bubbling*; the latter two have the potential to cause diagnostic confusion. Respondents who usually advised their patients to use sodium phosphate for colonic cleansing considered that *renal failure*, *heart failure*, *incomplete bowel obstruction*, and *extreme old age* were reasons for its non-use.

Mineral and fluid balance The efficacy and safety of oral sodium phosphate have been tested in 20 patients who required colonoscopy (44[C]). Colonic cleansing was satisfactory and most patients found the formulation acceptable. Nausea and vomiting were the most frequent adverse effects, and although they occurred in about half the patients only one graded them as severe. Significant *hyperphosphatemia*, *hypocalcemia*, and *hypokalemia* were observed in most patients, but tended to normalize subsequently. There were no changes in the serum sodium and chloride concentrations. Several case reports have also highlighted an association between phosphate enemas used for colonic preparation and hypocalcemia and hyperphosphatemia (45[c]), (46[c]), including one in a 3-year-old child who had such severe electrolyte imbalance as to cause acute mental and cardiorespiratory changes (47[c]). The commonly held notion that these enemas are not absorbed, and are therefore systemically inactive, seems to be incorrect.

AMINOSALICYLATES *(SED-13, 1082; SEDA-19, 329; SEDA-20, 320; SEDA-21, 364)*

Most of the adverse effects of sulfasalazine are associated with the sulfonamide moiety.

Modified formulations of mesalazine (5-aminosalicylic acid) are therefore gaining popularity in the maintenance treatment of inflammatory bowel disease. In a review of a large database drawn from general practices in the UK, 2894 patients taking treatment for ulcerative colitis were assessed (48[C]). The average duration of observation was 2.1 years per patient. Adverse effects reported were: *anemia*, *neutropenia*, *thrombocytopenia*, *other hematological disorders*, *hepatic effects*, *pancreatic effects*, and *renal effects* (*nephrotic syndrome*, *nephritis*, *renal insufficiency*); all were very rare and serious adverse effects did not affect management.

In a randomized open study of 242 patients, mesalazine suppositories 1 g/day were more effective than hydrocortisone acetate foam 100 mg/day in acute proctitis (49[c]). The frequencies of adverse effects were similar in the two groups. Common adverse effects with mesalazine included local effects (*rectal pain and irritation*) and systemic effects (*abdominal pain and bloating*, *diarrhea*, *headache*, *sleep disturbance*, *back pain*, and *skin rash*). In another randomized, double-blind, placebo-controlled study, mesalazine in an oral dosage of 3 g/day reduced the rate of relapse in Crohn's disease more effectively than placebo (50[c]). The frequency of adverse effects thought to be related to drug therapy were similar in the two groups. However, mesalazine-treated patients were more likely to have adverse effects characterized as moderate or severe compared with those receiving placebo. Of 141 patients taking mesalamine 18 discontinued it because of adverse effects: *diarrhea*, *headache*, *nausea*, *vomiting*, and in one case *pancreatitis*.

A meta-analysis of studies of the effectiveness of mesalazine in maintaining remission in Crohn's disease showed an adverse effect frequency of 13.7% in patients taking mesalazine and 14.9% in patients taking placebo (51[c]). The most frequent adverse effect attributable to mesalazine was *diarrhea*.

Respiratory A possible association has been described between mesalazine and *interstitial lung disease*, which resolved after withdrawal of the drug (52[c]), (53[c]).

Liver *Severe hepatic injury with biopsy-proven cholestasis* has been reported in a man who had taken mesalazine in a dose of 4 g/day for 4 months (54[c]). There was no evidence of general hypersensitivity, and the illness resolved completely on withdrawal.

Pancreas *Pancreatitis*, a rare adverse effect of mesalazine, usually occurs within a short time of starting treatment. Two unusual cases of delayed-onset pancreatitis occurring 3 months and 2 years after starting mesalamine therapy have been recently described (55[c]).

Urinary system A point prevalence study of renal dysfunction in patients with inflammatory bowel disease of at least 6 months duration showed that patients taking high dosages of mesalazine had an increased frequency of *proximal renal tubular proteinuria* (56[C]). However, the authors pointed out the difficulty in differentiating between the possible impact of chronic inflammation on the kidney from that of high-dosage mesalazine. Nevertheless, they stressed the importance of monitoring renal function in patients taking high dosages.

Renal dysfunction associated with mesalazine has been described in three cases. One patient developed *renal tubular acidosis* and reduced renal function (57[c]) and two others developed *interstitial nephritis*, a recognized but rare adverse effect (58[c]), (59[c]).

Immunological and hypersensitivity reactions A case of *severe systemic hypersensitivity* to mesalazine suppositories has been reported; the isomer 4-ASA was substituted without any further adverse effects (60[c]).

Six cases of *lupus-like syndrome* associated with mesalazine have been documented (61[c]), and it has now also been reported during treatment with olsalazine (62[c]).

ANTISPASMODIC AGENTS

(SED-13, 1084; SEDA-19, 329; SEDA-20, 320)

Glucagon is often used to inhibit duodenal motility and enhance cannulation during endoscopic retrograde cholangiopancreatography (ERCP). However, it is expensive. In a prospective double-blind study of 308 patients L-hyoscyamine sulfate was compared with glucagon to assess its inhibitory action on small bowel motility during ERCP (63[C]). L-Hyoscyamine was slightly less effective in inhibiting motility, but this did not make the procedure more difficult. L-Hyoscyamine was also associated with more minor adverse effects (*nausea*, *vomiting*, and *abdominal pain*) than glucagon, but there was no difference in the frequency of *pancreatitis*. The cost of glucagon was however nearly twice that of L-hyoscyamine. L-Hyoscyamine may provide a reasonable alternative to glucagon as an anti-motility agent during ERCP.

Immunological and hypersensitivity reactions From 1978 to 1997, 21 cases of adverse reactions to mebeverine were reported in The Netherlands; 12 of the patients had hypersensitivity reactions and recovered completely after withdrawal (64[r]). The reactions consisted of *skin rashes*, sometimes accompanied by *fever*, *polyarthritis*, *thrombocytopenia*, and *angio-edema*. They occurred from within minutes to 14 days of starting the drug.

CHOLELITHOLYTIC AGENTS–BILE ACIDS *(SED-13, 1085; SEDA-19, 330)*

In 413 patients with chronic hepatitis (18% HBsAg+, 58% anti-HCV+) and persistently raised aminotransferase activities, ursodeoxycholic acid in a dosage of 600 mg/day for 6 months produced significant improvement in the biochemical markers of chronic hepatitis (65[c]). Mild and transient adverse effects, such as *gastric discomfort*, *pyrosis*, and *diarrhea* were reported in a few patients (5.3%). In another study of the efficacy of a combination of ursodeoxycholic acid and interferon-α in the treatment of chronic hepatitis C in 80 patients, there were no significant adverse effects (including liver dysfunction) attributable to ursodeoxycholic acid (66[c]).

In a prospective, randomized, double-blind study of 25 patients a combination of ursodeoxycholic acid and methotrexate was not superior to ursodeoxycholic acid alone in primary biliary cirrhosis (67[c]). No adverse effects were reported among the patients who received ursodeoxycholic acid alone.

Contact dissolution of gall stones using nasobiliary infusions of a solvent containing sodium deoxycholate, ethylenediaminetetraacetic acid and dimethylsulfoxide gave good results in 44 patients with large gall stones after failed Dormia extraction (68[C]). Adverse effects occurred in a significant proportion of patients but were mild and transient, and consisted mainly of *abdominal pain*, *nausea*, *vomiting*, *diarrhea*, and *drowsiness*.

PANCREATIC ENZYME SUPPLEMENTS *(SED-13, 1086; SEDA-19, 330; SEDA-20, 322; SEDA-21, 366)*

The dosages of pancreatic supplements used to treat exocrine pancreatic failure in children with cystic fibrosis have tended to increase over the years. Excessive dosages have been reported to cause severe constipation and even colonic strictures (*fibrosing colonopathy*). In an age-matched case–control study of 29 patients with cystic fibrosis with fibrosing colonopathy and 105 controls with cystic fibrosis without colonopathy, there was a strong association between high daily doses of pancreatic enzyme supplements and fibrosing colonopathy (69[C]). These finding support the recommendation that the daily dose of pancreatic enzyme supplements for most patients should be below 10 000 units of lipase per kg body weight.

A similar analysis of treatment details in 14 patients with cystic fibrosis with fibrosing colonopathy and 56 age-matched controls without colonopathy in the UK showed that the development of colonopathy was strongly associated with the use of pancreatic enzyme supplements coated with methacrylic acid copolymer, taken for at least 6 months, but not with other pancreatic supplements (70[C]).

REFERENCES

1. Goldhill DR. Cisapride and the ICU patient. Care Crit Ill 1997;13:61–4.
2. Schutze K, Bigard MA, Van Waes L, Hinojosa J, Bedogni G, Hentschel E. Comparison of two dosing regimens of cisapride in the treatment of reflux oesophagitis. Aliment Pharmacol Ther 1997;11:497–503.
3. Hatlebakk JG, Johnsson F, Vilien M, Carling L, Wetterhus S, Thogerson T. The effect of cisapride in maintaining symptomatic remission in patients with gastro-oesophageal reflux disease. Scand J Gastroenterol 1997;32:1100–6.
4. Song CW, Um SH, Kim CD, Ryu HS, Hyun JH, Choe JG. Double blind placebo controlled study of cisapride in patients with non specific esophageal motility disorder accompanied by delayed esophageal transit. Scand J Gastroenterol 1997;32:541–6.
5. Zix JA, Geerdes-Fenge HF, Rau M, Vockler J, Borner K, Koeppe P, Lode H. Pharmacokinetics of sparfloxacin and interaction with cisapride and sucralfate. Antimicrob Agents Chemother 1997;41:1668–72.
6. Tierney MG, Uhthoff TL, Kravcik S, Wielgosz AT. Potential cisapride erythromycin interaction. Can J Clin Pharmacol 1997;4:82–4.
7. Soykan I, Sarosiek I, Shifflett J, Wooten GF, McCallum RW. Effect of chronic oral domperidone therapy on gastrointestinal symptoms and gastric emptying in patients with Parkinson's Disease. Mov Disord 1997;12:952–7.
8. Soykan I, Sarosiek I, McCallum RW. The effect of chronic oral domperidone therapy on gastrointestinal symptoms, gastric emptying and quality of life in patients with gastroparesis. Am J Gastroenterol 1997;92:976–80.
9. Madani S, Tolia V. Gynecomastia with metoclopramide use in paediatric patients. J Clin Gastroenterol 1997;24:79–81.
10. Sreevastava DK, Garcha PS, Prabhakar T, Mukherjee D, Divekar DS. Metoclopramide and respiratory arrest. J Anaesth Clin Pharmacol 1996;13:83–4.
11. Lebeau B, Depierre A, Giovannini M, Riviere A, Kaluzinski L, Votan B, Hedouin M, d'Allens H, and the French Ondansetron Study Group. The efficacy of a combination of ondansetron, methylprednisolone and metopimazine in patients previously uncontrolled with a dual antiemetic treatment in cisplastin-based chemotherapy. Ann Oncol 1997;8:887–92.
12. Mustacchi G, Ceccherini R, Leita ML, Sandri P, Milani S, Carbonara T. The combination of metoclopramide, methylprednisolone and ondansetron against antiblastic-delayed emesis: a randomised phase II study. Anticancer Res 1997; 17:1345–8.
13. Aass N, Hatun DE, Thoresen M, Fossa SD. Prophylactic use of tropisetron or metoclopramide during adjuvant abdominal radiotherapy of seminoma stage I: a randomised open trial in 23 patients. Radiother Oncol 1997;45:125–8.
14. Johannessen T, Kristensen P. On demand therapy in gastroesophageal reflux disease: a comparison of the early effects of single doses of fast dissolving famotidine wafers and ranitidine tablets. Clin Ther 1997;19:73–81.
15. Mann SG, Cottrell J, Murakami A, Stauffer L, Rao AN. Prevention of heartburn relapse by low dose famotidine: a test meal model for duration of symptom control. Aliment Pharmacol Ther 1997;11:121–7.
16. Rodriguez LAG, Wallander M-A, Stricker BHCh. The risk of acute liver injury associated with cimetidine and other acid suppressing drugs. Br J Clin Pharmacol 1997;43:183–8.
17. Rodriguez LAG, Ruigomez A, Jick H. A review of epidemiologic research on drug induced acute liver injury using the general practice research data base in the United Kingdom. Pharmacotherapy 1997;17:721–8.
18. Beaugerie L, Patey N, Brousse N. Ranitidine, diarrhoea, and lymphocytic colitis. Gut 1995;37:708–11.
19. Duncan HD, Talbot IC, Silk DBA. Collagenous colitis and cimetidine. Eur J Gastroenterol Hepatol 1997;9:819–20.
20. San Miguel P, Sancho M, Enriquez JL, Fernandez J, Gonzalez-Palacios F. Lobular carcinoma of the male breast associated with the use of cimetidine. Virchows Arch 1997;430:261–3.
21. Mills JG, Koch KM, Webster C, Sirgo MA, Fitzgerald K, Wood JR. The safety of ranitidine in over a decade of use. Aliment Pharmacol Ther 1997;11:129–37.
22. Kavula MP. Thrombocytopenia secondary to prophylactic use of ranitidine hydrochloride. J Pharm Pract 1997;10:5–6.
23. Labenz J, Peitz U, Leusing C, Tillenburg B, Blum AL, Borsch G. Efficacy of primed infusions with high dose ranitidine and omeprazole to maintain high intragastric pH in patients with peptic ulcer bleeding: a prospective randomised controlled study. Gut 1997;40:36–41.
24. Scott DR, Besancon M, Sachs G, Helander H. Effects of antisecretory agents on parietal cell structure and H/K-ATPase levels in rabbit gastric mucosa in vivo. Dig Dis Sci 1994;39:2118–26.
25. Nwokolo CU, Smith JT, Gavey C, Sawyer A, Pounder RE. Tolerance during 29 days of conventional dosing with cimetidine, nizatidine, famotidine or ranitidine. Aliment Pharmacol Ther 1990;4 Suppl 1:29–45.
26. Sontag SJ, Schnell TG, Chejfec G, Kurucar C, Karpf J, Levine G. Lansoprazole heals erosive oesophagitis in patients with Barrett's oesophagus. Aliment Pharmcol Ther 1997;11:147–56.
27. Sontag SJ, Kogut DG, Fleischmann R, Campbell DR, Richter J, Robinson M, McFarland M, Sabesin S, Lehman GA, Castell D. Lansoprazole heals erosive reflux oesophagitis reisist-

ant to histamine H_2 receptor antagonist therapy. Am J Gastroenterol 1997;92:429–37.
28. El-Zimaity HMT, Jackson FW, Graham DY. Fundic gland polyps developing during omeprazole therapy. Am J Gastroenterol 1997;92:1858–60.
29. Borum ML, Cannava M. Diffuse alopecia associated with omeprazole. Am J Gastroenterol 1997;92:1576.
30. Navarro JF, Gallego E, Aviles J. Recurrent severe acute hepatitis and omeprazole. Ann Intern Med 1997;127:1135–6.
31. Meeuwisse EJM, Groen FC, Dees A, Smit GH, Ottervanger JP. Lethargy and omeprazole. Br Med J 1997;314:481.
32. Badov D, Perry G, Lambert J, Dowling J. Acute interstitial nephritis secondary to omeprazole. Nephrol Dial Transplant 1997;12:2414–16.
33. Vreeburg EM, De Vlaam-Schluter GM, Trienekens PH, Snel P, Tytgat GNJ. Lack of effect of omeprazole on oral acenocoumarol anticoagulant therapy. Scand J Gastroenterol 1997;32:991–4.
34. Gionchetti P, Rizzello F, Venturi A, Ferretti M, Brignola C, Peruzzo S, Belloli C, Poggioli G, Miglioli M, Campieri M. Long-term efficacy of bismuth carbomer enemas in patients with treatment-resistant chronic pouchitis. Aliment Pharmacol Ther 1997;11:673–8.
35. Razafimahefa H, Mouterde O, Devaux AM. Bezoard oesophagien chez un enfant traite par sucralfate. Arch Pediatr 1997;4:659–61.
36. Goh KL, Parasakthi N, Chuah SY, Toetsch M. Combination amoxycillin and metronidazole with famotidine in the eradication of *Helicobacter pylori*: a randomised, double blind, comparison of a three times daily and twice daily regimen. Eur J Gastroenterol Hepatol 1997;9:1091–5.
37. Kung NNS, Sung JJY, Yuen NWF, Ng PW, Wong KC, Chung ECH, Lim BH, Choi CH, Li TH, Ma HC, Kwok SPY. Anti-*Helicobacter pylori* treatment in bleeding ulcers: randomized controlled trial comparing 2-day versus 7-day bismuth quadruple therapy. Am J Gastroenterol 1997; 92:438–41.
38. Rinaldi V, Zullo A, Pugliano F, Valente C, Diana F, Attili AF. The management of failed dual or triple therapy for *Helicobacter pylori*. Aliment Pharmacol Ther 1997;11:929–33.
39. Lerang F, Moum B, Ragnhildstveit E, Haug JB, Hauge T, Tolas P, Aubert E, Henriksen M, Efskind PS, Nicolaysen K, Soberg Y, Odegaard A, Berge T. A comparison between omeprazole-based triple therapy and bismuth-based triple therapy for the treatment of *Helicobacter pylori* infection: a prospective randomised 1-yr follow-up study. Am J Gastroenterol 1997;92:653–8.
40. Mitty RD, Wolfe GRZ, Cosman M. Initial description of gastric melanosis in a laxative-abusing patient. Am J Gastroenterol 1997;92:707–8.
41. Wanatabe A, Sakai T, Sato S, Imai F, Ohto M, Arakawa Y, Toda G, Kobayashi K, Muto Y, Tsujii T, Kawasaki H, Okita K, Tanikawa K, Fujiyama S, Shimada S. Clinical efficacy of lactulose in cirrhotic patients with and without subclinical hepatic encephalopathy. Hepatology 1997;26:1410–14.
42. Longnecker MP, Sandler DP, Haile RW, Sandler RS. Phenolphthalein-containing laxative use in relation to adenomatous colorectal polyps in three studies. Environ Health Perspect 1997;105:1210–12.
43. Chan A, Depew W, Vanner S. Use of oral sodium phosphate colonic lavage solution by Canadian colonoscopists: pitfalls and complications. Can J Gastroenterol 1997;11:334–8.
44. Bozkaya H, Ozturk H, Uzun Y, Ozden A. Efficiency and safety of oral sodium phosphate in colon cleansing. Turk J Gastroenterol 1997; 8:217–21.
45. Ehrenpreis ED, Weiland JM, Cabral J, Estevez V, Zaiman D, Secrest K. Symptomatic hypocalcemia, hypomagnesemia and hyperphophatemia secondary to Fleet's Phospho-Soda colonoscopy preparation in a patient with a jejunoileal bypass. Dig Dis Sci 1997;42:858–60.
46. Vukasin P, Weston LA, Beart RW. Oral Fleet Phospho-Soda laxative induced hyperphosphatemia and hypocalcemic tetany in an adult: report of a case. Dis Colon Rectum 1997;40:497–9.
47. Helikson MA, Parham WA, Tobias JD. Hypocalcemia and hyperphosphatemia after phosphate enema use in a child. J Paediatr Surg 1997;32:1244–6.
48. Walker AM, Szneke P, Bianchi LA, Field LG, Sutherland LR, Dreyer NA. 5-Aminosalicylates, sulphasalazine, steroid use and complications in patients with ulcerative colitis. Am J Gastroenterol 1997;92:816–20.
49. Lucidarme D, Marteau P, Foucault M, Vautrin B, Filoche B. Efficacy and tolerance of mesalazine suppositories vs. hydrocortisone foam in proctitis. Aliment Pharmacol Ther 1997;11:335–40.
50. Sutherland LR, Martin F, Bailey RJ, Fedorak RN, Poleski M, Dallaire C, Rossman R, Saibil F, Lariviere L, and the Canadian mesalamine for Remission of Crohn's Disease Study Group. A randomized, placebo-controlled, double-blind trial of mesalamine in the maintenance of remission of Crohn's disease. Gastroenterology 1997;112:1069–77.
51. Camma C, Giunta M, Rosselli M, Cottone M. Mesalamine in the maintenance treatment of Crohn's disease: a meta-analysis adjusted for confounding variables. Gastroenterology 1997; 113:1465–73.
52. Lazaro MT, Garcia-Tejero MT, Diaz-Lobato S. Mesalamine induced lung disease. Arch Intern Med 1997;157:462.
53. Sviri S, Gafanovich I, Kramer MR, Tsvang E, Ben-Chetrit E. Mesalamine induced hypersensitivity pneumonitis. J Clin Gastroenterol 1997; 24:34–6.
54. Stoschus B, Meybehm M, Spengler U, Scheurlen C, Sauerbruch T. Cholestasis asso-

ciated with mesalazine therapy in a patient with Crohn's disease. J Hepatol 1997;26:425–8.
55. Fernandez J, Sala M, Panes J, Feu F, Navarro S, Teres J. Acute pancreatitis after long-term 5-aminosalicylic acid therapy. Am J Gastroenterol 1997;92:2302–3.
56. Schreiber S, Hamling J, Zehnter E, Wowaldt S, Daerr W, Raedler A, Kruis W. Renal tubular dysfunction in patients with inflammatory bowel disease treated with aminosalicylate. Gut 1997; 40:761–6.
57. Hamling J, Raedler A, Helmchen U, Schreiber S. 5-Amino salicylic acid-associated renal tubular acidosis with decreased renal function in Crohn's disease. Digestion 1997;58:304–7.
58. Manenti L, De Rosa A, Buzio C. Mesalazine associated interstitial nephritis: twice in the same patient. Neprhol Dial Transplant 1997;12:2031.
59. De Broe ME, Stolear JC, Nouwen EJ, Elseviers MM. 5-Amino salicylic acid and chronic tubulointerstitial nephritis in patients with chronic inflammatory bowel disease: is there a link? Nephrol Dial Transplant 1997;12:1839–41.
60. Borum ML, Ginsberg A. Hypersensitivity to 5-ASA suppositories. Dig Dis Sci 1997;42:1076–8.
61. Timsit M-A, Anglicheau D, Liote F, Marteau P, Dryll A. Mesalazine induced lupus. Rev Rhum Engl Ed 1997;64:586–8.
62. Gunnarsson I, Pettersson E, Lindblad S, Ringertz B. Olsalazine-induced lupus syndrome. Scand J Rheumatol 1997;26:65–6.
63. Lahoti S, Catalano MF, Geenen JE, Hogan WJ. A prospective, double-blind trial of L-hyoscyamine versus glucagon for the inhibition of small intestinal motility during ERCP. Gastrointest Endosc 1997;46:139–42.
64. In'T Veld BA, Van Puyenbroek E, Striker BHCh. Overgevoeligheidsreacties bij gebruik van mebeverine. Ned Tijdschr Geneeskd 1997; 141:1392–5.
65. Sama C, Rusticali AG, Morselli-Labate AM, Malavolti M and participating physicians. Effect of ursodeoxycholic acid on liver tests in chronic hepatitis. Assessment of prognostic parameters. Clin Drug Invest 1997;13:192–8.
66. Kiso S, Kawata S, Tamura S, Imai Y, Inui Y, Nagase T, Maeda Y, Yamasaki E, Tsushima H, Igura T, Himeno S, Seki K, Matsuzawa Y. Efficacy of combination therapy of interferon alpha with ursodeoxycholic acid in chronic hepatitis C: a randomized controlled clinical trial. J Gastroenterol 1997;32:56–62.
67. Gonzalez-Koch A, Brahm J, Antezana C, Smok G, Cumsille MA. A combination of ursodeoxycholic acid and methotrexate for primary biliary cirrhosis is not better than ursodeoxycholic acid alone. J Hepatol 1997;27:143–9.
68. Takacs T, Lonovics J, Caroli-Bosc F-X, Montet A-M, Montet J-C. Litholyse de contact des calculs de la voie biliaire principale. Gastroenterol Clin Biol 1997;21:655–9.
69. FitzSimmons SC, Burkhart GA, Borowitz D, Grand RJ, Hammerstrom T, Durie PR, Lloyd-Still JD, Lowenfels AB. High-dose pancreatic-enzyme supplements and fibrosing colonopathy in children with cystic fibrosis. New Engl J Med 1997;336:1283–9.
70. Bakowski MT, Prescott P. Patterns of use of pancreatic enzyme supplements in fibrosing colonopathy: implications for pathogenesis. Pharmacoepidemiol Drug Saf 1997;6:347–58.

Thierry Vial, Guillaume Chevrel and Jacques Descotes

37 Drugs acting on the immune system

INTERFERONS

Interferon-α

Although interferon-α has a wide range of indications, most of the important recent studies have been performed in patients with chronic hepatitis C, in which prolonged therapeutic success is still low and the long-term benefit:risk ratio is uncertain (1[r]). Combination therapy is potentially promising. Recent large, placebo-controlled, randomized trials have shown that interferon-α_{2b}, in combination with oral ribavirin for 24 or 48 weeks, is more effective than interferon-α_{2b} alone for the initial treatment of chronic hepatitis C (2[C]), (3[C]) or in patients who have relapsed after an initial response to interferon-α (4[C]). Although dosage reduction or drug withdrawal was more often required with combination therapy (2[C]), (4[C]), there were no synergistic adverse effects in these studies.

There have been few comparisons of the safety of various commercially available formulations of interferon-α (SEDA-21, 369). In a study of 1071 patients with chronic hepatitis C, randomized to either lymphoblastoid interferon-α_{n1} or interferon-α_{2b} for 24 weeks, there was no significant difference in the adverse effects profile and frequency of treatment withdrawal because of adverse effects, but a sustained response was more common in patients treated with lymphoblastoid interferon-α_{n1} (5[C]).

The effects of interferon-α_2 have been studied in a multicenter study (10 centers in six countries) involving 249 patients aged 18 years and over with clinically visible condylomata acuminata on the external genitalia and/or perianal area, likely to be cleared by ablative therapy within 5 weeks, who had not received treatment within 1 month of study entry (6[C]). There were adverse effects in 118 patients (47%); 43 of these were being given interferon 1 MIU, 42 interferon 3 MIU, and 33 placebo. The most frequently reported adverse events in the interferon-treated patients were *headaches*, *fatigue*, *'flu-like symptoms*, *local erythema*, *dizziness*, and *myalgia*. The most common adverse events in placebo-treated patients were headache, fatigue, dizziness, nasal congestion, and 'flu-like symptoms. The majority of adverse events were mild and most were considered by the investigator to be probably or possibly related to the study drug.

Cardiovascular Severe cardiotoxicity is rare, and has usually caused subacute or chronic complications in isolated patients. Adjuvant high-dose interferon-α in malignant melanoma has been implicated in a case of acute fatal *non-cardiogenic shock* (7[c]).

A 47-year-old man received intravenous interferon-α (20 MU/m^2 per day) for malignant melanoma. Six hours after the third dose he became weak, dizzy, and short of breath, with metabolic acidosis, vascular congestion, and pulmonary edema. His condition deteriorated rapidly, and he died the next day. There were massive serous pleural and pericardial effusions with only minimum atherosclerotic heart disease at autopsy.

Raynaud's phenomenon has previously been recognized as a possible peripheral vascular complication, but the spectrum of interferon-α-induced *vascular toxicity* is broader.

The characteristic clinical features of asymptomatic acrocyanosis with worsening after exposure to cold temperature occurred in a 56-year-old woman

Side Effects of Drugs, Annual 22
J.K. Aronson, ed.

treated for mycosis fungoides and who had a raised titer of antinuclear antibody (8[c]).

Another case of peripheral arterial occlusion has been reported after long-term interferon-α treatment for chronic myelogenous leukemia (9[c]).

Nervous system Reversible *focal neurological symptoms* occurred in two patients treated for malignant melanoma, one of whom had confirmed ischemic areas on brain imaging (10[c]). However, the pathogenic mechanisms of these vascular effects are still unclear and may involve vasculitis, hypercoagulability, vasospasm, or an underlying cardiovascular disease (9[r]). In addition, a role of the underlying treated disease cannot be excluded, as these patients had malignant disease.

Interferon-α sometimes worsens cryoglobulinemia-associated neuropathy, but *peripheral neuropathy* can also occur in patients with no previous neurological history, as occurred in a 44-year-old man with chronic hepatitis C (11[c]). There was also an abnormally high level of expression of HLA-DR antigens on Schwann cells, predominantly in unmyelinated fibers, but the relevance of this finding is unknown.

Psychiatric Neuropsychiatric adverse effects of interferon-α are a matter of great concern (SED-13, 1091). Unfortunately, very few large, randomized, controlled trials have specifically addressed this issue. In a recent study, 67 patients with metastatic malignant melanoma were randomized to receive low-dose adjuvant interferon-α ($n = 37$) or no interferon-α ($n = 30$) (12[C]). Neurological and neuropsychological evaluations were performed at baseline and after 1, 3, 6, and 12 months. There was a *fluctuating action tremor* in eight patients taking interferon compared with none in the control group. Although *fatigue* and *anxiety* increased significantly with interferon-α, there was no measurable impact on the quality of life. Moreover, psychiatric evaluation and cognitive performance were similar in the groups.

Nevertheless, *depressive disorders* and *psychosis* remain major complications of interferon-α, and their clinical impact should be carefully taken into account in the patient's management. An unexpectedly high incidence of suicidal ideation or suicide attempts has previously been noted in patients treated for chronic viral hepatitis (SED-13, 1092). Similar results were found by other investigators, who also stressed that the risk persisted even after discontinuation of treatment (13[c]). Among 306 patients they observed one case of suicidal impulse, two suicide attempts, and two successful suicides within the 6 months after interferon-α withdrawal. One patient had another episode of suicidal impulse after interferon-α had been restarted. In another report of successful suicide, alcoholism was suggested as a possible disinhibitory co-factor (14[c]). Murderous impulses have also emerged as a possible complication in two patients, including one with a previous history of heroin abuse (15[c]).

Mania has been described during interferon-α treatment (SEDA-21, 370). In two other patients who had depressive symptoms during interferon-α therapy, the abrupt discontinuation of treatment was supposedly the cause of an acute manic state (16[c]).

More recently, *post-traumatic stress symptoms*, including vivid nightmares, intrusive memories, mood swings, anxiodepressive symptoms, and suicidal thoughts, have been described in three patients with a past history of trauma after they had taken interferon-α for hepatitis C (17[c]).

Unfortunately, predictive factors for the development of severe psychiatric adverse effects have not yet been clearly identified, and only the duration of treatment is known to play a significant role (18[R]). The mechanisms by which interferon-α produces neuropsychiatric symptoms are still debated. The release of secondary cytokines (19[R]) or a reduction in central dopaminergic activity through the binding of interferon to opioid receptors have been proposed as mechanisms for interferon-α-induced mood disorders (18[R]).

Endocrine, metabolic *Thyroid dysfunction* Thyroid dysfunction is one of the commonest late complications of interferon-α treatment (in about 6–8% of patients). There are many potential predisposing factors, including thyroid autoantibodies either before or during treatment, combination therapy with IL-2, and the underlying disease, namely cancer or hepatitis C.

Further prospective studies have been reported in patients with chronic hepatitis C. In the first study, 77 patients received lymphoblastoid interferon-α, and 7.5% developed thyroid abnormalities (20[C]). This incidence, which is similar to that noted with recombinant interferon-α, confirmed that thyroid disorders are not related to the type of interferon-α used. In addition, although 21% of the patients had a familial or personal thyroid history before treatment, this was not considered as a significant risk factor for further thyroid disorders. In a study of 59 patients with chronic hepatitis C, nine developed thyroid dysfunction, including five of 19 who had various abnormal thyroid findings before interferon compared with four of 40 with normal thyroid function before treatment (21[C]). Six of nine patients who developed thyroid disorders never had thyroid antibodies. This further suggests that the induction of an autoimmune reaction and/or the exacerbation of pre-existing latent thyroid autoimmunity may not be the primary mechanism of interferon-α-induced thyroid dysfunction. As a matter of fact, in 61 patients treated with interferon-α or interferon-β, either alone or in association with IL-2 or antineoplastic agents, the thyroid autoantibody pattern in seven patients who developed thyroid dysfunction during cytokine treatment was not different from that of 54 patients without thyroid dysfunction (22[C]). In addition, this autoantibody pattern was significantly different compared with 105 patients with various forms of spontaneous autoimmune thyroid disease.

It has been suggested that the hepatitis C virus genotype produces a different pattern of thyroid disorders (23[c]). In five of 19 patients who developed thyroid disorders during treatment with interferon-α, alone or in combination with ribavirin, three of 15 patients with genotype 1b had thyroid disorders and were thyroid antibody positive, whereas two of four patients with genotype 3 and thyroid disorders were thyroid antibody negative. Although the number of patients was small, this suggests that different hepatitis C virus genotypes cause thyroid disorders by different mechanisms, and that genotype 1b influences the development of thyroid antibodies.

Glucose tolerance The links between chronic viral hepatitis, interferon-α treatment, and disorders of glucose metabolism are still unclear. Patients with previously impaired glucose tolerance should be considered more predisposed. Interferon-α therapy for 2 weeks in 14 patients with chronic hepatitis C caused insulin resistance in the splanchnic or peripheral tissues, although there were no changes in plasma glucose and insulin profiles during this short time (24[C]). On the other hand, recovery of hepatic function was associated with an improvement in glucose metabolism in patients with chronic hepatitis B ($n = 11$) or hepatitis C ($n = 15$) treated with interferon-α (25[C]), (26[C]).

Very few cases of insulin-dependent diabetes mellitus have been reported. Interferon-α triggers, rather than causes, latent autoimmunity in patients who have a predisposition to insulin-dependent diabetes mellitus. This has again illustrated by the case of a 29-year-old man who developed insulin-dependent diabetes after 5 months of treatment (27[c]). Extensive retrospective evaluation for genetic susceptibility and markers of pancreatic autoimmunity yielded positive results either before or during treatment with interferon-α.

Hematological Interferon-α sometimes causes acute *autoimmune hemolytic anemia*. Direct anti-globulin (DAT) tests were positive in nine of 28 patients with chronic myeloid leukemia treated with interferon-α for a median of 1 year (28[c]). DAT-positive patients also had a significantly lower median hemoglobin, but most of them were women. There were other autoimmune phenomena in most of the nine DAT-positive patients, whereas only four of the 19 DAT-negative patients developed autoimmune disorders. In contrast, direct anti-globulin tests were negative in all of 50 patients with chronic myeloid leukemia not treated with interferon-α.

Hemolytic–uremic syndrome is a possible complication of interferon-α, but it has previously been reported only in patients with chronic myelogenous leukemia. A case of fatal *thrombotic thrombocytopenic purpura*, which shared many features of the hemolytic–uremic syndrome, has now been described in a patient with hepatitis C (29[c]).

A 57-year-old man with chronic hepatitis C received interferon-α 70 MU/week for 4 weeks and then 30 MU/week. After 16 weeks he developed headache and fever, and 1 week later severe thrombocytopenia, hemolytic anemia, proteinuria, and microhematuria. He rapidly deteriorated, with somnolence and two episodes of tonic convulsions. Despite plasma transfusion, antiplatelet drugs, and corticosteroids, he died of respiratory arrest.

Various bleeding complications have been attributed to interferon-α, in particular in patients with decompensated cirrhosis. *Meno-metrorrhagia*, which recurred on rechallenge, has also been reported in a patient with mild chronic hepatitis C who had a previous history of uterine bleeding leading to uterine curettage (30[c]).

Liver Interferon-α-induced *autoimmune hepatitis* has mostly been reported in patients with chronic hepatitis, and the underlying hepatic disease as well as the triggering of a latent autoimmune hepatitis have been presumed to be confounders. However, de novo autoimmune hepatitis still remains possible.

A 51-year-old woman receiving interferon-α for chronic myeloid leukemia developed severe type 1 autoimmune hepatitis together with autoimmune hypothyroidism (31[c]). Liver enzymes and antinuclear antibodies were normal before treatment, increased during the first 2 years of treatment, and subsequently normalized after interferon-α withdrawal.

There have been previous reports of *hepatic granulomas* due to interferon-α (SEDA-20, 329; SEDA-21, 372). Three other cases have been described in patients with chronic hepatitis C (32[c]). They had normal pretreatment liver biopsies and did not respond to interferon-α. In two patients, numerous non-necrotizing hepatic granulomas were found in liver biopsies performed during the sixth and seventh months of interferon-α treatment, and one had complete regression of the granulomas in a third biopsy 17 months after interferon-α discontinuation. In the last patient, granulomatous destruction of the bile duct in one portal tract and occasional granulomas in the remaining tracts were identified in a liver biopsy 2.5 years after interferon-α withdrawal, suggesting that persistent granulomas can occur.

Gastrointestinal Interferon-α can cause a mild-to-moderate stomatitis of early onset. In 124 patients with chronic hepatitis C randomly assigned to plautanol or no preventive treatment, oral plautanol started 2 weeks before interferon-α significantly reduced the symptoms of stomatitis, but only during the first 2 weeks of interferon-α treatment (33[C]).

Urinary system *Acute renal insufficiency* due to interferon-α has mostly been observed after several weeks of treatment in patients treated for malignancy and/or receiving relatively high dosages, as has again been reported in a 57-year-old man with idiopathic hypereosinophilic syndrome (34[cr]). In another case, lower dosages (9 MU/week) might have been the cause of short-term onset and severe renal insufficiency in a 38-year-old man who had nephrotic syndrome secondary to hepatitis B-induced membranous glomerulopathy (35[c]).

Skin and appendages Several types of skin disorders have been reported during interferon-α treatment. Of 120 patients receiving interferon-α for 6–18 months for chronic viral hepatitis, three developed *lichen planus* and one had relapsing *aphthous stomatitis* (36[c]). These rare lesions were not observed in a similar number of patients with non-viral chronic liver disease who had never received interferon-α. Two other reports of local cutaneous necrosis in patients receiving interferon-α have suggested that high-dose interferon-α (37[c]) or the concomitant presence of activated protein C resistance (38[c]) might be risk factors.

Several isolated reports have described new dermatological findings.

Worsening of previously stable *lichen myxedematosus* occurred in a 59-year-old woman treated for 1 month for chronic hepatitis C (39[c]).

Within 1 month of treatment, a 48-year-old woman with chronic granulocytic leukemia developed fever, and severe lesions of *pyoderma gangrenosum* at the site of interferon-α injection (40[c]). She was successfully treated with cyclosporin and corticosteroids.

Finally, papular lesions of *polymorphous light eruption* occurred several hours after sun exposure on the dorsal forearms and around the injection site in a 38-year-old woman who was given interferon-α for chronic hepatitis C (41[c]).

Special senses Several previously undescribed adverse effects of interferon-α treatment have been reported.

Interferon-α was suggested to have caused *anosmia* in a 55-year-old man, but he also had impaired glucose tolerance, and his anosmia persisted for 9 months after treatment discontinuation (42[c]).

After 5 days of treatment, a 26-year-old man suddenly developed spontaneous vertigo and nystagmus related to acute *unilateral vestibular dysfunction* (43[c]). He improved only after interferon withdrawal.

In a detailed prospective ophthalmological evaluation of 53 patients (mean age 52 years) with chronic viral hepatitis, 11 (15 eyes) of 45 patients who initially had normal baseline visual evoked responses developed abnormally long values after they had received interferon-α 9–15 MU/week for a median of 11 months (44[C]). There was also a significant *fall in central visual sensitivity*. Other potential risk factors included older age, chronic hepatitis B, and higher serum cholesterol concentrations. Although the clinical relevance of these subclinical abnormalities remains to be determined, another examination performed after a median of 9.8 months after interferon-α withdrawal showed that the neurovisual disorders slowly reversed (median of 4.8 months) in seven patients (10 eyes) and still persisted in five (five eyes).

Musculoskeletal Whereas interferon-α often causes reversible *myalgia* or *muscular weakness* during the first weeks of treatment, delayed muscular toxicity has been rarely reported.

There was delayed persistent muscular weakness and myalgia associated with electromyographic findings of severe myopathic changes in the upper and/or lower limbs in four women aged 46–50 years who were receiving interferon-α (9–27 MU/week) for various skin disorders (45[c]). Three of them slowly improved over 4–8 weeks after withdrawal.

A 41-year-old man developed proximal weakness and electromyographic findings consistent with a diagnosis of Lambert-Eaton syndrome after 4 months of treatment with interferon-α and hydroxyurea for leukemia; he also developed reversible bone marrow necrosis (46[c]). Although antibodies to voltage-gated calcium channels were undetectable, interferon-α was the postulated cause and his symptoms resolved with prednisolone.

Immunological and hypersensitivity reactions Previous studies in patients with chronic viral hepatitis receiving interferon-α have not shown a significant increase in overt autoimmune diseases, despite increased positivity of several autoantibodies (SEDA-20, 330; SEDA-21; 373). In another study of 214 patients with carcinoid or endocrine pancreatic tumors, 17 patients developed high-affinity dsDNA antibodies, but only one had signs of *polymyositis* (47[C]).

The clinical significance of the development of neutralizing anti-interferon-α antibodies has been debated (SED-13, 1097; SEDA-20, 331), and this issue has again been extensively reviewed (48[R]). In patients with chronic hepatitis C *neutralizing antibodies to interferon* developed in 13 of the 84 patients who had received recombinant interferon-α_{2a} and in none of the 78 patients who had received interferon-α_{2b} (49[C]). The prevalence of these antibodies was significantly higher in patients who experienced breakthrough after an initial response (5/13) compared with patients who had a complete response (2/71) or no response (6/78).

Of 37 patients with interferon-α-induced arthritis, mostly patients with leukemia, antinuclear antibodies were found in 72% and rheumatoid factor in 34% (50[cR]). *Symmetrical polyarthritis* was the most common clinical feature and there were additional autoimmune features in 27 patients. The arthritis resolved in most of the patients after withdrawal, either spontaneously or after the addition of anti-inflammatory or disease-modifying antirheumatic drugs. Arthritis recurred in five of eight patients who restarted interferon-α.

The possible deleterious effect of pretransplant interferon-α treatment on the outcome of bone marrow transplantation for chronic myelogenous leukemia is still controversial. Two retrospective analyses in 51 and 32 consecutive patients who had received an allogeneic bone marrow transplant from an HLA-identical familial donor showed no evidence of an adverse effect of prior interferon-α therapy ($n = 46$) on the incidence of acute and chronic graft-versus-host disease or on overall survival, compared with patients who had not received interferon-α ($n = 37$) (51[C])(52[C]). In contrast, in 184 patients who underwent unrelated donor transplantation, pretransplant interferon-α treatment for more than 6 months ($n = 48$) was associated with an increased risk of severe acute *graft-versus-host disease* and death compared with 136 patients who had not receive prior interferon or who had had less than 6 months of prior interferon treatment (53[C]).

Isolated cases of *acute graft failure* shortly after interferon-α treatment in renal transplant patients are often reported (54[c]), (55[c]), but clear evidence that interferon-α adversely affects the outcome of renal transplantation is still lacking. There were no significant differences in the incidence of rejection episodes, retransplantation, or mortality in 24 liver transplant patients who were randomized to prophylaxis with interferon-α for 6 months ($n = 12$) or to no prophylaxis ($n = 12$) (56[C]).

Infections Interferon-α has been suspected

to precipitate fatal Entamoeba histolytica infection (57[c]).

A 65-year-old woman was treated with daily interferon-α (6 MU) for chronic hepatitis C. She developed a fever (39°C) after 14 days. Although interferon-α was immediately withdrawn, her fever persisted and an abdominal scan showed features of multiple liver abscesses. Despite drainage, she subsequently died from disseminated intravascular coagulation. Trophozoites of *E. histolytica* in the liver abscess were found at autopsy.

The triggering of this amebic infection was suggested by the presence of asymptomatic and moderate increase in anti-*E. histolytica* antibodies 1 year before and at the start of treatment, with a subsequent dramatic increase in the number of liver abscesses at the time of diagnosis.

Miscellaneous *Cutaneous and/or pulmonary sarcoidosis* has again been reported after interferon-α therapy (58[c]), (59[c]), and the incidence may have been underestimated, at least in patients receiving additional immunomodulating drugs. Of 60 patients who entered a randomized comparison of interferon-α versus interferon-α plus ribavirin in chronic hepatitis C, three patients (two in the combination group) developed pulmonary sarcoidosis within 12–21 weeks of treatment (60[C]). There was spontaneous improvement within 5–8 months after withdrawal in all three cases.

Risk factors *Children* There are many neurological adverse effects of interferon-α and children with an immature central nervous system may be at extra risk. Among 26 infants treated for severe hemangiomas, five developed spastic diplegia (61[c]). All had been treated with interferon-α since the age of 5 weeks to 4 months and up to 8–33 months of age. In three infants, diplegia persisted with significant functional sequelae, whereas two infants improved after withdrawal of interferon.

Interactions Interferon-α often causes neutropenia, but agranulocytosis is exceptional. A synergistic effect of interferon-α has been suggested in a 29-year-old man who received *clozapine* for 5 years and developed agranulocytosis 7 weeks after interferon-α had been started for chronic hepatitis C (62[c]).

As noted before (SED-13, 1099), interferon-α can increase the anticoagulant effect of *coumarins*.

A 46-year-old woman on stable treatment with acenocoumarol had a reduced thrombotest (19%) and gingival bleeding 6 weeks after interferon-α (3 MU thrice weekly) had been introduced for chronic hepatitis C (63[c]). The thrombotest returned to the target range after reduction of the acenocoumarol dosage. When the dosage of interferon-α was reduced to 3 MU twice weekly 5 months later the thrombotest increased to 69% within 3 weeks.

Interferon-β

The results of two phase III trials have extended our knowledge of the safety of interferon-β_{1a} and interferon-β_{1b} in multiple sclerosis (64[C]), (65[C]). The first was a comparison of thrice-weekly interferon-β_{1a} (6 million IU (n = 189), or 12 million IU (n = 184)) with placebo (n = 187) in patients with relapsing-remitting multiple sclerosis (64[C]). *Lymphopenia, leukopenia, granulocytopenia*, and *increased transaminase activities* were significantly more frequent with interferon, and were more pronounced in those taking the higher dose. By contrast, reactions at the injection site had similar frequencies in the two dosage groups. Psychological assessments in 267 patients showed no differences among the three groups, and there were no differences in the incidences of depression, attempted suicide, or suicidal thoughts. The second trial, in 718 patients with secondary progressive multiple sclerosis randomized to interferon-β_{1b} (8 million IU every other day) or placebo, has largely confirmed the safety profile of interferon-β_{1b}: interferon caused significantly more *injection-site reactions, flu-like reactions, muscle hypertonia, hypertension, increases in transaminase activities*, and *reductions in leukocyte counts* (65[C]). Again, there were no differences in the numbers of patients with depression, suicide, or suicide attempts.

As in previous studies, *neutralizing antibodies to interferon-β_{1a}* were found in 24 and 13% of the 373 patients in the first study who received 6 or 12 million IU thrice a week, but their presence did not appear to affect efficacy, measured as relapse rate (64[C]). In contrast, neutralizing antibodies were found in 28% of the 360 patients in the second study who received interferon-β_{1b} and were associated with a significant reduction in relapse rate (65[C]). There were differences in the incidence and clinical significance of neutralizing antibodies to interferon-β_{1a} or -β_{1b} in a more comprehensive study (66[C]), but they are not yet understood and still a matter of debate (67[r]).

Flu-like symptoms are very common during the first weeks of treatment. In 71 patients treated with interferon-β_{1b}, paracetamol plus prednisone was more effective than paracetamol alone in reducing the frequency and severity of flu-like symptoms (68[C]).

Cardiovascular Interferon-β-induced *Raynaud's phenomenon* has not been previously reported.

A 35-year-old woman was given interferon-β_{1b} (8 MU every other day) for severe remitting-relapsing multiple sclerosis (69[c]). After about 1 year of treatment she had severe pain and whitish skin coloration at the tips of several fingers. Angiography showed multiple occlusions of digital arteries and screening for other possible causes was negative. Alprostadil was not effective and she finally improved slowly with oral prednisone, low-molecular weight heparin, and replacement of interferon-β by copolymer-I.

Urinary system The first case of *hemolytic–uremic syndrome* attributed to interferon-β has been reported (70[c]).

A 66-year-old woman received intravenous interferon-β (6 MU/day) for chronic hepatitis C. Six weeks later her serum creatinine was 177 μmol/l and she had proteinuria of 6.8 g/day. Anemia and thrombocytopenia developed rapidly, with increased lactate dehydrogenase (1092 IU/l) and reduced haptoglobin (43 mg/l). There was fragmentation of erythrocytes in peripheral blood smears and bone marrow, and the diagnosis was hemolytic–uremic syndrome. Interferon was withdrawn and she recovered within 6 weeks. Renal biopsy showed local mesangial interposition of the glomerular basement membrane with diffuse interstitial lymphocytic infiltration in the tubulointerstitium. Immunofluorescence and electron microscopy were suggestive of hemolytic–uremic syndrome.

Skin and appendages Reports to the FDA of reactions to interferon-β_{1b} at injection sites have been reviewed (71[R]), including 1443 *injection-site reactions*, 212 cases of *necrosis* at the injections site, and 10 of necrosis at other sites. These mostly occurred within the first month of treatment, but the longest time to onset was 29 months. Most of the cases were reported in women (87–100%). Patients who had injection-site reactions or necrosis often had two or more symptoms, namely erythema, pain, induration, bruising, edema, ulceration, infection. Antibiotics and/or surgery were, respectively, required in 31 and 21% of patients.

Immunological and hypersensitivity reactions There are still discrepant reports about the ability of interferon-β to cause autoimmune disorders in patients with multiple sclerosis. In one study in 26 patients treated with interferon-β_{1b}, there was no clear evidence for *an increased frequency or titers of several autoantibodies* (antinuclear, antithyroid, and various heterophilic antibodies), although most of the patients who were tested before the start of treatment were positive for one or more autoantibodies (72[C]). In addition, none of the 19 patients treated for at least 6 months had clinical features suggestive of an autoimmune disease. In contrast, of 17 patients without a family or personal history of thyroid disorders and receiving either interferon-β_{1a} ($n = 12$) or interferon-β_{1b} ($n = 5$), five developed antithyroid antibodies (73[C]). This was higher than the 10% prevalence of thyroid autoantibodies in 40 patients with multiple sclerosis not receiving interferon. In addition, one patient developed transient and spontaneously reversible *hyperthyroidism* after 15 months of treatment. Several isolated reports have also emphasized the risk of autoimmune disorders, such as transient *autoimmune hepatitis* (74[c]) or subacute *cutaneous lupus erythematosus* (75[c]) during treatment with interferon-β. In the second of these cases clinical improvement occurred within 3 months of withdrawal of interferon.

Interferon-γ

Cardiovascular The cardiovascular effects of interferon-γ are infrequent. Reversible *chest pain suggestive of coronary vasospasm* with normal coronary arteriography has been reported in a 68-year-old man treated for renal cell carcinoma (76[c]).

Endocrine, metabolic *Hyperglycemia* during interferon-γ therapy has not previously been described.

A 42-year-old man with a history of impaired glucose tolerance and renal cancer was treated with interferon-γ (300–600 MU/day) for metastatic lung disease (77[c]). After 7 days, his fasting blood glucose concentration was 31 mmol/l. Anti-islet cell antibody and anti-glutamic acid decarboxylase were negative. Other investigations (urinary C-peptide, insulin concentration, insulin tolerance test) suggested insulin resistance as the most likely mechanism. His fasting blood glucose concentration fell to 7.4 mmol/l with insulin, which he no longer needed after interferon-γ withdrawal.

Hematological Interferon-γ produces very few hematological adverse effects. Interferon-γ was supposedly the cause of *autoimmune thrombocytopenia* with an increased anti-nuclear antibody titer in a 9-year-old girl with hyperimmunoglobulin E (78[c]).

Miscellaneous *Enlargement of the thymus* with normal histology has been reported in a 7-year-old boy treated for 3 years with interferon-γ for chronic granulomatous disease (79[c]).

INTERLEUKINS

Interleukin-2 (IL-2)

In metastatic renal cell carcinoma, IL-2 or interferon-α alone are beneficial in a minority of patients. In the largest randomized trial so far performed, in 425 patients, the combination of these cytokines gave a significantly higher response rate (19%) and a longer event-free survival than either alone (6.5% with IL-2 and 7.5% with interferon-α) (80[C]). However, that was achieved at the cost of substantial toxicity, most of which was attributed to IL-2 and consisted of the *capillary leak syndrome* with hypotension resistant to vasopressors. In addition, overall survival did not differ between the groups. Factors that were identified as being useful to detect patients with little likelihood of benefit included more than one metastatic site, liver involvement, and the occurrence of metastases less than 1 year after the diagnosis of the primary tumor.

Cardiovascular Cardiovascular complications of IL-2 are well known (SED-13, 1102). However, myocarditis and cardiomyopathy have been seldom reported. *Fulminant myocarditis*, previously unreported, has been described and an autoimmune mechanism suggested.

A 61-year old woman with relapsed follicular lymphoma underwent autologous stem cell transplantation (81[c]). The myeloablation regimen included total body irradiation and cyclophosphamide (60 mg/kg), followed by transplantation with IL-2-activated peripheral blood stem cells. IL-2 (1.8×10^6 IU/m^2 per day) was initiated 13 days later, 3 days after granulocyte engraftment. Four days later she suddenly developed acute abdominal pain, dyspnea, rigors, fever, sinus tachycardia, and right bundle branch block, and died within minutes. Post-mortem examination showed a diffuse lymphocytic infiltrate of the myocardium with features of giant cell myocarditis.

Interleukin-6 (IL-6)

The neuroendocrine effects of a single low dose of IL-6 (0.5 μg/kg) have been compared with those of placebo in a double-blind, cross-over study in 16 healthy volunteers (82[C]). IL-6 caused *increased plasma concentrations of ACTH and cortisol and reduced TSH concentrations*. IL-6-treated patients complained of *mood changes* and had significant *alterations in sleep architecture*.

STEM CELL FACTOR

Stem cell factor, in combination with a lineage-specific hemopoietic growth factor (e.g. G-CSF, IL-3) amplifies the proliferation and mobilization of myeloid, erythroid, and megakaryocyte colonies. Stem cell factor is currently under clinical investigation. Transient allergic-type reactions resulting from a dose-dependent mast cell degranulation have been observed in the first trials and included *urticaria*, *respiratory symptoms*, and *injection-site reactions* (83[r]). Except for injection-site reactions, these adverse effects were prevented by premedication with H_1 or H_2 histamine receptor antagonists or inhaled β_2 adrenoceptor agonists.

TUMOR NECROSIS FACTOR-α (TNF-α)

Because systemic TNF-α is very toxic (SED-13, 1110), its use has been limited to direct administration into tumors. However, hyperthermic isolated limb perfusion of TNF-α, in addition to cytostatic drugs (e.g. melphalan), produces interesting results in patients with sarcoma, melanomas, and other tumors (84[C]). In this setting, systemic toxicity was moderate and easily manageable. However, there is still a risk of leakage of TNF-α into the systemic circulation, with clinical features of *septic shock-like syndrome* and direct, but reversible, *nephrotoxicity* (85[C]). In addition, the possibility of more severe *rhabdomyolysis* in patients receiving TNF-α compared with those receiving cytostatics alone should be kept in mind (86[C]).

TNF-α has been considered to have major neurotoxic effects after systemic administration, but these effects were very limited after hyperthermic isolated limb perfusion, with a frequent but mild and usually transient *sensory neuropathy* in the perfused limbs (87[C]). Adverse effects after the local treatment of malignant pleural effusion, are limited to a frequent '*flu-like syndrome*, *nausea and vomiting*, and *chest pain* (88[C]).

COLONY-STIMULATING FACTORS

Granulocyte colony-stimulating factor *(*G-CSF*;* filgrastim, lenograstim, marograstim, nartograstim*)*

Hemopoietic growth factors are being increasingly used to mobilize blood stem cells or granulocytes in normal allogeneic donors for collection by apheresis and infusion into transplant or neutropenic patients. G-CSF is usually given in dosages of 2–16 μg/kg per day for 4–6 days. A review of published data in about 400 healthy donors showed that G-CSF generally produced minor adverse effects, namely *bone pain*, *headache*, *fatigue*, and *nausea* (89[R]). The frequency and severity of adverse effects were influenced by the dose and duration of administration of G-CSF. They resulted in treatment withdrawal in 1–3% of patients. More severe adverse consequences have been identified in healthy donors, such as *spontaneous splenic rupture* (90[c]), *an anaphylactoid reaction* after the first subcutaneous injection (91[c]), *deep necrotizing toxic folliculitis with syringometaplasia* (92[c]), *a psoriasiform eruption* (92[c]), acute *gouty arthritis* (93[c]), and *episcleritis* (SEDA-21, 378).

Cardiovascular *Capillary leak syndrome* has been rarely reported in patients treated with G-CSF (SEDA-12, 1115), and a further case has illustrated the possible role of accelerated release of activated circulating granulocytes (94[c]).

A 15-year-old boy with a mediastinal granulocytic sarcoma received G-CSF (6 μg/kg per day) for chemotherapy-induced bone marrow aplasia. Fever (over 40°C) and raised acute phase proteins, suggesting septicemia, were noted within 36 h after G-CSF withdrawal, and he was given antibiotics. He subsequently developed generalized edema, a 22% increase in weight, anuria, severe hypotension, and a significant increase in circulating leukocytes with marked toxic granulations. He recovered fully with vigorous fluid therapy.

Respiratory The role of G-CSF in the development of *pulmonary toxicity* is still debated. It has again been studied in 52 consecutive patients with newly diagnosed non-Hodgkin's lymphoma who received cyclophosphamide, doxorubicin, vincristine, and prednisolone (CHOP) every 2 weeks and G-CSF (95[C]). Six patients developed moderate or severe symptoms of pulmonary toxicity, and some required assisted ventilation or continuous oxygen, whereas none of the 49 patients who received CHOP every 3 weeks before the availability of G-CSF had similar complications. All the patients recovered after treatment with antibiotics and high-dose corticosteroids, and there was no recurrence in two patients who were rechallenged with a lower dose of G-CSF and for a shorter period of time. A mean peak leukocyte count above 23×10^9/l in each cycle of therapy was suggested to account for the development of pulmonary toxicity. Although CHOP has infrequently been associated with pulmonary complications, the fact that chemotherapy was given every 2 weeks instead of every 3 weeks might also have accounted for this toxicity.

Hematological Severe narcotic-resistant generalized bone pain that occurred shortly after G-CSF pretransplant conditioning therapy for peripheral blood stem cell transplantation was attributed to *bone marrow necrosis* in a 38-year-old man with refractory acute myeloblastic leukemia (96[c]). Engraftment after transplant was not altered.

Skin and appendages The role of G-CSF in the development or exacerbation of *neutrophilic dermatosis* is continuously discussed, and there have been additional reports of reversible *neutrophilic eccrine hidradenitis* (97[c]), acute *exacerbation of pyoderma gangrenosum* (98[c]), and rapidly reversible *Sweet's syndrome* (99[c]).

Special senses Severe subretinal hemorrhage has previously been described (SEDA-21, 378), and *retinal hemorrhage* resulting from hyperleukocytosis has now been reported (100[c]).

A 49-year-old man with a non-Hodgkin's lymphoma received cyclophosphamide for 2 days and etoposide for 3 days, followed by filgrastim (10 μg/kg per day for 10 days). He had a blurred spot in his central vision with dizziness and fatigue on day 13 and underwent leukapheresis 2 days later. At this time, his leukocyte count was 87×10^9/l and he again reported similar symptoms. The leukocyte count increased further to 121×10^9/l and he developed papillary and macular retinal hemorrhages with reduced visual acuity. His symptoms and ophthalmological signs progressively improved after leukapheresis, and he recovered normal vision within 12 weeks after transplantation.

Musculoskeletal system *Exacerbation of pseudogout*, with sudden pain in both knee joints, has again been reported (101[c]).

Worsening of rheumatoid symptoms has sometimes been reported in patients with Felty's syndrome, as has severe neutropenia (SED-13, 1116), but potential benefit has also been suggested. Five of eight patients with Felty's syndrome had significant adverse effects (*severe generalized joint pain*, *vasculitic rash*, *'flu-like symptoms*, *severe nausea*) during the first 1–2 weeks of G-CSF treatment (102[C]). Two withdrew from treatment, but changes in the formulation and/or dosage of G-CSF allowed the rest to continue treatment for 4–40 months without further complications or deterioration of their rheumatoid arthritis.

Immunological and hypersensitivity reactions Based on the results of skin testing in two patients who had *anaphylaxis* to *E. coli*-derived PEG-asparaginase, the possibility of immune cross-reactivity with *E. coli*-derived G-CSF (filgrastim) has been suggested (103[c]). Both patients had negative skin test response to yeast-derived GM-CSF (sargramostim) and subsequently received it without complication.

Granulocyte-macrophage colony-stimulating factor (GM-CSF; molgramostim, sargramostim)

GM-CSF is usually considered to cause more adverse effects than G-CSF, but this view has been based on limited and not carefully controlled data. In a prospective randomized trial in 42 patients with breast cancer who underwent autologous peripheral blood stem cell transplantation, there were no major differences in efficacy or adverse effects between filgrastim and molgramostim (5 μg/kg per day for mean of 7 days) (104[C]).

Two patients treated with low-dose GM-CSF after autologous bone marrow transplantation for Hodgkin's disease developed clinical features of *capillary leak syndrome*, and extensive and persistent bone marrow histiocytosis (105[c]). This was considered to be the possible cause of failed engraftment, and both patients died 2 months after marrow transplantation.

Our limited knowledge about the safety of GM-CSF in patients with AIDS has been reviewed (106[R]). Most patients were studied in non-randomized, controlled trials or uncontrolled case series ($n = 228$ patients), and only two randomized, controlled trials ($n = 46$ patients) were retrieved. From these limited data, there was no convincing evidence that GM-CSF enhances viral replication or increases the risk of infections or neoplasms.

MONOCLONAL ANTIBODIES

Orthoclone OKT3

The first-dose effect of OKT3 typically causes a complex of symptoms that is referred to as the *cytokine-release syndrome* and includes fever, chills, headache, myalgias, tachycardia, and gastrointestinal symptoms. A 2-h intravenous infusion of OKT3 considerably reduced the incidence of this syndrome, compared with a single bolus injection, in 18 patients randomized to receive either scheme of administration (107[C]). Complement activation was also significantly less in the patients given OKT3 by 2-h infusion, suggesting that complement activation may play a role in the first-dose adverse effects of OKT3.

Sensitization to orthoclone OKT3 is frequent, and the presence of *elevated anti-OKT3 IgG antibody titers* may reduce its clinical efficacy, precluding further administration. Immunosuppressive regimens may play a part in causing OKT3 sensitization. In 62 patients with renal transplants who received prophylactic OKT3, the incidence of anti-OKT3 antibodies was 50, 19, and 0%, respectively, in patients whose primary immunosuppression consisted of azathioprine plus cyclosporin (standard formulation) ($n = 20$), azathioprine plus cyclosporin (microemulsion formulation) ($n = 31$), or mycophenolate mofetil plus cyclosporin (microemulsion formulation) ($n = 11$), (108[C]). However, the results were limited by the retrospective design of the study and the small number of patients who received mycophenolate mofetil.

Other monoclonal antibodies

Despite intensive research, albeit in a limited number of patients, a wide range of monoclonal antibodies (anti-pan T lymphocytes, anti-inactivated T lymphocytes, anti-adhesion molecule, or anti-TNF antibodies) have had questionable benefit in the management of steroid-resistant acute graft-versus-host disease (109[R]). Whereas adverse effects are usually limited to *'flu-like symptoms, thrombocytopenia*, and *leukopenia*, it is still not known whether these agents increase the risk of infection or leukemia relapse.

In the prophylaxis of acute renal transplant rejection, the incidence of adverse events and infections did not differ between patients randomized to basiliximab (a chimeric IL-2 receptor monoclonal antibody) 40 mg (190 patients) or placebo (186 patients) (110[C]). In particular, there were no signs of the cytokine-release syndrome and no increase in the incidence of infections in basiliximab-treated patients. Significantly fewer patients had acute rejection episodes in the basiliximab group.

T10B9, an anti-human pan T-lymphocyte monoclonal antibody, has been developed for the treatment of acute renal transplant rejection. Promising results have been obtained in a randomized trial in 76 patients allocated to T10B9 or OKT3 for 10 days (111[C]). Whereas graft and patient survival at 4 years did not differ between the two groups, the incidence of acute or delayed adverse effects, namely *fever and respiratory, gastrointestinal, or neurological symptoms*, was significantly lower in the T10B9 group. Although the difference was not significant, infectious complications were less frequent in patients treated with T10B9 compared with OKT3 (17 vs 28%), and only the latter experienced severe infections.

IMMUNOSUPPRESSIVE DRUGS

Azathioprine and 6-mercaptopurine

Prolonged treatment with azathioprine or 6-mercaptopurine is used in inflammatory and autoimmune diseases. Of 95 children (mean age 14 years at the start of therapy) treated for chronic inflammatory bowel disease, 51 tolerated the treatment, 27 had an adverse reaction that required dosage reduction or resolved spontaneously (mostly moderate *leukopenia* or *increased ALT activity*), and 17 had to discontinue treatment because of *hypersensitivity reactions* ($n = 8$), *pancreatitis* ($n = 4$), *gastrointestinal intolerance* ($n = 3$), *recurrent infections* ($n = 3$), progressive *hyperpigmentation*, and *thrombocytopenia* and *leukopenia* (one case each) (112[C]). Except for a higher incidence of hepatic toxicity (ALT activity, 80–396 IU), this adverse effects profile is very similar to that previously found in children and adults with inflammatory bowel disease.

In randomized and non-randomized trials of conversion from cyclosporin to azathioprine after renal transplantation, azathioprine had beneficial effects in selected closely monitored patients, improving renal function and reducing cardiovascular risk factors (hypertension and cholesterol concentrations) (113[R]). The incidence of chronic rejection or graft loss was not increased, and conversion resulted in significant cost reduction.

Skin and appendages The first case of *Sweet's syndrome* has been reported.

A 42-year-old woman with Crohn's colitis, uveitis, arthritis, and erythema nodosum developed a pruritic maculopapular rash after taking azathioprine for 10 days (114[c]). Histopathological examination showed characteristic lesions of Sweet's syndrome, with intense dermal neutrophilic infiltration. The rash resolved within 2 weeks of azathioprine withdrawal and recurred several months later within days of reintroduction.

This sequence of events strongly suggested azathioprine-induced Sweet's syndrome.

Immunological and hypersensitivity reactions Further reports of azathioprine-induced isolated *fever* (115[c]) or *hypersensitivity reactions*, with a wide range of clinical effects, have appeared (116[c]), (117[c]). From these new case reports, it appears that hypersensitivity to azathioprine is frequently misdiagnosed and should be promptly recognized to avoid unnecessary and costly investigations or antibiotic treatment, and further recurrence on reintroduction of azathioprine.

Tumor-inducing effects There is as yet no definite evidence for an increased incidence of cancer in patients who have had prolonged exposure to azathioprine or 6-mercaptopurine. In a case of fatal *acute myeloblastic leukemia*, diagnosed after 12 years of 6-mercaptopurine treatment for Crohn's disease, deletion of chromosome 7 on cytogenic bone-marrow examination strongly suggested treatment-related leukemia (118[c]).

Cyclophosphamide

Both daily oral or cyclic-pulse intravenous cyclophosphamide are used in the treatment of various inflammatory or autoimmune diseases. It is as yet unclear whether one route of administration should be preferred to another (119[r]). The cumulative dose of cyclophosphamide with an intravenous pulse regimen is consistently lower than the cumulative dose with daily oral administration, and the incidence of bladder cancer is therefore expected to be lower with the former mode of administration. However, the choice of maintenance regimen is still problematic, as has again been exemplified in 50 patients with newly diagnosed Wegener's granulomatosis (120[C]). After similar initial treatment with methylprednisolone and cyclophosphamide, they were randomized to receive either prednisone plus intravenous pulse cyclophosphamide (group A, 27 patients) or prednisone plus oral cyclophosphamide (group B, 23 patients) for at least 1 year. The overall incidence of adverse effects was similar in the two groups, but significantly more patients in group B had infectious complications (70 vs 41%), mostly *Pneumocystis carinii* pneumonia. As a result, more patients died from infection-related adverse effects in group B (6/23 vs 3/27). In contrast, although the remission rates at 6 months were identical, the cumulative relapse rates at 4.5 years was higher in group A (59 vs 13%).

Urinary system Hemorrhagic cystitis is a well-known complication of cyclophosphamide. *Upper renal tract disorders* have also been reported.

A 43-year-old woman with systemic lupus erythematosus had received 50 mg/day cyclophosphamide for 33 months when she had a typical cyclophosphamide-induced hemorrhagic cystitis (121[c]). Cystoscopy and biopsies performed 2, 3, and 4 years after cyclophosphamide withdrawal showed persistent hematuric cystitis. In addition, urodynamic studies showed high-pressure bladder with ureteric reflux and bilateral hydronephrosis.

Endocrine, metabolic Cyclophosphamide can cause *ovarian failure* (SEDA-20, 342). Risk factors have been investigated in a retrospective study in 274 women aged under 45 years with systemic lupus erythematosus, of whom 70 had received intravenous intermittent pulse or oral cyclophosphamide (group I), 84 azathioprine but not cyclophosphamide (group II), and 88 either no drug or hydroxychloroquine alone (group III) (122[C]). The overall incidence of ovarian failure, defined as sustained amenorrhea for at least 12 months, and documented by reduced estradiol concentrations, was 26% in group I, 1% in group II, and 0% in group III. The mean time interval between cyclophosphamide treatment and the first missed menses was 4.4 months. A higher age at the start of treatment and total cumulative dose were independent risk factors for cyclophosphamide-induced ovarian failure, with incidences of 14, 28, and 50% in patients aged under 30 years, 30–39 years, and over 40 years, respectively, and 4, 26, 31, and 70% for cumulative dose of under 10, 10–20, 20–30, and over 40 g, respectively.

Hematological There was a significant *increase in eosinophil count* (2–20%) in 32 patients with multiple sclerosis who received intravenous pulses of cyclophosphamide plus methylprednisolone compared with 15 patients treated with methylprednisolone alone (0–4%) (123[C]). The increase was correlated with increased IL-4 secretion and provided indirect evidence of an immune deviation toward a Th2 response in cyclophosphamide-treated patients.

Tumor-inducing effects An increased risk of *bladder cancer* may be the consequence of long-term oral cyclophosphamide treatment in patients with Wegener's granulomatosis (SEDA-20, 343). A retrospective analysis has identified an excess incidence of bladder cancer in 2351 patients with multiple sclerosis with indwelling catheters (124[C]). Seven (0.3%) had bladder cancer, of whom six had had an indwelling catheter for over 1 year. Five (5.7%) of the 70 patients who had received cyclophosphamide had bladder cancer, and all five had an indwelling catheter. Both factors were therefore suggested to have accounted for the bladder cancer. Cyclophosphamide-treated patients had received a mean total cumulative dose of 61 g and bladder cancer was diagnosed a mean of 5.8 years after the last dose.

Cyclosporin

A microemulsion formulation of cyclosporin (Neoral) seems to have significant advantages over the standard formulation. In a meta-analysis of 49 studies (including 16 blinded, 26 randomized, 24 with a longitudinal design, and 45 in adults) in 4024 patients treated with Neoral and 3133 treated with cyclosporin, the adverse event profiles were similar in both groups, but Neoral (as the primary immunosuppressive agent) produced significant benefit on the incidence of rejection (125[C]). In particular, patients with liver transplants treated with Neoral had a 2-fold lower incidence of adverse events compared with those who took the standard formulation. Because dosage adjustments are sometimes difficult to make, other investigators have considered that conversion to Neoral may be hazardous and of little benefit, at least in stable liver transplant patients, and found that 30 of 54 patients undergoing conversion required multiple dosage reduction, mostly because of increased cyclosporin blood concentrations and dose-related cyclosporin adverse effects, whereas six who underwent dosage reduction had biopsy-proven rejection (126[C]).

Nervous system Cyclosporin acute neurotoxicity is well known, but it had not been extensively studied in children. The clinical characteristics, EEG, brain imaging findings, and the outcome of cyclosporin-induced *acute encephalopathy* and *seizures* have been retrospectively analysed in 19 transplant patients aged 3–17 years, i.e. about 2.6% of patients taking cyclosporin (127[C]). Focal or generalized motor seizures associated with headache or cortical visual disturbances were identified after a median of 30 days after transplantation. Brain imaging showed typical lesions in 14 patients, predominantly bilateral parieto-occipital, cerebral cortical, and subcortical abnormalities, and EEG showed epileptiform discharges and focal or diffuse slowing in all patients. After a median follow-up period of 49 months in 13 patients, brain imaging abnormalities usually disappeared or improved, whereas there were persistent EEG abnormalities in 70% of patients. Seizures recurred at 3–14 months in six patients, all of whom had persistent EEG abnormalities.

After allogeneic bone marrow transplantation, eight of 87 patients developed cyclosporin neurotoxicity, namely visual abnormalities, cortical blindness, or seizures (128[C]). Patients with HLA-mismatched and unrelated donor transplants (6/8) were more predisposed, and had symptoms earlier after transplantation. All eight patients who developed neurotoxicity lived less than 6 months after toxicity.

Endocrine, metabolic *Hyperlipidemia* is a major issue in long-term survivors of transplantation, as it may produce atherogenic changes with increased cardiovascular morbidity, chronic nephropathy, and graft loss. Many factors contribute to the occurrence of hyperlipidemia after transplantation, including the immunosuppressive regimen, in particular cyclosporin and steroids. However, the individual contribution of these drugs is still being debated.

Several recent studies have provided striking evidence that cyclosporin causes lipid abnormalities more often than tacrolimus. In the European multicenter FK-506 study, cholesterol and LDL concentrations were significantly lower with tacrolimus than cyclosporin after 1 year of treatment (129[C]). At that time, with tacrolimus the number of patients initially classified as having normal, borderline, or high cholesterol concentrations was unchanged, whereas with cyclosporin there was a 2-fold reduction in the number of patients with initially normal cholesterol concentrations and a 2-fold increase in those with initially high cholesterol concentrations. Analysis of risk factors for hypercholesterolemia confirmed that treatment was the most important.

In another study, 65 patients with stable renal function for at least 12 months after transplantation and hypercholesterolemia (6.2 mmol/l) were randomized to continue cyclosporin or to convert to tacrolimus without changes in steroid dosage or the lipid-lowering drug regimen (130[C]). During the 6-month observation period, there were significant falls in total cholesterol (16%), LDL cholesterol (25%), and apolipoprotein B (23%) in tacrolimus-treated patients, whereas renal function or serum glucose concentrations remained unchanged. Another study in 27 patients randomized to tacrolimus or cyclosporin showed significantly lower total and LDL cholesterol serum concentrations with tacrolimus, but the steroid-sparing effect of tacrolimus was thought to have fully accounted for these findings (131[C]).

However, the concept of the steroid dosage as a confounding factor for these differences has been challenged in a retrospective study involving renal transplant patients whose serum cholesterol concentrations were below 5.2 mmol/l before transplantation (132[C]). Cumulative steroid dose and hypercholesterolemia risk factors were matched in 20 patients taking tacrolimus and 40 taking cyclosporin. After 1 year there was hypercholesterolemia (over 5.2 mmol/l) in 67% of patients taking cyclosporin compared with 26% taking tacrolimus, with definitive hypercholesterolemia (over 6.2 mmol/l) in 29 and 0%, respectively. As expected, the cumulative doses of steroid were not significantly different in the groups. Taken together, these results suggest a major role for cyclosporin in the development of lipid metabolism disturbances.

Urinary system A considerable amount of information on chronic cyclosporin *nephropathy* appears each year, but its long-term prognosis remains a source of conflicting opinions. It is still unclear whether chronic nephropathy is irreversible or can improve after dosage reduction. The latter possibility has been investigated in 23 patients with renal transplants and histologically proven chronic cyclosporin nephropathy, i.e. 6% of the whole renal transplant population (133[C]). These patients had taken cyclosporin for a mean of 27 months at diagnosis and were regularly followed up after immediate cyclosporin dosage reduction (18 patients) or withdrawal (five patients). Although renal vascular resistance, filtration fraction, and albumin excretion were unchanged, glomerular filtration rate and effective renal plasma flow increased significantly at 2 years, showing that renal improvement can be obtained rapidly. There was a 26% fall in serum creatinine concentration at 12 months, and this was sustained after a further 60 months in 17 patients. Histological lesions also improved markedly in six patients who underwent renal biopsy after 6–58 months. Overall, these data suggest that chronic nephropathy can be reversed if the dosage of cyclosporin is reduced early after diagnosis, but this possibility should be carefully evaluated, because of the risk of chronic rejection, which occurred in three patients within 35–58 months.

The possibility of irreversible chronic nephropathy is also a major outcome of cyclosporin maintenance in non-transplant patients, in whom the benefit:risk ratio should be carefully evaluated. A meta-analysis of 18 controlled, randomized trials of cyclosporin dosages below 10 mg/kg per day (mean dosage 4.8 mg/kg per day) during at least 2 months (mean duration 6.4 months) in the treatment of autoimmune diseases showed that the overall weighted percentage increase in serum creatinine concentration was 17% in the 852 patients taking cyclosporin, compared with 1.7% in the 763 control patients at the end of treatment (134[C]). Renal dysfunction normalized partially (seven studies, 223 patients) or completely (six studies, 483 patients) after cyclosporin withdrawal, but long-term outcomes were rarely described. Serum creatinine concentrations (available in 13 studies), increased by more than 50% of the pre-treatment value at least once in 102 of 474 patients with cyclosporin compared with five of 393 controls, a corrected risk difference of 21% (95% CI 12–30). The possible progression of cyclosporin nephrotoxicity to irreversible renal injury in non-transplant patients remains debatable (SEDA-20, 345; SEDA-21, 384).

Long-term follow-up of patients with psoriasis who had taken low-dose cyclosporin for an average of 10 years (group I, seven patients) or six years (group II, 20 patients) suggested that the time to occurrence and the speed of progression of cyclosporin-induced nephrotoxicity varied greatly from one patient to another (135[C]). There was a persistent increase in serum creatinine concentrations of more than 30% from baseline in all seven patients in group I and in nine of 20 patients in group II; four and five patients, respectively, had increases of more than 50%. The glomerular filtration rate was reduced by more than 30% in two of seven and in five of 18 patients. Repeat renal biopsies at 5 and 10 years in two patients showed features of progressive nephropathy. About half of the patients in the two groups had to take antihypertensive treatment after 5 years. Finally, there was an improvement in renal function after 5 years in two other patients who discontinued cyclosporin because of biopsy-proven nephrotoxicity after 5 years of treatment.

Hemolytic–uremic syndrome is another severe complication of cyclosporin. Symptoms usually appear early after transplantation, but can be delayed for up to 5–9 months (136[c]). Although rare, its incidence may have been underestimated. Clinical and histological features have been detailed in seven of 201 patients (3.5%) who developed hemolytic–uremic syndrome within 2 weeks after renal transplantation (137[C]). These patients had high cyclosporin blood concentrations at diagnosis, and the clinical course was more severe in recipients of cadaveric kidneys. In this and another study (138[c]) there was no recurrence after initial withdrawal when cyclosporin was reintroduced, or even despite cyclosporin continuation with dosage reduction. However, as suggested by a meta-analysis, the use of cyclosporin or tacrolimus as immunosuppressive drugs after transplantation was a significant risk factor for the recurrence of hemolytic–uremic syndrome in patients who underwent renal transplantation for end-stage renal disease associated with hemolytic–uremic syndrome (139[C]).

Skin and appendages *Worsening of subcutaneous sarcoidosis* has been reported (140[c]).

A 52-year-old man took cyclosporin 5 mg/kg per day for biopsy-proven pyoderma gangrenosum on the pretibial area. He also had sarcoidosis. Although the pretibial lesions disappeared completely, he developed numerous tender nodules on his arms and trunk 3 months later. Biopsies showed subcutaneous sarcoidosis. After cyclosporin withdrawal, the pyoderma gangrenosum reappeared, but the subcutaneous nodules resolved. A further course of cyclosporin with prednisone produced healing of the pyoderma without recurrence of the nodules; cyclosporin was resumed and prednisone tapered over 1 month. His pretibial lesions reappeared, and a third course of cyclosporin was given without prednisone. The pyoderma resolved but the subcutaneous nodules reappeared, and were more numerous. There was spontaneous healing after cyclosporin withdrawal.

Teeth and gums *Gingival hyperplasia* is a common adverse effect of cyclosporin, with significant cosmetic and functional sequelae. Dental hygiene with plaque control is often sufficient, but surgical treatment is sometimes required. Since the appearance of preliminary reports, azithromycin has received considerable attention as medical management. Four recent studies in 87 patients have confirmed that azithromycin (250–500 mg/day for 3–5 days) produced rapid and significant improvement of cyclosporin-induced gingival overgrowth in most patients (141[C])–(144[C]). The beneficial effect was more marked in patients with less initial hyperplasia (141[C]).

Assessment of quality of life in 303 of 412 renal transplant patients showed moderately but significantly lower scores with cyclosporin compared with tacrolimus, possibly associated with a higher incidence of *hirsutism* (8.7 vs 0.5%), *gingivitis* (8.7 vs 1.5%), and *gum hyperplasia* (5.3 vs 0.5%) (145[C]).

Musculoskeletal system Cyclosporin rarely causes muscular disorders. A 35-year-old man had a 38-fold *increase in serum creatinine kinase activity* without any clinical symptoms, and reversal was observed only after cyclosporin dosage reduction (146[c]). However, a drug interaction with the patient's multidrug regimen could not be ruled out.

Immunological and hypersensitivity reactions The mechanism of the well-known immediate *hypersensitivity reactions* to intravenous cyclosporin is still unclear, and skin tests were performed in only three of the 22 previously published cases. In a further report of an anaphylactic reaction, intradermal tests to the intravenous formulation were positive, suggesting a possible IgE-mediated reaction, most probably directed against Cremophor EL, the solvent of the intravenous solution (147[cR]). Indeed, the patient subsequently tolerated a soft gelatin formulation based on corn oil.

Miscellaneous *Fever*, a previously unreported adverse effect of cyclosporin, occurred in a 31-year-old woman with atopic dermatitis (148[c]). After 1 month of treatment, recurrent episodes of isolated fever occurred within 90 min after each dose of cyclosporin and completely resolved after withdrawal.

Use in pregnancy In a retrospective review of the outcome of 14 pregnancies in 13 liver transplant recipients treated with tacrolimus ($n = 5$) or cyclosporin ($n = 8$) during their pregnancy, cyclosporin was suggested to have caused more frequent maternal *renal dysfunction* or *pre-eclampsia*, suggesting that tacrolimus might be preferred in pregnant women with transplants (149[c]).

Use in lactation Breast-feeding is commonly contraindicated in patients taking cyclosporin. After follow-up for 12–36 months, none of seven breast-fed infants whose mothers had taken cyclosporin while breast-feeding had long-term adverse consequences (150[c]). In particular, serum creatinine concentrations were normal at the end of follow-up. The duration of breast-feeding was 4–12 months, and cyclosporin concentrations in random blood samples of infants were always below the detection limit. Cyclosporin concentrations measured in the breast milk of six mothers were close to those measured in blood samples, and it was calculated that the infants ingested less than 300 μg/day. However, more information is needed with more careful and longer follow-up, because the effects of even very low doses of cyclosporin on the developing infant are unknown.

Tumor-inducing effects There is much concern about the risk of cancer in patients taking long-term immunosuppressives. Cancers in cyclosporin-treated patients are thought to be dose related. In a single-center trial, 231 stable renal transplant patients treated with cyclosporin were randomized at 1 year to receive low-dosage cyclosporin (trough concentrations of 75–125 μg/l) or a normal dosage (trough concentrations of 150–250 μg/l) (151[C]). After a mean follow-up period of 66 months the overall frequency of cancers, mostly *skin cancers*, was significantly higher in the normal than in the low-dosage group (37 vs 23). *Viral infections* were also more common in the normal-dosage group. Although renal function and graft survival did not differ between the groups, acute rejection was more frequent in the low-dosage group (nine vs one patient), suggesting that the potential benefit of a low dosage of cyclosporin should be carefully evaluated.

Long-term cyclosporin treatment in non-transplant patients also carries a potential risk of malignancies, but the results of studies have been conflicting. Compared with the expected incidence rate of cancer in patients with psoriasis, the relative risk of malignancies was 5.6 (95% CI 3.9–8) in 1223 patients with psoriasis enrolled to receive cyclosporin in clinical trials (152[c]). This was comparable to the increased risk of cancer in patients treated with other immunosuppressants. By contrast, a retrospective, matched cohort study in patients with rheumatoid arthritis showed no increased risk of malignancies in 208 patients taking cyclosporin compared with 415 patients who had never taken cyclosporin (153[C]). However, the median duration of follow up in the cyclosporin group was only 4.7 years.

Interactions Papers on drug interactions involving cyclosporin often appear. Only previously unreported interactions will be discussed here.

Anticancer drugs In a phase I trial in 18 children with cancers, high-dosage cyclosporin (15–30 mg/kg per day) produced an 89% increase in etoposide AUC and a 48% reduction in clearance, suggesting that etoposide dosage should be reduced by 50% during co-administration of cyclosporin (154[C]).

Antidepressants Fluvoxamine and nefazodone, which are potent inhibitors of CYP3A4, caused 3- and 1.5-fold increases, respectively, in trough cyclosporin concentrations in two patients (155[c]). Both had an increase in serum creatinine concentrations and subsequently required a 33–50% reduction in cyclosporin dosage. In contrast, cyclosporin blood concentrations were not affected in heart or lung transplant patients treated with sertraline, paroxetine, or fluoxetine, but only six patients were studied (156[c]).

Azithromycin Two studies have shown that azithromycin does not alter cyclosporin blood concentrations (141[C]), (143[C]).

Carvedilol The effects of carvedilol on the pharmacokinetic of cyclosporin have been studied in 21 renal transplant patients with chronic vascular rejection (157[C]). After progressive carvedilol titration to 50 mg/day over 90 days, the cyclosporin dosage had to be reduced by an average of 20% to maintain therapeutic cyclosporin concentrations.

Chloroquine In a randomized double-blind study in 88 patients, the addition of low-dosage cyclosporin to chloroquine in patients with rheumatoid arthritis was associated with an unfavorable benefit:risk ratio (158[C]). Whereas none of the 29 patients who took chloroquine and placebo discontinued treatment, premature withdrawal was required because of adverse events in three of 29 and four of 30 patients randomized to cyclosporin 1.25 and 2.5 mg/kg per day, respectively. The reasons for withdrawal were gastrointestinal disorders ($n = 5$), folliculitis ($n = 1$), and an increase in serum creatinine concentration ($n = 1$). Compared with placebo, there was a significant increase in serum creatinine concentrations in those who took cyclosporin 2.5 mg/kg per day, of whom 11 had an increase of more than 30% in serum creatinine concentrations.

Paclitaxel and sirolimus Cyclosporin inhibits the multidrug transporter P-glycoprotein and produced a 9-fold increase in the oral absorption of paclitaxel, a poorly available drug with a high affinity for P-glycoprotein, compared with oral paclitaxel alone (159[c]). Whether these results can be extrapolated to other drugs with low oral availability and a high affinity for P-glycoprotein is unknown, but the increase in AUC and trough concentrations of sirolimus when administered with cyclosporin (160[C]) might be partly explained by this mechanism.

Troglitazone The introduction of troglitazone in two patients with stable cyclosporin concentrations dramatically reduced serum cyclosporin concentrations (161[c], 162[c]). One patient developed signs of moderate acute cellular rejection. That troglitazone can induce cyclosporin metabolism was further supported by the retrospective identification of a 15–48% reduction in cyclosporin trough concentrations soon after the introduction of troglitazone in seven stable renal transplant patients (162[c]).

Methotrexate

Methotrexate is one of the most widely used disease-modifying antirheumatic drugs. Although adverse effects are very common, they are rarely severe enough to require drug withdrawal, even after very long-term treatment. In a long-term prospective study (11 years) of 26 patients with rheumatoid arthritis, adverse effects were attributed to low-dosage methotrexate in 70% of patients, including *gastrointestinal toxicity* (42%), *alopecia* (27%), *headache* (19%), *rheumatoid-like nodules* (12%), and *pulmonary toxicity* (8%) (163[C]). These adverse effects usually occurred during the first 84 months of treatment and treatment was withdrawn in three patients (two with pneumonitis and one with alopecia). Only 10 patients completed the 132 months of the study.

Methotrexate produces similar benefits to gold sodium thiomalate, and drug withdrawal is required less often because of adverse effects (16% of 87 patients vs 53% of 87 patients) (164[C]). In addition, adverse effects occurred significantly later with methotrexate. The most frequent were *liver enzyme rises* (30%), *nausea* (19%), *alopecia* (12%), and *hematological* (10%), *mucocutaneous* (9%), *gastrointestinal* (7.6%), and *bronchopulmonary* events (4.8%).

Respiratory Methotrexate-induced lung disease is rare but potentially serious, and confirmatory diagnosis is sometimes difficult to obtain. Over 5 years, 10 of 1162 patients treated with low-dosage methotrexate developed definite or probable *pneumonitis* after 1–72 months of treatment (165[c]). The estimated prevalence in this population was 0.86%. Shortness of breath (100%) and dry cough (60%) were the most common initial clinical features, and three patients died. Patients with pre-existing pleuropulmonary involvement were more likely to develop this complication. Although corticosteroids were commonly used in management, there is not yet evidence that they positively affect the outcome.

A previous history of drug-induced pulmonary disorders is also a risk factor, as suggested by the development of methotrexate pneumonitis in a 64-year-old man who had had aminorex-induced primary pulmonary hypertension (166[c]).

Hematological Isolated *thrombocytopenia*, an uncommon feature of methotrexate-induced hematological toxicity, has been reported (167[c]).

A 36-year-old woman taking ibuprofen for rheumatoid arthritis took a single oral dose of methotrexate (7.5 mg) for sarcoidosis. One week later she developed numerous limb petechiae and her platelet count fell from 195 to 25×10^9/l, while her hemoglobin and leukocyte count remained normal. Her platelet count normalized after both drugs had been withdrawn.

Liver Although methotrexate *hepatotoxicity* is well-known, no additional hepatotoxic effects were evidenced in 48 patients with primary biliary cirrhosis. After 2 years of methotrexate treatment, and compared with the initial liver biopsy, the histological stage of the disease and fibrosis continue to progress, but inflammation and bile duct injury were reduced (168[C]).

Urinary system Low-dosage methotrexate very rarely causes renal damage. Generalized edema and severe proteinuria with minimal change disease on biopsy occurred after a second injection of methotrexate in a 39-year-old man, but this *nephrotic syndrome* could not be conclusively attributed to methotrexate because it resolved after corticosteroid treatment and withdrawal of other drugs (169[c]).

Skin and appendages Methotrexate can cause histologically proven *leukocytoclastic vasculitis*, and two further cases have been carefully reported (170[c]), (171[c]). An immediate hypersensitivity reaction was suggested as a possible mechanism, because one patient had a prompt recurrence of vasculitis after methotrexate rechallenge (170[c]), whereas the second patient, who had had an episode of methotrexate-induced urticaria 2 years before, rapidly developed severe necrotic skin lesions after a second weekly injection (171[c]). In addition, one patient had a positive mast cell degranulation test to methotrexate, suggesting the presence of specific IgE antibodies against methotrexate (170[c]).

Methotrexate-induced *skin ulceration* has previously been described in patients with psoriasis, but now it has been described in a 67-year-old man taking methotrexate for rheumatoid arthritis (172[c]).

Musculoskeletal system Whether methotrexate can cause changes in bone metabolism is still controversial. A 65-year-old woman with scleroderma developed four *stress fractures* within a period of 13 months. She had none of the classical risk factors for osteoporosis and had never taken steroids (173[cr]). There have been 12 other previously published cases, including 10 women and three men who had taken methotrexate for a mean of 5 years and a mean cumulative dose of 4 g.

Tumor-inducing effects Although the oncogenic potential of low-dose methotrexate has never been convincingly demonstrated, low-dose methotrexate has been sometimes associated with the development of various type of cancers. However, the relation with methotrexate is far from demonstrated, and most of the cases have been described in sporadic reports (174[R]).

The possible increased incidence of *lymphoma* in patients taking low-dosage methotrexate treatment is the most consistently discussed, but the pathophysiological mechanisms are still unclear. It is as yet unknown whether this is due to direct methotrexate toxicity, a typical complication of immunosuppression resulting in Epstein-Barr virus-associated lymphoproliferative disease, or a delayed complication of the underlying disease, in particular in patients with rheumatoid arthritis. In addition, although spontaneous regression can occur after methotrexate withdrawal, other patients need chemotherapy. These features of methotrexate-associated lymphoma have again been illustrated.

A 64-year-old woman developed non-Hodgkin's lymphoma after 2 years of methotrexate, and Epstein-Barr virus RNA was detected in the lymphoma cells (175[c]). Methotrexate withdrawal resulted in spontaneous remission.

In contrast, a 6-year-old girl with juvenile rheumatoid arthritis developed Epstein-Barr virus-negative Hodgkin's disease while taking methotrexate, and combination chemotherapy was required to obtain complete resolution (176[c]).

Of four patients who took methotrexate for 1–7 years and developed B cell lymphomas, only one of three tested was positive for Epstein-Barr virus (177[c]). All four underwent chemotherapy after methotrexate withdrawal failed to cause improvement.

Finally, four lesions of *malignant melanoma* occurred simultaneously in a 64-year-old man taking methotrexate without predisposing factors (178[c]).

Infections The increased risk of infections (usually common bacterial infections, *Herpes zoster*, and more rarely opportunistic infections) in methotrexate-treated patients is considered to be low (174[R]), (179[c]). The most severe complications usually occur in patients who are also taking steroids, as shown by further reports of *septic arthritis* with *Listeria monocytogenes* (180[c]), *cavitary lung tuberculosis* (181[c]), disseminated cutaneous *Herpes zoster* infection complicated by *Staphylococcus aureus* induced subacute *necrotizing fasciitis* (182[c]), *Pneumocystis carinii* pneumonia (183[c]), and acute reactivation of a presumed quiescent *chronic hepatitis B infection* after methotrexate withdrawal (184[c]). In this last case, T-cell-mediated immunological rebound was the presumed cause of the rapid destruction of infected hepatocytes.

Use in pregnancy Most of our limited knowledge on the consequences to the embryo and fetus of methotrexate exposure during pregnancy is derived from patients treated for cancer, and only a few reports have documented the outcome of pregnancies after exposure to low-dosage methotrexate (185[R]). Previous data have suggested that the critical period of exposure for the *fetal methotrexate syndrome* is 6–8 weeks after conception, and 10 mg weekly is the minimal dose. A description of three other patients with a complete or partial form of the fetal methotrexate syndrome has emphasized the risk of congenital abnormalities associated with high-dosage methotrexate and suggested that the critical period may extend to week 11 (186[c]). Two patients were exposed in an attempt to induce abortion at 6 weeks and at 11–23 weeks after conception; the other was given methotrexate for breast cancer from 7 to 30 weeks after conception.

Interactions The additional risk of myelosuppression when methotrexate is added to *co-trimoxazole*, both of which have antifolate effects, is well known, and this should also be taken into account in patients taking trimethoprim alone.

A 81-year-old woman took methotrexate (7.5 mg/week) for rheumatoid arthritis (187[c]). Her erythrocyte folate concentration was normal before methotrexate treatment and fell to 76 ng/ml (reference range 95–570). Two months after prophylactic trimethoprim (100 mg/day) had been added for an inoperable bladder carcinoma, and 2 weeks after the trimethoprim dosage had been increased to 200 mg/day for a urinary tract infection, she became acutely septic with pancytopenia. She died 1 week later, despite treatment with folinic acid and granulocyte colony-stimulating factor.

Mycophenolate mofetil

Respiratory Mycophenolate mofetil has previously been associated with *lung fibrosis and respiratory failure* in one patient (SEDA-21, 389), and there has been another report of severe pulmonary toxicity (188[c]).

A 61-year-old man underwent renal transplantation and took cyclosporin, mycophenolate mofetil (2 g/day), steroids, and prophylactic ketoconazole, aciclovir, and co-trimoxazole. Four weeks later he developed progressive dyspnea with pulmonary edema, and required intubation because of rapid pulmonary deterioration. Mycophenolate mofetil was withdrawal and the dosage of cyclosporin was reduced. There was no improvement after 14 days of broad-spectrum antibiotics, fluconazole, and ganciclovir. His renal function remained stable and cyclosporin was withdrawn. Tracheostomy and open lung biopsy showed severe interstitial fibrosis without evidence of infection. Methylprednisolone produced no benefit and he died 3 months after transplantation, from respiratory failure.

Because other drugs, in particular anti-infective drugs, were used the role of mycophenolate mofetil in this case was uncertain.

Italian investigators have suggested that *dry cough* and *dyspnea* are possible adverse effects and might be considered as early symptoms of pulmonary toxicity (189[c]). Among 45 renal transplant recipients (26 men, 19 women) who received mycophenolate mofetil (2 g/day) together with cyclosporin and steroids, five women developed a non-productive cough after 36–84 days. Three had no past history of respiratory disease. One had exacerbation of asthma, and another, a heavy smoker, dyspnea and hypoxia. Symptoms resolved only after mycophenolate mofetil withdrawal, within 3–4 weeks in all five patients.

Gastrointestinal Mycophenolate mofetil often causes gastrointestinal disorders, such as gastric and duodenal ulceration. *Colonic ulceration and lower gastrointestinal bleeding* have also been noted in four patients within 16–78 days of treatment, with no recurrence after withdrawal (190[c]).

Urinary system Nephrotoxicity has not been observed in clinical trials reported so far and mycophenolate mofetil was successfully used to replace cyclosporin in six patients with biopsy-proven nephrotoxicity, with significant improvement in renal function, blood pressure, and hyperlipidemia (191[C]).

Skin and appendages Although hair loss has not been found in large trials, *alopecia* has been noted in two patients converted from cyclosporin to mycophenolate mofetil (192[c]).

Infections Data from three large multicenter trials have shown an increased risk of leukopenia and *cytomegalovirus disease* in renal transplant patients taking the highest dose of mycophenolate mofetil (3 g/day). In a more careful analysis of the European Mycophenolate Mofetil Cooperative study, the incidence of cytomegalovirus disease after transplantation was 36, 7.4, and 3.7% in patients taking either mycophenolate mofetil 3 g/day (n = 27), 2 g/day (n = 27), or placebo (n = 28) in combination with standard dose cyclosporin and prednisone (193[C]). In 15 other patients who took mycophenolate mofetil 3 g/day plus low-dose cyclosporin only one patient had cytomegalovirus disease, but there was a comparable incidence of mycophenolate mofetil-associated leukopenia (40%). This confirmed that over-immunosuppression rather than mycophenolate mofetil per se is associated with an increased incidence of cytomegalovirus disease. These results are in accordance with those of a case–control study that found no association between the use of mycophenolate mofetil and cytomegalovirus infection in 31 renal transplant patients (194[C]). In this study, the odds ratio for cytomegalovirus infection was 1.0 when mycophenolate mofetil was compared with azathioprine as part of cyclosporin/prednisone-based immunosuppression. Other investigators have found that mycophenolate mofetil in addition to tacrolimus-based immunosuppression is not associated with an increased risk of infectious complications in liver transplant recipients (195[C]).

Tumor-inducing effects In a 3-year follow-up of 503 patients the incidence of *lymphoproliferative disorders* was 1.2, 1.8, and 0.6% in patients taking mycophenolate mofetil 2 g/day, mycophenolate mofetil 3 g/day, or azathioprine, each in combination with cyclosporin and prednisone (196[C]). The respective incidences of *skin carcinoma* were 14, 11, and 4.3%, and of *other malignancies* 2.3, 5.5, and 3.7%. Longer follow-up periods are awaited to provide more accurate analysis of the risk and type of malignancy in patients taking mycophenolate.

Tacrolimus

Although the adverse effects profiles of cyclosporin and tacrolimus, particularly the pattern of nephrotoxicity, are remarkably similar (197[R]), (198[R]), conversion from cyclosporin to tacrolimus can be a therapeutic alternative in patients with cyclosporin adverse effects. The beneficial effect of doing this has again been emphasized in 15 patients with cyclosporin-induced severe gingival hyperplasia or hypertrichosis, and there was a significant improvement or complete regression of both disorders within the first 3 months of conversion to tacrolimus (199[C]). There were additional benefits on the lipid profile, serum creatinine concentrations, arterial blood pressure, and the reduction in concomitant use of antihypertensive therapy, during a 6-month follow-up of 50 patients switched from cyclosporin to tacrolimus (200[C]). Only five patients had to change again to cyclosporin because of severe *alopecia*.

However, changing from cyclosporin to tacrolimus is not always successful. Two patients who developed cyclosporin-induced cortical blindness after bone marrow transplantation were switched to tacrolimus (201[c]). Although visual abnormalities promptly resolved, both rapidly developed *thrombotic thrombocytopenic purpura* and *graft-versus-host disease* requiring high-dose steroids, and finally died 33 days after transplantation, from presumed brain-stem compression with diffuse cerebellar edema, hydrocephalus, and herniation.

Cardiovascular *Cardiomyopathy* is a rare but severe cardiac complication of tacrolimus. *QT interval prolongation and torsade de pointes* have also emerged as potentially life-threatening consequences of tacrolimus. Electrocardiographic analysis at baseline and at least 4 days after tacrolimus was started in 33 transplant patients showed a small but significant increase in mean QT_c interval (21 ms) (202[c]). Seven patients had a QT_c interval over 500 ms and four had QT dispersion over 100 ms. The QT_c interval prolongation was more marked in patients with organic heart disease. The potential risk of severe dysrhythmias has been illustrated in a case report (203[c]).

A 35-year-old woman underwent a second kidney transplantation and received intravenous tacrolimus (0.25 mg/h) to prevent rejection. Twelve hours later, the QT and QT_c intervals were 664 and

776 ms, respectively (vs 408 and 476 ms preoperatively) and the T waves were wide and inverted. A few minutes later she had recurrent episodes of torsade de pointes, which persisted for 6 h despite magnesium, potassium, lidocaine, and 50 electrical cardioversions. The dysrhythmia subsided after treatment with phenytoin and temporary pacing. There was a linear relation between serum tacrolimus concentrations and QT/QT_c interval prolongation.

Nervous system Neurological toxicity in the early post transplant period is well known and sometimes severe, particularly in liver transplant recipients. Several of these neurological disorders have been attributed to immunosuppressive drugs. Three patients with liver transplants had *headache*, *bilateral visual blurring*, *confusion*, and generalized *seizures*, which resolved after tacrolimus withdrawal (204[c]) or dosage reduction (205[c]). Brain imaging suggested a reversible posterior *leukoencephalopathy* in two patients.

A fatal complication has also been reported (206[c]).

A 39-year-old woman underwent liver transplantation and took tacrolimus for 5 months. She suddenly developed paresthesia and sphincter dysfunction, and her serum tacrolimus concentrations were at the upper end of the target range (13–15 μg/l). Despite a switch to cyclosporin, her neurological condition progressively deteriorated, with aphasia, left-sided sensorimotor deficits, and coma, and she died. Brain biopsy ruled out infection.

In this case, autopsy showed multiple cerebral hemispheric infarcts due to *cerebral vasculitis*.

Endocrine, metabolic Abnormal glucose metabolism and subsequent diabetes mellitus occurs in transplant patients, and has been recognized as a potential complication of tacrolimus, particularly in adults and in patients taking high doses (SEDA 20, 347). Children can also be very sensitive to the diabetogenic effects of tacrolimus, as shown by additional reports of five renal transplant patients aged 10–18 years who developed *insulin-dependent diabetes mellitus* within 20–180 days of treatment (207[C]). Both concomitant steroid treatment and sustained tacrolimus concentrations between 10–20 ng/ml probably contributed.

Hematological New reports have strongly suggested that tacrolimus may be associated with *pure red cell aplasia*. Two children, aged 6 months and 1.5 years, treated with tacrolimus and prednisone as primary immunosuppressive agents for liver transplantation, were investigated for severe anemia (hemoglobin concentrations 5.2 and 5.8 g/dl) 8–47 months after transplantation (208[c]). Both had typical features of pure red cell aplasia, with low reticulocyte counts, increased erythropoietin concentrations, and bone marrow biopsy findings of severe erythroid hypoplasia. As there was no improvement after repeated blood transfusions over 8–14 weeks, cyclosporin was substituted. The hemoglobin concentrations normalized within 3 weeks and further blood transfusion was not required.

Urinary system The morphological features of tacrolimus nephrotoxicity are very similar to those of cyclosporin, i.e. *tubular lesions*, *arteriopathy*, and *hemolytic–uremic syndrome-like changes in glomeruli and vessels*. *Isolated glomerular microthrombosis*, not previously described, has also been identified in three of 13 patients who underwent renal biopsy (209[c]). The lesions reversed in all patients, despite unchanged tacrolimus dosage in two.

Tacrolimus has been associated with more frequent and more pronounced *distal tubular acidosis* than cyclosporin 6 months after renal transplantation (210[C]), but the study included only eight patients in each group.

Musculoskeletal system Tacrolimus has been suggested to cause *reduced bone mineral density* in seven patients studied before and after an average of 3 months after heart transplantation, but all were also taking azathioprine and steroids (211[c]).

Tumor-inducing effects The incidence of tacrolimus-induced *lymphoproliferative disease* after transplantation is similar to that with other immunosuppressive agents, but long-term experience is still limited in children, who are often Epstein-Barr virus negative. It occurs in up to 22% of children taking tacrolimus after liver transplantation (212[R]), and risk factors have recently been studied. Of 89 children with liver transplants and primary or rescue tacrolimus treatment, 18 (20%) had lymphoproliferative disease after a mean delay of 263 days (213[C]). Sixteen had concomitant Epstein-Barr virus infection and six died (33% of patients with lymphoproliferative disease and 6.7% of all tacrolimus-treated patients). Previous OKT3 or antithymocyte globulin and a higher mean tacrolimus blood concentration during the period before Epstein-Barr virus infection were significantly associated with the development of lymphoproliferative disease, confirming that a high degree of immunosuppression is likely to be involved. An increase in total γ-globulin and the appearance of oligoclonal or polyclonal immunoglobulins were thought to be preliminary signs of this syndrome. These results emphasized the need to obtain low trough tacrolimus concentrations a month after transplantation.

Interactions *Chloramphenicol* Chloramphenicol increased the tacrolimus concentration in a 13-year-old girl, who required a 83% reduction in tacrolimus dosage (214[c]).

Itraconazole A pharmacokinetic interaction of tacrolimus with itraconazole, predicted in vitro, has been confirmed. Two patients had toxic tacrolimus blood concentrations during itraconazole treatment, and both required a dramatic reduction in tacrolimus dosage to maintain therapeutic blood concentrations (215[c]), (216[c]). The interaction also resulted in increased serum creatinine concentrations in one patient. Moreover, a retrospective analysis showed that the mean dosage of tacrolimus was three times lower in seven patients who took tacrolimus alone compared with seven patients who took both drugs simultaneously (216[c]).

Mycophenolate mofetil The serum concentrations of mycophenolic acid were significantly higher in 18 patients taking tacrolimus compared with patients taking cyclosporin and similar doses of mycophenolate mofetil (217[C]). This resulted in a greater degree of the in vitro immunosuppressive effects, and should probably be taken into account to avoid the adverse consequences of excess immunosuppression or to reduce the adverse effects of mycophenolate mofetil.

IMMUNOENHANCING DRUGS

Thymosin

Thymosin α_1 is an immunomodulatory peptide that has been used as a vaccine stimulant or in the treatment of heritable immunodeficiency disorders. It has also been studied in patients with chronic hepatitis B or to enhance the antiviral response of interferon-α in chronic hepatitis C. There were no significant adverse effects, except moderate *injection-sites reactions*, in 98 patients with chronic hepatitis B randomized to thymosin α-1 alone (1.6 mg twice a week for 26 or 52 weeks) or placebo (218[C]).

In a double-blind, placebo-controlled trial, patients with chronic hepatitis C were randomized to receive either thymosin α_1 plus interferon-α ($n = 35$), placebo plus interferon-α ($n = 37$), or double placebo ($n = 37$) for 26 weeks (219[C]). Whereas the biochemical response was significantly better in patients taking both drugs, the adverse effects profile was similar in both interferon-α groups. In particular, there was no evidence of more frequent autoimmune and thyroid disorders in those taking thymosin α_1/interferon-α compared with interferon-α alone.

REFERENCES

1. Malnick SDH, Schmilovitz-Weiss H. Interferon therapy for chronic HCV hepatitis: trick or treat? J Clin Gastroenterol 1997;25:310–13.
2. McHutchison JG, Gordon SC, Schiff ER, Shiffman ML, Lee WM, Rustgi VK, Goodman ZD, Ling MH, Cort S, Albrecht JK, for the Hepatitis Interventional Therapy Group. Interferon alfa-2b alone or in combination with ribavarin as initial treatment for chronic hepatitis C. New Engl J Med 1998;339:1485–92.
3. Poynard T, Marcellin P, Lee SS, Niederau C, Minuk GS, Ideo G, Bain V, Heathcote J, Zeuzem

S, Trepo C, Albrecht J, for the International Hepatitis Interventional Therapy Group. Randomised trial of interferon alfa2b plus ribavarin for 48 weeks or for 24 weeks versus interferon alfa2b plus pacebo for 48 weeks for treatment of chronic infection with hepatitis C virus. Lancet 1998;31:1426–32.

4. Davis GL, Esteban-Mur R, Rustgi V, Hoefs J, Gordon SC, Trepo C, Shiffman ML, Zeuzem S, Craxi A, Ling MH, Albrecht J, for the International Hepatitis Interventional Therapy Group. Interferon alfa-2b alone or in combination with ribavarin for the treatment of relapse of chronic hepatitis C. New Engl J Med 1998;339:1493–9.
5. Farrell GC, Bacon BR, Goldin RD, and the Clinical Advisory Group for the Hepatitis C Comparative Study. Lymphoblastoid interferon alfa-n1 improves the long-term response to a 6-month course of treatment in chronic hepatitis C compared with recombinant interferon alfa-2b: results of an international randomized controlled trial. Hepatology 1998;27:1121–7.
6. Armstrong DKB, Maw RD, Dinsmore WW, Blaakaer J, Correa MAG, Falk L, Ferenczy AS, Fortier M, Frazer I, Law C, Moller BM, Oyakawa N. Combined therapy trial with interferon alpha-2 and ablative therapy in the treatment of anogenital warts. Genitourin Med 1996;72:103–7.
7. Carson JJ, Gold LH, Barton AB, Biss RT. Fatality and interferon-alfa for malignant melanoma. Lancet 1998;352:1443–4.
8. Campo-Voegeli A, Estrach T, Marti RM, Corominas N, Tuset M, Mascaro JM. Acrocyanosis induced by interferon-alfa2a. Dermatology 1998; 196:361–3.
9. Penninger C, Heidrich H. Peripheral arterial occlusion induced by interferon-alpha. Onkologie 1998;21:240–3.
10. Herbst RA, Gutzmer R, Jung EG, Kapp A, Weiss J. Focal neurological signs and symptoms induced by interferon-alpha in two patients with malignant melanoma. Br J Dermatol 1997;137:1011–31.
11. Quattrini A, Comi G, Nemni R, Martinelli V, Villa A, Caimi M, Wrabetz L, Canal N. Axonal neuropathy associated with interferon-alfa treatment for hepatitis C: HLA-DR immunoreactivity in Schwann cells. Acta Neuropathol 1997;94:504–8.
12. Caraceni A, Gangeri L, Martini C, Belli F, Brunelli C, Baldini M, Mascheroni L, Lenisa L, Cascinelli N. Neurotoxicity of interferon-alfa in melanoma therapy. Results from a randomized controlled trial. Cancer 1998;83:482–9.
13. Rifflet H, Vuillemin E, Oberti F, Duverger P, Laine P, Garre JB, Calès P. Pulsions suicidaires chez des malades atteints d'hépatite chronique C au cours ou au décours du traitement par l'interféron alpha. Gastroenterol Clin Biol 1998;22:353–7.
14. Bacq Y, Tantaoui Elaraki A, Metman EH. Suicide chez un malade atteint d'hépatite chronique virale C traité par interféron alpha: rôle favorisant de l'alcool? Gastroenterol Clin Biol 1997;21:797–8.
15. Rifflet H, Pol S, Vuillemin E, Oberti F, Duverger P, Laine P, Garre JB, Calès P. Pulsions meurtrières chez deux malades atteints d'hépatite chronique C traités par interféron alpha. Gastroentérol Clin Biol 1998;22:105–6.
16. Carpiniello B, Orrl MG, Baita A, Pariante CM. Mania induced by withdrawal of treatment with interferon alfa. Arch Gen Psychiatry 1998; 55:88–9.
17. Maunder RG, Hunter JJ, Feinman SV. Interferon treatment of hepatitis C associated with symptoms of PTSD. Psychosomatics 1998;39:461–4.
18. Valentine AD, Meyers CA, Kling MA, Richelson E, Hauser P. Mood and cognitive side effects of interferon-alfa therapy. Semin Oncol 1998;25 (Suppl 1):39–47.
19. Licinio J, Kling MA, Hauser P. Cytokines and brain function: relevance to interferon-alfa-induced mood and cognitive changes. Semin Oncol 1998;25 (Suppl 1):30–8.
20. Benelhadj S, Marcellin P, Castelnau C, Colas-Linhart N, Benhamou JP, Erlinger S, Bok B. Incidence of dysthyroidism during interferon therapy in chronic hepatitic C. Horm Res 1997; 48:209–14.
21. Amenomori M, Mori T, Fukuda Y, Sugawa H, Nishida N, Furukawa M, Kita R, Sando T, Komeda T, Nakao K. Incidence and characteristics of thyroid dysfunction following interferon therapy in patients with chronic hepatitis C. Intern Med 1998;37:246–52.
22. Schuppert F, Rambusch E, Kirchner H, Atzpodien J, Kohn LD, Von Zur MHhlen A. Patients treated with interferon-alfa, interferon-β, and interleukin-2 have a different thyroid autoantibody pattern than patients suffering from endogenous autoimmune thyroid disease. Thyroid 1997;7:837–42.
23. Sachithanandan S, Clarke G, Crowe J, Fielding JF. Interferon-associated thyroid dysfunction in anti-D related chronic hepatitis C. J Interfer Cytokine Res 1997;17:409–11.
24. Imano E, Kanda T, Ishigami Y, Kubota M, Ikeda M, Matsuhisa M, Kawamori R, Yamasaki Y. Interferon induces insulin resistance in patients with chronic active hepatitis C. J Hepatol 1998;28:189–93.
25. Tanaka H, Shiota G, Kawasaki H. Changes in glucose tolerance after interferon-alfa therapy in patients with chronic hepatitis C. J Med 1997;28:335–46.
26. Tanaka H, Shiota G, Kawasaki H. Interferon-alfa therapy alters glucose metabolism in patients with chronic hepatitis B. J Med 1997;28:325–34.
27. Fabris P, Betterle C, Greggio NA, Zanchetta R, Bosi E, Biasin MR, de Lalla F. Insulin-dependent diabetes mellitus during alpha-interferon therapy for chronic viral hepatitis. J Hepatol 1998;28:514–17.
28. Steegmann JL, Pinilla I, Requena MJ, de la Camara R, Granados E, Fernandez Villalta MJ, Fernandez-Ranada JM. The direct antiglobulin test is frequently positive in chronic myeloid leu-

kemia patients treated with interferon-alpha. Transfusion 1997;37:446.
29. Iyoda K, Kato M, Nagawa T, Kakiuchi Y, Sugiyasu Y, Fujii E, Fujimoto K, Michida T, Kaneko A, Hayashi N, Yamamoto K, Kurosawa K, Ikeda M, Masuzawa M. Thrombotic thrombocytopenic purpura developed suddenly during interferon treatment for chronic hepatitis C. J Gastroenterol 1998;33:588–92.
30. Uberti-Foppa C, Finazzi R, De Bona A. Recombinant interferon-alpha therapy and menometrorrhagia. Br J Obstet Gynaecol 1998; 105:367–8.
31. Steegmann JL, Requena MJ, Garcia-Buey ML, Granados E, Romero R, Fernandez-Ranada JM, Moreno R. Severe autoimmune hepatitis in a chronic myeloid leukemia patient treated with interferon alpha and with complete genetic response. Am J Hematol 1998;59:95–7.
32. Ryan BM, McDonald GSA, Pilkington R, Kelleher D. The development of hepatic granulomas following interferon-alfa2b therapy for chronic hepatitis C infection. Eur J Gastroenterol Hepatol 1998;10:349–51.
33. Nomura H, Kawasaki A, Mizuno Y, Kouyama T, Nakamura M, Iwao T. The effect of plaunotol on stomatitis induced by interferon. Curr Ther Res Clin Exp 1997;58:428–33.
34. Nassar GM, Pedro P, Remmers RE, Mohanty LB, Smith W. Reversible renal failure in a patient with the hypereosinophilia syndrome during therapy with alpha interferon. Am J Kidney Dis 1998;31:121–6.
35. Al Harbi A, Al Ghamdi S, Subaity Y, Khalil A. Interferon-induced acute renal failure in nephrotic syndrome. Nephrol Dial Transplant 1998;13:1316–18.
36. Dalekos GN, Hatzis J, Tsianos EV. Dermatologic disease during interferon-alfa therapy for chronic viral hepatitis. Ann Intern Med 1998;128:409–10.
37. Sickler JB, Simmons RA, Cobb DK, Sherman KE. Cutaneous necrosis associated with interferon alfa-2b. Am J Gastroenterol 1998; 93:463–4.
38. Le Lostec Z, Mornet P, Lampert A, Peltier JY, Glaser C, Dray Suied N, De Mazancourt P, Pauwels C. Nécrose cutanée localisée après injection d'interféron alpha révélatrice d'une résistance à la protéine C activée. Rev Med Interne 1998;19 (Suppl 1):198.
39. Rongioletti F, Rebora A. Worsening of lichen myxedematosus during interferon alfa-2a therapy for chronic active hepatitis C. J Am Acad Dermatol 1998;38:760–1.
40. Montoto S, Bosch F, Estrach T, Blade J, Nomdedeu B, Nontserrat E. Pyoderma gangrenosum triggered by alfa2b-interferon in a patient with chronic granulocytic leukemia. Leuk Lymphoma 1998;30:199–202.
41. Nikkels AF, Delwaide J, Letawe C, Piérard GE. Polymorphous light eruption-like lesions on sun-protected injection sites of recombinant IFN-alfa-2b. J Dermatol Treatment 1997;8:285.
42. Maruyama S, Hirayama C, Kadowaki Y, Sagayama A, Omura H, Nakamoto M. Interferon-induced anosmia in a patient with chronic hepatitis C. Am J Gastroenterol 1998;93:122–3.
43. Murofuschi T, Takeuchi N, Ozeki H, Mizuno M. Acute vestibular dysfunction associated with interferon-alpha therapy. Eur Arch Otorhinolaryngol 1998;255:77–8.
44. Manesis EK, Moschos M, Brouzas D, Kotsiras J, Petrou C, Theodosiadis G, Hadziyannis S. Neurovisual impairment: a frequent complication of alpha-interferon treatment in chronic viral hepatitis. Hepatology 1998;27:1421–7.
45. Dippel E, Zouboulis CC, Tebbe B, Orfanos CE. Myopathic syndrome associated with long-term recombinant interferon alfa treatment in 4 patients with skin disorders. Arch Dermatol 1998;134:880–1.
46. Kumakura S, Ishikura H, Kobayashi S. Bone marrow necrosis and the Lambert-Eaton syndrome associated with interferon alfa treatment. New Engl J Med 1998;338:199–200.
47. Kälkner KM, Rönnblom L, Karlsson-Parra AK, Bengtsson M, Olsson Y, Oberg K. Antibodies against double-stranded DNA and development of polymyositis during treatment with interferon. Q J Med 1998;91:393–9.
48. Hanley JP, Haydson GH. The biology of interferon-alfa and the clinical significance of anti-interferon antibodies. Leuk Lymphoma 1998; 29:257–68.
49. Leroy V, Baud M, De Traversay C, Maynard-Muet M, Lebon P, Zarski JP. Role of anti-interferon antibodies in breakthrough occurence during alpha 2a and 2b therapy in patients with chronic hepatitis C. J Hepatol 1998;28:375–81.
50. Nesher G, Ruchlemer R. Alpha-interferon-induced arthritis: clinical presentation, treatment, and prevention. Semin Arthritis Rheum 1998; 27:360–5.
51. Tomas JF, Lopez-Lorenzo JL, Requena MJ, Aguilar R, Steegmann JL, Camara R, Alegre A, Arranz R, Figuera A, Fernandez-Ranada JM. Absence of influence of prior treatment with interferon on the outcome of allogenic bone marrow transplantation for chronic myeloid leukemia. Bone Marrow Transplant 1998;22:47–51.
52. Zuffa E, Bandini G, Bonini A, Santucci MA, Martinelli G, Rosti G, Testoni N, Zaccaria A, Tura S. Prior treatment with alpha-interferon does not adversely affect the outcome of allogenic BMT in chronic phase chronic myeloid leukemia. Haematologica 1998;83:231–6.
53. Morton AJ, Gooley T, Hansen JA, Appelbaum FR, Bruemmer B, Bjerke JW, Clift R, Martin PJ, Petersdorf EW, Sanders JE, Storb R, Sullivan KM, Woolfrey A, Anasetti C. Association between pretransplant interferon-alfa and outcome after unrelated donor marrow transplantation for chronic myelogenous leukemia in chronic phase. Blood 1998;92:394–401.
54. Bren A, Kandus A, Fergula D. Rapidly progressive renal graft failure associated with interferon-alfa treatment in a patient with chronic

myelogenous leukemia. Clin Nephrol 1998; 50:266–7.

55. Munoz De Bustillo E, Ibarrola C, Andrés A, Colina F, Morales JM. Hepatitis-B-virus related fibrosing cholestatic hepatitis after renal transplantation with acute graft failure following interferon-alpha therapy. Nephrol Dial Transplant 1998;13:1574–6.
56. Singh N, Gayowski T, Wannstedt CF, Obaid Shakil A, Wagener MM, Fung JJ, Marino IR. Interferon-alfa for prophylaxis of recurrent viral hepatitis C in liver transplant recipients. A prospective, randomized, controlled trial. Transplantation 1998;65:82–6.
57. Matsuo T, Shinzawa H, Sugahara K, Mitsuhashi H, Watanabe H, Abe T, Ohno S, Terashita M, Saito K, Saito T, Misawa H, Togashi H, Takahashi T. Case report: a patient who developed an amoebic liver abscess during treatment with interferon. J Gastroenterol Hepatol 1998;13: 1068–71.
58. Kikawada M, Ichinose Y, Kunisawa A, Yanagisawa N, Minemura K, Kasuga I, Yonemaru M, Kawanishi K, Takasaki M, Toyama K. Sarcoidosis induced by interferon therapy for chronic myelogenous leukaemia. Respirology 1998;3:41–4.
59. Yavorkovsky LL, Carrum G, Bruce S, McCarthy PL. Cutaneous sarcoidosis in a patient with Philadelphia-positive chronic myelogenous leukemia treated with interferon-alpha. Am J Hematol 1998;58:80–1.
60. Hoffmann RM, Jung MC, Motz R, Gobl C, Emslander HP, zachoval R, Pape GR. Sarcoidosis associated with interferon-alfa therapy for chronic hepatitis C. J Hepatol 1998;28:1058–63.
61. Barlow CF, Priebe CJ, Mulliken JB, Barnes PD, MacDonald D, Folkman J, Ezekowitz AB. Spastic diplegia as a complication of interferon alfa-2a treatment of hemangiomas of infancy. J Pediatr 1998;132:527–30.
62. Hoffmann RM, Ott S, Parhofer KG, Bartl R, Pape GR. Interferon-alfa induced agranulocytosis in a patient on long-term clozapine therapy. J Hepatol 1998;29:170.
63. Serratrice J, Durand JM, Morange S. Interferon-alpha 2b interaction with acenocoumarol. Am J Hematol 1998;57:89.
64. Ebers GC, Hommes O, Hughes RAC, Kappos L, Sandberg-Wolheim M, Palace J, Paty D, for the PRISMS Study Group. Randomised double-blind placebo-controlled study of interferon beta-1a in relapsing/remitting multiple sclerosis. Lancet 1998;352:1498–504.
65. Kappos L, Polman C, Pozzilli C, Thompson A, Dahlke F, for the European Study Group on Interferon beta-1b in Secondary Progressive MS. Placebo-controlled multicentre randomised trial of interferon beta-1b in treatment of secondary progressive multiple sclerosis. Lancet 1998; 352:1491–7.
66. Rudick RA, Simonian NA, Alam JA, Campion M, Scaramucci JO, Jones W, Coats ME, Goodkin DE, Weinstock-Guttman B, Herndon RM, Mass MK, Richert JR, Salazar AM, Munschauser FE, Cookfair DL, Simon JH, Jacobs LD, and the Multiple Sclerosis Collaborative Research Group. Incidence and significance of neutralizing antibodies to interferon beta-1a in multiple sclerosis. Neurology 1998;50:1266–72.
67. Cross AH, Antel JP. Antibodies to beta-interferons in multiple sclerosis. Can we neutralize the controversy? Neurology 1998;50:1206–8.
68. Rio J, Nos C, Marzo ME, Tintoré M, Montalban X. Low-dose steroids reduce flu-like symptoms at the initiation of IFN-beta-1b in relapsing-remitting MS. Neurology 1998;50:1910–12.
69. Linden D. Severe Raynaud's phenomenon associated with interferon-beta treatment for multiple sclerosis. Lancet 1998;352:878–9.
70. Ubara Y, Hara S, Takedatu H, Katori H, Yamada K, Yoshihara K, Matsushita Y, Yokoyama K, Takemoto F, Yamada A, Takagawa R, Endo Y, Hara M, Koida I, Kumada H. Hemolytic uremic syndrome associated with beta-interferon therapy for chronic hepatitis C. Nephron 1998;80:107–8.
71. Gaines AR, Varricchio F. Interferon beta-1b injection site reactions and necroses. Multiple Sclerosis 1998;4:70–3.
72. Kivis kk P, Lundahl J, von Heigl Z, Fredrikson S. No evidence for increased frequency of autoantibodies during interferon-beta1b treatment of multiple sclerosis. Acta Neurol Scand 1998;97:320–3.
73. Martinelli V, Gironi M, Rodegher M, Martino G, Comi G. Occurrence of thyroid autoimmunity in relapsing remitting multiple sclerosis patients undergoing interferon-beta treatment. Ital J Neurol Sci 1988;19:65–7.
74. Durelli L, Bongiovanni MR, Ferrero B, Oggero A, Marzano A, Rizzetto M. Interferon treatment for multiple sclerosis: autoimmune complications may be lethal. Neurology 1998;50:570–1.
75. Nousari HC, Kimyai-Asadi A, Tausk FA. Subacute cutaneous lupus erythematosus associated with interferon beta-1a. Lancet 1998; 352:1825–6.
76. Yamamoto N, Nishigaki K, Ban Y, Kawada Y. Coronary vasospasm after interferon administration. Br J Urol 1998;81:916–17.
77. Shiba T, Higashi N, Nishimura Y. Hyperglycaemia due to insulin resistance caused by interferon-gamma. Diabetic Med 1998;15:435–6.
78. Aihara Y, Mori M, Katakura S, Yokota S. Recombinant IFN-gamma treatment of a patient with hyperimmunoglobulin E syndrome triggered autoimmune thrombocytopenia. J Interfer Cytokine Res 1998;18:561–3.
79. Kourtis AP, Abramowsky C, Ibegbu C, Kobrynski L. Enlargement of the thymus in a child with chronic granulomatous disease receiving interferon-α therapy. Arch Pathol Lab Med 1998;122:562–5.
80. Négrier S, Escudier B, Lasset C, Douillard JY, Savary J, Chevreau C, Ravaud A, Mercatello A, Peny J, Mousseau M, Philip T, Tursz T, for the Groupe Français d'Immunothérapie. Recom-

binant human interleukin-2, recombinant human interferon alfa-2a, or both in metastatic renal-cell carcinoma. New Engl J Med 1998;338:1272–8.
81. Truica CI, Hansen CH, Garvin DF, Meehan KR. Idiopathic giant cell myocarditis after autologous hematopoietic stem cell transplantation and interleukin-2 immunotherapy. A case report. Cancer 1998;83:1231–6.
82. Späth-Schwalbe E, Hansen K, Schmidt F, Schrezenmeier H, Marshall L, Burger K, Fehm HL, Born J. Acute effects of recombinant human interleukin-6 on endocrine and central nervous sleep functions in healthy men. J Clin Endocrinol Metabol 1998;83:1573–9.
83. Maslak P, Nimer SD. The efficacy of IL-3, SCF, IL-6, and IL-11 in treating thrombocytopenia. Semin Hematol 1998;35:253–60.
84. Eggermont AMM, Schraffordt Koops H, Klausner JM, Kroon BBR, Schlag PM, Liénard D, Van Geel AN, Hoekstra HJ, Meller I, Nieweg OE, Kettelhack C, Ben-Ari G, Pector JC, Lejeune FJ. Isolated limb perfusion with tumor necrosis factor and melphalan for limb salvage in 186 patients with locally advanced soft tissue extremity sarcomas. The Cumulative Multicenter European experience. Ann Surg 1996;224:756–65.
85. Zwaveling JH, Hoekstra HJ, Maring JK, Ginkel RJV, Schrafford Koops H, Smit AJ, Girbes ARJ. Renal function in cancer patients treated with hyperthermic isolated limb perfusion with recombinant tumor necrosis factor-alfa and melphalan. Nephron 1997;76:146–52.
86. Hohenberger P, Haier J, Schlag PM. Rhabdomyolysis and renal function impairment after isolated limb perfusion. Comparison between the effects of perfusion with rhTNFalfa and 'triple drug' regimen. Eur J Cancer 1997;33:596–601.
87. Drory VE, Lev D, Groozman GB, Gutmann M, Klausner JM. Neurotoxicity of isolated limb perfusion with tumor necrosis factor. J Neurol Sci 1998;158:1–4.
88. Rauthe G, Sitstermanns J. Recombinant tumour necrosis factor in the local therapy of malignant pleural effusion. Eur J Cancer 1997; 33:226–31.
89. Anderlini P, Przepiorka D, Champlin R, Korbling M. Biologic and clinical effects of granulocyte colony-stimulating factor in normal individuals. Blood 1996;88:2819–25.
90. Becker PS, Wagle M, Matous S, Swanson RS, Pihan G, Lowry PA, Stewart FM, Heard SO. Spontaneous splenic rupture following administration of granulocyte colony-stimulating factor (G-CSF): occurrence in an allogeneic donor of peripheral blood stem cells. Biol Blood Marrow Transplant 1997;3:45–9.
91. Adkins DR. Anaphylactoid reaction in a normal donor given granulocyte colony-stimulating factor. J Clin Oncol 1998;16:812–13.
92. Paul C, Giachetti S, Pinquier L, Flageul B, Dubertret L, Calvo F. Cutaneous effects of granulocyte colony-stimulating factor in healthy volunteers. Arch Dermatol 1998;134:111–12.
93. Spitzer T, McAfee S, Poliquin C, Colby C. Acute gouty arthritis following recombinant human granulocyte colony-stimulating factor therapy in an allogeneic blood stem cell donor. Bone Marrow Transplant 1998;21:966–7.
94. Heitger A, Maurer K, Neu N, Fink FM. Capillary leak syndrome in a patient with septicemia and granulocyte-colony-stimulating factor (G-CSF)-induced accelerated granulopoiesis. Med Pediatr Oncol 1998;31:126–9.
95. Yokose N, Ogata K, Tamura H, An E, Nakamura K, Kamikubo K, Kudoh S, Dan K, Nomura T. Pulmonary toxicity after granulocyte colony-stimulating factor-combined chemotherapy for non-Hodgkin's lymphoma. Br J Cancer 1998; 77:2286–90.
96. Katayama Y, Deguchi S, Shinagawa K, Teshima T, Notohara K, Taguchi K, Omoto E, Harada M. Bone marrow necrosis in a patient with acute myeloblastic leukemia during administration of G-CSF and rapid hematologic recovery after allotransplantation of peripheral blood stem cells. Am J Hematol 1998;57:238–40.
97. Bachmeyer C, Chaibi P, Aractingi S. Neutrophilic eccrine hidradenitis induced by granulocyte colony-stimulating factor. Br J Dermatol 1998; 139:354–5.
98. Takagi S, Ohsaka A, Taguchi H, Kusama H, Matsuoka T. Pyoderma gangrenosum following cytosine arabinoside, aclarubicin and granulocyte colony-stimulating factor combination therapy in myelodysplastic syndrome. Intern Med 1998; 37:316–19.
99. Hasegawa M, Sato S, Nakada M, Nitta H, Shirasaki H, Kasahara K, Takehara K. Sweet's syndrome associated with granulocyte colony-stimulating factor. Eur J Dermatol 1998;8:503–5.
100. Salloum E, Stoessel KM, Cooper DL. Hyperleukocytosis and retinal hemorrhages after chemotherapy and filgrastim administration for peripheral blood progenitor cell mobilization. Bone Marrow Transplant 1998;21:835–7.
101. Teramoto S, Yamamoto H, Ouchi Y. Increased synovial interleukin-8 and interleukin-6 levels in pseudogout associated with granulocyte colony-stimulating factor. Ann Intern Med 1998;129:424 5.
102. Stanworth SJ, Bhavnani M, Chattopadhya C, Miller H, Swinson DR. Treatment of Felty's syndrome with the haemopoietic growth factor granulocyte colony-stimulating factor (G-CSF). Q J Med 1998;91:49–56.
103. Stone HD, DiPiro C, Davis PC, Meyer CF, Wray BB. Hypersensitivity reactions to *Escherichia coli*-derived polyethylene glycolated-asparaginase associated with subsequent immediate skin test reactivity to *E. coli*-derived granulocyte colony-stimulating factor. J Allergy Clin Immunol 1998;101:429–31.
104. Caballero MD, Vasquez L, Barragan JM, Cruz JJ, Gomez A, Nieto MJ, Corral M, Fonseca E, San Miguel JF. Randomized study of filgrastim versus molgramostin after peripheral stem cell transplant in breast cancer. Haematologica 1998;83:514–8.

105. Al-Homaidhi A, Prince HM, Al-Zahrani H, Doucette D, Keating A. Granulocyte-macrophage colony-stimulating factor-associated histiocytosis and capillary-leak syndrome following autologous bone marrow transplantation: two case reports and a review of the literature. Bone Marrow Transplant 1998;21:209–14.
106. Ross SD, DiGeorge A, Connelly JE, Whiting GW, McDonnell N. Safety of GM-CSF in patients with AIDS: a review of the literature. Pharmacotherapy 1998;18:1290–7.
107. Buysmann S, Hack CE, Van Dieppen FNJ, Surachno J, Ten Berge IJM. Administration of OKT3 as a two-hour infusion attenuates first-dose side effects. Transplantation 1997;64:1620–3.
108. Broeders N, Wissing KM, Crusiaux A, Kinnaert P, Vereerstraeten P, Abramowicz D. Mycophenolate mofetil, together with cyclosporin A, prevents anti-OKT3 antibody response in kidney transplant recipients. J Am Soc Nephrol 1998; 9:1521–5.
109. Tse JC, Moore TB. Monoclonal antibodies in the treatment of steroid-resistant acute graft-versus-host disease. Pharmacotherapy 1998; 18:988–1000.
110. Nashan B, Moore R, Amlot P, Schmidt AG, Abeywickrama K, Soulillou JP. Randomised trial of basiliximab versus placebo for control of acute cellular rejection in renal allograft recipients. Lancet 1997;350:1193–8 (erratum 1484).
111. Waid TH, Lucas BA, Thompson JS, McKeown JW, Brown S, Kryscio R, Skeeters LJ. Treatment of renal allograft rejection with T10B9.1A31 or OKT3. First analysis of a phase II clinical trial. Transplantation 1997;64:274–81.
112. Kirschner BS. Safety of azathioprine and 6-mercaptopurine in pediatric patients with inflammatory bowel disease. Gastroenterology 1998;115:813–21.
113. Hollander AAMJ, Van der Woude FJ. Efficacy and tolerability of conversion from cyclosporin to azathioprine after kidney transplantation. A review of the evidence. BioDrugs 1998;9:197–210.
114. Padda S, Ramirez F, Berggreen PJ. Sweet's syndrome associated with the use of azathioprine in a patient with Crohn's colitis. Am J Gastroenterol 1998;93:1735.
115. Sabeel A, Al Meshari K, Abutaleb N, Al Shaibani K. Drug fever induced by azathioprine in a haemodialysis patient. Nephrol Dial Transplant 1998;13:1004–5.
116. Fields CL, Robinson JW, Roy TM, Ossorio MA, Byrd RP. Hypersensitivity reaction to azathioprine. South Med J 1998;91:471–4.
117. Garey KW, Streetman DS, Rainish MC. Azathioprine hypersensitivity reaction in a patient with ulcerative colitis. Ann Pharmacother 1998;32:425–8.
118. Heizer WD, Peterson JL. Acute myeloblastic leukemia following prolonged treatment of Crohn's disease with 6-mercaptopurine. Dig Dis Sci 1998;43:1791–3.
119. Werth VP. Pulse intravenous cyclophosphamide for treatment of autoimmune blistering disease. Is there an advantage over oral routes? Arch Dermatol 1997;133:229–30.
120. Guillevin L, Cordier JF, Lhote F, Cohen P, Jarrousse B, Royer I, Lesavre P, Jacquot C, Bindi P, Bielefeld P, Desson JF, Détrée F, Dubois A, Hachulla E, Hoen B, Jacomy D, Seigneuric C, Lauque D, Stern M, Longy-Boursier M. A prospective, multicenter, randomized trial comparing steroids and pulse cyclophosphamide versus steroids and oral cyclophosphamide in the treatment of generalized wegener's granulomatosis. Arthritis Rheum 1997;40:2187–98.
121. Sweeney JP, Fan CW, Keogh JAB, Thornhill JA. Upper renal tract deterioration after cyclophosphamide-induced cystitis: the case for monitoring after cyclophosphamide therapy. Br J Urol 1998;81:639–40.
122. Mok CC, Lau CS, Wong RWS. Risk factors for ovarian failure in patients with systemic lupus erythematosus receiving cyclophosphamide therapy. Arthritis Rheum 1998;41:831–7.
123. Smith DR, Balashov KE, Hafler DA, Khoury SJ, Weiner HL. Immune deviation following pulse cyclophosphamide/methylprednisolone treatment of multiple sclerosis: increased interleukin-4 production and associated eosinophilia. Ann Neurol 1997;42:313–18.
124. De Ridder D, Van Poppel H, Demonty L, D'Hooghe B, Gonsette R, Carton H, Baert L. Bladder cancer in patients with multiple sclerosis treated with cyclophosphamide. J Urol 1998;159:1881–4.
125. Shah MB, Martin JE, Schroeder TJ, First MR. Evaluation of the safety and tolerability of Neoral and Sandimmune: a meta-analysis. Transplant Proc 1998;30:1697–700.
126. Shield CF, McGrath M, Goss TF, for the FK506 Kidney Transplant Study Group. Assessment of health-related quality of life in kidney transplant patients receiving tacrolimus (FK506)-based versus cyclosporine-based immunosuppression. Transplantation 1997;64:1738–43.
127. Gleeson JG, DuPlessis AJ, Barnes PD, Riviello JJ. Cyclosporin A acute encephalopathy and seizure syndrome in childhood: clinical features and risk of seizure recurrence. J Child Neurol 1998;13:336–44.
128. Zimmer WE, Hourihane JM, Wang HZ, Schriber JR. The effect of human leukocyte antigen disparity on cyclosporine neurotoxicity after allogeneic bone marrow transplantation. Am J Neuroradiol 1998;19:601–8.
129. Claesson K, Mayer AD, Squifflet JP, Grabensee B, Eigler FW, Behrend M, Vanrenterghem Y, Van Hooff J, Morales JM, Johnson RWG, Buchholz B, Land W, Forsythe JLR, Neumayer HH, Ericzon BG, MHhlbacher F. Lipoprotein patterns in renal transplant patients: a comparison between FK506 and cyclosporine A patients. Transplant Proc 1998;30:1292–4.
130. McCune TR, Thacker LR II, Peters TG, Mulloy L, Rohr MS, Adams PA, Yium J, Light JA, Pruett T, Gaber AO, Selman SH, Jonsson J,

Hayes JM, Wright FH, Armata T, Blanton J, Burdick JF. Effects of tacrolimus on hyperlipidemia after successful renal transplantation. Transplantation 1998;65:87–92.
131. Fernandez-Miranda C, Guijarro C, De La Calle A, Loinaz C, Gonzalez-Pinto I, Gomez-Izquierdo T, Larumbe S, Moreno E, Del Palacio A. Lipid abnormalities in stable liver transplant recipients-effects of cyclosporin, tacrolimus, and steroids. Transplant Int 1998;11:137–42.
132. Satterthwaite R, Aswad S, Sunga V, Shidban H, Bogaard T, Asai P, Khetan U, Akra I, Mendez RG, Mendez R. Incidence of new-onset hypercholesterolemia in renal transplant patients treated with FK506 or cyclosporine. Transplantation 1998;65:446–9.
133. Mourad G, Vela C, Ribstein J, Mimran A. Long-term improvement in renal function after cyclosporine reduction in renal transplant recipients with histologically proven chronic cyclosporine nephropathy. Transplantation 1998;65:661–7.
134. Vercauteren SB, Bosmans JL, Elseviers MM, Verpooten GA, De Broe ME. A meta-analysis and morphological review of cyclosporine-induced nephrotoxicity in auto-immune diseases. Kidney Int 1998;54:536–45.
135. Powles AV, Hardman CM, Porter WM, Cook T, Hulme B, Fry L. Renal function after 10 years' treatment with cyclosporin for psoriasis. Br J Dermatol 1998;138:443–9.
136. Roberts P, Follette D, Allen R, Katznelson S, Albertson T. Cyclosporine A-associated thrombotic thrombocytopenic purpura following lung transplantation. Transplant Proc 1998;30:1512–13.
137. Bren AF, Kandus A, Buturovic J, Koselj M, Pavlovcic SK, Ponikvar R, Kovac D, Lindic J, Vizjak A, Ferluga D. Cyclosporine-related hemolytic-uremic syndrome in kidney graft recipients: clinical and histomorphologic evaluation. Transplant Proc 1998;30:1201–3.
138. Guella A, Daoud M, Al Dayel A. Uneventful re-treatment with cyclosporin in two cases of cyclosporin-induced haemolytic uraemic syndrome. Nephrol Dial Transplantation 1998; 13:1864–5.
139. Ducloux D, Rebibou JM, Semhoun-Ducloux S, Jamali M, Fournier V, Bresson-Vautrin C, Chalopin JM. Recurrence of hemolytic-uremic syndrome in renal transplant recipients. Transplantation 1998;65:1405–7.
140. Losada A, Garcia-Doval I, De La Torre C, Cruces MJ. Subcutaneous sarcoidosis worsened by cyclosporin treatment for pyoderma gangrenosum. Br J Dermatol 1998;138:1103–4.
141. Gomez E, Sanchez-Nunez M, Sanchez JE, Corte C, Aguado S, Portal C, Baltar J, Alvarez-Grande J. Treatment of cyclosporin-induced gingival hyperplasia with azithromycin. Nephrol Dial Transplant 1997;12:2694–7.
142. Jucgla A, Moreso F, Sais G, Gil-Vernet S, Grealls J, Grinyo JM, Peyri J. The use of azithromycin for cyclosporin-induced gingival overgrowth. Br J Dermatol 1998;138:198–9.
143. Nash MM, Zaltzman JS. Efficacy of azithromycin in the treatment of cyclosporine-induced gingival hyperplasia in renal transplant recipients. Transplantation 1998;65:1611–15.
144. Wirnsberger GH, Pfragner R, Mauric A, Zach R, Bogiatzis A, Holzer H. Effect of antibiotic treatment with azithromycin on cyclosporine A-induced gingival hyperplasia among renal transplant recipients. Transplant Proc 1998; 30:2117–19.
145. Freise CE, Galbraith CA, Nikolai BJ, Ascher NL, Lake JR, Stock PG, Roberts JP. Risks associated with conversion of stable patients after liver transplantation to the microemulsion formulation of cyclosporine. Transplantation 1998;65:995–7.
146. Budak-Alpdogan T, Kalayoglu-Besisik S, Sargin D, Tangün Y. Cyclosporin-related reversible muscular toxicity. Bone Marrow Transplant 1998;22:115–16.
147. Volcheck GW, Van Dellen RG. Anaphylaxis to intravenous cyclosporine and tolerance to oral cyclosporine: case report and review. Ann Allergy Asthma Immunol 1998;80:159–63.
148. Thomas MD, Cook LJ. Fever associated with cyclosporin for treating atopic dermatitis. Br Med J 1998;314:1291.
149. Casele HL, Laifer SA. Association of pregnancy complications and choice of immunosuppressant in liver transplant patients. Transplantation 1998;65:581–3.
150. Nyberg G, Haljamäe U, Frisenette-Fich C, Wennergren M, Kjellmer I. Breast-feeding during treatment with cyclosporine. Transplantation 1998;65:253–5.
151. Dantal J, Hourmant M, Cantarovich D, Giral M, Blancho G, Dreno B. Effect of long-term immunosuppression in kidney-graft recipients on cancer incidence: randomised comparison of two cyclosporin regimens. Lancet 1998;351:623–8.
152. Arellano F. Risk of cancer with cyclosporine in psoriasis. Int J Dermatol 1997;36:15–17.
153. Van Den Borne BEEM, Landewé RBM, Houkes I, Schild F, Van Der Heyden PCW, Hazes JMW, Vandenbroucke JP, Zwinderman AH, Goei The HS, Breedveld FC, Bernelot Moens HJ, Kluin PM, Dijkmans BAC. No increased risk of malignancies and mortality in cyclosporin A-treated patients with rheumatoid arthritis. Arthritis Rheum 1998;41:1930–7.
154. Bisogno G, Cowie F, Boddy A, Thomas HD, Dick G, Pinkerton CR. High-dose cyclosporin with etoposide toxicity and pharmacokinetic interaction in children with solid tumours. Br J Cancer 1998;77:2304–9.
155. Vella JP, Sayegh MH. Interactions between cyclosporine and newer antidepressant medications. Am J Kidney Dis 1998;31:320–3.
156. Markowitz JS, Gill HS, Hunt NM, Monroe RR, DeVane CL. Lack of antidepressant-cyclosporine pharmacokinetic interactions. J Clin Psychopharmacol 1998;18:91–3.
157. Kaijser M, Johnsson C, Zezina L, Backman

U, Dimény E, Fellström B. Elevation of cyclosporin A blood levels during carvedilol treatment in renal transplant patients. Clin Transplant 1997;11:577–81.

158. Van Den Borne BEEM, Landewé RBM, Goei The HS, Rietveld JH, Zwinderman AH, Bruyn GAW, Breedveld FC, Dijkmans BAC. Combination therapy in recent onset rheumatoid arthritis: a randomized double blind trial of the addition of low dose cyclosporine to patients treated with low dose chloroquine. J Rheumatol 1998;25:1493–8.
159. Terwogt JMM, Beijnen JH, Bokkel Huinink WWt, Rosing H, Schellens JHM. Co-administration of cyclosporin enables oral therapy with paclitaxel. Lancet 1998;352:285.
160. Kaplan B, Meier-Kriesche HU, Napoli KL, Kahan BD. The effects of relative timing of sirolimus and cyclosporine microemulsion formulation coadministration on the pharmacokinetics of each agent. Clin Pharmacol Ther 1998;63:48–53.
161. Frantz RP, Nguyen TT. Rezulin (troglitazone) greatly increases cyclosporine metabolism. J Heart Lung Transplant 1998;17:1037–8.
162. Kaplan B, Friedman G, Jacobs M, Viscuso R, Lyman N, DeFranco P, Bonomini L, Mulgaonkar SP. Potential interaction of troglitazone and cyclosporine. Transplantation 1998;65:1399–400.
163. Weinblatt ME, Maier AL, Fraser PA, Coblyn JS. Long-term prospective study of methotrexate in rheumatoid arthritis: conclusion after 132 months of therapy. J Rheumatol 1998;25:238–42.
164. Menninger H, Herborn G, Sander O, Blechschmidt J, Rau R. A 36 month comparative trial of methotrexate and gold sodium thiomalate in the treatment of early active and erosive rheumatoid arthritis. Br J Rheumatol 1998;37:1060–8.
165. Bartram SA. Experience with methotrexate-associated pneumonitis in Northeastern England: comment on the article by Kremer et al. Arthritis Rheum 1998;41:1327–8.
166. Leeb BF, Scheinecker C, Schweitzer H, Smolen JS. Two different drug-induced pulmonary complications in a patient suffering from rheumatoid arthritis. Br J Rheumatol 1998;37:586–7.
167. Jih DM, Werth VP. Thrombocytopenia after a single test dose of methotrexate. J Am Acad Dermatol 1998;39:349–51.
168. Bach N, Thung SN, Schaffner F. The histologic effects of low-dose methotrexate therapy for primary biliary cirrhosis. Arch Pathol Lab Med 1998;122:342–5.
169. Jean G, Ouesis E, Chazot C, Charra B. Nephrotic syndrome following initiation of methotrexate therapy for rheumatoid arthritis. Clin Nephrol 1998;50:198.
170. Halevy S, Giryes H, Avinoach I, Livni E, Sukenik S. Leukocytoclastic vasculitis induced by low-dose methotrexate: in vitro evidence for an immunologic mechanism. J Eur Acad Dermatol Venereol 1998;10:81–5.
171. Simonart TH, Durez P, Margaux J, Van Geertruyden J, Goldschmidt D, Parent D. Cutaneous necrotizing vasculitis after low dose methotrexate therapy for rheumatoid arthritis: a possible manifestation of methotrexate hypersensitivity. Clin Rheumatol 1997;16:623–5.
172. Ben-Amitai D, Hodak E, David M. Cutaneous ulceration: an unusual sign of methotrexate toxicity:first report in a patient without psoriasis. Ann Pharmacother 1998;32:651–3.
173. Singwe M, Le Gars L, Karneff A, Prier A, Kaplan G. Multiple stress fractures in a scleroderma patient on methotrexate therapy. Rev Rhum (Engl Ed) 1998;65:508–10.
174. Kanik KS, Cash JM. Does methotrexate increase the risk of infection or malignancy. Rheum Dis Clin North Am 1997;4:955–67.
175. Le Goff P, Chicault P, Saraux A, Baron D, Valls-Bellec I, Leroy JP. Lymphoma with regression after methotrexate withdrawal in a patient with rheumatoid arthritis. Role for the Epstein-Barr virus. Rev Rhum (Engl Ed) 1998;65:283–6.
176. Londino AV, Blatt J, Knisely AS. Hodgkin's disease in a patient with juvenile rheumatoid arthritis taking weekly low dose methotrexate. J Rheumatol 1998;25:1245–6.
177. Kleiman KS, Mahowald ML. Methotrexate and lymphoma: a presentation of four cases and review of the literature. J Clin Rheumatol 1998;4:254–9.
178. Potter T, Hardwick N, Mulherin D. Multiple malignant melanomas in a patient with RA treated with methotrexate. J Rheumatol 1998;25:2282–3.
179. Duncan KO, Imaeda S, Milstone LM. *Pneumocystis carinii* pneumonia complicating methotrexate treatment of pityriasis rubra pilaris. J Am Acad Dermatol 1998;39:276–8.
180. Jansen TL, Van Heereveld HA, Laan RF, Barrera P, Van de Putte LB. Septic arthritis with *Listeria monocytogenes* during low-dose methotrexate. J Intern Med 1998;244:87–90.
181. Di Girolamo C, Pappone N, Melillo E, Rengo C, Giuliano F, Melillo G. Cavitary lung tuberculosis in a rheumatoid arthritis patient treated with low-dose methotrexate and steroid pulse therapy. Br J Rheumatol 1998;37:1136–7.
182. Jarrett P, Ha T, Oliver F. Necrotizing fasciitis complicating disseminated cutaneous *Herpes zoster*. Clin Exp Dermatol 1998;23:87–8.
183. Rolland Y, Cantagrel A, Laroche M, Mazières B. Pneumopathie à *Pneumocystis carinii* au cours d'une polyarthrite rhumatoïde traitée par méthotrexate chez un patient souffrant d'asbestose pulmonaire. Rev Med Interne 1998;19:581–3.
184. Narvaez J, Rodriguez-Moreno J, Martinez-Aguila MD, Clavaguera T. Severe hepatitis linked to B virus infection after withdrawal of low dose methotrexate therapy. J Rheumatol 1998;25:2037–8.
185. Ostensen M, Ramsey-Goldman R. Treatment of inflammatory rheumatic disorders in pregnancy. What are the safest treatment options? Drug Saf 1998;19:389–410.
186. Bawle EV, Conard JV, Weiss L. Adult and

two children with fetal methotrexate syndrome. Teratology 1998;57:51–5.

187. Steuer A, Gumpel JM. Methotrexate and trimethoprim: a fatal interaction. Br J Rheumatol 1998;37:105–6.

188. Morrissey P, Gohh R, Madras P, Monaco AP. Pulmonary fibrosis secondary to administration of mycophenolate mofetil. Transplantation 1998;65:1414–16.

189. Elli A, Aroldi A, Montagnino G, Tarantino A, Ponticelli C. Mycophenolate mofetil and cough. Transplantation 1998;66:409.

190. Golconda M, Valente J, Bejarano P, Gilinsky N, First MR. Colonic ulceration. A previously unreported adverse effect of mycophenolate mofetil. Transplantation 1998;65:S148.

191. Ducloux D, Fournier V, Bresson-Vautrin C, Rebibou JM, Billerey C, Saint Hillier Y, Chalopin JM. Mycophenolate mofetil in renal transplant recipients with cyclosporin-associated nephrotoxicity. A preliminary report. Transplantation 1998;65:1504–6.

192. Smak Gregoor PJH, Hesse CJ, Van Gelder T, Van der Mast BJ, Ijzermans JNM, Van Besouw NM, Weimar W. Relation of mycophenolic acid trough levels and adverse events in kidney allograft recipients. Transplant Proc 1998;30:1192–3.

193. Moreso F, Seron D, Morales JM, Cruzado JM, Gil-Vernet S, Pérez JL, Fulladosa X, Andrès A, Grinyo JM. Incidence of leukopenia and cytomegalovirus disease in kidney transplants treated with mycophenolate mofetil combined with low cyclosporine and steroid doses. Clin Transplant 1998;12:198–205.

194. Sarmiento JM, Munn SR, Paya CV, Velosa JA, Nguyen H. Is cytomegalovirus infection related to mycophenolate mofetil after kidney transplantation? A case-control study. Clin Transplant 1998;12:371–4.

195. Paterson DL, Singh N, Panebianco A, Wannstedt CF, Wagener MM, Gayowski T, Marino IR. Infectious complications occurring in liver transplant recipients receiving mycophenolate mofetil. Transplantation 1998;66:593–8.

196. Mathew TH for the Tricontinental Mycophenolate Mofetil Renal Transplantation Study Group. A blinded, long-term, randomized multicenter study of mycophenolate mofetil in cadaveric renal transplantation. Results at three years. Transplantation 1998;65:1450–4.

197. Ader JL, Rostaing L. Cyclosporin nephrotoxicity: pathophysiology and comparison with FK-506. Curr Opin Nephrol Hypertens 1998; 7:539–45.

198. Mihatsch MJ, Kyo M, Morozumi K, Yamaguchi Y, Nickeleit V, Ryffel B. The side-effects of cyclosporin-A and tacrolimus. Clin Nephrol 1998;49:356–63.

199. Busque S, Demers P, St-Louis G, Boily JG, Tousignant J, Lemieux F, Smeesters C, Corman J, Daloze P. Conversion from neoral (cyclosporine) to tacrolimus of kidney transplant recipients for gingival hyperplasia or hypertrichosis. Transplant Proc 1998;30:1247–8.

200. Friemann S, Feuring E, Padberg W, Ernst W. Improvement of nephrotoxicity, hypertension, and lipid metabolism after conversion of kidney transplant recipients from cyclosporine to tacrolimus. Transplant Proc 1998;30:1240–2.

201. Tezcan H, Zimmer W, Fenstermaker R, Herzig GP, Schriber J. Severe cerebellar swelling and thrombotic thrombocytopenic purpura associated with FK506. Bone Marrow Transplant 1998;21:105–9.

202. Sanoski CA, Vasquez EM, Bauman JL. QT interval prolongation associated with the use of tacrolimus in transplant recipients. Pharmacotherapy 1998;18:427.

203. Hodak SP, Moubarak JB, Rodriguez I, Gelfand MC, Alijani MR, Tracy CM. QT prolongation and near fatal cardiac arrhythmia after intravenous tacrolimus administration. A case report. Transplantation 1998;66:535–7.

204. Nakamura M, Fuchinoue S, Sato S, Hoshino T, Sawada T, Sageshima J, Kitajima K, Tojinbara T, Fujita S, Nakajima I, Agishi T, Tanaka K. Clinical and radiological features of two cases of tacrolimus-related posterior leukoencephalopathy in living related liver transplantation. Transplant Proc 1998;30:1477–8.

205. Idilman R, De Maria N, Kugelmas M, Colantoni A, Van Thiel DH. Immunosuppressive drug-induced leukoencephalopathy in patients with liver transplant. Eur J Gastroenterol Hepatol 1998;10:433–6.

206. Pizzolato GP, Sztajzel R, Burkhardt K, Megret M, Borisch B. Cerebral vasculitis during FK506 treatment in a liver transplant patient. Neurology 1998;50:1154–7.

207. Moxey-Mims MM, Kay C, Light JA, Kher KK. Increased incidence of insulin-dependent diabetes mellitus in pediatric renal transplant patients receiving tacrolimus (FK506). Transplantation 1998;65:617–19.

208. Misra S, Moore TB, Ament ME, Busuttil RW, McDiarmid S. Red cell aplasia in children on tacrolimus after liver transplantation. Transplantation 1998;65:575–7.

209. Antoine C, Thakur S, Daugas E, Fraoui R, Boudjeltia S, Julia P, Nochy D, Glotz D. Vascular microthrombosis in renal transplant recipients treated with tacrolimus. Transplant Proc 1998; 30:2813–14.

210. Heering P, Ivens K, Aker S, Grabensee B. Distal tubular acidosis induced by FK506. Clin Transplant 1998;12:465–71.

211. Stempfle HU, Werner C, Echtler S, Assum T, Meiser B, Angermann CE, Theisen K, Gartner R. Rapid trabecular bone loss after cardiac transplantation using FK506 (tacrolimus)-based immunosuppression. Transplant Proc 1998;30:1132–3.

212. McDiarmid SV. The use of tacrolimus in pediatric liver transplantation. J Pediatr Gastroenterol Nutr 1998;26:90–102.

213. Sokal EM, Antunes H, Beguin C, Bodeus M, Wallemacq P, Ville De Goyet JD, Reding R, Janssen M, Buts JP, Otte JB. Early signs and risk

factors for the increased incidence of Epstein-Barr virus-related posttransplant lymphoproliferative diseases in pediatric liver transplant recipients treated with tacrolimus. Transplantation 1997; 64:1438–42.
214. Schulman SL, Shaw LM, Jabs K, Leonard MB, Brayman KL. Interaction between tacrolimus and chloramphenicol in a renal transplant recipient. Transplantation 1998;65:1397–8.
215. Billaud EM, Guillemain R, Tacco F, Chevalier P. Evidence for a pharmacokinetic interaction between itraconazole and tacrolimus in organ transplant patients. Br J Clin Pharmacol 1998;46:271.
216. Furlan V, Parquin F, Penaud JF, Cerrina J, Le Roy Ladurie F, Dartevelle P, Taburet AM. Interaction between tacrolimus and itraconazole in a heart-lung transplant recipient. Transplant Proc 1998;30:187–8.
217. Zucker K, Rosen A, Tsaroucha A, DeFaria L, Roth D, Ciancio G, Esquenazi V, Burke G, Tzakis A, Miller J. Unexpected augmentation of mycophenolic acid pharmacokinetics in renal transplant patients receiving tacrolimus and mycophenolate mofetil in combination therapy, and analogous in vitro findings. Transplant Immunol 1997;5:225–32.
218. Chien RN, Liaw YF, Chen TC, Yeh CT, Sheen IS. Efficacy of thymosin alfa1 in patients with chronic hepatitis B: a randomized, controlled trial. Hepatology 1998;27:1383–7.
219. Sherman KE, Sjogren M, Creager RL, Damiano MA, Freeman S, Lewey S, Davis D, Root S, Weber FL, Ishak KG, Goodman ZD. Combination therapy with thymosin alpha1 and interferon for the treatment of chronic hepatitis C infection: a randomized, placebo-controlled double-blind trial. Hepatology 1998;27:1128–35.

H.D. Reuter

38 Vitamins

℞ *Vitamin supplementation therapy in old age*

Vitamin supplementation in large dosages has become common in older people, who mostly self-prescribe, because they want to prevent diseases and take responsibility for their own health. Vitamin enthusiasts and vitamin manufacturers motivated by profits often advocate large dosages of vitamins as a means of disease prevention. To date the scientific community has failed to educate the general public about the potential adverse effects of excessive vitamin use. The potential benefits and detriments of vitamin supplementation in elderly people have therefore been reviewed (1[R]).

Ascorbic acid *Antioxidant vitamins are the most commonly self-prescribed vitamins. Ascorbic acid supplementation in elderly patients with non-insulin-dependent diabetes mellitus results in significant falls in fasting insulin concentrations, glycosylated hemoglobin, and low density lipoprotein cholesterol (2[C]). In patients with diabetes mellitus or impaired glucose tolerance, ascorbic acid supplementation can improve carbohydrate metabolism, enhance the action of insulin, and increase non-oxidative glucose disposal (3[C]). Ascorbic acid also improves vascular integrity in patients in nursing homes (4[C]). In order to avoid potential adverse effects it has been recommended that supplemental ascorbic acid ingestion should be under 500 mg/day (5[C]).*

However, large doses of ascorbic acid have relatively few adverse effects. As dosages in excess of 1 g are largely unabsorbed, gastrointestinal pooling leads to the most common adverse effects, namely abdominal bloating and osmotic diarrhea (6[R]). Although the most common dosage of over-the-counter ascorbic acid supplements (500 mg, which is about 10-fold higher than the recommended daily allowance) is well tolerated, it may have insidious adverse effects. For example, supplementation may falsely lower blood and urine glucose concentration readings on common testing strips, leading to a perceived improvement in the control of diabetes (7[c]). Ascorbic acid can also affect stool occult blood test results and deplete serum cyanocobalamin (vitamin B_{12}) (8[R]), (9[R]). Rarely ascorbic acid precipitates acute hemolysis in patients with glucose-6-phosphate dehydrogenase deficiency (10[c]). The abrupt discontinuation of ascorbic acid in patients who take megadoses causes a relative deficiency of vitamin C, presenting with the classical features of scurvy, including gum and subperiosteal bleeding (1[R]).

Cholecalciferol (vitamin D) *The current recommended daily allowance for cholecalciferol is 200 IU. Dietary supplementation with at least 200 IU/day alleviates seasonal parathyroid hormone variations and maintains normal vitamin D concentrations. Continuous low-dosage supplementation with 400 IU/day of oral vitamin D is a simple and well tolerated way of reducing the incidence and sequelae, such as osteopenia, of vitamin D deficiency. Adverse effects were not mentioned (1[R]).*

Cyanocobalamin (vitamin B_{12}) *The current recommended daily allowance of cyanocobalamin is 2.0 μg. Despite large body stores, deficiency is common, because the ability to absorb dietary cyanocobalamin falls with age (11[R]). Serious adverse effects have not been reported.*

Folic acid *The current recommended daily allowance for folic acid in elderly people is about 200 μg. However, a folic acid intake of over 400 μg/day is required for optimal suppression of high concentrations of homocysteine, which have been correlated with the risk of vascular disease in elderly people. High-dos-*

Side Effects of Drugs, Annual 22
J.K. Aronson, ed.

age supplementation with folic acid is well tolerated and largely without adverse effects (12[R]). In 130 nursing-home residents who were taking folic acid (400 μg/day) serum folate concentrations were not reduced, even in those taking phenytoin; of the 325 residents not taking a folate supplement, nine had low folic acid concentrations (below 2.5 ng/ml) (13[C]).

Nicotinic acid Nicotinic acid, but not nicotinamide, is often used in large dosages (2–3 g/day) for hyperlipidemia. Unfortunately, because of prostaglandin-mediated flushing, caused by high dosages of nicotinic acid, many patients do not tolerate therapy (14[R]). However, this effect is often self-limiting and can be alleviated by the co-administration of aspirin (14[R]). Modified-release formulations of nicotinic acid may lessen the flushing, but they increase the risk of hepatotoxicity or fulminant liver failure (15[C]). Headache, postural hypotension, nausea, diarrhea, increased serum uric concentration and gout, and an increased need for liver function monitoring have been reported (14[R]). Because of the association of nicotinic acid therapy with myositis or myopathy, ophthalmological disorders, reduced serum thyroid hormone concentrations, and glucose intolerance, patients who take nicotinic acid should be followed closely for symptoms of toxicity (16[c])–(18[c]), (19[C]).

Phytomenadione (vitamin K_1) Phytomenadione supplementation reduces urinary calcium loss in postmenopausal women and has potential for the prevention or treatment of osteoporosis (20[C]). However, prospective studies of the effect of long-term vitamin K supplementation on the pathogenesis of osteoporosis are necessary.

Pyridoxine Pyridoxine is well tolerated in elderly people in dosages of under 100 mg/day. The dosage limit is 50 times the current recommended daily allowance (i.e. an RDA of 2 mg/day). Mega-dosage pyridoxine (in excess of 200 mg/day) is associated with a progressive sensory ataxia and impairment of distal vibratory and positional sensation (21[R]). Tendon reflexes can be diminished or abolished (22[c]). Large dosages of pyridoxine cause dysfunction of large and small nerve fibers (23[C]). High-dosage pyridoxine can cause photosensitivity (24[c]).

Retinoids and carotenoids (vitamin A) The current recommended daily allowance for retinol is about 5000 IU/day for individuals aged over 50 years. Retinol is available without a prescription in capsules containing 25 000 IU. Although there is no proof that retinol supplementation is beneficial, mean intake in elderly people is nearly double the recommended daily allowance. Acute retinol overdosage can result in an increased intracranial pressure, pseudotumor cerebri, and headache (25[C]). Chronic toxicity with retinol dosages of 5000–10 000 IU/day is associated with liver toxicity, dry skin, or desquamation (26[R]).

Unlike preformed retinol, β-carotene supplementation is largely without adverse effects, except hypercarotenosis, characterized by yellowing of the skin, including the palms, but not the sclerae (26[R]), (27[R]).

Riboflavin The current recommended daily allowance for riboflavin is 1.2–1.4 mg. Supplementation is advisable when adequate dietary intake is not possible, and it is well tolerated. Adverse effects have not been reported.

Thiamine Supplementation with thiamine may be beneficial in patients who are prone to deficiency and who have co-existing cardiac failure (28[C]). Oral thiamine supplementation has not been associated with toxicity, since excess thiamine is rapidly cleared by the kidneys (29[R]).

Tocopherols (vitamin E) Vitamin E may have beneficial effects on LDL-cholesterol by inhibition of LDL oxidation by free radicals. Long-term supplementation of vitamin E in dosages well above the recommended daily allowance is generally well tolerated and apparently free from adverse effects. However, vitamin E supplementation can worsen vitamin K deficiency (e.g. in patients treated with warfarin) (30[C]). However, the authors of the review stated that before high-dosage vitamin E can be accepted as a therapeutic agent, further long-term studies must be undertaken to examine its efficacy and potential for adverse effects (1[R]).

Table 1. *Recommended daily dietary allowances of vitamins for individuals aged over 50 years in the US (adapted from Ref.* (31[R]).

Vitamin	Men	Women
Folic acid (μg)	200	180
Nicotinic acid (niacin) (mg)	15	13
Vitamin A (retinol) (mg)	1000	800
Vitamin B_1 (thiamine) (mg)	1.2	1.0
Vitamin B_2 (riboflavin) (mg)	1.4	1.2
Vitamin B_6 (pyridoxine) (mg)	2.0	1.6
Vitamin B_{12} (cyanocobalamin) (μg)	2.0	2.0
Vitamin C (ascorbic acid) (mg)	60	60
Vitamin D (cholecalciferol) (IU)	200	200
Vitamin E (tocopherols) (IU)	15	12
Vitamin K (mg)	80	65

Conclusions *From published data the authors concluded that apart from the legitimate use of mega-dosages of vitamins for therapeutic measures (e.g. the use of retinol or its analogs in the treatment of dermatological disorders such as psoriasis and ichthyosis, the use of nicotinic acid to lower serum cholesterol, and the use of vitamin D for the management of osteomalacia and hypoparathyroidism), at the present time there is no conclusive evidence that supports recommending the use of large dosages of any vitamin in elderly patients. The current recommended dietary allowances per day for individuals over 50 years in the USA are presented in Table 1 (31[R]).*

Future studies should focus on the long-term safety and efficacy of large doses of various vitamins that have putative beneficial effects.

VITAMIN A (RETINOL) *(SED-13, 1167; SEDA-18, 380; SEDA-21, 405)*

All-trans retinoic acid

Recently many studies on the treatment and prevention of cancer with all-*trans* retinoic acid have been conducted. A major obstacle is the substantial dose-related toxicity of the retinoids. Several adverse effects have been reported after the use of all-*trans* retinoic acid in acute promyelocytic leukemia. Except for severe adverse effects, including the *retinoic acid syndrome*, the mechanisms remain unclear.

A phase I clinical trial of all-*trans* retinoic acid has been conducted to establish the maximum tolerable daily dose in 49 patients with solid tumors (32[C]). The maximum tolerable dose was 269 mg/m^2 per day. Although adverse effects of at least grade 3 occurred with lower doses, there was no consistent dose-limiting toxicity at these doses. The dose-limiting adverse effect was *hyperlipidemia*. Grade 3 hypertriglyceridemia occurred in one patient at daily doses of 110, 138, and 269 mg/m^2. Grade 4 hypertriglyceridemia occurred in three patients with daily doses of 88, 215, and 269 mg/m^2. Grade 3 hypercholesterolemia occurred in one patient at a daily dose of 269 mg/m^2. Other grade 3 and 4 effects occurred sporadically, e.g., a localized desquamative scrotal *rash* (45 and 138 mg/m^2; $n = 2$), *staphylococcal bacteremia* (110 mg/m^2; $n = 1$), *pseudotumor cerebri* (110 and 309 mg/m^2; $n = 2$), *shortness of breath* on minimal exertion (110 and 138 mg/m^2; $n = 2$), severe *cough* (110 and 138 mg/m^2; $n = 2$), *dehydration and transient renal insufficiency* (56 mg/m^2; $n = 1$), grade 3 *myalgias* (172 and 215 mg/m^2; $n = 2$), and grade 3 *headache* (110, 110, and 215 mg/m^2; $n = 3$). The following grade 3 adverse effects were observed in one patient each, without relation to dose: *anorexia*, *fatigue*, *dysphagia*, *nausea*, and *vomiting*; there were transient *increases in transaminases* in four patients at dosages over 56 mg/m^2 per day. Frequent grade 2 effects included *anemia* ($n = 8$), *anorexia* ($n = 6$), *dyspnea* ($n = 4$), *depression* ($n = 4$), *fatigue* ($n = 8$), *dry skin and/or eyes* in the majority of patients, '*stuffy ears*' in several patients, *fever* ($n = 4$), transient *headache* ($n = 9$), *hypertriglyceridemia* ($n = 4$), *raised transaminases* ($n = 4$), *nausea* ($n = 7$), and *vomiting* ($n = 6$). Grade 2 infections included one patient with a *paronychia*, two with *urinary tract infections*, and one with *vaginal candidiasis*. One patient had *acidosis, burning of the skin, acute transient renal failure*, and *shortness of breath*. All adverse effects resolved on drug withdrawal.

Some rare adverse effects and their management have been reviewed (Table 2) (33[R]).

Retinoic acid syndrome The retinoic acid syndrome presents with symptoms including

Table 2. *List of rare adverse effects of retonic acid* (33[R]).

Cardiovascular	Thromboembolic events
Endocrine and metabolic	Male infertility
Mineral and fluid balance	Hypercalcemia
Hematological	Bone marrow necrosis
	Bone marrow fibrosis
Pancreas	Acute pancreatitis
Skin and appendages	Sweet's syndrome
	Erythema nodosum
	Hyperhistaminemia
	Granulomatous proliferation

pleuropericardial effusion and respiratory distress after the start of treatment with all-*trans* retinoic acid. In nine of 25 patients with acute promyelocytic leukemia treated with oral all-*trans* retinoic acid, 45 mg/m^2 per day, the retinoic acid syndrome developed at 2–25 days after the start of therapy (34[C]). Seven of them had a raised temperature (over 38°C). One patient with a normal ECG before treatment developed complete atrioventricular block. In seven patients the syndrome occurred shortly before the peak white cell count had been reached, but in one it happened when there was obvious differentiation of leukemic cells and relative leukopenia. With the exception of one patient, who possibly died of both the retinoic acid syndrome and co-existent *Staphylococcus aureus* sepsis, all the patients were successfully treated with dexamethasone for 3–5 days.

Cardiovascular Reported *thrombotic events* were fatal thromboembolism without leukocytosis, thromboembolic events shortly after the start of treatment, pulmonary embolism, multiple thrombosis of the brachycephalic, popliteal, and forearm veins after withdrawal (35[C]), and multivisceral failure due to multiple thrombosis (36[C]). All-*trans* retinoic acid may not rapidly correct hyperfibrinolysis, and thrombin generation may persist for a long time.

Pulmonary embolism occurred in a patient with acute promyelocytic leukemia treated with all-*trans* retinoic acid (37[c]).

A 32-year-old patient with acute promyeloytic leukemia, but no clinical or laboratory evidence of coagulopathy, was given all-*trans* retinoic acid (45 mg/m^2 per day); on day 8 daunorubicin was added. On day 27, when he was in complete remission, he developed acute dyspnea and chest pain, with signs of acute venous thrombosis in both legs; perfusion scintigraphy confirmed pulmonary embolism. Improvement in perfusion in both lungs was achieved by fibrinolytic therapy.

Respiratory Two patients with retinoic acid syndrome complicating *pleural effusion and pulmonary infiltrates* were successfully treated with diuretics (38[c]).

Endocrine, metabolic The effects of all-*trans* retinoic acid on serum lipids (32[C]) have been noted above. *Hyperlipidemia* is one of the common adverse effects of all-*trans* retinoic acid. In one case hyperlipidemia after all-*trans* retinoic acid treatment progressed to acute pancreatitis (39[c]).

A 49-year-old man with acute promyelocytic leukemia was given two courses of chemotherapy, followed by severe complications, including bacterial liver abscess and extensive fistula formation. Intensive therapy was replaced by all-*trans* retinoic acid (45 mg/m^2 per day). Before this his serum cholesterol and triglyceride concentrations had been in the reference ranges, except for occasional increases in triglycerides up to 2.0 g/l. After 20 weeks of treatment with all-*trans* retinoic acid he developed severe abdominal pain. He had raised C-reactive protein, lipase, and elastase and marked increases in serum cholesterol (5.25 g/l) and triglycerides (14.25 g/l). Abdominal CT showed a low-density area around the pancreas and confirmed the diagnosis of acute pancreatitis. Retinoic acid was withdrawn and he was given bezafibrate and probucol. His serum lipid concentration returned to normal after 2 weeks.

Hyperlipidemia developed in 10 of 25 patients with acute promyelocytic leukemia treated with all-*trans* retinoic acid (34[C]). About 20% of patients treated with all-*trans* retinoic acid had raised serum concentrations of total cholesterol and triglycerides (40[C]). Hyperlipidemia was treated with a protease inhibitor and pravastatin.

Mineral and fluid balance In five patients with acute promyelocytic leukemia all-*trans* retinoic acid may have caused *hypercalcemia* by stimulating osteoclastic activity (41[c]).

In multiple myeloma all-*trans* retinoic acid increased the serum interleukin-6 concentration, leading to advanced bone absorption (42[C]). Apoptosis was the main mechanism of action of all-trans retinoic acid in reducing the number of myeloma cells. Three of six patients had increased calcium concentrations, which normalized after withdrawal.

Hematological *Bone marrow necrosis* occurred in a case of acute promyelocytic leukemia during treatment with all-*trans* retinoic acid (43[c]). The patient subsequent recovered and achieved complete remission. Two other patients developed leukocytosis after the administration of all-*trans* retinoic acid; this was successfully treated with hydroxyurea. However, hydroxyurea must be used with caution, because in combination with all-*trans* retinoic acid it can cause bone marrow necrosis.

Bone marrow fibrosis occurred in 13 of 15 patients who received all-trans retinoic acid for acute promyelocytic leukemia (44[C]). Collagenous fibrosis also occurred. The fibrotic changes were common and reversible. Collagen synthesis may have been stimulated by TGF-β.

A marked *basophil leukocytosis* occurred during treatment with all-*trans* retinoic acid, associated with severe symptoms due to hyperhistaminemia (45[C]). One patient out of 10 had hypotension and a large gastric ulcer resulting from hyperhistaminemia. The symptoms of hyperhistaminemia were prevented by the administration of a histamine H_2 receptor antagonist.

All-*trans* retinoic acid has caused exacerbation of a *coagulopathy* (46[c]).

A 22-year-old woman with acute promyelocytic leukemia presented with extensive lower abdominal bruising after being struck by a heavy crate. She was treated with all-*trans* retinoic acid 45 mg/m^2 and prednisolone 25 mg tds. Five days later she developed extensive skin and subcutaneous bleeding and a rigid abdomen with reduced bowel sounds. The worsening coagulopathy was complicated by bone marrow necrosis, parenchymal liver damage, and acute tubular necrosis. Temporary withdrawal of the drug and subsequent dosage reduction controlled the coagulopathy. After 12 days hepatic and renal function returned to normal.

The authors recommended daily monitoring of clinical and laboratory parameters during induction therapy with all-*trans* retinoic acid in patients with coagulopathies.

Thrombocytosis has been associated with all-*trans* retinoic acid (47[c]).

A 45-year-old patient presented with a 2-month history of progressive weakness, followed by spontaneous cutaneous hemorrhages. Acute promyelocytic leukemia was diagnosed and he was given idarubicin 45 mg/m^2 per day orally every 2 days for 8 days. On day 7 he complained of headache and blurred vision, suggestive of pseudotumor cerebri. All-*trans* retinoic acid was withdrawn and re-administered on day 12, after the recovery of normal vision and disappearance of the headaches. On day 42, laboratory tests showed thrombocytosis (platelet count 1071×10^9/l) All-*trans* retinoic acid was suspected of causing thrombocytosis and was withdrawn. The platelet count fell to 960×10^9/l after 2 days and became normal on day 56.

Pancreas Acute *pancreatitis* with hyperlipidemia has been attributed to all-*trans* retinoic acid (39[c]). The patient had high serum activities of lipase and amylase.

Urinary system The occurrence of *acute renal insufficiency* due to occlusion of renal vessels further supports the concern about thromboembolic complications associated with all-*trans* retinoic acid in patients with acute promyelocytic leukemia (48[c]).

A 43-year-old man presented with acute promyelocytic leukemia and was given all-*trans* retinoic acid. After 10 days he developed acute renal failure, which resolved after complete remission of the leukemia had been achieved and therapy withdrawn.

The authors suggested that thrombotic events could be avoided by using prophylactic low-dose heparin.

Skin and appendages Six cases of *Sweet's syndrome* (neutrophil infiltration of the skin and internal organs) have been reported (49[C]). The onset was at 7–34 days. In one case erythema nodosum developed during treatment with all-*trans* retinoic acid. All cases responded well to glucocorticoids.

Skin dryness was seen in nine of 25 patients with acute promyelocytic leukemia treated with all-*trans* retinoic acid (34[C]).

Sexual function The effects of all-*trans* retinoic acid on the male reproductive system include *gynecomastia*, *discomfort*, *potency dis-*

orders, *reduced fertility*, and *ejaculatory failure* (50[C]). Their frequencies are very high.

Tumor-inducing effects In one patient a *myeloblastoma* developed in the oral and buccal mucosa 29 days after the administration of retinoic acid (51[c]). The growth of the tumor depended on the administration of all-*trans* retinoic acid and was controlled by low-dose cytosine arabinoside.

Effects in pregnancy 13-*Cis* retinoic acid (Accutane) causes a characteristic retinoid embryopathy. Its isomer, all-*trans* retinoic acid (tretinoin) is teratogenic in animals. The outcomes of 291 pregnancy have been reported; there was no difference in the malformation rates between exposed and unexposed fetuses. A prospective, observational controlled study has compared the rate of malformations among fetuses exposed (94) and unexposed (133) to all-*trans* retinoic acid (52[C]). There were no differences between cases and controls in the rates of live births, miscarriages, or elective terminations of pregnancy. Among exposed live-born babies the incidence of major malformations did not differ from controls, and none was consistent with the retinoic acid embryopathy.

In a pilot trial 13 patients with Philadelphia chromosome-positive chronic myeloid leukemia were treated with all-*trans* retinoic acid 175 mg/m^2 per day in two divided doses (53[C]). Seven patients had *headache*, which was severe in three; one patient required a 50% dosage reduction. Four patients had *nausea*, which was severe in one. Three patients had *dry skin* and three had *dry mucous membranes*. There were no changes in liver function tests or triglycerides.

A *fetal dysrhythmia* during treatment of pregnancy-associated promyelocytic leukemia has been associated with all-*trans* retinoic acid (54[c]).

A 37-year-old Japanese primigravida developed promyelocytic leukemia and was given all-*trans* retinoic acid 5 mg/m^2 per day at 30 weeks gestation. Her total thrombocyte count gradually increased on day 81 and fibrin degradation products fell to within the reference range on day 22. There was no leukocytosis. However, fetal growth was retarded, and a fetal dysrhythmia was noted during the 34th week. Echocardiography showed abnormal systolic anterior motion of the fetal mitral valve and the child was delivered by cesarean section. A neonatal electrocardiogram showed blocked atrial extra beats, which disappeared by the next morning.

The authors recommended close fetal monitoring during all-*trans* retinoic acid administration, with special attention to the risk of dysrhythmias. Further trials and long-term follow-up of neonates are needed to confirm the safety of all-trans retinoic acid for the fetus.

VITAMINS OF THE B GROUP

(SED-13, 1171; SEDA-18, 381; SEDA-19, 369; SEDA-20, 364; SEDA-21, 407)

Nicotinic acid (niacin), nicotinamide

The American Society of Health-System Pharmacists has issued a therapeutic statement on the safe use of niacin in the management of dyslipidemias and has reviewed its adverse effects (55[R]).

Modified-release formulations The efficacy, safety, and tolerability of a regimen of regular niacin, 500 mg qds, lovastatin 20 mg bd, and colestipol 10 g bd for 8 months have been evaluated in 29 men with hyperlipidemia and coronary artery disease (56[C]). During a second 8-month course regular niacin was replaced by a polygel modified-release formulation. The modified-release formulation was preferred by 21 patients and the regular niacin by four, and compliance was 95 and 85%, respectively. The modified-release niacin and regular niacin regimens did not differ in terms of uric acid, glucose, or insulin concentrations or aspartate aminotransferase activities. The two niacin formulations did not differ in adverse effects.

Cardiovascular *Vasodilatation* can lower the blood pressure and rarely precipitate angina in patients with pre-existing coronary heart disease (55[R]).

Endocrine, metabolic *Glucose tolerance* Niacin reduces glucose tolerance dose dependently, possibly by causing or aggravating insulin resistance. In diabetes mellitus niacin can worsen glycemic control.

Uric acid Niacin reduces the urinary secretion of uric acid dose dependently, increasing plasma uric acid concentrations. Niacin should be avoided in patients with a recent history of acute gout and who are taking uric acid-lowering drugs, and in patients who have frequent attacks of gout despite treatment.

Liver Although hepatotoxicity is probably the most serious adverse effect of niacin, its frequency is not known. An *increase in serum hepatic transaminases* is dose related and occurs with both immediate-release and modified-release niacin. Niacin should be withdrawn in patients with asymptomatic rises in enzymes three times the upper limit. Rises in hepatic transaminases less than three times the upper limit can occur early in therapy and usually resolve with continued therapy or dosage reduction. The enzymatic changes are usually reversible on withdrawal, although the frequency of hepatotoxicity is greater with certain modified-release products and there have been a few reports of *fulminant hepatitis*. Because of this increased risk with modified-release products, the maximum dosage recommended by the NCEP (National Cholesterol Education Program) is 2 g/day. On the other hand, modified-release niacin is more than twice as potent in lowering cholesterol as immediate-release products. Patients should be instructed to report any signs or symptoms of hepatotoxicity (e.g. nausea, vomiting, malaise, loss of appetite, right upper quadrant pain, jaundice, and dark urine).

Gastrointestinal Niacin-related gastrointestinal adverse effects include *nausea*, *vomiting*, *abdominal pain*, *indigestion*, *heartburn*, *anorexia*, and *diarrhea*. The frequency of adverse effects is higher in users of modified-release niacin. Niacin should be avoided in patients with active peptic ulcer disease. Gastrointestinal distress can be minimized by the administration of divided doses and by instructing patients to take niacin on a full stomach.

In two trials patients with head and neck cancer were given nicotinamide in addition to radiotherapy (57[C]), (58[C]). The first study (57[C]) included 35 patients who were treated with accelerated radiotherapy, carbogen, and nicotinamide. Adverse effects in 15 patients given tablets of nicotinamide (80 mg/kg) 90 min before irradiation were nausea ($n = 7$), vomiting ($n = 10$), headache and blurred vision ($n = 1$), headache and diarrhea ($n = 1$), headache ($n = 1$), and hypotension ($n = 1$).

In the second study (58[C]) nicotinamide was given in a daily dose of 80 mg/kg to a maximum of 6 g as a liquid formulation to 40 patients receiving a 5–7-week course of radiotherapy. With prolonged administration, nausea with or without vomiting occurred in 65% of the patients and was often unresponsive to antiemetics. In 14 patients nicotinamide had either to be withdrawn or the dosage had to be reduced. There was a significant correlation between adverse effects and some pharmacokinetic parameters. In particular high plasma concentrations over days were associated with severe adverse effects, whereas daily dose was not. Thus, apart from direct topical irritation of the gastrointestinal mucosa, nicotinamide probably also has a systemic effect, and alternative routes of administration may fail to solve the problem of nausea.

Skin and appendages Skin reactions due to niacin include *flushing*, *pruritus*, *dry skin*, and reversible *acanthosis nigricans* (55[R]). Flushing results from PGD_2-mediated vasodilatation. Tolerance to these effects may develop and is associated with reduced mediator release.

Thiamine

Wernicke's encephalopathy, a disorder with a high morbidity and mortality, is common among alcoholics. Thiamine deficiency plays a key role, and parenteral high-dose thiamine is effective in prophylaxis and treatment. Unfortunately, reports of rare *anaphylactoid reactions* have led to a dramatic reduction in the use of parenteral thiamine, and it is possible that this change in treatment has led, or will lead, to an increase in morbidity and mortality. There is a particular risk of anaphylactoid reactions with formulations that contain polyethoxylated castor oil. Doctors who treat alcoholics need to be educated, in order to ensure the appropriate use of parenteral thiamine (59[r]).

VITAMIN C (ASCORBIC ACID) *(SED-13, 1175; SEDA-18, 382; SEDA-21, 407)*

A double-blind, randomized, controlled trial of vitamin C supplementation (50 mg/day) in premature neonates (birth weights 1000–1500 g) showed no evidence of increased erythrocyte destruction, hyperbilirubinemia, or other morbidity (60[C]).

VITAMIN D (CALCIFEROL) AND ANALOGS *(SED-13, 1177; SEDA-19, 371; SEDA-20, 366; SEDA-21, 408)*

Calcitriol (1,25-dihydroxycholecalciferol)

A prospective randomized comparison of calcitriol treatment with etidronate–calcitriol and calcitonin–calcitriol combinations in 30 Turkish women with postmenopausal osteoporosis for 1 year showed no improvement in spinal bone mineral density but a high rate of adverse events, such as hypercalciuria, in almost all patients and hypercalcemia in about half (61[C]). In order to avoid serious nephrotoxicity, treatment with calcitriol requires close monitoring of serum and urine calcium concentrations.

To improve growth failure, bowed legs, and biochemical and radiological abnormalities in patients with X-linked hypophosphatemic vitamin D-resistant rickets, combined therapy with phosphate and calcitriol is currently the best approach. However, the complications of combined therapy, such as hypercalcemia, nephrocalcinosis, and hyperparathyroidism, have not been solved. To achieve better control, new therapeutic approaches have recently been reported, for example, growth hormone or new vitamin D analogs (62[R]). Growth hormone improved linear growth, reduced phosphate reabsorption, and increased 1α-hydroxylase activity. Furthermore, 24,25-dihydroxycholecalciferol improved the bone lesions in hypophosphatemic mice and also in patients with X-linked hypophosphatemic vitamin D-resistant rickets, without adverse effects such as hypercalcemia or hypercalciuria, compared with 1,25-dihydroxycholecalciferol. These new approaches should be considered for the treatment of patients with X-linked hypophosphatemic vitamin D-resistant rickets.

Hypoparathyroidism is a rare disease, whose main symptom is hypocalcemia. In adults, hypocalcemia is mainly due to postoperative hypoparathyroidism (by accidental parathyroidectomy during thyroidectomy). Hypoparathyroidism requires life-long therapy with vitamin D or metabolites. Genuine vitamin D_3 (cholecalciferol, Vigantol) is the most economic treatment; however, cholecalciferol has a very long half-life, with the danger of chronic vitamin D intoxication. Dihydrotachysterol (AT10), an analogue of vitamin D, acts similarly and can be used as an alternative. 1,25-Dihydroxycholecalciferol (Rocaltrol), an active metabolite of cholecalciferol, is very potent, but can cause acute intoxication; it has a short half-life and is more expensive than cholecalciferol. A further metabolite, 1-hydroxycholecalciferol (alfacalcidol, Doss, EinsAlpha) is available for therapeutic use.

There have been no clinical intervention trials on the best therapy and management of hypoparathyroidism. Therefore, German physicians treating hypoparathyroidism have been surveyed to examine whether the measurement of 25-hydroxycholecalciferol is helpful in managing hypoparathyroidism (63[C]). Data from 59 children and 270 adults were obtained, including 45 patients whom the authors had treated during the previous 8 years. 1,25-Dihydroxycholecalciferol was the only form of vitamin D that had been administered to children, whereas 32% of adults had been treated with dihydrotachysterol, 28% with cholecalciferol, and 20% with 1,25-dihydroxycholecalciferol. There was a positive correlation between serum 25-hydroxycholecalciferol concentrations and the dose of cholecalciferol. In patients treated with cholecalciferol, serum calcium concentrations correlated significantly with serum 25-hydroxycholecalciferol concentrations, but not with calcium dose.

VITAMIN K (PHYTOMENADIONE) *(SED-13, 1182; SEDA-17, 441; SEDA-18, 383; SEDA-19, 372; SEDA-20, 409)*

Cardiovascular collapse has been reported after the use of vitamin K to aid postoperative hemostasis (64[c]).

A 62-year-old patient who underwent a partial right hepatic lobectomy for adenocarcinoma of the colon with metastases in the liver experienced sudden and severe hypotension, bradycardia, and asystole 6 h later. Differential diagnoses included acute myocardial infarction, hemorrhage from the surgical site, and pulmonary embolism. As these complications were ruled out, an allergic reaction to vitamin K (10 mg in crystalloid intravenously over 10 min) was suggested.

REFERENCES

1. Thurman JE, Mooradian ID. Vitamin supplementation therapy in the elderly. Drugs Aging 1997;11:433–49.
2. Paolisso G, Balbi V, Volpe C, Varricchio G, Gambardella A, Saccomanno F, Ammendola S, Varricchio M, D'Onofrio F. Metabolic benefits deriving from chronic vitamin C supplementation in aged non-insulin dependent diabetics. J Am Coll Nutr 1995;14:387–92.
3. Paolisso G, D'Amore A, Balbi V, Volpe C, Galzerano D, Giugliano D, Sgambato S, Varricchio M, D'Onofrio F. Plasma vitamin C affects glucose homeostasis in healthy subjects and in non-insulin-dependent diabetics Am J Physiol 1994;266:E261–8 (with errata in 267 (4 Pt 1 and 6 Pt 3): section E following tables of contents).
4. Schorah CJ, Tormey WP, Brooks GH, Robertshaw AM, Young GA, Talukder R, Kelly JF. The effect of vitamin C supplements on body weight, serum proteins, and general health of an elderly population. Am J Clin Nutr 1981;34:871–6.
5. Levine M, Dhariwal KR, Welch RW, Wang Y, Park JB. Determination of optimal vitamin C requirements in humans. Am J Clin Nutr 1995;62 (Suppl):1347–56S.
6. Jacob RA. Vitamin C. In: Shils ME, Olson JA, Shike, M, editors. Modern Nutrition in Health and Disease, 8th edition. Philadelphia: Lea and Febiger, 1994:342–8.
7. Strijdom JG, Marais BJ, Koeslag JH. Ascorbic acid causes spuriously low blood glucose measurements. S Afr Med J 1993;83:64–5.
8. Herbert, V, Jacob E. Destruction of vitamin B_{12} by ascorbic acid. J Am Med Assoc 1974; 230:241–2.
9. Herbert V, Jacob E, Wong KT, Scott J, Pfeffer RD. Low serum vitamin B_{12} levels in patients receiving ascorbic acid in megadoses: studies concerning the effect of ascorbate on radioisotope vitamin B_{12} assay. Am J Clin Nutr 1978;31:253–8.
10. Rees DC, Kelsey H, Richards JDM. Acute haemolysis induced by high dose ascorbic acid in glucose-6-phosphate dehydrogenase deficiency. Br Med J 1993;306:841–2.
11. Rosenberg ICH, Miller JW. Nutritional factors in physical and cognitive functions of elderly people. Am J Clin Nutr 1992;55:1237–43S.
12. Oakley GP, Adams MJ, Dickinson CM. More folic acid for everyone, now. J Nutr 1996;126 (Suppl):751–5S.
13. Drinka PJ, Langer EH, Voeks SK, Goodwin JS. Low serum folic acid levels in a nursing home population: a clinical experience. J Am Coll Nutr 1993;12:186–9.
14. Durrington PN. Drug therapy of hyperlipidaemia. In: Hyperlipidaemia: Diagnosis and Management, 2nd edition. Cambridge: Cambridge University Press, 1995:258–90.
15. Dalton TA, Berry RS. Hepatotoxicity associated with sustained-release niacin. Am J Med 1992;93:102–4.
16. Gharavi AG, Diamond A, Smith DA, Phillips RA. Niacin-induced myopathy. Am J Cardiol 1994;74:841–2.
17. Fraunfelder FW, Fraunfelder FT, Illingworth DR. Adverse ocular effects associated with niacin therapy. Br J Ophthalmol 1995;79:54–6.
18. Shakir KM, Kroll S, Aprill BS, Drake AJ 3rd, Eisold JF. Nicotinic acid decreases serum thyroid hormone levels while maintaining an euthyroid state. Mayo Clin Proc 1995;70:556–8.
19. Wahlberg G, Walldius G, Efendic S. Effects of nicotinic acid on glucose tolerance and glucose incorporation into adipose tissue in hypertriglyceridaemia. Scand J Clin Lab Invest 1992;52:537–45.
20. Knapen MH, Jie KS, Hamulyak K, Vermeer C. Vitamin K-induced changes in markers for osteoblast activity and urinary calcium loss. Calcif Tissue Int 1993;53:81–5.
21. Leklem JE. Vitamin B_6 reservoirs, receptors and red-cell reactions. Ann NY Acad Sci 1992;669:34–41.
22. Schaumburg H, Kaplan J, Windebank A, Vick N, Rasmus S, Pleasure D, Brown MJ. Sensory neuropathy from pyridoxine abuse: a new megavitamin syndrome. New Engl J Med 1983;309:445–8.
23. Berger AR, Schaumburg HH, Schroeder C, Schroeder C, Apfel S, Reynolds R. Dose response, coasting, and differential fiber vulnerability in human toxic neuropathy: a prospective study of neurotoxicity. Neurology 1992;42:1367–70.
24. Morimoto K, Kawada A, Hiruma M, Ishibashi A. Photosensitivity from pyridoxine hydrochlor-

ide (vitamin B_6). J Am Acad Dermatol 1996; 35:304–5.
25. Hathcock JN, Hattan DG, Jenkins MY, McDonald JT, Sundaresan PR, Wilkening VL. Evaluation of vitamin A toxicity. Am J Clin Nutr 1990;52:183–202.
26. Olson JA. Vitamin A, retinoids, and carotenoids. In: Shils ME, Olson JA, Shike M, editors. Modern Nutrition in Health and Disease, 8th edition. Philadelphia: Lea and Febiger, 1994:287–307.
27. Garewal HS, Diplock AT. How 'safe' are antioxidant vitamins? Drug Saf 1995;13:8–14.
28. Kwok T, Falconer-Smith JF, Potter JHF, and Ives DR. Thiamine status of elderly patients with cardiac failure. Age Ageing 1992;21:67–71.
29. National Research Council. Recommended Dietary Allowances, 10th edition. Washington, DC: National Academy Press, 1989.
30. Corrigan JJ. The effect of vitamin E on warfarin-induced vitamin K deficiency. Ann NY Acad Sci 1982;393:361–8.
31. Posner BM, Jette A, Smigelski C, Miller D, Mitchell P. Nutritional risk in New England elders. J Gerontol 1994;3 (Suppl):M123–32.
32. Conley BA, Egorin MJ, Sridhara R, Finley R, Hemady R, Wu S, Tait NS, Van Echo DA. Phase I clinical trial of all-*trans*-retinoic acid with correlation of its pharmacokinetics and pharmacodynamics. Cancer Chemother Pharmacol 1997;39:291–9.
33. Hatake K, Uwai M, Ohtsuki T, Tomizuka H, Izumi T, Yoshida M, Miura Y. Rare but important adverse effects of all-*trans* retinoic acid in acute promyelocytic leukemia and their management. Int J Hematol 1997;66:13–9.
34. Chou W-C, Tang JL, Yao M, Liang YJ, Lee FY, Lin MT, Wang CH, Shen MC, Chen YC, Tien HF. Clinical and biological characteristics of acute promyelocytic leukemia in Taiwan: a high relapse rate in patients with high initial and peak white blood cell counts during all-*trans*-retinoic acid treatment. Leukemia 1997;1:921–8.
35. Forjaz De Lacerda J, Alves Do Carmo J, Lurdes Guerra M, Geraldes J, Forjaz De Lacerda JM. Multiple thrombosis in acute promyelocytic leukemia after tretionin. Lancet 1993;342:114.
36. Fenaux P, Castaigne S, Dombret H. All-*trans* retinoic acid (ATRA) as first-line therapy of acute promyelocytic leukemia (APL). A report of 31 cases. Br J Haematol 1991;77:51.
37. Jimenez-Yuste V, Martin MP, Canales M, Ojeda E. Pulmonary embolism in a patient with acute promyelocytic leukemia treatment with all-*trans* retinoic acid. Leukemia 1997;11:1988–9.
38. Yokokura, Hatake K, Komatsu N, Miura Y. Toxicity of tretionin in acute promyelocytic leukemia. Lancet 1994;344:361–2.
39. Yutsudo Y, Imoto S, Ozuru R, Kajimoto K, Itoi H, Koizumi T, Nishimura R, Nakagawa T. Acute pancreatitis after all-*trans* retinoic acid therapy. Ann Hematol 1997;74:295–6.
40. Warrell RP Jr, de The H, Wang ZY, Degos L. Acute promyelocytic leukemia. New Engl J Med 1994;329:177–89.
41. Akiyama H, Makamura N, Nagasaka S, Sakamaki H, Onozawa Y. Hypercalcaemia due to all-*trans* retinoic acid. Lancet 1992;1:338.
42. Niesvizky R, Siegel DS, Busquets X, Nichols G, Muindi J, Warrell RP, Michaeli J. Hypercalcemia and increased serum interleukin-6 levels induced by all-*trans* retinoic acid in patients with multiple myeloma. Br J Haematol 1995;89:217–8.
43. Limentani SA, Pretell JO, Potter D, Dubois JS, Daoust PR, Spieler PS, Miller KB. Bone marrow necrosis in two patients with acute promyelocytic leukemia during treatment with all-*trans* retinoic acid. Am J Hematol 1994;47:50–5.
44. Hatake K, Ohtsuki T, Uwai M, Takahashi H, Izumi T, Yoshida M, Kanai N, Saito K, Harigaya K, Miura Y. Tretinoin induces bone marrow collagenous fibrosis in acute promyelocytic leukemia: new adverse, but reversible effect. Br J Haematol 1996;93:646–9.
45. Shimamoto Y, Suga K, Yamaguchi M, Kuriyama K, Tomonaga M. Prophylaxis of symptoms of hyperhistaminemia after the treatment of acute promyelocytic leukemia with all-*trans* retinoic acid. Acta Haematol 1994;92:109–12.
46. Cull GM, Eikelboom JW, Cannell PK. Exacerbation of coagulopathy with concurrent bone marrow necrosis, hepatic and renal dysfunction secondary to all-*trans* retinoic acid therapy for acute promyelocytic leukemia. Hematol Oncol 1997;5:13–7.
47. Kentos A, Le Moine F, Crenier L, Capel P, Meyer S, Muus P, Mandelli F, Feremans W. All-*trans* retinoic acid induced thrombocytosis in a patient with acute promyelocytic leukaemia. Br J Haematol 1997;97:685.
48. Pogliani EM, Rossini F, Casaroli I, Maffe P, Corneo G. Thrombotic complications in acute promyelocytic leukemia during all-*trans*-retinoic acid therapy. Acta Haematol 1997;97:228–30.
49. Christ E, Linka A, Jacky E, Speich R, Marincek B, Schaffner A. Sweet's syndrome involving the musculoskeletal system during treatment of promyelocytic leukemia with all-*trans* retinoic acid. Leukemia 1996;10:731–4.
50. Coleman R, MacDonald D. Effects of isotretionin on male reproductive system. Lancet 1994; 344:198–9.
51. Izumi T, Hatake K, Imagawa S, Yoshida M, Ohta M, Sasaki P, Miwa A, Suda T, Sakamoto S, Miura Y. A case of acute promyelocytic leukemia (APL) with myeloblastoma in the oral cavity developing after receiving all-*trans* retinoic acid. Jpn J Clin Hematol 1994;35:598–602.
52. Shapiro L, Pastuszak A, Curto G, Koren G. Safety of first-trimester exposure to topical tretinoin: prospective cohort study. Lancet 1997; 350:1143–4.
53. Cortes J, Kantarjian H, O'Brien S, Beran M, Estey E, Keating M, Talpaz M. A pilot study of all-*trans* retinoic acid in patients with Philadelphia chromosome-positive chronic myelogenous leukemia. Leukemia 1997;11:929–32.
54. Terada Y, Shindo T, Endoh A, Watanabe M,

Fukuya T, Yajima A. Fetal arrhythmia during treatment of pregnancy-associated acute promyelocytic leukemia with all-*trans* retinoic acid and favorable outcome. Leukemia 1997;11:454–5.
55. Britton ML, Bradberry JC, Letassy NA, McKenney JM, Sirmans SM. ASHP therapeutic position statement on the safe use of niacin in the management of dyslipidemias. Am J Health Syst Pharm 1997;54:2815–19.
56. Brown BG, Bardsley, Poulin D, Hillger LA, Dowdy A. Moderate dose, three-drug therapy with niacin, lovastatin, and colestipol to reduce low-density lipoprotein cholesterol <100 mg/dl in patients with hyperlipidemia and coronary artery disease. Am J Cardiol 1997;80:111–15.
57. Saunders MI, Hoskin PJ, Pigott K, Powell MEB, Goodchild K, Dische S, Denekamp J, Stratford MRL, Dennis MF, Rojas AM. Accelerated radiotherapy, carbogen and nicotinamide (ARCON) in locally advanced head and neck cancer: a feasibility study. Radiother Oncol 1997;45:159–66.
58. Kaanders JHAM, Stratford MRL, Liefers J, Dennis MF, Van Der Kogel AJ, Van Daal WAJ, Rojas A. Administration of nicotinamide during a five- to seven-week course of radiotherapy: pharmacokinetics, tolerance, and compliance. Radiother Oncol 1997;43:67–73.
59. Thomson AD, Cook CCH. Parenteral thiamine and Wernicke's encephalopathy: the balance of risks and perception of concern. Alcohol Alcoholism 1997;32:207–9.
60. Doyle J, Vreman HJ, Stevenson DK, Brown EJ, Schmidt B, Paes B, Ohlsson A, Boulton J, Kelly E, Gillie P, Lewis N, Merko S, Shaw D, Zipursky A. Does vitamin C cause hemolysis in premature newborn infants? Results of a multicenter double-blind, randomized, controlled trial. J Pediatr 1997;130:103–9.
61. Gürlek A, Bayraktar M, Gedik O. Comparison of calcitriol treatment with idronate-calcitriol and calcitonin-calcitriol combinations in Turkish women with post-menopausal osteoporosis: a prospective study. Calcif Tissue Int 1997;61:39–43.
62. Ono T, Seino Y. Medical management and complications of X-linked hypophosphatemic vitamin D resistant rickets. Acta Paediatr Jpn 1997;39:503–7.
63. Schilling T, Ziegler R. Current therapy of hypoparathyroidism—a survey of German endocrinology centers. Exp Clin Endocrinol Diabetes 1997;105:237–41.
64. Songy KA Jr, Layon AJ. Vitamin K-induced cardiovascular collapse. J Clin Anesth 1997; 9:514–19.

J. Costa and M. Farré

39 Corticotrophins, corticosteroids, and prostaglandins

CORTICOTROPHINS

Adrenocorticotropic hormone

(SED-13, 1990; SEDA-19, 374; SEDA-20, 368; SEDA-21, 412)

Adrenocorticotropic hormone (ACTH) is the treatment of choice of infantile spasms. ACTH (depot formulation 10 IU/day) has been compared with vigabatrin (100–150 mg/kg per day) in a recent randomized trial in 42 infants (22 boys and 20 girls) aged 2–9 months with newly diagnosed spasms (1[C]). Although ACTH was more effective than vigabatrin, abolishing spasms in 14 patients (74%) compared with 11 patients (48%), the incidence of adverse effects was also higher. *Drowsiness*, *hypotonia*, and *irritability* were observed in 13 and 37% of infants given vigabatrin and ACTH, respectively. In another trial in infantile spasms due to tuberous sclerosis, vigabatrin was more effective that hydrocortisone and caused a lower incidence of adverse effects (2[C]). Vigabatrin could be an alternative to steroids in the treatment of infantile spasm, but more evidence is needed.

Nervous system The administration of ACTH to children with infantile spasm is often associated with *brain shrinkage*. Magnetic resonance spectroscopy was used to determine brain water content and concentrations of *N*-acetylaspartate, creatine + phosphocreatine, and choline in nine patients (seven boys and two girls) treated with ACTH (mean dose 69 units) (3[C]). Only the *N*-acetylaspartate concentration changed significantly, suggesting a catabolic effect of ACTH on the brain.

Special senses *Central serous retinopathy* is a disease that predominantly affects men in their fourth or fifth decade of life, causing detachment of the neurosensory retina and/or the retinal epithelium in the posterior pole. It has been linked to the therapeutic use of ACTH or corticosteroids or to endogenous ACTH hypersecretion. Bilateral central serous retinopathy has been reported in a woman treated with a synthetic ACTH analog intramuscularly (4[c]).

A 35-year-old woman developed acute reduction in vision in the right eye and the impression that a light bulb was shining in the lower visual field of the left eye. She had a chronic relapsing seronegative arthritis and enthesiopathy, affecting the ankles, knees, and elbows asymmetrically and had been taking non-steroidal anti-inflammatory drugs until 3 weeks before. Six days before the occurrence of her ocular symptoms she had received an intramuscular injection of tetracosactrin 1 mg and 4 days later a second dose. She had visual acuities of 6/12 in the right eye and 6/7.5 in the left. The anterior segment was normal and the intraocular pressure was 12 mmHg in both eyes. There were no cells or flare in the anterior chambers of the vitreous, and the lenses were clear. The pupils were equal and briskly reactive. In the right eye there was a well-demarcated, round, serous detachment of the central macula, approximately four disc diameters in size. In the left eye there was a similar but smaller detachment in the area of the lower temporal vascular arcade. Fluorescein angiography showed early leakage in the inferior part of the lesion in the right eye, increasing in size, and showing a late 'ink-blot' pattern. The left eye showed a smaller but similar process in the upper temporal vascular arcade area. A diagnosis of bilateral central serous retinopathy was made. The tetracosactrin was withdrawn and after 2 months she was asymptomatic, with visual

Side Effects of Drugs, Annual 22
J.K. Aronson, ed.

acuities of 6/7.5 in both eyes and resolution of the serous detachments.

Based on reported experimental and clinical evidence, the author suggested that ACTH had had a direct independent effect, through the melanotrophic part of the molecule, on retinal pigmented epithelial cells.

GLUCOCORTICOSTEROIDS

(SED-13, 1193; SEDA-19, 374; SEDA-20, 368; SEDA-21, 412)

Cardiovascular Myocardial hypertrophy is an adverse effect of dexamethasone in preterm infants. *Hypertrophic cardiomyopathy* has been reported in two preterm neonates; both recovered after withdrawal of steroids (5^c).

A girl born at 35 weeks of gestation was given dexamethasone (1 mg/kg per day i.v. for 7 days; 0.5 mg/kg per day for 3 days) for bronchopulmonary dysplasia, with good effect. At 21 days of age she progressively worsened and had a systolic ejection murmur. Echocardiography showed thickening of the interventricular septum and mild thickening of the posterior left ventricular free wall. Repeat echocardiography 27 days after steroid withdrawal was normal.

A girl born prematurely at 25 weeks was given dexamethasone (0.5 mg/kg per day for 3 days, 0.25 mg/kg per day for 3 days, 0.15 mg/kg per day on the 7th day, and 0.08 mg/kg per 48 h up to 16 days) for bronchopulmonary dysplasia. At 30 days a systolic murmur was detected. Echocardiography showed interventricular septum thickening, moderate mid-ventricular trapping without left ventricle tract outflow obstruction, and mild mitral valve regurgitation. Corticosteroids were discontinued. Echocardiography 23 days later was normal.

In a study of 23 patients who received cyclosporin and azathioprine, 26 who received cyclosporin, azathioprine, and prednisone (duration of therapy over 6 months), and 25 healthy controls, heart transplant recipients who received prednisone developed significant *impairment of fibrinolysis* compared with those who did not and with controls (6^C). Fibrinolysis was significantly impaired, owing to high concentrations of plasminogen activator inhibitor-1 in 69% (18/26) of the patients who received prednisone compared with 35% (8/23) of those who did not. An increase in plasminogen activator inhibitor-1 is an independent risk factor for cardiovascular disease. The researchers concluded that in heart transplant recipients, corticosteroid-induced impairment of fibrinolysis may constitute a risk factor for thrombotic disease.

A previously healthy girl developed disseminated *varicella* and staphylococcal *pericarditis* after a single application of triamcinolone cream 0.1% to relieve pruritus associated with *varicella* skin lesions (7^c).

The mother of a 17-month-old girl applied triamcinolone cream once to *varicella* lesions on her daughter's groin and buttocks. A day later new lesions erupted on the child's face, limbs, and abdomen and she became dehydrated, with a fever of 39.3°C, tachycardia, hypotension, and a raised leukocyte count (28×10^9/l). She had over 1000 lesions on her body. Despite intravenous fluids and acyclovir her condition worsened over the next 48 h. Her leukocyte count increased to 46×10^9/l, she had hepatomegaly, poor peripheral perfusion, bilateral interstitial pulmonary infiltrates, a pericardial effusion, and poor myocardial contractility. *Staphylococcus aureus* was isolated from the pericardial fluid.

A controlled study has been carried out in 16 ventilator-dependent neonates of very low birth weights treated with dexamethasone for bronchopulmonary dysplasia, in order to determine the incidence and time-course of *hypertension* (8^C). Systolic and diastolic blood pressures before dexamethasone correlated with corrected gestational age. When dexamethasone was given, the blood pressure increased significantly from days 1 to 2. Mean systolic pressure was 51 mmHg before dexamethasone, compared with 64 mmHg during therapy; diastolic pressure was 29 mmHg compared with 41 mmHg. After the end of therapy, the blood pressure continued to increase: systolic, 67 mmHg; diastolic, 42 mmHg. Both systolic and diastolic pressures increased as a function of weight and age. When the authors controlled for these co-variates, there was an independent effect of dexamethasone. Of 2182 individual systolic pressure readings, 9.4% were in the hypertensive range. Six infants treated with hydralazine had significantly higher mean systolic pressures before dexamethasone than infants without hydralazine (56 vs 46 mmHg) and were 2 weeks older at the start of therapy. The authors concluded that blood pressure increases significantly during dexamethasone therapy, particularly in the first 48 h, and does not return to baseline after therapy. Infants who are most likely to be labelled hypertensive tend to be older at the start of therapy but do not have any other risk factors.

Nervous system Glucocorticoids are used to treat edema associated with cerebral tumors, and can cause a fall in intracranial pressure. In 13 patients with various cerebral tumors given methylprednisolone (1.4 mg/kg per day for 5 days) intracranial pressure only fell in patients with malignant tumors and with initial intracranial pressures over 15 mmHg (9[c]).

Psychiatric Neuropsychiatric effects of steroids can result from intra-articular administration.

Hallucinations occurred in a 72-year-old man who had taken oral prednisone 5 mg/day for about a year, and who had increased the dosage to 10 mg/day because of a flare-up of his rheumatoid arthritis (10[c]). About 1 month later, he was given an intra-articular injection of triamcinolone 80 mg and 24 h later had an episode of visual hallucinations lasting 4 days. About 3 months later he received another intra-articular injection of triamcinolone 80 mg and had further visual hallucinations, which resolved after 4 days. He had previously received intra-articular triamcinolone before taking oral prednisone and had not had hallucinations.

The high dosage of triamcinolone could have played a part in this case, as could the continuous low-dose oral prednisone.

Lithium has been used in the treatment and prophylaxis of steroid-induced psychosis and has been proposed as an alternative for the treatment of steroid-induced depression after its successful use in two patients who developed depression after the administration of high dosages of prednisolone (50–60 mg/day) (11[c]).

Acute mania has been reported to be related to an interaction between prednisone and clarithromycin (12[c]).

A 30-year-old woman took clarithromycin 1000 mg/day and prednisone 20 mg/day for acute sinusitis and increased the dosage of prednisone to 40 mg/day after 2 days. After 3 days she developed delusional paranoia, disorganized thoughts and behavior, pressured speech, increased energy, a reduced need for sleep, impaired functioning at work, and a labile affect. After withdrawal of the two drugs her mental status gradually normalized and she returned to work within 2 weeks.

Prednisone alone may have been responsible for the development of mania in this patient. However, an interaction between prednisone and clarithromycin was considered, because clarithromycin inhibits CYP3A4, which is responsible for the metabolic clearance of prednisolone, the biologically active metabolite of prednisone.

Endocrine, metabolic *Pituitary gland* Two patients developed *hypopituitarism* and *empty sella syndrome* during corticosteroid pulse therapy for nephrotic syndrome (13[c]).

A 50-year-old woman received intravenous methylprednisolone 1 g/day for 3 days. Two weeks later, she developed severe lethargy, malaise, headache, amenorrhea, and cold intolerance. She had low concentrations of TSH, free T_3, free T_4, FSH, LH, GH, and ACTH. TSH and GH did not respond to TRH provocation. An MRI scan showed atrophy of the pituitary gland and an empty sella. She was treated with thyroid replacement and prednisolone and her symptoms improved within 3 weeks.

A 19-year-old man received corticosteroid pulse therapy seven times between the ages of 7 and 16 years (details not given). After each pulse, he took prednisolone 50–60 mg for 2–3 weeks, tapering the dosage to 15 mg/day for maintenance. He subsequently received further corticosteroid pulse therapy, consisting of prednisolone 10 mg/day (duration not stated). One year later he was investigated for short stature and had no response to GH. An MRI scan showed an empty sella.

Adrenal gland Inhaled fluticasone produced almost 2-fold greater *adrenal suppression*, judged by the 08:00 h plasma cortisol concentration, than microgram-equivalent doses of triamcinolone in a single-blind, randomized, crossover study in 12 volunteers (mean age 28 years) who took triamcinolone 800 μg bd, fluticasone 875 μg in the morning and 750 μg at night, or placebo via a metered dose inhaler with a spacer (14[C]). The authors suggested that the 2-fold difference in adrenal suppression between fluticasone and triamcinolone was likely to be even greater with long-term dosing at steady state.

The effects of fluticasone on adrenal function have been studied in 34 children taking high dosages (400–909 μg/m^2 per day) of inhaled beclomethasone, dipropionate, or budesonide with a spacer, in a double-blind, crossover study (15[C]). A comparison of the effects of fluticasone and beclomethasone on 24-h excretion rates of total cortisol and cortisol metabolites reached significance only after correction for urinary creatinine excretion (tetrahydrocortisol and 5′-α-tetrahydrocortisol geometric means: 424 vs 341 μg/m^2 per day). The baseline data showed adrenal suppression in the children taking beclomethasone (total cortisol geometric means: 975 vs 1542 μg/day) and dose-related suppression in the children taking budesonide. Suppressed adrenal function in the children who were taking beclomethasone at baseline subsequently improved with fluticasone and beclomethasone. Fluticasone is less likely to suppress adrenal function than beclomethasone at therapeutically equivalent doses. The baseline data also supported the claim that spacers should be used for the administration of high doses of inhaled steroids.

Gestational diabetes mellitus was more common in 50 women who had received corticosteroids with or without β-adrenoceptor agonists for threatened preterm delivery compared with 1985 controls (16[C]). Of the women in the study group, 21 with preterm labor received intravenous magnesium sulfate followed by oral terbutaline, 2.5–5 mg every 3–6 h, plus intramuscular betamethasone 12 mg/day; the other 29 received only betamethasone for threatened preterm delivery without a diagnosis of preterm labor. Of the women treated with corticosteroids plus β-agonists, 24% had an abnormal 3-h glucose tolerance test compared with 4% of the controls. There were abnormal 1-h glucose tolerance tests in 76% of those given a corticosteroid plus a β-agonist, 48% of those given a corticosteroid only, and 25% of the control group. The researchers commented that the high rate of abnormal 1-h glucose tolerance tests suggested that this screening test is of limited value in this setting.

It is important for physicians to be alert to the possibility of rapidly developing *ketoacidosis* with atypical biochemical features in pregnant women who require high doses of glucocorticoids (17[c]).

A 40-year-old woman with mild gestational diabetes developed ketoacidosis at 31 weeks after the administration of betamethasone 12 mg bd to assist fetal lung maturation in premature labor. She had a metabolic acidosis with a raised anion gap. Her blood glucose concentration was 8.3 mmol/l and urinalysis showed a lot of ketones but no glucose. There was no evidence of lactic acidosis. She responded to glucose and insulin.

It is well known that long-term steroids play an important role in the development of glucose intolerance and diabetes mellitus. Deflazacort, an oxazoline derivative of prednisolone, has been introduced as a potential substitute for conventional steroids in order to ameliorate glucose intolerance. In a randomized study in kidney transplant recipients with pre-transplantation or post-transplantation diabetes mellitus, 42 patients who switched from prednisone to deflazacort (in the ratio 5:6 mg) were prospectively compared with 40 patients who continued to take prednisone (18[C]). During the mean follow-up period of 13 months, neither graft dysfunction nor acute rejection developed in the conversion group, and there was improvement in blood glucose control. When the conversion group was stratified into those with pre- or post-transplantation diabetes, there were promising effects in the patients with post-transplantation diabetes. More than a 50% dosage reduction of hypoglycemic drugs was possible in 42% of those with post-transplantation diabetes. It was therefore possible to control blood glucose better in recipients with post-transplantation diabetes without seriously affecting immunosuppressive activity by converting to deflazacort.

Hematological A *leukemoid reaction* occurred in a neonate after the mother had received betamethasone for fetal lung maturation (19[c]).

A 34-year-old mother developed abdominal and low back pain and slight vaginal bleeding at 25 weeks. Subchorionic haemorrhage was diagnosed and she received antibacterial prophylaxis and tocolysis: two injections of betamethasone 12 mg, 12 h apart. Three days later she gave birth to a baby girl whose leukocyte count was 57×10^9/l. Blood culture was negative. The leukocyte count reached a maximum of 159×10^9/l on day 4, and by day 17 had fallen to 17×10^9/l.

Gastrointestinal Abdominal tenderness is the most common and often the only early sign of *perforated diverticula* in patients taking

Table 1. *The risks of ocular hypertension or open-angle glaucoma associated with duration of oral corticosteroid use*

Duration of use	Adjusted odds ratio (95% CI)
Not used	1.00
No continuous use	0.98 (0.86, 1.12)
1–2 months	1.29 (0.93, 1.80)
3–5 months	1.63 (1.16, 2.30)
6–11 months	1.87 (1.34, 2.60)
over 12 months	1.52 (1.13, 2.05)

corticosteroids. However, in some cases even abdominal tenderness is absent (20[c]).

An 85-year-old woman took prednisone 60 mg/day with gradual tapering. While taking 30 mg/day she developed fever and died, despite treatment with antibacterial drugs for presumed sepsis. Autopsy showed extensive diverticulitis, fecal peritonitis, and ulceration and perforation of the cecum. She had had no history of abdominal pain or distension or change in bowel habit and her bowel sounds had been normal.

Special senses *Ocular hypertension* and *open-angle glaucoma* are well-known adverse effects of ophthalmic administration of corticosteroids. A large case–control study, in which 9793 elderly patients with ocular hypertension or open-angle glaucoma were compared with 38 325 controls, has now shown an increased risk of these complications with oral corticosteroids (21[C]). The risk of ocular hypertension or open-angle glaucoma increased with increasing dose and duration of use of the oral corticosteroid (Table 1). There was no significant increase in the risk of ocular hypertension or open-angle glaucoma in patients who had stopped taking oral corticosteroids 15–45 days before. The researchers suggested that monitoring of intraocular pressure may be justified in long-term users of oral corticosteroids, as it is in long-term users of topical corticosteroids. They estimated that the excess risk of ocular hypertension or open-angle glaucoma with current oral corticosteroid use is 43 additional cases per 10 000 patients per year. However, in patients taking over 80 mg/day of hydrocortisone equivalents, the excess risk is 93 additional cases per 10 000 patients per year.

Prolonged use of high doses of inhaled corticosteroids also increases the risk of ocular hypertension and open-angle glaucoma (22[C]). In a case–control study of the records of 9793 elderly patients with ocular hypertension or open-angle glaucoma over a 6-year period there was a significantly increased risk of ocular hypertension and open-angle glaucoma in patients who had taken high doses of inhaled corticosteroids (1500–1600 μg) for 3 months or longer (OR = 1.44; 95% CI 1.01, 2.06). Both a high dosage of inhaled corticosteroid and prolonged continuous duration of therapy had to be present to increase the risk. The continuous use of intranasal corticosteroids was relatively rare, and only continuous exposure to intranasal corticosteroids irrespective of dose was analysed; there was no increased risk of ocular hypertension or open-angle glaucoma. The researchers suggested that if patients are to take high doses of inhaled corticosteroids for several months, their ocular pressure should be monitored.

The ocular hypertensive response in adults to topical ocular corticosteroids is well established. In contrast, descriptions of this phenomenon in children are scarce. The effects on intraocular pressure of topical dexamethasone have been compared with those of fluorometholone in 16 Chinese children under 10 years of age who underwent bilateral strabismus surgery (23[C]). They received 0.1% dexamethasone to one eye and 0.1% fluorometholone to the other six times per day for up to 4 weeks. The peak intraocular pressure in dexamethasone-treated eyes was 31 (range 13–48) mmHg, and in fluorometholone-treated eyes significantly lower at 21 (range 11–36) mmHg. The ocular-hypertensive response to topical dexamethasone in children occurs more frequently, more severely, and more rapidly than that reported in adults. It should be avoided in children if possible and it is desirable to monitor the intraocular pressure when it is being used. Fluorometholone may be more acceptable.

The use of inhaled corticosteroids was associated with a dose-dependent increased risk of *posterior subcapsular and nuclear cataracts* in a study of 6454 patients aged 49–97 years (24[C]). Data on corticosteroid use were available for 3313 of these patients; corticosteroid use was classified as 'none' in 2784 patients, inhaled only in 241, systemic only in 177, and both inhaled and systemic in 111. Compared with non-use, current or prior use of inhaled corticosteroids was associated with a significant increase in the prevalence of nuclear cataracts (adjusted relative prevalence 1.5; 95% CI 1.2, 1.9) and posterior subcapsular cataracts (1.9; 1.3, 2.8), but not cortical cataracts. The increased prevalence of posterior subcapsular cataracts was significantly associated with current use of inhaled corticosteroids (2.6; 1.7, 4.0); there was no association with past use. Current use of inhaled corticosteroids was also associated with an increased prevalence of cortical cataracts (1.4; 1.1, 1.7). The highest prevalences of posterior subcapsular and grade 4 or 5 nuclear cataracts were found in patients who had taken a cumulative dose of beclomethasone over 2000 mg.

An active contribution of deflazacort to the progression of posterior subcapsular cataracts in a child has been described (25[c]).

An 8-year-old girl developed extensive posterior subcapsular opacities and severe vision impairment after taking high doses of deflazacort for 30 months for type 1 mesangiocapillary glomerulonephritis. Initially, she was treated with methylprednisolone 40 mg on alternate days. After 4 months she developed muscle weakness, Cushing's syndrome, and a 10% increase in body weight. Routine eye examination showed mild opacities in her posterior capsule. Methylprednisolone was changed to deflazacort 0.8–1 mg (frequency of administration not stated). Her visual acuity worsened and the opacities of her posterior capsule grew. During the first 2 years of deflazacort therapy her growth curve paralleled the 97th percentile, but in the last year it fell to the 75th percentile. Deflazacort was withdrawn over a 3-month period. The outcome was not stated.

Musculoskeletal *Osteoporosis* and *related fractures* are among the most serious adverse effects of glucocorticosteroids, which are the most common cause of drug-related osteoporosis. Each year new data are published about the incidence of these reactions and prophylactic therapy.

Inhaled corticosteroids reduce spinal bone mineral density in women, but not in men. The size of this effect has been documented for the first time in patients aged 20–40 years with asthma who had never taken inhaled or systemic corticosteroids ($n = 34$) or who had used inhaled corticosteroids (beclomethasone or budesonide 100–3000 μg/day) for at least 5 years (mean duration, 7.8 years) with only limited exposure to systemic corticosteroids ($n = 47$) (26[C]). There were no overall differences in mean bone mineral density between those using and those not using inhaled corticosteroids. However, multivariate analysis showed a statistically significant reduction in bone mineral density in the lumbar spine in women with increasing dosages of inhaled corticosteroid, equivalent to a 0.11 SD reduction for every year's use of 1000 μg/day of inhaled corticosteroid. The analysis was adjusted for potential confounding factors, such as physical activity, body weight, smoking, alcohol consumption, oral contraceptive use, and parity. Women who used inhaled corticosteroids also had lower serum concentrations of osteocalcin than those who did not, but this effect was not dose-related. The authors pointed out that although such a small reduction in bone mineral density is unimportant in the short term, it may become very important during long-term treatment. For example, several studies have shown that the risk of vertebral fracture doubles for each SD reduction in bone mineral density.

In an analysis of 24 published prospective studies (1966–95), in which bone loss induced by corticosteroids in rheumatic arthritis was assessed, the authors concluded that bone loss is limited and influenced by interaction with the disease characteristics and the dosage of corticosteroid. In patients treated with steroids, bone mass change per year in the lumbar spine had a weighted mean of 0.0% (CI −0.6, 0.7), and in the femoral neck of −3.0% (CI −1.8, 4.4). In the patients who did not take steroids, bone mass change per year in lumbar spine had a weighted mean of −0.6% (CI −2.0, 0.2), and in the femoral neck of −0.7% (CI −1.0, −0.3) (27[R]).

Useful recommendations has been published for the prevention of corticosteroid-induced osteoporosis (28[R]).

Contradictory results have been published about the prophylactic use of two different bisphosphonates in patients treated with steroids. A group of 27 patients (21 women, mean age 70 years) with giant cell arteritis were randomized double-blind to intermittent cyclic clodronate (800 mg as a single dose in months 1, 3, 5, 7, 9, and 11) or placebo. A calcium supplement (500–750 mg/day) was given to all participants. Prednisolone was taken as a single morning dose (mean 40, range 16–60 mg) and adjusted during the trial to the lowest maintenance dosage. There were no bone losses after therapy, and no differences in bone density or biochemical bone markers between placebo and clodronate (29[C]).

Pamidronate disodium has been compared with calcium supplementation in an open trial of primary prevention of glucocorticoid-induced osteoporosis in 27 patients (22 women, mean age 60 years) with different rheumatic conditions, randomly assigned to pamidronate (90 mg intravenously every 3 months) plus calcium (800 mg calcium carbonate) or calcium only for 1 year (30[C]). The corticosteroids were given in a starting dosage of 10–80 mg/day. With pamidronate there was a significant increase in bone density (3.6% lumbar, 2.2% femoral neck), but there was a significant reduction with calcium (−5.3% in both spine and femoral neck).

Salmon calcitonin nasal spray prevented bone loss in the lumbar spine of 31 patients (18 woman, mean age 70 years) treated with prednisone for polymyalgia rheumatica (31[C]). They were randomized to salmon calcitonin nasal spray (200 IU/day) or matched placebo for 1 year. Both groups were treated with calcium supplements if their dietary intake was below 800 mg/day. With calcitonin the mean bone mineral density in the lumbar spine fell by 1.3% and with placebo by 5% after 1 year. There were no differences in the hip, including the femoral neck and trochanter, or in total body bone density.

Osteonecrosis Of 103 patients with systemic lupus erythematosus, 31 developed osteonecrosis and were compared with those who did not (32[C]). Osteonecrosis was associated with maximal prednisone doses (60 vs 37 mg/day), Cushingoid changes, the presence of anticardiolipin antibodies, clinical evidence of venous thrombosis, and vasculitis.

Avascular necrosis has been investigated in 285 patients who received renal transplants (33[C]). Four patients developed avascular necrosis; two had received additional pulses of intravenous methylprednisolone for the treatment of acute rejection. The prevalence of avascular necrosis was lower than has previously been described. Possible explanations were careful attention to and control of renal osteodystrophy before and after regular dialysis treatment and the use of low dosages of steroids after transplantation.

Necrotizing fasciitis occurred in a woman who received an intra-articular injection of methylprednisolone for a painful left shoulder (34[c]).

A 41-year-old woman was given an injection of methylprednisolone 40 mg with lidocaine; 2 days later, she experienced malaise, diarrhea, and vomiting, became sweaty and confused, and eventually collapsed. She was cyanosed and had a blood pressure of 90/40 mmHg. There was a fine petechial rash over her trunk, shoulders, and groin, and a well-demarcated purple area over her left arm, with skin peeling and edema. She had hyponatremia, hypoglycemia, metabolic acidosis, and raised urea and creatinine concentrations. Septic shock secondary to necrotizing fasciitis was diagnosed. At necropsy a group A streptococcus was identified.

Necrotizing fasciitis after steroid injection has been previously reported. Steroids inhibit leukocyte function, both locally and systemically, and may have been a predisposing factor in this patient. She had also recently started taking oral diclofenac, and NSAIDs have also been implicated in the pathogenesis of necrotizing fasciitis.

Immunological and hypersensitivity reactions
Anaphylactic reactions to corticosteroids are rare. In the majority of cases the reaction is so severe that rechallenge is not performed. In two recent cases rechallenge was performed to assess the causality of anaphylactic/anaphylactoid reactions to dexamethasone (35[c]) and methylprednisolone (36[c]).

A 48-year-old woman had an anaphylactic reaction after the intramuscular administration of Dalamon, a product containing dexamethasone 1.5 mg, lidocaine, co-carboxylase, pyridoxal 5-phosphate, cobamide, cyanocobalamin, and hydroxocobalamin. Skin tests (prick and intradermal) were negative with all the compounds. Controlled challenge tests were negative with all except dexamethasone. Subcutaneous administration of dexamethasone 0.4 mg caused an anaphylactic reaction. Skin tests were negative to 6-methylprednisolone, prednisolone, hydrocortisone, and betamethasone. She tolerated a challenge with 6-methylprednisolone (40 mg subcutaneously), but had another anaphylactic reaction after hydrocortisone (20 mg subcutaneously).

A 44-year-old woman was given high doses of intravenous methylprednisolone for progressive multiple sclerosis. A day after the first dose of 1000 mg she developed urticaria. The second dose was given under close supervision, and there was reactivation of a skin rash and difficulties in swallowing and breathing. Skin tests and IgE measurements were inconclusive, but large concentrations of methylprednisolone resulted in basophilic histamine release in vitro, suggesting an anaphylactoid reaction.

Acute laryngeal obstruction has been described for the first time after the intravenous administration of hydrocortisone (37[c]).

A 73-year-old man underwent direct laryngoscopy to rule out recurrence of carcinoma of the larynx. Because of mild stridor after the bronchoscopy he was given hydrocortisone hemisuccinate 100 mg intravenously. Within 15–20 s he become totally obstructed, and his oxygen saturation fell to 50%. An intradermal test was negative, suggesting an anaphylactoid reaction.

Anaphylaxis occurred in a 31-year-old woman after an intra-articular injection of methylprednisolone. She had received an intra-articular injection of methylprednisolone on a previous occasion without complications. The author concluded that the anaphylaxis had been caused by methylprednisolone, based on the finding of no allergic skin reactions to any of the individual components of the commercially available product (38[c]).

Infections and infestations Fatal cases of *Strongyloides stercolaris superinfection* have been well documented in asymptomatic carriers of the parasite taking corticosteroids for various conditions. Suppression of cell-mediated immunity by corticosteroids is believed to play a role in the development of hyperinfection. In addition, corticosteroids and their metabolites may have a direct stimulatory effect on intraintestinal larvae, promoting autoinfection. Fatal strongyloidiasis has been described after corticosteroid therapy for ulcerative colitis (39[c]).

A 60-year-old man presented with a 2-week history of progressive bloody diarrhea, abdominal distension, and pain. No infection was discovered, and he was given intravenous hydrocortisone 100 mg qds and parenteral nutrition for toxic megacolon due to ulcerative colitis, followed by maintenance therapy with prednisolone 20 mg/day and mesalazine. Two weeks later he developed a recurrence of bloody diarrhea and abdominal pain. Blood cultures grew *Escherichia coli* and *Klebsiella aerogenes* and at necropsy there was heavy infestation with *Strongyloides stercoralis* in his stomach and intestine.

Aspergillosis is an uncommon fungal infection that can occur in immunodeficient patients. Two reviews have addressed the role of corticosteroids in this opportunistic infection. Of 2496 recipients of bone marrow transplants, 214 had *Aspergillus* identified. Of these, 158 had invasive aspergillosis, 44 were colonized, and 12 had contaminated cultures. In a comparison of cases of infection with matched controls, the use of corticosteroids resulted in an increased risk in those who presented with the infection more than 40 days after transplantation (RR = 3.1; 90% CI 1.7, 5.0) (40[R]).

Of 473 HIV-infected children, seven (1.5%) developed invasive aspergillosis during the study period (1987–95) (41[R]). Sustained neutropenia or corticosteroid therapy as predisposing factors for invasive aspergillosis were found in only two patients.

Invasive pulmonary aspergillosis with cerebromeningeal involvement has been described after short-term intravenous administration of methylprednisolone (42[c]).

A 74-year-old woman, who had been taking inhaled salbutamol and beclomethasone and oral theophylline for several years, was given intravenous methylprednisolone 120 mg/day and amoxicillin during an acute attack. Her respiratory symptoms improved and the dosage of methylprednisolone was reduced to 80 mg/day after 8 days, then to 40 mg/day after 14 days, when X-rays showed diffuse, nodular, densities throughout her lung fields, and *Aspergillus fumigatus* and *Acinetobacter baumanii* were found in her lungs. At necropsy her lungs contained abscesses with numerous *Aspergillus* hyphae and in the brain there was subcortical blood vessel and meningeal invasion by *Aspergillus*.

The authors commented that there have been very few reports of invasive pulmonary aspergillosis in asthmatic patients. Corticosteroid therapy, even short-term parenteral administration, was probably a risk factor in this patient. It seems doubtful that her prehospital treatment with inhaled corticosteroids could have been responsible, since she had no fungal hyphae in her sputum at the time of admission.

Four cases of fulminant *Pneumocystis carinii* pneumonia in patients with dermatomyositis have been described. The most relevant feature was that in three cases the pneumonia occurred in the first month of treatment with prednisone in the usual doses (1–1.5 mg/kg per day), and the other occurred 58 days after starting steroid therapy (43[c]).

Oropharyngeal candidiasis is a well-described adverse effect of inhaled corticosteroids. However, few cases of *esophageal candidiasis* have been reported (44[c]).

A 70-year-old woman developed esophageal candidiasis after long-term use of inhaled triamcinolone 400 mg qds for asthma. She had a history of gastritis and peptic ulceration and when she noted worsening upper abdominal dyspeptic pain and heartburn, an endoscopy was performed; it showed esophageal candidiasis. Triamcinolone was withdrawn and replaced with nedocromil sodium. There was suppression of the delayed-type hypersensitivity reaction in vivo, although there was no evidence of underlying cellular immunodeficiency and her lymphocytes were highly reactive in vitro to *Candida*.

Primary *esophageal histoplasmosis* must be considered in patients who have a history of gastro-esophageal reflux disease and are immunosuppressed by long-term corticosteroids (45[c]).

A 61-year-old man, who had been taking an unidentified corticosteroid for 10 years for rheumatoid arthritis, developed dysphagia for solids. Endoscopy showed areas of diffuse ulceration with nodules in the distal esophagus. *Histoplasma capsulatum* was identified.

Although infection with *varicella* organisms is a common problem in immunosuppressed patients, it remains a relatively unusual complication in inflammatory bowel disease. Four patients developed severe *varicella zoster* virus infections while they were taking immunosuppressive therapy for inflammatory bowel disease (46[c]).

Three men (aged 71–77 years) with temporal arteritis were infected with opportunistic pathogens during treatment with prednisone (47[c]). The organisms involved were *Clostridium difficile*, *Pseudomonas aeruginosa*, and enterococci in the first case, *Pneumocystis carinii* in the second, and *Listeria monocytogenes* in the third. These patients were at risk of opportunistic infections for at least three reasons: it is likely that the most important risk factor was the use of corticosteroids; all were over 65 years; and the presence of temporal arteritis may have contributed to dysregulation of their immune systems with increased susceptibility to infection.

Tumor-inducing effects Immunosuppression induced by prednisone is a risk factor for the development of *Kaposi's sarcoma*, probably in genetically susceptible people. A 63-year-old woman developed disseminated Kaposi's sarcoma following long-term treatment with prednisone for bronchial asthma (48[c]).

A 63-year-old woman developed painful disseminated skin lesions on her limbs. She had taken prednisone 15–60 mg/day for 35 years and had developed corticosteroid-related diabetes mellitus 9 years before. There were multiple, hard, painful nodules and infiltrates, red-violet to brown in colour on her limbs, merging into larger and irregular plaques, and she had lymphedema of her hands and legs. Later, similar lesions appeared on her tongue and upper eyelids. Histological examination was consistent with Kaposi's sarcoma.

Miscellaneous Dexamethasone (40 mg qds orally) caused *hiccups* at a frequency of 4–8 times/min in a 47-year-old white man with multiple myeloma (49[c]). Withdrawal of dexamethasone led to prompt resolution, and rechallenge twice caused the reappearance of hiccups within 12 h. However intravenous dexamethasone did not cause hiccups. The authors suggested that local gastrointestinal effects had led to reflex arc stimulation.

Risk factors Prolonged use of corticosteroids in *elderly people* can exacerbate diabetes, hypertension, congestive heart failure, and osteoporosis or cause depression. In a recent retrospective controlled study the risks of high-dose intravenous or oral corticosteroid therapy were assessed in 55 patients with Crohn's disease who were over the age of 50 years (50[C]). They had a higher risk of developing hypertension, hypokalemia, and changes in mental state.

Interactions Dexamethasone reduced the clearance of *albendazole* and increased the elimination half-life; plasma concentrations almost doubled (51[C]).

Pneumocystis carinii pneumonia 1 month after he began high-dose cyclosporin has been reported in a man who was also taking prednisone and was attributed to additive immunosuppression (52[c]).

A 63-year-old man took oral cyclosporin 200 mg bd for ulcerative colitis plus prednisolone, mesalazine, and hydrocortisone enemas. His trough blood cyclosporin concentration rose to 410 μg/l, and his cyclosporin dosage was reduced to 100 mg bd. Six days later he developed dyspnea, fever (39°C), and right-sided lung consolidation. Despite treatment with intravenous ampicillin and erythromycin and discontinuation of cyclosporin, he developed respiratory failure and died of *P. carinii* pneumonia.

The authors suggest that *P. carinii* prophylaxis should always be considered when high-dose cyclosporin is combined with corticosteroids.

SPECIAL ROUTES OF ADMINISTRATION OF CORTICOSTEROIDS *(SED-13, 1204; SEDA-19, 379; SEDA-20, 378; SEDA-21, 419)*

Epidural Symptoms consistent with *complex regional pain syndrome* have been reported after a cervical epidural steroid injection (53[c]).

A 49-year-old woman was given a cervical epidural injection of methylprednisolone 80 mg for cervical radiculopathy and 2 days later reported spontaneous lancinating pain in the distal portion of the right first finger, radiating to the elbow. Carbamazepine had no effect, but she obtained relief from stellate ganglion block with lidocaine.

Epidural steroid therapy is a commonly used 'conservative' therapy, but it is not inherently benign. Although arachnoiditis, infection, and meningitis have been reported, *acute paraplegia* has not been reported as a complication of either caudal or spinal epidural steroid injection. A unique case of transient profound paralysis after epidural steroid injection has now been reported (54[c]). The procedure was carried out without fluoroscopic control and was complicated by puncture of the thecal sac. Radiography showed a focal space-occupying lesion in the spinal canal at the level corresponding to the neurological deficit, which spontaneously resolved over the next 2–3 h, with recovery of motor, sensory, and bowel and bladder function over the next 48 h, consistent with an acute compressive injury and inconsistent with an anesthetic effect. Radiographic studies suggested three possible explanations: (a) inadvertent thecal penetration during injection may have produced atypical anesthetic block; (b) loculation of the injected fluid may have caused a transient compressive lesion; (c) intrathecal injection may have produced an iatrogenic arachnoid cyst. Although pathological confirmation of the cause was not possible, the potential for this alarming complication should be recognized by physicians who prescribe epidural steroid therapy.

Intrathecal Two women developed *cerebral venous thrombosis* after intrathecal injections of dexamethasone or hydrocortisone to treat sciatica (55[c]).

A 34-year-old woman, who was taking a combined oral contraceptive, was given an intrathecal injection of dexamethasone 15 mg. The next day she had an occipital headache, and on the fourth day developed partial seizures, followed by generalized status epilepticus, leading to coma. Cerebral arteriography showed extensive thrombosis of the superior sagittal sinus and the right and left transverse sinuses.

A 47-year-old woman had postural frontal and occipital headache for 3 weeks after an intrathecal injection of hydrocortisone 125 mg. She was taking a low-dose combined oral contraceptive. MRI angiography failed to show the right transverse sinus and thrombosis was diagnosed.

Oral contraceptives can cause sinus thrombosis and may have been implicated in these cases; however, there was a strong temporal association with corticosteroid administration.

Peridural *Diplopia* associated with the peridural or intrathecal infiltration of prednisolone have not been previously reported (56[c]).

Two women developed diplopia after being given prednisolone 50 mg by peridural or intrathecal infiltration for mechanical sciatica. The first, aged 44 years, had headaches and diplopia, associated with paralysis of the sixth left cranial nerve, 2 days after receiving peridural prednisolone. The second developed post-lumbar puncture syndrome 2 days after receiving intrathecal prednisolone; 5 days later she developed diplopia associated with paralysis of the sixth right cranial nerve. In both cases the symptoms resolved over the next 6 months.

PROSTAGLANDINS *(SED-13, 1316; SEDA-18, 422; SEDA-21, 420)*

Alprostadil (Prostaglandin E_1)

Gastrointestinal The radiographs of nine neonates with congenital heart disease who had received prostaglandins during the first week of life have been reviewed for comparison with 18 matched controls (nine healthy neonates and nine infants with non-cyanotic congenital heart disease) who had not received prostaglandins (57[C]). Within 48 h of initial prostaglandin therapy, there was persistent *gastric distension* in four infants, all of whom had received high-dose prostaglandin therapy (0.1 μg/kg per min). No infants developed feeding intolerance during the first week of life, but two (both with initial asymptomatic gastric distension) developed feeding intolerance with prolonged prostaglandin therapy. In all cases, gastric distension resolved on withdrawal of prostaglandins. The radiographs of the control infants were unremarkable.

Prostaglandin-induced *foveolar hyperplasia of the gastric mucosa* is a new entity, to which radiologists have recently paid special attention. Most patients described in previous reports have had only mild abdominal symptoms. A boy born at 37 weeks had 2600 g of acute gastric outlet obstruction, which developed after the cumulative infusion of prostaglandin E_1 2914 μg/kg for hypoplastic left heart syndrome (58[c]). Histology showed gastric foveolar hyperplasia with impacted interfoveolar mucin products and dilated mucosal glands.

Skin and appendages A case of *toxic pustuloderma* has been described after the administration of a single intracavernous dose of PGE_1 (59[c]).

A 63-year-old man with Peyronie's disease received an intracavernous injection of PGE_1 to define penile morphology before surgery. Six days later he developed generalized pruritic erythema involving 80% of the skin. Within 48 h multiple pustules appeared on the background erythema and he became febrile. Laboratory finding included leukocytosis with eosinophilia, hypoalbuminemia, and hypocalcemia. Skin biopsy showed urticaria with superficial pustulosis. Complete resolution was obtained within a week with antihistamines and topical corticosteroids.

Dinoprost (prostaglandin $F_2\alpha$)

Extra-amniotic saline (121 women) has been compared with intra-amniotic prostaglandin $F_2\alpha$ (123 women) in inducing labor in pregnancies with intrauterine fetal death in a randomized controlled trial (60[C]). The methods were equally effective in achieving delivery but there were more complications with intra-amniotic prostaglandin: five women developed hypertonic contractions compared with none given extra-amniotic saline. In addition 23% of the women given intra-amniotic prostaglandin developed acute distressing vasovagal-like symptoms (*chest pain/discomfort* 7%, *nausea or vomiting* 11%, *diarrhea* 7%, *feeling hot* 13%, *sweating* 12%, or *hypotension* 11%) lasting for 10–15 min.

Dinoprostone (prostaglandin E_2)

Dinoprostone causes uterine contractions at any stage of pregnancy and is used principally for induction of labor and termination of pregnancy. *Hypotension* followed by ventricular fibrillation occurred in a woman after she had been given intramyometrial dinoprostone during a cesarean section (61[c]).

After cesarean section a 21-year-old woman received dinoprostone 1 mg because of poor uterine contraction; 30 s later her heart rate increased from 85 to 140 beats/min and her blood pressure fell from 120/60 to 60/25 mmHg. Her end-tidal CO_2 fell from 35 to 20 mmHg and her SaO_2 could not be measured. Shortly afterwards, she developed ventricular fibrillation. Resuscitation restored sinus rhythm, and severe bronchospasm responded to aminophylline and methylprednisolone.

The authors attributed hypotension in this case to the vasodilatory effect of dinoprostone, but anaphylaxis cannot be ruled out.

Iloprost

The prostacyclin analog iloprost, a potent inhibitor of platelet function and a vasodilator, has been used for the treatment of peripheral arterial occlusive disease. Iloprost can be beneficial in patients with pulmonary hypertension and Raynaud's phenomenon. Its use has been proposed in patients with systemic sclerosis, a disease that is often characterized by pulmonary hypertension and Raynaud's phenomenon. Eight patients with severe Raynaud's phenomenon secondary to systemic sclerosis received a 7-h infusion (1 ng/kg per min) of iloprost for 5 consecutive days and then for 1 day 3 months later (62[C]). There were beneficial effects on the peripheral microcirculation after 5 days of infusion, but they lasted for less than 4 weeks. The reported adverse effects were *headache*, *flushing*, and *nausea*; in one case the authors had to reduce the infusion rate to 0.5 ng/kg per min and gave metoclopramide because of severe nausea and vomiting. In another case there were typical symptoms of *angina pectoris* during infusion, with ST segment depression although coronary arteriography show no evidence of coronary artery disease.

Latanoprost

Latanoprost is an ester analogue of prostaglandin $F_{2\alpha}$. It reduces intraocular pressure and is marketed in some countries for the topical treatment of primary open-angle glaucoma or ocular hypertension.

Skin and appendages New adverse reactions have been described after the topical use of latanoprost: *hypertrichosis* and *increased pigmentation of the eyelashes*. These adverse effects occurred in a 65-year-old woman, firstly when the drug was administered to her left eye and later to her right eye. The color of the eyelashes changed from grey to dark and a higher density was reported (63[c]).

All of 43 patients using unilateral topical latanoprost developed *hypertrichosis* and *pigmentation of eyelashes*. The mean duration of treatment was 20 weeks (range 11–40). Differences between the latanoprost-treated eye and the untreated eye included an increased number, length, thickness, curvature, and pigmentation of eyelashes (64[c]).

Special senses Latanoprost can cause ocular inflammatory effects. The incidence of *cystoid macular edema* and *anterior uveitis* has been studied in 94 patients (163 eyes) treated with topical latanoprost. Six patients (eight of the 163 eyes) had anterior uveitis, and two of 94 patients (two of 163 eyes) had cystoid macular edema while using latanoprost (65[C]).

Similar reactions has been described in three patients within 1–4 weeks after starting topical latanoprost (66[c]). Latanoprost should be avoided in patients with history of, or currently active, iritis.

As commented in the last Annual (SEDA-21, 422), latanoprost can causes *changes in iris pigmentation*. In a new study of 779 patients from three countries, iris pigmentation was observed in 12, 23, and 11% of patients in the US, UK, and Scandinavia, respectively. The highest incidence was in green-brown, yellow-brown, and blue/grey-brown eyes. Eyes with uniformly blue, grey, green, or brown colours were seldom affected. If both eyes were treated, they became pigmented to the same degree. If only one eye was treated, the other eye was always unaffected. The change, a concentric increase in iris pigmentation, appeared after 6 months (range, 3–17) and was noticed by the patient in about two-thirds of cases. After withdrawal of latanoprost for 2 years, the pigmentation did not resolve (67[C]).

A similar effect occurs in monkeys after the administration of different prostaglandins. Over 18–44 weeks one eye of each primate was treated daily with a drop (30 μl) of $PGF_{2\alpha}$-isopropyl ester, PGE_2-isopropyl ester, or latanoprost (68[C]). The other eye served as a control. All the prostaglandins caused increased melanogenesis in the melanocytes in the iris. The first sign of this effect was seen after about 2 months.

Misoprostol

Complete abortions were obtained in 265 of 287 patients when misoprostol (800 μg intravaginally) was administered 3, 4, or 5 days after intramuscular methotrexate 50 mg/m^2. The adverse effects of misoprostol were: *nausea* 19%, *vomiting* 22%, *diarrhea* 63%, *dizziness* 15%, *migraine* 15%, *fever* (subjective) 25%, *chills* 56%, *rashes* 0.7%, and *pelvic pain* 96%; the symptoms, except pain, were mild and of short duration, disappearing in 1–2 h (69[C]). In another prospective multicenter study complete abortion occurred in 273 of 299 women who received methotrexate (50 mg orally) followed 5–6 days later by misoprostol (800 μg intravaginally). The adverse effects of methotrexate and misoprostol were: *nausea* (37 and 33%), *vomiting* (11 and 18%), *diarrhea* (12 and 18%), and subjective *fever or chills* (15 and 31%) (70[c]).

Hematological Aggravation of gastrointestinal bleeding due to *impaired platelet function* occurred in a man who had been given misoprostol 200 μg qds (71[c]).

A 70-year-old man took misoprostol 200 μg qds for chronic bleeding from multiple gastrointestinal telangiectases. He had a prolonged bleeding time (15 min) and severely impaired platelet aggregation on testing with adrenaline, collagen, ristocetin, and adenosine diphosphate. Misoprostol was withdrawn. One week later his bleeding time and platelet aggregation normalized. His bone marrow showed mild myelodysplasia.

Gastrointestinal *Diarrhea* is a common adverse effect of misoprostol. To study its effects on chronic refractory constipation, misoprostol was given in dosages of 800–2400 μg/day to 18 patients as adjuvant therapy for 4 weeks (72[C]). Misoprostol augmented colonic motility and reduced constipation. However, six patients withdrew owing to adverse effects, which included *headache* and *abdominal cramps* and *bloating*. Adverse effects especially at high doses can limit the use of misoprostol in constipation.

Sexual function *Uterine rupture* has been described after the use of misoprostol for induction of labor (73[c]).

A healthy 34-year-old woman, admitted for labor induction at 39 weeks, was given misoprostol 25 μg into the posterior vaginal fornix every 3 h. The first dose produced mild and irregular contractions. Three hours after the second dose, misoprostol was withheld because of intermittent tachycardia. Five hours after the second dose, the fetus developed bradycardia, and uterine hyperstimulation was refractory to terbutaline. There was blood in the vagina, a floating fetal head, and cervical dilatation of 2 cm. At cesarean section there was a 15 cm linear rupture of the left posterior uterine wall.

Miscellaneous *Severe hyperthermia* occurred after the administration of misoprostol for prophylaxis against postpartum hemorrhage (74[c]).

A 20-year-old woman received oral misoprostol 800 μg postpartum, and 13 min later developed chills and rigors and became restless and disorientated. Her core temperature increased to 41.9°C. Her serum creatine phosphokinase activity peaked at 4715 IU/l (reference range, 60–375) on the first day postpartum and then normalized.

Unoprostone

Unoprostone is related to prostaglandin $F_{2\alpha}$ and has similar therapeutic properties to latanoprost. *Change in iris color* has been described after the administration of unoprostone to a 64-year-old Japanese man with normal-tension glaucoma (75[c]). His right eye was treated with unoprostone drops (0.12%) and a year later the iris of the treated eye had darkened. There were no changes in the other eye.

PROSTACYCLIN ANALOGS

Epoprostenol

Pulmonary hypertension is a life-threatening disease that can require treatment with prostacyclin. One of the difficult problems in sustaining a patient receiving prostacyclin before lung transplantation is the high occurrence of adverse effects, especially *nausea* and *vomiting*. Nausea and vomiting can be very severe (76[c]) and can limit the physician's ability to maximize prostacyclin therapy, minimize right-sided heart failure, and maintain an adequate nutritional status.

A 38-year-old woman treated with prostacyclin developed severe nausea and vomiting after prostacyclin treatment. Promethazine, prochlorperazine, and metoclopramide were ineffective, but her symptoms responded to ondansetron 8 mg tds.

REFERENCES

1. Vigevano F, Cilio MR. Vigabatrin versus ACTH as first-line treatment for infantile spasms: a randomized prospective study. Epilepsia 1997;38:1270–4.
2. Chiron C, Dumas C, Jambaqué I, Mumford J, Dulac O. Randomized trial comparing vigabatrin and hydrocortisone in infantile spasm due to tuberous sclerosis. Epilepsy Res 1997;26:389–95.
3. Maeda H, Furune S, Normura K, Kitou O, Ando Y, Negoro T, Watanabe K. Decrease of *N*-acetylaspartate after ACTH therapy in patients with infantile spasms. Neuropediatrics 1997; 28:262–7.
4. Zamir E. Central serous retinopathy associated with adrenocorticotrophic hormone therapy. A case report and a hypothesis. Graefes Arch Clin Exp Ophthalmol 1997;235:339–44.
5. Miranda-Mallea J, Pérez-Verdú J, Gascó-Lacalle B, Sáez-Palacios JM, Fernández-Gilino C, Izquierdo-Macián I. Hypertrophic cardiomyopathy in preterm infants treated with dexamethasone. Eur J Pediatr 1997;156:394–6.
6. Patrassi GM, Sartori MT, Livi U, Casonato A, Danesin C, Vettore S, Girolami A. Impairment of fibrinolytic potential in long-term steroid treatment after heart transplantation. Transplantation 1997;64:1610–14.
7. Brumund MR, Truemper EJ, Lutin WA, Pearson-Shaver AL. Disseminated *Varicella* and staphylococcal pericarditis after topical steroids. J Pediatr 1997;131:162–3.
8. Marinelli KA, Burke GS, Herson VC. Effects of dexamethasone on blood pressure in premature infants with bronchopulmonary dysplasia. J Pediatr 1997;130:594–602.
9. Skjoeth J, Bjerre SJ. Effects of glucocorticoids on ICP in patients with a cerebral tumour. Acta Neurol Scand 1997;96:167–70.
10. Daragon A, Vittecopq O, Le Loêt X. Visual hallucinations induced by intraarticular injection of steroids. J Rheumatol 1997;24:411.
11. Terao T, Yoshimura R, Shiratuchi T, Abe K. Effects of lithium on steroid-induced depression. Biol Psychiatry 1997;41:1225–6.
12. Finkenbine R, Gill HS. Case of mania due to prednisone–clarithromycin interaction. Can J Psychiatry 1997;42:778.
13. Kobayashi S, Warabi H, Hashimoto H. Hypopituitarism with empty sella after steroid pulse therapy. J Rheumatol 1997;24:236–8.
14. Wilson AM, Clark DJ, McFarlane L, Lipworth BJ. Adrenal suppression with high doses of inhaled fluticasone propionate and triamcinolone acetonide in healthy volunteers. Eur J Clin Pharmacol 1997;53:33–7.
15. Yiallouros PK, Milner AD, Conway E, Honour JW. Adrenal function and high dose inhaled corticosteroids for asthma. Arch Dis Child 1997;76:405–10.
16. Fisher JE, Smith RS, Lagrandeur R, Lorenz RP. Gestational diabetes mellitus in women receiving beta-adrenergics and corticosteroids for threatened preterm delivery. Obstet Gynecol 1997;90:880–3.
17. Bedalov A, Balasubramanyam A. Glucocorticoid-induced ketoacidosis in gestational diabetes: sequela of the acute treatment of preterm labor. A case report. Diabetes Care 1997;20:922–4 (erratum 1343).
18. Kim YS, Kim MS, Kim SI, Lim SK, Lee HY, Han DS, Park K. Post-transplantation diabetes is better controlled after conversion from prednisone to deflazacort: a prospective trial in renal transplants. Transplant Int 1997;10:197–201.
19. Hoff DS, Mammel MC. Suspected betamethasone-induced leukemoid reaction in a premature infant. Pharmacotherapy 1997;17:1031–4.
20. Sharma R, Gupta KL, Ammon RH, Gambert SR. Atypical presentation of colon perforation related to corticosteroid use. Geriatrics 1997; 52:88–90.
21. Garbe E, LeLorier J, Boivin J-F, Suissa S. Risk of ocular hypertension or open-angle glaucoma in elderly patients on oral glucocorticoids. Lancet 1997;350:979–82.
22. Garbe E, LeLorier J, Boivin J-F, Suissa S. Inhaled and nasal glucocorticoids and the risks of ocular hypertension or open-angle glaucoma. J Am Med Assoc 1997;277:722–7.
23. Kwok AKH, Lam DSC, Ng JSK, Fan DSP, Chew S-J, Tso MOM. Ocular hypertensive response to topical steroids in children. Ophthalmology 1997;104:2112–16.
24. Cumming RG, Mitchell P, Leeder SR. Use of inhaled corticosteroids and the risk of cataracts. New Engl J Med 1997;337:8–14.
25. Krmar RT, Ramirez JA, Torres CG, Ferraris JR. Posterior subcapsular cataracts associated with deflazacort therapy. Clin Nephrol 1997; 47:205.
26. Wisniewski AF, Lewis SA, Green DJ, Maslanka W, Burrell H, Tattersfield AE. Cross sectional investigation of the effects of inhaled corticosteroids on bone density and bone metabolism in patients with asthma. Thorax 1997;52:853–60.
27. Verhoeven AC, Boers M. Limited bone loss due to corticosteroids; a systematic review of prospective studies in rheumatic arthritis and other diseases. J Rheumatol 1997;24:1495–503.
28. Bijlsma JWJ. Prevention of glucocorticoid induced osteoporosis. Ann Rheum Dis 1997; 56:507–9.

29. Nordborg E, Schaufelberger C, Andersson R, Bosaeus I, Bengtsson BA. The ineffectiveness of cyclical oral clodronate on bone mineral density in glucocorticoid-treated patients with giant-cell arteritis. J Intern Med 1997;242:367–71.
30. Boutsen Y, Jamart J, Essenlincks W, Stoffel M, Devogelaer JP. Primary prevention of glucocorticosteroid-induced osteoporosis with intermittent intravenous pamidronate: a randomized trial. Calcif Tissue Int 1997;61:266–71.
31. Adachi JD, Bensen WG, Bell MJ, Bianchi FA, Cividino AA, Craig GL, Sturtridge WC, Sebaldt RJ, Steele M, Gordon M, Themeles E, Tugwell P, Roberts R, Gent M. Salmon calcitonin nasal spray in the prevention of corticosteroid-induced osteoporosis. Br J Rheumatol 1997; 36:255–9.
32. Mont MA, Glueck CJ, Pacheco IH, Wang P, Hungerford DS, Petri M. Risk factors for osteonecrosis in systemic lupus erythematosus patients. J Rheumatol 1997;24:654–62.
33. Jagose JT, Bailey RR. Avascular necrosis of bone after renal transplantation. Nephrology 1997;3:207–10.
34. Birkinshaw R, O'Donnell J, Sammy I. Necrotising fasciitis as a complication of steroid injection. J Accident Emerg Med 1997;14:52–4.
35. Figueredo E, Cuesta-Herranz J, De Las Heras M, Lluch-Bernal M, Umpierrez A, Sastre J. Anaphylaxis to dexamethasone. Allergy 1997;52:877.
36. Van Den Berg JSP, Van Heikema OR, Wuis EW, Stapel S, Van Der Valk PGM. Anaphylactoid reaction to intravenous methylprednisolone in a patient with multiple sclerosis. J Neurol Neurosurg Psychiatry 1997;62:813–14.
37. Srinivasan V, Lanham PRW. Acute laryngeal obstruction-reaction to intravenous hydrocortisone? Eur J Anaesthesiol 1997;14:342.
38. Mace S, Vadas P, Pruzanski W. Anaphylactic shock induced by intraarticular injection of methylprednisolone acetate. J Rheumatol 1997; 24:1191–4.
39. Leung VKS, Liew CT, Sung JJY. Fatal strongyloidiasis in a patient with ulcerative colitis after corticosteroid therapy. Am J Gastroenterol 1997; 92:1383–4.
40. Wald A, Leisenring W, Van Burik, Bowden RA. Epidemiology of *Aspergillus* infections in a large cohort of patients undergoing bone marrow transplantation. J Infect Dis 1997;175:1459–66.
41. Shetty D, Giri N, Gonzalez CE, Pizzo PA, Walsh TJ. Invasive aspergillosis in human immunodeficiency virus-infected children. Pedriatr Infect Dis J 1997;16:216–21.
42. Monlun E, De Blay F, Berton C, Gasser B, Jaeger A, Pauli G. Invasive pulmonary aspergillosis with cerebromeningeal involvement after short-term intravenous corticosteroid therapy in a patient with asthma. Respir Med 1997;91:435–7.
43. Bachelez H, Schremer B, Cadranel J, Mouly F, Sarfatt C, Aghaliba F, Schlemmer B, Mayaud CM, Dubertret L. Fulminant *Pneumocystis carinii* pneumonia in 4 patients with dermatomyositis. Arch Intern Med 1997;157:1501–3.
44. Simon MR, Houser WL, Smith KA, Long PM. Esophageal candidiasis as a complication of inhaled corticosteroids. Ann Allergy Asthma Immunol 1997;79:333–8.
45. Fucci JC, Nightengale ML. Primary esophageal histoplasmosis. Am J Gastroenterol 1997;92:530–1.
46. Mouzas IA, Greenstein AJ, Giannadaki E, Balasubramanian S, Manousos ON, Sachar DB. Management of *Varicella* infection during the course of inflammatory bowel disease. Am J Gastroenterol 1997;92:1534–7.
47. Hedderwick SA, Bonilla HF, Bradley SF, Kauffman CA. Opportunistic infections in patients with temporal arteritis treated with corticosteroids. J Am Geriatr Soc 1997;45:334–7.
48. Starzycki Z, Bogdaszewska Czabanowska J, Zeman J, Szmigie Michalak K. Disseminated Kaposi's sarcoma after long-term prednisone therapy. Eur J Dermatol 1997;7:307–10.
49. Lossos IS. Comment: drug-induced hiccups. Ann Pharmacother 1997;31:1264–5.
50. Akerkar GA, Peppercorn M, Hamel MB, Parker RA. Corticosteroid associated complications in elderly Crohn's disease patients. Am J Gastroenterol 1997;92:461–4.
51. Takayanagui OM, Lanchote VL, Marques MPC, Sueli P. Therapy of neurocysticercosis: pharmacokinetic interaction of albendazole sulfoxide with dexamethasone. Ther Drug Monit 1997;19:51–5.
52. Quan VA, Saunders BP, Hicks BH, Sladen GE. Cyclosporin treatment for ulcerative colitis complicated by fatal *Pneumocystis carinii* pneumonia. Br Med J 1997;314:363–4.
53. Siegfried RN. Development of complex regional pain syndrome after a cervical epidural steroid injection. Anesthesiology 1997;86:1394–6.
54. McLain RF, Fry M, Hecht ST. Transient paralysis associated with epidural steroid injection. J Spinal Disord 1997;10:441–4.
55. Ergan M, Hansen Von Bunau F, Courtheoux P, Viader F, Prouzeau S, Marcelli C. Cerebral vein thrombosis after an intrathecal glucocorticoid injection. Rev Rhum (Engl Ed) 1997;64:513–16.
56. Brocq O, Breuil V, Grisot C, Flory P, Ziegler G, Euller Ziegler L. Diplopia after peridural and intradural prednisolone infiltrations. Presse Med 1997;26:271.
57. Kriss VM, Desai NS. Relation of gastric distention to prostaglandin therapy in neonates. Radiology 1997;203:219–21.
58. Kobayashi N, Aida N, Nishimura G, Kashimura T, Ohta M, Kawataki M. Acute gastric outlet obstruction following the administration of prostaglandin: an additional case. Pediatr Radiol 1997;27:57–9.
59. Gallego I, Badell A, Notario J, Gallardo F, Servitje O, Peyri J. Toxic pustuloderma induced by intracavernous prostaglandin E1. Br J Dermatol 1997;136:975–6.
60. Mahomed K, Jayaguru AS. Extra-amniotic saline infusion for induction of labour in antepartum fetal death: a cost effective method worthy of

wider use. Br J Obstet Gynaecol 1997;104:1058–61.
61. Marcus MAE, Vertommen JD, Van Aken H, Swinnen G. Prostaglandin-induced ventricular fibrillation during cesarean section. Int J Obstet Anesth 1997;6:130–1.
62. Ceru S, Pancera P, Sansone S, Sfondrini G, Codella O, De Sandre G, Lechi A, Lunardi C. Effects of five-day versus one-day infusion of iloprost on the peripheral microcirculation in patients with systemic sclerosis. Clin Exp Rheumatol 1997;15:381–5.
63. Wand M. Latanoprost and hyperpigmentation of eyelashes. Arch Ophthalmol 1997;115:1206–8.
64. Johnstone MA. Hypertrichosis and increased pigmentation of eyelashes and adjacent hair in the region of the ipsilateral eyelids of patients treated with unilateral topical latanoprost. Am J Ophthalmol 1997;124:544–7.
65. Warwar RE, Bullock JD, Ballal D. Cystoid macular edema and anterior uveitis associated with latanoprost use. Ophthalmology 1997; 105:263–8.
66. Rowe JA, Hattenhauer MG, Herman DC. Adverse side effects associated with latanoprost. Am J Ophthalmol 1997;124:683–5.
67. Wistrand PJ, Stjernschantz J, Olsson K. The incidence and time-course of latanoprost-induced iridial pigmentation as a function of eye color. Surv Ophthalmol 1997;41 (Suppl 2):S129–38.
68. Selén G, Stjernschantz J, Resul B. Prostaglandin-induced iridial pigmentation in primates. Surv Ophthalmol 1997;41 (Suppl 2):S125–8.
69. Carbonell JL, Esteve I, Velazco A, Varela L, Cabezas E, Fernández C, Sánchez C. Misoprostol 3, 4, or 5 days after methotrexate for early abortion: a randomized trial. Contraception 1997; 56:169–74.
70. Creinin MD, Vittinghoff E, Schaff E, Klaisle C, Darney PD, Dean C. Medical abortion with oral methotrexate and vaginal misoprostol. Obstet Gynecol 1997;90:611–16.
71. Beales ILP, Clemons M, Kong WM. Misoprostol-associated platelet aggregation dysfunction and increased gastrointestinal blood loss. Eur J Gastroenterol Hepatol 1997;9:91–2.
72. Roarty TP, Weber F, Soykan I, McCallum RW. Misoprostol in the treatment of chronic refractory constipation: results of a long-term open label trial. Aliment Pharmacol Ther 1997; 11:1059–66.
73. Bennett BB. Uterine rupture during induction of labor at term with intravaginal misoprostol. Obstet Gynecol 1997;89:832–3.
74. Chon YS, Chua S, Arulkumaran S. Severe hyperthermia following oral misoprostol in the immediate postpartum period. Obstet Gynecol 1997;90:703–4.
75. Yamamoto T, Kitazawa Y. Iris-color change developed after topical isopropyl unoprostone treatment. J Glaucoma 1997;6:430–2.
76. Lawhorn S, Lawhorn CD, Davison C. Ondansetron eliminates nausea and vomiting associated with prostacyclin in a patient awaiting lung transplantation. J Heart Lung Transplant 1997;16:472–3.

A. Buitenhuis and C.J. van Boxtel

40 Sex hormones and related compounds, including hormonal contraceptives

ESTROGENS AND PROGESTOGENS *(SED-13, 1255; SEDA-19, 386; SEDA-20, 381; SEDA-21, 426)*

The authors of a recent review have pointed out that today women are exposed to exogenous hormones from a much younger age, and have mentioned the need for discussion of the dangers with them (1[r]).

Estrogens

Delivering estradiol by a vaginal ring eliminates irregular administration intervals, variable absorption, and potential problems with vaginal leakage of estradiol cream. A low-dose estradiol vaginal ring has been compared with a conjugated estrogen cream for postmenopausal urogenital atrophy (2[C]). The incidences of adverse events considered to have been related to treatment were comparable. The most frequent adverse events were breast tenderness with the cream and vaginitis with the ring. There was at least one drug-related adverse event in 42 (33%) of the subjects treated with the vaginal ring and 24 (36%) of those treated with the vaginal cream.

Side Effects of Drugs, Annual 22
J.K. Aronson, ed.

Hormone replacement therapy (HRT)

Cardiovascular The risk of deep vein thrombosis with HRT has been reviewed (3[R]). Recent publications have suggested that the risk of venous thromboembolism may be increased by up to 3-fold during HRT. Some individuals may have a pre-existing risk (environmental or genetic) high enough for the effect of HRT to trigger thrombosis at an early stage in treatment. A personal or family history of venous thromboembolism probably justifies screening for thrombophilia. Any detected risk must be weighed against the woman's personal risk factors: a personal history of venous thromboembolism or superficial thrombophlebitis, smoking, obesity, or varicose veins. The relative risk of venous thromboembolism may be 2 or 3. The absolute increase in risk is low: one case of venous thromboembolism per 5000 woman-years of HRT use.

In epidemiological studies of HRT and thrombosis, of 68 deaths from pulmonary embolism 22 were in women currently taking HRT and 19 in previous users (3[R]). The odds ratios (95% CI) for the first year, years 2–3, and after 3 years were, respectively 7.0 (2.1, 22.8), 4.6 (1.6, 12.9) and 1.7 (NS). These studies have suggested an increased risk in the early phase of HRT use, with a reduction in risk to a non-significant level after a few years. The risk of thrombosis reflects the balance of thrombosis and fibrinolysis in the individual. Immobilization, venous stasis, vessel damage, and surgery can tip the balance towards thrombosis. Genetic predisposition to venous thromboembolism is mainly due to deficiency of the coagulation inhibitors antithrombin III, protein C, or protein S, and activated protein C resistance (Factor V Leiden mutation). The effect of HRT on the risk of deep vein thrombosis is of limited importance compared with its beneficial effects on coronary artery disease, bone turnover, and possibly Alzheimer's disease, and with the increase in the risk of breast cancer. Before giving a woman HRT her risk of venous thromboembolism should be assessed from her history of relevant family and personal factors.

The association between HRT and the risk of idiopathic venous thromboembolism has been evaluated in 292 women admitted to hospital with a first episode of pulmonary embolism or deep venous thrombosis (4[R]). Women with a previous history of venous thromboembolism or other risk factors for thromboembolism were excluded. The results were consistent with those of Barlow (3[R]) and three other recent epidemiological studies (5[C])–(7[C]) with different methods, and showed 2–4-fold increases in risk among current users of HRT. The authors concluded that current use of HRT is associated with a higher risk of venous thromboembolism, but restricted to the first year of use. This higher risk could not be explained by factors such as age, bilateral oophorectomy, a history of superficial phlebitis or varicose veins, obesity, or smoking.

HRT has been associated with cardiac dysrhythmias (8[cr]).

A 51-year-old lady was admitted to the hospital with a supraventricular tachycardia. She had had bouts of palpitation before but not during menstruation for about 14 years. After starting combined HRT her palpitation had returned. She was taking no other medications. She was cardioverted with 6 mg of adenosine intravenously. After discharge she continued to take HRT and to have minor episodes of palpitation.

There is a positive correlation between plasma progesterone concentration and the number of episodes and duration of supraventricular tachycardia in women. Estrogens inhibit the release of adrenaline, and there is a significant inverse correlation between plasma estradiol-17 and the number of episodes and duration of supraventricular tachycardia. However, progesterone-opposed estrogen effects can result in increased adrenergic activity and potentiation of dysrhythmias.

Endocrine, metabolic The effects of HRT on lipoproteins have been reviewed (9[R]). Estrogen replacement therapy (ERT) reduces the risk of coronary heart disease by about 50% and by 80–90% in women with established coronary heart disease. Premature menopause in women not taking ERT and aged over 55 years is a risk factor. The incidence of coronary heart disease increases with age and is rare in women before the age of 55 years. There are no significant differences in risk for naturally versus surgically menopausal women. HDL cholesterol and triglycerides are independent predictors of cardiovascular disease mortality after adjusting for a history of heart disease, smoking, estrogen use, age, diabetes mellitus, and hypertension.

HDL cholesterol is a stronger predictor of cardiovascular disease risk than other lipids in women aged 50–69 years. Raised triglycerides are a particular risk factor in women with low HDL concentrations. Contraindications to HRT therapy are a history of breast cancer and triglyceride concentrations over 8.5 mmol/l (absolute contraindication) and 3.4 mmol/l (relative contraindication). Adding progestogens to ERT maintains the reduction in LDL cholesterol, attenuates the increase in HDL cholesterol, and does not significantly change triglycerides. Compliance with ERT and HRT depends on adverse effects: resumption of menstruation, breast tenderness, and bloating. Long-term administration of unopposed conjugated equine estrogen results in a reduction in LDL cholesterol and an increase in triglycerides and HDL cholesterol. HDL cholesterol concentrations rise during the first 6–12 months of treatment and, although they gradually fall over the next 24 months, they do not return to baseline. ERT and HRT may have no effect on triglycerides or may cause increases of up to 11–40% (9[R]).

Liver Chronic liver disease can cause osteodystrophy, causing pain, immobility, deformity, and fracture of the long bones and vertebrae, and loss of bone density. The problem is greatest with primary sclerosing cholangitis and primary biliary cirrhosis. Liver patients with osteodystrophy often have osteoporosis, especially when they have taken corticosteroids for a long time and take excessive amounts of alcohol (10[R]). The osteoporosis is caused by reduced bone formation, rather than increased resorption. Women with liver disease who took combined HRT (estradiol and conjugated estrogens, but not ethinylestradiol) did not have cholestasis or hepatotoxicity as judged by changes in serum alkaline phosphatase, aminotransferases, or bilirubin. The benefits of HRT have the same value to women with or without liver disease, including prevention or reversal of vaginal atrophy, psychofunctional disturbances, hot flushes, breast atrophy. and ischemic heart disease. HRT can be continued if the serum bilirubin has remained normal and if the serum γ-glutamyltranspeptidase and alkaline phosphatase have not risen by more than 100%. In patients with liver disease, first choices for the route of administration are transdermal patches and gels and subcutaneous implants. This maintains physiological blood estrogen concentrations without exposing the liver to a high concentration of conjugated estrogens in the portal blood. Transdermal estradiol is not lithogenic in bile. This is an advantage in cholestatic liver disease, especially primary biliary cirrhosis, in which gallstones are common. The first choice is estradiol (rather than ethinylestradiol), and a dose of 50 μg/day is sufficient to stabilize bone mineral density in most postmenopausal women.

Skin and appendages Three patients developed erythema nodosum complicating estrogen replacement therapy (11[c]). Since 1980 only two other similar reports have been published (12[c]), (13[c]). The recent cases developed after estrogen dosages equivalent to the physiological norm. The amount of estrogen taken during estrogen replacement is about one-quarter of that found in oral contraceptives. This dose should restore physiological concentrations of endogenous estrogens.

Musculoskeletal system Estrogen replacement can prevent osteoporosis both before and after the age of 75 years in daily doses of 50 μg of transdermal estrogen, 25 μg of ethinylestradiol, 2 mg of estradiol, or 0.625 mg of conjugated estrogens (14[R]). The prevention and treatment of osteoporosis with estrogen has been reviewed (15[R]).

Osteoporosis is noted first in the spine. Osteoporosis in peripheral bone, such as the hips, is also accelerated after the menopause, but it occurs much more slowly. Osteoblasts have estrogen receptors and can secrete insulin-like growth factor 1 and transform growth factor β. These growth factors inhibit activation of the osteoclasts. Estrogens also inhibit the production of interleukins 1 and 6, two cytokines that are important in the activation of osteoclasts.

Trabecular bone accounts for 20% of skeletal mass. It has a larger ratio of surface area to volume than cortical bone and also has a higher rate of metabolic activity. Women 65 years of age or older who are current users of HRT have a 60% reduction in wrist fractures and a 40% reduction in all non-spinal fractures. The effect of estrogen repletion is stabilization of bone mass; lost bone is not regained. Hypo-estrogenism results in accelerated bone loss, regardless of etiology, and affects not only the quantity of bone but also its quality. The goal of therapy is the maintenance of a circulating estradiol concentration of 60 pg/ml.

Other hormone replacement therapy

Women with an intact uterus who take estrogen replacement therapy require a progestogen to prevent endometrial hyperplasia, regardless of whether they use androgens or not (16[R]). The combined use of estradiol and dydrogesterone has been reviewed (17[R]). Cyclical vaginal bleeding occurs in 83–93% of treatment cycles and lasts for an average of 5–6 days. Non-cyclical bleeding occurs in under 10% of cycles. Endometrial hyperplasia develops in under 1%. There has been no evidence of malignancy in any study. Contraindications to use of the combination are pregnancy, abnormal genital bleeding, an acute venous thromboembolic disorder, lactation, a hormone-dependent neoplasm (e.g. carcinoma of the breast or endometrium), liver disease, and a persistent liver function test abnormality. Caution is required in patients with a past history of epilepsy, stroke, endometriosis, hemoglobinopathies, migraine, thromboembolic disorder, uterine leiomyoma, porphyria, deep vein thrombosis, otosclerosis, cardiac failure, or hypertension. The estrogenic effect of estradiol can be reduced by drugs that induce liver enzymes. Adverse events leading to treatment withdrawal are breast tenderness, vaginal bleeding, headache, and bloating. The combination reduces the percentage of women bothered by vaginal dryness from 55 to 30% and those bothered by dyspareunia from 35 to 20%. The use of HRT for less than 5 years is not associated with an increased risk of breast cancer.

Estrogen plus androgen therapy

Psychiatric Depression and anxiety improve significantly in women using an oral estrogen–androgen combination, but not in women using an estrogen alone (16[R]).

Endocrine, metabolic Estrogen alone increases HDL cholesterol concentrations by 7%, whereas combined treatment reduces the HDL cholesterol by 16%. The question remains whether these changes in lipoproteins prevent the impact of estrogen on coronary artery disease, but androgen replacement demands clinical and lipoprotein monitoring. Transdermal sex steroid administration is associated with less change in lipoproteins than oral therapy (16[R]).

Liver Oral androgen therapy in high dosages can be toxic to the liver; however, there were no clinically significant changes in liver function tests in a 2-year study of daily esterified estrogen 1.25 mg combined with methyltestosterone 2.5 mg (16[R]).

Skin and appendages In a 2-year study methyltestosterone 2.5 mg with 1.25 mg esterified estrogen was associated with a 36% incidence of hirsutism and a 30% incidence of acne (16[R]). However, not all clinical trial data suggest that combined estrogen–androgen replacement causes hirsutism.

Sexual function In two clinical trials of oral estrogen–androgen formulations there were no cases of enlarged clitoris (16[R]), (18[C]), (19[C]).

Miscellaneous Deepening of the voice occurred in some participants who took the estrogen–androgen formulation (16[R]).

Transdermal estrogen therapy

New developments in topical estrogen therapy (vaginal estrogen creams and rings, subcutaneous implants, percutaneous estrogen gel, and transdermal therapeutic systems) have been reviewed (20[R]). Compliance with vaginal creams can be poor, because these creams are messy and unpleasant to use. Vaginal vascularization and secretions can change from day to day, and so serum concentrations can be unstable. In dosages that provide therapeutic concentrations of estradiol, both conjugated equine estrogen and estradiol creams significantly increase liver protein synthesis. Lower dosages can reverse atrophic vaginal changes. The estrogenic effects of subcutaneous implants last for 4–12 months. In the case of overdose or intolerance, removal may be technically difficult.

Absorption of percutaneous estrogen gel is proportional to the intensity of rubbing-in, the surface area of application, and the extent of removal by clothing; accurate administration is therefore difficult to achieve. With this route of administration estradiol serum concentrations can be extremely variable. The gel must be spread on to a large area of the skin and allowed to dry for 2 or 3 min before activities can be resumed. Some women find this inconvenient. The gel can relieve climacteric symptoms, achieve physiological estradiol:estrone ratios, and improve vaginal cytology, without altering liver protein production.

Women who have headache or nausea with oral estrogens may tolerate transdermal estradiol. For example, the adverse effects of an investigational low-dose patch (20 g/day) were similar to those of placebo (20[R]). The incidence of adverse effects in double-blind trials has been similar with oral and transdermal administration. In the manufacturer's pooled data from 11 562 women, 14% of patients treated with Estraderm patches reported skin reactions and 6.3% discontinued treatment for this reason (20[R]). Safety analyses in 11

562 women treated with 50 or 100 g/day of transdermal estradiol showed a less than 5% incidence of nausea, flushing, breast tenderness, depression, headache, fluid retention, and weight gain (20[R]).

Transdermal vs oral estrogen therapy Women who use oral estrogens and who are at risk of gall-bladder disease can be treated with transdermal estradiol, and about 70–80% of women prefer the transdermal route over previous ERT (20[R]). Estrogens reduce the synthesis of bile acids and increase the concentration of cholesterol, which may cause bile to become more lithogenic. Oral estrogens increase cortisol-binding globulin, sex hormone-binding globulin, thyroxine binding globulin, and angiotensinogen (but hypertension has not been associated with the use of oral estrogens). These changes are not observed with transdermal administration. Transdermal estradiol is significantly more effective than placebo; there is improvement in sleep, somatic complaints, sexual function, and health-related complaints. The large first-pass effect through the liver is associated with alterations in lipid profile, hepatic protein synthesis, and bile composition. The risk of cholecystectomy increases with duration of estrogen use and does not completely resolve after withdrawal, suggesting that gallstones formed during oral estrogen use do not necessarily dissolve after discontinuation.

However, the majority of postmenopausal women are still not using this potentially bone-conserving cardioprotective intervention.

Progestogens

Minimizing the dosage of progestogen in HRT is important to avoid adverse effects on coagulation, carbohydrate and lipid metabolism, and vasodilatation, especially in patients with a cardiovascular risk. Maybe in these patients a intermittent regimen is best; however, this can result in an increased risk of endometrial hyperplasia (21[C]).

The frequency of hyperplasia with intermittent progestogen therapy is similar to the prevalence of endometrial hyperplasia in postmenopausal women without any hormonal treatment. The effects of transdermal estradiol (0.05 mg/day) and oral norethisterone acetate (2.5 mg/day) for 12 days every 2 months (group A, $n = 83$) or every 3 months (group B, $n = 89$) have been studied in patients whose menopause had begun at least 4 years earlier (22[C]). Even patients with severe symptoms responded within 8–12 weeks, with a good overall result in about 90%. About 88% of the women wanted to continue at the end of the study. Reasons for discontinuation (groups A/B) were systemic adverse effects (4/1), breakthrough bleeding (1/2), skin irritation (1/2), preference for hormonal tablets (0/1) or injections (0/1), severe withdrawal bleeding (2/1), and other non-medical objections (2/3). There were no differences in adverse effects, patient acceptance, bleeding pattern, or urogenital complaints. Overall systemic tolerability was judged good or very good in more than 90% of the patients in both groups. The adverse effects in group A were weight gain (3), edema (1), raised blood pressure (1), skin irritation (6), a systemic allergic reaction (1), and central nervous system effects (7) such as depression, migraine, and headache. Adverse effects in group B were skin irritation (3), edema (2), central nervous system effects (4), and mastodynia (6). There were major skin reactions due to the patch in about 5% in both groups. There was endometrial hyperplasia in 6.2% of the women during long-cycle treatment and in only 0.8% with monthly progestogen addition.

Oral contraceptives *(SED-13, 1211; SEDA-19, 381; SEDA-20, 384)*

Outcomes have been studied in 56 adolescents aged 18 years who used a Norplant implant compared with 56 age-matched controls who used an oral contraceptive (23[C]). One year later 91% of those who had used an implant and 34% of those who had used an oral contraceptive were still using their chosen method. Adverse effects were reported by over 80% of the women in both groups. Menstrual irregularities were significant more frequent in those who used Norplant (73 vs 5%). Norplant users gained more weight (4 vs 2 kg) and were twice as likely to have an abnormal Papanicolaou smear. There was a low rate of consistent condom use, resulting in a high rate of sexually transmitted diseases: gonorrhea 11% and *Chlamydia* 27%. Other adverse effects with Norplant and oral contraceptives, respectively, were: breast tenderness (31 vs 37%), amenorrhea (6 vs 0%), nausea and vomiting (18 vs 16%), abnormal hair growth or loss (18 vs 11%), weight gain (60 vs 53%), headaches (26 vs 42%), and increased appetite (33 vs 42%).

Cardiovascular The risk of cardiovascular disease with oral contraceptives has been reviewed (24[R]). First-generation oral contraceptives increased the risk of myocardial infarction, stroke, and venous thromboembolism. The risk of venous thrombosis among carriers of the factor V Leiden mutation is increased 8-fold overall and 30-fold among carriers who take an oral contraceptive. Oral contraceptives containing second- and third-generation progestogens and less than 50 μg of estrogen are associated with a smaller increase in the incidence of venous thromboembolism than first-generation drugs, although the risk with third-generation drugs is higher than with second-generation drugs (SEDA-19, 383). The increase with formulations containing the third-generation progestogens gestodene and desogestrel is about 1.5–2 times that for second-generation formulations.

There is a smaller increase in the risk of myocardial infarction associated with modern formulations: a 3-fold increase with second-generation progestogens and no increase with the third-generation progestogens. There is little or no increase in the risk of stroke with modern formulations among women without risk factors.

Pregnancy is accompanied by a reduction in sensitivity to activated protein C, which may explain the increased risk of venous thrombosis in oral contraceptive users (25[C]). About 4% of West Europeans are heterozygous for activated protein C resistance, and this abnormality is found in 20–50% of patients with venous thrombosis.

A mutation in factor V (factor V Leiden) also results in resistance to activated protein C. This mutation potentiates the prothrombotic effect of oral contraceptives. Women taking third-generation progestogens are significantly less sensitive to activated protein C than women taking second-generation progestogens (25[C]).

Skin and appendages Oral contraceptives lower androgen concentrations and have been used to treat patients with acne vulgaris. The effectiveness of a triphasic combination oral contraceptive in moderate acne has been studied in 257 healthy women, aged 15–49 years, in a multicenter, randomized, double-blind, placebo-controlled trial (26[C]). The oral contraceptive was more effective than placebo. The three adverse events reported by the greatest percentage of subjects were nausea, upper respiratory tract infections, and headache with the oral contraceptive, and headache, upper respiratory infections, and dysmenorrhea with placebo. The progestogen norgestimate has a lower androgen activity than other currently available progestogens. The combination of norgestimate with ethinylestradiol increases sex hormone-binding globulin and reduces free testosterone in healthy women, leading to reduced activity of acne vulgaris.

ANDROGENIC AND ANABOLIC STEROIDS AND RELATED COMPOUNDS *(SED-13, 1265; SEDA-20, 386; SEDA-21, 434)*

In patients with hereditary angio-edema treated with the 17-alkylated androgens danazol ($n = 5$) or danazol plus stanozolol ($n = 31$) hypertension can develop after a few months, but also after many years (27[C]), and is not related to higher doses or longer treatment. Other adverse effects in this study were menstrual irregularities (in 50% of women taking danazol and 10% taking stanozolol), increased body weight in men and women (20% with danazol and 17% with stanozolol), acne, hypothyroidism, and myocardial infarction; menstrual irregularities and increased body weight were dose related

Adverse effects of testosterone implants for androgen replacement therapy are infections and bleeding. In a study of 973 men the most common adverse effect was extrusion of the implant (in 8.5%) (28[C]).

In 23 impotent hypogonadal men treated with oral testosterone undecanoate for no less than 60 days adverse effects (acne, breast tenderness, urticaria, and weight gain) occurred in one patient each (29[C]).

Endocrine, metabolic Anabolic steroids have an anticatabolic effect, improving the utilization of protein and inhibiting the catabolic effects of glucocorticoids. These effects may lead to gains in strength by reducing an athlete's sense of fatigue during training, by increasing aggressiveness, and by producing euphoria. Of particular concern is premature epiphyseal closure, which results in a reduction in adult height (30[R]).

In men, anabolic steroid use reduces concentrations of follicle-stimulating hormone and luteinizing hormone. This leads to reduced spermatogenesis, reduced production of endogenous testosterone, and testicular atrophy (30[R]).

Gynecomastia reaching the size of a normal female breast has been reported in a 25-year-old man who had taken cyproterone 300 mg/day for 2 years (31[c]).

Skin and appendages Scrotal and non-scrotal transdermal systems for the administration of testosterone have been compared (32[C]). The advantage of rate-controlled transdermal therapy over oral administration is that it mimics the natural endogenous pattern of serum testosterone. This has positive effects on sexual function, mood, and fatigue, and significantly increases sexual activity. Other advantages are a sustained reliable plasma concentration and improved systemic availability. Frequently reported topical effects of a non-scrotal transdermal system are erythema (7%), blistering (12%), a burning sensation (3%), pruritus (37%), induration (3%), allergic contact dermatitis (4%), and vesicles (6%). There was irritation after removal in 5% of patients using the scrotal system and in 32% of patients using the non-scrotal system. Scrotal systems did not cause contact allergy.

ANTIANDROGENS *(SED-13, 1267; SEDA-20, 387)*

Bicalutamide

Bicalutamide, a new antiandrogen developed for the treatment of prostate cancer has been reviewed (33[R]). The expected adverse effects, gynecomastia, breast pain, and hot flushes, occurred in at least 5% of patients. Adverse events reported by at least 10% of patients treated with a combination of bicalutamide and an LHRH analogue are hot flushes (49%), general pain (27%), constipation (17%), back pain (15%), weakness (15%), pelvic pain (13%), nausea (11%), infections (10%), and diarrhea (10%).

Liver Hepatic failure has been attributed to bicalutamide (34[c]).

A 60-year-old man with adenocarcinoma of the prostate received androgen blockade with flutamide 250 mg tds and monthly subcutaneous goserelin acetate. This was well tolerated. After 3 months it was discontinued and bicalutamide 50 mg/day was introduced instead. After the second dose he developed jaundice, confusion, and encephalopathy.

Another similar case of fulminant hepatic failure associated with bicalutamide has been described; however, the author thought that it was probably not due to the drug (35[c]).

Finasteride

In 44 women with polycystic ovary syndrome treated with finasteride or flutamide for 6 months the adverse effects of flutamide were reduced libido, gastrointestinal disorders, and dry skin (36[C]). Finasteride caused reduced libido, headache, and dry skin. Dry skin was reported in 68% of users of flutamide and only in 27% of users of finasteride.

Musculoskeletal Reversible severe myopathy during treatment with finasteride has been described in a 70-year-old patient (37[c]).

Flutamide

The adverse effects of flutamide in 44 women with polycystic ovary syndrome treated with flutamide for 6 months (36[C]) have been mentioned above.

Hematological Flutamide-induced methemoglobinemia has been described (38[c]).

Nilutamide

The use of nilutamide, a non-steroidal anti-androgen, in the treatment of prostate cancer has been reviewed (39[R]). Its most common adverse effects are gastrointestinal (nausea and vomiting) and ophthalmic effects.

In a dose of 300 mg/day nilutamide caused disorders of light–dark adaptation (67%), alcohol intolerance (4–19%), and a reversible intestinal pneumonia (1–3%). Bright illumination had a recovery time of 9 min (0.3–25) the normal upper limit being 1–2 min. This is a problem for patients who drive at night. Symptoms of interstitial pneumonia coccurred after a cumulative dose of 3–38 g and a treatment duration of 10 days to 4 months. Libido and potency were preserved in 50% of patients.

Psychiatric A 77-year-old man with prostate carcinoma treated with nilutamide developed acute depression (40[c]).

Interactions Nilutamide is metabolized by the cytochrome P450 system, and should therefore interact with other agents metabolized by this system (39[R]).

GONADOTROPHINS AND OVULATION-INDUCING DRUGS *(SED-13, 1259; SEDA-20, 388)*

The fertility drugs have been reviewed (41[R]).

Immunological and hypersensitivity reactions A woman with long-standing quiescent SLE died of a severe neurological exacerbation after a second cycle of hormonal drugs administered for in vitro fertilization and embryo transfer (42[c]).

Tumor-inducing effects of sex hormones

R

Breast cancer *Current users of estrogens when breast cancer is diagnosed survive 5 years longer than non-users do (43[R]). Current users of estrogens also have an increased incidence of breast cancer. The increased survival disappears when it is corrected for stage at diagnosis. Estrogen use relates most strongly to early-stage tumors. One would expect that these tumors would be less aggressive and be associated with increased survival after diagnosis. Patients with breast cancer who have discontinued estrogen treatment less than 1 year before diagnosis have a significantly higher survival rate.*

The use of combined estrogen–progestogen therapy has increased recently. The addition of a progestogen does not seem to reduce the risk of breast cancer associated with estrogen use alone. Whether combined therapy carries a greater risk of breast cancer than estrogens alone has yet to be determined. Two case–control studies involving 537 (44[C]) and 3130 (45[C]) patients showed no increase in risk among users of either estrogens alone or combined therapy.

In 435 Swedish women aged 40–74 years attending mammography screening, progestogen-combined regimens used for more than 10 years were associated with higher risk estimates, OR = 2.4 (95% CI 0.7, 8.6), compared with equally long treatment with medium-potency estrogens only, OR = 1.3 (95% CI 0.5, 3.7); the two estimates were not significantly different (46[C]). Cases had on average had a more frequent family history of breast cancer, were older at the time of their first birth, had a higher ever use of HRT, and were of lower parity. Use of HRT for many years is associated with a moderately increased risk of breast cancer and hypothetically a further enhancement of the risk with added progestogens. Multivariate analyses showed an increased risk among users of any type of HRT for more than 10 years, the odds ratio being 2.1 (95% CI 1.1, 4.0).

Estrogen replacement increases the of risk breast cancer predominantly in lean women. The possible effects of HRT on tumor biology have been studied in 477 consecutive patients with breast cancer (47[C]). There was a trend towards a higher proportion of localized tumors in HRT users. A less advanced clinical stage in breast cancer was associated with better survival and lower mortality. HRT caused a lower proliferation rate in established breast tumors, and proliferation rate and tumor size were significantly correlated.

The effect of HRT on breast cancer mortality may even be beneficial (48[C]), (49[C]). Indicators of biological aggressiveness are c-erb B_2 oncoprotein, ploidy, tumor proliferation rate, estrogen receptors, and progesterone receptors (47[C]).

Endometrial cancer *Postmenopausal women who take combined estrogen and cyclic progestogen have an increased risk of endometrial cancer in comparison with women not taking HRT (50[C]). This is so even when a progestogen is added for 10 or more days per month. However, this increase is much smaller than that associated with unopposed estrogen. The use of combined therapy is not associated with an increased risk, unless the progestogen is added for fewer than 10 days each month.*

The relation between hormone replacement therapy (HRT) and endometrial cancer has been reviewed (51[R]). Exogenous unopposed estrogen replacement therapy is a predisposing factor in endometrial cancer. Therefore, if the uterus is present, progestogen therapy is recommended as a component of HRT. The progestogen component can be given every day with the estrogen or in a cyclic fashion on 12–14 days each month. This regimen is usually associated with regular predictable bleeding after the progestogen has been taken. When patients have adverse effects during HRT it is necessary to determine whether the progestogen or the estrogen is causing the problem. If heavy bleeding or breast tenderness is the primary complaint, the estrogen component is probably the problem, and the dosage should be reduced. If the patient complains of irritability, depression, or headaches, the problems are probably due to the progestogen component, and the progestogen should be changed or the dosage adjusted. The disadvantage of continuous progestogen administration is irregular bleeding; the advantage is amenorrhea. There are no benefits and sometimes disadvantages in giving an estrogen on only 25 days a month, particularly estrogen withdrawal symptoms, such as reduced well-being, headaches, and hot flushes. The most commonly used progestogens are norethindrone, norethindrone acetate, medroxyprogesterone acetate, and micronized progesterone.

If irregular bleeding is persistent, transvaginal sonography and/or endometrial sampling should be performed to rule out endometrial cancer. Risk estimates for this show a summary relative risk (RR) of 2.3 for estrogen users in comparison with non-users and a much higher RR of 9.5 associated with a prolonged duration of 10 or more years. The increased risk persists for years after discontinuation of the unopposed estrogen. There is also an increased risk of endometrial tumors with the use of tamoxifen in patients with breast cancer. Patients with endometrial cancer often have upper abdominal obesity, an increase in estrogen production, oligo-ovulation and a lower sex-hormone-binding globulin concentration, resulting in high concentrations of unbound estrogen.

Ovarian cancer *A possible association between drugs that induce ovulation and ovarian cancer has been discussed (41[R]). The relative risk of ovarian cancer falls significantly with the number of pregnancies. A direct causal effect of infertility treatment on ovarian cancer seems unlikely. Oral contraceptives taken for more than 3 years protect women from ovarian cancer (RR = 0.5–0.7). This protection is maintained for more than 10 years after withdrawal and also depends on the duration of use. A woman with primary infertility has an increased risk of ovarian carcinoma, independent of nulliparity, and must be examined with great care before and after the administration of fertility drugs. When childbirth is followed by breast-feeding, maximal protection against ovarian carcinoma is gained.*

Prostate cancer *A 58-year-old man treated with exogenous testosterone for impotence was subsequently diagnosed with prostate cancer (52[c]). However, prostate cancer is very common, and there was no evidence of a cause-and-effect association, particularly since prostate cancer in this case probably antedated the use of testosterone.*

Other tumors *A 35-year-old woman developed a bile duct hamartoma in association with long-term treatment with danazol (53[c]).*

REFERENCES

1. Price EH, Little HK, Grant ECG, Steel CM. Women need to be warned about dangers of hormone replacement therapy. Br Med J 1997; 314:376–7.
2. Bachmann G, Notelovitz M, Nachtigall L, Birgerson L. A comparative study of a low-dose estradiol vaginal ring and conjugated estrogen cream for post menopausal urogenital atrophy. Prim Care Update Ob/Gyn 1997;4:109–15.
3. Barlow DH. HRT and the risk of deep vein thrombosis. Int J Gynecol Obstet 1997;59 (Suppl 1):S29–33.
4. Pérez-Gutthann S, Garcia-Rodriguez LA, Castellsague J, Duque-Oliart A. Hormone replacement therapy and risk of venous thromboembolism: population based case-control study. Br Med J 1997;314:796–800.
5. Grodstein F, Stampfer MJ, Goldhaber SZ, Manson JE, Colditz GA, Speizer FE, Willett WC, Hennekens CH. Prospective study of exogenous hormones and risk of pulmonary embolism in women. Lancet 1996;348:983–7.
6. Daly E, Vessey MP, Hawkins MM, Carson JL, Gough P, Marsh S. Risk of venous thromboembolism in users of hormone replacement therapy. Lancet 1996;348:977–80.
7. Jick H, Derby LE, Myers MW, Vasilakis C, Newton KM. Risk of hospital admission for idiopathic venous thromboembolism among users of postmenopausal oestrogens. Lancet 1996; 348:981–3.
8. Taylor AD, Smith DR. Cyclical paroxysmal superventricular tachycardia related to hormone replacement therapy. Br J Cardiol 1998;5:394–6.
9. Plushner SL. Lipoprotein disorders in women: which women are the best candidates for hormone replacement therapy? Ann Pharmacother 1997; 301:98–107.
10. O'Donohue J, Williams R. Hormone replacement therapy in women with liver disease. Br J Obstet Gynaecol 1997;104:1–3.
11. Yang SG, Han KH, Cho KH, Lee AY. Development of erythema nodosum in the course of oestrogen replacement therapy. Br J Dermatol 1997;137:319–20.
12. Touboul JL, Beaumont V, Meyniel D, Pieron R. Erytheme noueux et contraception orale. Mise en evidence d'un anticorps anti-ethinyl-estradiol. Nouv Presse Med 1981;10:712.
13. Muller-Ladner U, Kaufmann R, Adler G, Scherbaum WA. Rezidivierendes Erythema nodosum nach Einnahme eines niedrig dosierten oralen Antikonzeptivums. Med Klin 1994;89:100–2.
14. Fitzsimmons A, Freundlich B, Bonner F. Osteoporosis and rehabilitation. Crit Rev Phys Rehabil Med 1997;9:331–53.
15. Battistini M. Estrogen and the prevention and treatment of osteoporosis. J Clin Rheumatol 1997;3 (Suppl):S28–33.
16. Kaunitz AM. The role of androgens in menopausal hormone replacement. Endocrinol Metab Clin North Am 1997;26:391–7.
17. Foster RH, Balfour JA. Estradiol and dydrogesterone. A review of their combined use as hormone replacement therapy in postmenopausal women. Drugs Aging 1997;11:309–32.
18. Hickok LR, Toomey C, Speroff L. A comparison of esterified estrogens with and without methyltestosterone: effects on endometrial histology and serum lipoproteins in postmenopausal women. Obstet Gynecol 1993;82:919–24.
19. Watts NB, Notelovitz M, Timmons MC, Addison WA, Wiita B, Downey LJ. Comparison of oral estrogens and estrogens plus androgen on bone mineral density, menopausal symptoms, and lipid-lipoprotein profiles in surgical menopause. Obstet Gynecol 1995;85:529–37 (erratum 668).
20. Jewelewicz R. New developments in topical estrogen therapy. Fertil Steril 1997;67:1–12.
21. Cerin A, Heldaas K, Moeller B. Adverse endometrial effects of long-cycle estrogen and progestagen replacement therapy. New Engl J Med 1996;334:668–9.
22. Rabe T, Mueck AO, Deuringer FU, Vladescu E, Runnebaum B. Spacing-out of progestin-efficacy, tolerability and compliance of two regimens for hormonal replacement in the late postmenopause. Gynecol Endocrinol 1997;11:383–92.
23. Berenson AB, Wiemann CM, Rickerr VI, McCombs SL. Contraceptive outcomes among adolescents prescribed Norplant implants versus oral contraceptives after one year of use. Am J Obstet Gynecol 1997;176:586–92.
24. Rosenberg L, Palmer JR, Sands MI, Grimes D, Bergman U, Daling J, Mills A. Modern oral contraceptives and cardiovascular disease. Am J Obstet Gynecol 1997;177:707–15.
25. Rosing J, Tans G, Nicolaes GAF, Thomassen MCLGD, Van Oerle R, Van Der Ploeg PMEN, Heijnen P, Hamulyak K, Hemker HC. Oral contraceptives and venous thrombosis: different sensitivities to activated protein C in women using

second- and third-generation oral contraceptives. Br J Haematol 1997;97:233–8.
26. Lucky AW, Henderson TA, Olson WH, Robisch DM, Lebwohl M. Effectiveness of norgestimate and ethinyl estradiol in treating moderate acne vulgaris. J Am Acad Dermatol 1997;37:746–54.
27. Cicardi M, Castelli R, Zingale LC, Agostoni A. Side effects of long-term prophylaxis with attenuated androgens in hereditary angioedema: comparison of treated and untreated patients. J Allergy Clin Immunol 1997;99:194–6.
28. Handelsman DJ, Mackey MA, Howe C, Turner L, Conway AJ. An analysis of testosterone implants for androgen replacement therapy. Clin Endocrinol 1997;47:311–16.
29. Morales A, Johnston B, Heaton JPW, Lundie M. Testosterone supplementation for hypogonadal impotence: assessment of biochemical measures and therapeutic outcomes. J Urol 1997;157:849–54.
30. Anderson SJ, Bolduc SP, Coryllos E, Griesemer B, Mclain L, Rowland TW, Tanner SM, Keely K, Malacrea R, Young JC, Washington RL, Reed FE, Bar Or O, Risser WL. Adolescents and anabolic steroids: a subject review. Pediatrics 1997;99;904–8.
31. Ren GS, Julien JP, Raoust I. Cyproterone-induced large gynaecomastia. Breast 1997;6:306.
32. Jordan WP Jr. Allergy and topical irritation associated with transdermal testosterone administration: a comparison of scrotal and non-scrotal transdermal systems. Am J Contact Dermatitis 1997;8:108–13.
33. Blackledge GRP, Cockshott ID, Furr BJA. Casodex (Bicalutamide): overview of a new antiandrogen developed for treatment of prostate cancer. Eur Urol 1997;31 (Suppl 2):30–9.
34. Dawson LA, Chow E, Morton G. Fulminant hepatic failure associated with bicalutamide. Urology 1997;49:283–4.
35. Schellhammer PF. Fulminant hepatic failure associated with bicalutamide. Urology 1997; 50:827.
36. Falsetti L, De Fusco D, Eleftheriou G, Rosina B. Treatment of hirsutism by finasteride and flutamide in women with polycystic ovary syndrome. Gynaecol Endosc 1997;6:251–7.
37. Haan J, Hollander JMR, van Duinen SG, Saxena PR, Wintzen AR. Reversible severe myopathy during treatment with finasteride. Muscle Nerve 1997;20:502–4.
38. Khan AM, Singh NT, Bilgrami S. Flutamide induced methemoglobinemia. J Urol 1997;157:1363.
39. Dole EJ, Holdsworth MT. Nilutamide: an antiandrogen for the treatment of prostate cancer. Ann Pharmacother 1997;31:65–75.
40. Maroy B, Pitrou P. Acute depression probably due to nilutamide. Thérapie 1997;52:79–81.
41. Artini PG, Fasciani A, Cela V, Battaglia C, De Micheroux AA, D'Ambrogio G, Genazzani AR. Fertility drugs and ovarian cancer. Gynecol Endocrinol 1997;11:59–68.
42. Casoli P, Tumiati B, La Scala G. Fatal exacerbation of systemic lupus erythematosus after induction of ovulation. J Rheumatol 1997;24:1639–40.
43. Brinton LA. Hormone replacement therapy and risk for breast cancer. Endocrinol Metab Clin North Am 1997;26:361–78.
44. Stanford JL, Weiss NS, Voigt LF, Daling JR, Habel LA, Rossing MA. Combined estrogen and progestin hormone replacement therapy in relation to risk of breast cancer in middle-aged women. J Am Med Assoc 1995;274:137–42.
45. Newcomb PA, Longnecker MP, Storer BE, Mittendorf R, Baron J, Clapp RW, Bogdan G, Willett WC. Long-term hormone replacement therapy and risk of breast cancer in postmenopausal women. Am J Epidemiol 1995;142:788–95.
46. Persson I, Thurfjell E, Bergström R, Holmberg L. Hormone replacement therapy and risk of breast cancer. Nested case-control study in a cohort of Swedish women attending mammography screening. Int J Cancer 1997;72:758–61.
47. Holli K, Isola J, Cuzick J. Hormone replacement therapy and biological aggressiveness of breast cancer. Lancet 1997;350:1704–5.
48. Willis DB, Calle EE, Miracle-McMahill H, Heath CW Jr. Estrogen replacement therapy and risk of fatal breast cancer in a prospective cohort of postmenopausal women in the United States. Cancer Causes Control 1996;7:449–57.
49. Grodstein F, Stampfer MJ, Colditz GA, Willett WC, Manson JE, Joffe M, Rosner B, Fuchs C, Hankinson SE, Hunter DJ, Hennekens CH, Speizer FE. Postmenopausal hormone therapy and mortality. New Engl J Med 1997;336:1769–75.
50. Beresford SAA, Weiss NS, Voigt LF, McKnight B. Risk of endometrial cancer in relation to use of oestrogen combined with cyclic progestagen therapy in postmenopausal women. Lancet 1997;349:458–61.
51. Sulak PJ. Endometrial cancer and hormone replacement therapy: appropriate use of progestins to oppose endogenous and exogenous estrogen. Endocrinol Metab Clin North Am 1997; 26:399–412.
52. Loughlin KR, Richie JP. Prostate cancer after exogenous testosterone treatment for impotence. J Urol 1997;157:1845.
53. Elmadbouh HM, Douglas-Jones M. Bileduct hamartoma occurring in association with long-term treatment with danazol. Br J Clin Pract 1997;51:179–80.

J.A. Franklyn

41 Thyroid hormones and antithyroid drugs

THYROID HORMONES *(SED-13, 1275; SEDA-19, 391; SEDA-20, 393; SEDA-21, 437)*

The development and routine use of sensitive assays for measurement of serum thyrotrophin (TSH) has led to increased awareness of the fact that many patients taking standard doses of thyroxine have biochemical evidence of over-treatment, indicated by reduced TSH concentrations. The literature continues to address the question of whether there are any significant consequences of these minor degrees of *'subclinical' hyperthyroidism*, with particular emphasis on cardiovascular and skeletal effects. The evidence supporting adverse effects of thyroxine on the heart and on bone metabolism has been reviewed (1^R).

Nervous system There have been case reports of *pseudotumor cerebri*, a rare occurrence in children and adolescents taking thyroxine replacement therapy (1^R), (2^c).

Interactions It is generally considered that drug interactions with thyroxine are few and clinically unimportant. There have been three reports of hypothyroidism, confirmed biochemically by a rise in serum TSH, in patients who had been clinically and biochemically euthyroid before the addition of a new drug.

One of these reports described a series of nine patients who required an increase in thyroxine dosage of 11–50% after the introduction of *sertraline*, which was postulated to increase the clearance of thyroxine by an unspecified mechanism (3^C).

The second described a marked increase in serum TSH in the same patient on two occasions after several weeks of antimalarial prophylaxis with *chloroquine* and *proguanil*, the likely mechanism being enzyme induction and increased thyroxine catabolism (4^c).

A further case report has described biochemical hypothyroidism in a patient taking thyroxine after the introduction of *ferrous sulfate*, probably resulting from reduced absorption of thyroxine (5^c).

ANTITHYROID DRUGS *(SED-13, 1279; SEDA-19, 391; SEDA-20, 394; SEDA-21, 437)*

Effects in pregnancy Treatment with thionamides in pregnancy can result in *fetal hypothyroidism and goiter*, and maternal doses of thionamides should be reduced as much as possible while maintaining serum thyroid hormone concentrations within the reference range. Propylthiouracil is generally considered the drug of choice in pregnancy, because it has been believed to cross the placenta to a lesser extent than carbimazole or its active metabolite methimazole. However, this view has not previously been subjected to scientific scrutiny.

The effects of maternal propylthiouracil and methimazole on fetal thyroid function at delivery (measured in cord blood) have therefore been compared in 77 euthyroid Japanese women with Graves' disease (6^C). There were no significant differences between mean free thyroxine and TSH concentrations in fetal serum at delivery; the prevalence of biochemical hypothyroidism (high serum TSH) was also similar in the two groups (23 vs 14%). These 13 cases of hypothyroidism occurred in women taking low doses of thionamides (propylthiouracil 100 mg/day or less or methimazole 10 mg/day or less), emphasizing the fact that fetal hypothyroidism is a relatively

Side Effects of Drugs, Annual 22
J.K. Aronson, ed.

common finding in infants born to hyperthyroid women, either because of transplacental passage of antithyroid drugs or because of transplacental passage of TSH receptor-blocking antibodies. It also appears that there is little support for the view that propylthiouracil is the drug of choice in pregnancy because of less marked transplacental passage and hence fetal hypothyroidism.

The fact that thionamides can result in severe complications in pregnancy has been highlighted by a case report of congenital hypothyroidism and goiter in an infant born to a mother treated with propylthiouracil 100 mg bd or tds from the eighth week of pregnancy (7[c]).

Aside from the induction of fetal hypothyroidism and goiter, thionamides are considered to be safe in pregnancy, although debate has surrounded the possible rare association of carbimazole with *aplasia cutis* (8[C]). Severe congenital abnormalities, including *choanal atresia*, *esophageal atresia with tracheo-oesophageal fistula*, and *multiple ventricular septal defects* have been described in an infant born to a mother with severe hyperthyroidism presenting in early pregnancy and treated with methimazole (30 mg/day) before subtotal thyroidectomy (9[c]). However, the mother had also taken metoprolol and used budesonide and salmeterol inhalers, so that no single drug could be implicated. Hyperthyroidism itself has also been thought to be associated with an increased risk of congenital abnormality.

Immunological and hypersensitivity reactions While agranulocytosis remains the most recognised and feared complication of thionamide therapy, there has been an increasing number of reports of *vasculitic illnesses* affecting either the kidney or skin in patients taking methimazole or propylthiouracil. These include a description of three patients who developed severe cutaneous vasculitis within the first few weeks of treatment with propylthiouracil (10[C]), and cases of diffuse proliferative lupus nephritis associated with antineutrophil cytoplasmic antibodies (11[cR]), (12[c]). These cases emphasize the importance of considering the role of thionamides in patients with hyperthyroidism who develop vasculitic illnesses, not least because such vasculitic syndromes may be severe but reversible after thionamide withdrawal.

IODINE AND THE IODIDES

(SED-13, 1281; SEDA-19, 392; SEDA-21, 438)

Iodine deficiency is a major problem world wide, with an estimated one billion people affected. While iodine replacement programs have been successful in many developing countries in reducing the incidence of iodine deficiency-associated goiter and mental retardation, mild iodine deficiency remains a problem in many parts of the world, including Europe. Iodine supplementation can lead to *an increase in the incidence of thyroid dysfunction* in the population in the short term, although this has not been studied prospectively in a controlled fashion.

The efficacy and adverse effects of low-dose iodine supplementation (potassium iodide 200 mg/day) have been evaluated in a double-blind placebo-controlled study of 62 subjects with euthyroid diffuse endemic goiter in a moderately iodine deficient area of Germany (13[C]). Iodine substantially reduced thyroid volume, and the therapeutic effect persisted after iodine withdrawal. However, three of 31 subjects taking iodine developed *positive antithyroid antibodies* and a further two developed iodine-induced *hyper- or hypothyroidism*, abnormalities that disappeared within 2 years of follow-up. This result supports the view that iodine supplementation, while effective in combating the potentially serious effects of iodine deficiency, is associated with an increased likelihood of autoimmune thyroid dysfunction, a factor that must be taken into account when iodine replacement programs are initiated.

REFERENCES

1. Williams JB. Adverse effects of thyroid hormones. Drugs Aging 1997;11:460–9.
2. Raghavan S, DiMartino-Nardi J, Saenger P, Linder B. Pseudotumor cerebri in an infant after L-thyroxine therapy for transient neonatal hypothyroidism. J Pediatr 1997;1130:47–80.
3. McCowen KC, Garber JR, Spark R. Elevated serum thyrotropin in thyroxine-treated patients with hypothyroidism given sertraline. New Engl J Med 1997;337:1010–11.
4. Munera Y, Hughes FC, Le Jeune C, Pays JF. Interaction of thyroxine sodium with antimalarial drugs. Br Med J 1997;314:1593.
5. Shakir KMM, Chute JP, Aprill BS, Lazarus AA. Ferrous sulphate-induced increase in requirement for thyroxine in a patient with primary hypothyroidism. South Med J 1997;90:637–9.
6. Momotani N, Yoshimura Noh J, Ishikawa N, Ito K. Effects of propylthiouracil and methimazole on fetal thyroid status in mothers with Graves' hyperthyroidism. J Clin Endocrinol Metab 1997;82:3633–6.
7. Giardino AA, Foley C. Radiological case of the month. Arch Adolesc Med 1997;151:199–200.
8. Vogt T, Stolz W, Landthaler M. Aplasia cutis congenita after exposure to methimazole: a causal relationship? Br J Dermatol 1995;133:994–6.
9. Johnsson E, Larsson G, Ljunggren M. Severe malformations in infant born to hyperthyroid woman on methimazole. Lancet 1997;350:1520.
10. Yarman S, Sandalci O, Tanakol R, Azizlerli H, Oguz H, Alagol F. Propylthiouracil-induced cutaneous vasculitis. Int J Clin Pharmacol Ther 1997;35;282–6.
11. Prasad GVR, Bastacky S, Johnson JP. Propylthiouracil-induced diffuse proliferative lupus nephritis: review of immunological complications. J Am Soc Nephrol 1997;8:1205–10.
12. Kudoh Y, Kuroda S, Shimamoto K, Iimura O. Propylthiouracil-induced rapidly progressive glomerulonephritis associated with antineutrophil cytoplasmic autoantibodies. Clin Nephrol 1997; 48:41–3.
13. Kahaly G, Dienes HP, Beyer J, Hommel G. Randomized, double blind, placebo-controlled trial of low dose iodide in endemic goiter. J Clin Endocrinol Metab 1997;82:4049–53.

H.M.J. Krans

42 Insulin, glucagon, and hypoglycemic drugs

The Diabetes Control and Complications Trial (DCCT; SEDA-18, 409) showed that strict control delayed the development of secondary complications in type 1 diabetes. The recently published UK Prospective Diabetes Study (UKPDS) in 3867 patients with type 2 diabetes has shown a substantial reduction (25%) in microvascular complications when blood glucose (HbA1c) was lower, although there was no clear effect on death rate ([1R]). As in the DCCT this was accompanied by more instances of *hypoglycemia* and *increased body weight*.

INSULIN *(SED-13, 1290; SEDA-19, 393; SEDA-20, 396; SEDA-21, 440)*

Modes of administration of insulin Insulin, its various sources, methods of administration, ways of mixing insulins, new formulations, and allergic reactions have recently been reviewed ([2R]). The American Diabetes Association has published a position statement on insulin administration ([3R]).

In a retrospective study of metabolic control in children and adolescents it was concluded that metabolic control improved with the use of two or more daily injections rather than one ([4cr]); three or four daily injections improved metabolic control when HbA1c was over 9% but worsened it when HbA_{1c} was below 7%. The duration of diabetes only had an effect in the first 5 years. The authors concluded that multiple injection therapy was most indicated for poor control or adolescents.

Hypoglycemia Workloads were performed by 10 patients with type 1 diabetes the day after hypoglycemia (2.3–2.7 mmol/l) had been induced for 1 h or after an identical period during which hypoglycemia was not induced ([5r]). The sense of well-being was affected but not cerebral function. Fatigue after hypoglycemia could not be explained by biochemical changes.

Pontine myelinolysis has been reported after a severe attack of hypoglycemia ([6C]).

A 24-year-old woman, whose diabetes was difficult to control and who had many secondary complications, had slurred speech and mild cerebellar ataxia of the limbs during a prolonged period of hypoglycemia. An MRI scan showed signs typical of the effects of central pontine myelinolysis. By 6 months her speech was normal but she still had some impairment on heel/toe walking.

Hypoglycemia in elderly people Attention has been paid to symptoms of hypoglycemia in elderly people in a study of 132 insulin-treated patients over 70 years ([7r]). Lightheadedness and unsteadiness were prominent symptoms. Neurological symptoms were more commonly reported and could be misinterpreted as cerebrovascular disease. Three separate groups of symptoms could be distinguished: (1) symptoms related to impairment of co-ordination and articulation; (2) neuroglycopenic symptoms; (3) autonomic symptoms.

Hypoglycemia in elderly people has been retrospectively studied from admissions over 3 years in a large Singapore hospital ([8c]). There were 45 cases, of which 13 were drug related (seven glibenclamide, one chlorpropamide, two tolbutamide, one insulin, one unknown, and one low caloric diet, in six cases combined with a missed meal); nine were due to diseases other than diabetes, and 23 to a combination of drug and disease (10 glibenclamide, five tolbutamide, one chlorpropamide, one glipizide, two insulin). The majority had

Side Effects of Drugs, Annual 22
J.K. Aronson, ed.

psychiatric diseases and poor diet. There were neuroglycopenic symptoms in 40 patients and adrenergic symptoms in five. One patient had an irreversible stroke and one suffered a fall.

There was no increase in incidence, severity, or unawareness of hypoglycemia in 46 older people with long-standing diabetes who were transferred from animal to human insulin compared with 48 patients who remained on animal insulin (9[c]).

Hypoglycemia in children In 150 children and adolescents (2–16 years), who took their insulin and evening meal at home (10[r]) and of whom 130 had conventional therapy, blood glucose was monitored every hour from 22:00 to 08:00 h. There was nocturnal hypoglycemia in 47% and about 50% were asymptomatic. Predictive values for hypoglycemia were a blood sugar under 5.3 mmol/l at dinner-time or under 6.8 mmol at 07:00 h. Values at 22:00 h had only weak predictive value. Other risk factors were two or more serious episodes of hypoglycemia, more than five blood glucose concentrations below 3.3 mmol/l during the last month, or an insulin dosage over 0.85 U/kg.

There were 287 hypoglycemic attacks (blood glucose below 3 mmol/l) during 3 months in 83 of 161 young patients who kept a diary; 81% were treated with multiple-dose therapy; 221 attacks were mild and two resulted in coma and/or convulsions (11[c]). Of the predominant symptoms 39% were classified as autonomic, 20% as neuroglycopenic, and 41% as non-specific. In children under 6 years autonomic symptoms were less common.

In 31 boys and 30 girls (2.6–8.5 years) taking conventional therapy (insulin twice a day) blood glucose was tested before the evening meal, before supper/bedtime, at 23:00 and 02:00 h, and before breakfast (12[r]). Blood glucose concentrations were below 3.5, 3.0, 2.5, and 2.0 mmol/l, respectively, in 38, 17, 13, and 8% of the children. In children aged 5 years or less, but not in the older group, the frequency of low blood glucose concentrations increased during the night. Carbohydrate intake during supper had no effect. The symptoms of nocturnal hypoglycemia were less well recognized when the children were young, in those with a low HbA_{1c}, and when hypoglycemia occurred at breakfast. A glucose determination at 23:00 h had little predictive value for subsequent hypoglycemia. The question of possible neurocognitive consequences of hypoglycemia was raised. The dangers of both hyperglycemia and hypoglycemia in young people were discussed in a parallel editorial (13[r]).

Immunological and hypersensitivity reactions A 63-year-old man with type 2 diabetes had a 5 year history of five to nine daily periods of anxiety, sweating, confusion, and weakness (14[Cr]). He had not taken hypoglycemic drugs during that time, although he had previously used insulin and tolazamide. His total insulin concentration was 1345 mU/l, his unbound insulin concentration 76 mU/l, and there was 77% insulin autoantibody binding. This prompted a study into the relation between insulin antibody concentrations and hypoglycemia in six patients. Two types of binding sites were found: high and low affinity; a high percentage saturation of low-affinity binding sites was related to a risk of hypoglycemia.

Urticaria occurred in a 22-year-old woman secondary to crystalline insulin during pump treatment after 8 years of treatment with recombinant NPH insulin; she could not be desensitized with porcine or human Actrapid insulin but she responded to lispro insulin (15[c]).

A 34-year-old obese woman with type 2 diabetes was treated for 6 months with human insulin and for 18 months with glibenclamide (glyburide) only. She required insulin but developed insulin allergy. Lispro caused a 50% less intensive wheal-and-flare response (16[c]). The IgE and IgG binding antibody titers fell within a year. In vitro lispro and human insulins showed complete cross-reactivity.

Local complications of insulin injection Further cases of *lipodystrophy* and other local complications of insulin injection have been reported.

Membranous lipodystrophy, consisting of two annular coin-sized depressed atrophic lesions, combined with insulin atrophy occurred in a 60-year-old woman (17[C]). A biopsy showed lobules of small adipocytes with capillaries, degenerative loss of adipose tissue, and multiple irregular cysts. She first used beef insulin and later purified pork insulin. She had not rotated the injection sites, although she had been advised to do so.

A 23-year-old man with a 20 year history of diabetes had had lipohypertrophy for 9 years (18[C]). Recombinant human insulin had not been effective. After transfer to lispro no new hypertrophy developed. This may have been due to the shorter action of lispro, but he also changed his night-time insulin from ultralente to Insulatard.

A 59-year-old woman who had used insulin for over a year developed pruritic patches that became minimally elevated plaques at injection sites (19[C]). Histology showed cellular infiltration with histiocytes and scattered Langerhans-type giant cells only in the dermis and not in the subcutis. She had been using a pen injection device with human insulin. When the same insulin was given by a conventional pen and needle no lesions occurred. The problem was solved by educating her to give deeper injections by vertical instead of angular insertion of the needle, in order to avoid intradermal injection.

A 30-year-old woman stopped using a continuous subcutaneous insulin infusion because of poor tolerance of the needles (20[C]). A small nodular erythematous lesion developed in the last needle site. The abscess grew over 8 weeks, despite antibiotic therapy, and *Mycobacterium peregrinum* was found.

In a follow-up of 548 implantable insulin pumps in 352 patients during 1180 patient years 84 patients had problems: local inflammation 35%, subcutaneous atrophy and skin erosion 44% (with temporary disconnection of the pump in 16%), chronic seromas 16%, and local infections 9.5% (21[r]).

Interactions It is a matter of debate whether *ACE inhibitors* aggravate or generate hypoglycemia in patients using hypoglycemic drugs. Over a period of 16 months there were 64 cases of serious hypoglycemia (42 with insulin, 22 with oral hypoglycemic drugs) among 6649 diabetic patients (22[Cr]). Seven had used ACE inhibitors. In a case–control comparison with other patients using ACE inhibitors, β-blockers, or calcium antagonists, there was an increased risk of hypoglycemia with ACE inhibitors (OR = 3.2; 95% CI 1.2, 8.3). However, this finding was debated, on the grounds that serum creatinine concentrations had been available in under 50% of cases (23[r]), that data on glycemic control and duration of diabetes had been missing (24[r]), and that in the EURODIAB Lisinopril trial there had been no effect of lisinopril on metabolic regulation (24[r]). The authors replied that clinical studies often do not include people at high risk (25[r]). An association between ACE inhibitors and hypoglycemia was also found in an earlier study (26[r]).

Insulin aspart

In insulin aspart the amino acid in the 28 position of the B-chain, proline, has been exchanged for aspartate. When three daily injections of human regular insulin were given as insulin aspart, blood glucose excursions during 24 h were reduced and there was less hypoglycemia (27[r]). However, control during the night was less good.

A modified-release formulation of insulin aspart has been made by binding it to protamine. A formulation containing 30% aspart and 70% modified-release aspart had a much faster metabolic effect in the first 4 h compared with a regular/NPH formulation (28[r]). After 8 h, when aspart insulin has lost its activity, the glucose lowering effect of the modified-release formulation was reduced. The efficacy of insulin aspart in regular treatment still has to be established.

Lispro insulin

Several papers have been published on lispro insulin, an analog in which the amino acids lysine at position 28 and proline at position 29 of the B-chain of insulin have switched positions. This insulin has a reduced tendency to aggregate, is more quickly absorbed, and acts more rapidly. Compared with other insulins it improves postprandial hyperglycemia (SEDA 21, 442). The frequency of severe hypoglycemic coma is reduced (29[r]), (30[r]). It can be given immediately before a meal with a high carbohydrate content or immediately after a meal with a high solid fat content (31[r]). However, owing to its shorter action, preprandial blood glucose concentrations (32[r]) and glucose concentrations during the night (33[r]) are often higher, which makes lispro less suitable. Extra administration of NPH insulin with reduction of lispro during lunch-time improves interprandial blood glucose control (34[r]). Frequent administration of long-acting insulin as an extra injection with lispro has been proposed (35[r]), but this increases the number of daily injections.

Lispro seems to be safe when used in pumps (36[r]). To reduce the tendency to an increased glucose concentration during the night, neutral protamine lispro (NPL) has been developed, but there were no major differences between NPL and NPH in the control of night-time hyperglycemia (37[r]).

In two adolescent children, aged 15 and 11 years, transferred to lispro insulin at breakfast and at dinner and to lispro plus intermediate insulin at lunch-time and intermediate insulin in the late evening, there was severe *hypoglycemia* before breakfast on three occasions (38[c]). Blood glucose concentrations were not measured before insulin injection; this means that a contribution from a pre-existing low blood glucose concentration cannot be excluded.

SULFONYLUREAS *(SED-13, 1297; SEDA-19, 395; SEDA-20, 398; SEDA-21, 443)*

The UKPDS did not find that the use of sulfonylureas increased sudden death, myocardial infarction, or diabetes-related deaths (1[R]).

Hypoglycemia The combination of reduced caloric intake, stimulation of insulin secretion, and the long half-life of the hypoglycemic effect of glibenclamide can result in hypoglycemia in older patients who develop intercurrent illnesses. Five patients developed serious hypoglycemia after starting to take glibenclamide in dosages of 2.5–7 mg/day (39[C]). Four patients died, but in three the main cause was the accompanying illness (sepsis, uremia, cirrhosis); one died from hypoglycemia.

A 71-year-old woman with congestive heart failure, chronic obstructive pulmonary disease, hyperthyroidism, hypercholesterolemia, type 2 diabetes, and a coronary artery bypass, became hypoglycemic and developed congestive cardiac failure and renal failure. She was taking glibenclamide 5 mg/day, enalapril 10 mg/day, levothyroxine 100 μg/day, and digoxin 125 μg/day (40[C]). It took 36 h to achieve a blood glucose concentration outside the hypoglycemic range, despite continuous glucose infusion and glucose boluses.

Renal insufficiency is accompanied by reduced insulin secretion and glibenclamide inactivation. It is not clear whether enalapril played a role in this case (see Interactions under Insulin above).

In a prospective study 52 patients with type 2 diabetes took placebo, glibenclamide 10 mg/day, and glibenclamide 20 mg/day sequentially for 1 week each, or glipizide GITS 10 mg/day and glipizide GITS 20 mg/day sequentially for 1 week each [GITS, glipizide gastrointestinal system, is a type of tablet that uses the principle of osmotic release to effect steady release over 24 h] (41[Cr]). They fasted for 23 h at the end of each week. There were no cases of hypoglycemia (glucose below 3.33 mmol/l). C-Peptide and adrenaline concentrations during fasting were increased in those who took glibenclamide. The authors concluded that older age is not a contraindication to sulfonylureas as long as other defects, such as heart, liver, or renal insufficiency, are excluded.

There was increased sensitivity to dosages of glibenclamide as low as 0.5 mg/day, leading to hypoglycemia in a family with MODY type 3 (caused by a mutation in the hepatic nuclear factor-1α gene) (42[c]).

Skin and appendages In a review of *photosensitization* by sulfonamide-derived drugs (43[R]) the author stated that photosensitivity reactions to sulfonylureas are very rare and have only been reported for four sulfonylureas: carbutamide, chlorpropamide, glibenclamide, and tolbutamide.

Interactions Of 29 patients taking glibenclamide who used *rifampicin* for 10 days, 17 developed uncontrollable diabetes, suggesting that rifampicin reduces the effect of glibenclamide (44[r]).

The reported effect of *ACE inhibitors* in exacerbating the effect of hypoglycemic drugs, mentioned above, involved patients taking oral therapy as well as insulin (22[Cr]).

BIGUANIDES *(SED-13, 1301; SEDA-19, 396; SEDA-20, 398; SEDA-21, 445)*

Metformin

Reviews of metformin (45[R])–(48[R]), (49[r]) and of metformin in combination with insulin (50[R]), (51[r]) have recently been published. The most frequent adverse effects are *gastrointestinal complaints*, sometimes leading to *deficiency of vitamin B_{12} and folic acid*. Metformin reduces bile salt resorption, leading to increased colonic bile salt concentrations, which contributes to the *liquidity of the stools* (52).

In the UKPDS study in 1704 patients with over 120% of their ideal body weight, metformin produced better results than the other therapies, with less hypoglycemia and less increase in body weight (53[C]). Both the general death rate and the death rate due to diabetes were lower when metformin was compared with diet only. It is not clear why the combination of metformin with glibenclamide caused a higher number of deaths than the other treatments.

Endocrine, metabolic The most serious adverse effect, lethal in about 50%, is *lactic acidosis*, for which abnormal renal or liver function or cardiac insufficiency and old age are high risk factors. Radiocontrast media can cause acute renal insufficiency in patients taking metformin (SEDA-20, 399; SEDA-21, 445; and see below).

Lactic acidosis occurred regularly in patients with type 2 diabetes before the introduction of metformin in the US, although much less often than in metformin users (54[r]). From May 1995, when metformin was introduced into the US, to June 1996 (14 months) the FDA received 66 reports of lactic acidosis in patients taking metformin; 47 were confirmed by serum lactate concentrations over 5 mmol/l (55[R]). There were one or more risk factors in 43: pre-existing cardiac disease (n = 30), renal disease (13, including two on dialysis), chronic pulmonary disease with hypoxia (n = 3), or over the age of 80 (n = 8); 20 patients died, but the four patients with no risk factors all recovered. The authors estimated that the incidence was five cases per 100 000 users (in Saskatchewan nine per 100 000).

Other anecdotal reports have appeared.

A 62-year-old woman on renal dialysis for 1 month was given metformin 500 mg bd by a physician who was unaware of her renal impairment; she survived (56[C]).

A 67-year-old man with cardiac failure who had been using O_2 and insulin, developed lactic acidosis after taking metformin 1000 mg bd for 15 weeks; he survived with dialysis (57[C]).

A 66-year-old man taking metformin 500 mg/day developed pneumonia and lactic acidosis (10.5 mmol/l) postoperatively and died; dialysis was not possible because his circulation was unstable (58[C]).

In a 71-year-old woman taking metformin 500 mg and enalapril 5 mg, lactic acidosis was precipitated by dehydration and a urinary tract infection (59[C]). The authors speculated that enalapril had contributed to the metabolic changes.

A 40-year-old woman had taken glibenclamide 10 mg bd, metformin 1000 mg bd, and lisinopril 5 mg/day (60[C]). The metformin was increased to 850 mg tds and 14 days later she developed respiratory distress. Her serum lactic acid concentration was 6.9 mmol/l (normal below 1.7), and there was no ketoacidosis. Her serum metformin concentration was 0.9 mg/l (within the target range). Her lactic acidosis resolved rapidly after the metformin had been withdrawn and was within the reference range on the third day; the lisinopril was continued.

Recently 13 cases of metformin intoxication in France have been studied (61[R]). The authors concluded that it was hemodynamic status and not metformin concentration that determined the degree and outcome of lactic acidosis. However, their conclusion that metformin can no longer be considered in itself a toxic drug was an overstatement. In certain circumstances, of which the physician is not always aware, metformin contributes to life-threatening toxic effects.

Skin and appendages An association between metformin and *lichen ruber planus* has been reported (62[c]).

A 35-year-old woman developed lichen ruber planus 2 weeks after she started to take metformin 1700 mg/day. It disappeared after metformin was withdrawn. She had a positive macrophage migration inhibiting factor test for metformin only.

Interactions The use of *radiographic contrast media* caused near-fatal lactic acidosis in a 68-year-old man taking metformin 850 mg bd (63[c]). Whether theophylline can prevent or treat this effect of contrast media is not clear (64[c]), (65).

Phenformin

Further reports of *lactic acidosis* due to phenformin have appeared.

A 64-year-old Haitian woman developed unexplained lactic acidosis four times (66[C]). On a fifth occasion it was discovered that for several years she had taken bidiab, an Italian drug that contains chlorpropamide 125 mg and phenformin 50 mg, which she had bought in Haiti without the knowledge of her physician. She died despite hemodialysis, insulin, sodium bicarbonate, and antibiotics.

Two men, aged 46 and 63 years, with renal insufficiency developed lactic acidosis while taking phenformin, which is still available in Italy; they survived (67[C]). The authors made a plea for the withdrawal of phenformin from all European countries (68).

ALDOSE REDUCTASE INHIBITORS *(SED-13, 1302; SEDA-19, 398; SEDA-20, 400; SEDA-21, 447)*

Tolrestat

Liver A 41-year-old woman taking tolrestat 200 mg/day developed hepatic symptoms without a history of previous hepatitis, hepatic enzyme changes, or alcohol abuse. Tests for hepatitis A, B, and C and for Epstein-Barr virus were negative. She was treated for 50 days and died 30 days after stopping treatment (69[C]). Tolrestat had poor efficacy in clinical trials and was withdrawn in October 1996 after reports of two other deaths from hepatic necrosis (70[r]).

α-GLUCOSIDASE INHIBITORS *(SED-13, 1302; SEDA-19, 397; SEDA-20, 399; SEDA-21, 446)*

Acarbose

Clinical experience with acarbose in the US has been reviewed (71[R]). Adverse effects caused more withdrawals among patients taking acarbose than placebo, but the percentage of patients who stopped taking placebo because of lack of effectiveness was greater. Most of the adverse effects were related to gastrointestinal symptoms: *abdominal discomfort*, *flatulence*, and *diarrhea*. The symptoms occurred early and gradually mitigated after 4–8 weeks. Rises in serum transaminases were comparable with acarbose and placebo; however, changes in transaminases occurred more often in people weighing more than 60 kg and taking dosages over 100 mg tds.

Liver *Rises in serum transaminases*, sometimes with rises in alkaline phosphatase, have been reported in several patients taking acarbose: a 51-year-old woman (72[c]), a 45-year-old man and a 54-year-old woman (73[C]). In the last two cases, there was no evidence of viral or autoimmune liver disease; both had normal transaminases 4 and 5 months after withdrawal of acarbose.

Serious hepatotoxicity has also been reported (74[c]).

A 40-year-old woman developed a tender liver and became icteric after taking acarbose 100 mg tds for 2 months. Her serum transaminases, alkaline phosphatase, and bilirubin were substantially increased but became normal 2.5 months after acarbose withdrawal. Rechallenge resulted in an increase in transaminases, which returned to normal 1 month after withdrawal.

Gastrointestinal In a multicenter study in 97 patients, 10 of 33 patients who took acarbose 100 mg tds had *gastrointestinal adverse effects* (75[r]).

In eight patients with type 2 diabetes acarbose reduced *carbohydrate malabsorption* by about 70% after 2–4 months (76[r]).

In an open 16-week study of acarbose in 91 patients with type 1 diabetes, the most frequent adverse effects were *flatulence* (43%), *diarrhea* (27%), *abdominal pain* (11%), and *flu-like symptoms* (9%); 16 patients withdrew because of adverse events, 13 while taking acarbose (77[r]). Other adverse effects were as reported in other studies. HbA_{1c} fell but increased again after the study. Insulin dosages remained the same, and there were no changes in lipids. There were no cases of serious hypoglycemia.

Interactions Acarbose can increase the availability of *warfarin* (78[C]).

Miglitol

There have been three recent studies of the effects of miglitol: miglitol 50–200 mg tds (n = 220) versus placebo (n = 120) (79[r]); miglitol 50–100 mg tds (n = 228) versus placebo (n = 117) for a year (80[r]); and miglitol 100 mg tds (n = 60) for 24 weeks in addition to insulin (81[c]). In all the studies miglitol caused *diarrhea* and *flatulence* and in the last study there were cases of mild *hypoglycemia*.

Voglibose

Voglibose is a new α-glucosidase inhibitor, which should be 20 times more potent than acarbose or miglitol in inhibiting small intestine disaccharides. When it was given to 14 of 27 patients, alone or in combination with glibenclamide, intrinsic insulin secretion was reduced and blood glucose concentrations were lower (82[Cr]). The rate of gastric emptying did not affect the efficacy of voglibose (83[c]).

THIAZOLIDINEDIONES *(SED-13, 1302; SEDA-19, 398; SEDA-20, 399; SEDA-21, 446)*

Thiazolidinedione drugs reduce insulin resistance by binding to an intracellular receptor, the peroxisome proliferator-activated receptor (PPAR), in adipose cells (84[R]), specifically PPAR-γ, activation of which results in the expression of adipocyte-specific genes and differentiation of various cell types in mature adipocytes capable of active glucose uptake and energy storage in the form of lipids (85[R]).

The effects of the long-term use of these drugs are not known (86[r]). In studies in which troglitazone (200–800 mg/day) has been substituted for other hypoglycemic drugs, added as a new drug (87[r]), or added to insulin (84[R]), (88[r]), a sulfonylurea (89[r]), or metformin (90[r]), HbA_{1c}, fasting blood glucose and insulin resistance were generally reduced. Adverse effects were dose related, but it was often not clear whether an adverse effect was caused by troglitazone or the combination. *Hypoglycemia* has been reported almost only in studies of a combination of drugs. There were temporary *reductions in mean erythrocyte count, hematocrit, and hemoglobin by 5%* (88[r]). Two patients became *hyperbilirubinemic and jaundiced* and one developed concomitant *congestive heart failure*. *Gastrointestinal complaints*, *gastric reflux*, and *anorexia* also occur.

Respiratory A 47-year-old man developed pleuropulmonary disease after taking troglitazone 200 mg bd for 1 week; it resolved 48 h after withdrawal (91[C]). All cultures were negative. There were no similar cases in the manufacturer's clinical trials database of over 2700 patients nor in postmarketing reports of adverse events in 1.3 million patients.

Liver The most important adverse effect of troglitazone is *liver insufficiency*, and deaths have been reported (92[C]). This has led to its withdrawal. Trials in Europe have been terminated (SEDA-20, 446) and US clinical trials have been reviewed (93[r]). Of 2510 patients, 48 (1.6%) had serum transaminase activities more than three times the upper limit of the reference range, compared with only three of 475 patients (0.6%) treated with placebo. Three more serious cases of liver damage have been reported recently (94[C]), (95[C]), although a causative relation has not clearly been proven. In many of the studies reported earlier some patients were withdrawn because of raised transaminases which later returned to normal, although sometimes similar rises are found with the same frequency in placebo-treated patients.

In 229 older patients (69–85 years) troglitazone 200–800 mg/day or placebo was added to the diet or substituted for other hypoglycemic drugs (96[r]). There were 65 withdrawals, 43 of them due to lack of efficacy or gastrointestinal symptoms. However, the latter was similar with placebo and troglitazone, and there were no major adverse effects. Changes in ALT and AST were more marked at the higher dosages.

Interactions Troglitazone interferes with the lipid-lowering action of *gemfibrozil* (97[r]). Although gemfibrozil binds to PPAR-α and troglitazone to PPAR-γ it may be that troglitazone binds to both PPARs.

MISCELLANEOUS DRUGS

Repaglinide

Repaglinide is a new oral hypoglycemic drug of the meglitidine family. Like the sulfonylureas, from which it differs in structure, it stimulates insulin secretion. It is well absorbed and has a half-life of less than 1 h. In a phase II multicenter trial for 12 weeks, after a run-in period of 6 weeks to adjust the dosage, 66 patients used repaglinide and 33 placebo (98[r]). Non-severe *hypoglycemia* was the most frequent adverse effect. Of 25 patients who did not complete the study, 10 of the 15 placebo users and three of 10 drug users withdrew because of ineffective therapy; other reasons was withdrawal were myocardial infarction (repaglinide) and foot ulcer (placebo).

REFERENCES

1. Turner RC, UK Prospective Diabetes Study Group (UKPDS). Intensive blood-glucose control with sulphonylureas or insulin compared with conventional treatment and risk of complications in patients with type II diabetes (UKPDS 33). Lancet 1998;352:8537–53.
2. Burge MR, Schade DS. Insulins. Endocrinol Metab Clin North Am 1997;26:575–98.
3. American Diabetes Association. Insulin administration. Diabetes Care 1997;209 (Suppl 1):S46–9.
4. Salardi S, Cacciari E, Zucchini S, Donati S, Steri L, Gualandi S, Mazzanti L, Calliva R. Modifications of metabolic control in type I diabetic childeren and adolescents: experience over the last 20 years. J Pediatr Endocrinol Metab 1997;10:569–78.
5. King P, Kong M-F, Parkin H, Macdonald IA, Tattersall RB. Well-being, cerebral function, and physical fatigue after nocturnal hypoglycemia in IDDM. Diabetes Care 1998;21:341–5.
6. Rajbhandari SM, Powell T, Davies-Jones GAB, Ward JD. Central pontine myelinolysis and ataxia: an unusual manifestation of hypoglycaemia. Diabetic Med 1998;15:259–61.
7. Jaap JA, Jones GC, McCrimmon RJ, Deary IJ, Frier BM. Perceived symptoms of hypoglycaemia in elderly type II diabetic patients treated with insulin. Diabetic Med 1998;15:398–401.
8. Teo SK, Ee CH. Hypoglycaemia in the elderly. Singapore Med J 1997;38:432–4.
9. Feldman S, Bonnemaire M, Elian N, Altman J-J, TRANSFERT study. Transferring aged type I diabetic patients from animal to human insulin. Diabetes Care 1998;21:196–7.
10. Beregszàszi M, Tubiana-Rufi N, Benali K, Noël M, Bloch J, Czernichow P. Nocturnal hypoglycemia in children and adolescents with insulin-dependent diabetes mellitus: prevalence and risk factors. J Pediatr 1997;131:27–33.
11. Tupola S, Rajantie J. Documented symptomatic hypoglycaemia in children and adolescents using multiple daily insulin injection therapy. Diabetic Med 1998;15:492–6.
12. Porter PA, Keating B, Byrne G, Jones TW. Incidence and predictive criteria of nocturnal hypoglycemia in young children with insulin-dependent diabetes mellitus. J Pediatr 1997; 130:366–72.
13. Sperling MA. The Scylla and Charybdis of blood glucose control in children with diabetes mellitus. J Pediatr 1997;130:339–41.
14. Kim MR, Sheeler LR, Mansharamani N, Haug MT, Faiman C, Gupta MK. Insulin antibodies and hypoglycemia in diabetic patients: can a quantitative analysis of binding predict the risk of hypoglycemia? Endocrine 1997;6:285–91.
15. Frigerio C, Aubry M, Gomez F, Graf I, Dayer E, de Kalbermatten R, Gaillard RC, Spertini F. Desensitization-resistant insulin allergy. Allergy Eur J Allergy Clin Immunol 1997;52:238–9.
16. Kumar D. Lispro Analog for treatment of generalized allergy to human insulin. Diabetes Care 1997;20:1357–9.
17. Kim KT, Ahn SK, Choi EH, Lee SH. Membranous lipodystrophy associated with insulin lipoatrophy. Int J Dermatol 1997;36:299–301.
18. Resolution of lipohypertrophy following change of short-acting insulin to insulin lispro (Humalog®). Diabetic Med 1998;15:1063–4.
19. Winkler G, Sápi Z, Pál B, Molnár L. Injection-site skin lesions following pen-injection treatment in a 59-year-old woman with insulin-treated type II diabetes mellitus. Diabetic Med 1997; 14:1078–9.
20. Pagnoux C, Nassie X, Bottard C, Timsit J. Infection of continuous subcutaneous insulin iunfusion site with *Mycobacterium peregrinum*. Diabetes Care 1998;21:191–2.
21. Bélicar P, Lassmann-Vague V, the EVADIAC Study Group. Local adverse events associated with long-term treatment by implantable insulin pumps. Diabetes Care 1998;21:325–6.
22. Morris AD, Boyle DIR, McMahon AD, Pearce H, Evans JMM, Newton RW, Jung RT, MacDonald TM, The DARTS/MEMO Collaboration. ACE inhibitor use is associated with hospitaliz-

ation for severe hypoglycemia in patients with diabetes. Diabetes Care 1997;20:1363–7.
23. Strachan MWJ, Frier BM. Risk of severe hypoglycemia in diabetic patients taking ACE inhibitors. Diabetes Care 1998;21:470.
24. Chaturvedi N, Fuller JH. ACE inhibitors and risk of hypoglycemia in people with diabetes. Diabetes Care 1998;21:470–1.
25. Morris AD, McMahon AD, Boyle DIR, Evans JMM, Newton RW, Jung RT, MacDonald TM, The DARTS/MEMO Collaboration. Response to Strachan and Frier and to Chaturvedi and Fuller. Diabetes Care 1998;21:471–2.
26. Herrings RMC, De Boer A, Stricker BHC, Leufkens HGM, Porsius A. Hypoglycaemia associated with the use of angiotensin-converting enzyme. Lancet 1996;345:1195–8.
27. Home PD, Lindholm A, Hylleberg B, Round P, UK Insulin Aspart Study Group. Improved glycemic control with insulin aspart. Diabetes Care 1998;21:1904–9.
28. Weyer C, Heise T, Heinemann L. Insulin aspart in a 30/70 premixed formulation. Diabetes Care 1997;20:1612–14.
29. Holleman F, Schmitt H, Rottiers R, Rees A, Symanowski S Anderson JH, The Benelux-UK insulin lispro study group. Reduced frequency of severe hypoglycemia and coma in well-controlled IDDM patients treated with insuli lispro. Diabetes Care 1997;20:1827–32.
30. Brunelle RJ, Llewelyn J, Anderson JH Jr, Gale EAM, Koivisto VA. Meta-analysis of the effect of insulin lispro on severe hypoglycemia in patients with type I diabetes. Diabetes Care 1998;21:1726–31.
31. Strachan MWJ, Frier BM. Optimal time of administration of insulin lispro. Diabetes Care 1998;21:26–31.
32. Bartsocas CS. A word of caution on the use of lispro. Diabetes Care 1998;21:462.
33. Ahmed ABE, Home PD. The effect of the insulin analog lispro on nighttime bloodglucose control in type I diabetic patients. Diabetes Care 1998;21:32–7.
34. Ahmed ABE, Home PD. Optimal provision of daytime NPH insulin in patients using the insulin analog lispro. Diabetes Care 1998;21:1707–14.
35. Del Sindaco B, Ciofetta M, Lalli C, Perriello G, Pampanelli S, Torlone E, Brunetti P, Bolli GB. Use of the short-acting insulin analogue lispro in intensive treatment of type I diabetes mellitus: importance of appropriate replacement of basal insulin and time-interval injection meal. Diabetic Med 1998;15:592–600.
36. Schmausz S, König A, Landgraf R. Human insulin analogue [lys(B28),pro(B29)]: the ideal pump insulin? Diabetic Med 1998;15:247–9.
37. Janssen MMJ, Casteleijn S, Devillé W, Popp-Snijders C, Roach P, Heine RJ. Nighttime insulin kinetics and glycemic control in type I diabetes patients following administration of an intermediate-acting lispro preparation. Diabetes Care 1997;20:1870–3.
38. Iafusco D, Angius E, Prisco F. Early preprandial hypoglycemia after administration of insulin lispro. Diabetes Care 1998;21:1777–8.
39. Carlsen SM. Sulfonylureaindusert hypoglykemi. En iatrogen og potensielt dodelig tilstand. Tidskr Nor Lægeforen 1997;117:3079–82.
40. Sills MN, Ogu CC, Maxa J. Prolonged hypoglycemic crisis associated with glyburide. Pharmacotherapy 1997;17:1338–40.
41. Burge MR, Schmitz-Fiorentino K, Fischette C, Qualls CR, Schade DS. A prospective trial of risk factors for sulfonylurea-induced hypoglycemia in type II diabetes. J Am Med Assoc 1998;279:137–43.
42. Søvik O, Njølstad P, Følling I, Sagen J, Cockburn BN, Bell GI. Hyperexcitability to sulphonylurea in MODY 3. Diabetologia 1998; 41:607–8.
43. Selvaag E. Photosensitivity to sulfonamide-derived oral antidiabetic and diuretic drugs. Dermatosen Beruf Umwelt 1997;45:56–9.
44. Surekha V, Peter JV, Jeyaseelan L, Cherian AM. Drug interaction: rifampicin and glibenclamide. Natl Med J India 1997;10:11–12.
45. Pugh J. Metformin monotherapy for type II diabetes. Adv Ther 1997;14:338–47.
46. Wildasin EM, Skaar DJ, Kirchain WR, Hulse M. Metformin, a promising oral antihyperglycemic for the treatment of noninsulin-dependent diabetes mellitus. Pharmacotherapy 1997;17:62–73.
47. Haupt E, Panten U. Metformin and its role in the management of type-2 diabetes. Med Klin 1997;92:472–9.
48. Guthrie R. Treatment of non-insulin-dependent diabetes mellitus with metformin. J Am Board Fam Pract 1997;10:213–21.
49. Garber AJ, Duncan TG, Goodman AM, Mills DJ, Rohlf JL. Efficacy of metformin in type II diabetes: results of a double-blind, placebo-controlled, dose-response trial. Am J Med 1997;103:491–7
50. Daniel JR, Hagmeyer KO. Metformin and insulin: is there a role for combination therapy. Ann Pharmacother 1997;31:474–80.
51. Pumar A, Losada F, Mangas MA, Acosta D, Astorga R. Adding metformin versus insulin dose increase in insulin-treated but poorly controlled type II diabetes mellitus: an open-label randomized trial. Diabetic Med 1998;15:997–1002.
52. Scarpello JHB, Hodgson E, Howlett HCS. Effect of metformin on bile salt circulation and intestinal motility in type II diabetes mellitus. Diabetic Med 1998;15:651–6.
53. UKPDS Group. Effect of intensive blood-glucose control with metformin on complications in overweight patients with type II diabetes (UKPDS 34). Lancet 1998;352:854–65.
54. Brown JB, Pedula K, Barzilay J, Herson MK, Latare P. Lactic acidosis rates in type II diabetes. Diabetes Care 1998;21:1659–63.
55. Misbin RI, Green L, Stadel BV, Gueriguian JL, Gubbi A, Fleming GA. Lactic acidosis in patients with diabetes treated with metformin. New Engl J Med 1998;338:265–6.

56. Schmidt R, Horn E, Richards J, Stamatakis M. Survival after metformin-associated lactic acidosis in peritoneal dialysis-dependent renal failure. Am J Med 1997;102:486–8.
57. Jurovich MR, Wooldridge JD, Force RW. Metformin-associated nonketotic metabolic acidosis. Ann Pharmacother 1997;31:53–5.
58. Mercker SK, Maier C, Neumann G, Wulf H. Lactic acidosis as a serious perioperative complication of antidiabetic biguanide medication with metformin. Anaesthesiology 1997;87:1003–5.
59. Franzetti I, Paolo D, Marco G, Emanuela M, Elisabetta Z, Renato U. Possible synergistic effect of metformin and enalapril on the development of hyperkaliemic lactic acidosis. Diabetes Res Clin Pract 1997;38:173–6.
60. Al-Jebawi AF, Lassman MN, Abourizk NN. Lactic acidosis with therapeutic metformin blood level in a low-risk diabetic patient. Diabetes Care 1998;21:1364–5.
61. Lalau JD, Mourlhon C, Bergeret A, Lacroix C. Consequences of metformin intoxication. Diabetes Care 1998;21:2036–7.
62. Azzam H, Bergman R, Friedman-Birnbaum R. Lichen planus associated with metformin therapy. Dermatology 1997;194:376.
63. Zandijk E, Demey HE, Bossaert LL. Lactic acidosis due to metformin. Tijdschr Geneeskd 1997;53:543–6.
64. Nolan DB. Theophylline option for attenuating contrast media-induced nephrotoxicity in patients on metformin. Am J Health Syst Pharm 1997;54:587–8.
65. Quasny H, Nolan DB. Metformin, contrast media and theophylilline. Am J Health Syst Pharm 1997;54:2007–8.
66. Rosand J, Friedberg JW, Yang JM. Fatal phenformin-associated acidosis. Ann Intern Med 1997;127:170.
67. Enia G, Garozzo M, Zoccali C. Phenformin induced lactic acidosis: an underestimated problem. G Ital Nefrol 1997;14:403–5.
68. Enia G, Garozzo M, Zoccali C. Lactic acidosis induced by phenformin is still a public health problem in Italy. Br Med J 1997;315:1466–7.
69. Foppiano M, Lombardo G. Worldwide pharmacovigilance systems and tolrestat withdrawal. Lancet 1997;349:399–400.
70. Anonymous. Tolrestat: hepatic necrosis. WHO Drug Inf 1997;11:21–2.
71. Coniff R, Krol A. Acarbose: a review of US clinical experience. Clin Ther 1997;19:16–26.
72. Anonymous. ADR reviews: two years on the Swedish market: acarbose. Bull SADRAC 1997:66.
73. Andrade RJ, Lucena M, Vega JL, Torres M, Salmerón FJ, Bellot V, García-Escaño D, Moreno P. Acarbose-associated hepatotoxicity. Diabetes Care 1998;21:2029–30.
74. Carrascosa M, Pascual F, Aresti S. Acarbose-induced acute severe hepatotoxicity. Lancet 1997;349:698–9.
75. Kovacevic I, Profozic V, Skrabalo Z, Cabrijan T, Zjacic-Rotkvic V, Goldoni V, Jovic-Paskvalin Lj. Crncevic-Orlic Z, Koseij M, Metelko Z. Multicentric clinical trial to assess efficacy and tolerability of acarbose (Bay G 5421) in comparison to glibenclamide and placebo. Diabetol Croat 1997;26:83–9.
76. Sobajima H, Mori M, Niwa T, Muramatsu M, Sugimoto Y, Kato K, Naruse S, Kondo T, Hayakawa T. Carbohydrate malabsorption following acarbose administration. Diabetic Med 1998;15:393–7.
77. Sels JPJE, Verdonk HER, Wolffenbutel BHR. Effects of acarbose (Glucobay) in persons with type I diabetes: a multicentre study. Diabetes Res Clin Pract 1998;41:139–45.
78. Morreale AP, Janetzky K. Probabale interaction of warfarin and acarbose. Am J Health Syst Pharm 1997;54:1551–2.
79. Johnston PS, Feig PU, Coniff RF, Krol A, Davidson JA, Haffner SM. Long-term titrated-dose alpha-glucosidase inhibition in non-insulin-requiring hispanic NIDDM patients. Diabetes Care 1998;21:409–15.
80. Johnston PS, Feig PU, Coniff RF, Krol A, Kelley DE, Mooradian AD. Chronic treatment of African-American type II diabetic patients with alpha-glucosidase inhibition. Diabetes Care 1998;21:416–22.
81. Mitrakou A, Tountas N, Raptis AE. Bauer RJ, Schulz H, Raptis SA. Long-term effectiveness of a new alpha-glucosidase inhibitor (BAY m1099-miglitol) in insulin-treated type II diabetes mellitus. Diabetic Med 1998;15:657–60.
82. Matsumoto K, Yano M, Miyake S, Ueki Y, Yamaguchi Y, Akazawa S, Tominaga Y. Effects of voglibose on glycemic excursions, insulin secretion and insulin sensitivity in non-insulin-treated NIDDM patients. Diabetes Care 1998;21:256–60.
83. Kawagishi T, Nishizawa Y, Taniwaki H, Tanaka S, Okuno Y, Inaba M, Ishimura E, Emoto M, Morii H. Relationship between gastric emptying and an alpha-glucosidase inhibitor effect on postprandial hyperglycemia in NIDDM patients. Diabetes Care 1997;20:1529–35.
84. Spiegelman BM. PPAR gamma: adipogenic regulator and thiazolidinedione receptor. Diabetes 1998;47:507–14.
85. Komers R, Vrana A. Thiazolidinediones—tools for the research of metabolic syndrome X. Physiol Res 1998;47:215–25.
86. Riddle MC. Learning to use troglitazone. Diabetes Care 1998;21:1389–90.
87. Horton ES, Whitehouse F, Ghazzi MN, Venable TC, Whitcomb RW. Troglitazone in combination with sulfonylurea restores glycemic control in patients with type II diabetes. The Triglitazone Study Group. Diabetes Care 1998;21:1462–9.
88. Schwartz S, Raskin P, Fonseca V, Graveline JF, Troglitazone, Exogenous Insulin Study Group. Effect of troglitazone in insulin-treated patients with type II diabetes mellitus. New Engl J Med 1998;338:861–6.
89. Buse JG, Gumbiner B, Mathias NP Nelson DM, Faja BW, Withcomb RW, Troglitazone use in insulin-treated type II diabetic patients. The

Troglitazone Study Group. Diabetes Care 1998; 21:1455–61.

90. Inzucchi SE, Maggs DG, Spollett GR, Page SL, Rife FS, Walton V, Shulman GI. Efficacy and metabolic effects of metformin and troglitazone in type II diabetes mellitus. New Engl J Med 1998;338:867–72.

91. Koshida H, Shibata K, Kametani T. Pleuropulmonary disease in a man with diabetes who was treated with troglitazone. New Engl J Med 1998;339:1400–1.

92. Anonymous. FDA Talk Paper. Patient labeling and testing strengthened for rezulin. US Department of Health and Human Services 1997.

93. Imura H. A novel antidiabetic drug, troglitazone—reason for hope and concern. New Engl J Med 1998;338:908–9.

94. Galin N, Julie NL, Spurr CL, Lim KM, Juarbe HM. Two cases of severe clinical and histological hepatotoxicity associated with troglitazone. Ann Intern Med 1998;129:36–8.

95. Neuschwander-Tetri BA, Isley WL, Oki JC, Ramrakhiani S, Quiason SG, Philips NJ, Brunt EM. Troglitazone induced hepatic failure leading to liver transplantation: a case report. Ann Intern Med 1998;129:38–41.

96. Kumar S. Prange A, Schulze J, Lettis S, Barnett AH. Troglitazone, an insulin action enhancer, improves glycaemic control and insulin sensitivity in elderly type II diabetes patients. Diabetic Med 1998;15:772–9.

97. Bell DSH, Ovalle F. Troglitazone interferes with gemfibrozil's lipid-lowering action. Diabetes Care 1998;21:2028–9.

98. Goldberg RB, Einhorn D, Lucas CP, Rendell MS, Damsbo P Huang W-C, Strange P, Brodows RG. A randomized placebo-controlled trial of repaglinide in the treatment of type II diabetes. Diabetes Care 1998;21:1897–903.

P. Coates

43 Miscellaneous hormones

CALCITONIN *(SED-13, 1307; SEDA-19, 402; SEDA-20, 402; SEDA-21, 451)*

Calcitonin is well established in the treatment of disorders of increased bone turnover, including Paget's disease and postmenopausal osteoporosis. Salmon calcitonin is more potent than human calcitonin, and the latter is reserved for patients with antibody-mediated resistance to salmon calcitonin (1[R]). If used continuously at high doses, its therapeutic effect is sustained for only a few months (SED-13, 1307). Clinical studies in osteoporosis extend to 2 years, and there is no information as to whether benefit is sustained beyond this.

The systemic availability of the intranasal formulation is 3% that of the subcutaneous form, and it is associated with a lower incidence of adverse effects. This difference may be dose related.

Adverse effects are usually mild (SED-13, 1308). *Flushing* and *nausea* are common and may be reduced by giving calcitonin at bedtime.

In a recent review (1[R]) it has been estimated that with subcutaneous calcitonin gastrointestinal effects (*nausea*, *cramps*, and *vomiting*) occur in 10% of patients, *dizziness and flushing* in 2–5%, and *injection site reactions* in 10%. Intranasal calcitonin is associated with local symptoms in 11–12%, including *rhinitis*, *dryness*, *sneezing*, and *epistaxis*.

An additional indication for calcitonin is as analgesia after pathological fracture due to osteoporosis or malignancy. Subcutaneous and intranasal calcitonin have been compared after vertebral crush fracture (2[C]). Both formulations were effective in relieving pain within 15 days but there were more *gastrointestinal adverse effects* in the subcutaneous group. One patient developed *neutropenia*, which was not severe and which resolved when treatment was withdrawn.

Interactions In a 2-year study of osteoporotic women treated with calcitonin in combination with nandrolone decanoate there was a negative interaction between the two agents, with a fall in lumbar spine bone mineral content, which was unexplained (3[C]).

GONADOTROPIN-RELEASING HORMONE (GnRH, GONADORELIN) *(SED-13, 1311; SEDA-19, 403; SEDA-20, 404; SEDA-21, 451)*

The effects of gonadorelin differ according to the duration of use. When given continuously, it first stimulates gonadotropin release, then inhibits it by down-regulation of hypophyseal receptors. Its therapeutic indications have been summarized previously (SED-13, 1311). In a recent randomized controlled trial of 415 patients, combined goserelin and radiotherapy improved survival in men with locally advanced prostate cancer compared with radiotherapy alone (4[C]). Adverse effects are the same for short-acting and depot formulations.

Nervous system *Headache* has been reported in up to a third of recipients (5[C]).

Psychiatric *Depression* has been infrequently reported. Four patients treated with leuprolide developed psychiatric disorders, including *panic disorder* and *depression* with and without psychotic features in one report (6[c]). These symptoms improved with sertraline.

Endocrine, metabolic Symptoms of hypo-

Side Effects of Drugs, Annual 22
J.K. Aronson, ed.

estrogenism occur in almost all women who receive long-term GnRH and include *hot flushes*, *vaginal dryness*, *reduced libido*, and *mood changes*. Men experience *reduced libido and impotence* in almost all cases, and *flushing* in 35–70% (7[R]). These often improve with continued treatment. *Testicular atrophy* is common after administration for more than 8 months. There has been one report of *increased prolactin concentrations* and *male-pattern alopecia* in five of 22 children treated with triptorelin (8[c]). *Pituitary apoplexy* (severe headache followed by pituitary hormone deficiency) has now been described in three elderly patients who had both prostate cancer and pituitary gonadotropinoma (9[c])–(11[c]).

Musculoskeletal Gonadorelin commonly causes *osteoporosis* in both sexes, mainly affecting trabecular bone. The treatment period in premenopausal women has been limited to 6 months for this reason, but is reversible if treatment is stopped after this period. In a randomized controlled trial of 40 women given leuprolide for endometriosis (12[C]), treatment with equine estrogen and medroxyprogesterone acetate relieved flushing and preserved bone density, without impairing the effectiveness of the treatment. A similar effect on vasomotor and bone adverse effects was achieved in a randomized trial of 29 patients with the synthetic estrogenic steroid tibolone (13[C]).

Immunological and hypersensitivity reactions Flare-ups in the activity of *systemic lupus erythematosus* have been reported in patients receiving ovulation induction, probably secondary to surges in estrogen concentrations (14[c]), (15[cr]). Only one case of hypersensitivity has been reported to date (SEDA-21, 451).

Tumor-modifying effects In patients with prostate cancer, biochemical tumor flare-up with an increase in tumor markers can be seen in all patients during the first 1–2 weeks of therapy. Symptoms, including *worsening bone pain*, *anorexia*, or *urinary obstruction*, occur in 10% of patients (7[R]). Gonadorelin is not recommended as monotherapy in patients with impending spinal cord compression or renal failure from metastases. To reduce the incidence of these life-threatening complications, pretreatment with androgen receptor blockers (e.g. flutamide, nilutamide, or bicalutamide) or drugs that suppress luteinizing hormone release (e.g., cyproterone acetate) has been used (7[R]).

HUMAN GROWTH HORMONE (hGH, SOMATOTROPIN) *(SED-13, 1307; SEDA-19, 402; SEDA-20, 402; SEDA-21, 451)*

The indications for treatment with recombinant human growth hormone continue to increase. It is well accepted as treatment in childhood growth hormone deficiency, Turner's syndrome, and chronic renal failure. Treatment should be begun before growth is severely limited in order to maximize final height, and it has been suggested that it should be continued even after target height has been reached, in order to maximize peak bone mass (SEDA-21, 451). Other well-studied indications include idiopathic short stature in children, adult growth hormone deficiency, osteoporosis, and critical illnesses and chronic wasting conditions. Treatment of children with Prader-Willi syndrome promoted linear growth, but there was no improvement in body composition, and the indication is experimental only (16[C]). A novel use for growth hormone still under investigation is the treatment of patients with chronic congestive heart failure. Short-term studies have shown hemodynamic improvements in small groups of patients (17[C]), (18[C]). However, in a controlled trial there was no survival benefit (19[C]).

Cardiovascular *Hypertension* and *peripheral edema* are commoner in adults and patients with adult onset hGH deficiency (20[C]), (21[C]), (22[R]) (SEDA-21, 452). Increased left ventricular thickness has been described in adults (SEDA-21, 453).

Nervous system *Carpal tunnel syndrome* is more frequent in adults than in children and appears to be dose related. Headache or visual disturbance early in treatment may be an early manifestation of *idiopathic intracranial hypertension* (pseudotumor cerebri), and requires further investigation. Children with chronic renal failure are at the highest risk (15/1670 treated patients), but it is also seen in other children (9/10 540) (23[R]), (24[C]). Most cases occur during the first 8 weeks of treatment, and withdrawal or dosage reduction gives complete resolution.

Endocrine, metabolic Glucose metabolism should be assessed regularly in all patients receiving hGH, as treated patients develop *hyperinsulinism* and *reduced insulin sensitivity* (21[C]), (25[C]). Although short-term studies of hGH-treated patients did not show an increased incidence of diabetes, in the KIGS database of 20 055 patients the incidence of type I diabetes was slightly higher and of type II diabetes three times higher than expected. This may represent earlier onset of diabetes rather than an increase in de novo cases (26[R]).

A randomized controlled trial of 173 patients has shown different effects on plasma lipids and body composition in growth hormone-deficient adults, depending on the age of onset of hormone deficiency (20[C]). The waist:hip ratio decreased in patients with adult-onset but not childhood-onset deficiency, and the ratio of HDL to total cholesterol increased more in the former group of patients. Adverse effects were mainly present in the adult-onset group.

Thyroid function tests are altered with increased conversion of T_4 to T_3: this is not clinically significant at low dosages (SEDA-21, 453).

Growth hormone increases plasma and urinary calcium with a concomitant slight fall in parathyroid hormone concentrations, probably via IGF-1-mediated increase in 1,25-dihydroxyvitamin D (27[C]), (28[C]). In most patients this is not clinically significant, although it may account for *increases in bone mass* in short-term trials of hGH in osteoporosis.

Prepubertal *gynecomastia* is rarely seen in boys treated with hGH, with only 30 cases reported to date. In elderly men, gynecomastia was more frequent in patients with IGF-1 concentrations above 1.0 U/ml (26[R]).

Mineral and fluid balance There has been one report of *hypercalcemia* in a patient with AIDS (29[c]), which resolved after hGH was withdrawn.

Hematological In patients treated with hGH 44 new cases of *leukemia* have now been reported (24[C]). However, only 12 of these patients had no other risk factors, and this was no higher than the expected population incidence. Groups of patients at higher risk include those with a past history of craniopharyngioma or cranial irradiation. There is no increase in tumor recurrence in treated patients, despite the potential mitogenic action of hGH (SEDA-21, 452). It is still suggested, however, that where there is a pre-existing malignancy treatment be delayed for 1 year after tumor therapy is finished (26[R]).

Musculoskeletal *Myalgia and arthralgia* are commoner in patients with adult-onset hGH deficiency and are probably dose related.

Slipped capital femoral epiphysis has been reported in 0.27–0.57 cases per 1000 treatment years (26[R]), about three to four times the expected incidence in an age-matched population. The risk is significantly increased in children who have previously been given chemotherapy or radiotherapy for leukemia. Girls with Turner's syndrome, renal failure, and idiopathic hGH deficiency are also at increased risk. Children with unfused epiphyses who develop pain or limping require further investigation (30[R]).

Pre-existing *scoliosis* progressed rapidly in six of 250 children who received hGH in a recent study (31[C]). Most of them had accelerated growth rates at the time of diagnosis. Previous spinal radiation may have been an additional risk factor.

Risk Factors *Age* Adverse effects differ in adults and children and have been summarized before (SEDA-21, 453). In adults adverse effects are more commonly reported in patients with adult onset growth hormone deficiency, heavier patients, and those with the greatest increases in IGF-1 and IGFBP-3 after 1 month of therapy (SEDA-21, 452; 21[C]). These patients received the highest dose of hGH, as it is calculated according to body weight, but efficacy was no different. The ideal dose regimen for adult patients is still being evaluated. Adverse effects are often transient, are more common with rapid dosage escalation, and are reversible after dosage reduction. To minimize adverse effects it is recommended that treatment be started at a low dose, i.e., approximately 1 IU/day, increase upwards by approximately 0.5 IU/month, and titrate according to the age-specific normal IGF-1 concentration (32[C]). In general, the dosage should not exceed 3.0 IU/day in young adults or 2.0 IU/day in middle-aged and elderly patients (22[R]).

GROWTH HORMONE RELEASE-INHIBITING HORMONE (SOMATOSTATIN) AND ANALOGS *(SED-13, 1309; SEDA-19, 403; SEDA-20, 403; SEDA-21, 453)*

Somatostatin has several sites of action, including as a neurotransmitter, as a regulator for hGH and thyrotropin release, in the gastrointestinal tract and pancreas, and as an immune modulator. Synthetic analogs have longer half-lives and have been selected to have a greater effect on growth hormone secretion relative to the native hormone, while attempting to minimize other effects. The indications have been summarized before (SEDA-21, 453).

Octreotide, an octapeptide analog of somatostatin, has been available for several years. Lanreotide (33[C]), (34[C]) and a modified-release version of octreotide (35[C]) have now been studied in patient groups for up to 3 years. Injection is once every 10–14 days for lanreotide or every 4 weeks for modified-release octreotide, compared with three times daily for octreotide. The indications for longer-acting analogs appear to be identical to octreotide. Adverse effects are common early in treatment but usually resolve spontaneously after the first 10–14 days.

Endocrine, metabolic *Slight increases in plasma glucose and glycated hemoglobin* have been noted, but did not reach clinical significance (33[C]), (36[C]). Conversely, *hypoglycemia* has been reported in a few patients (37[R]).

Biliary *Gallstones* occur in up to 40% of patients due to reduced gall-bladder contractility (SEDA-21, 453) (38[C]), and are more common in some racial groups, particularly the Chinese. However, only 1% become symptomatic per year of treatment.

Gastrointestinal *Nausea, abdominal cramps, diarrhea,* and *flatulence* are common at the start of treatment but usually subside within 10–14 days despite continued treatment. *Gastritis* has occasionally been described during long-term treatment with octreotide (37[R]). The therapeutic effects of octreotide on the gastrointestinal tract also lessen over time.

Skin and appendages *Loss of scalp hair* has been reported in patients treated with octreotide (39[c]) or its modified-release form (35[C]). This was transient in one patient.

Use in pregnancy Under 15 patients world wide have been treated with octreotide during pregnancy. There is maternal–fetal transfer of octreotide, presumed to be by diffusion across the placenta (40[c]). One patient treated with octreotide during pregnancy had a child with an *imperforate anus* (37[R]).

THYROTROPIN-RELEASING HORMONE (PROTIRELIN, TRH) *(SED-13, 1311; SEDA-20, 404; SEDA-21, 454)*

Use in pregnancy Early studies of TRH therapy suggested better neonatal survival in women at risk of preterm delivery. However, a large randomized trial failed to confirm this, and also showed a significant increase in *hypertension* in the treated group (41[C]). A rapid *increase in blood pressure* without tachycardia during TRH infusion responded to hydralazine (42[c]). In 1042 infants from the ACTOBAT study who were assessed at 12 months of age there were minor but consistent *delays in motor and social development* (43[C]).

VASOPRESSIN (ANTIDIURETIC HORMONE) AND ANALOGS
(SED-13, 1310; SEDA-19, 403; SEDA-20, 403; SEDA-21, 454)

Vasopressin has both antidiuretic and vasoconstrictor properties. Its short half-life necessitates continuous administration or frequent dosing, and several longer-acting analogs have been developed, including terlipressin (triglycyl-lysine vasopressin).

Desmopressin (*N*-deamino-8-D-arginine vasopressin, ddAVP) has little vasoconstrictor effect but potent antidiuretic action. It also has significant hemostatic properties, although the mode of action is not understood. Adverse effects include mild *flushing* and *headache* in up to 30% of patients (SEDA-21, 454). Systemic availability in the oral form is low (0.1–0.2%) compared with the intranasal form (3–5%), although the oral form has been studied in patients with enuresis (44[C]). The use of ddAVP in von Willebrand's disease has recently been reviewed (45[R]). Adverse effects are usually mild and include *flushing*, mild *tachycardia*, and *headache* in up to 30% of patients. *Tachyphylaxis* may develop after prolonged continuous use, due to depletion of stored clotting factors (SEDA-21, 454).

Cardiovascular Desmopressin should be used with caution with elderly patients with significant atherosclerosis, as a few cases of *myocardial infarction* and *stroke* have been reported in hemophiliac and uremic patients (45[R]). There are also reports of *reversible myocardial ischemia* secondary to terlipressin (SEDA-21, 454; 46[C]).

Mineral and fluid balance *Hyponatremia*, which may be severe enough to cause seizures in some patients, can occur if water intake is not controlled after administration of either vasopressin or its analogs. Infants, unconscious patients, and those receiving intravenous fluids need to be monitored carefully (47[cr]), (48[c]), (49[c]).

Skin and appendages *Gangrene* and *skin necrosis* have been reported in a few cases. A warning sign may be a white line over the injection site (50[cr]).

REFERENCES

1. Sewell KL. Calcitonin. J Clin Rheumatol 1997; 3 (Suppl 2):S40–5.
2. Combe B, Cohen C, Aubin F. Equivalence of nasal spray and subcutaneous formulations of salmon calcitonin. Calcif Tissue Int 1997;61:10–15.
3. Flicker L, Hopper JL, Larkins RG, Lichtenstein M, Buirski G, Wark JD. Nandrolone decanoate and intranasal calcitonin as therapy in established osteoporosis. Osteoporosis Int 1997;7:29–35.
4. Bolla M, Gonzalez D, Warde P, Dubois JB, Mirimanoff R-O, Storme G, Bernier J, Kuten A, Sternberg C, Gil T, Collette L, Pierat M. Improved survival in patients with locally advanced prostate cancer treated with radiotherapy and goserelin. New Engl J Med 1997;337:295–300.
5. Donnez J, Vilos G, Gannon MJ, Stampe-Sorensen S, Klinte I, Miller RM. Goserelin acetate (Zoladex) plus endometrial ablation for dysfunctional uterine bleeding: a large randomized, double-blind study. Fertil Steril 1997;68:29–36.
6. Warnock JK, Bundren JC. Anxiety and mood disorders associated with gonadotropin-releasing hormone agonist therapy. Psychopharmacol Bull 1997;33:311–16.
7. Sharifi R, Ratanawong C, Jung A, Wu Z, Browneller R, Lee M. Therapeutic effects of leuprorelin microspheres in prostate cancer. Adv Drug Deliv Rev 1997;28:121–38.
8. Kauschansky A, Lurie R, Ingber A. Hair loss in children on long-acting gonadotropin-releasing hormone agonist triptorelin treatment. Acta Dermatol Venereol 1997;77:333.
9. Morsi A, Jamal S, Silverberg JDH. Pituitary apoplexy after leuprolide administration for carcinoma of the prostate. Clin Endocrinol 1996; 44:121–4.
10. Ando S, Hoshino T, Mihara S. Pituitary apoplexy after goserelin. Lancet 1995;345:458.
11. Chanson P, Schaison G. Pituitary apoplexy caused by GnRH-agonist treatment revealing gonadotroph adenoma. J Clin Endocrinol Metab 1995;80:2267–8.
12. Grigoriou O, Konidaris S, Vitoratos N, Papadias C, Papoulias I, Chryssicopoulos A. Gonadotropin-releasing hormone analogue plus hormone replacement therapy for the treatment of endometriosis: a randomized controlled trial. Int J Fertil Women's Med 1997;42:406–11.
13. Taskin O, Yalcinoglu AI, Kucuk S, Uryan I, Buhur A, Burak F. Effectiveness of tibolone on

hypoestrogenic symptoms induced by goserelin treatment in patients with endometriosis. Fertil Steril 1997;67:40–5.

14. Metcalfe W, Boulton-Jones JM. Exacerbation of lupus nephritis in association with leuprorelin injection for uterine leiomyoma. Nephrol Dial Transplant 1997;12:1699–700.
15. Huong DL, Wechsler B, Piette J-C, Arfi S, Gallinari C, Darbois Y, Frances C, Godeau P. Risks of ovulation-induction therapy in systemic lupus erythematosus. Br J Rheumatol 1996; 35:1184–6.
16. Hauffa BP. One-year results of growth hormone treatment of short stature in Prader-Willi syndrome. Acta Paediatr 1997;423 (Suppl):63–5.
17. Fazio S, Sabatini D, Capaldo B, Vigorito C, Giordano A, Guida R, Pardo F, Biondi B, Sacca L. A preliminary study of growth hormone in the treatment of dilated cardiomyopathy. New Engl J Med 1996;334:809–14.
18. Volterrani M, Desenanzi P, Lorusso R, D'Aloia A, Manelli F, Giustina A. Haemodynamic effects of intravenous growth hormone in congestive heart failure. Lancet 1997;349:1067–8.
19. Osterziel KJ, Strohm O, Schuler J, Friedrich M, Hanlein D, Willenbrock R, Anker SD, Poole-Wilson PA, Ranke MB, Dietz R. Randomised, double-blind, placebo-controlled trial of human recombinant growth hormone in patients with chronic heart failure due to dilated cardiomyopathy. Lancet 1998;351:1233–7.
20. Attanasio AF, Lamberts SWJ, Matranga AMC, Birkett MA, Bates PC, Valk NK, Hilsted J, Bengtsson B-A, Strasburger CJ, Charbonnel B, Chiumello G, Fossati P, Lokkgaard N, Jung RT, Scriba PC, Trygstad OE, Webb S, Wuster C. Adult growth hormone (GH)-deficient patients demonstrate heterogeneity between childhood onset and adult onset before and during human GH treatment. J Clin Endocrinol Metab 1997;82:82–8.
21. Chipman JJ, Attanasio AF, Birkett MA, Bates PC, Webb S, Lamberts SWJ. The safety profile of GH replacement therapy in adults. Clin Endocrinol 1997;46:473–81.
22. De Boer H, Van Der Veen E. Guidelines for optimizing growth hormone replacement therapy in adults. Horm Res 1997;48 (Suppl 5):21–30.
23. Koller EA, Stadel BV, Malozowski SN. Papilledema in 15 renally compromised patients treated with growth hormone. Pediatr Nephrol 1997; 11:451–4.
24. Blethen SL, Allen DB, Graves D, August G, Moshang T, Rosenfeld R. Safety of recombinant deoxyribonucleic acid-derived growth hormone: The National Cooperative Growth Study experience. J Clin Endocrinol Metab 1996;81:1704–10.
25. Heptulla RA, Boulware SD, Caprio S, Silver D, Sherwin RS, Tamborlane WV. Decreased insulin sensitivity and compensatory hyperinsulinemia after hormone treatment in children with short stature. J Clin Endocrinol Metab 1997; 82:3234–8.
26. Frisch H. Pharmacovigilance: the use of KIGS (Pharmacia and Upjohn International Growth Database) to monitor the safety of growth hormone treatment in children. Endocrinol Metab 1997;4 (Suppl B):83–6.
27. Wei S, Tanaka H, Kubo T, Ono T, Kanzaki S, Seino Y. Growth hormone increases serum 1,25-dihydroxyvitamin D levels and decreases 24,25-dihydroxyvitamin D levels in children with growth hormone deficiency. Eur J Endocrinol 1997; 136:45–51.
28. Wright NM, Papadea N, Wentz B, Hollis B, Willi S, Bell NH. Increased serum 1,25-dihydroxyvitamin D after growth hormone administration is not parathyroid hormone-mediated. Calcif Tissue Int 1997;61:101–3.
29. Sakoulas G, Tritos NA, Lally M, Wanke C, Hartzband P. Hypercalcemia in an AIDS patient treated with growth hormone. AIDS 1997; 11:1353–6.
30. Blethen SL, MacGillivray MH. A risk-benefit assessment of growth hormone use in children. Drug Saf 1997;17:303–16.
31. Wang ED, Drummond DS, Dormans JP, Moshang T, Davidson RS, Gruccio D. Scoliosis in patients treated with growth hormone. J Pediatr Orthop 1997;17:708–11.
32. Johansson G, Rosen T, Bengtsson B-A. Individualized dose titration of growth hormone (GH) during GH treatment of hypopituitary adults. Clin Endocrinol 1997;47:571–81.
33. Giusti M, Gussoni G, Cuttica CM, Giordano G, Camanni F, Ciccarelli E, Dallabonzana D, Strada S, Delitala G, Porcu L, Faglia G, Arosio M, Liuzzi A, Ghiggi MR. Effectiveness and tolerability of slow release lanreotide treatment in active acromegaly: six-month report on an Italian multicenter study. J Clin Endocrinol Metab 1996;81:2089–97.
34. Caron P, Morange-Ramos I, Cogne M, Jaquet P. Three-year follow-up of acromegalic patients treated with intramuscular slow-release lanreotide. J Clin Endocrinol Metab 1997;82:18–22.
35. Flogstad AK, Halse J, Bakke S, Lancranjan I, Marbach P, Bruns C, Jervell J. Sandostatin LAR in acromegalic patients: long-term treatment. J Clin Endocrinol Metab 1997;82:23–8.
36. Ippoliti C, Champlin R, Bugazia N, Przepiorka D, Neumann J, Giralt S, Khouri I, Gajewski J. Use of octreotide in the symptomatic management of diarrhea induced by graft-versus-host disease in patients with hematologic malignancies. J Clin Oncol 1997;15:3350–4.
37. Van Der Lely AJ, de Herder WW, Lamberts SWJ. A risk-benefit assessment of octreotide in the treatment of acromegaly. Drug Saf 1997; 17:317–24.
38. Cheung NW, Taylor L, Boyages SC. An audit of long-term octreotide therapy for acromegaly. Aust New Zealand J Med 1997;27:12–18.
39. Nakauchi Y, Kumon Y, Yamasaki H, Tahara K, Kurisaka M, Hashimoto K. Scalp hair loss caused by octreotide in a patient with acromegaly: a case report. Endocr J 1995;42:385–9.

40. Caron P, Gerbeau C, Pradayrol L. Maternal-fetal transfer of octreotide. New Engl J Med 1995;333:601–2.
41. Crowther CA, Hiller JE, Haslam RR, Robinson JS, Giles W, Gill A, and 13 other authors. Australian Collaborative Trial of Antenatal Thyrotropin-releasing Hormone (ACTOBAT) for prevention of neonatal respiratory disease. Lancet 1995;345:877–81.
42. Tan ASA, Hsu C-D, Marder S, Copel JA. Is maternal thyrotropin releasing hormone administration safe in the pregnant woman with preeclampsia? Am J Perinatol 1997;14:5–6.
43. Crowther CA, Hiller JE, Haslam RR, Robinson JS, Giles W, Gill A, et al. (70 authors). Australian Collaborative Trial of Antenatal Thyrotropin-Releasing Hormone: adverse effects at 12-month follow-up. Pediatrics 1997;99:311–17.
44. Janknegt RA, Zweers HMM, Delaere KPJ, Kloet AG, Khoe SGS, Arendsen HJ, De Pagter GF, Leenarts JAF, Nijman JM, Simoons HA, Tummers RFHM, van Capelle JW, van Weel TF, Vegt PDJ, Vrijhof HJEJ, Ypma AFGVM. Oral desmopressin as a new treatment modality for primary nocturnal enuresis in adolescents and adults: a double-blind, randomized, multicenter study. J Urol 1997;157:513–17.
45. Mannucci PM. Treatment of von Willebrand's disease. J Intern Med 1997;242 (Suppl 740):129–32.
46. Cervoni J-P, Lecomte T, Cellier C, Auroux J, Simon C, Landi B, Gadano A, Barbier J-P. Terlipressin may influence the outcome of hepatorenal syndrome complicating alcoholic hepatitis. Am J Gastroenterol 1997;92:2113–14.
47. Robson WLM, Norgaard JP, Leung AKC. Hyponatremia in patients with nocturnal enuresis treated with DDAVP. Eur J Pediatr 1996; 155:959–62.
48. Schwab M, Ruder H, Hyponatremia and cerebral convulsion due to DDAVP administration in patients with enuresis nocturna or urine concentration testing. Eur J Pediatr 1997;156:668.
49. Robson WLM, Shashi V, Nagaraj S, Norgaard JP. Water intoxication in a patient with the Prader-Willi syndrome treated with desmopressin for nocturnal enuresis. J Urol 1997;157:646–7.
50. Lin R-Y, Du S-L, Yeh H-S, Wang W-M. Vasopressin-induced amber-like skin necrosis. Dermatology 1997;195:271–3.

I. Aursnes

44 Drugs affecting lipid metabolism

FIBRATES *(SED-13, 1324; SEDA-18, 426; SEDA-19, 407)*

The frequency of adverse effects with the newly developed micronized fenofibrate is comparable with the frequency with the usual formulation. In 7235 patients with dyslipidemia of types IIa, IIb, or IV, treated with micronized fenofibrate 200 mg/day for 12 weeks, 335 adverse events were reported by a total of 289 patients (4%) (1[R]). The most frequently reported adverse events were those affecting the digestive system (2%), followed by adverse events associated with the skin and appendages (0.7%), nervous system (0.5%), or the body as a whole (0.5%). A total of 34 adverse events (10% of all adverse events) were classified as serious. Three of the serious events were reported to be possibly related to the study drug (two cases of *cholelithiasis*, one case of *jaundice*). In another study of 1334 patients in the same review, there was one case of *epistaxis* with concomitant oral anticoagulant therapy, two episodes of *acute pancreatitis*, and one of *hepatitis*. Hepatic enzyme activities were increased in under 2% of 1334 patients in another series after 6 months of treatment (1[R]).

Skin *Photosensitivity* is a problem with the fibrates (SEDA-21, 458) and there is cross-reactivity between ketoprofen and fenofibrate, believed to be due to chemical similarities between these two drugs (2[C]).

Risk factors *Hypothyroidism* predisposes to rhabdomyolysis in patients taking hypolipidemic drugs and it has been suggested that one should screen thyroid function before starting therapy (SEDA-21, 458). This has been recently supported by a report of thyroid myopathy in a 69-year-old man taking fenofibrate 200 mg/day, when his hyperthyroidism was treated with radioiodine (3[c]).

Interactions Acute renal insufficiency has been seen in a 29-year-old man taking ciprofibrate 100 mg and *ibuprofen* 400 mg (4[c]). Both drugs are highly protein bound and contain propionic acid groups; ibuprofen may therefore displace ciprofibrate.

Several interactions of *warfarin* with hypolipidemic drugs have been described (SEDA-21, 459). This now also includes a clinically important potentiation of bezafibrate by warfarin (5[C]).

HMG COENZYME-A REDUCTASE INHIBITORS (STATINS) *(SED-13, 1327; SEDA-19, 408; SEDA-20, 408; SEDA-21, 459)*

Musculoskeletal Symptoms, predominantly *stiffness and tenderness of proximal limb muscles* and *difficulty in rising from a low chair*, can develop within a month of starting statin therapy and most cases develop within 3 months. Most patients recover after withdrawal. Sometimes a corticosteroid is needed to reverse the *myopathy*. In a 42-year-old man muscle biopsies showed that the myopathy was at least partly due to an inflammatory reaction (6[C]).

Skin and appendages A case of *ichthyosiform eruptions* on the abdomen and back was observed in a 42-year-old Korean woman after 3 months of lovastatin therapy and disappeared on withdrawal (7[c]).

Side Effects of Drugs, Annual 22
J.K. Aronson, ed.

Interactions With the exception of fluvastatin and pravastatin, the statins are metabolized by CYP3A4. Other drugs metabolized by this enzyme can greatly enhance the concentrations of statins in the body and can thereby precipitate rhabdomyolysis, for example the macrolide antibiotic erythromycin (SED-13, 1328). This has now also been observed when patients taking long-term statins were given a course of the similar drugs *clarithromycin* and *azithromycin* (8[C]). It has also been observed with the antidepressant *nefazodone* (9[c]). Other drugs that are metabolized by CYP3A4, such as cimetidine, have not been reported to cause this effect.

Cyclosporin also increases the risk of rhabdomyolysis, the risk varying from statin to statin. This effect is at least partly due to differences in kinetic interactions. For example, cyclosporin increased the AUC of pravastatin (20 mg/day) 5-fold and the AUC of lovastatin (20 mg/day) 20-fold (10[C]). Furthermore, lovastatin accumulated during steady-state therapy and pravastatin did not.

Hepatotoxicity is another problem when various drugs are combined. In one study of 389 patients, combined pravastatin or simvastatin with gemfibrozil or ciprofibrate for 29 months in patients with refractory familial combined hyperlipidemia, five patients (1.3%) were withdrawn because their transaminase activities were increased more than 3-fold. The investigators concluded that rare drug-induced reversible hepatotoxicity calls for close monitoring (11[C]).

Potassium-depleting diuretics, but not indapamide, have been reported to attenuate the effect of lovastatin on blood lipid concentrations (12[C]).

INDIVIDUAL STATINS

Although there may be differences in the degree of interaction with, for instance, cyclosporin (see above), the general impression is that the frequencies of adverse effects connected with the various statins are the same.

Atorvastatin *((SEDA-20, 409)*

There was no difference in adverse effects in 177 patients randomized for 52 weeks to either simvastatin or atorvastatin (13[C]).

Musculoskeletal *Myopathy* has not been reported in patients taking atorvastatin, but experience with it has been limited (14[R]). *Myalgia* was reported in 3% of the atorvastatin group in one study of 133 patients, but no patient had persistent increases in creatine phosphokinase activity over 10 times the normal limit (14[R]).

Special senses After 1 year of treatment with atorvastatin, there was no evidence of lens opacities.

Interactions Mean prothrombin times fell slightly in 12 patients taking maintenance *warfarin* who took atorvastatin 80 mg/day for 2 weeks, but only during the first few days (15[C]). Thus, atorvastatin had no consistent effect on the *anticoagulant activity* of warfarin and adjustments in warfarin dosing should not be necessary.

Cerivastatin

Cerivastatin is the most potent statin mg for mg. Rhabdomyolysis, myoglobinemia, and acute renal insufficiency have not been reported, but it has only recently been introduced. Serum aminotransferase activities rose more than 3-fold in under 1% of patients, a figure similar to that found with other statins (16[R]). In other respects too the tolerability of this drug is similar to that of other statins (17[R]).

Fluvastatin *(SEDA-19, 408; SEDA-20, 409; SEDA-21, 460)*

Experience with fluvastatin in over 1800 patients treated for an average of 61 weeks has shown it to be safe and well tolerated (SEDA-19, 408).

Musculoskeletal There have been no reports of myopathy with fluvastatin in any studies. Some cases of *myalgia* have been reported, mainly after exercise, but the increases in creatine kinase were less than 3-fold, rather than the 10-fold change that is used to define myopathy (SEDA-19, 408). There are, however, good reasons to believe that myopathy is a class effect and should be expected even with this drug. Indeed, of 85 spontaneous reports about fluvastatin in Australia in 1996, 30 described muscle disorders (18[c]).

Interactions Three patients who had taken warfarin and fluvastatin 20 mg/day for 1–2 weeks had raised international normalized ratios (19[C]).

Simvastatin *(SED-13, 1329; SEDA-18, 428)*

Skin and appendages A hypersensitivity *purpura-like eruption* occurred in a 62-year-old man with cirrhosis of the liver who took simvastatin 20 mg/day (20[c]).

Interactions Severe *rhabdomyolysis* occurred in a 52-year-old woman who took a combination of gemfibrozil and simvastatin (21[c]).

NICOTINIC ACID DERIVATIVES

Niacin *(SED-13, 1329)*

A wide range of adverse effects have been reported with niacin (22[R]). In a recent comparison of modified-release with normal-release niacin in 29 men with hyperlipidemia and coronary artery disease, there were differences in tolerability but not in adverse effects (23[C]). The men took daily regular niacin 1 g, lovastatin 40 mg, and colestipol 20 g for 1 year, followed by two random-sequence crossover phases (8 months each) alternating regular with modified-release niacin. Compliance was significantly higher with modified-release niacin (95 vs 85%). The modified-release niacin was preferred by 21 patients and the regular niacin by four. There were no differences in uric acid, glucose, or insulin concentrations or aspartate aminotransferase activities. The two niacin formulations did not differ in extent of toxicity.

MISCELLANEOUS DRUGS

Probucol

Altogether 16 cases of *tachydysrhythmias*, especially *torsade de pointes*, have been reported in association with probucol, 15 in women; prolongation of the QT interval is seen (SEDA-21, 460). Since the Probucol Quantitative Regression Swedish Trial (PQRST) showed no improvement in lumen volume of the femoral artery in patients given probucol plus cholestyramine compared with those given cholestyramine alone, doubts have been raised about its efficacy (24[R]).

REFERENCES/

1. Adkins JC, Faulds D. Micronised fenofibrate: a review of its pharmacodynamic properties and clinical efficacy in the management of dyslipidaemia. Drugs 1997;54:615–33.
2. Leroy D, Dompmartin A, Szczurko C, Michel M, Louvet S. Photodermatitis from ketoprofen with cross-reactivity to fenofibrate and benzophenones. Photodermatol Photoimmunol Photomed 1997;13:93–7.
3. Schlienger JL, Goichot B, Grunenberger F, Pradignac A. Revelation d'une myopathie thyroidienne par un fibrate. Rev Med Interne 1997; 18:169–70.
4. Ramachandran S, Giles PD, Hartland A. Acute renal failure due to rhabdomyolysis in presence of concurrent ciprofibrate and ibuprofen treatment. Br Med J 1997;314:1593.
5. Beringer TRO. Warfarin potentiation with bezafibrate. Postgrad Med J 1997;73:657–8.

6. Giordano N, Senesi M, Mattii G, Battisti E, Villanov M, Gennari C. Polymyositis associated with simvastatin. Lancet 1997;349:1600–1.
7. Soeong-Jea-Jeong, Young-Tae-Kim. A case of acquired ichthyosis developed during cholesterol-lowering treatment. Korean J Dermatol 1997; 35:546–50.
8. Grunden JW, Fisher KA. Lovastatin-induced rhabdomyolysis possibly associated with clarithromycin and azithromycin. Ann Pharmacother 1997;31:859–63.
9. Jacobson RH, Wang P, Glueck C J, Jody DN. Myositis and rhabdomyolysis associated with concurrent use of simvastatin and nefazodone. J Am Med Assoc 1997;277:296–7.
10. Olbricht C, Wanner C, Eisenhauer T, Kliem V, Doll R, Boddaert M, O'Grady P, Krekler M, Mangold B, Christians U. Accumulation of lovastatin, but not pravastatin, in the blood of cyclosporine-treated kidney graft patients after multiple doses. Clin Pharmacol Ther 1997; 62:311–21.
11. Athyros VG, Papageorgiou AA, Hatzikonstandinou HA, Didangelo TP, Carina MV, Kranitsas DF, Kontopoulos AG. Safety and efficacy of long-term statin-fibrate combinations in patients with refractory familial combined hyperlipidemia. Am J Cardiol 1997;80:608–13.
12. Aruna AS, Akula SK, Sarpong DF. Interaction between potassium-depleting diuretics and lovastatin in hypercholesterolemic ambulatory care patients. J Pharm Technol 1997;13:21–6.
13. Dart A, Jerums G, Nicholson G, D'Emden M, Hamilton-Craig I, Tallis G, Best J, West M, Sullivan D, Bracs P, Black D. A multicenter, double-blind, one-year study comparing safety and efficacy of atorvastatin versus simvastatin in patients with hypercholesterolemia. Am J Cardiol 1997;80:39–44.
14. Lea AP, McTavish D. Atorvastatin. A review of its pharmacology and therapeutic potential in the management of hyperlipidaemias. Drugs 1997;53:828–47.
15. Stern R, Abel R, Gibson GL, Besserer J. Atorvastatin does not alter the anticoagulant activity of warfarin. J Clin Pharmacol 1997;37:1062–4.
16. Anonymous. Cerivastatin for hypercholesterolemia. Med Lett Drugs Ther 1998;40:13–14.
17. McLellan KJ, Wisemann LR, McTavish D. Cerivastatin. Drugs 1998;55:415–20.
18. Anonymous. WHO Drug Information 1997; 11:68.
19. Kline SS, Harrell CC. Potential warfarin-fluvastatin interaction. Ann Pharmacother 1997; 31:790.
20. Horiuchi Y, Maruok H. Petechial eruptions due to simvastatin in a patient with diabetes mellitus and liver cirrhosis. J Dermatol 1997;24:549–51.
21. Tal A, Rajeshawari M. Isley W. Rhabdomyolysis associated with simvastatin-gemfibrozil therapy. South Med J 1997;90:546–7.
22. Britton ML, Bradberry JC, Letassy NA, McKenney JM, Sirman SM. ASHP therapeutic position statement on the safe use of niacin in the management of dyslipidemias. Am J Health Syst Pharm 1997;54:2815–19.
23. Brown B G, Bardsley J, Poulin D, Hillger LA, Dowdy A, Maher V M G, Zhao XQ, Albers JJ, Knopf RH. Moderate dose three-drug therapy with niacin, lovastatin, and colestipol to reduce low-density lipoprotein cholesterol <100 mg/dl in patients with hyperlipidema and coronary artery disease. Am J Cardiol 1997;80:111–15.
24. Sasich LD, Sukkar SR. Probucol—lack of efficacy and market withdrawals. Saudi Pharm J 1997;5:72–3.

Andrew Stanley

45 Cytostatic drugs

Author's note: *The wide range of cytostatic drugs, the multitude of their toxic effects, and the fact that they are generally used in combinations of several agents all make it impossible to provide as detailed an overview of adverse reactions in this field as the annual gives in others. For this reason, in this chapter I present only salient points that appear to provide entirely new data, or increase the understanding of known but uncommon adverse effects. I have paid particular attention to incidents in which it seems possible to attribute particular effects to individual agents. Because of the methods used to identify toxic effects for inclusion, far fewer potential sources of information have been reviewed; thus, the information in this year's chapter may not be as comprehensive as in some previous years.*

Finally, I should like to thank those clinicians and researchers who have sent me copies of their original research papers.

While cancer is not being cured with existing cytostatic drugs (and in certain cases many combinations have been tested), some researchers are examining the effects of different doses or dosage schedules on both responses and toxic effects. For example, vinorelbine toxicity, but not efficacy, can be reduced by using a continuous infusion (1[C]). Some authors have studied a particular toxic effect, such as cardiovascular complications across the complete range of chemotherapeutic agents (2[C]), whilst others have reviewed the effect of a single agent (for example, megestrol acetate (3[C])) across a number of toxic effects. Yet others have taken a particular patient population and considered the use and toxic effects of chemotherapy in that population; of particular note are several articles on cancer in the elderly in volumes of *Clinics in Geriatric Medicine* (4), (5).

The effect of busulfan plasma concentration on the outcome of transplantation from HLA identical family members for the treatment of chronic myelogenous leukemia has been studied in 45 patients, who received busulfan 16 mg/kg orally and cyclophosphamide 120 mg/kg intravenously (6[C]). The mean steady-state plasma busulfan concentration was 917 ng/ml (range 642–1749; median 917 ng/ml). Of patients with a steady-state plasma busulfan concentration below the median, seven developed persistent relapse, of whom three died. There were no relapses in patients with plasma busulfan concentrations above the median. The authors concluded that low plasma busulfan concentrations are associated with an increased risk of relapse.

CARDIOVASCULAR

Anthracyclines It is well documented that anthracyclines cause *heart failure*. The etiology and clinical course are extremely variable, and so it is preferable that cardiotoxicity be detected early and preferably by non-invasive measures. Thoracic electrical bioimpedance cardiography has been used for such a purpose (7[C]).

Patients with low doxorubicin exposure (mean dose less than 300 mg/m^2) have been shown to have a *lower stroke index* and *higher heart rate* for any given value of oxygen uptake, despite normal resting systolic function, compared with age-matched controls 5 years after low-dose therapy (8[C]). This has confirmed a previous result (9[C]).

Fluorouracil Fluorouracil *cardiotoxicity* has been reviewed (10[R]). The consensus is that cardiotoxicity with fluorouracil is much more common and clinically significant than has previously been thought.

Side Effects of Drugs, Annual 22
J.K. Aronson, ed.

Chest pain and electrocardiographic changes diagnostic of *acute cardiac ischemia* occurred in a 67-year-old man with no cardiac history, who had been given intravenous fluorouracil; he was subsequently discovered to have otherwise asymptomatic coronary artery disease (11[c]). The authors reinforced the message that an association between fluorouracil and myocardial ischemia should be made sooner rather than later, so as to avoid potentially fatal consequences.

RESPIRATORY

Carmustine The risk factors for *idiopathic pneumonia syndrome* after high-dose chemotherapy for relapsed Hodgkin's disease have been further defined (12[C]). The chances of death are related to the total dose of carmustine, the threshold dose being 475 mg/m^2. Above this dose women are at significantly greater risk than men.

Methotrexate A significant *reduction in oxygen transfer factor* has been reported in 16 low-risk patients receiving methotrexate 50 mg intravenously, four doses per cycle for a mean of 7.5 cycles; three of the patients had pleuritic chest pain and dyspnea (13[C]).

NERVOUS SYSTEM

The *neurotoxicity* of the combination of docetaxol and cisplatinum was more severe than either alone at similar doses in 55 patients, 29 of whom had measurable neurotoxicity, which correlated significantly with the cumulative doses of both drugs (14[C]).

ENDOCRINE, METABOLIC

Clinical *adrenal insufficiency* developed in 13 of 89 patients who had taken oral megestrol acetate 160 mg/day for advanced breast cancer; the mean time to onset was 17 months (15[C]).

HEMATOLOGICAL

A predictive model for radiotherapy-associated *neutropenia* and *thrombocytopenia* has been proposed (16[R]). Because radiotherapy is now an integral part of the multimodality treatment of cancer, this type of work is of use in helping to predict possible additive or cumulative toxic effects.

The relation between hematological toxicity (*leukopenia*) and survival (distant disease-free survival and overall survival) has been studied in 211 patients with node-positive stage II and III breast cancer treated with eight cycles of cyclophosphamide, doxorubicin, and ftorafur, with and without tamoxifen (17[C]). Patients with a lower leukocyte nadir during chemotherapy had significantly better survival, suggesting that the leukocyte nadir is a biological marker of the efficacy of chemotherapy. The authors suggested that this presents the possibility of establishing an optimal dose for each patient.

Chlorodeoxyadenosine Of 16 patients with hairy cell leukemia treated with 2-chlorodeoxyadenosine, five had severe *neutropenic infections* and/or required prolonged blood transfusion; patients with low tumor mass and moderate cytopenias were more likely to achieve complete remission, whereas those with high tumor burden and severe bone-marrow impairment during treatment were at increased risk of severe infections and blood transfusion requirements (18[C]). Since all of these unfavorable features can be corrected by short-term therapy with interferon-α, the authors suggested that such patients might benefit from interferon-α before being given 2-chlorodeoxyadenosine.

Hydroxyurea Fatal *thrombotic microangiopathy* occurred in a 57-year-old woman with chronic myelogenous leukemia taking hydroxyurea alone (19[c]).

URINARY SYSTEM

Contrary to popular opinion, the severity of the *nephrotoxicity* precipitated by ifosfamide and commonly experienced by children was not altered by the dosage schedule in 16 children given either 9 g/m^2 as a 72-h continuous infusion or 3 g/m^2 over 1 h on three consecutive days (20[C]).

SKIN AND APPENDAGES

Ten cases of *eccrine squamous syringometaplasia* have been reported during or after pretransplant high-dose chemotherapy and have been highlighted as alternative reactions to the erythematous reactions associated with graft-versus-host disease (21[C]).

A case of the self-limiting inflammatory dermatosis *neutrophilic eccrine hidradenitis* has been reported in a 43-year-old patient treated with cytarabine, daunorubicin, and thioguanine for acute myelogenous leukemia (22[c]). The authors suggested that it was due to accumulation of the chemotherapeutic drugs in the secretary epithelia of the sweat glands.

SPECIAL SENSES

Paclitaxel The previously fairly rare effect of *dry eyes* (grade 3) has been reported in 3% of 36 patients who received single-agent paclitaxel 225 mg/m^2 over 3 h (23[C]).

MUSCULOSKELETAL

Paclitaxel Grade 3 *bone pain* occurred with an incidence of 22% in 36 patients who received single-agent paclitaxel 225 mg/m^2 over 3 h (23[C]).

SEXUAL FUNCTION

Cyclophosphamide Intramuscular testosterone, 100 mg intramuscularly every 15 days, prevented the azoospermia induced by cyclophosphamide in five men with the nephrotic syndrome, compared with 10 who did not receive testosterone (24[C]). The men received cumulative doses of cyclophosphamide of between 27 and 36 g over 6–8 months.

TUMOR-INDUCING EFFECTS

Fludarabine In a 72-year-old man with chronic lymphocytic leukemia, who was given fludarabine 25 mg/m^2 for 5 days for relapsed chronic lymphocytic leukemia, there was a *flare-up of scalp lesions of squamous cell carcinoma*, which had initially been noted 4 years before (25[c]). The lesions were multiple and grew rapidly. The authors suggested that the flare-up and exacerbation of the lesions had been triggered by fludarabine, which suppresses T lymphocytes.

REFERENCES

1. Gasco M, Gardin G, Repetto L, Campora E, Rosso R. Vinorelbine as palliative therapy in advanced breast cancer. Anticancer Res 1997; 17:1431–4.
2. Ferrari E, Taillan B, Morand P, Baudouy M. Cardiovascular complications of anticancer chemotherapy. Sang Throm Vaiss 1996;8:112–18.
3. Strang P. The effect of megestrol acetate on anorexia, weight loss and cachexia in cancer and AIDS patients. Anticancer Res 1997;17:657–62.
4. Cancer in the elderly. Part I. Clin Geriatr Med 1997;13(1).
5. Cancer in the elderly. Part II. Clin Geriatr Med 1997;13(2).
6. Slattery JT, Clift RA, Buckner CD, Radich J, Storer B, Bensinger WI, Soll E, Anasetti C, Bowden R, Bryant E, Chauncey T, Deeg HJ, Doney KC, Flowers M, Gooley T, Hansen JA, Martin PJ, McDonald GB, Nash R, Petersdorf EW, Sanders JE, Schoch G, Stewart P, Storb R, Appelbaum FR, et al. Marrow transplantation for chronic myeloid leukemia: the influence of plasma busulfan levels on the outcome of transplantation. Blood 1997;89:3055–60.
7. Massidda B, Fenu MA, Ionta MT, Tronci M, Foddi MR, Montaldo C, Montaldo PL. Early detection of the anthracycline induced cardiotoxicity. A non-invasive haemodynamic study. Anticancer Res 1997;17:663–8.
8. Johnson D, Perrault H, Fournier A, Leclerc JM, Bigras JL, Davignon A. Cardiovascular responses to dynamic submaximal exercise in chil-

dren previously treated with anthracyclines. Am Heart J 1997;133:169–73.
9. Lipshultz SE, Colan SD, Gelber RD, Perez Atayde AR, Sallan SE, Sanders SP. Late cardiac effects of doxorubicin therapy for acute lymphoblastic leukemia in childhood. New Engl J Med 1991;324:808–15.
10. Anand A. Fluorouracil cardiotoxicity. Ann Pharmacother 1994;28:374–8.
11. Farooqi IS, Aronson JK. Iatrogenic chest pain: a case of 5-fluorouracil cardiotoxicity. Q J Med 1996;89:953–5
12. Rubio C, Hill ME, Milan S, O'Brien ME, Cunningham D. Idiopathic pneumonia syndrome after high dose chemotherapy for relapse Hodgkin's disease. Br J Cancer 1997;75:1044–8.
13. Gillespie AM, Lorigan PC, Radstone CR, Waterhouse JC, Coleman RE, Hancock BW. Pulmonary function in patients with trophoblastic disease treated with low-dose methotrexate. Br J Cancer 1997;7:1382–6.
14. Hilkens PH, Pronk LC, Verweij J, Vecht CJ, Van Putten WL, Van Den Bent MJ. Peripheral neuropathy induced by combination chemotherapy of docetaxel cisplatin. Br J Cancer 1997;75:417–22.
15. Subramanian S, Goker H, Kanji A, Sweeney H. Clinical adrenal insufficiency in patients receiving megestrol therapy. Arch Intern Med 1997; 157:1008–11.
16. MacManus M, Lamborn K, Khan W, Varghese A, Graef L, Knox S. Radiotherapy associated neutropenia and thrombocytopenia: analysis of factors and development of a predictive model. Blood 1997;89:2303–10.
17. Saarto T, Blomqvist C, Rissanen P, Auvinen A, Elomaa I. Haematological toxicity: a marker of adjuvant chemotherapy in stage II and III breast cancer. Br J Cancer 1997;75:301–5.
18. Legrand O, Vekhoff A, Marie JP, Zittoun R, Delmer A. Treatment of hairy cell leukaemia (HCL) with 2-chlorodeoxyadenosine (2-CdA): identification of parameters predictive of adverse effects. Br J Haematol 1997;99:165–7.
19. Shammas F, Meyer P, Heikkila R, Apeland T, Goransson L, Berland J, Kjellevold K. Thrombotic microangiopathy in a patient with chronic myelogenous leukemia on hydroxyurea. Acta Haematol 1997;97:184–6.
20. English MW, Skinner R, Pearson AD, Price L, Wyllie R, Craft AW. The influence of ifosfamide scheduling on acute nephrotoxicity in children. Br J Cancer 1997;75:1356–9.
21. Valks R, Fraga J, Porras-Luque J, Figuera A, Garcia-Diez A, Fernandez-Herrera J. Chemotherapy-induced eccrine squamous syringometaplasia: a distinctive eruption in patients receiving hematopoietic progenitor cells. Arch Dermatol 1997;133:873–8.
22. Brehler R, Reimann S, Bonsmann G, Metze D. Neutrophilic hidradenitis induced by chemotherapy involves eccrine and apocrine glands. Am J Dermatopathol 1997;19:73–8.
23. Gore ME, Rustin G, Slevin M, Gallagher C, Penson R, Osborne R, Ledermann J, Cameron T, Thompson JM. Single-agent paclitaxel in patients with previously untreated stage IV epithelial ovarian cancer. London Gynaecological Oncology and North Thames Gynaecological Oncology Groups. Br J Cancer 1997;75:710–14.
24. Masala A, Faedda R, Alagna S, Satta A, Chiarelli G, Rovasio PP, Ivaldi R, Taras MS, Lai E, Bartoli E. Use of testosterone to prevent cyclophosphamide-induced azoospermia. Ann Intern Med 1997;126:292–5.
25. Davidovitz Y, Ballin A, Meytes D. Flare-up of squamous cell carcinoma of the skin following fludarabine therapy for chronic lymphocytic leukemia. Acta Haematol 1997;98:44–6.

Sameh K. Morcos and Peter Brown

46 Radiological contrast agents

Intravascular radiological contrast agents include iodinated water-soluble contrast agents used for X-ray imaging, gadolinium-based contrast agents for magnetic resonance imaging (MRI), and contrast agents that can be used to enhance the diagnostic information provided by ultrasound imaging. Oral contrast agents based on barium sulfate suspension are widely used for imaging the gastrointestinal tract; adverse reactions to these agents are rare.

Four different classes of iodinated contrast media for X-ray imaging are currently available: high osmolar ionic monomers, low osmolar ionic dimers, low osmolar non-ionic monomers, and iso-osmolar non-ionic dimers. Adverse reactions to iodinated contrast media are few and serious reactions are uncommon.

For MRI there are high osmolar ionic and low osmolar non-ionic contrast agents. Clinical experience so far suggests that they have even better tolerance and safety profiles than iodinated contrast agents. MRI is being increasingly used for abdominal imaging, and various agents are being evaluated to provide suitable bowel contrast. However, satisfactory bowel contrast requires the ingestion of a large volume of contrast agent, which patients can find difficult to tolerate. Furthermore, positive bowel contrast agents (e.g., oral gadolinium chelates) are not as useful as negative contrast agents, as bowel peristalsis can cause hyperintense ghost artefacts, reducing image quality. Negative contrast agents are increasingly popular and include perflubron (SEDA-21, 484), oral magnetic particles and barium sulfate.

Ultrasound contrast agents use microbubbles to provide acoustic enhancement and are extremely safe.

INTRAVASCULAR IODINATED CONTRAST AGENTS *(SED-13, 1391; SEDA-19, 425; SEDA-20, 416; SEDA-21, 476)*

Modern iodinated water-soluble contrast agents differ in osmolarity and viscosity but all have essentially the same pharmacokinetics. Most adverse reactions to contrast media are either idiosyncratic or toxic, although some reactions are difficult to categorize so specifically. Toxic effects of contrast media are more likely to occur in patients who are debilitated or medically unstable, such as those with renal impairment or severe cardiovascular or respiratory diseases.

Incidence of reactions Acute reactions to contrast media can be divided into minor, intermediate, and severe life-threatening reactions. The minor reactions include *flushing*, *nausea*, *arm pain*, *pruritus*, *vomiting*, *headache*, and *urticaria*. They are usually mild in severity, of short duration, and self-limiting; they generally require no specific treatment. The incidence of these reactions to high osmolar contrast media is 5–15%.

Intermediate reactions are more serious degrees of the above effects, plus moderate degrees of *hypotension* and *bronchospasm*. They usually respond to appropriate therapy. The incidence of these reactions to high osmolar contrast media is about 1–2%.

Severe life-threatening reactions include severe manifestations of all of the above effects, plus *convulsions*, *coma*, *laryngeal edema*, *severe bronchospasm*, *pulmonary edema*, *severe cardiac dysrhythmias and arrest*, and *cardiovascular and pulmonary collapse*. The incidence of serious reactions with high osmolar contrast media is around 0.06–0.4%. Reactions to low osmolar contrast media are about five times less common than reactions to high osmolar agents.

An analysis of safety reports received by

Side Effects of Drugs, Annual 22
J.K. Aronson, ed.

the FDA from 1990 to 1994 on reactions to contrast media has shown that the incidence (per million examinations) comparing high with low osmolar agents was 194 vs 44 for all reactions, 37 vs 11 for severe reactions and 3.9 vs 2.1 for fatal reactions (1[Cr]). When high osmolar agents were compared with ioxaglate (a low osmolar ionic dimer) the incidence of total reactions was higher (194 vs 143), the incidence of severe reactions was almost the same (37 vs 34), and the incidence of fatal reactions was lower (3.9 vs 6.4). Although the introduction of new low osmolar agents has caused an overall reduction in the number of contrast reactions, there has been no definite reduction in fatal reactions. A review of fatal reactions with ionic and non-ionic media reported to the UK Committee on Safety of Medicines from 1963 to 1991 also failed to show any statistically significant difference in the incidence of deaths associated with ionic compared with non-ionic media (1[Cr]).

A study conducted by the Society of Cardiovascular and Interventional Radiology in over 60 000 patients showed that overall adverse events and events requiring treatment after the administration of contrast media were significantly more common with high osmolar contrast agents, with the exception of arterial interventional procedures (2[Cr]). Serious adverse events were not different between the two classes of agents, except for cardiac procedures. A previous reaction to contrast media was the most important risk factor in predicting an adverse event. This study had similar findings to the previous report. The results suggest that there are statistically significant differences between high and low osmolar contrast agents. These differences are most marked when all adverse events related to contrast media are considered. They are less apparent with events for which treatment is necessary and are absent (except in cardiac and interventional procedures) with serious events related to contrast media. The authors concluded that low osmolar contrast agents offer statistically significant advantages in certain situations and little or no advantage in others. They suggested that high-risk patients (those with a history of previous reactions to contrast media or those with NYHA Class III or IV congestive heart failure) and patients undergoing certain cardiac intervention procedures will benefit from the use of low osmolar contrast agents. Other patients without risk factors and those who undergo arterial intervention procedures are unlikely to benefit from the use of low osmolar contrast agents (2[Cr]).

Another study from the US in 2166 patients has shown that the universal use of low osmolar contrast agents would not eliminate the risks of contrast-related reactions in cardiac angiography. The results suggested that there is a definite advantage in using low osmolar rather than high osmolar agents only in relation to mild reactions. The authors concluded that high osmolar contrast agents are reasonably safe in patients with stable left main coronary artery disease (i.e. without pulmonary edema, angina, or significant dysrhythmias), but that low osmolar agents should be used in unstable patients (3[C]).

At a time when reductions in the costs of medical care are critical, decisions about which class of contrast media to use are not determined purely on clinical grounds but by a consideration of the cost:benefit ratio. Concern about financial implications has been the major factor in preventing the universal conversion to non-ionic contrast agents, which are better tolerated. However, an assessment of the cost and potential benefits of making this change in radiology departments in the UK has shown no increase in cost and a lower incidence of adverse reactions with non-ionic low osmolar contrast media (2.7%) compared with high osmolar agents (17%). This was mainly because substantial discounts on the price of low osmolar contrast media can be negotiated by bulk ordering (4[C]).

Delayed reactions Delayed reactions to both ionic and non-ionic media are much more common than has previously been appreciated. Most reactions are not serious or life threatening, and include *flu-like illness*, *parotitis*, *nausea and vomiting*, *abdominal pain*, and *headache*. Delayed *allergy-like reactions* with skin reactions to non-ionic dimers have also been reported. Delayed reactions to iso-osmolar dimers are twice as common as delayed reactions to low osmolar non-ionic monomers and are higher in Japan and the US than in Europe (by a factor of two). The pathophysiology of these delayed reactions is unknown.

Adverse reactions after the intravenous administration of contrast media during CT examination has been evaluated in 472 Japanese patients who received ioxaglate (a low osmolar ionic dimer) and 512 who received iopamidol (a low osmolar non-ionic monomer). Immediate reactions (within 1 h of injection) occurred in 6.4% of the patients given iopamidol and in 24% of those given ioxaglate; there was no significant difference in the incidence of delayed reactions (occurring more than 1 h after the injection) between the two groups (17% for ioxaglate and 15% for iopamidol) (5[C]). However, it was not clear for how long the patients were monitored for delayed reactions, and it is possible that the incidence of delayed adverse effects may have been underestimated. Previous reports have suggested that some adverse reactions may be delayed for several days after the administration of contrast media. Delayed adverse reactions may occur in as many as 20% of injected patients, a higher incidence than that of immediate reactions. The prevalence of delayed skin reactions is 0.42–3.4%.

Cardiovascular The molecular toxicity and physicochemical characteristics of these agents, i.e., osmolality, viscosity, hydrophilicity, calcium binding properties, and sodium content, account for some of their cardiovascular adverse effects.

Contrast media, particularly the ionic agents, are vasoactive, and clinical observations have suggested that they can induce vasodilatation in most vascular beds, with the exception of the kidney, in which there is sustained vasoconstriction. There has been a report of *peripheral vasoconstriction* attributed to diatrizoate, a high osmolar agent (6[c]).

A 74-year-old man with intermittent claudication underwent lower limb angiography. Immediately after the injection of a high osmolar contrast agent (diatrizoate) 100 ml, he developed a sudden pain in the small of the back, radiating to both legs. This was followed by cold, marmoreal, livid skin, suggesting severe prolonged vasospasm. His femoral pulses were weak and vasodilators (nifedipine, sodium nitroprusside) and analgesics were ineffective. A CT scan excluded aortic dissection. During the next 12 h he developed paraplegia, disseminated intravascular coagulation, and adult respiratory distress syndrome, and died. Post-mortem examination showed generalized arteriosclerosis without organ damage.

The authors suggested that the contrast agent had caused severe prolonged vasospasm and that death had been the consequence of massive tissue hypoxia. Alternatively, he may have suffered massive cholesterol embolism, owing to catheter manipulation, although histological proof was absent.

Coronary artery spasm has been attributed to ioversol, a low osmolar non-ionic monomer (7[c])

A 75-year-old man with no previous history of heart disease or symptoms of angina pectoris and with an ulcer on the right foot underwent angiography to assess arterial flow and received 30 ml of ioversol injected into the lower part of the abdominal aorta. After 5 min he developed severe chest pain and 5 min later had a cardiac arrest. Resuscitation was successful. His electrocardiogram showed features suggestive of acute inferior myocardial ischemia. The chest pain abated and the cardiographic abnormalities returned to normal 1 h later. Left coronary arterial angiography a week later (with 7 ml of ioversol) was normal. However, he gradually developed chest pain and the electrocardiogram showed ischemic changes compatible with right coronary artery spasm. Right coronary angiography showed severe spasm, which was relieved by an intra-arterial infusion of glyceryl trinitrate 1.5 mg. The chest pain subsided and the electrocardiogram returned to normal. Right coronary angiography 5 min later was normal.

Coronary artery spasm after contrast administration is rare. All previously reported cases have developed after direct intracoronary injection. The mechanism is not clear but could be due to the stress of the angiographic procedure itself. Electrocardiographic monitoring during all angiographic procedures should be mandatory. Electrocardiographic abnormalities suggestive of ischemic changes in the heart should be treated rapidly with intravenous glyceryl trinitrate to prevent a fatal outcome.

Nervous system Patients undergoing myelography may develop a variety of adverse reactions after subarachnoid administration of contrast media. Complications range from mild transient systemic reactions to severe meningeal reactions and death. Common adverse reactions include *headache*, *nausea*, *vomiting*, *vertigo*, and *spinal pain*. More serious adverse effects, such as *convulsions* and *neuropsychiatric reactions*, are uncommon. A recently reported case has suggested that some neurological adverse effects may be due to the development of *hydrocephalus* (8[c]).

A 33-year-old Chinese woman developed acute hydrocephalus 20 h after lumbar myelography with iotrolan (a water-soluble iso-osmolar non-ionic dimer). She developed headache, drowsiness, and neck stiffness, and her level of consciousness deteriorated. A CT scan of the head showed contrast medium in the subarachnoid space, with mild dilatation of the cerebral ventricles. After shunting her level of consciousness improved, and 3 days later a CT scan showed normal sized ventricles, although contrast medium was present in the brain parenchyma.

The pathogenesis of hydrocephalus in this patient was not clear. Hydrocephalus after myelography was previously mainly due to arachnoiditis caused by the oily contrast agents that were widely used in the past. However, it is a rare complication of myelography with modern non-ionic water-soluble contrast media.

In contrast, ionic media are extremely neurotoxic and should not be introduced into the subarachnoid space; however, accidental administration (SEDA-20, 418: SEDA-21, 478) continues to be reported (9[c]).

Hypaque (a high osmolar ionic contrast agent) 10 ml was inadvertently introduced into the subarachnoid space in a 65-year-old man during intraoperative myelography performed to confirm complete decompression of disc prolapse. After the operation, he recovered from the anesthesia and was awake, alert, and recovering normally. However, 3 h later he developed painful myoclonic spasms about every 90 s in his legs. The spasms became gradually more frequent and ascended to involve the trunk, arms, and face. He also became pyrexic (39°C). Severe rhabdomyolysis occurred, with myoglobinuria. He required aggressive intensive treatment for 3 days and made a full recovery with no further complications.

Prevention of inadvertent administration of ionic contrast media into the subarachnoid space is extremely important. If it occurs, the flow of the agent into the subarachnoid space around the brain should be minimized. Intubation and mechanical ventilation with neuromuscular blockade are also important. Rhabdomyolysis and subsequent multisystem organ failure commonly cause death. Rhabdomyolysis is particularly associated with renal failure and disseminated intravascular coagulation. Treatment involves the maintenance of adequate blood volume and urine output. Diuretics should be used to maintain a high urine output. Alkalinization of the urine has been advocated to prevent the dissociation of myoglobin into ferrihemate, a nephrotoxic metabolite.

Hematological The hematological adverse effects of contrast media have been extensively evaluated over the last decade, and in particular their effects on blood coagulation and platelet aggregation. It has been suggested that ionic contrast media have antiplatelet activity and that non-ionic agents do not.

Recurrent acute *thrombocytopenia* has been reported in a 50-year-old Japanese man who was given iopamidol (a low osmolar non-ionic contrast agent) for coronary angiography (10[c]). The authors suggested that the thrombocytopenia may have resulted from platelet aggregation induced by iopamidol, which was observed in vitro after the addition of iopamidol to the patient's whole blood. This effect was not observed with ioxaglate (a low osmolar ionic contrast medium). This report supports the view that non-ionic low osmolar contrast agents can cause platelet aggregation. However, this issue remains contentious, and although non-ionic agents are viewed as being less anticoagulant than ionic contrast media, they are not considered to be procoagulant.

Urinary system *Nephrotoxicity* due to contrast media has been difficult to demonstrate in patients with normal renal function. However, it is well established that pre-existing renal insufficiency is a major risk factor.

There has been a recent large prospective study of 1826 patients undergoing coronary intervention with renal insufficiency (11[Cr]). The incidence of acute renal failure after contrast administration was 15%, and 0.8% of patients required dialysis. The threshold dose for the development of contrast nephrotoxicity requiring dialysis was 100 ml. No patient with a creatinine clearance above 47 ml/min developed nephrotoxicity requiring dialysis. Hospital mortality of those who required dialysis was 36%. This large study documented the incidence of nephrotoxicity due to contrast media in patients with pre-existing renal insufficiency, and showed that the dose of the contrast agent and baseline renal function are important predictors of renal failure. The need for dialysis is rare (<1%) but it is associated with high mortality.

Renal impairment can follow intravenous urography, even if low osmolar non-ionic agents are used. In a prospective study of renal function after intravenous urography with iopromide (mean dose 0.9 ml/kg) in 39 patients there was an increase in serum creatinine concentration in six patients within 48 h and normalization within a week (12[C]). The incidence of renal impairment was 15%. This study has confirmed that mild renal impairment can occur after the intravascular administration of a contrast agent; in most cases renal function recovers spontaneously without intervention.

The effectiveness of hemodialysis in preventing nephrotoxicity due to contrast media has been investigated in 15 patients with impaired renal function (13[C]). Despite dialysis the patients had significant increases in serum creatinine after contrast administration. The authors concluded that hemodialysis does not offer effective prophylaxis against this complication.

It has been suggested that retention of contrast media in the renal cortex, demonstrated on CT scanning of the abdomen performed beyond 12 h after administration of contrast, is a predictor of the nephrotoxicity due to contrast media. However, a recent study in Japan has shown that there is retention of contrast media in the renal cortex in patients who maintain normal renal function after administration, not consistently associated with the development of contrast nephrotoxicity (14[C]).

Although the pathophysiology of renal impairment due to contrast media has not been fully explained, recent studies have suggested that endothelin plays an important role. In 77 children there was an increase in the urinary excretion of endothelin after angiography, in agreement with the results of previous studies; the urinary concentrations of tubular markers were also increased, and these changes correlated with changes in endothelin excretion (15[Cr]).

Skin and appendages *Urticaria* can occur after the intravascular administration of contrast agents and has an incidence of 0.5–3%. It is often mild and responds well to an antihistamine. A case of fixed drug eruption due to contrast media, a rare event, has been reported (16[c]).

A 41-year-old woman with a long history of systemic lupus erythematosus and requiring hemodialysis developed a fixed drug eruption a few hours after the intra-vascular administration of iopamidol (a non-ionic monomeric low osmolar contrast agent) to investigate a malfunctioning dialysis fistula. The eruption was characterized by patchy erythema of the skin of the arms, legs, and trunk. Some lesions progressed to bullae and erosions. Biopsy showed broad epidermal necrosis with pronounced eosinophilic degeneration. The skin lesions improved with prednisolone (30 mg/day).

Miscellaneous *Pain* and *a sensation of heat* are often experienced during angiographic procedures under local anesthetic when high osmolar contrast media are used. These adverse effects are reduced with the use of low osmolar contrast agents. The recently developed iso-osmolar dimeric contrast media are often not associated with feelings of heat and pain during angiography. However, delayed allergy-like reactions after the intravascular use of these agents have been a source of concern.

The incidence of pain associated with injection of the iso-osmolar dimer iodixanol has recently been compared with the incidence of pain with the low osmolar non-ionic monomer iopromide in a large multicenter study (17[C]). Iodixanol caused pain in significantly fewer subjects (0.9% of 1125) than iopromide (9.5% of 1227). It was disappointing that patients were not assessed for delayed contrast reactions, as some reports have suggested that delayed allergic-like skin reactions are twice as common with non-ionic dimers than with non-ionic monomers.

ORAL CONTRAST AGENTS

Barium sulfate

Of 16 patients who received high-density barium sulfate before abdominal MRI, only five drank the total volume of barium requested (450 ml), seven drank 300 ml, and four could only tolerate 150 ml (18[C]). Four patients reported a dislike of the taste, nausea, and abdominal cramping. The authors suggested that barium sulfate should be reserved for MRI of the pancreas and lesions of the gastrointestinal tract, as these areas require specific bowel enhancement.

Immunological and hypersensitivity reactions Adverse drug reactions during barium examinations are uncommon, although there has been a report of *anaphylaxis* (19[c]).

A 48-year-old man with no significant past medical history and no known allergies underwent a barium meal examination. He took E-Z Gas carbon dioxide effervescent crystals, followed by barium sulfate suspension. About 35 min later he developed diffused facial urticaria and edema and complained of progressive dizziness, chest tightness, and shortness of breath. His pulse rate was 60–80 beats/min and his systolic blood pressure 60 mmHg. He eventually recovered but required systemic corticosteroids.

Hypersensitivity reactions to products used during barium meal examinations are extremely rare. Barium sulfate is generally regarded as an inert insoluble compound that is neither absorbed nor metabolized and is eliminated unchanged. However, some studies have shown that very small amounts of barium sulfate can be absorbed from the gastrointestinal tract and that barium can be detected in the plasma and urine after the oral administration of barium sulfate. In addition, there are many additives in commercial barium products, and they are essentially the same as many additives used in food products, some of which can cause an immune response. It is unclear whether the barium itself or the additives in the barium suspension and in the effervescent granules were responsible for this unusual reaction. A patient with a history of a severe reaction to barium products should not receive barium again.

Magnetic particles

In a study of the effects of hyoscine butyl bromide (an antiperistaltic agent) on 33 patients given oral magnetic particles before abdominal MRI, only 27 patients took the full 800 ml, four took only 500–750 ml, and two could not tolerate the particles owing to *vomiting* (this may have been disease related in one of the patients); 27 found the taste of the particles acceptable, three found it unpleasant, and two classified the taste as bad (20[C]).

GADOLINIUM

Gadolinium chelates in MRI

(SEDA-20, 419; SEDA-21, 483)

Widespread monitoring of the use of gadolinium-based contrast agents in MRI has confirmed an overall adverse reaction rate of around 2% to gadolinium DTPA at a dose of 0.1 mmol/kg. It is unclear whether the frequency of adverse effects is higher at higher doses.

The adverse effects of a 'triple dose' (0.3 mmol/kg) have been assessed in a study of gadolinium dose, magnetization transfer contrast, and delayed imaging in the detection of lesions in multiple sclerosis (21[C]). There were seven adverse events with high-dose gadolinium DTPA in 50 patients compared with one with the standard dose (0.1 mmol/kg) in 48. Adverse effects at 0.3 mmol/kg included *urticaria*, *vomiting*, *diarrhea*, *flushing*, *paresthesia*, and *headache*, which have previously been reported with standard doses. The authors suggested that the use of bolus administration in this study rather than an infusion contributed to the increased frequency of adverse events at the higher dose.

An adverse reaction rate of 1.9% has been confirmed in 479 patients given a non-ionic gadolinium chelate (gadodiamide) 0.1 mmol/kg (22[C]). All adverse events were minor and lasted less than 5 min. The most common adverse effects were *nausea* and *a metallic taste*. No adverse effects were recorded in 79 patients given 0.3 mmol/kg.

Gadolinium chelates are proving to be safer in every respect than even non-ionic iodinated X-ray contrast agents. This may be because of the smaller volume of contrast required for MRI examination. However, despite their safety there are still occasional case reports of unusual adverse events.

Cardiovascular A case of delayed *thrombophlebitis* has been reported after the administration of gadolinium DTPA for cranial MRI (23[C]).

A 58-year-old woman received 16 ml of gadolinium DTPA into a dorsal hand vein, without extravasation. Four minutes after the scan she developed red streaking in the distribution of the draining veins extending from the injection site to the wrist. This resolved, but 12 h later she complained of forearm swelling and erythema with multiple erythematous nodules. Superficial thrombophlebitis was diagnosed and treated with simple analgesics and antibiotics. Her symptoms resolved 4 days after injection.

Endocrine, metabolic There has been a report of *pituitary apoplexy* with spontaneous cure of acromegaly following gadolinium DTPA administration for cranial MRI (24[c]).

A 44-year-old man developed a severe headache during an injection of gadolinium DTPA, and a repeat scan suggested hemorrhagic infarction of a growth hormone-producing macroadenoma. There was no clinical or endocrinological evidence of florid acromegaly 14 months later.

The authors suggest a causal link between the gadolinium injection and the infarction, possibly because of a cardiovascular reaction to the contrast media and associated hypotension.

Gadolinium compounds used as contrast agents apart from MRI

Gadolinium has a relatively high rate of X-ray attenuation and there has been recent interest in using the gadolinium chelates as specific CT contrast agents. Gadoxetic acid disodium was developed as a tissue-specific contrast agent for the liver and biliary system to be used in MRI and is a derivative of gadolinium DTPA with higher lipophilicity. It is taken up into hepatocytes and undergoes biliary excretion. Intravenous gadoxetic acid disodium has been used to assess liver enhancement and detect lesions in CT scanning of 15 patients with known liver metastases (25[C]). The contrast was administered as an intravenous infusion over 20 or 30 min in doses of 0.2, 0.35, and 0.5 mmol/kg. There were three mild and one moderate adverse reactions. Two patients reported *a burning sensation at the site of infusion or retrosternally*, which resolved when the flow rate of the infusion was reduced. Two other patients reported *right upper quadrant pain*, which began 4 h after the infusion; this resolved spontaneously after a few hours. There were also minor reversible *alterations in liver enzymes* in some patients. Overall patient tolerance was acceptable and the images showed good or excellent liver enhancement, liver to tumor attenuation difference, and tumor visualization in the majority of cases with doses of 0.35 and 0.5 mmol/kg.

Urinary system Gadolinium compounds show little evidence of nephrotoxicity. The use of gadolinium DTPA as a suitable contrast agent in two patients with renal insufficiency undergoing vascular intervention with standard X-ray screening has been reported (26[C]). Two patients, who each received 50–60 ml of gadolinium DTPA, were treated without alterations in serum creatinine or any other adverse effect.

ULTRASOUND CONTRAST AGENTS *(SEDA-20, 418)*

Contrast agents for enhancing ultrasound images and Doppler signals continue to be developed. The ideal ultrasound contrast agent would be non-toxic and ready to use, injectable intravenously, capable of crossing the pulmonary capillary bed, stable for the duration of the ultrasound examination, and would provide both Doppler and grey scale enhancement (27[C]).

Galactose microparticles

A safety analysis of phase 3 trials of Levovist (SHU508A, Schering, Berlin, Germany), an agent that contains galactose microparticles and palmitic acid, involving 1255 patients has been reported (28[C]). Levovist 200, 300, and 400 mg/ml was well tolerated with no significant changes in physical examination or standard laboratory tests. There were no serious adverse effects and no events required specific medical intervention. Adverse effects were reported in 11% of patients, the majority being *transient heat or pain* lasting less than 30 s.

Echovist (SHU454 Schering, Berlin, Germany) is another agent that contains galactose microparticles. There has been a meta-analysis of the use of Echovist in 986 patients in the assessment of fallopian tube patency (29[R]). Echovist was well tolerated, although there were adverse events in 47%. By far the most common adverse effect was *abdominal pain* during the examination (38%). This correlated with tubal patency and was most severe in patients with blockage of both fallopian tubes, presumably because of increased intraluminal pressure. The only other common adverse events were *vasovagal reactions* (2.8%) and *nausea* (1.5%), which also may not have been directly related to contrast administration.

Perflenapent

The safety of a new agent, perflenapent emulsion (Echogen, SONUS Pharmaceuticals, Bothell, WA), has been assessed (30[Cr]). Perflenapent emulsion contains dodecafluoropentane, which is converted to gaseous microbubbles before intravenous administration. The microbubbles cross the lung capillary bed and persist in solution much longer than microbubbles of air or other gases of similar size, providing prolonged contrast enhancement. A review of 21 clinical studies involving 743 patients who received perflenapent emulsion and 151 patients who received placebo, showed no clinically important abnormalities in laboratory tests, pulse oximetry, vital signs, or electrocardiography. There were adverse events in 6.7% of patients after perflenapent emulsion and 2.6% of patients after placebo. The most frequent adverse effects considered relevant to perflenapent emulsion were *vasodilatation* (2.8%) and *taste disturbances* (1.2%). Adverse events were generally mild to moderate, started within 10–20 min of contrast administration, and resolved spontaneously within 10–20 min. These reassuring findings are in keeping with safety reports about other ultrasound contrast agents.

REFERENCES

1. Lasser EC, Lyon SG, Berry CC. Reports on contrast media reactions: analysis of data from reports to the US Food and Drug Administration. Radiology 1997;203:605–10 (erratum 876).
2. Bettmann MA, Heeren T, Greenfield A, Goudey C. Adverse events with radiographic contrast agents: results of the SCVIR Contrast Agent Registry. Radiology 1997;203:611–20.
3. Kussmaul WG III, Mishra JP, Matthai WH, Hirschfeld JW Jr. Complications of cardiac angiography using low- or high-osmolarity contrast agents in patients with left main coronary stenosis. Cathet Cardiovasc Diagn 1997;42:376–9.
4. Thomas SM, Williams JE, Adam EJ. Intravascular contrast media: can we justify the continued use of ionic contrast agents? Clin Radiol 1997;52:59–61.
5. Oi H, Yamazaki H, Matsushita M. Delayed vs. immediate adverse reactions to ionic and non-ionic low osmolality contrast media. Radiat Med 1997;15:23–7.
6. Vucicevic Z, Suskovic T, Delic-Bikljacic D. Severe vasospasm and death following angiography with a high osmolar contrast medium. Acta Clin Croat 1997;36:123–4.
7. Sakamoto I, Uchida T, Hayashi K. Case report: cardiac arrest due to coronary artery spasm during angiographic procedure. Clin Radiol 1997;52:798–800.
8. Tseng SH, Tseng WS. Acute hydrocephalus after iotrolan lumbar myelography. Neuroradiology 1997;39:863–4.
9. Killeffer JA, Kaufman HH. Inadvertent intraoperative myelography with Hypaque: case report and discussion. Surg Neurol 1997;48:70–3.
10. Ogasawara T, Takenaka T, Horimoto M,

Baba C, Sakuma K. Thrombocytopenia induced by non-ionic radiographic contrast medium. Jpn J Clin Radiol 1997;42:393–6.
11. McCullough PA, Wolyn R, Rocher LL, Levin RN, O'Neill WW. Acute renal failure after coronary intervention: incidence, risk factors, and relationship to mortality. Am J Med 1997;103:368–75.
12. Krasteva R, Andreev E, Kiroycheva M, Kundurdjiev A, Kiperova B. Contrast induced nephropathy following intravenous urography with iopromide. Roentgenol Radiol 1997;36:20–2.
13. Schaffner T, Gondolf K, Lehnert T, Keller E. Nephrotoxicity of radio contrast agents. Nieren-Hochdruckkr 1997;27:283–91.
14. Yamazaki H, Oi H, Matsushita M, Inoue T, Teshima T, Koizumi M, Nose T, Tanaka E, Nakamura H, Inoue T, Kim T, Elbaradie MM. Renal cortical retention on delayed CT after angiography and contrast associated nephropathy. Br J Radiol 1997;70:897–902.
15. Nattyus I, Zimmerhackl LB, Schwarz A, Brandis M, Miltenyi M. Renal excretion of endothelin in children. Pediatr Nephrol 1997;11:513–21.
16. Yamauchi R, Morita A, Tsuji T. Fixed drug eruption caused by iopamidol, a contrast medium. J Dermatol 1997;24:243–5.
17. Justesen P, Downes M, Grynne BH, Lang H, Rasch W, Seim E. Injection associated pain in femoral arteriography: a European multi-centre study comparing safety, tolerability and efficacy of iodixanol and iopromide. Cardiovasc Intervent Radiol 1997;22:251–6.
18. Burton SS, Leibig T, Frazier SD, Ros PR. High-density oral barium sulphate in abdominal MRI: efficacy and tolerance in a clinical setting. Magn Reson Imaging 1997;15:147–53.
19. Seymour PC, Kesack CD. Anaphylactic shock during a routine upper gastrointestinal series. Am J Roentgenol 1997;168:957–8.
20. Laniado M, Gronwaller E, Kopp AF, Kaminsky SF, Hamm B. The value of hyoscine butylbromide in abdominal MR imaging with and without oral magnetic particles. Abdom Imaging 1997; 22:381–8.
21. Silver NC, Good CD, Barker GJ, MacManus DJ, Thompson AJ. Sensitivity of contrast enhanced MRI in multiple sclerosis. Effects of gadolinium dose, magnetization transfer contrast and delayed imaging. Brain 1997;120:1149–61.
22. Thomsen HS. Frequency of acute adverse events to a non-ionic low osmolar contrast medium: the effect of a verbal interview. Pharmacol Toxicol 1997;80:108–10.
23. Murphy KJ, Hansen R, Prince MR. Cutaneous nodules, pain, and thrombophlebitis as an adverse reaction to gadolinium contrast media. Am J Roentgenol 1997;169:318–19.
24. Wichers M, Kristof RA, Springer W, Schramm J, Klingmuller D. Pituitary apoplexy with spontaneous cure of acromegaly and its possible relation to Gd-DTPA-administration. Acta Neurochir Wien 1997;139:992–4.
25. Schmitz SA, Haberle JH, Balzer T, Shamsi K, Boese-Landgraf J, Wolf K-J. Detection of focal liver lesions: CT of the hepatobiliary system with gadoxetic acid disodium, or Gd-EOB-DTPA. Radiology 1997;202:399–405.
26. Hatrick AG, Jarosz JM, Irvine AT. Gadopentate dimeglumine as an alternative contrast agent for use in interventional procedures. Clin Radiol 1997;52:948–52.
27. Correas J-M, Quay SC. EchoGen emulsion: a new ultrasound contrast agent based on phase shift colloids. Clin Radiol 1996;51:11–41.
28. Schlief R. The use of Levovist (SHU508A) for echo-enhancement of vascular Doppler imaging in clinical diagnosis. Angiology 1996;47:S3–8.
29. Holz K, Becker R, Schurmann R. Ultrasound in the investigation of tubal patency. A meta-analysis of comparitive studies of Echovist-200 including 1007 women. Zentralbl Gynäkol 1997; 119:366–73.
30. Quay SC, Eisenfield AJ. Safety assessment of the use of perflenapent emulsion for contrast enhancement of echocardiography and diagnostic radiology ultrasound studies. Clin Cardiol 1997;20 (Suppl 1):1.19–26.

B.C.P. Polak

47 Drugs used in ocular treatment

R ## *Risk factors for adverse effects of drugs used in ocular treatment*

In this review I shall discuss the specific problems of risk factors for the adverse effects of topical ocular drugs, concentrating on the increased risks run by elderly people. Old people are at increased risk of adverse effects of ocular drugs for several reasons.

(1) Between 30 and 80% of a drug given as eye drops can be absorbed directly into the bloodstream, following transfer from the eye to the nose, and avoiding first-pass hepatic metabolism in the same manner as an intravenous injection. The systemic drug concentrations that result from this mode of entry tend to be higher in older people, because of altered volumes of distribution, reduced protein binding, impaired metabolism, and reduced renal excretion.

(2) Old people are sometimes also more susceptible to the pharmacological actions of drugs.

(3) Chronic ophthalmic diseases, requiring long-term topical ocular treatment, are more prevalent among older people. Older people are also likely to have other medical conditions (e.g., cardiac, respiratory, or neurological diseases) that can be induced or exacerbated by topical ophthalmic agents.

(4) Polypharmacy is common in elderly people, and is associated with an increased risk of drug interactions.

Phenylephrine

Topical phenylephrine eye drops can increase the blood pressure, although the risk appears to be small in most patients (1[R]). Dramatic rises, however, can occur in elderly patients with phenylephrine 5% and 10% eye drops. The risk of hypertension is probably lower with 2.5% drops, but it is still present (2[R]). After topical ophthalmic use phenylephrine can cause myocardial infarction, as well as tachycardia, headache, tremor, and sweating.

One has to be aware that over-the-counter ophthalmic decongestants are commonly used to control ocular redness and discomfort. The principal active ingredient in these eye drops is an α-adrenergic, vasoconstrictor amine, such as naphazoline, tetrahydrozoline, or phenylephrine. Decongestant eye drops containing vasoconstrictors can cause acute and chronic conjunctival redness by pharmacological, toxic, and allergic mechanisms, mydriasis, blurred vision, acute angle closure, and increased intraocular pressure, nervousness, headache, dizziness, nausea, hypotension, hypertension, and cardiac dysrhythmias (3[c]).

Phenylephrine should be avoided in patients with hypertension, cardiac diseases, aneurysms, and advanced arteriosclerosis. It should also be used with caution in elderly people and in patients taking monoamine oxidase inhibitors, tricyclic antidepressants, or atropine (2[R]).

Anticholinergic drugs

Atropine, homatropine, cyclopentolate, and tropicamide paralyse the musculus sphincter pupillae and the ciliary body, dilating the pupil and immobilizing the lens, producing cycloplegia. The systemic adverse effects of these

Side Effects of Drugs, Annual 22
J.K. Aronson, ed.

drugs are generally dose dependent, but an idiosyncratic effect is occasionally seen with atropine. Topical ophthalmic anticholinergic agents can cause central nervous system abnormalities, including cerebellar signs, ataxia, dysarthria, hallucinations, incoherent speech, restlessness, confusion, and seizures, which can especially develop in older patients (1[R]), (4[c]).

DRUGS USED IN GLAUCOMA

Glaucoma and its treatment can have an enormous impact on a patient's quality of life. Open-angle glaucoma is now the commonest cause of blindness world wide, affecting 7% of people over the age of 75, and twice as often in patients with diabetes mellitus. Treatment, whether topical, oral, or surgical, can have adverse effects with significant consequences. Topical agents used in the treatment of glaucoma lower intraocular pressure, either by reducing aqueous humor production or by increasing aqueous outflow through the trabecular meshwork or uveoscleral pathway.

β-Blockers

β-Adrenoceptor antagonists are effective in glaucoma without notable effects on pupillary size or refraction. They act by blocking β-adrenoceptors in the iris and ciliary body, reducing aqueous humour production and intraocular pressure. Timolol, levobunolol, metipranolol, and carteolol are non-selective β_1- and β_2-adrenoceptor antagonists, while betaxolol is β_1-selective. Non-selective topical β-blockers can cause bronchospasm and asthma in patients with obstructive airways disease by blocking pulmonary β_2-adrenoceptors: non-selective β-blockers should therefore be avoided in these patients. Elderly people are at greater risk (1[R]). Selective β-blockers block β_1-adrenoceptors at concentrations below those required to block β_2-adrenoceptors in the bronchi, and may be less likely to precipitate bronchospasm: these pulmonary adverse reactions and other systemic effects can nevertheless occur after topical treatment with selective β-blockers.

Local effects *Dry eyes can occur after the systemic or ocular use of β-blockers. The sensation of dry eyes is usually transitory and there can be reduced tear production (Schirmer test) and tear film break-up time. Symptomatic superficial punctate keratitis in association with complete corneal anesthesia has been observed (SED-13, 1418). Dry eyes develop especially in older women, owing to a menopausal reduction in tear production: treatment with β-blockers can produce more severe keratoconjunctivitis sicca in such patients.*

Cardiovascular *Non-selective topical β-blockers can cause hypotension and a reduction in resting heart rate, and are therefore contraindicated in patients with second- or third-degree heart block or cardiac failure (1[R]). There can be an additive effect in combination with systemic β-blockers, and in older patients who are already using systemic agents β-blocking eye drops should be avoided (5[r]). Topical β-blockers can interact with other systemic agents, including calcium antagonists, to give profound hypotension, and with adrenergic psychotropic agents (e.g., phenothiazines) to produce confusion. β-Blockers can increase pulmonary edema secondary to heart failure (6[c]). Of 32 deaths attributed to the use of topical timolol since its introduction in the US, 13 were of cardiovascular origins (1[R]). Half of them occurred at 2–48 h after starting therapy. Bradycardia can be followed by profound lethargy (7[c]). The effect of betaxolol on pulse rate and blood pressure is not great and certainly less than that associated with timolol.*

Respiratory *Pulmonary adverse reactions can occur in patients who are prone to subclinical disease and who are predisposed to respiratory obstruction, but who do not give this information on direct questioning. Although betaxolol does not significantly affect pulmonary β_2-receptors it has occasionally been reported to cause bronchospasm and should be used with caution in patients with a history of respiratory disease. It is prudent to measure and record the pretreatment FEV_1 in elderly patients not known to have obstructive airways disease, so that asymptomatic deterioration during treatment can be recognized (5[r]).*

Nervous system *CNS adverse effects, such as headaches, dizziness, anxiety, depression, memory loss, psychosis, dementia, and hallucinations, occur in 3–10% of patients using topical β-blockers and are usually dose dependent and reversible on withdrawal. Patients may be unaware of the symptoms until the drug is withdrawn. Older patients, however, have short-term memory loss and are disorientated and confused before starting to use a topical β-blocker. Central nervous adverse reactions can easily be attributed to old age.*

Endocrine, metabolic *β-Blockers can mask the tachycardia that otherwise provides warning hypoglycemia in patients with insulin-dependent diabetes mellitus. In addition, β-blockers can oppose the hypoglycemic effect of oral hypoglycemic drugs by reducing insulin secretion, causing hyperglycemia.*

Skin and appendages *Betaxolol-associated hyperpigmentation of the fingers has been described in a patient with unrelated contact dermatitis (8[c]).*

Excessive sweating occurred in a 73-year-old man with non-insulin-dependent diabetes mellitus and normal glycemia tests after he had used topical carteolol for 2 years for glaucoma: carteolol was withdrawn and in a few days his sweating decreased dramatically (9[c]).

Special senses *Glaucoma-induced visual field loss requiring non-miotic topical treatment was a major risk factor for falls in elderly people, and the effect of medication was more important than the visual field loss (10[r]).*

Musculoskeletal *Aggravation of myasthenia gravis has been observed during ophthalmic timolol therapy. Elderly patients are at greater risk (1[R]).*

Sexual function *Impotence and loss of libido may be experienced with ophthalmic β-blocking treatment. Elderly patients are at greater risk (1[R]).*

Carbonic anhydrase inhibitors

Dorzolamide is the first topical carbonic anhydrase inhibitor. It penetrates the cornea and acts on the ciliary body, reducing the secretion of aqueous humor. Although experience with this drug is limited, it can cause similar adverse effects to oral acetazolamide, including hypokalemia and renal calculi.

Carbonic anhydrase inhibitors should be used with caution in patients with respiratory acidosis or loss of respiratory capacity and in patients with diabetes mellitus. These drugs are contraindicated in patients with hepatic disease or insufficiency, reduced serum sodium or potassium concentrations, adrenocortical insufficiency, hyperchloremic acidosis, or severe renal disease or insufficiency (SED-13, 1423).

Cholinoceptor agonists

Pilocarpine increases aqueous humor outflow via the trabecular meshwork. Its systemic adverse effects include headaches and periorbital pain, nausea, vomiting, sweating, hypersalivation, lacrimation, hypotension, bradycardia, bronchial constriction, respiratory failure, and nightmares. Urinary urgency and frequency, abdominal cramping, diarrhea, ataxia, and confusion can occur and elderly people are at particular risk (SED-13, 1422).

Clonidine analogs

Apraclonidine and brimonidine are β_2-adrenoceptor agonists, related to clonidine, that act by reducing aqueous humor production. Their systemic adverse effects include dry mouth, hypotension, dizziness, gastrointestinal symptoms, and headache. These drugs should be used with caution in patients with angina pectoris, myocardial infarction, heart failure, and depression, and are contraindicated in patients taking monoamine oxidase inhibitors or tricyclic antidepressants, since the antidepressants can influence the uptake of circulating amines (SEDA-19, 433). Elderly patients are at greater risk (1[R]).

Prostaglandin analogs

Latanoprost is a prostaglandin analog with limited use. In patients with asthma or cardiovascular disease it is thought to be well tolerated. Iris pigmentation can be increased in patients with green/brown irises.

REFERENCES

1. Diamond JP. Systemic adverse effects of topical ophthalmic agents. Implications for older patients. Drugs Aging 1997;11:352–60.
2. Fraunfelder FT. Drug-induced Ocular Side Effects, 4th edition. Baltimore: Williams and Wilkins, 1996:281–3.
3. Soparkar CNS, Wilhelmus KR, Koch DD, Wallace GW, Jones DB. Acute and chronic conjunctivitis due to over-the-counter ophthalmic decongestants. Arch Ophthalmol 1997;115:34–8.
4. Falbe WJ, Boyd DL. Homatropine-associated confusion in an elderly patient. J Am Geriatr Soc 1988;36:649.
5. Brooks AMV, Gillies WE. Ocular beta-blockers in glaucoma management. Drugs Aging 1992;2:208–21.
6. Backlund M, Kirvela M, Lindgren L. Cardiac failure aggravated by timolol eye drops: preoperative improvement by changing to pilocarpine. Acta Anaesthesiol Scand 1996;40:379–81.
7. Vahidasser MD, Foy CJ, O'Malley T, Passmore AP. Eye drops and lethargy. J R Soc Med 1997;90:155.
8. Adams DR, Marks JG. Betaxolol-associated hyperpigmentation of the fingers in a patient with unrelated contact dermatitis. Am J Contact Dermatitis 1997;8:183–4.
9. Schmutz JL, Barbaud A, Reichert S, Vasse JP, Trechot Ph. First report of sweating associated with topical beta-blocker therapy. Dermatology 1997;194:197–8.
10. Glynn RJ, Seddon JM, Krug JH Jr. Falls in elderly patients with glaucoma. Arch Ophthalmol 1991;109:205–10.

E. Ernst and J. Barnes

48 Treatments used in complementary medicine

Contrary to public opinion, promotion, and media coverage, treatments used in complementary/alternative medicine are not without adverse effects. This issue has recently received much attention in medical publications. In particular, several articles have focused on safety issues associated with herbal remedies (1[R]), (2[R]), including monitoring the safety of such products (3[R]), (4[R]), plant toxicity (5[R]), (6[R]), including hepatotoxicity (7[R]), (8[r]), (9[R]), the regulation of herbal medicines in various countries (10[R]), risks associated with the consumption of herbal teas (11[R]), potential interactions between herbs and conventional drugs (12[R]), the use of herbal remedies during pregnancy (13[R]), (14[R]), and methods of reducing the risks associated with the use of herbal products (15[r]). Other problems related to the use of herbal treatments are product contamination, adulteration, and botanical misidentification. Safety aspects of other treatments used in complementary medicine, such as acupuncture and spinal manipulation, have also been highlighted.

Incidence of adverse effects Despite the attention that herbal safety has received in the medical literature, research into the incidence of adverse effects associated with herbal remedies remains scarce.

During a 5-year study designed to assess toxicological problems associated with the use of traditional and herbal remedies and food supplements, a London-based toxicology unit received 1297 reports from medical professionals in the UK (16[C]). Of these, a confirmed association (12 cases), a probable association (35), or a possible association (38) with use of the product was made in 785 cases; 10 of the 12 confirmed cases related to Chinese/Indian remedies. Reports of adverse effects were not limited to ethnic traditional remedies: reports of adverse effects associated with the long-term use of valerian, a herb widely used across Europe for insomnia, were also reported.

A similar study has been conducted by a Taiwan-based poison center (17[C]). Over a 2-year period the center received 318 enquiries about Chinese herbal medicines; 273 cases were classified as poisoning and there were 22 deaths. All of the poisonings occurred as a result of suicide attempts, accidents, or erroneous or improper use or processing.

Of 229 women in early labor interviewed in a South African hospital, 55% reported taking traditional herbal remedies during pregnancy (18[C]). Of these, 56% had grade II–III meconium staining of liquor, while in those women who did not report herbal use during pregnancy the figure was 15%. The proportions of cesarean deliveries were 39 and 22%, respectively.

A review of 165 papers on adverse drug reactions published in a Chinese pharmaceutical journal reported that 11% of these papers referred to reports of reactions related to traditional Chinese medicines (19[r]).

WESTERN HERBALISM

Cat's claw

A case of acute *allergic interstitial nephritis* has been described after the use of cat's claw capsules, one qds, as an adjunctive treatment for arthritic symptoms by a 35-year-old Peruvian woman with systemic lupus erythematosus (20[c]). Her serum creatinine rose to 256 μmol/l and later to 318 μmol/l, but she had no other abnormal signs or symptoms. Her creatinine

Side Effects of Drugs, Annual 22
J.K. Aronson, ed.

concentration normalized after withdrawal of this Peruvian herbal treatment.

Ephedra *(SED-13, 1434)*

A formulation called 'Fen-Phen' is increasingly being promoted as a dietary supplement and a herbal alternative to the prescription drug commonly known as 'fen-phen', a combination of fenfluramine and phentermine (21[c]). The so-called 'herbal fen-phen' products are being marketed over the Internet and through weight-loss clinics, as well as other outlets, and do not contain fenfluramine or phentermine. The FDA considers these products to be non-approved drugs because their names reflect that they are intended for the same use as the anti-obesity drugs, fenfluramine and phentermine, and is warning consumers that these drugs have not been shown to be safe or effective and may contain ingredients that have been associated with injuries. Fenfluramine and dexfenfluramine have recently been withdrawn from the market because of safety concerns. The FDA believes that the use of non-approved alternative products may increase as a result of this withdrawal.

The main ingredient of 'herbal fen-phen' is ephedra, commonly known as Ma-huang. Ephedra contains the alkaloid ephedrine a sympathomimetic compound that stimulates the central nervous system and increases cardiac output. The FDA has investigated more than 800 reports of adverse events associated with the use of ephedrine alkaloid-containing products since 1994. These events ranged from episodes of high blood pressure, heart rate irregularities, insomnia, nervousness, tremors, and headache, to seizures, heart attack, stroke, and death.

Other contents of fen-phen products include *Hypericum perforatum*, a herb commonly known as St John's wort and sometimes referred to as 'herbal Prozac', and 5-hydroxytryptophan. St John's wort has been investigated in about 30 controlled trials in patients with depression, and its adverse effects have been reviewed (22[R]); 5-hydroxytryptophan is a derivative of tryptophan, a dietary supplement formerly used primarily as a sleep aid that was withdrawn from the market in 1990 after it was found to be linked to more than 1500 cases (some fatal) of a disorder known as eosinophilia myalgia syndrome (SEDA-13, 1447). The FDA is taking appropriate action to remove these products from the market.

Eucalyptus

Eucalyptus oil products, available in a variety of formulations, are commonly used in vaporizers for symptomatic relief in upper respiratory tract infections. The toxicity of such products in young children has been well documented. From an analysis of four Australian databases, it has been estimated that eucalyptus oil was a leading cause of hospital admission for childhood poisoning in Victoria, Australia (23[C]). Furthermore, over a 9-month period, 149 cases of ingestion or suspected ingestion of eucalyptus oil by children were reported to the Victorian Poisons Information Centre or presented to the emergency departments of hospitals participating in the Victorian Injury Surveillance System. Of 109 of these cases that could be included in a telephone survey, 90 involved vaporizer solutions, 15 eucalyptus oil formulations, and the remainder other products containing eucalyptus oil. As a result of these studies, a selection of measures has been suggested to prevent similar incidents with eucalyptus oil formulations.

Jimson weed (*Datura stramonium*)

Jimson weed (thorn apple, devil's apple) is often abused for its hallucinogenic properties; parts of the plant are chewed, eaten, or made into a tea. The plant is related to *Atropa belladonna* (deadly nightshade), and its toxic properties are due to its tropane alkaloid constituents, mainly hyoscyamine, hyoscine, and atropine. Adverse effects of jimson weed include *tachycardia*, *dry mouth*, *dilated pupils*, *blurred vision*, *hallucinations*, *confusion*, *coma*, and *seizures*.

Nine teenagers (eight male) were treated in hospital after taking jimson weed (24[C]). The majority presented with *tachycardia*, *halluci-*

nations, and *confusion*; all had *pupillary dilatation*. Treatment comprised supportive care, including intravenous fluids, activated charcoal, and gastric lavage. The average length of hospital stay was 1–2 days.

A 20-year-old man with thorn apple intoxication had *restlessness*, *hallucinations*, *euphoria*, and *pupil dilatation* (25[C]).

For mild cases, treatment consists of activated charcoal and gastric lavage; when there are severe symptoms, such as *seizures*, *severe hypertension*, and *life-threatening dysrhythmias*, treatment with the anticholinesterase inhibitor physostigmine is indicated.

Kava (*Piper methysticum*)

Kava is made from the root of the pepper plant and is used as a recreational drink by Pacific Islanders. Recently it has become a popular anxiolytic drug and is marketed in many countries as a food supplement.

Nervous system A male Aboriginal Australian 'kava binger' repeatedly presented with severe generalized *choreoathetosis* involving the limbs, trunk, neck, and facial muscles, associated with the ingestion of large amount of kava (26[c]). His symptoms were always successfully treated with intravenous diazepam and on each occasion he was aysmptomatic within 12 h.

Plantain

The FDA has issued a warning against dietary products purporting to contain 'plantain' (sometimes also called 'Chomper' or 'Uriseptic tea'), because the products may contain digitalis (27[r]). The FDA conducted an investigation after receiving information about a young woman who experienced an abnormal heart rate with heart block after consuming a dietary supplement product labelled as containing plantain. The agency's laboratory analysis confirmed the presence of lanatosides, constituents of Digitalis lanata in samples of the raw material used in the product. Since then, other products containing digitalis have been identified.

EASTERN HERBALISM

In addition to Western herbalism, various other traditional systems of herbal medicine have gained popularity outside their Asian countries of origin. Examples are traditional Chinese herbalism, Japanese Kampo medicine, and Ayurvedic medicine from India. There have been many reports relating to safety issues with such types of treatment.

Chinese herbal combinations

Cardiovascular *Heart failure* has been attributed to a Chinese herbal mixture (28[c]).

A 42-year-old woman consulted a London-based Chinese herbalist for long-standing severe atopic eczema and was given a herbal tea consisting of multiple unknown herbal ingredients. She took a 2-week course of the tea and also took herbal tea baths. Three weeks after starting the treatment she developed signs and symptoms of congestive heart failure. She had a dilated cardiomyopathy which progressed rapidly despite withdrawal of the herbal treatment. However, she made a full recovery in 3 weeks with standard therapy. One ingredient of the tea was identified as liquorice, but causal attribution was impossible.

Liver There have been reports of *liver damage* due to two different Chinese herbal combinations, dai-saiko-to (da-chai-hu-tang) and sho-saiko-to.

A 55-year-old Japanese woman took dai-saiko-to for fatty cell infiltration of the liver (29[c]). Dai-saiko-to is often prescribed in Japan for this condition and for chronic viral hepatitis. Two weeks later, she developed worsening signs of liver disease. A diagnosis of autoimmune hepatitis was made.

Dai-saiko-to for autoimmune dermatitis was associated with interstitial pneumonitis and hepatitis in a man (30[c]). He developed dyspnea and greatly raised liver function tests after having used dai-saiko-to daily for 6 weeks. He recovered after withdrawal.

Sho-saiko-to is a Chinese herbal combination similar, but not identical, to Dai-saiko-to. Sho-saiko-to is used predominantly as a treatment for chronic liver disease due to hepatitis C virus infection. In Japan 72 cases of sho-saiko-to-induced *pneumonia* have been reported (31[C]). Most of the patients developed acute cough, dyspnea, and fever after taking the drug. Pneumonia was confirmed by radiography. In all, 64 patients survived after withdrawal of sho-saiko-to only or with steroid therapy; the other eight patients died despite high-dose steroid therapy.

Danshen

Danshen, the root of *Salvia miltiorrhiza*, is a Chinese medical herb used for a variety of indications, particularly cardiovascular.

Interaction An interaction of danshen with *warfarin* has been described (32[c]).

A 48-year-old woman with rheumatic heart disease complicated by atrial fibrillation and mitral stenosis, who was taking warfarin, digoxin, and furosemide, also obtained danshen from a herbalist for treatment of a flu-like illness. Several weeks later she developed general malaise, dyspnea, and fever. Her prothrombin time was in excess of 60 s, her INR was over 5.6, and she had a microcytic anemia; over-anticoagulation, a chest infection, and gastrointestinal blood loss were diagnosed. Danshen and warfarin were withdrawn, but the clotting abnormality persisted for 5 days.

Danshen is thought to potentiate the anticoagulant effects of warfarin, but the mechanism is not known.

Tripterygium wilfordii

Tripterygium wilfordii is used for rheumatoid arthritis and for male contraception in Japan. Its high level of toxicity has been described repeatedly.

Use in pregnancy A Japanese woman took the remedy during early pregnancy for rheumatoid arthritis (33[c]). After an uncomplicated delivery at 38 weeks, the infant suffered from occipital meningoencephalocele and cerebellar agenesis. The authors considered that *Tripterygium wilfordii* was the most likely cause of this infant's anomalies.

CONTAMINATION WITH HEAVY METALS

Arsenic

Of 17 Chinese patients with *skin lesions* related to chronic arsenicism, 14 (82%) had taken Chinese herbal medicines known to contain inorganic arsenic (three had environmental arsenic exposure from well water) (34[C]). The mean duration of arsenic intake in the 14 patients exposed to Chinese herbal medicines was 6.4 years.

Lead

In the United Arab Emirates, 19 infants (mean age 3.8 months) were shown to suffer from *lead encephalopathy* after the use of 'traditional medicines' (*Bint al Thahab* and surma/kohl) (35[C]). All presented with convulsions, four had signs of brain edema on CT scan, and four had signs of brain atrophy; 13 developed brain damage during follow-up. The median lead concentration in the cerebrospinal fluid of all 19 infants was 3.6 μmol/l.

An unusual case of lead poisoning occurred in Japan, where a 33-year-old woman was diagnosed as having signs and symptoms of a raised lead burden (36[c]). She had self administered herbal medicines for hematuria for several years. The undefined herbal mixture, which itself was not significantly contaminated with lead, had a high lead concentration when boiled in an earthen tea pot, suggesting that a component of the herbs acted as a chelating agent extracting lead from the teapot into the tea.

ADULTERATION WITH THERAPEUTIC DRUGS

In order to determine how often Chinese medicines sold in Taiwan were adulterated with synthetic therapeutic substances, 2609 samples were collected over a 1-year period from eight major general hospitals (37). Physicians were instructed to request samples of such remedies from outpatients whose symptoms were suggestive of the use of adulterated traditional Chinese medicines. Samples were analysed using methods established by the National Laboratories of Food and Drugs. 618 (24%) of the samples proved to be adulterated. Four samples contained six different adulterants, and more than 50% of the adulterated samples contained two or more adulterants. The adulterants found included paracetamol, hydrochlorothiazide, indomethacin, phenobarbital, theophylline, and corticosteroids. Corticosteroids have also been found in Chinese herbal formulations for topical use sold in New Zealand for $30 per tube (38[c]).

BOTANICAL SUBSTITUTION

Botanical substitution can be either accidental, e.g., when one plant species is mistakenly identified as a similar species, or intentional, e.g. when an expensive plant is replaced by a similar-looking but inexpensive substitute. Safety problems obviously arise if the substitute is toxic.

A 31-year-old man took an unknown quantity of mandrake, purchased from a health food store, for its hallucinogenic properties (39[c]). He abruptly developed severe paroxysmal vomiting and was treated with standard supportive measures, including activated charcoal and intravenous fluids. He was discharged without symptoms the following day.

It appeared likely that he had intended to take *Mandragora officinarum*. However, based on chromatographic identification of podophyllotoxin, it was strongly suspected that he had instead taken *Podophyllum peltatum* (also known as mandrake). Podophyllotoxin is used topically in the treatment of condylomata accuminata and has severe systemic toxic effects, including *bone marrow suppression*, *renal failure*, *hepatotoxicity*, and *central and peripheral nervous system effects*, which can result from excessive transdermal absorption or direct ingestion.

One of the most dramatic incidents of botanical substitution relates to the use of a slimming regimen, including Chinese herbs, resulting in what has become known as 'Chinese herb nephropathy'. One of the constituents of the slimming aid *Stephania tetrandra* was substituted by *Aristolochia fangchi*. The latter contains the nephrotoxin aristolochic acid, which is thought to be the cause of severe *interstitial nephritis* in a proportion of individuals, mainly women, who have followed the slimming regimen. In Belgium alone, about 100 women were affected, about 30 of whom died (40[R]). Other cases of Chinese herb *nephropathy* have been reported in Japan (41[C]), (42[C]). In a case–control study it was reported that compared with nephropathies of other origin Chinese herb nephropathy is associated with a faster deterioration in renal function, more severe anemia, and a higher prevalence of aortic insufficiency and urothelial carcinoma (43[C]).

MISCELLANEOUS MEDICATIONS

Kombucha tea

Kombucha, also known as Manchurian or Kargasok 'mushroom', is not a fungus but a yeast–bacteria aggregate surrounded by a permeable membrane. It is used for making a tea that is said to cure cancer, ease arthritis, reduce wrinkles, and alleviate constipation and a host of other medical conditions. Kombucha is particularly popular in the US.

Kombucha tea has been reported to have been associated with toxicity in four cases (44[c]).

A 53-year-old woman with a history of heavy alcohol consumption developed jaundice 2 weeks after she began drinking two glasses of Kombucha tea per day. Liver function tests were abnormal and hepatitis serology was negative. Seven weeks after discontinuation of the tea, her liver function tests had normalized.

A 51-year-old woman taking thyroid hormone and estrogen replacement, complained of xerostomia, dizziness, nausea, vomiting, headache, and neck pain. She had taken half a glass of Kombucha tea per day for several months. The tea was discontinued, she was treated symptomatically, and her symptoms abated. On taking the tea again her symptoms recurred. The only abnormal finding was a caffeine concentration of 3.8 mg/l. Analysis of the 'mushroom' showed that it only contained caffeine.

The third patient presented with shaking, shortness of breath, and akathisia after consumption of tea and no other medication and the fourth had

Table 1. *Adverse effects of acupuncture*

Condition	Causality established by	Risk factor(s)	Outcome	Reference
Pneumothorax	Chest X-ray	Elderly, chronic bronchitis	Full recovery	(47[C])
Pneumothorax	Chest X-ray	Cystic fibrosis	Full recovery	(47[C])
Pneumothorax	Chest X-ray	None	Full recovery	(48[C])
Cardiac tamponade	Dislodged needle seen in right ventricle	Indwelling needle	Surgery, full recovery	(49[C])
Drop foot	Clinically; nerve conduction studies	None	Physiotherapy, residual weakness after 6 years	(50[C])
Bacterial meningitis	Analysis of cerebrospinal fluid	Needled through clothing	Full recovery	(51[C])
Pyarthrosis	Analysis of joint fluid	None	Full recovery	(52[C])
Auricular perichondritis	Clinically	Indwelling needle	Disfigurement	(53[C])

shortness of breath and throat tightness after drinking tea 1 h before and ephedrine 5 min before. Both patients had hypotension, tachycardia, and tachypnea. In both cases an allergic reaction was assumed, symptomatic treatment was successful, and the patients were discharged the same day.

MISCELLANEOUS PROCEDURES

Acupuncture

A systematic review of all serious adverse reactions associated with acupuncture and reported in the medical literature (1969–96) has been published (45[R]). Infections and tissue trauma were the most frequently reported serious adverse effects. A total of five deaths had been associated with acupuncture. It was concluded that acupuncture is not free from serious adverse effects and that reliable incidence figures are currently not available.

When 100 Japanese individuals were randomly selected from a sample of 420 people who were screened for liver disease and were tested for hepatitis G virus/GB virus C, 80% of those who tested positive had a history of using folk remedies such as acupuncture, compared with only 43% in those who tested negative (46[C]).

There have been eight case reports (47[c])–(53[c]) of adverse effects of acupuncture (Table 1). Five were due to traumatic tissue injury through the use of acupuncture needles (47[c])–(50[c]), of which *pneumothorax* was the most common result. The other three cases were due to *infections* introduced via acupuncture needles (51[c])–(53[c]). It is notable that all of these adverse events would not have occurred if acupuncture had been carried out properly.

Aromatherapy

Aromatherapy is a popular treatment, in which plant essential oils are applied usually by gentle massage techniques on the body surface. Essential oils can cause *allergic reactions*.

A 39-year-old woman had a 10-week history of a pruritic, erythematous, eruption on her face and chest (54[c]). She had been using aromatherapy for the past 2–3 years. Patch testing was positive for neomycin, fragrance mix, and benzoylperoxide. Discontinuation of aromatherapy led to rapid resolution.

Similar cases of allergic contact dermatitis have been associated with tea tree oil (55[C]), (56[c]) and black cumin oil (57[C]).

Chiropractic

The most common causes of malpractice lawsuits against chiropractors in the US have been reviewed (58[R]). Between 1991 and 1995 the National Chiropractic Mutual Insurance Company (NCMIC) paid over $73 million for 1403 lost cases at an average of $52 000 per case. Claims were most often made (in decreasing order) for disc problems (27%), fractures, failure to make a diagnosis, aggravation of a prior condition, strokes, vicarious liability, and burns (3.5%).

In a prospective survey, adverse effect data on 12 consecutive new patients of 102 Norwegian chiropractors have been collected (59[C]), covering 4712 treatments on 1058 patients. At least one adverse effect was reported by 55% of these patients at some time during the course of a maximum of six treatments. *Local discomfort* (53%), *headache* (72%), *tiredness* (11%), or *radiating discomfort* (10%) were the most frequent symptoms. Reactions were mostly transient and mild to moderate and 74% had resolved within 24 h.

Special senses Some serious adverse effects on vision have been reported.

A 39-year-old woman was treated with cervical manipulation by a chiropractor (60[c]). She subsequently developed sudden left peripheral visual field loss. An MRI scan performed on the day of the event showed acute infarction of the ventromedial aspect of the inferior right occipital lobe. The authors assumed that the incident had been caused by cervical manipulation.

A 45-year-old woman received chiropractic treatment for tension headache and experienced sudden retro-orbital pain on her left side (61[c]). Over the next 36 h, she developed complete ophthalmoplegia and the pain increased. Angiography of the intracranial vessels showed an aneurysm of the posterior communicating artery. This had apparently been asymptomatic before the high velocity rotational thrust of the chiropractor. The patient made an uneventful recovery after operation.

Delays in diagnosis Two case reports (62[c]) have provided impressive examples of the indirect risks of complementary medicine. Both cases relate to children who had been in prolonged chiropractic care for back and leg pains. This treatment was not successful and they were eventually seen by a pediatrician, who diagnosed a large choriocarcinoma in the child with back pain and an aggressive osteosarcoma in the patient with leg pain. In both cases valuable time had been lost owing to failure to diagnose.

Massage

A 51-year-old woman with a left ureteral stent to relieve the symptoms of a ureteral stricture consulted a Rolfing therapist, who treated her with a deep body massage according to the Rolfing technique (63[c]). The massage included the patient's abdomen, pelvis, and lower back. Towards the end of the session she felt left flank pain and had urinary incontinence. X-ray examination showed displacement of the stent. Surgical restoration of the stent quickly resolved her symptoms.

REFERENCES

1. Drew AK, Myers SP. Safety issues in herbal medicine: implications for the health professions. Med J Aust 1997;166:538–41.
2. Thompson CA. Adverse reactions to alternative medicine. Am J Health Syst Pharm 1997; 54:1707.
3. Chan TYK. Monitoring the safety of herbal medicines. Drug Saf 1997;17:209–15.
4. Castot A, Djezzar S, Deleau N, Guillot B, Efthymiou ML. Une pharmacovigilance hors des sentiers battus: la phytovigilance ou la pharmacovigilance des plantes médicinales. Thérapie 1997;52:97–103.
5. De Smet PAGM. Adverse effects of herbal remedies. Adv Drug React Bull 1997;183:695–8.
6. Furbee B, Wermuth M. Life-threatening plant poisoning. Crit Care Clin 1997;13:849.
7. Kaplowitz N. Hepatotoxicity of herbal remedies: insights into the intricacies of plant-animal warfare and cell death. Gastroenterology 1997; 113:1408–11.
8. Lee AU, Farrell GC. Drug-induced liver disease. Curr Opin Gastroenterol 1997;13:199–205.
9. Larrey D. Hepatotoxicity of herbal remedies. J Hepatol 1997;26 (Suppl 1):47–51.
10. Benzi G, Ceci A. Herbal medicines in European regulation. Pharmacol Res 1997;35:355–62.
11. Manteiga R, Park DL. Risks associated with consumption of herbal teas. Rev Environ Contam Toxicol 1997;150:1–30.
12. Brown R. Potential interactions of herbal medicines with antipsychotics, antidepressants and hypnotics. Eur J Med 1997;3:25–8.
13. Lepik K. Safety of herbal medications in pregnancy. Can Pharm J 1997;130:29–33.
14. Varga CA, Veale DJH. Isihlambezo: utilization patterns and potential health effects of pregnancy-related traditional herbal medicine. Soc Sci Med 1997;44:911–24.
15. Anonymous. Phytotherapy: how to minimise risks. Prescrire Int 1997;6:25–6.
16. Shaw D, Leon C, Kolev S, Murray V. Traditional remedies and food supplements. A 5-year toxicological study (1991–1995). Drug Saf 1997; 17:342–56.
17. Deng J-F, Lin T-J, Kao W-F, Chen S-S. The

difficulty in handling poisonings associated with Chinese traditional medicine: a poison control centre experience for 1991–1993. Vet Human Toxicol 1997;39:106–14.
18. Mabina MH, Pitsoe SB, Moodley J. The effect of traditional herbal medicines on pregnancy outcome. S Afr Med J 1997;87:1008–10.
19. Ma JW. Review of the literature about adverse drug reactions published in the Chinese Pharmaceutical Journal. Clin Pharm J (China) 1997;32:308–11.
20. Hilepo JN, Bellucci AG, Mossey RT. Acute renal failure caused by 'Cat's claw' herbal remedy in a patient with systemic lupus erythematosus. Nephron 1997;77:361.
21. Anonymous. Herbal 'Fen-Phen' warning concerning 'natural' anti-obesity alternatives. WHO Pharm Newslett 1977;9110:2.
22. Ernst E, Rand JI, Barnes J, Stevenson C. Adverse effects profile of the herbal antidepressant St John's wort (*Hypericum perforatum* L.). Eur J Clin Pharmacol 1998;54:589–94.
23. Parsons BJ, Dobbin M, Tibballs J. Eucalyptus oil poisoning among young children: mechanisms of access and the potential for prevention. Aust New Zealand J Publ Health 1997;21:297–302.
24. Dewitt MS, Swain R, Gibson LB. The dangers of Jimson weed and its abuse by teenagers in the Kanawha Valley of West Virginia. West Va Med J 1997;93:182–5.
25. Koevoets PF, van Harten PN. Doornappelintoxicatie. Ned Tijdschr Geneesk 1997;141:888–9.
26. Spillane PK, Fisher DA, Currie BJ. Neurological manifestations of kava intoxication. Med J Aust 1997;167:172–3.
27. Anonymous. Herbal products mislabelled as 'plantain'—warning: may contain digitalis. WHO Pharm Newslett 1997;11112:6.
28. Ferguson JE, Chalmers RJG, Rowlands DJ. Reversible dilated cardiomyopathy following treatment of atopic eczema with Chinese herbal medicine. Br J Dermatol 1997;136:592–3.
29. Kamiyama T, Nouchi T, Kojima S, Murata N, Ikeda T, Sato C. Autoimmune hepatitis triggered by administration of an herbal medicine. Am J Gastroenterol 1997;92:703–4.
30. Matsuda R, Takahashi D, Chiba E, Kawana I, Tomiyama M, Ebira H, Ikegami T, Kitamura H, Ishii M. A case of drug induced hepatitis and interstitial pneumonia caused by a herbal drug, dai saiko-to. Jap J Dig Med 1997;94:787–91.
31. Sato A, Toyoshima M, Kondo A, Ohta K, Sato H, Ohsumi A. Pneumonitis induced by the herbal medicine sho-saiko-to in Japan. Jpn J Thorac Dis 1997;35:391–5.
32. Yu CM, Chan JCN, Sanderson JE. Chinese herbs and warfarin potentiation by 'danshen'. J Int Med 1997;241:337–9.
33. Takei A, Nagashima G, Suzuki R, Hokaku H, Takahashi M, Miyo T, Asai J, Sanada Y, Fujimoto T. Meningoencephalocele associated with *Tripterygium wilfordii* treatment. Pediatr Neurosurg 1997;27:45–8.
34. Wong SS, Tan KC, Goh CL. Cutaneous manifestations of chronic arsenicism: review of seventeen cases. J Am Acad Dermatol 1998;38:179–85.
35. Khayat AA, Menon NS, Alidini MR. Acute lead encephalopathy in early infancy-clinical presentation and outcome. Ann Trop Paediatr 1997;17:39–44.
36. Hasegawa S, Nakayama K, Iwakiri K, An E, Gomi S, Dan K, Katsumata M, Minami M, Wakabayashi W. Herbal medicine-associated lead intoxication. Int Med 1997;36:56–8.
37. Huang WF, Wen K-C, Hsiao M-L. Adulteration by synthetic therapeutic substances of traditional Chinese medicines in Taiwan. J Clin Pharmacol 1997;37:344–50.
38. Wood B, Wishart J. Potent topical steroid in a Chinese herbal cream. NZ Med J 1997;110:420–1.
39. Frasca T, Brett AS, Yoo SD. Mandrake toxicity. Arch Intern Med 1997;157:2007–9.
40. Violon C. Belgian (Chinese herb) nephropathy: why? J Pharm Belg 1997;52:7–27.
41. Tanaka A, Nishida R, Sawai K, Nagae T, Shinkai S, Ishikawa M, Mueda K, Murata M, Seta K, Okuda J, Yoshida T, Sugawara A, Kuwahara T. Chinese herbs nephropathy. Jpn J Nephrol 1997;39:794–7.
42. Tanaka A, Shinkai S, Kasuno K, Maeda K, Murata M, Seta K, Okuda J, Sugawara A, Yoshida T, Nishida R, Kuwahara T. Chinese herbs nephropathy. Jpn J Nephrol 1997;39:438–40.
43. Reginster F, Jadoul M, Van Ypersele de Strihou C. Chinese herbs nephropathy presentation, natural history and fate after transplantation. Nephrol Dial Transplant 1997;12:81–6.
44. Breenbaum D, Smolinske S, Srinivasan R. Probable gastrointestinal toxicity kombucha tea, 'Is this beverage healthy or harmful?' J Gen Intern Med 1997;12:643–4.
45. Ernst E, White A. Life-threatening adverse reactions after acupuncture? A systematic review. Pain 1997;71:123–6.
46. Tanaka E, Nakatsuji Y, Kobayashi M, Iijima A, Ichijo T, Imai H, Yoshizawa K, Sodeyama T, Kiyosawa K. Hepatitis G virus/GB virus C infection in an area of high endemic hepatitis C virus infection. Hepatol Res 1997;7:130–5.
47. Vilke M. Case reports of two patients with pneumothorax following acupuncture. J Emerg Med 1997;15:155–7.
48. Mansuri I, Olusanya O. Pneumothorax following acupuncture. J Am Board Fam Pract 1997;10:296–7.
49. Kataoka H. Cardiac tamponade caused by penetration of an acupuncture needle into the right ventricle. J Thorac Card Surg 1997;114:674–6.
50. Huang EY, Sobel E, Wieting CB. Drop foot as a complication of acupuncture injury and intragluteal injection. J Am Podiatr Med Assoc 1997;87:52–9.
51. Chen CY, Huang CL, Liu GC, Sheu RS. Bacterial meningitis and lumbar epidural hematoma due to lumbar acupunctures: a case report. Kaohsiung J Med Sci 1997;13:328–31.

52. Kirschenbaum AE, Rizzo C. Glenohumeral pyarthrosis following acupuncture treatment. Orthopedics 1997;20:1184–6.
53. Pinto LF, Ramos RF, Ramos S. Auricular perichondritis due to acupuncture. Rev Bras Otorrinol 1997;63:589–92.
54. James WD, Weiss RR. Allergic contact dermatitis from aromatherapy. Am J Contact Dermatitis 1997;8:250–1.
55. Beck BM. Allergic contact dermatitis from tea tree oil in a wart paint. Am J Contact Dermatitis 1997;36:117–18.
56. Kranke B. Allergy inducing potency of tea tree oil. Hautarzt 1997;48:203–4.
57. Agothos M, Breit R, Schatzle M, Steinmann A. Allergic contact dermatitis from black cumin (*Nigella sativa*) oil after topical use. Am J Contact Dermatitis 1997;36:268–9.
58. Jagbandhansingh MP. Most common causes of chiropractic malpractice lawsuits. J Manip Physiol Ther 1997;20:60–4.
59. Senstad O, Leboeuf-Yde C, Borchgrevink C. Frequency and characteristics of side effects of spinal manipulative therapy. Spine 1997;22:435–41.
60. Donzis PB. Visual field loss resulting from cervical chiropractic manipulation. Am J Ophthalmol 1997;123:851–2.
61. Simnad VI. Alerts, notices, and case reports. Acute onset of painful ophthalmoplegia following chiropractic manipulation of the neck. Initial sign of intracranial aneurysm. West J Med 1997; 166:207–10.
62. Turow VD. Chiropractic for children. Arch Pediatr Adolesc Med 1997;151:527–8.
63. Kerr HD. Ureteral stent displacement associated with deep massage. Wisconsin Med J 1997;12:57–8.

N.H. Choulis

49 Miscellaneous drugs, materials, and medical devices

DRUGS

Ammoniated mercury

Health Canada has warned consumers not to use Diana Cream (Diana de Beaut®), a product that is used for skin lightening, mainly by Afro-Caribbean communities. The product, which is manufactured in the Lebanon, has not been approved for sale in Canada and is being illegally imported. It contains ammoniated mercury, bismuth subnitrate, and salicylic acid, and the mercury content poses a high risk of mercury poisoning in adults and a serious health hazard to unborn and nursing infants of women who use the product (1[r]).

The Directorate General of Pharmaceutical Affairs and Drug Control has prohibited the registration, import, and sale of Diana Cream. The product is not registered as a drug in Oman, but it is available on the market as a cosmetic product. After the warning had been issued in Canada, an analysis carried out by the Directorate's Quality Control Laboratory confirmed that it contains ammoniated mercury.

Bisphosphonates and aminobisphosphonates *(SEDA 10, 444)*

The development of bisphosphonates for clinical purposes began with the discovery that inorganic pyrophosphate is present in blood and urine and inhibits the precipitation of calcium and phosphate (2[R]). Derivatives of pyrophosphate had been widely used for industrial purposes, because they inhibit the precipitation of calcium carbonate. Their principal use was as antiscaling additives in washing powders, water, and oil brines, to prevent deposition of calcium carbonate scale. It was then found that pyrophosphate binds strongly to calcium phosphate, prevents both the formation and dissolution of calcium phosphate crystals, and inhibits calcification in vitro. Furthermore, ectopic calcification was prevented by parenteral, but not oral, pyrophosphate (3[R]). The bisphosphonates are an important class of drugs for treating postmenopausal osteoporosis.

The beneficial effect of orally administered bisphosphonates on bone mineral density has been firmly established. Placebo-controlled double-blind studies of intermittent cyclical etidronate treatment of postmenopausal women showed an approximate 5% gain in lumbar bone mineral density. Most of the gain was achieved in the first year, but extension studies have confirmed additional slight increments in bone mineral density. Etidronate was given orally for only the first 2 weeks of each 3-month period, since prolonged daily administration of etidronate causes osteomalacia.

But gains come at a price. Besides causing osteomalacia, etidronate causes gastrointestinal problems in a few patients. The aminobisphosphonates cause more severe gastrointestinal adverse effects but do not cause osteomalacia; however, of greatest concern is their capacity to cause esophageal lesions. A recent report identified three patients with severe esophagitis from alendronate (an aminobisphosphonate) (4[r]).

The efficacy and safety of amidronate in recalcitrant reflex sympathetic dystrophy have been assessed in 10 women and 13 men, mean age 44 years (5[C]). The involved sites were the

Side Effects of Drugs, Annual 22
J.K. Aronson, ed.

ankle ($n = 10$), the foot ($n = 7$), the hand ($n = 3$), the hip ($n = 2$), the knee ($n = 2$), and the shoulder ($n = 1$). Some patients had more than one site involved. Mean duration of the disease was 15 months. The disease was in the pseudoinflammatory phase in 16 patients and in the ischemic phase in seven. It was post-traumatic in 17 cases; 11 patients have been previously treated unsuccessfully by sympathetic blockades. Amidronate was given intravenously in a dose of 1 mg/kg per day for 1–3 days. There were adverse events in 14 patients: transient fever ($n = 6$), venous inflammation ($n = 2$), transient symptomless hypocalcemia ($n = 3$), nausea ($n = 1$), lymphopenia ($n = 1$), transient hypertension ($n = 1$).

In 57 patients with advanced prostate cancer resistant to first-line hormonal therapy treated with estramustine and clodronate (300 mg/day intravenously for 5 days followed by 1.6 g/day orally for 12 months), the main adverse effect was nausea (6[C]). However, therapeutic efficacy was small.

Disulfiram *(SED-13, 1465)*

Disulfiram (tetraethylthiurum disulfide), a quaternary ammonium compound, acts as a deterrent against drinking.

Cardiovascular Cardiac dysrhythmias occurred during a disulfiram-alcohol test in a 48-year-old man who had been an alcoholic for 5 years (7[c]). He was a well-motivated, cooperative patient with no other illnesses and normal laboratory examinations including electrocardiography. He was given disulfiram 250 mg bd, and a week later came to the clinic, where he was allowed to drink alcohol under close supervision. After drinking a small amount of alcohol, he developed flushing, nausea, vomiting, sweating, dyspnea and hyperventilation, palpitation, tremor, confusion, and syncope. The electrocardiogram showed atrial fibrillation and non-sustained bouts of ventricular tachycardia of 7–8 beats/-min. He also had severe hypotension (BP 140/60 mmHg).

Psychiatric Of 52 patients (51 men) with alcohol dependence/abuse who were given disulfiram 250 mg bd after food, six developed psychotic symptoms; all had a mood disorder but no thought disorder (8[C]). The psychotic symptoms remitted completely after withdrawal and a short course of antipsychotic therapy, except in one patient who had to be given lithium.

Skin and appendages A 55-year-old man developed yellow palms and soles while taking disulfiram (9[c]). The authors speculated that the mechanism was inhibition of carotene metabolism by disulfiram.

γ-Hydroxybutyric acid

The FDA has reiterated its warning against the use of γ-hydroxybutyric acid for body building and 'recreational' uses. This product is unapproved and potentially dangerous, and its use can lead to symptoms such as vomiting, dizziness, tremors, and seizures, frequently requiring hospitalization; some deaths have occurred (10[r]).

Despite enforcement actions against manufacturers, distributors, and importers, as well as public education campaigns, there appears to be a resurgence in the abuse of γ-hydroxybutyric acid. Virtually all the products now encountered have been produced in clandestine laboratories.

Nicotine *(SED-13, 1468; SEDA-19, 443; SEDA-20, 439)*

The FDA has recently approved the use of nicotine inhalers, available by prescription only, for smoking cessation. In one study of 123 participants, after 3–5 days, 33 (27%) reported coughing and 18 (15%) had irritation of the mouth or throat (11[C]). At 3 weeks, 7% reported coughing and 10% mouth and throat irritation.

In another study (12[C]) 18 healthy subjects who inhaled nicotine for 20 min (80 inhalations) every hour for 10 h at three different environmental temperatures of 20, 30, and 40°C, the adverse experiences reported were twice as frequent at 40°C as at 20°C. Most often reported were coughing, a lump in the throat, and a sore or irritated throat. Belching, hiccups, pressure over the chest, headache, and heartburn were reported only occasionally. About one-fifth of the subjects experienced coughing after the first five to 10 inhalations.

Cardiovascular Nicotine patches have been reported to be associated with acute myocardial infarction (13[r]), (14[r]) and dysrhythmias (15[r]).

A 33-year-old woman presented with chest and abdominal pain shortly after using a nicotine patch twice (16[c]). A type A aortic dissection was diagnosed and repaired. Pathological examination showed cystic medial necrosis and subacute and acute dissection, with no evidence of chronic aortic insufficiency.

The close temporal relation between the use of the nicotine patch and the onset of symptoms compatible with dissection followed by extension raised the possibility that the nicotine patch was implicated in or precipitated this woman's aortic dissection.

Musculoskeletal Myasthenia gravis was worsened by a nicotine transdermal system in a man who usually smoked 40 cigarettes per day without effect on his myasthenia (17[c]). Two hours after applying a nicotine transdermal system he noted increased bilateral ptosis, total ophthalmoplegia, difficulty in chewing, and generalized weakness; the symptoms improved after he removed the patch. Cholinergic receptors involved in myasthenia gravis are nicotinergic, and their number at the neuromuscular junction is reduced in myasthenia gravis. That led to a functional overdosage after the use of nicotine, similar to a cholinergic crisis. This case can be compared with myasthenic syndromes described during the Second World War in tobacco chewers without any muscle impairment.

Phenol *(SED-13, 1468)*

Chemical neurolysis with phenol is commonly used in chemical denervation for the treatment of hypertonia and related motor disorders. Many of these disorders are amenable to this form of treatment, although the likelihood of success depends to some extent on the nature of the motor disorder. The physiological and therapeutic effects, technique, safety, and toxicology and adverse effects and complications have been reviewed (18[R]).

Other reports have suggested that intramuscular injections of phenol can result in pain and swelling in the muscle (19[r]), (20[r]). Sometimes a firm nodular swelling develops in the calf 1–3 weeks after intramuscular neurolysis (21[r]), particularly when larger quantities of phenol are injected into the intramuscular branches of the tibial nerve. This can usually be avoided by limiting the quantity of phenol injected to the minimum necessary and by applying cold packs to the injected area after the procedure.

Muscle necrosis and round cell infiltrates have also been seen in histological studies of animal muscle recently injected with phenol, but are not seen after a few months have passed (21[r]).

Otherwise, the complications of motor and mixed sensorimotor chemical denervation are similar. Peripheral edema may develop when tone in an extremity is reduced, particularly in blocks affecting the triceps surae.

Finally, loss of voluntary motor strength or sensory loss are not uncommon in the first few days after chemical neurolysis with phenol (22[r]), but permanent loss, other than motor changes associated with the reduction in hypertonia, are unusual (23[r]), (24[r]). A muscle that is already weak is more susceptible to further weakening with chemical neurolysis (25[r]). There has been only one report of loss of all sensation and strength after chemical neurolysis. This occurred in the distribution of the posterior tibial nerve following mixed sensorimotor block of this nerve, in this case after five blocks of the nerve or its motor branches over many years. Some strength and partial sensation returned after surgical lysis of excessive fibrous tissue at the site where the injection had been performed (26[r]).

Polyvinylpyrrolidone storage disease

Polyvinylpyrrolidone was formerly used as a plasma expander (27[r]) and has been inappro-

priately used for intravenous injection as a 'blood tonic'. It is a polymer with a variable molecular weight. Molecules that weigh less than 20 kDa can be excreted by a normal functioning kidney, whereas larger polymers are phagocytosed and permanently stored in the mononuclear phagocytic system, causing so-called polyvinylpyrrolidone storage disease. The first cutaneous case of polyvinylpyrrolidone storage disease, reported in 1964 (28[c]), was caused by local injection of polyvinylpyrrolidone-containing posterior pituitary extracts for the treatment of diabetes insipidus. Similar cases, including those following local injection of porcine polyvinylpyrrolidone to treat neuralgia, were documented, mostly in European reports (29[c]), (30[c]). Localized cutaneous polyvinylpyrrolidone storage disease was then known as Dupont-Lachapelle disease (31[c]).

Five cases of polyvinylpyrrolidone storage disease with cutaneous involvement have been studied (32[C]). Two patients presented with skin eruptions mimicking collagen vascular disease and chronic pigmented purpuric dermatosis. Two other cases were found incidentally: in one, polyvinylpyrrolidone was found in a metastatic tumor, and in the other in a pemphigus lesion. The fifth case was seen in a blind skin biopsy specimen taken to exclude Niemann-Pick disease after examination of a bone marrow smear. The latter patient and the patient with a collagen vascular-like disease also had severe anemia and serious orthopedic and neurological complications due to massive infiltration of polyvinylpyrrolidone-containing cells in the bone marrow, with destruction of the bone. Severe irreversible anemia due to polyvinylpyrrolidone storage disease has not been reported before.

Polyvinylpyrrolidone storage disease can be diagnosed by its histopathological features. The skin biopsy specimens all showed a variable number of characteristic blue-gray vacuolated cells around blood vessels and adnexal structures and stained positively with mucicarmine, colloidal iron, and alkaline Congo red, and negatively with periodic acid Schiff and alcian blue. The polyvinylpyrrolidone storage cells were CD68+ macrophages. The presence of polyvinylpyrrolidone in the skin induced little or no inflammatory reaction. Only the pelvic mass in one patient had a foreign body granuloma formation.

This study showed that parenteral administration of polyvinylpyrrolidone could result in the accumulation of polyvinylpyrrolidone storage cells in the skin, with or without clinical eruptions. The diagnosis of systemic polyvinylpyrrolidone storage disease can be established by skin biopsy. It is important for pathologists and clinicians to be aware of this iatrogenic storage disease to avoid misdiagnosis of hereditary storage disease, osteomyelitis, or signet-ring cell carcinoma. Serious hematological and orthopedic complications can be caused by repeated massive intravenous injection of polyvinylpyrrolidone. Polyvinylpyrrolidone should therefore be strictly prohibited for systemic administration.

Sorbitol

Kayexalate (sodium polystyrene sulfonate) in sorbitol is commonly used to treat hyperkalemia in patients with renal insufficiency. Isolated case reports have documented intestinal necrosis after the administration of kayexalate in sorbitol (33[c]). In one study there was an incidence of 1.8%, and the authors concluded that sorbitol-associated complications may not be uncommon postoperatively (34[c]). Furthermore, it has been suggested that some cases of idiopathic colonic ulcers in patients with renal failure are due to the effects of sorbitol. While kayexalate crystals, which are purple, irregular, and jagged, can be an incidental finding and are not known to cause injury, they are a helpful histological clue to the possibility that sorbitol has been administered. It must be remembered that kayexalate crystals can be found in normal mucosa and must be distinguished from cholestyramine crystals. Kayexalate crystals are less basophilic and opaque than cholestyramine crystals and stain red with acid-fast stain (35[C]).

Five cases of extensive mucosal necrosis and transmural infarction of the colon have been reported after the use of kayexalate and sorbitol enemas to treat hyperkalemia in uremic patients (36[C]). The authors studied the effects of kayexalate sorbitol enemas in normal and uremic rats and concluded that sorbitol was responsible for colonic damage and that the injury was potentiated in uremic rats.

When sorbitol alone or kayexalate sorbitol were given, extensive transmural necrosis developed in 80% of normal rats and in all the uremic rats. The pathogenesis was unclear but it was speculated that the osmotic load could cause vascular shunting, resulting in intestinal ischemia, or that the osmotic load from sorbitol could cause direct toxic damage by disrupting mechanisms that regulate cell volume.

Finally sorbitol has been used for treating raised intracranial pressure (37[r]). The hazards of intravenous fructose loading (hyperlactatemia, lactic acidosis, hyperuricemia, depletion of intracellular ATP and ADP, and depletion of inorganic phosphate) are well known (38[R]). Although in humans sorbitol is converted to fructose, the hazards of sorbitol administration are less well recognized.

In an otherwise healthy 56-year-old man who underwent a craniotomy, sorbitol loading caused severe electrolyte and acid–base disturbances (39[c]). He developed lactic acidosis, hypophosphatemia, and hyperglycemia, and had a reduced inorganic phosphate and an increased uric acid, which could have been explained by sorbitol metabolism.

Sorbitol is oxidized to fructose by sorbitol dehydrogenase, and thereafter its metabolism is the same as that of fructose. The main sites of sorbitol oxidation are the liver (40[r]) and to a lesser extent the kidney (41[r]).

Sterile water

The FDA is aware of four cases of hemolysis that have occurred since 1994, during or after plasmapheresis when human albumin 25% was diluted to a 5% final protein concentration using sterile water for injection (42[C]). Hemolysis, which was observed in all four cases and which was followed by acute renal failure in two, resulted from infusion, during plasmapheresis, of varying amounts of hypotonic albumin solutions that had been prepared with sterile water for injection. Human albumin solutions of all concentrations are formulated to have a sodium concentration of 130–160 mmol/l. Thus, a 5-fold dilution in sterile water would produce about one-fifth that of 0.9% sodium chloride (isotonic saline). The large volumes used in plasmapheresis/-plasma exchange were likely a contributing factor, in view of the fact that the hypotonic plasma replacement mixture would have accounted for a significant fraction of the patient's calculated blood volume. In the hypotonic environment, shear forces in the plasmapheresis device may have contributed to the hemolysis.

It is not known how often this dilution error occurs in pharmacies. However, the current short supply of human albumin may lead to increasingly frequent instances of dilution of more concentrated solutions, creating an increased potential for error. The FDA is recommending to manufacturers of human albumin 25% that the package inserts for their products be revised to include: (1) a warning statement about the risk of potentially fatal hemolysis and acute renal failure when sterile water for injection is used as a diluent for albumin; and (2) information on acceptable diluents, such as 0.9% saline or 5% dextrose in water. The importance of consulting up-to-date references is also emphasized. The risk of serious morbidity and mortality can be reduced by remembering that whenever drugs for intravenous infusion are diluted, the tonicity of the final solution must be considered.

DIETARY PRODUCTS

Grapefruit juice

The UK Committee on Safety of Medicines has cautioned against the concurrent consumption of grapefruit juice with cyclosporin, terfenadine, and calcium antagonists (except amlodipine and diltiazem), since the metabolism of these drugs is inhibited by a substance, possibly a psoralen, in grapefruit juice, with a resultant increase in plasma concentrations, which could be clinically important (43[r]).

The duration of the effect is not known and it is unclear how long patients should leave between drinking grapefruit juice and taking the drugs. Although the Committee has not received any reports of adverse reactions as a consequence of interactions between these medicines and grapefruit juice, patients are advised to avoid drinking grapefruit juice when taking these drugs.

MEDICAL DEVICES

Chlorhexidine-impregnated medical devices

The FDA has alerted health-care professionals to a potential for serious hypersensitivity reactions to chlorhexidine-impregnated medical devices (44[r]). Three types of medical devices have been approved recently that incorporate chlorhexidine: intravenous catheters, topic antimicrobial skin dressings, and implanted antimicrobial surgical mesh.

Although the antimicrobial properties of chlorhexidine are well known, it is less well known that chlorhexidine has been associated with hypersensitivity reactions. Anaphylactoid and other types of reactions have been reported with chlorhexidine used topically, and intraurethrally, as a lubricant on urinary catheters and with chlorhexidine-impregnated catheters.

Medical telemetry systems

The FDA and the Federal Communications Commission have issued a joint statement concerning incidents involving digital television transmissions interfering with medical telemetry systems, such as cardiac monitors, that use TV channels (45[r]). In one case, the telemetry system was operating on a TV channel that had been unused for many years but had been recently reassigned by the Federal Communications Commission to a TV station in the vicinity of the hospital. The new TV signal interfered with the hospital's telemetry system and rendered it unusable. Another hospital in the same city was also affected.

Medical telemetry devices have long shared the TV broadcast spectrum on a secondary basis. However, television stations are now beginning to use these formerly unoccupied TV channels as the transition to digital television proceeds. The sharing can continue during the implementation of digital television; however, it is important to ensure that broadcasters, the health care community and manufacturers of medical devices have adequate information and take appropriate steps to avoid radio frequency interference.

'Stimulator'

The FDA has issued a consumer alert about a device called the 'Stimulator', which has been widely promoted for relieving pain and treating a variety of other medical problems; this product has not been approved by the FDA (46[r]). The 'Stimulator' is essentially an electric gas barbecue grill igniter fitted with a finger grip. Another product, the 'Xtender', connects to the Stimulator so that it can be used on hard-to-reach parts of the body. When pressed against the skin, the Stimulator sparks and causes a small electric shock. Makers of the device claim that it can relieve headaches, back pain, arthritis, stress, menstrual cramps, earaches, sinus pain, nosebleeds, influenza, and other ailments. Because of these claims, the Stimulator is considered to be a medical device. The manufacturers, however, have not complied with any FDA regulations that govern the marketing of medical devices and have submitted no information showing that the device is either safe or effective, or substantially equivalent to any other legally marketed medical device.

SURGICAL MATERIALS AND DEVICES

Collagen *(SED-13, 1456)*

One of the minimally invasive treatment options for urinary incontinence is the injection of bulking agents such as collagen (47[r]) into the suburethral tissues. Glutaraldehyde cross-linked bovine purified collagen was approved by the FDA in 1993 for the management of urinary incontinence. The procedure is relatively simple and can be performed under local anesthesia. Few complications have been reported, including a delayed hypersensitivity response, urinary tract infection, bleeding, and transient urinary retention.

A 76-year-old woman was referred for evaluation of persistent urgency, increased urinary frequency, nocturia, and urge incontinence 18 months after repeated transurethral collagen injections (48[c]). She had a history of retropubic bladder neck suspension

Table 1. *Miscellaneous reports*

Drug/material	Adverse effect(s)	Reference
Cremophor EL	Anaphylactoid reactions	(51[r])
Cyanamide	Granulocytopenia	(52[r])
Fluorescein	Anaphylactic shock	(53[r])
Magnesium lactate and citrate	Digestive problems	(54[c])
Methylene blue	Anaphylactic shock	(55[c])
Nitric oxide (animals)	Hypotension, bradycardia	(56)
Paraffin	Paraffinoma	(57[r])
Royal jelly	Allergic reactions	(58[r])
Silicone	Fibromyalgia	(59[c])
Sodium phosphate	Hypokalemia	(60[c])
Tea tree oil	Skin reactions, contact allergic eczema	(61[r])
Zirconium	Hypersensitivity granulomas	(62[C])

and an anterior repair combined with a Starney suspension performed, respectively, 6 and 2 years before presentation. After the last operation she had been re-evaluated for recurrent stress urinary incontinence and was offered periurethral collagen injections. There were numerous collagen deposits obstructing the bladder outlet and the proximal urethra. A transurethral resection of the collagen was performed, and her symptoms and flow pattern improved.

Although irritating lower urinary tract symptoms after collagen injection could be related to local inflammatory changes, persistence and eventual worsening of these symptoms should suggest the presence of iatrogenic bladder outlet obstruction.

Condoms

The FDA has issued a final regulation requiring that the labelling of latex condoms shall contain an expiration date based on physical and mechanical testing performed after exposing the product to varying conditions that age latex, both on the outside packaging and on the individual packaging (49[r]).

Latex condoms degrade over time. Such degradation has a significant effect on the product's ability to provide a barrier to sexually transmitted agents, including human immunodeficiency virus (HIV).

The agency has also stipulated that if a latex condom contains spermicide, and if the expiry date based upon spermicidal stability testing is different from the expiry date based on latex integrity testing, the product shall bear only the earlier expiry date.

Latex *(SED-13, 1463)*

In response to reports of allergic reactions to some medical devices, the FDA is requiring all medical devices containing latex to be labelled as such and to carry a caution that latex can cause allergic reactions (50[r]).

The following statement will be required on the labelling of devices that contain natural rubber latex and their packaging: Caution: this product contains natural rubber latex which may cause allergic reactions. Products and packaging that contain dry natural rubber will have to be identified as containing dry natural rubber.

Over the past decade, the FDA has received more than 1700 reports of severe allergic reactions, including 16 deaths, related to medical devices containing latex. The deaths all occurred in 1989 among children with spina bifida and were caused by a reaction to the latex cuffs used on the tip of barium enema catheters. The manufacturer voluntarily recalled all the enema tips on the market and started using tips with silicon tips instead.

Allergic reactions have been reported to a wide range of medical devices that contain latex, including latex surgical gloves, adhesive bandages, intravenous catheters, and anesthesia equipment. Two groups are at greater risk than the general public, because of constant exposure to latex: health-care workers and children with spina bifida and other conditions that require multiple surgical procedures.

The FDA is also requiring that all 'hypoallergenic' claims on medical devices be removed, because they incorrectly imply that the devices may be safely used by people sensitive to latex. Such claims are currently found on many medical devices that contain reduced amounts of latex protein. However, these products may still cause allergic reactions in people who are latex sensitive.

MISCELLANEOUS

Reports of adverse effects of other miscellaneous substances are listed in Table 1.

REFERENCES

1. Anonymous. Ammoniated mercury in skin lightening cream—warning against use and prohibition. WHO Pharm Newslett 1998;5/6 (May/June):1.
2. Vitte C, Fleisch H, Guenther HL. Bisphosphonates induce osteoblasts to secrete an inhibitor of osteoclast-mediated resorption. Endocrinology 1966;137:2324–33.
3. Papapulos SE. Osteoporosis. New York: Academic Press, 1996:1212–15.
4. Dreyfuss BJ, Rai DS. Biophosphonates in the treatment of osteoporosis. West J Med 1997; 167:177–8.
5. Cortet B, Flipo R-M, Coquerelle P, Duquesnoy B, Delcambre B. Treatment of severe, recalcitrant reflex sympathetic dystrophy: assessment of efficacy and safety of the second generation biphosphonate pamidronate. Clin Rheumatol 1997;16:51–6.
6. Kylmala T, Taube T, Tammela TLJ, Risteli L, Elomaa I. Concomitant i.v. and oral clodronate in the relief of bone pain: a double-blind placebo-controlled study in patients with prostate cancer. Br J Cancer 1997;76:939–42.
7. Savas MC, Gullu IH. Disulfiram-ethanol test reaction: significance of supervision. Ann Pharmacother 1997;31:374–5.
8. Murthy KK. Psychosis during disulfiram therapy for alcoholism. J Indian Med Assoc 1997; 95:80–1.
9. Santonastaso M, Cecchetti E, Pace M, Piccolo D. Yellow palms with disulfiram. Lancet 1997;350:266.
10. Anonymous. γ-Hydroxybutyric-acid: warning. WHO Pharm Newslett 1997;11/12 (Nov/Dec):6.
11. Hjalmarson A, Nilsson F, Sjostrom L, Wiklund O. Nicotine inhaler in smoking cessation. Arch Intern Med 1997;157:1721–8.
12. Lunell E, Molander L, Andersson S-B. Temperature dependency of the release and bioavailability of nicotine from a nicotine vapour inhaler; in vitro/in vivo correlation. Eur J Clin Pharmacol 1997;52:495–500.
13. Orleans CT, Ockene JK. Routine hospital-based quit-smoking treatment for the postmyocardial infarction patient: an idea whose time has come. J Am Coll Cardiol 1993;22:1703–5.
14. Warner JG Jr, Little WC. Myocardial infarction in a patient who smoked while wearing a nicotine patch. Ann Intern Med 1994;120:695.
15. Arnaot MR. Treating heart disease. Nicotine patches may not be safe. Br Med J 1995;310:663–4.
16. Ropchan GV, Sanfilippo AJ, Ford SE. Aortic dissection and use of the nicotine patch: a case involving a temporal relationship. Can J Cardiol 1997;13:525–8.
17. Moreau T, Vukusic S, Vandenabeele S, Confavreux C. Nicotine et aggravation de la myasthenie. Rev Neurol 1997;153:141–3.
18. Glenn MB, Elovic E. Chemical denervation for the treatment of hypertonia and related motor disordrers: phenol and Botulinum toxin. J Head Trauma Rehabil 1997;12:40–62.
19. Halpern D, Meelhuysen FE. Phenol motor point block in the management of muscular hypertonia. Arch Phys Med Rehabil 1966;47:659–64.
20. Garland DE, Lilling M, Keenan MA. Percutaneous phenol blocks to motor points of spastic forearm muscles in head-injured adults. Arch Phys Med Rehabil 1984;65:243–5.
21. Halpern D, Meelhuysen FE. Duration of relaxation after intramuscular neurolysis with phenol. J Am Med Assoc 1967;200:1152–4.
22. Khalili AA, Betts HB. Peripheral nerve block with phenol in the management of spasticity: indications and complications. J Am Med Assoc 1967;200:1155–7.
23. Tardieu G, Tardieu C, Hariga J, Gagnard L. Treatment of spasticity by injection of dilute alcohol at the motor point or by epidural route. Dev Med Child Neurol 1968;10:555–68.
24. Copp EP, Harris R, Keenan J. Peripheral nerve block and motor point block with phenol in the management of spasticity. Proc R Soc Med 1970;63:937–8.
25. Khalili AA, Benton JG. A physiologic approach to the evaluation and the management of spasticity with procaine and phenol nerve block. Clin Orthop 1966;47:97–104.
26. Glenn MB. Nerve blocks for the treatment of spasticity. Phys Med Rehabil State of the Art Rev 1994;3:481–505.
27. Weese HG, Periston H. Ein never Blutluessigkeitsersatz. MHnch Med Wochenschr 1943;90:11–15.
28. Dupont A, Lachapelle JM. Dermite due à un depot medicamenteux au cours du traitement d'un diabète insipide. Bull Soc Fr Dermatol Syphilol 1964;71:508–9.
29. Lachapelle JM. Thesaurismose cutanée par polyvinylpyrrolidone. Dermatologica 1966;132: 476–89.

30. Mensing H, Koster W, Schaeg O, Nasemann T. Clinical variability of the polyvinylpyrrolidone dermatosis. Z Hautkr 1983;59:1027–37.
31. Bazex A, Geraud J, Guilhem A, Dupre A, Rascol A, Cantala P. Maladie de Dupont et Lachapelle (thesaurismose cutanée par polyvinylpyrrolidone) Arch Belg Dermatol Syphiligr 1966; 22:227–33.
32. Kuo TT, Hu S, Huang CL, Chan HL, Chang MJM, Dunn P. Cutaneous involvement in polyvinylpyrrolidone storage disease: a clinicopathologic study of five patients, including two patients with severe anemia. Am J Surg Pathol 1997; 21:1361–7.
33. Gardiner GW. Kayexalate (sodium polystyrene sulphonate) in sorbitol associated with intestinal necrosis in uremic patients. Can J Gastroenterol 1997;11:573–7.
34. Gerstman BB, Kirkman K, Platt R. Intestinal necrosis associated with postoperative orally administered sodium polystyrene sulfonate in sorbitol. Am J Kidney Dis 1992;20:159–61.
35. Rashid A, Hamilton SR. Necrosis of the gastrointestinal tract in uremic patients as a result of sodium polystyrene sulfonate (kayexalate) in sorbitol. Am J Surg Pathol 1997;21:60–9.
36. Lillimoe KD, Romolo JL, Hamilton SR, Pennington LR, Burdeck JF, Williams GM. Intestinal necrosis due to sodium polystyrene (Kayexalate) in sorbitol enemas. Clinical and experimental support for the hypothesis. Surgery 1987;101:266–72.
37. Panning B, Stolke D. Cerebraler perfusionsdruck bei akuter Blutdrucksenkung mit hyperosmolalem Sorbit unter Narkosebedingungen. Neurochirurgia 1990;33:37–41.
38. Woods HF, Alberti KG. Dangers of intravenous fructose. Lancet 1972;ii:13547.
39. Buijs EJ, Van Zuylen HJ. Metabolic consequences of a sorbitol overdose during neurosurgery. J Neurosurg Anesthesiol 1997;9:17–20.
40. Krebs HA. Some general considerations concerning the use of carbohydrates in parenteral nutrition. In: Johnston IDA, editor. Advances in Parenteral Nutrition. Lancaster: MTP Press, 1978:23–8.
41. Newton D, Connor H, Woods HF. Metabolic pathways for carbohydrates in parenteral nutrition. In: Johnston IDA, editor. Advances in Parenteral Nutrition. Lancaster: MTP Press, 1978:29–44.
42. Anonymous. Hemolysis and renal failure associated with inappropriate use of sterile water to dilute 25% albumin solution. FDA Med Bull 1998;28:5.
43. Anonymous. Grapefruit juice—drug interactions. WHO Pharm Newslett 1997;9/10 (Sept/Oct):12.
44. Anonymous. Chlorhexidine-impregnated medical devices: hypersensitivity reactions. WHO Pharm Newslett 1997;3/4 (Mar/Apr):11.
45. Anonymous. Medical telemetry systems: interference from digital TV. WHO Pharm Newslett 1997;5/6 (May/June):14.
46. Anonymous. 'Stimulator' device—consumer alert. WHO Pharm Newslett 1997;9/10 (Sept/Oct):18.
47. Winters JC, Apell R. Periurethral injection of collagen in the treatment of intrinsic sphincteric deficiency in the female patient. Urol Clin N Am 1995;22:673–8.
48. Bernier PA, Zimmern PE, Saboorian MH, Chassagne S. Female outlet obstruction after repeated collagen injections. Urology 1997;50:618–21.
49. Anonymous. Latex condoms—expiry date. WHO Pharm Newslett 1998;1/2 (Jan/Feb):14.
50. Anonymous. Latex containing devices—labelling required. WHO Pharm Newslett 1997;1/2 (Jan/Feb):16–17.
51. Michaud LB. Methods for preventing reactions secondary to cremophor EL. Ann Pharmacother 1997;31:1402–4.
52. Ajima M, Usuki K, lgarashi A, Okazaki R, Hamano K, Urabe A, Totsuka Y. Cyanamide-induced granulocytopenia. Intern Med 1997; 36:640–2.
53. Moneret-Vautrin DA. À propos des chocs anaphylactiques par application de fluoresceine sur la conjonctive oculaire. Presse Med 1997;26:420.
54. Zartarian M, Perez J-P, Gelas B, Thomas J-L.Étude comparative de l'acceptabilité et de la tolerance a court terme d'une nouvelle formulation orale de magnesium (TX 1341) et d'un magnésium de reférence. J Gynecol Obstet Biol Reprod 1997;26:182–6.
55. Evora PRB, Roselino CHC, Schiaveto PM. Methylene blue in anaphylactic shock. Ann Emerg Med 1997;30:240.
56. Verma S, Raghubir R, Patnaik GK. Nitric oxide modulation of cardiovascular responses from ventral surface of medulla in cat. Indian J Pharmacol 1997;29:125–8.
57. Mounios-Perchenet AS, Le Fourn B, Hepner-Lavergne D, Pannier M. Les paraffinomes: historique, aspects cliniques et traitement. À propos d'une observation. Ann Chir Plast Estet 1997; 42:27–30.
58. Anonymous. Royal jelly: warning concerning severe allergic reactions. WHO Pharm Newslett 1998;1/2 (Jan/Feb):7.
59. Huerkamp C, Schubert-Sollberg E, Schulze H-J, Sollberg S. Fibromyalgia syndrome in silicone breast implants. HGZ Hautkr 1997;72:212–13.
60. Anonymous. Oral sodium phosphate bowel preparations—electrolyte disturbances. WHO Pharm Newslett 1998;1/2 (Jan/Feb):4.
61. Beermann B. Tea tree oil: skin reactions. Bull SADRAC 1997;66:4.
62. Montemarano AD, Sau O, Johnson FB, James WD. Cutaneous granulomas caused by an aluminum-zirconium complex: an ingredient of antiperspirants. J Am Acad Dermatol 1997; 37:496–8.

The WHO International Drug Monitoring Programme

History

The Programme was established in 1968 as a pilot project with the participation of 10 countries that had organized national pharmacovigilance systems at that time. The intent was to develop international collaboration to make it easier to detect rare adverse drug reactions not revealed during clinical trials. The international drug monitoring centre was moved from WHO headquarters in Geneva, Switzerland, to a WHO Collaborating Centre for International Drug Monitoring in Uppsala, Sweden, in 1978. This was the result of an agreement between WHO and the government of Sweden by which Sweden assumed the operational responsibility for the Programme. WHO headquarters, Geneva, retained the responsibility for policy matters.

Present programme structure

At present 54 countries are active members of the WHO Programme. Additional nine countries have formally applied for membership and they are considered associated members while the issue of technical compatibility of their reports with the WHO requirements is established. Member countries and associated member countries are listed in the table below.

In each country a national centre, designated by the competent health authority, is responsible for the collection, processing, and evaluation of adverse reaction case reports submitted by health professionals. Information obtained from these reports is passed back to the professionals on a national basis, but is also submitted to the WHO-centre for inclusion in the international database. Collectively the centres annually provide 150 000–200 000 individual reports to WHO of reactions suspected of being drug-induced. The cumulative database of the WHO Programme now comprises two million case reports.

Case reports submitted to the WHO-centre according to an agreed format, are checked for technical correctness and then incorporated in the international database in a weekly routine. The material is screened at least four times a year for new and serious reactions as well as the reporting frequencies of associations of particular interest. Many additional examinations of the data are made on an ad hoc basis.

The WHO centre in Uppsala presently has 18 staff members. Director is Professor I. Ralph Edwards, clinical toxicologist. This staff is supported by people from various national centres, about 50 consultants of various kinds, as well as companies that provide particular specialist services. The Centre's strategy is to create a global network to optimally tackle drug safety issues.

Signal generation

A combination of automatic signalling devices and scanning by experienced medical personnel is considered most advantageous to successfully fulfil the original aim of the programme, i.e., the early identification of new adverse drug reactions. National centres are provided with a variety of signalling documents four times a year, automatically generated by the WHO

Country	Year of entry	Country	Year of entry
ARGENTINA	1994	JAPAN	1972
AUSTRALIA	1968	KOREA, REP OF	1992
AUSTRIA	1991	MALAYSIA	1990
BELGIUM	1977	MOROCCO	1992
BULGARIA	1975	NETHERLANDS	1968
CANADA	1968	NEW ZEALAND	1968
CHILE	1996	NORWAY	1971
CHINA, PR	1998	OMAN	1995
COSTA RICA	1991	PHILIPPINES	1995
CROATIA	1992	POLAND	1972
CUBA	1994	PORTUGAL	1993
CZECH REPUBLIC	1992	ROMANIA	1976
DENMARK	1968	RUSSIA	1998
ESTONIA	1998	SINGAPORE	1993
FINLAND	1974	SLOVAK REPUBLIC	1993
FRANCE	1986	SOUTH AFRICA	1992
GERMANY	1968	SPAIN	1984
GREECE	1990	SWEDEN	1968
HUNGARY	1990	SWITZERLAND	1991
ICELAND	1990	TANZANIA	1993
INDIA	1998	THAILAND	1984
INDONESIA	1990	TUNISIA	1993
IRAN	1998	TURKEY	1987
IRELAND	1968	UNITED KINGDOM	1968
ISRAEL	1973	USA	1968
ITALY	1975	VENEZUELA	1995
ZIMBABWE	1998		

Associated member countries

Armenia	Pakistan
Cyprus	Sri Lanka
Egypt	Vietnam
Macedonia	Yugoslavia
Mexico	

computer system. In addition a panel of experts has been established to analyse reactions pertaining to particular body systems. Short summaries of their findings are circulated to participating national centres in a memorandum called "Signal". A recent investigation has demonstrated that the WHO Programme is successful in finding new drug-adverse reaction associations at an early stage and in providing useful information about them to national centres (1).

In 1998 a new methodology (2) developed at the Uppsala Monitoring Centre, using a Bayesian ConfidencePropagation Neural Network (BCPNN) in analysing the database, was put into routine use.

Case reports are received within the WHO Programme, but the intention is that other sources of drug safety information should also be considered.

When the new data has been processed and entered into the ADR database, a BCPNN scan is run to generate statistical measurements for each drug-ADR combination. The resulting Combinations database (Combination: *Adverse drug reaction (ADR) data elements occuring together in ADR reports*) will be made available to national centres, and to pharmaceutical companies, in the latter case including only information on the company's own patented products.

The database will be presented in a computerised form which facilitates searching and sorting of the information.

An associations database (Association: *Combinations selected from a database on a quantitative basis.*) is generated by selecting those combinations that pass a pre-set threshold. Based on the results of the test runs of the BCPNN the threshold level for associations is that of the lower 95% confidence limit of the IC value crossing zero when a new batch of reports is added.

All associations are followed automatically for two years, the data being checked at 6-monthly intervals. After the final listing, an association may be reintroduced for another 2-year follow-up. The associations are also copied to a cumulative log file (history file), which will serve as a filter to exclude combinations that have in previous quarters passed the threshold level. This will prevent drug-ADR combinations with a confidence limit fluctuating around zero from being fed into the review process repetitiously.

The database is also sent to the expert review panel for evaluation as well as in the Collaborating Centre. Before distributing the database, associations are checked against standard reference sources (e.g. Physician's Desk Reference (PDR), Martindale), and the published literature (using e.g. Med-line and Reactions). This facilitates the review and identifies those associations that are, if not generally known, at least identified previously. Searching and sorting of the associations data can be done, not only on drug, ADR and the various statistical measurements, but also on System Organ Class and on therapeutic drug groups using the Anatomical-Therapeutic-Chemical (ATC) classification. To ensure that there are at least two reviewers per SOC, we intend to extend the panel of reviewers from today's 30 experts to around double over the next few years.

To the Associations stage, the process is purely quantitative, but clinical knowledge and judgement is necessary for the evaluation of associations, and is provided by the national centres and expert reviewers.

The signals that have been identified will be published as before in the Signal document and sent to national centres. Individualised sections of the Signal document will be provided to companies on a subscription basis (only on their patented products).

To aid the expert reviewers, and also to facilitate interpretation of the information presented in the Signal document, a set of guidelines is being established.

As with the associations, all signals will be automatically reassessed on a 6-monthly basis, for two years, with a possibility of re-introduction for follow-up, and also copied to a history file for easy tracking. With the new follow up procedures we have introduced a mechanism by which signals can be re-evaluated following new information. This enables, for example, renewed consideration of associations for which there initially was not enough information to merit signalling. Signals that are later supported by new evidence can also be highlighted. The nature of the signal will determine what measures need be taken in terms of follow up.

A larger number of variables than the routine drug-ADR combinations can also be considered using the Bayesian approach, as described above. For example, a specific pair of adverse reactions can be highly associated with a specific drug, or the effects can be determined of any other report variable or combination of variables on the 'information component' values. Also the effects of including drugs reported as 'concomitant medication' can be studied using the BCPNN.

One of the outcomes of these analyses may be to identify patient subgroups that may be at particularly high risk of getting a specific adverse reaction when they have taken a specific drug. Another possibility is to establish that a drug safety problem is related to a particular country, or region, or a certain time period. It should, however, be pointed out that, in order for these data to be useful, there needs to be a substantial number of cases reported.

Reference source

The data base of the WHO Programme is a unique reference source used in many different situations. When a national centre receives the first report of an unfamiliar drug-reaction association the WHO data base is often consulted to find out whether a similar observation has been made elsewhere in the world. If so, the initial signal may be strengthened. National centres are provided with an annual reference document providing summary figures of suspected drug-reaction associations reported to WHO. On-line search facilities are also at the disposal of national centres for up-to-date checking of the reporting situation.

From the data base cohorts of patients affected by similar kinds of drug associated reactions may be retrieved. By looking for common features in these reports, risk factors and hypothesis for underlying mechanisms may be revealed.

Quantification

There is a general need to quantify adverse reaction information. Under-reporting of adverse reactions in routine monitoring is the norm. However, the degree of under-reporting differ from time-to-time, place-to-place and between drugs. The WHO-centre is working jointly with IMS International, to analyse adverse reaction reports together with drug use data from different countries. This allows national differences in reporting rates to be further analysed for reasons that may be due to differences in indications for use, medical practice and demographics etc. (3), (4). It is hoped that this type of analysis of international data will serve as a guide to the need of more precise pharmacoepidemiological investigations.

A clearing house for information

The Uppsala Monitoring Centre has an important role to play as a communication centre—a clearing house for information on drug safety at the service of drug regulatory agencies, pharmaceutical industry, researchers and other groups in need of drug safety information. Requests for special data base searches and investigations are received from these parties at a rate of around 250 per year. In addition flexible on-line retrieval programmes are made available by which the data base users may perform a variety of standardized searches by themselves. Access for non-member parties is subjected to confidentiality restrictions agreed by Programme members. Some countries maintain the right to refuse the release of their own information if they so wish. Use of the information released is subject to a caveat document as to its proper use. Detailed manuals for the or-line service and the customized retrievals on request are available from the Uppsala centre.

National centres are provided with an Adverse Reactions Newsletter on a three-monthly basis since 1982. The Newsletter contains reviews of national adverse reaction bulletins and news of drug problems being investigated in various countries, supplemented by figures from the WHO register. A new type of bulletin, freely available to all interested parties, was recently introduced under the name "Uppsala Reports". It provides an easy-to-read account of news about the WHO Programme, its members and services.

Communications within the WHO Programme has improved with the increasing use of electronic communications media. In the 1980s an electronic mail and conferencing system, DISNET, was introduced for communications between national centres. Since Internet in the 1990s has become more widely spread, the DISNET system has been replaced by e-mail. The Uppsala Monitoring Centre is now maintaining an e-mail discussion group called 'Vigimed', which allows for rapid exchange of information around the world on drug safety matters. Membership is restricted to persons connected to national pharmacovigilance centres.

The Internet home page of the WHO Programme (http://www.who-umc.org) was introduced in 1996. It is intended to be developed into a dynamic tool for communications with all clients of the Uppsala Monitoring Centre.

Terminologies and standards

The WHO Programme has assumed responsibility for developing a standardized adverse reaction terminology (WHO-ART) and a comprehensive index of reported drugs (WHO-DD), both of which have a utility beyond their importance to the monitoring system. These tools are used in the pre-marketing safety area, as well as for post-marketing studies by many pharmaceutical companies. WHO-ART has also been adopted by the International Programme on Chemical Safety as the medical terminology to describe poisoning incidents.

The WHO Drug Dictionary is unique in its coverage of drugs marketed throughout the world. It is available in paper print, as computer files or on a diskette together with user friendly software. The Uppsala Centre is developing it further to incorporate more detailed information and make it compatible with the pre-standard proposed by the European Committee for Standardisation (CEN).

The Centre is also working with XML standards for its terminologies and dictionaries, as well as supporting such work with ICD10. The use of XML versions of terminologies will greatly enhance their combined utility and availability, for example, by internet.

Within the WHO Programme a number of definitions of commonly used terms like adverse reaction, side effect, adverse event, signal etc. have been worked out (5). These definitions contribute to a harmonized way of communicating both inside and outside the Programme.

Education

In order to foster education and communication in pharmacovigilance, the WHO Centre offers every second year, a two week training course in Adverse Reactions and Adverse Reaction Monitoring in Uppsala to which 25 health care professionals are accepted. The course is in three consecutive modules. The first offers some insight into the clinical aspects and diagnosis of adverse drug reactions, the second is about spontaneous monitoring and the practicalities of managing a drug monitoring centre. This section also offers hands on experience in using the data base of the WHO Programme. The final module is an introduction to wider issues in pharmacoepidemiology.

There is an increasing trend towards local and regional meetings and courses in pharmacovigilance. The WHO Programme often takes part in such meetings, particularly those organized in developing countries, to provide support and technical advise.

Annual meetings

Every year representatives of national centres are invited to a meeting arranged jointly by WHO and one of the participating countries. At these meetings technical issues are being discussed, both in relation to how to improve global drug monitoring in general and concerning individual drug safety problems. Since the meetings have very high attendance rates they are important for the establishment and maintenance of personal relationships subsequently contributing to good communications.

Programme development

The Uppsala Monitoring Centre is currently exploring a number of leads to further improve the use of the information collected and to develop the services of the Programme.

- By further developing the methodology of Bayesian artificial neural networks (see above) for the analysis of the large amount of data in the WHO data base it is expected that hitherto unrevealed risk factors for the development of drug related ailments will be possible to detect.
- In response to the challenge to safety monitoring offered by traditional herbal remedies the

WHO-centre has taken initiatives to improve the classification systems for such medicines. In a joint project with institutions in the UK and the Netherlands, a system compatible with the ATC-system used for modern, synthetic medicines is being developed. Input from experts from all parts of the world, representing different therapeutic traditions, will be indispensable for this project.
- In collaboration with the computer service company PharmaSoft, assisting the Uppsala Monitoring Centre, a new, extended, adverse reaction data base is being developed based on the recommendations of the CIOMS 1A and the ICH E2B working parties. In this data model much more detailed information on each case may be stored and case reports may also, in principle, be received directly from drug companies. Other software to support the functions of national centres is also being developed.
- With the aim of improving communications in pharmacovigilance initiatives have been taken to call together representatives of all major groups involved in the provision of drug safety information. The so called Erice declaration on communicating drug safety information sets out the basis for further development in this area (6). The Uppsala Monitoring Centre is collaborating with the Council for International Organizations of Medical Sciences (CIOMS) to work out detailed recommendations on good communication practices in pharmacovigilance.

Collaboration with other organizations

Reports of patient injuries caused by drugs used in doses above "normal" are usually referred to poison control centres and not to ADR centres. Experience gained in the WHO Programme has been used to assist also the International Programme on Chemical Safety (IPCS) in the collection of information on poisoning cases from all over the world. A separate data base for severe drug intoxication cases is being maintained by the Uppsala centre on a pilot basis.

Co-operation with organizations interested in developing early signals of significance is of importance to achieve a safer drug therapy. The International Society for Pharmacoepidemiology (ISPE) is specifically interested in the science of pharmacovigilance and the Council for International Organizations of Medical Sciences (CIOMS) is pivotal in bringing interested parties together to mount various collaborative projects. Much support has been given to the European Society of Pharmacovigilance (ESOP) which is gaining increasing international status. The Centre also supports the European Pharmacovigilance Research Group which has allowed regulators and drug safety specialists from a variety of European countries to come together to plan coordinated drug safety exercises. Initiatives like these may pave the way for a much more logical development and investigation of drug safety signals world wide.

Joining the WHO Programme

Considering the sensitive nature of the data being collected within the Programme, countries contributing such data to the scheme have agreed on certain requirements that should be complied with by countries wishing to join. Collaborating with WHO, being an organization for cooperation between member states, also requires a certain administrative structure of the drug monitoring activity. The basic requirements are:

- General acquaintance with the methodology of spontaneous monitoring. A country joining the WHO Programme must have a programme for collection of spontaneous adverse reaction reports in place.
- A national centre for pharmacovigilance must be designated and recognized by Ministry of Health (or equivalent).
- Technical competence to fulfill reporting requirements to WHO. Case reports collected in

the national drug monitoring programme must be submitted to the WHO Programme in a defined format.

For further information please contact:

World Health Organization
Division of Drug Management and Policy
CH-1211 Geneva 27
Switzerland
telephone +41-22 7912111
telefax +41-22 7910746
e-mail tenhamm@who.ch

WHO Collaborating Centre for
International Drug Monitoring
Stora Torget 3
S-753 20 Uppsala
Sweden
telephone +46-18 656060
telefax +46-18 656080
e-mail who.drugs@who.pharmasoft.se

References

1. Fucik H, Edwards IR. Impact and credibility of the WHO adverse reaction signals. Drug Information Journal 1996;30:461–464.
2. Bate A, Lindquist M, Edwards IR, Olsson S, Orre R, Lansner A, De Freitas RM. A Bayesian neural network method for adverse drug reaction signal detection. Eur J Clin Pharmacol 1998;54:315–21.
3. Lindquist M, Sanderson J, Claesson C, Imbs J-L, Rohan A, Edwards IR. New pharmacovigilance information on an old drug; an international study of spontaneous reports on digoxin. Drug Invest 1994;8:73–80.
4. Stahl MMS, Lindquist M, Pettersson M, Edwards IR, Sanderson JH, Taylor NFA, Fletcher AP, Schou J. Withdrawal reactions with selective serotonin re-uptake inhibitors as reported to the WHO system. Eur J Clin Pharmacol 1997;53:163–9.
5. Biriell C, Edwards IR. Harmonisation in pharmacovigilance. Drug Saf 1994;10:93–102.
6. Olsson S. The role of the WHO Programme on International Drug Monitoring in coordinating worldwide drug safety efforts. Drug Saf 1998;19:1–10.

Address list of national centres participating in the WHO drug monitoring programme

Argentina (ARG)

Dr. Mabel Teresa Foppiano
Tel. +54-1-340 0866
Fax +54-1-340 0866
E-mail: snfvg@anmat.gov.ar

Administración Nacional de Medicamentos,
Alimentos y Tecnologia Medica (ANMAT)
Sistema Nacional de Farmacovigilancia
Avenida de Mayo 869, piso 11o
(1084) BUENOS AIRES
Argentina

Australia (AUS)

Dr. Patrick Purcell
Tel. +61-6-289 8671
Fax +61-6-232 8392
E-mail:
patrick.purcell@health.gov.au

Therapeutic Goods Administration
Dept of Community Services and Health
Australian Drug Evaluation Committee
P.O. Box 100
WODEN, A.C.T. 2606
Australia

Austria (AUT)

Ms. Eva Hofbauer
Tel. +43-1-711 72, ext. 4641
Fax +43-1-712 0823
E-mail: viiia3@bmg.gv.at

Federal Ministry of Health and
Consumer Protection
Pharmacovigilance Department II/A/3
Radetzkystraße 2
A-1030 VIENNA
Austria

Belgium (BEL)

Mr. Thierry Roisin
Tel. +32-2-227 5533
Fax +32-2-227 5528

Ministry of Health
Pharmacy General Inspectorate
Centre National de Pharmacovigilance
Vesale Building, 20 rue Montagne de l'Oratoire
B-1010 BRUSSELS
Belgium

Bulgaria (BUL)

Dr. Jasmina Mircheva
Tel. +359-2-446 566, 434 71
Fax +359-2-442 697
E-mail: pharmacovig@ndi.bg400.bg

National Drug Institute
Committee on Adverse Drug Reactions
26, Yanko Sakazov Boulevard
BG-1504 SOFIA
Bulgaria

Canada (CAN)
Dr. Philippe Duclos
Tel. +1-613-957 0325
Fax +1-613-998 6413
E-mail: pduclos@hpb.hc-sc.gc.ca

Health Canada, Division of Immunization
Vaccine-Associated Adverse Events Surveillance Progr.
Laboratory Centre for Disease Control (LCDC), Bldg 0603EI
Tunney's Pasture
OTTAWA, Ontario K1A 0L2
Canada

Canada (CAN)
Ms. Heather Sutcliffe
Acting Head
Tel. +1-954 1541, 957 0337
Fax +1-957 0335
E-mail: Heather_Sutcliffe@hc-sc.gc.ca

ADR. Reporting Unit
Bureau of Drug Surveillance
Health Canada
Address Locator
K1A 1B9 Ottawa, Ontario
Canada

Chile (CHL)
Dr. Q F Cecilia Morgado-Cadiz
Tel. +56-2-239 8769, 1105
Fax +56-2-239 8760, 6960
E-mail: cmorgado@ispch.cl

Instituto de Salud Publica de Chile
Centro Nacional de Información de Medicamentos y Farmacovigilancia – CENIMEF
Avenida Marathon 1000, 3 piso, Nuñoa-Casilla 48
SANTIAGO
Chile

China, People's Rep of (CHN)
Prof. Zhu Yonghong
Tel. +86-10-701 7755, ext. 339
Fax +86-10-6511 3987

National Centre for ADR. Monitoring
c/o National Institute for Drug Control
Temple of Heaven
BEIJING P.R.C. 100050
China, People's Rep of

Costa Rica (COR)
Dr. Albin Chaves Matamoros
Coordinador
Tel. +506-222 1878
Fax +506-257 7004
E-mail: farmaco@info.ccss.sa.cr

Caja Costarricense de Seguro Social
Centro Nacional de Farmacovigilancia
Apartado 10-105
SAN JOSê 1000
Costa Rica

Croatia (CRO)
Prof. Bozidar Vrhovac
Tel. +385-1-213 861
Fax +385-1-213 861
E-mail: vrhovac@rebro.mef.hr

National Adverse Drug Reactions Monitoring Centre
Section of Clinical Pharmacology
Department of Medicine, University Hospital Centre
12 Kispaticeva
41000 ZAGREB
Croatia

Cuba (CUB)
Dr. Julian Perez Peña
Tel. +53-7-240 924
Fax +53-7-247 227
E-mail: cdf@infomed.sld.cu

Centro para el Desarrollo de la Farmacoepidemiología
calle 44 # 502
Quinta Avenida y Quinta B
Miramar, Playa
CIUDAD DE LA HABANA C.P. 11300
Cuba

Czech Republic (CZE)
MUDr. Dana Stolbova
Tel. +420-2-732 335, 6708 1111
Fax +420-2-7173 2377
E-mail: sukl@sukl.anet.cz

Centre for Monitoring of Adverse Drug Reactions
State Institute for Drug Control
Státni ústav pro Kontrolu Léciv
Srobárova 48, post. prihr. 87
100 41 PRAHA 10
Czech Republic

Denmark (DEN)
Mrs. Kirsten G. Astrup
Head
Tel. +45-4-488 9111
Fax +45-4-491 7373
E-mail: dkma@dkma.dk

Danish Medicines Agency
Department of Medicines Evaluation
378, Frederikssundsvej
DK-2700 BRONSHOJ
Denmark

Estonia (EST)
Dr. Maia UuskÅla
Tel. +372-7-441 219
Fax +372-7-441 549
E-mail: maia@sam.ee

Riigi Ravimiamet
State Agency of Medicines
Kalevi 4, P.O. Box 150
EE-2400 TARTU
Estonia

Finland (FIN)
Dr. Erkki Palva
Research Director
Tel. +358-9-4733 4288
Fax +358-9-4733 4297
E-mail: erkki.palva@ll.nam.fi

National Agency for Medicines (NAM)
Lääkelaitos
Drug Information Centre
P.O. Box 55
Mannerheimintie 166
SF-00301 HELSINKI
Finland

France (FRA)
Dr. Anne Castot
Tel. +33-1-481 322 85
Fax +33-1-481 322 83

Agence du Médicament
Unité de Pharmacovigilance
143–145, boulevard Anatole France
F-93285 SAINT-DENIS, Cedex
France

France (FRA)
Dr. Claude Larousse
Tel. +33-240-084 096
Fax +33-240-084 097

CHR Institut de Biologie
Centre Regional Pharmacovigilance
BP 1005
F-44035 NANTES, Cedex
France

Germany (GFR)
Dr. Jürgen Beckmann
Tel. +49-30-454 830 00, 454 833 11
Fax +49-30-454 835 15

Federal Institute for Drugs and Medical Devices
Bundesinstitut für Arzneimittel und Medizinprodukte
Seestraße 10
D-13353 BERLIN
Germany

Germany (GFR)
Dr. Karl-Heinz Munter
Secretary-General
Tel. +49-221-400 4525
Fax +49-221-400 4510, 400 4539

Drug Commission of the German Medical Profession
Arzneimittelkommission der Deutschen Ärzgeschaft
P.O. Box 41 01 25, Aachener Straße 233–237
D-50931 KÖLN
Germany

Greece (GRC)
Ms. Antonia Pandouvaki
Tel. +30-1-654 9585
Fax +30-1-654 9585
E-mail: helpdesk@eof.gr

National Drug Organization (EOF)
Adverse Drug Reactions Section
284 Messogion Av.
GR-155 62 HOLARGOS
Greece

Hungary (HUN)
Dr. János Borvendég
Tel. +36-1-215 8977
Fax +36-1-215 8977

National Institute of Pharmacy
Adverse Drug Reactions Monitoring Centre
Zrínyi u. 3, Box 450
H-1372 BUDAPEST
Hungary

Iceland (ICE)
Dr. Olafur Olafsson
Director
Tel. +354-5-627 555
Fax +354-5-623 716

Director General of Public Health
Landlæknir
Laugavegi 116
IS-150 REYKJAVIK
Iceland

India(IND)
Prof. Suresh K Gupta
Tel. +91-11-659 3633, 686 4930
Fax +91-11-686 2663

National Pharmacovigilance Centre
All India Institute of Medical Sciences
Department of Pharmacology
Ansari Nagar
NEW DELHI 110029
India

Indonesia(INO)
Dr. Andajaningsih
Chairman
Tel. +62-21-424 4755
Fax +62-21-426 5927
E-mail: regobpom@indo.net.id

Ministry of Health
Directorate General of Drug and Food Control
National Centre for Monitoring of Adverse Drug Reactions
Jalan Percetakan Negara No. 23
JAKARTA 10560
Indonesia

Ireland (IRE)
Ms. Niamh Arthur
Pharmacovigilance Co-ordinator
Tel. +353-1-676 4971
Fax +353-1-676 7836
E-mail: imb@imb.ie

Irish Medicines Board
Pharmacovigilance Unit
Earlsfort Centre
Earlsfort Terrace
DUBLIN 2
Ireland

Islamic Republic of Iran (IRN)
Dr. Mohammad Sharifzadeh
Tel. +98-21-640 5569, 641 9306
Fax +98-21-675 868

Iranian Drug Information Center, ADR. unit
Under-secretary for Curative and Drug Affairs
Building no. 3
Fakhre Razi, Enghlab Ave
TEHRAN 13145
Islamic Republic of Iran

Israel (ISR)
Dr. Dina Hemo
M.Sc. Pharm
Tel. +972-2-568 1219
Fax +972-2-672 58 20

Ministry of Health
Clinical Pharmacology Department
Drug Monitoring Center
Rivka Street 29
JERUSALEM 91010
Israel

Italy (ITA)
Dr. Dina De Stefano
Tel. +39-6-5994 32 12
Fax +39-6-5994 33 65

National Pharmacovigilance Center
Pharmacovigilance Department
Ministry of Health
Via Civiltà Romana 7
I-00144 ROMA
Italy

Japan (JPN)
Dr. Michiharu Abe
Director, Safety Division
Tel. +81-3-359 524 35
Fax +81-3-350 843 64
E-mail: MA-TGR@mhw.go.jp

Ministry of Health and Welfare
Pharmaceutical and Medical Safety Bureau
1-2-2, Kasumigaseki, Chiyoda-ku
TOKYO 100-8045
Japan

Korea, Rep of (KOR)
Dr. Joon-Shik Chang
Director
Tel. +82-2-503 7585, 500 3041
Fax +82-2-503 7591, 504 1456
E-mail:
bokji12@nownuri.nowcom.co.kr

Ministry of Health & Welfare
Pharmaceutical Affairs Bureau
Pharmaceutical Development Division
1, Chung-ang Dong, Government Complex II
KWACHUN-SHI, KYUNGKIDO 427-760
Korea, Rep of

Malaysia (MAL)
Ms. Abida Haq Bt Syed M Haq
Principal Assistant Director
Tel. +60-3-757 3611, ext. 258
Fax +60-3-758 1312
E-mail: ah@bpfk.gov.my

Ministry of Health Malaysia
National Pharmaceutical Control Bureau
National Adverse Drug Reaction Committee
Jalan University, P.O. Box 319
MA-46730 PETALING JAYA
Malaysia

Morocco (MOR)
Dr. Rachida Soulaymani-Bencheikh
Tel. +212-7-770 137
Fax +212-7-772 067

Institut National d'Hygiène
Centre Anti Poisons et de Pharmacovigilance
Avenue Ibn Batouta 27
B.P. 769, Agdal
M-11400 RABAT
Morocco

Netherlands (NET)
Dr. Arthur P Meiners
Senior Drug Safety Officer
Tel. +31-70-356 7400
Fax +31-70-356 7515
E-mail: ap.meiners@cbg-meb.nl

Medicines Evaluation Board
P.O. Box 16229
Kalvermarkt 53
NL-2500 BE THE HAGUE
Netherlands

Netherlands (NET)
Dr. A.C. van Grootheest
Tel. +31-73-646 9700
Fax +31-73-642 6136
E-mail: ac.vangrootheest@lareb.nl

Netherlands Pharmacovigilance Foundation LAREB
Goudsbloemvallei 7
NL-5237 MH S-HERTOGENBOSCH
Netherlands

New Zealand (NEZ)
Dr. David Coulter
Tel. +64-3-479 7249
Fax +64-3-477 0509
E-mail:
david.coulter@stonebow.otago.ac.nz

University of Otago Medical School
National Toxicology Group
P.O. Box 913
DUNEDIN
New Zealand

Norway (NOR)
Ms. Elena Kvan
Tel. +47-22-897 700
Fax +47-22-897 799
E-mail: elena.kvan@slk.no

Norwegian Medicines Control Authority
Statens Legemiddelkontroll (SLK)
Adverse Drug Reaction Section
Sven Oftedals vei 6
N-0950 OSLO 9
Norway

Oman (OMN)
Dr. Ph Sawsan Ahmad Jaffar
Tel. +968-694 744
Fax +968-602 287, 604 684

Ministry of Health
Directorate General of Pharmaceutical Affairs and Drug Control
P.O. Box 393
113 MUSCAT
Oman

Philippines (PHL)
Mrs. Nazarita T Lanuza
Tel. +63-2-807 0725, 807 0731
Fax +63-2-807 0725, 807 0721, 807 0751

Bureau of Food and Drugs
Filinvest Corporate City
Alabang, Muntinlupa
METRO MANILA 1770
Philippines

Philippines (PHL)

Dr. Kenneth Hartigan-Go
Tel. +63-2-521 8450 loc 3948
Fax +63-2-526 0062
E-mail: hartigan@kulog.upm.edu.ph

University of the Philippines
UP College of Medicine
Department of Pharmacology
547 Pedro Gil St., Ermita
P.O. Box 593
MANILA 1000
Philippines

Poland (POL)

Ms. Agata Maciejczyk
Tel. +48-22-416 742
Fax +48-22-651 4366
E-mail: magat@il.waw.pl

Institute for Drug Research and Control
Centre for Monitoring of Adverse Effects to Drugs
30/34 Chelmska Street
PL-00725 WARSAW
Poland

Portugal (POR)

Dr. António M.N. Faria Vaz
Tel. +351-1-790 8558
Fax +351-1-795 9116, 795 9069
E-mail: infarmed@mail.telepac.pt

Centro Nacional de Farmacovigilancia
Instituto Nacional da Farámcia e do Medicamento (INFARMED)
Parque de Saúde de Lisboa, Avenida do Brasil, no. 53
P-1700 LISBOA
Portugal

Romania (ROM)

Dr. Stanciu Juliana Daniela
Tel. +40-1-224 1102, 224 1710
Fax +40-1-230 5083
E-mail: rb@ns.icsmcf.ro

State Institute for Drug Control and
Pharmaceutical Research
Str Aviator Sanatescu no 48, Sector 1
R-71 324 BUCURESTI
Romania

Russia (RUS)

Prof. V.K. Lepakhin
Tel. +7-095-433 5600, 434 5244
Fax +7-095-434 0292
E-mail: lepakh@pfu.med.edu.ru

Ministry of Health of the Russian Federation
Federal Centre for Adverse Reactions Study
Miklucho-Maklaya str 8
117198 MOSCOW
Russia

Singapore (SIN)

Ms. Cheng Leng Chan
Head (Information & Research)
Tel. +65-325 5604, 325 5610
Fax +65-325 5448, 325 5604, 325 5610
E-mail:
chan_cheng_leng@moh.gov.sg

Ministry of Health
Adverse Drug Reaction Monitoring Unit
Pharmaceutical Department
Information & Research Unit
No. 2 Jalan Bukit Merah
SINGAPORE 169547
Singapore

Slovakia (SVK)
Dr. Pavol Gibala
Tel. +421-7-566 5075, 542 1860
Fax +421-7-566 4127, 566 4026
E-mail: kevicka@NZBA.sk

National Centre for Monitoring Adverse Reactions to Drugs
State Institute for Drug Control
Kvetná 11
852 08 BRATISLAVA
Slovakia

South Africa (SOA)
Ms. Ushma Mehta
Tel. +27-21-471 618
Fax +27-21-448 6181
E-mail: umehta@uctgsh1.uct.ac.za

National Adverse Drug Event Monitoring Centre
c/o Department of Pharmacology
Faculty of Medicine
University of Cape Town
OBSERVATORY 7925
South Africa

Spain (SPA)
Dr. Fransisco José de Abajo
Tel. +34-1-509 7947, 509 7902
Fax +34-1-509 7948
E-mail: fvigilan@isciii.es

Centro Coordinador del Sistema Español de Farmacovigilancia
Instituto de Salud "Carlos III"
Centro Nacional de Farmacobiología
Carretera a Pozuelo, Km 2
E-28220 MAJADAHONDA (MADRID)
Spain

Sweden (SWE)
Dr. Bengt-Erik Wiholm
Tel. +46-18-17 46 00
Fax +46-18-54 85 66
E-mail: beje.wiholm@mpa.se

Medical Products Agency
Div of Drug Epidemiology, Information & Inspection
Adverse Drug Reaction Section
P.O. Box 26, Husargatan 8
S-751 03 UPPSALA
Sweden

Switzerland (SCH)
Dr. Rudolf Stoller
Tel. +41-31-322 0211, 322 0352
Fax +41-31-322 0212, 322 0418
E-mail:
IKS.pharmacovigilance@hin.ch

Interkantonale Kontrollstelle fÅr Heilmittel
Pharmacovigilance Centre
Erlachstraße 8
CH-3000 BERN 9
Switzerland

Tanzania (TAN)
Mr. Henry Irunde
Tel. +255-51-450 512
Fax +255-51-462 29
E-mail: tadatis@tan.healthnet.org

Tanzania Drug and Toxicology Information Service (TADATIS)
P.O. Box 77150
DAR ES SALAAM
Tanzania

Thailand (THA)
Mrs. Suboonya Hutangkabodee
Tel. +66-2-590 7281
Fax +66-2-591 8457, 590 7282
E-mail:
suboonya@health.moph.go.th

Drug Information Center and NADRM, Techn Div.
National Adverse Drug Reaction Monitoring Centre
Ministry of Public Health
Food and Drug Administration
Ti-wa-nondh Rd
NONTHABUREE 11000
Thailand

Tunisia (TUN)
Prof. Chelbi Belkahia
Tel. +216-1-264 763
Fax +216-1-571 390

Centre National de Pharmacovigilance
Sis Hôpital Charles Nicolle
TUNIS 1006
Tunisia

Turkey (TUR)
Ms. Sevgi Öksüz
Chemist
Tel. +90-312-230 1674, 230 2769
Fax +90-312-230 1610
E-mail: tadmer@iegm.gov.tr

Ministry of Health
General Directorate of Drugs and Pharmacy
Ilkiz Sokak No 4
Sihhiye
ANKARA
Turkey

United Kingdom (UNK)
Dr. Susan Wood
Head
Tel. +44-171-273 0400
Fax +44-171-273 0282, 273 0675
E-mail: susan.wood@mca.gov.uk

Medicines Control Agency
Pharmacovigilance, Department of Health
Market Towers, 1 Nine Elms Lane
Vauxhall
LONDON SW8 5NQ
United Kingdom

United States of America (USA)
Dr. Ralph Lillie
Tel. +1-301-443 4227
Fax +1-301-443 5161

Food and Drug Administration
Center for Drug Evaluation and Research
Office of Epidemiology and Biostatics
Room 15B-31 (HFD-730)
5600 Fishers Lane
ROCKVILLE, MD 20857
United States of America

United States of America (USA)
Dr. Marcel Salive
Tel. +1-301-827 3974
Fax +1-301-827 3529
E-mail: salive@cber.fda.gov

Food and Drug Administration
Center for Biologics Evaluation and Research
Adverse Reaction Section, HFM-220
1401 Rockville Pike
ROCKVILLE, MD 20852
United States of America

Venezuela (VEN)
Dr. Carman Lozada A
Tel. +58-2-662 4797
Fax +58-2-662 4797, 693 1455
Instituto Nacional de Higiene "Rafael Rangel"
Sección de Farmacología Clinica Sanitaria
Centro Nacional de Vigilancia Farmacológia
Apartado Postal 60.412 – Oficina del Este
Ciudad Universitaria
CARACAS
Venezuela

Zimbabwe (ZIM)
the Registrar
Tel. +263-4-792 165
Fax +263-4-736 980
Drugs Control Council
P.O. Box UA 599, 106 Baines Avenue
Union Avenue
HARARE
Zimbabwe

Associate member countries

Armenia
Dr. Samvel Azatyan
Tel. +374-2-528 615, 529 523, 529 691
Fax +374-2-151 697
E-mail: pharmag@ns.r.am
Department of Pharmacovigilance and Rational Drug Use
Armenian Drug and Medical Technology Agency
15, Moskowian Street
YEREVAN 375001
Armenia

Cyprus
Dr. Eftychios Kkolos
Director
Tel. +357-2-302 001
Fax +357-2-302 721
Ministry of Health
Pharmaceutical Services
44 Kimonos Street
NICOSIA 138
Cyprus

Egypt
Dr. Gamila Mohamed Moussa
Tel. +20-2-354 9802
Fax +20-2-354 2627
Ministry of Health
Directorate General of Drug Control
CAIRO
Egypt

Macedonia
Ms. Vesna Nasteska-Nedanovska
Tel. +389-91-237 669
Fax +389-91-230 857
Ministry of Health
50 Divizija B.B.
91 000 SKOPJE
Macedonia

Macedonia
Prof. Stojmir Petrov
Director
Tel. +389-91-111 828, 235 966
Fax +389-91-111 828
E-mail: pharma@lotus.mpt.com.mk
Institute of Preclinical and Clinical Pharmacology and Toxicology
National Center for Adverse Drug Reaction Monitoring
50 Divizija br 6
91 000 SKOPJE
Macedonia

Pakistan
Prof. M Sultan Farooqui
President
Tel. +92-21-588 2997, 589 2801
Fax +92-21-589 3062, 588 7513
E-mail:
whocpsp%paknetbbs@sdnpk.undp.org

College of Physicians & Surgeons Pakistan (CPSP)
Department of Clinical Pharmacology
7th Central Street
Phase II, Defence Housing Authority
KARACHI 75500
Pakistan

Sri Lanka
Dr. U Ajith Mendis
Director
Tel. +94-1-695 173
Fax +94-1-695 173

Ministry of Health
Medical Technology and Supplies Division
No. 120, Norris Canal Road
COLOMBO 10
Sri Lanka

Vietnam
Prof. Hoang Tich Huyên
Tel. +84-4-245 292
Fax +84-4-823 1253

Adverse Drug Reaction Centre
Institute for Drug Quality Control
Ministry of Health
48 Hai Ba Trung street
HANOI
Vietnam

Yugoslavia, Fed Rep of
Prof. Vaso Antunovic
Tel. +381-11-361 5531

Clinical Centre of Serbia
National Centre for Adverse Drug Reactions
Visegradska 26
YU-11000 BELGRADE
Yugoslavia, Fed Rep of

Institutions

EU
Dr. Ana de Vasconcelos Batalha
Tel. +32-2-296 7072
Fax +32-2-296 1520
E-mail: ana.batalha@dg3.cec.be

European Commission
Directorate General III—Industry
Rue de la Loi 200
B-1049 BRUSSELS
Belgium

WHO
Dr. Martijn ten Ham
Chief
Tel. +41-22-791 2111, 791 3638
Fax +41-22-791 4730, 791 0746
E-mail: tenhamm@who.ch

World Health Organization
Drug Safety Unit
10 Avenue Appia
CH-1211 GENEVA 27
Switzerland

EMEA
Ms. Priya Bahri
Tel. +44-171-418 8454
E-mail:
priya.bahri@emea.eudra.org

EMEA—The European Agency for the Evaluation of Medicinal Products
Pharmacovigilance Section
7, Westferry Circus, Canary Wharf
LONDON E14 4HB
United Kingdom

Index of drugs

Page numbers in **bold** indicate where the given drug is discussed in detail.

Index of side effects